Pediatric Kidney Disease

Denis F. Geary • Franz Schaefer
Editors

Pediatric Kidney Disease

Volume 1

Second Edition

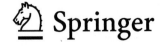

Editors
Denis F. Geary
Division of Nephrology
The Hospital for Sick Children
Toronto, ON
Canada

Department of Paediatrics
University of Toronto
Toronto, ON
Canada

Franz Schaefer
Division of Pediatric Nephrology
University of Heidelberg
Heidelberg
Germany

Previously published as COMPREHENSIVE PEDIATRIC NEPHROLOGY with Elsevier, The Netherlands, 2008
ISBN 978-3-662-52970-6   ISBN 978-3-662-52972-0   (eBook)
DOI 10.1007/978-3-662-52972-0

Library of Congress Control Number: 2016960670

Printed on acid-free paper

This Springer imprint is published by Springer Nature
The registered company is Springer-Verlag GmbH Germany
The registered company is Heidelberger Platz 3, 14197 Berlin, Germany

Preface

We are delighted to welcome you to this new book. Although certainly related to our previous text, *"Comprehensive Pediatric Nephrology"*, we believe you will find this book sufficiently different to justify the change in title to *Pediatric Kidney Disease*. As with our previous textbook, *Pediatric Kidney Disease* is not intended to compete with any other textbooks, but is an attempt to bridge the gap between the three-volume set of *Pediatric Nephrology*, and the several much briefer handbooks that exist in our specialty. It is hoped that *Pediatric Kidney Disease* will be the standard textbook for reference to busy clinicians, who need to obtain an up-to-date, easy-to-read, review of virtually all renal disorders that occur in children.

There are substantial differences between *Pediatric Kidney Disease* and the earlier *Comprehensive Pediatric Nephrology*. Although approximately half of the authors also contributed to our earlier text, an equal number of new authors are included here. These authorship changes reflect the evolution of our field and recognition of the emergence of new leaders in various subspecialty areas. For chapters that were included previously with the same authorship, each author was specifically asked to thoroughly update the material, and most of the authors have made extensive revisions.

Multiple new chapters have been included on recent advances in diagnostic tools which have developed increasing importance since our last book. One example is the emerging science of proteomics/metabolomics as tools for diagnosis which is acknowledged by the inclusion of a chapter dedicated to this subject.

To foster clinicians' understanding of scientific methodology in clinical research and encourage studies in rare kidney diseases, a special chapter covers the concept of evidence-based medicine, applied biostatistics, and ethical principles in pediatric research.

To reflect our increased understanding of the role of complement in the pathogenesis of an increasing number of renal disorders, we have devoted a complete section to this subject. We are grateful for the assistance of Christoph Licht in selecting the subject matter and authors as well as the editorial assistance for this section.

For all chapters, we have requested the authors to ensure the relevance of their chapter for busy pediatric and pediatric nephrology clinicians as well as the multidisciplinary team members. We hope the included material and its presentation is of value and will contribute to expansion of knowledge in the field of pediatric nephrology.

Toronto, ON, Canada   Denis F. Geary
Heidelberg, Germany   Franz Schaefer

Contents

Part I

Investigative Techniques in Pediatric Nephrology

Jeffrey Traubici and Ruth Lim

Introduction

Imaging plays an important role in the diagnosis and follow-up of many diseases of the pediatric urinary tract [1–3]. In the pediatric age group both congenital and acquired diseases of the urinary tract are imaged using a number of different modalities and in many cases it is the imaging study that offers a diagnosis or at least narrows what may begin as a fairly lengthy differential diagnosis. Radiography, excretory urography, contrast fluoroscopy, sonography, computed tomography, magnetic resonance imaging and nuclear scintigraphy have all been used to assess the urinary tract, each possessing its own relative strengths and weaknesses. In some cases, a combination of two or more complementary modalities will be necessary to narrow the differential diagnosis. It is of fundamental importance not only to know the most appropriate modality for the investigation of a particular patient but also to understand the risks and benefits associated with the various available modalities. Several of the modalities used in urinary tract imaging employ ionizing radiation. It has long been understood that exposure to radiation has deleterious effects, with recent evidence suggesting a strong association between exposure to radiation (particularly at doses reached in computed tomography (CT)) and subsequent development of neoplastic disease [4, 5]. Other risks to be considered relate to the administration of intravenous contrast agents and mainly involve contrast-induced nephropathy and adverse contrast reactions [6–8]. Finally, because some children will require sedation or general anesthesia in order to undergo an examination, the risk associated with the administration of anesthesia must also be considered [9, 10].

This chapter serves as an overview of these imaging modalities and presents examples of their application in the evaluation of children with urinary tract abnormalities.

J. Traubici
Department of Diagnostic Imaging, Hospital for Sick Children, 555 University Ave, Toronto, ON M5G1X8, Canada
e-mail: jeffrey.traubici@sickkids.ca

R. Lim (✉)
Department of Radiology, Massachusetts General Hospital, 55 Fruit Street, ELL237, Boston, MA 02114, USA
e-mail: rlim@mgh.harvard.edu

Ultrasound

Sonography has become an important part of the pediatric imaging armamentarium – perhaps the most important. Its strengths are many. To begin with, it does not use ionizing radiation. In addition ultrasound does not require the administration of intravenous contrast agents; although several ultrasound contrast agents have been recently developed that can increase the accuracy

© Springer-Verlag Berlin Heidelberg 2016
D.F. Geary, F. Schaefer (eds.), *Pediatric Kidney Disease*, DOI 10.1007/978-3-662-52972-0_1

of the imaging examination [11]. Furthermore sedation is very rarely required.

The most common indications for sonographic imaging of the kidneys include: urinary tract infection [12–14], follow-up of antenatally diagnosed hydronephrosis, evaluation of a palpable mass, assessment for vascular abnormalities (including renal artery stenosis), assessment of medical renal diseases, screening of patients at known risk to develop renal neoplasms (for instance Beckwith-Wiedemann Syndrome and other cancer predisposing syndromes) [15], and assessment for possible urinary obstruction. Ultrasound can also assess other findings noted on antenatal imaging such as renal agenesis, ectopia, dysplasia or mass.

The ultrasound examination can be tailored in many ways to suit the patient and clinical situation. A patient who is upset or frightened can be scanned lying next to a parent or in the arms of a parent, which can alleviate some anxiety. Coupled with a calm and reassuring environment and various distractions (e.g., toys, music, videos, computer tablets), this setting often allows for the performance of a satisfactory diagnostic study. The need for sedation is extremely rare but may be considered on a case-by-case basis.

The patient can be scanned in various positions (supine, prone, decubitus) depending on the scenario. In fact altering position can at times be helpful particularly in determining if a structure such as a calculus is mobile. In some situations the ultrasound examination can be repeated after an intervention has been performed in order to determine whether it was successful or resulted in a complication. One can study the urinary tract prior to or after voiding, after placement of a bladder catheter, ureteral stent or nephrostomy catheter or after biopsy. These repeated examinations can be done without concern for the effects of radiation.

By and large the small body habitus of children allows for excellent sonographic imaging of the urinary tract. There are cases of larger teenagers and obese children in which sonography of the urinary system can be suboptimal. Scanning of the kidneys is performed mainly with curved array transducers for assessment of kidney length, status of the renal parenchyma, the pelvo-caliceal system, ureters and the bladder. These images can be supplemented with those obtained with a high-resolution linear transducer, which offers a superior level of spatial resolution but is limited in terms of the depth to which the transducer can penetrate. For that reason high resolution sonography is particularly well suited to neonates, infants and younger children. In older children, the distance between the transducer and the kidneys may preclude this type of higher resolution examination.

The kidneys are ovoid organs that typically lie in the retroperitoneal renal fossae, although they can be ectopic. Their lengths can be measured and compared with published nomograms [16–18] (Fig. 1.1a–d). Growth of the kidneys can be followed on serial examinations; however, it is important to keep in mind that the kidney can occasionally be overmeasured or undermeasured depending on the circumstances of the examination. Retardation in renal growth can be a sign of ongoing insult such as vesicoureteral reflux [19].

In healthy children there is a difference in echogenicity between normal renal cortex and the medullary pyramids, with the former more echogenic and the latter more hypoechoic (Fig. 1.2). This difference, termed *cortico-medullary differentiation*, is most pronounced in the neonatal period when the cortex is slightly more echogenic than later in childhood and the renal pyramids are often profoundly hypoechoic [20]. The echogenicity of the renal cortex can be compared to an internal and adjacent standard – in the case of the right kidney, that being the liver. One must, however, ensure that this reference organ (the liver) is normal. Alteration in liver echogenicity due to hepatic disease negates its use as a reference in some cases. The pattern of normal renal echogenicity does vary in childhood. In the neonate the renal cortex can be isoechoic or even hyperechoic compared to the liver (Fig. 1.3) and the cortico-medullary differentiation can be quite marked. By the time the child is several months of age the renal cortex should be hypoechoic compared to the echogenicity of the liver [20, 21]. Any alteration in echogenicity at that point suggests renal

Fig. 1.1 Nomograms delineate the predicted mean and 95 % prediction limits of renal length as a function of age (**a**), height (**b**), weight (**c**), and total body surface area (**d**)

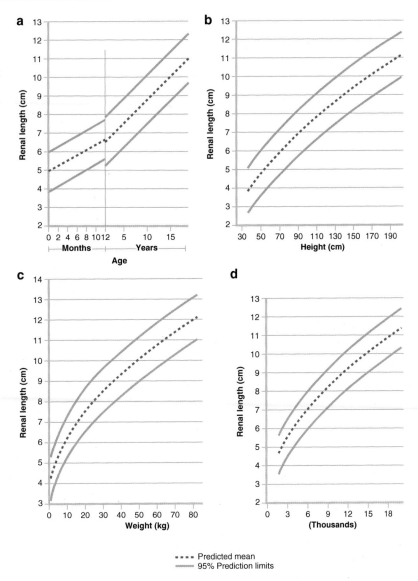

- ▪▪▪▪ Predicted mean
- ——— 95% Prediction limits

disease. The pyramids, particularly in the neonate, can be so hypoechoic that they can be mistaken for a dilated collecting system. There are exceptions to the hypoechogenicity of the renal pyramids, the majority of which relate to disease states (such as medullary nephrocalcinosis) or interventions (such as Lasix administration). The most common exception, however, seen in many neonates may be the transient increase in pyramidal echogenicity, which has been attributed to precipitation of Tamm Horsfall proteins [22]. In addition, there may be lobulation of the renal outline, especially in neonates. This should not be confused with scarring. The notching of normal lobulation tends to be seen in the portion of the cortex between pyramids; whereas focal scarring tends to occur in portions of the cortex directly overlying the pyramid.

The degree of renal collecting system dilatation can be assessed both qualitatively and quantitatively. Measurement of pelvic dilatation can be assessed at the level of the renal hilum – or just beyond it in the case of an extrarenal pelvis. A full bladder can exaggerate the degree of dilatation. It therefore may be prudent to assess the pelvic diameter after voiding if the urinary

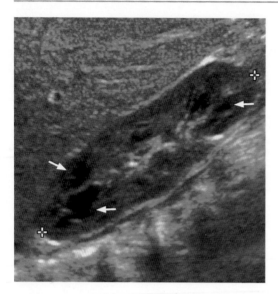

Fig. 1.2 Ultrasound of the normal kidney (length outlined with calipers) demonstrates renal pyramids which are nearly anechoic (*arrows*) and which can be mistaken for dilatation of the renal collecting system

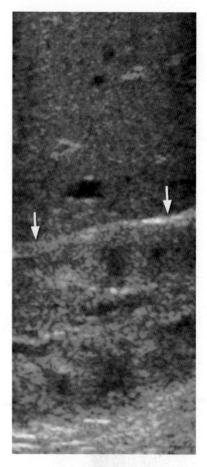

Fig. 1.3 Ultrasound of the normal neonatal kidney in which the renal cortex is more echogenic than the adjacent liver. This can be a normal finding in the neonate. After several months the renal cortex should be less echogenic than the liver

bladder is over-distended. If the ureter is dilated, its diameter can be assessed along its course, although it can be visualized most reliably proximally and distally (Fig. 1.4a–c). Overlying bowel gas often obscures the midportion of the ureter. The thickness of the wall of the intrarenal collecting system, ureter or bladder can also be assessed. Thickening of the urothelium anywhere along the urinary tract can be associated with, though is not pathognomonic for, infection or inflammation. Urolithiasis can be diagnosed as an echogenic focus with distal acoustic shadowing [23]. The degree of obstruction caused by a calculus can also be assessed with sonography.

Colour Doppler and pulsed Doppler interrogation of the kidneys can be used to assess vascularity of the kidneys. The study can assess the vessels from the ostia of the main renal arteries and veins through the arcuate vessels in the renal parenchyma. Indications for Doppler evaluation include suspicion of renal arterial or venous thrombosis [24], arterial stenosis [25], trauma [26], infection [27], acute tubular necrosis and transplant rejection [28] – though the role in the evaluation of rejection remains controversial [29].

Voiding Cystourethrography

Voiding cystourethrography is the study of choice for diagnosing vesicoureteral reflux and assessing the anatomy of the bladder and urethra. Indications for this investigation include urinary tract infection [14], antenatally or postnatally diagnosed hydronephrosis, and suspected posterior urethral valves, among others. A catheter is placed into the bladder using aseptic technique. At most institutions sedation is not administered. In our experience, the examination can be performed without sedation in the vast majority of children, given proper explanation and reassurance. The bladder is filled with water soluble

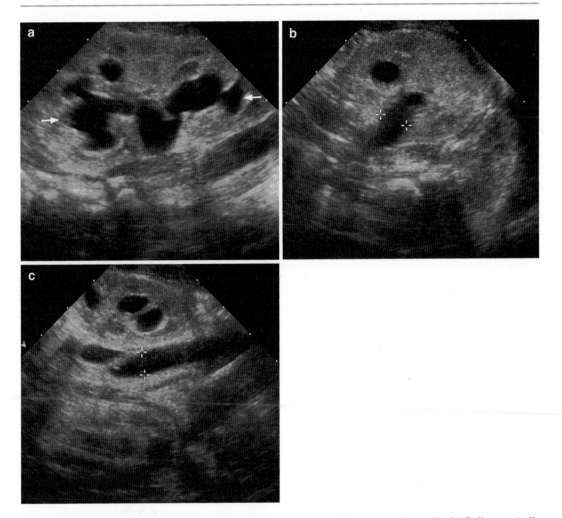

Fig. 1.4 (a) Ultrasound of the kidney in the longitudinal plane demonstrates moderate pelvocaliceal dilatation (*arrows*). (b) In the transverse plane the renal pelvis is measured with respect to its maximal AP diameter (calipers). (c) Scanning along the flank, one can often visualize the ureter if it is dilated (calipers)

contrast under the pressure of gravity until pressure within the bladder induces micturition. The amount of contrast used will vary according to the patient's age and bladder capacity. At some institutions a single cycle of filling and voiding is performed. At others, two or three cycles are the routine [30]. This latter method, termed *cyclic VCUG*, has demonstrated greater sensitivity in detecting reflux, but results in a higher radiation dose than does the single cycle method.

Exact views obtained will vary from institution to institution but all will include images of the bladder that will allow for assessment of its wall characteristics, and detect structural abnor-malities such as diverticula, ureteroceles or urachal abnormalities. These images should demonstrate whether there is any reflux into the ureters. Images of the urethra will be obtained during voiding either with the catheter in place or after its removal. Whether the urethra is imaged with a catheter in place or not depends on the practice of the institution and the individual radiologist. At our institution an image of the urethra is obtained with the catheter in place as well as after its removal, thus ensuring an image of the urethra in cases in which the child stops voiding just as the catheter is removed. An image of the renal fossae will assess for any reflux to the level of the kidney, characterize the collecting system anatomy (duplex or not) and assign a grade to that reflux, based on a 5-point international VCUG grading system [31].

Here, as with the other modalities, the study is tailored to the individual child. The bladder can be filled via a suprapubic catheter or a Mitrofanoff diversion if present. If a child is unable to void on his own, the bladder can be drained via the catheter in situ. If the child is reticent or unable to void, warm water applied to the perineum can induce voiding. Despite a variety of maneuvers there are children who will not void on the fluoroscopy table. In these cases the micturition phase of the study is not possible and the sensitivity of the study to detect reflux is diminished. In some institutions an image is taken after the child has been allowed to void in the washroom. In all cases care is given to minimizing the dose of ionizing radiation [32].

Complications related to the study can occur and are similar to those encountered in any catheterization of the bladder, with infection and trauma being the most common. At our institution, we do not administer prophylactic antibiotics unless there is a clinical indication for procedure related prophylaxis. If the examination is positive and the patient is not on long term antibiotic prophylaxis, a prompt communication of the results to the referring clinician is appropriate. One can also encounter urinary retention post-procedure.

Nuclear Medicine

Nuclear Medicine is a modality that comprises a variety of examinations for evaluating the pediatric urinary tract. Nuclear medicine techniques differ from other imaging modalities in that they focus on function rather than detailed anatomic structure. As a result, nuclear imaging plays an important complementary role to other modalities, particularly to the structural evaluation obtained with ultrasound.

The physical principles of how scintigraphic images are generated also differ from those of other imaging modalities. Rather than transmitting x-rays through the patient as is done with fluoroscopy, radiography and CT, nuclear medicine introduces a radioactive tracer into the patient's body. An Anger camera is then positioned adjacent to the patient, and images are created by detecting the gamma-rays emitted from the patient's own body. In nuclear urinary tract imaging, depending on the specific examination being performed, the radiopharmaceutical can be injected intravenously to be extracted by the kidneys, or can be instilled via catheter into the bladder. Radiation doses in nuclear medicine examinations of the urinary tract are lower than those encountered in CT and lower or comparable to those in fluoroscopy.

Most pediatric patients are either co-operative in lying still on the scintigraphy imaging table, or are infants small enough to be safely restrained with swaddling. Therefore the majority of patients will not require any form of sedation when undergoing a nuclear medicine examination. However, if it is anticipated that a child will have difficulty in lying still for at least 30 min, sedation can be considered. Rarely, general anaesthesia is necessary to perform a successful examination.

Urinary tract imaging comprises over half of the examinations performed in a typical pediatric nuclear medicine department. The most common clinical indications for performing nuclear renal imaging examinations include urinary tract infection, ante- or post-natally detected hydronephrosis, vesicoureteral reflux, suspected urinary obstruction, and suspected impairment of renal function.

Overview of Radiopharmaceuticals

Technetium-99m (99mTc) is the radionuclide (i.e., gamma-emitting isotope) that is used to label the overwhelming majority of radiopharmaceuticals in urinary tract imaging. It emits a 140 keV gamma-ray and has a physical half-life of 6 h.

Technetium-99m pertechnetate is the base form of 99mTc that is obtained from a portable generator unit found in any nuclear medicine radiopharmacy. 99mTc-pertechnetate can be used to radiolabel other pharmaceuticals through the use of commercially-available labeling kits. Other radiopharmaceuticals routinely used in nuclear urinary tract imaging are described below.

Glomerular Filtration Agents

99mTc-diethylenetriaminepentaacetic acid (DTPA) is used to calculate glomerular filtration function. Measuring its rate of extraction from plasma via serial blood sampling provides an accurate estimate of the glomerular filtration rate (GFR). Approximately 90 % of DTPA is filtered by the kidneys into the urine within 4 h after intravenous injection [33]. Renal imaging can also be performed using 99mTc-DTPA, providing additional information on excretion and drainage, as well as the ability to plot dynamic renogram time-activity curves.

51Cr-ethylenediaminetetraacetate (EDTA) is also used for calculation of glomerular filtration rate, and is the standard GFR agent used in Europe. Due to better radioisotope binding to the tracer, 51Cr-EDTA produces slightly higher values for GFR than 99mTc-DTPA. However, this difference is small (5 % or less) and is not considered to be clinically relevant [34]. Renal imaging is not performed with 51Cr-EDTA as it does not emit gamma-rays of suitable energy levels for imaging.

Tubular Secretion Agents

99mTc-mercaptoacetyltriglycine (MAG3) is injected intravenously, and cleared predominantly by the renal tubules (95 %) [33]. The extraction fraction of MAG3 is more than twice that of DTPA, resulting in a much higher target-to-background ratio. It is for this reason that image quality is more satisfactory with 99mTc-MAG3 than with 99mTc-DTPA, particularly in the setting of impaired renal function or urinary obstruction. 99mTc-MAG3 has become the radiopharmaceutical of choice for performing functional renal imaging (except when performing GFR measurement), which can assess renal function, detect obstructive uropathy, and evaluate renal transplant allografts. The clearance of MAG3 by the kidneys is proportional to effective renal plasma flow.

Iodine-123- or iodine-131-orthoiodohippuran (OIH) has been used in the past for nuclear renal imaging. The use of 123/131I-OIH for clinical imaging has been replaced by 99mTc-MAG3, which produces nearly identical renogram time-activity curves. 99mTc-MAG3 has the advantages of markedly better image resolution than 131I-OIH, and is easier to produce and thus less expensive than 123I-OIH. The radioisotope 123I is supplied by only a small handful of facilities worldwide, as its production requires a specialized cyclotron (particle accelerator) facility.

Renal Cortical Agents

99mTc-dimercaptosuccinic acid (DMSA) binds to the sulfylhydryl groups of the proximal renal tubules after filtration [33]. It is usually the cortical imaging agent of choice, as only 10 % is excreted into the urine during the first several hours after intravenous injection. Therefore 99mTc-DMSA produces excellent high-resolution images of the renal cortex without interference from urinary activity.

99mTc-glucoheptonate (GH) is cleared by the kidneys through both tubular secretion and glomerular filtration, with 10–15 % remaining bound to the renal tubules at one hour after injection. Therefore early imaging can be performed to evaluate renal perfusion, urinary excretion and drainage. Late imaging at 1–2 h will visualize the renal cortex. 99mTc-DMSA is the preferred cortical imaging agent, as its cortical binding is much higher than that of 99mTc-GH.

Direct Radionuclide Cystogram (DRC)

Direct radionuclide cystography (DRC) detects vesicoureteral reflux (VUR) with great sensitivity. It is used as a complementary modality to voiding cystourethrography (VCUG) [35–37]. Typically, patients who present with a first-time febrile urinary tract infection, or with newly-discovered hydronephrosis will initially undergo VCUG to diagnose reflux [38]. Subsequently, DRC is used as a follow-up examination to determine if reflux has resolved or is persistent, including post-operative evaluation after ureteral reimplantation surgery or minimally-invasive sub-trigonal injection procedure. Additionally, DRC is commonly performed as a primary screening examination to detect reflux in asymptomatic patients with a small kidney or solitary kidney, or who have a family history of VUR (first degree relative, i.e., parent or sibling).

VCUG vs. DRC

Since image acquisition during DRC is continuous, it is more sensitive for detecting brief intermittent episodes of VUR that may be missed with VCUG. DRC is also more sensitive in detecting small amounts of VUR, as there is no interference to the images from overlying stool and bowel gas, unlike VCUG. Additionally, and importantly, the radiation dose to the patient is approximately 1/12th to 1/100th of the dose received during VCUG [39, 40].

DRC, however, provides very little anatomic detail, and is not effective in detecting structural abnormalities such as ureteroceles, ectopic ureteral insertions, bladder diverticula, urethral abnormalities including posterior urethral valves, or duplicated collecting systems. These structural abnormalities require VCUG, and sometimes ultrasound, to be adequately demonstrated.

DRC is performed in much the same manner as voiding cystourethrography. The bladder is catheterized with a 5–8 French catheter and drained of urine, which is usually sent for microbiology culture. The bladder is then instilled with a 99mTc-based radiopharmaceutical, which can be any of: 99mTc-pertechnetate, 99mTc-DTPA, or 99mTc-sulphur colloid (a radio-labeled particulate material). The patient lies supine on the imaging table, with the camera positioned posteriorly. Continuous dynamic images are acquired while the bladder is filling and while the patient voids on the table. The bladder capacity is recorded, and radioactivity count data can subsequently be used to calculate the post-void residual bladder volume. As with VCUG, some institutions choose to perform a cyclic DRC with two or three cycles of bladder filling and thereby increase the sensitivity in detecting reflux.

A DRC examination is considered positive for reflux when radiotracer can be seen in the ureter and/or renal pelvis in one or both kidneys (Fig. 1.5). VUR can occur during bladder filling phase or during voiding phase, and the tracer may or may not clear completely from the renal pelvis by the completion of voiding. The severity of reflux is usually characterized by one of the following: Minimal (DRC Grade 1) = reflux into ureter only; Moderate (DRC Grade 2) = reflux reaches renal pelvis; or Severe (DRC Grade 3) = reflux reaches renal pelvis with dilatation of the pelvis and/or ureter. Please note that this 3-point DRC grading scale should not be confused the 5-point international VCUG grading system; these scales are not interchangeable. Minimal reflux is very difficult to detect on DRC, and false-negative examinations are not uncommon when reflux reaches only the distal ureter. However, this minimal form of reflux usually resolves early in childhood, and these false-negatives examinations are doubtful to be of clinical significance.

Indirect Radionuclide Cystogram

An alternative test for the detection of vesicoureteral reflux is the indirect radionuclide cystogram (IRC) [41–50]. This examination should be reserved for children in whom bladder catheterization is impossible [51] and who are older than 3 years of age [39]. To perform IRC, 99mTc-MAG3 is injected intravenously. Continuous dynamic images of the kidney and bladder are obtained during bladder filling and voiding (Fig. 1.6a). It is essential that the patient remains motionless during imaging and can void on command after the bladder has filled. Regions of interest are drawn over the intrarenal collecting systems and the ureters, and time-activity curves

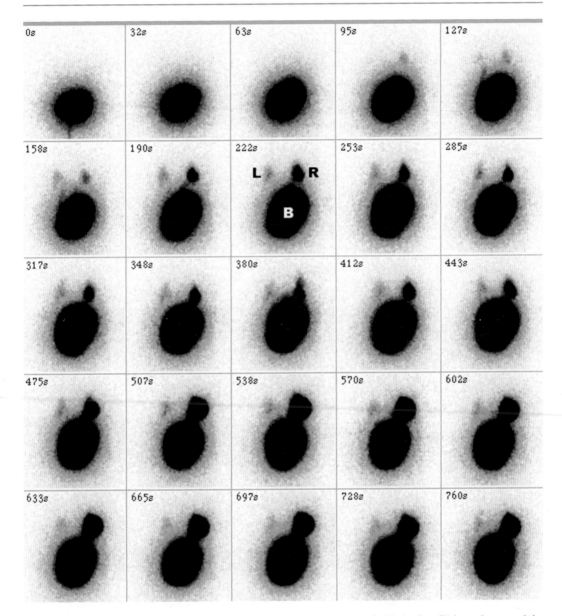

Fig. 1.5 Dynamic posterior images from a direct radionuclide cystogram (DRC). This patient demonstrates bilateral vesicoureteral reflux that occurs during bladder (B) filling. The left-sided reflux (L) is moderate, and the right-sided reflux (R) is severe and compatible with a dilated intrarenal collecting system and ureter

are plotted. A sudden increase in activity in the renal pelvis and ureter indicates the presence of VUR (Fig. 1.6b).

There is ongoing debate regarding whether direct vs. indirect radionuclide cystography is the preferable examination for detecting VUR. In theory, IRC is the better physiologic mimicker, with slow antegrade filling of the bladder. In con-

trast, DRC involves rapid retrograde bladder filling via a catheter, which some believe induces artificial reflux. Others assert that this higher sensitivity of DRC, as high as 95 % [52] is an advantage; and when comparing DRC results to prior VCUG results, the comparison is more valid when the same method of bladder filling has been used. DRC proponents also point out that patients

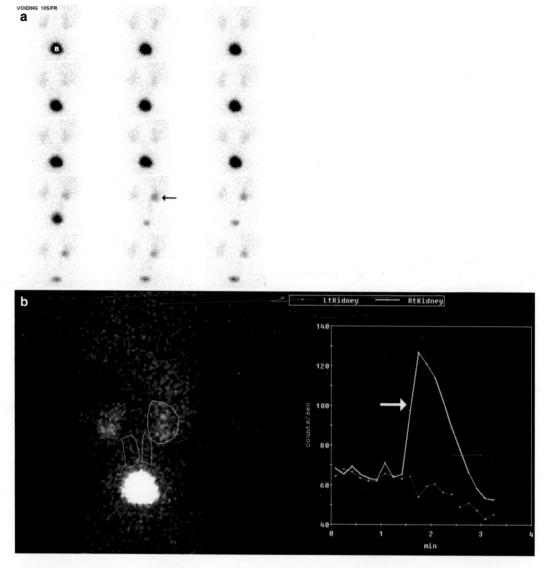

Fig. 1.6 (a) Dynamic posterior images from an indirect radionuclide cystogram (IRC). Initially there is normal drainage of radiotracer activity from the intrarenal collecting systems bilaterally. However, during bladder (b) voiding, there is a sudden and dramatic increased in the radiotracer activity in the right renal pelvis (*arrow*), consistent with vesicoureteral reflux. Dynamic renogram curve (b) confirms this finding; a sudden increase in activity in the right renal pelvis is observed (*arrow*). There is no evidence of reflux in the *left* kidney

with impaired renal function may have insufficient excretion of radiotracer during IRC, resulting in lower sensitivity ranging between 32 % and 81 % according to the literature [42, 45, 52–54]. In practice, there is also a high rate of failure of the IRC because of the inability of children to remain motionless during voiding, and often the inability to void at all during image acquisition [51]. In the case of a negative IRC examination, a subsequent DRC or VCUG is mandatory to confidently exclude vesicoureteral reflux [39].

Renal Cortical Scan

Cortical scintigraphy with 99mTc-DMSA is a highly sensitive examination for the detection of both acute lesions (i.e., pyelonephritis) and late sequelae (i.e., permanent parenchymal scarring) in children with urinary tract infections. It is important to understand that acute lesions of pyelonephritis can take as long as 6 months to resolve scintigraphically. Therefore permanent scarring can only be reported when the DMSA scan is performed at least 6 months after the acute infection. If less than 6 months have elapsed since the acute infection, any defects seen on DMSA scan should be interpreted as either resolving pyelonephritis or potential scar. Therefore it is not routinely recommended to perform renal cortical scintigraphy within 6 months of an acute infection, unless there is an acute need to document renal involvement, as a repeat scan will likely be needed later to exclude permanent scarring [14, 39, 55–57]. When requesting a DMSA scan, it is helpful for the referring physician to note the date of the most recent urinary tract infection.

Renal scarring tends to occur at the upper and lower poles of the kidney due to the round-shaped orifices of the compound papillae at these locations. The simple papillae at the mid-poles have slit-like orifices that are less prone to reflux of infected urine. Renal defects are reported as unilateral or bilateral, single or multiple, small or large, with or without loss of parenchymal volume. Permanent scarring tends to cause loss of parenchymal volume, whereas acute infection does not. If present, a dilated renal pelvis can also be visualized (Fig. 1.7a, b). DMSA cortical scintigraphy is more sensitive than intravenous pyelography and ultrasound for the detection of both acute lesions and permanent scarring [27, 56, 58, 59].

Other causes of cortical defects on DMSA scan include renal cysts and masses. Normal variations in appearance of the renal cortex can include indentation by the adjacent spleen, fetal lobulation, column of Bertin, duplex kidney, and malrotated kidney. Renal cortical scans are often useful in confirming the diagnoses of horseshoe kidney, ectopic kidney, or cross-fused renal ectopia when ultrasound is equivocal (Fig. 1.8a–c).

Images are acquired 2–3 h after injection of 99mTc-DMSA. Planar images are acquired in the posterior, and right and left posterior oblique positions (Fig. 1.9). In infants, additional pinhole images may be acquired that offer higher spatial resolution (Fig. 1.10). In older, sufficiently co-operative children, additional single photon emission computed tomography (SPECT) images may be acquired, again improving spatial resolution [60–64] (Fig. 1.11). The use of recently-developed SPECT iterative reconstruction algorithms can further improve spatial resolution, or maintain spatial resolution with a lower administered dose of radiopharmaceutical [65]. The utility of these additional views is not yet precisely known [66, 67]. Although they have been shown to improve sensitivity for detection of very small cortical defects, there is concern that many false-positive results are obtained [68]. Furthermore, what risk these very small defects pose for long-term clinical sequelae (i.e., hypertension and renal failure) is the subject of continued debate [69–71].

Functional Renal Imaging and Renography

Functional renal imaging uses dynamic image acquisition to evaluate renal perfusion, uptake, excretion, and drainage of radiotracer by the urinary system. Renography refers to the process of plotting the radiotracer activity in the urinary system as a function of time, resulting in renogram (time-activity) curves. The potential amount of information that can be acquired with functional renal imaging is large. Abnormal perfusion can suggest arterial stenosis or occlusion. Delayed uptake and excretion of radiotracer suggest parenchymal disease/dysfunction. Poor drainage of radiotracer into the bladder can suggest obstructive uropathy or over-compliance of the collecting system. Functional renal imaging can be custom-tailored for specific clinical problems. For example, a diuretic challenge can be administered to more sensitively evaluate for urinary obstruction (see below).

Although 99mTc-DTPA is widely used for functional renal imaging, 99mTc-MAG3 is preferred due to its higher extraction fraction and better target-to-background ratio. This advantage is

Fig. 1.7 DMSA Renal cortical scan in a patient with right hydronephrosis and a normal scan as comparison. (**a**) The right kidney is asymmetrically large in size, and demonstrates areas of central photopenia corresponding to the enlarged renal pelvis and calyces. The left kidney is normal. The differential function of the kidneys remains within normal limits (*left* = 45 %, *right* = 55 %). (**b**) Normal DMSA scan

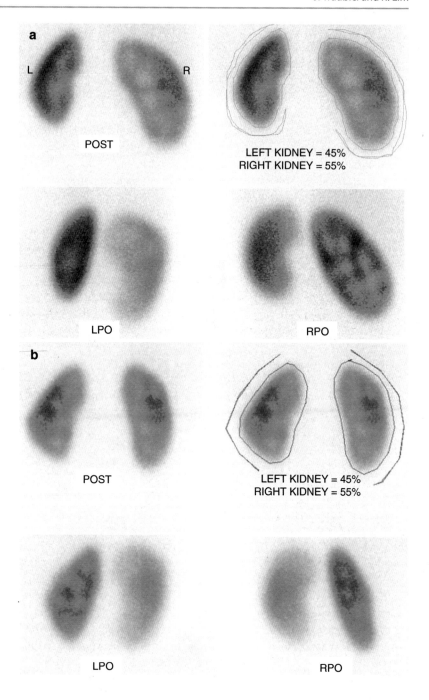

particularly important in patients with impaired renal function or urinary obstruction, and also in very young patients with immature renal function.

Immediately after the injection of radiotracer, imaging of renal perfusion can be performed. The patient lies supine with the camera positioned posteriorly. Radiotracer activity should reach the kidneys about 1 s after the tracer bolus in the abdominal aorta passes the renal arteries; there should be symmetric perfusion of the kidneys [33]. Over the next 20–30 min, imaging of renal function is performed. Maximal parenchymal activity is seen normally at 3–5 min after injection (T_{max}) [33]. Urinary activity in the renal pelvis is

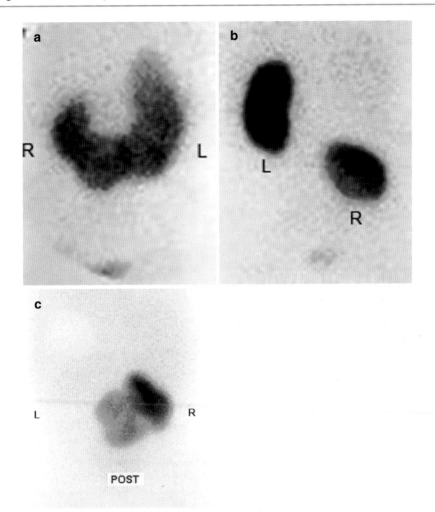

Fig. 1.8 DMSA Renal cortical scans in three different patients with anatomic renal variants. (**a**) Anterior image of a horseshoe kidney. (**b**) Posterior image of a pelvic ectopic right kidney. The left kidney is normal. (**c**) Posterior image of cross-fused renal ectopia

typically seen by 2–4 min after injection (calyceal transit time); however, there is no widespread consensus on what constitutes a normal calyceal transit time [72]. There should be prompt drainage of tracer into the urinary bladder, with less than half of the activity at T_{max} remaining in the renal pelvis by 8–12 min after injection ($T_{1/2}$) [33].

Renogram curves are generated by plotting the activity within regions of interest drawn around each kidney. The renogram is a graphic representation of the uptake, excretion, and drainage phases of renal function, and the curves for each kidney should be reasonably symmetric. Patients should be well-hydrated, preferably with intravenous fluids, when functional renal imaging is performed, as dehydration will result in an abnormal renogram with globally delayed function and slow drainage.

Diuretic Renogram

In the setting of urinary collecting system dilatation not due to vesicoureteral reflux, the possibility of urinary tract obstruction must be considered. Diuretic renography performed with furosemide, is useful in determining the presence of a high grade obstruction at the ureteropelvic junction (UPJ) or

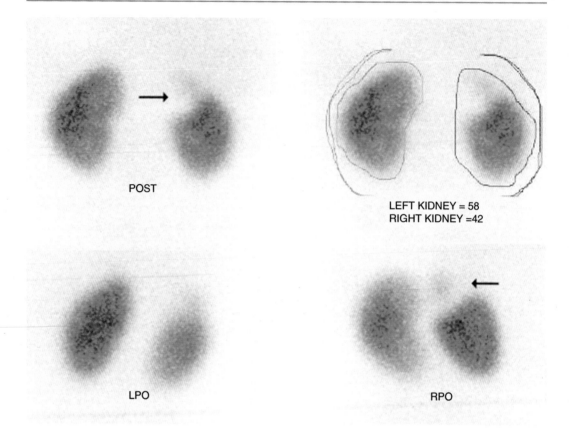

Fig. 1.9 DMSA Renal cortical scan in the posterior (*POST*), left posterior oblique (*LPO*), and right posterior oblique (*RPO*) projections. This patient has a large cortical defect (*arrows*) that represents an extensively scarred upper pole moiety in a duplex kidney. The left kidney is normal. The differential function of the kidneys is at the outer limits of normal (*left* 58 %, *right* 42 %), suggesting that the remaining *right lower* pole moiety has hypertrophied to somewhat compensate for the loss of *upper* pole function

the ureterovesical junction (UVJ). Diuretic renography is commonly used to evaluate the results of surgery in patients who have undergone pyeloplasty for ureteropelvic junction obstruction.

Diuretic renography is performed as described above for dynamic renal imaging, with the additional step of administering intravenous hydration and furosemide to cause maximal urine flow through the collecting system. The dose of furosemide is usually 1 mg/kg, with a maximum dose of 40 mg [73]. The timing of the furosemide administration varies among institutions, as several diuretic protocols have been described, validated, and debated in the literature [39, 74, 75]. The most commonly used protocols are: "F+20" (furosemide is given 20 min after radiotracer if normal spontaneous drainage has not occurred

[76]; this protocol is endorsed by the American Society of Fetal Urology); "F-15" (furosemide is injected first, followed 15 min later by radiotracer; this protocol is the widely-used European standard) [73]; and "F0" (radiotracer and furosemide are injected one immediately following the other) [77, 78].

Bladder catheterization is not always necessary, but should be performed in patients who are not toilet-trained, or who have known hydroureter, vesicoureteral reflux, bladder dysfunction, or posterior urethral valves. In this particular subset of patients, back pressure from urine in the bladder may cause a false-positive result.

The patient lies supine with the camera posterior, and dynamic images are acquired from the time of radiotracer injection for approximately

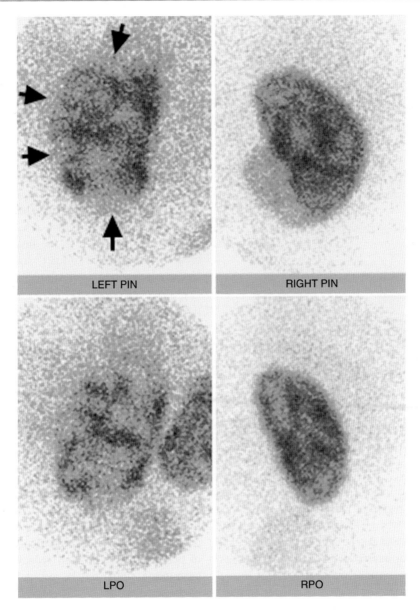

Fig. 1.10 DMSA Renal cortical scan images obtained with a pinhole collimator. This patient demonstrates numerous defects in the left kidney involving the *upper*, *mid*, and *lower* poles (*arrows*). The right kidney is normal

20 min. In the case of the F+20 protocol, an additional 20 min of imaging is performed after injection of furosemide.

In the absence of urinary obstruction, there is rapid drainage of radiotracer from the renal pelvis into the bladder to a minimal residual by 20 min. In quantitative terms, a drainage half-time, $T_{1/2}$, of less than 10 min usually means the absence of obstruction (Fig. 1.12a, b).

In an obstructed system, the drainage of radiotracer from the collecting system will be slow. In this case, a $T_{1/2}$ of greater than 20 min indicates obstruction (Fig. 1.13a–c). When $T_{1/2}$ ranges between 10 and 20 min, this is usually considered an equivocal result, and a follow-up examination will typically be performed to see if the drainage remains unchanged, normalizes, or becomes frankly obstructed.

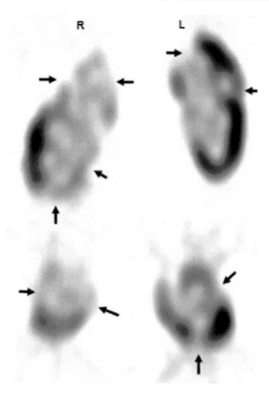

R   L

Fig. 1.11 DMSA Renal cortical scan images obtained with SPECT. This patient demonstrates numerous cortical defects in both kidneys (*arrows*). The right kidney is more extensively scarred than the left kidney

The above drainage parameters are used when analyzing a region of interest drawn around the renal pelvis, when UPJ obstruction is suspected. These values can also be applied to the ureter and to a region of interest combining the ureter and renal pelvis when ureterovesical junction obstruction is suspected.

If at the end of dynamic imaging, there remains a large amount of radiotracer in the renal pelvis and/or ureter, it is useful to position the patient upright and void if possible, followed by a final static image. Sometimes the postural/gravitational effect will cause additional drainage to occur [39].

Pitfalls are common in the interpretation of diuretic renography. Poor renal function from prolonged, severe obstruction can result in poor accumulation of radiotracer in the collecting system, making the renogram difficult or impossible to interpret. A very dilated, overly-compliant, but non-obstructed collecting system may have a prolonged $T_{1/2}$ because the capacious collecting system easily accommodates a large urine volume [73, 75]. This "reservoir effect" can be observed in the setting of primary megaureter, and in patients who have undergone successful pyeloplasty for UPJ obstruction.

Computed Tomography

Although rarely the initial imaging modality in the work-up of urinary tract disease, CT does contribute significantly to the imaging of children with suspected urinary tract disorders. Indications include neoplasia [79], trauma [80, 81], severe infections [82] and occasionally complex questions regarding anatomy [83] (although MRI often would be the preferred modality). Though ultrasound is the mainstay of imaging urolithiasis in children, CT can be useful in cases that on ultrasound are equivocal or non-diagnostic.

CT allows for cross sectional imaging of the urinary tract, and has the ability to reconstruct images in any plane for analysis. CT also provides excellent resolution of the urinary tract structures. The addition of intravenous contrast to the CT imaging allows for even greater accuracy in the detection of disease. Newer generations of CT technology provide higher spatial and temporal resolution and importantly can be done in many instances without sedation or general anaesthesia, which may be required for magnetic resonance imaging.

On unenhanced scans the kidneys demonstrate attenuation similar to the normal liver or spleen. They are surrounded by a variable amount of retroperitoneal fat depending on the age and health status of the child. Administration of contrast results in a reliable pattern of enhancement beginning in the renal cortex, followed by enhancement of the renal pyramids, and later by opacification of the pelvocaliceal system, ureters and bladder.

The ability of CT to differentiate between tissues of various densities allows for the detection of hydronephrosis, renal calcifications (Fig. 1.14)

volume of contrast, using an iso-osmolar contrast medium (e.g., iodixanol), and administering IV fluids before and after the administration of contrast. Prophylactically administered N-acetylcysteine has been shown to reduce contrast-induced nephropathy in certain adult populations; however, it is not routinely used at our institution because its benefit has not yet been proven in the pediatric population [84].

Risk factors for contrast-induced nephropathy include the following:

- Renal impairment
- Congestive Heart Failure
- Diabetes Mellitus
- Dehydration/volume depletion
- Nephrotoxic Drugs: (NSAIDs, ACE inhibitors, aminoglycosides, Metformin)

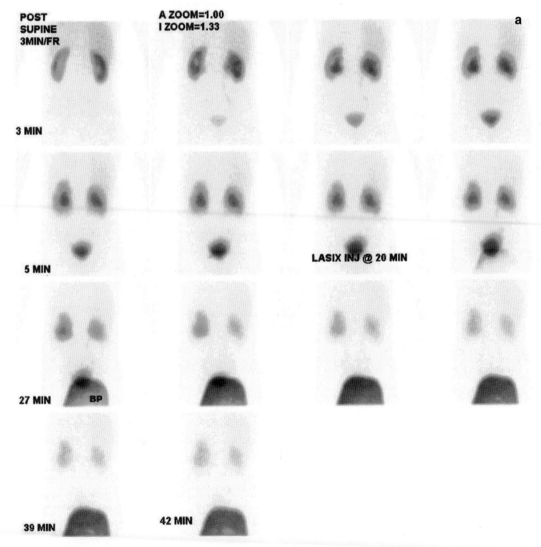

Fig. 1.12 Diuretic MAG3 scan in a patient with bilateral hydronephrosis. (a) After injection of MAG3, dynamic imaging demonstrates radiotracer accumulating in bilateral dilated intrarenal collecting systems, and there is some spontaneous drainage of tracer into the bladder. After injection of furosemide at 20 min (F + 20 protocol), bilateral collecting systems drain rapidly as the patient voids into a bedpan (BP). (b) The renogram curve is a graphic representation of the renal activity. The calculated drainage half-time (T1/2) of both kidneys is within normal limits, indicating the absence of a high-grade urinary obstruction

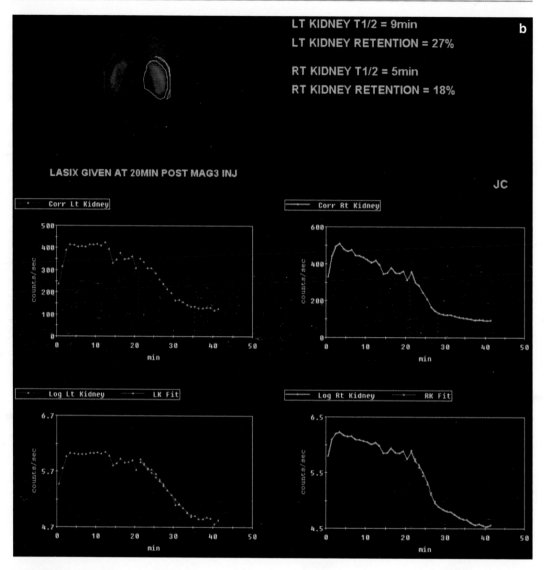

LT KIDNEY T1/2 = 9min
LT KIDNEY RETENTION = 27%

RT KIDNEY T1/2 = 5min
RT KIDNEY RETENTION = 18%

LASIX GIVEN AT 20MIN POST MAG3 INJ

Fig. 1.12 (continued)

and diseases extending into the perirenal fat even without the administration of intravenous contrast. With the addition of intravenous contrast, however, one can detect individual lesions of the renal parenchyma, such as cysts, tumours or nephroblastomatosis; focal areas of diminished enhancement, such as foci of pyelonephritis or contusion/laceration (Fig. 1.15); and global abnormalities of enhancement, such as is evident in renal artery stenosis or thrombosis).

Issues of contrast allergy and contrast induced nephropathy relate more to the iodinated compounds administered in CT than to other contrast agents used in diagnostic imaging. It is important to consider these issues when ordering a CT examination and to discuss the indications and risks with the radiologist involved. Strategies for reducing the risk of adverse contrast reactions include considering an alternative imaging modality, performing a non-contrast-enhanced CT, or administering pre-medication (typically corticosteroids and antihistamines). Other strategies for reducing the risk of contrast-induced nephropathy include reducing the administered

- Dose, frequency and route of contrast media administration
- Comorbid events
- Hypotension, hypertension, sepsis, and cardiac disease
- Structural kidney disease or damage

In diagnostic imaging, CT contributes significantly to the radiation dose imparted to patients, and its deleterious effects are becoming better understood. Recent evidence points to a potential increased risk of cancer in patients who undergo examinations using ionizing radiation, particularly CT [4, 85]. The risk is felt to be greatest in children, who have the greatest sensitivity to these deleterious effects and who have a longer lifespan during which to manifest these effects.

Magnetic Resonance Imaging

Magnetic Resonance Imaging (MRI), like ultrasound, is uniquely suited to the imaging of children in that the child is not exposed to ionizing radiation. Although radiofrequency energy is imparted during performance of the study, MRI has not been shown to have the deleterious

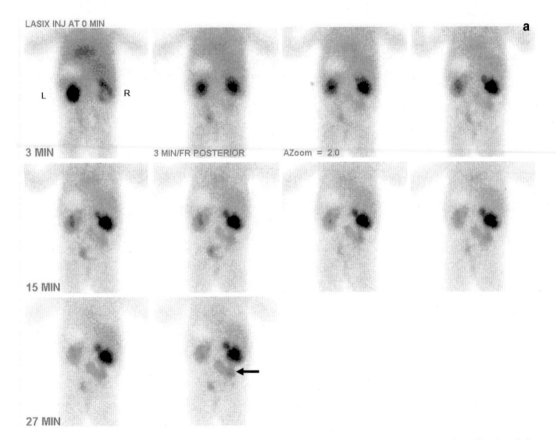

Fig. 1.13 Diuretic MAG3 scan in a patient with right hydronephrosis. In this patient, MAG3 and furosemide were injected at the same time (F0 protocol). (**a**) Dynamic imaging demonstrates normal drainage of radiotracer from the left intrarenal collecting system. However, the right kidney shows progressive accumulation of tracer in a dilated intrarenal collecting system and also in a dilated right ureter (*arrow*), suggestive of urinary obstruction at the ureterovesical junction (UVJ). (**b**) Renogram *curve* shows an abnormally prolonged T1/2 = 153 min of the intrarenal collecting system, compatible with high-grade obstruction. A renogram *curve* plotted from a region of interest drawn around the right ureter (not shown) also demonstrates a prolonged T/12, supportive of obstruction at the UVJ. (**c**) Differential renal function is abnormally asymmetric (*left* 69 %, *right* 31 %) suggesting that parenchymal damage has occurred as a result of the urinary obstruction

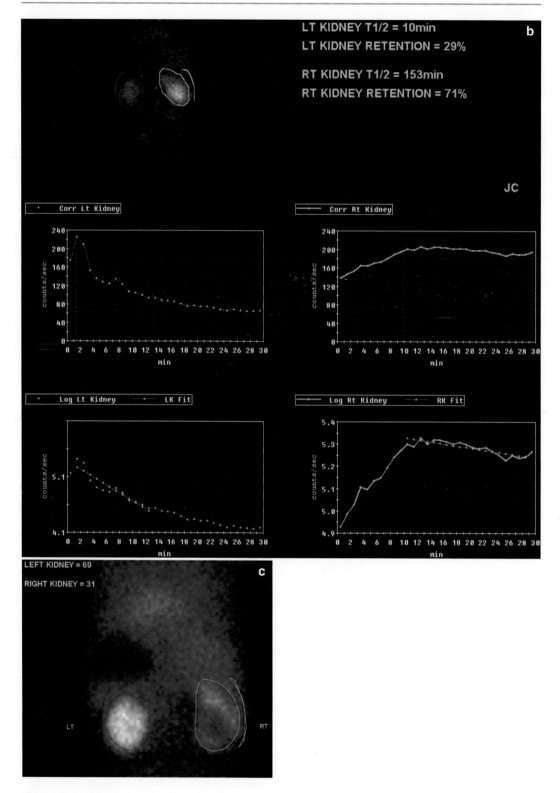

Fig. 1.13 (continued)

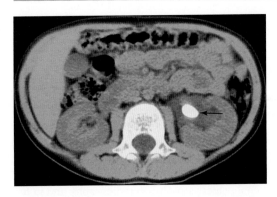

Fig. 1.14 Unenhanced CT at the level of the kidneys demonstrates a calculus (*arrow*) in the left renal pelvis with some pelvic dilatation

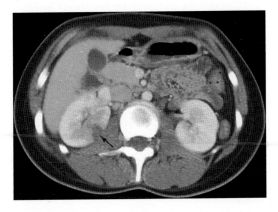

Fig. 1.15 Enhanced CT at the level of the kidneys demonstrates an area in the posteromedial aspect of the right kidney with diminished enhancement (*arrow*), consistent with the clinical suspicion of pyelonephritis

potential of CT. For that reason MRI is often preferred over CT for children. At the same time the examination length and reliance on a cooperative and still patient means that in some situations, particularly in children younger than 5 or 6 and in those with development delay or claustrophobia, sedation or general anaesthesia must be administered and the children carefully monitored [86]. In addition, access to an MR scanner remains limited in some regions of the world.

The superior tissue characterization of MRI makes it a powerful tool in assessing diseases of the urinary tract. Here too intravenous contrast can be administered to help in arriving at the correct diagnosis. Although generally considered safe, adverse reactions to gadolinium-based MRI contrast agents can occur. Although these reactions are by and large mild., severe reactions have been reported with MR contrast agents [87]. Recent reports have also demonstrated that Gadolinium based contrast agents have the potential to be nephrotoxic [88]. In addition recent reports have described an association between administration of Gadolinium based contrast agents and the development of Nephrogenic Fibrosing Dermopathy, a condition described in patients with kidney disease, who have indurated and erythematous plaques of the skin though other organs are also involved [89, 90]. For patients in whom gadolinium contrast is contraindicated, MRI without contrast can still provide detailed structural imaging of the urinary system.

MRI is particularly well suited in assessing neoplasms and tumour-like conditions of the kidneys [91, 92] including nephroblastomatosis [92]. MR can assist in lesion characterization by demonstrating necrosis and hemorrhage in lesions such as Wilms tumor or renal cell carcinoma. Areas of fat can be demonstrated in angiomyolipomas [93, 94]. The demonstration of calcification, however, is not as reliable with MRI as it is with CT.

As in adults, MR can be applied in the assessment of the renal arteries and the renal veins in children. Bland (non-tumour) thrombosis can readily be demonstrated as can tumor extension into the vessels [95, 96]. Renal artery stenosis can be assessed in the investigation of hypertension [97–100] (Fig. 1.16), although the role of MR in renal artery stenosis has been questioned in adult studies [101]. In addition, MR angiography can be a challenging examination in children because of the small size of their arteries. MRI has been applied, too, in the assessment of infection [102–104] and trauma [105, 106].

The ability of MR to assess fluid-containing structures allows for MR urography (MRU) in assessing the renal collecting systems both in terms of anatomical abnormalities (congenital and acquired) [107–109], and more recently in terms of demonstrating the level and degree of

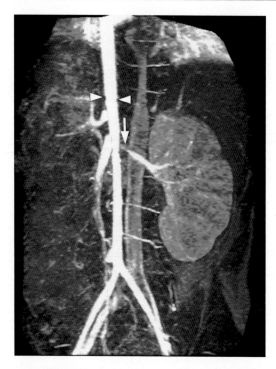

Fig. 1.16 Magnetic resonance angiography (MRA) demonstrates irregularity of the aortic wall and a stenosis (*arrow*) of the proximal aspect of the main renal artery supplying a solitary kidney. This patient was known to have neurofibromatosis

urinary obstruction [110–113] (Fig. 1.17a–c). Research is ongoing into the application of diffusion weighted MRI and MR elastography in renal disease in adults and children [114, 115].

Radiography

Radiography is the oldest modality used in the evaluation of urinary tract disease, but its utility is limited. The normal urinary tract is not sufficiently different in tissue density compared to the surrounding abdominal and pelvic structures to be properly evaluated using radiography alone. There may, however, be cases in which there is sufficient retroperitoneal fat to outline the kidneys on plain radiographs and even assess their relative sizes. A renal mass or severely hydronephrotic kidney might be detected by the presence of a soft tissue mass, calcification or fat, and displacement of adjacent structures (Fig. 1.18). A full bladder can also be seen as a

midline structure in the pelvis, which will occasionally displace bowel loops out of the pelvis (Fig. 1.19).

Calculi in the urinary collecting system can at times be seen on radiography depending on their composition [116–118] (Fig. 1.20). Nephrocalcinosis, cortical or medullary, can also be detected depending on the degree of involvement [119]. In instances of renal failure, particularly if chronic, there may be signs of renal osteodystrophy on radiography and in fact radiography remains the mainstay of imaging the osseous changes associated with renal failure [120].

Radiographs can also be beneficial in determining the correct positioning of various drainage catheters and stents. Ureteral stents in particular can migrate thereby mitigating their effectiveness. Most catheters and stents are sufficiently radio-opaque to be visible on radiographs (Fig. 1.21a, b).

Overall, however, the role of radiography has largely been supplanted by the cross-sectional imaging modalities (ultrasound, CT and MRI) and by nuclear medicine.

Excretory Urography

Excretory urography (intravenous pyelography) relies on the administration of intravenous contrast to enhance the urinary tract and thereby have it stand out against the remainder of the abdominal tissues [121–124]. As other modalities have been applied to the study of urinary tract disorders, the use of excretory urography has fallen off sharply. Ultrasound, CT, MRI and scintigraphy, have to a degree replaced excretory urography [125–128]. At this point, if used at all, excretory urography is performed to delineate and characterize the anatomy of the urinary tract. Congenital variants in ureteral anatomy including ectopic ureters and collecting system duplication can be delineated in this manner. For instance urinary dribbling in girls remains in many institutions and for many urologists an indication for excretory urography in assessing for variant insertion of the ureter [129, 130].

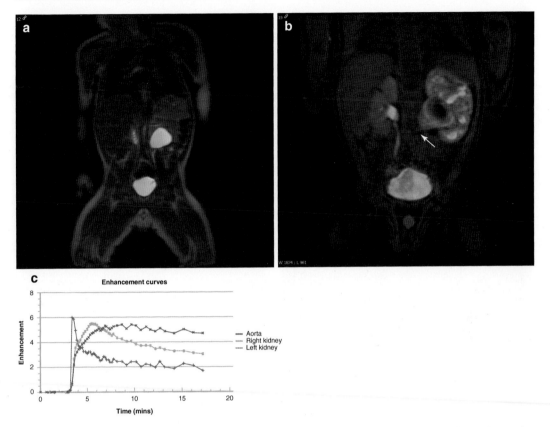

Fig. 1.17 An 8-month-old boy with left UPJ obstruction. (**a**) Coronal T2-WI and (**b**) post-contrast coronal VIBE images show left hydronephrosis with transition at the level of left UPJ (*arrow*). (**c**) Signal intensity versus time curve demonstrates asymmetric perfusion and excretion of contrast agent. The *curve* of the right kidney (*yellow line*) is normal and the left kidney (*purple line*) reveals a dense delayed nephrogram and also delayed excretion

Diseases of the urothelium and papillary necrosis can also be accurately diagnosed and followed with excretory urography [131].

Certainly if excretory urography is performed, care must be taken with respect to administration of intravenous contrast. Issues of nephrotoxicity and allergy to intravenous contrast must be considered. To minimize the radiation dose, the number of radiographs obtained as part of the study should be kept to a minimum, but without sacrificing the diagnostic performance of the test.

Retrograde Urethrography

Though retrograde urethrography is an examination that is not frequently performed, there are indications for this study that have remained constant for many years. In the setting of suspected acute trauma to the male urethra, retrograde urethrography remains the study of choice to assess for a disrupted urethra [132]. One can also assess for other urethral abnormalities both congenital (anterior urethral valves and diverticula) as well as acquired (post-traumatic, post-surgical or infectious) [133–135] (Fig. 1.22a, b). The examination involves placement of a balloon tipped catheter into the distal urethra and careful inflation of a balloon in the fossa navicularis. Images of the urethra are taken in an oblique projection during a hand injection of water-soluble contrast. Due to the presence of the external sphincter, the posterior urethra is usually not optimally assessed as part of this study but rather can be imaged during voiding after filling the bladder directly.

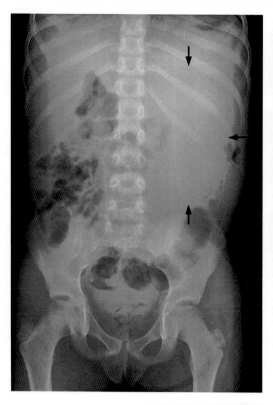

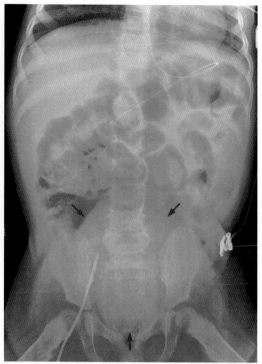

Fig. 1.18 Radiograph of the abdomen demonstrates soft tissue density in the region of the left renal fossa with displacement of bowel (*arrows*). A renal cell carcinoma was discovered on cross sectional imaging

Fig. 1.19 Radiograph of the abdomen demonstrates soft tissue in the pelvis displacing bowel out of the pelvis (*arrows*). Ultrasound demonstrated a full bladder was the cause of the imaging findings

Applications of Diagnostic Imaging

Diseases of the Neonate

With the increase in antenatal imaging (ultrasound and to a much lesser degree MRI) and the detection of abnormalities prenatally, there has been a commensurate increase in postnatal imaging in the work-up of antenatal findings. The most common indication for assessment of the urinary tract in these situations is the follow-up of antenatally diagnosed pelvocaliceal dilatation, renal ectopia, agenesis or dysplasia. The pathologies encountered in these children range from mild to severe and life-threatening. The initial postnatal examination will almost always be an ultrasound to determine whether two kidneys are present, their location and the status of the parenchyma and collecting system. An increase in parenchymal echogenicity or loss of corticomedullary differentiation can be a sign of renal abnormality. Parenchymal loss, scarring and cyst formation can be other signs of renal damage.

In many institutions, the initial postnatal ultrasound will be done after the first week of life so as not to miss hydronephrosis during the relative dehydrated state of the newborn period and the non-distended state of the collecting system. If dilatation is present and involves only the pelvocaliceal system, then there may be an obstruction at the ureteropelvic junction [136] (Fig. 1.23a, b). If the ureter is also dilated, an obstruction may be present at the ureterovesical junction [137]. If the bladder is distended and perhaps trabeculated, the obstruction may involve the bladder outlet or urethra (Fig. 1.24a–c) [138]. At the same time any degree of pelvocaliceal and/or ureteral dilatation can be due to vesicoureteral reflux.

The presence of a duplicated collecting system can be inferred on ultrasound when the renal

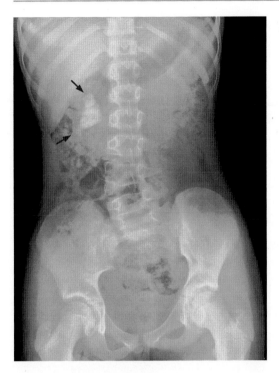

Fig. 1.20 Radiograph of the abdomen demonstrates a calcific density in the region of the right renal fossa (*arrows*). A staghorn calculus was found on ultrasound. Incidental note was made of a tripediculate vertebra in the lower lumbar spine

junction are termed *orthotopic or simple ureteroceles* and like ectopic ureteroceles can be obstructive or non-obstructive [141].

Thereafter the work-up of a dilated collecting system may vary among institutions. In brief, the investigations assess for the known pathologies that affect the neonate and infant. If the dilatation is indeed determined to be present and persistent on postnatal ultrasound, a VCUG can assess for vesicoureteral reflux and its degree. The VCUG can also assess for urethral obstruction due to posterior urethral valves in a male. If the child is found not to have reflux or valves, nuclear medicine diuretic renography can assess for any degree and level of urinary obstruction.

A number of other congenital abnormalities can be diagnosed in the antenatal or neonatal period. Failure of the ureteric bud to join the metanephric blastema is thought to be the inciting factor in the development of the multicystic dysplastic kidney (MCDK). In this case normal renal parenchyma is not present. Rather, the kidney is replaced by multiple non-communicating cysts with dysplastic parenchymal tissue [142, 143]. Demonstration of the lack of communication among the cysts differentiates this process from pelvocaliceal dilatation. Imaging can also demonstrate renal agenesis, ectopia, horseshoe and cross fused kidneys. Again, ultrasound is the preferred initial imaging modality, although in some cases the findings are discovered incidentally on other modalities (including DMSA renal cortical scintigraphy).

Conditions affecting the renal vasculature in the neonate, including thrombosis of the renal arteries or veins, can be assessed with Doppler ultrasound imaging of the vessels and the kidneys. Associated thrombosis of the aorta and IVC can also be assessed. If a central catheter is present, which can predispose a patient to thrombosis, its position can best be assessed with radiographs of the abdomen, although the catheters can certainly be resolved with ultrasound as well. If a thrombus has occurred, recanalization can be assessed sonographically after anticoagulation or thrombolysis. Occasionally residual thrombus can calcify and be visible as a linear hyperechoic structure along the vessel wall either

sinus echo complex is interrupted by a band of renal cortical tissue, though it can be difficult to distinguish this pattern from a prominent column of Bertin [139]. The presence of a duplex collecting system may be associated with obstruction (usually of the upper moiety) and/or reflux (usually of the lower moiety) according to the Meyer-Weigert rule. This rule states that in a duplicated collecting system, the upper moiety is drained by a ureter, which inserts ectopically and the lower moiety is drained by a ureter that inserts orthotopically – with the former often obstructed by a ureterocele and the latter demonstrating reflux. These entities (obstruction and reflux) can coexist in the same patient. With respect to ureteroceles, the diagnosis can be made on almost any modality, though most commonly it is diagnosed on ultrasound or VCUG [140]. One must bear in mind that not all ectopic ureters end in a ureterocele. Similarly not all ureteroceles are ectopic. Ureteroceles at the normal ureterovesical

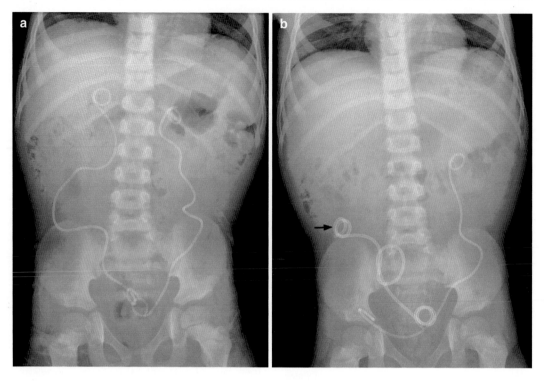

Fig. 1.21 (a) Radiograph of the abdomen demonstrates double J stents overlying the urinary tracts. Proximal and distal loops overlie the renal pelves and bladder respectively although the ureteral courses appear tortuous. (b) Several days later, both stents have changes in position most evident on the *right* where the proximal aspect of the stent appears to be in the right ureter (*arrow*)

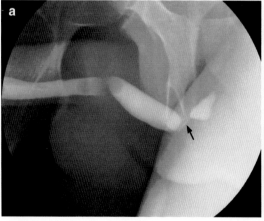

Fig. 1.22 (a) Retrograde urethrogram demonstrates a stricture of the bulbous urethra (*arrow*) post trauma (straddle injury). (b) In order to precisely determine the length and degree of the stricture the bladder was filled via a suprapubic tube. With voiding and simultaneous retrograde urethrography, one can precisely delineate the stricture length and severity. Posterior urethra (*black arrow*). Stricture (*white arrow*)

in the major vessels or within the renal parenchyma, in the case of small vessel thrombosis. Follow-up renal ultrasound can also assess for any long term sequelae of thrombosis, such as atrophy, abnormal parenchymal echogenicity or cyst formation.

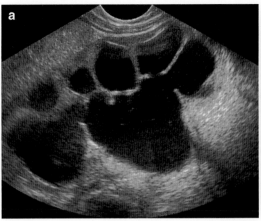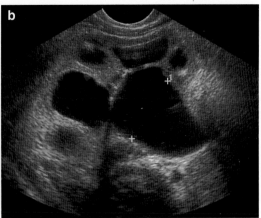

Fig. 1.23 (**a, b**) Longitudinal and transverse images of the kidney demonstrate a dilated collecting system with no ureteral dilatation noted in this patient in whom diuretic renal scintigraphy confirmed severe obstruction at the uretero-pelvic junction. Calipers measure the renal pelvis on the transverse image

Vesicoureteral Reflux and Infection

The topic of vesicoureteral reflux and infections of the urinary tract will be discussed more fully in subsequent chapters. There are numerous contributions that can be made by imaging in these conditions. Again ultrasound, VCUG and nuclear medicine will be the modalities most used in order to assess for findings suggestive of obstruction or reflux – although abnormal findings can be seen with other modalities. Typically ultrasound will be used to look for hydronephrosis that may suggest obstruction or reflux, as well as for signs of either acute infection or sequelae of previous infection (focal scarring or global volume loss). DMSA renal cortical scintigraphy remains the most sensitive modality for detection of pyelonephritis and scars. In the case of global volume loss, the contralateral kidney may undergo compensatory hypertrophy.

VCUG will assess for the presence of reflux, whether it occurs during filling or with voiding, and its grade. The system of the International Reflux Study in Children classifies reflux into five grades (Fig. 1.25). Reflux into the ureter alone is classified as Grade I. When contrast fills the intrarenal collecting system but without dilatation, it is classified as Grade II. Grades III–V demonstrate progressive dilatation of the ureter,

pelvis and calyces [31]. VCUG will also assess the anatomy of any opacified structure. The renal collecting system can be assessed for duplication. Parenchymal loss can be inferred by the opacification of the intrarenal system if the calyces appear convergent. The bladder can be assessed for capacity, thickening and trabeculation. Diverticulation and urachal opacification can be seen in some cases. Valves, diverticula and the overall morphology of the urethra particularly in the male can be assessed.

In cases of known VUR, follow-up evaluation can be performed with direct radionuclide cystogram to assess for resolution or persistence of reflux. In the case of a hydronephrotic kidney on ultrasound and a negative VCUG, a diuretic renogram can be used to evaluate for the presence of urinary tract obstruction.

There can be imaging findings for acute infection as well, though they are not always specific. With diffuse infection of the renal parenchyma, the entire kidney may be enlarged [144]. This enlargement may be reflected in an increase in renal length, although the entire volume should be assessed in order to detect increases in transverse diameter. Infection can also involve a portion of the kidney and, in some cases, can simulate a renal mass [145]. The echogenicity of the affected region can be increased or decreased [146, 147]. Increased echogenicity of the renal

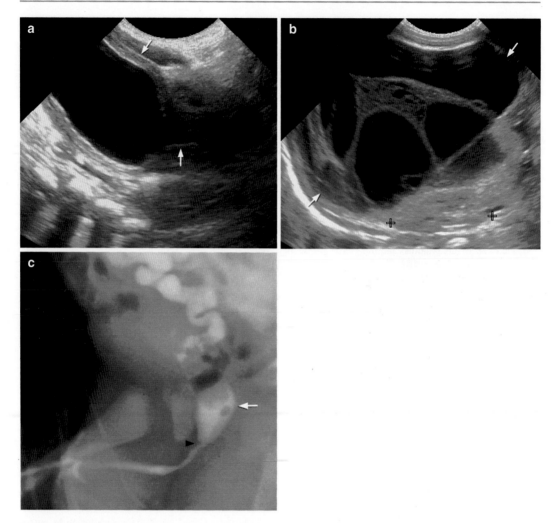

Fig. 1.24 (a) Ultrasound of the bladder in the longitudinal plane demonstrates thickening of the bladder wall (*black arrow*) and dilatation of the posterior urethra just beyond the bladder neck (*white arrow*) in this patient with posterior urethral valves. (b) In the same patient a complex appearing urinoma (*arrows*) is seen adjacent to an abnormally echogenic kidney (calipers). (c) Voiding cystourethrogram confirms dilatation of the posterior urethra (*white arrow*) to the level of obstruction (*black arrowhead*) just distal to the verumontanum. Vesicoureteral reflux into a tortuous ureter is also present

sinus has also been described in cases of infection [148]. The urothelial wall of the pelvis, ureter or bladder can also be thickened. One can also look at the appearance of the fluid in the urinary tract. Echogenic debris in the collecting system can suggest, though it is not pathognomonic for, infection.

Infected areas of the kidney are often relatively hypoperfused and may demonstrate diminished enhancement after the administration of intravenous contrast on CT or MRI and diminished flow on Doppler interrogation on ultrasound (Fig. 1.15). The area, however, can also be hyperperfused on sonography. Acute pyelonephritis will appear as cold defects on DMSA renal cortical scan. If cortical defects persist beyond 6 months after clinical resolution of the acute infection, they are considered to be permanent scars that can predispose to renal failure and hypertension.

Fungal infection of the kidneys represents a special situation where imaging can play an

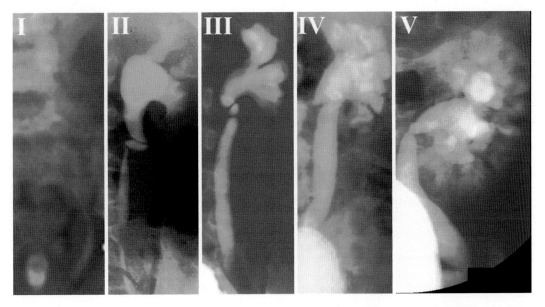

Fig. 1.25 International Grading System of vesicoureteral reflux, illustrating VCUG grades I through V

important role. In patients who are immunosuppressed or have indwelling catheters, ultrasound may demonstrate infection of the renal parenchyma and assess for the presence of fungal balls of the collecting systems. One must, however, exercise caution as blood clots or other tumefactive material can mimic fungal balls in the renal collecting system.

Neoplasm

Most renal neoplasms in children present as a palpable mass detected by the parent or physician. In cases such as these the mass is often very large and the first imaging modality requested is an ultrasound, though occasionally a radiograph might be obtained first. Ultrasound can suggest the renal origin of an abdominal mass by demonstrating extension of renal tissue around the mass – the so-called "claw sign" (Fig. 1.26a–c). It can also differentiate solid from cystic or necrotic areas and demonstrate if any hemorrhage or calcification is present. Ultrasound also is useful in determining whether the tumor involves the renal vein or IVC or extends into the heart. Once it is determined that a tumor is present, CT or MRI can assess the lesion further and better assess the

size, extent, involvement of adjacent structures, and spread [149, 150]. In fact it has been shown in Wilms tumor patients that cross-sectional imaging (CT or MRI) will add additional information over ultrasound alone in over half of patients [151]. Although CT and MRI would be roughly equivalent in assessing the primary renal mass, CT is the modality of choice to assess the lungs for metastatic disease. If the tumor has a propensity to metastasize elsewhere, then appropriate imaging modalities (CT or MRI of the brain, bone scan, etc.) can be performed.

Trauma

Imaging of trauma to the urinary tract has been studied extensively and remains a topic of debate [152]. In the acute setting, the imaging evaluation of the injured child is determined by the extent and type of injury as well as the practice of the particular institution [80, 153]. In some institutions evaluation of trauma to the abdomen begins with sonography of the abdomen to assess for free fluid and obvious visceral injuries [154, 155]. At other institutions, CT is the modality of choice in the initial assessment [38, 81, 152]. The decision as to which modality is used will depend

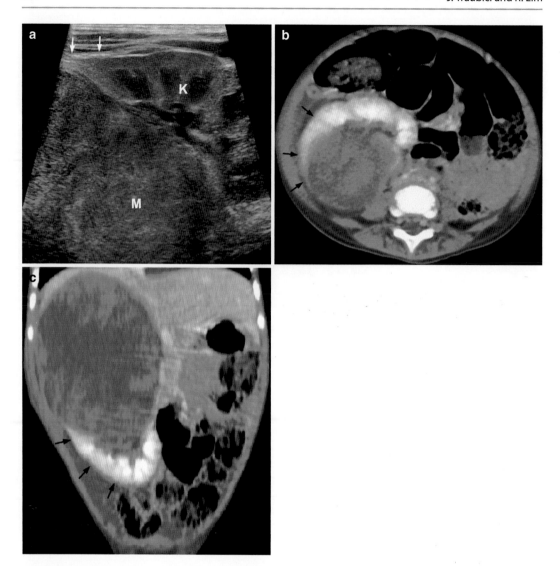

Fig. 1.26 (**a**) Ultrasound of the kidney demonstrates a mass arising from the kidney. A rim of renal tissue surrounds a portion of the mass – an appearance that has been given the term "claw sign." Kidney (*K*), Mass (*M*). (**b**, **c**) CT axial images and coronal reformations demonstrate a claw sign is present (*arrows*), confirming the renal origin of this mass, which was found to be a Wilms tumour

on the clinical situation. Ultrasound has a high sensitivity in detecting intraperitoneal fluid; however, in the setting of trauma, the presence of fluid is not an absolute indication for surgery. At the same time, there can be injury to the urinary tract without the presence of free fluid [156]. CT, on the other hand, can accurately assess for the presence of free fluid and at the same time assess the solid and hollow viscera of the abdomen.

Sonography can depict a renal laceration or contusion as a focal area of abnormal echotexture. The area can be hypoechoic, isoechoic or hyperechoic to the remainder of the kidney depending on the contents of the area and the stage of the evolution of the injury. Sonography can also depict the quality and amount of perirenal fluid (blood, urine or both) and follow the appearance so as to assess whether the collection is diminishing, remaining stable or increasing in size. Doppler interrogation of the kidneys can assess both for areas of the renal parenchyma that are ischemic due to vascular interruption and for arterial or venous thrombosis and

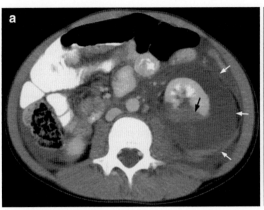 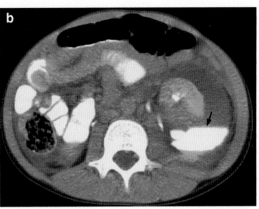

Fig. 1.27 (**a**) Enhanced CT demonstrates a large perinephric hematoma around the left kidney (*white arrows*) and a portion of the posterior aspect of the kidney, which demonstrates diminished enhancement consistent with an area of laceration/contusion (*black* *arrow*). (**b**) Delayed images obtained through the same area demonstrate accumulation of the intravenous contrast in the perinephric space (*arrow*), confirming an injury to the renal collecting system

pseudoaneurysm formation. Renal vascular injury can also be visualized with nuclear medicine functional renal imaging, with non-perfused regions of the kidney appearing as cold defects.

As mentioned, CT is the current modality of choice in assessing abdominal trauma in children and offers much in the evaluation of urinary tract trauma. The appearance of the kidneys and particularly their patterns of enhancement on CT can allow for the diagnosis of renal contusions and lacerations. Areas devoid of enhancement particularly if they are geographic, suggest infarction. Perinephric and/or periureteral fluid can also be assessed. Delayed imaging may show disruption of the collecting system if dense contrast is seen outside of the collecting system (Fig. 1.27a, b). CT cystography has also been used to assess for injuries to the urinary bladder and urethra.

In the past intravenous urography was used extensively in the evaluation of urinary tract trauma, but is seldom used today. Fluoroscopic studies (retrograde urethrography and cystography) are, however, still used extensively in the imaging of bladder and urethral injury.

Renal Failure

The appearance of the kidneys in cases of renal failure has been touched on in other parts of this chapter. There may be findings on imaging which point to the etiology of the disease if it is not yet known. In some cases, the failing kidneys will appear normal despite meticulous imaging. In many cases, however, there will be some detectable abnormality that will at least suggest a renal abnormality. In acute renal failure the kidneys may appear normal or increased in size on ultrasound and there may be an increase in parenchymal echogenicity. Diminution or loss of corticomedullary differentiation may also be present. If the changes involve mainly the cortex, then the corticomedullary differentiation may be accentuated. In chronic renal failure, the kidneys tend to be small and echogenic with diminished corticomedullary differentiation. Scarring and dysplastic cysts may be present depending on the etiology of the renal insult.

Differential Renal Function

During nuclear medicine functional renal imaging (i.e., 99mTc-MAG3 scintigraphy), renal uptake measured between 1 and 2 min after radiotracer injection is used to calculate differential renal function, also known as split function or relative function. Differential renal function refers to the percentage of total renal function that is contributed by each of the kidneys. Differential renal function can also be calculated based on renal uptake measured on DMSA cortical scintigraphy. In general, unilaterally reduced function to less than 44–45 % [66] is considered abnormal; however, cut-off values anywhere from 40 % to 45 % are widely used [39, 74, 157–161].

Differential function should be measured based on images acquired immediately before radiotracer enters the collecting system. Occasionally, the function in one kidney may be so delayed that its parenchyma is not yet visualized by the time the contralateral kidney has begun excretion of tracer. In this situation, an accurate differential function measurement is not possible.

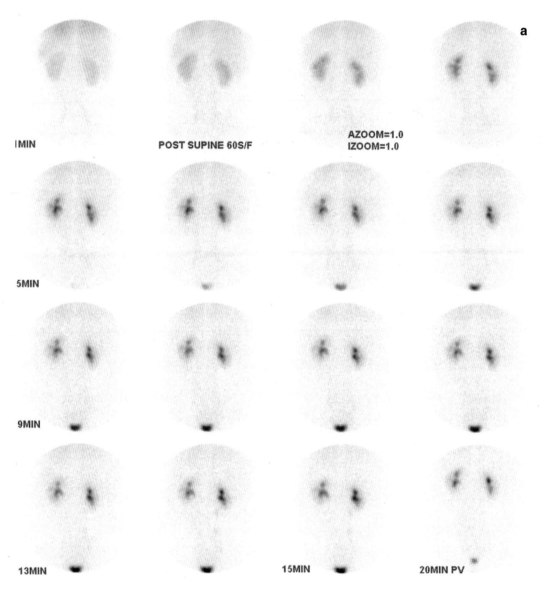

Fig. 1.28 DTPA GFR calculation. When 99mTc-DTPA is used to calculate GFR, dynamic renal imaging and differential function calculation can also be performed. (**a**) Dynamic renal imaging performed immediately after injection of radiotracer demonstrates normal uptake, excretion, and drainage in both kidneys. (**b**) Differential renal function is symmetric and normal (*left* 56 %, *right* 44 %). (**c**) Static image of the injection site in the antecubital fossa demonstrates that no extravasation of tracer has occurred. Calculations based on serial blood plasma sampling demonstrate normal GFR (GFR/1.73 m^2 = 127 mL/min)

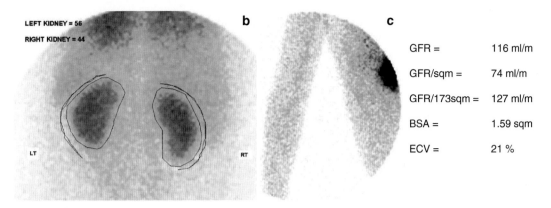

Fig. 1.28 (continued)

Anatomic abnormalities are another potential source of error. Attenuation effects due to severe hydronephrosis, a large renal cyst or mass, or an ectopically positioned kidney may artifactually lower the differential function value of the affected kidney. These attenuation effects can be reduced to some degree by using geometric-mean correction techniques, which utilize images acquired from both the anterior and posterior aspects of the patient's body. In the case of a duplicated collecting system, the scintigraphic images of the kidney can be divided into upper and lower pole regions of interest so that the relative contribution of each moiety can be reported.

Glomerular Filtration Rate

Measurement of glomerular filtration rate is discussed also in Chap. 3, "Laboratory Evaluation at of Renal Disease in Childhood." Either chromium 51 (51Cr) EDTA, or 99mTc-DTPA can be used to calculate GFR (see Glomerular Filtration Agents, above). If 99mTc-DTPA is used, functional renal imaging and calculation of differential renal function can also be performed (Fig. 1.28a–c).

Renal Transplant Evaluation

Imaging of the renal allograft has become an integral part of renal transplantation particularly in the immediate post-operative period. Given its non-invasive character, sonography is a mainstay of allograft imaging and can be performed in the operating room if the surgeon requests. The location of the allograft, in the iliac fossa, allows for close examination with grey scale and Doppler techniques. Sonography can assess for the overall echogenicity of the kidney and the presence of corticomedullary differentiation. It can also accurately assess the degree of hydronephrosis, if present. In addition, sonography plays an important role in assessing for perinephric fluid collections. When large, these collections may compromise drainage of urine, or blood flow to and from the kidney.

Doppler techniques can assess for renal artery or renal vein thrombosis or thrombus in the vessels to which the renal artery and vein are anastomosed, usually the iliac vessels. It can also assess for other causes of compromise to flow, such as stenosis or kinking of the vessel. In addition, Doppler interrogation of the allograft can detect arteriovenous fistulae, a not uncommon complication of allograft biopsy [162].

Although sonography, can assess for signs of acute and chronic rejection, the role of Doppler interrogation of the allograft remains controversial [29] and clinical findings and biopsy remain the mainstay of diagnosis. Later complications such as stone formation and neoplasm, including post transplant lymphoproliferative disorder (PTLD), can also be assessed with imaging (ultrasound, CT or MRI).

Nuclear medicine functional renal scintigraphy is another modality liberally utilized in many institutions. Patients who have undergone renal transplantation typically have renal scintigraphy performed within 24 h of surgery to assess the baseline perfusion and function of the allograft. The camera is positioned anteriorly in these patients to better image the kidney in the iliac fossa. If renal function deteriorates or post-operative complications are suspected, follow-up imaging can be performed and compared.

During the perfusion phase, radiotracer should reach the renal allograft at almost the same time it is seen in the iliac vessels. The uptake, excretion, and drainage phases should appear similar to those of a normal native kidney with maximal parenchymal activity at 3–5 min. Tracer should be seen in the bladder 4–8 min post-injection [33] (Fig. 1.29a, b).

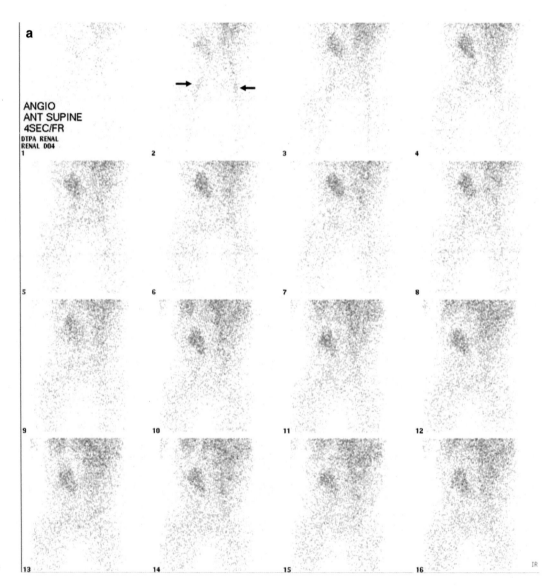

Fig. 1.29 Normal MAG3 renal transplant scan compared to normal native kidney scan. (**a**) Perfusion phase imaging demonstrates radiotracer reaching the renal allograft at the same time the iliac arteries (*arrows*) are visualized. (**b**) There is normal uptake, excretion and drainage of radiotracer, with activity seen in the bladder (**B**) and Foley catheter (*F*) by 2–3 min post-injection. No parenchymal defects or urine extravasation are seen

b

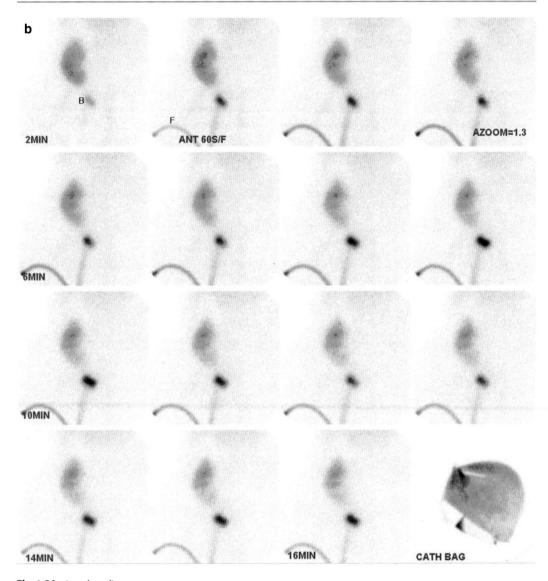

Fig. 1.29 (continued)

Possible complications of renal transplantation include acute tubular necrosis (ATN), rejection, cyclosporine toxicity, urinoma, urinary obstruction, lymphocele, hematoma, and arterial or venous thrombosis [163–170].

Acute tubular necrosis is characterized by preserved renal perfusion, but also by progressive parenchymal retention of radiotracer with decreased or absent urine production (Fig. 1.30a–c). It typically resolves within a few weeks after transplantation. ATN occurs more commonly in cadaveric transplants than in living-related donor transplants, and is related to the elapsed time between harvesting and transplantation. Cyclosporine toxicity has a similar appearance to ATN, but differs in time course and occurs many weeks after transplantation. It usually resolves after withdrawal of cyclosporine therapy.

Rejection is characterized by poor perfusion and poor excretion of radiotracer. Hematoma, urinoma and lymphocele can appear as a photopenic defect on early blood pool images. A suffi-

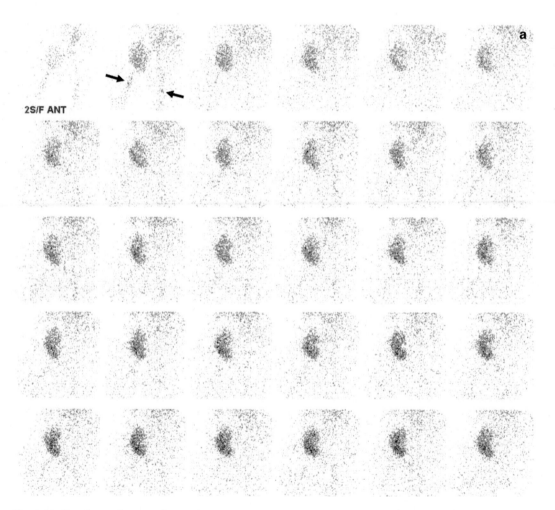

Fig. 1.30 Renal transplant scan in a patient with acute tubular necrosis (ATN). (**a**) Perfusion phase images show relatively preserved perfusion with radiotracer reaching the renal allograft at the same time as the iliac arterial vessels (*arrows*). (**b**) There is relatively preserved uptake into the renal parenchymal without focal defect. However, there is poor clearance of tracer from soft tissues, and there is no detectable excretion of tracer into the renal pelvis, ureter, or bladder consistent with ATN. (**c**) Delayed images obtained 30 min post-injection show prolonged retention of radiotracer in soft tissues and kidney parenchyma (*arrow*). There continues to be no excretion of radiotracer into the urinary collecting system, and no urine activity is detected in the Foley catheter bag (*right*)

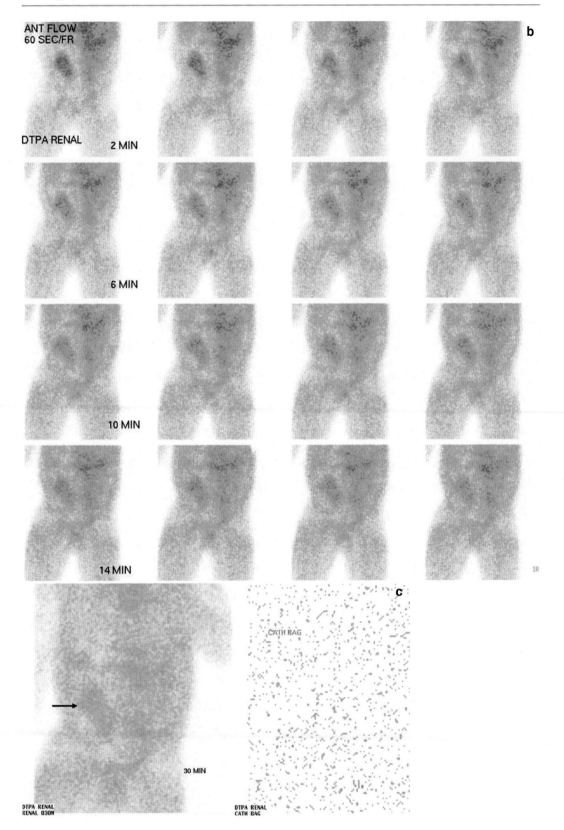

Fig. 1.30 (continued)

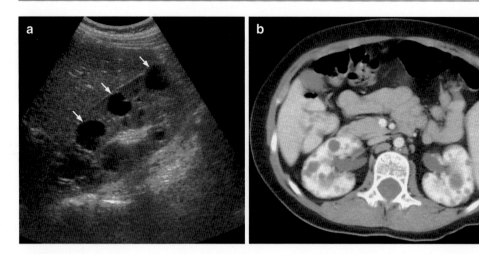

Fig. 1.31 (**a**) Ultrasound of the right kidney demonstrates multiple cysts (*arrows*) in a patient with autosomal dominant polycystic kidney disease. (**b**) Enhanced CT in the same patient demonstrated multiple cysts of varying sizes scattered throughout both kidneys

ciently large urine leak may result in extrarenal accumulation of radiotracer. Vascular occlusion will appear as a large reniform photopenic region. Urinary obstruction will appear as accumulation of radiotracer in the renal pelvis with poor drainage into the bladder. Postural drainage maneuvers and diuretic challenge (see above) should be considered when urinary obstruction is suspected [166, 171].

Renal Cystic Diseases

Cysts in the kidney can be seen at any age in the pediatric group and can be associated with a wide array of disease states as well as sporadically and unassociated with any other pathology. It can be difficult to differentiate a renal cyst from a caliceal diverticulum. This can be assessed if necessary by using a modality in which contrast is administered such as CT or MR, as contrast will fill a diverticulum but not a cyst.

A number of systems of classification of cysts have been proposed and are discussed elsewhere in this text. Cysts of the kidneys can broadly be divided into those with hereditary causes and those with non-hereditary causes [172]. The imaging appearance can in some cases point to an etiology and in some cases cannot. Simple renal cysts can be seen in children, just as in adults, though the reported incidence is as low as 0.2 % [173]. Solitary cysts can also be seen as the sequela of previous insult to the kidney, such as trauma or infection. In most cases of solitary cysts the appearance of the remainder of the kidney is often normal.

On ultrasound, a renal cyst will appear anechoic with an imperceptible wall. Increased through transmission can be seen deep to the cyst. On CT the cyst will have an attenuation equal or near that of simple fluid and again will have an imperceptible wall. There should be little to no change in the attenuation of the cyst after contrast administration. If there is enhancement (either on CT or MRI) or any other complex feature to the structure, then one should consider the possibility that what may appear to be a simple cyst may in fact be a neoplastic lesion, which may require further evaluation.

Imaging has proven useful in the evaluation of non-hereditary renal cystic disease including multicystic dysplastic kidney [174], solitary simple and acquired cysts [173], and medullary sponge kidney [175]. Imaging has also proven its utility in the evaluation of hereditary cystic renal disease both in the diagnosis and in follow-up. Several authors have described the specific features of these renal cystic diseases. Autosomal dominant polycystic kidney disease [176] (Fig. 1.31a, b) can evolve as the child grows. There may be macroscopic cysts at the initial examination, be it in infancy or childhood, with the cysts increasing in number and size as the child grows. Autosomal recessive polycystic kidney disease can have a number of findings, which are best seen when the kidneys are assessed with a high resolution transducer. Macroscopic cysts, dilated tubules, crystal deposition, preservation of a normal appearing cortical rim and overall nephromegaly have been described in children with ARPKD [177]. In juvenile nephronophthisis cysts are seen in the medullary pyramids [178]. The appearance of glomerulocystic disease [179] is one of enlarged and hyperechoic kidneys with cortical cysts particularly in the periphery.

Imaging can not only assess the cysts in these scenarios but also other associated findings, which may be present. Examples would include assessing for angiomyolipomas in children with tuberous sclerosis or assessing for liver disease in children with autosomal recessive polycystic kidney disease [180].

Nephrocalcinosis, Urolithiasis and Miscellaneous Calcifications

There are a number of imaging findings in the pediatric urinary tract, which have been classified under the broad term renal calcification. Most are detected on ultrasound by virtue of the fact that ultrasound remains the most commonly used modality and is the most sensitive to these changes.

Urolithiasis can be relatively easy to diagnose with imaging and with ultrasound in particular. Renal stones can range from a few millimeters in size in a renal calyx to several centimeters in size filling the renal pelvis (staghorn calculus) (Fig. 1.32). They are most reliably detected when present in the kidney or bladder, but can also be seen in the ureter when not obscured by overlying bowel gas. On ultrasound, they present as echogenic foci, often with distal acoustic shadowing. When small they can be difficult to differentiate from vessels or portions of renal sinus fat – particularly if the distal shadowing is not present. The

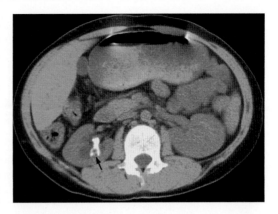

Fig. 1.32 Unenhanced CT demonstrates a calculus (*arrow*) in the right renal collecting system extending into the calyces. The attenuation differences between calculi and the renal parenchyma are sufficient to allow for the diagnosis of urolithiasis without the administration of intravenous contrast

stones can be assessed in terms of their size and any associated collecting system dilatation. As stated earlier, ultrasound remains the modality of choice in imaging urolithiasis in children, with CT performed when the ultrasound examination is equivocal or non-diagnostic. Some have advocated a role for CT in predicting the success of extracorporeal shock wave lithotripsy based on stone size and using the Hounsfield attenuation values to infer composition [181].

Nephrocalcinosis can also be assessed with imaging and again ultrasound is often the modality of choice. While cortical nephrocalcinosis can be seen, it is a rare finding in children [182]. Medullary nephrocalcinosis is well described in children and can be accurately diagnosed and followed – again preferably with ultrasound. The appearance is typically one of echogenic pyramids, often outlining the rim of the pyramid and a normal appearing cortex (Fig. 1.33a, b). A pattern of peripheral increased echogenicity followed by progression toward the center of the pyramid has been described as the Anderson Carr progression of nephrocalcinosis [119].

Lastly with the improvement in high resolution imaging of the kidneys in children, smaller echogenic foci are being detected. While the precise etiology of these findings is being

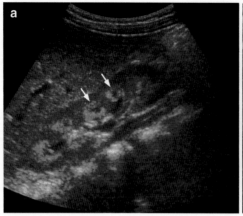 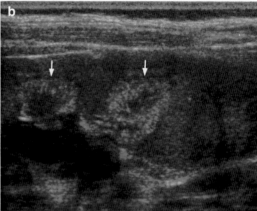

Fig. 1.33 (**a**) Ultrasound of the right kidney demonstrates increased echogenicity of the periphery of the renal pyramids. The renal cortex is normal. (**b**) High resolution image demonstrates this pattern of echogenicity, known as the Anderson Carr progression of nephrocalcinosis, to better advantage

worked out, they almost certainly represent small or early deposition of calcified or crystalline material. This deposition can be in the pelvocaliceal system, in the normal nephron, or in a pathologically dilated portion of the nephron [177].

Conclusion

Over many decades the role of radiology in the diagnosis and treatment of diseases of the urinary tract has evolved. Modalities such as radiography and excretory urography have diminished in utility and at the same time newer modalities and their refinements such as ultrasound, computed tomography, magnetic resonance imaging and nuclear medicine have reached the forefront. What remains constant is the close collaboration required among radiologists, nephrologists and urologists in the care of children with urinary tract abnormalities.

Acknowledgement The authors express their gratitude to Dr. Paul Babyn and Dr. Martin Charron for their valuable assistance in the preparation and review of this chapter.

References

1. Kirks DR, Griscom NT. Practical pediatric imaging : diagnostic radiology of infants and children. 3rd ed. Philadelphia: Lippincott-Raven; 1998. p. 1226: xx.

2. Aaronson IA, Cremin BJ. Clinical paediatric uroradiology. Edinburgh: Churchill Livingstone; 1984. p. 441.
3. Kuhn JP, et al. Caffey's pediatric diagnostic imaging. 10th ed. Philadelphia: Mosby; 2004. p. 2 v.
4. Brenner D, et al. Estimated risks of radiation-induced fatal cancer from pediatric CT. AJR Am J Roentgenol. 2001;176(2):289–96.
5. Costello JE, et al. CT radiation dose: current controversies and dose reduction strategies. AJR Am J Roentgenol. 2013;201(6):1283–90.
6. Morcos SK, Thomsen HS. Adverse reactions to iodinated contrast media. Eur Radiol. 2001;11(7):1267–75.
7. Lameier NH. Contrast-induced nephropathy – prevention and risk reduction. Nephrol Dial Transplant. 2006;21(6):i11–23.
8. McClennan BL. Adverse reactions to iodinated contrast media. Recognition and response. Invest Radio. 1994;29 Suppl 1:S46–50.
9. Malviya S, et al. Sedation and general anaesthesia in children undergoing MRI and CT: adverse events and outcomes. Br J Anaesth. 2000;84(6):743–8.
10. Frush DP, Bisset 3rd GS, Hall SC. Pediatric sedation in radiology: the practice of safe sleep. AJR Am J Roentgenol. 1996;167(6):1381–7.
11. Robbin ML. Ultrasound contrast agents: a promising future. Radiol Clin North Am. 2001;39(3):399–414.
12. Peratoner L, et al. Kidney length and scarring in children with urinary tract infection: importance of ultrasound scans. Abdom Imaging. 2005;30(6):780–5.
13. Dacher JN, et al. Imaging strategies in pediatric urinary tract infection. Eur Radiol. 2005;15(7):1283–8.
14. Practice parameter: the diagnosis, treatment, and evaluation of the initial urinary tract infection in febrile infants and young children. American Academy of Pediatrics. Committee on Quality Improvement. Subcommittee on Urinary Tract Infection. Pediatrics. 1999;103(4 Pt 1):843–52.

15. Monsalve J, et al. Imaging of cancer predisposition syndromes in children. Radiogra. 2011;31(1):263–80.

16. Chen JJ, et al. The renal length nomogram: multivariable approach. J Urol. 2002;168(5):2149–52.

17. Blane CE, et al. Sonographic standards for normal infant kidney length. AJR Am J Roentgenol. 1985;145(6):1289–91.

18. Rosenbaum DM, Korngold E, Teele RL. Sonographic assessment of renal length in normal children. AJR Am J Roentgenol. 1984;142(3):467–9.

19. Ginalski JM, Michaud A, Genton N. Renal growth retardation in children: sign suggestive of vesicoureteral reflux? AJR Am J Roentgenol. 1985;145(3): 617–9.

20. Hricak H, et al. Neonatal kidneys: sonographic anatomic correlation. Radiology. 1983;147(3):699–702.

21. Haller JO, Berdon WE, Friedman AP. Increased renal cortical echogenicity: a normal finding in neonates and infants. Radiology. 1982;142(1):173–4.

22. Starinsky R, et al. Increased renal medullary echogenicity in neonates. Pediatr Radiol. 1995;25 Suppl 1:S43–5.

23. Nimkin K, et al. Urolithiasis in a children's hospital: 1985–1990. Urol Radiol. 1992;14(3):139–43.

24. Ricci MA, Lloyd DA. Renal venous thrombosis in infants and children. Arch Surg. 1990;125(9):1195–9.

25. Brun P, et al. Value of Doppler ultrasound for the diagnosis of renal artery stenosis in children. Pediatr Nephrol. 1997;11(1):27–30.

26. Fang YC, et al. A case of acute renal artery thrombosis caused by blunt trauma: computed tomographic and Doppler ultrasonic findings. J Formos Med Assoc. 1993;92(4):356–8.

27. Hitzel A, et al. Color and power Doppler sonography versus DMSA scintigraphy in acute pyelonephritis and in prediction of renal scarring. J Nucl Med. 2002;43(1):27–32.

28. Irshad A, et al. An overview of renal transplantation: current practice and use of ultrasound. Semin Ultrasound CT MR. 2009;30(4):298–314.

29. Sharma AK, et al. Utility of serial Doppler ultrasound scans for the diagnosis of acute rejection in renal allografts. Transpl Int. 2004;17(3):138–44.

30. Fotter R. Pediatric uroradiology. Medical radiology. Berlin: Springer; 2001. p. 431.

31. Lebowitz RL, et al. International system of radiographic grading of vesicoureteric reflux. International Reflux Study in Children. Pediatr Radiol. 1985;15(2):105–9.

32. Ward VL. Patient dose reduction during voiding cystourethrography. Pediatr Radiol. 2006;36 Suppl 2:168–72.

33. Mettler FA. Essentials of nuclear medicine imaging. 5th ed. Philadelphia: Saunders Elsevier; 2006.

34. Fleming JS, et al. Guidelines for the measurement of glomerular filtration rate using plasma sampling. Nucl Med Commun. 2004;25(8):759–69.

35. Unver T, et al. Comparison of direct radionuclide cystography and voiding cystourethrography in detecting vesicoureteral reflux. Pediatr Int. 2006;48(3):287–91.

36. Sukan A, et al. Comparison of direct radionuclide cystography and voiding direct cystography in the detection of vesicoureteral reflux. Ann Nucl Med. 2003;17(7):549–53.

37. Fettich J, et al. Guidelines for direct radionuclide cystography in children. Eur J Nucl Med Mol Imaging. 2003;30(5):B39–44.

38. Carpio F, Morey AF. Radiographic staging of renal injuries. World J Urol. 1999;17(2):66–70.

39. Piepsz A, Ham HR. Pediatric applications of renal nuclear medicine. Semin Nucl Med. 2006;36(1): 16–35.

40. Ward VL, et al. Pediatric radiation exposure and effective dose reduction during voiding cystourethrography. Radiology. 2008;249(3):1002–9.

41. Peters AM, Morony S, Gordon I. Indirect radionuclide cystography demonstrates reflux under physiological conditions. Clin Radiol. 1990;41(1):44–7.

42. Gordon I, Peters AM, Morony S. Indirect radionuclide cystography: a sensitive technique for the detection of vesico-ureteral reflux. Pediatr Nephrol. 1990;4(6):604–6.

43. Gordon I. Indirect radionuclide cystography – the coming of age. Nucl Med Commun. 1989;10(7):457–8.

44. Pollet JE, Sharp PF, Smith FW. Comparison of "direct" and "indirect" radionuclide cystography. J Nucl Med. 1985;26(12):1501–2.

45. Bower G, et al. Comparison of "direct" and "indirect" radionuclide cystography. J Nucl Med. 1985; 26(5):465–8.

46. Pollet JE, et al. Intravenous radionuclide cystography for the detection of vesicorenal reflux. J Urol. 1981;125(1):75–8.

47. Conway JJ, Kruglik JD. Effectiveness of direct and indirect radionuclide cystography in detecting vesicoureteral reflux. J Nucl Med. 1976;17(02):81–3.

48. Conway JJ, et al. Direct and indirect radionuclide cystography. J Urol. 1975;113(5):689–93.

49. Conway JJ, Belman AB, King LR. Direct and indirect radionuclide cystography. Semin Nucl Med. 1974;4(2):197–211.

50. Gordon I, et al. Guidelines for indirect radionuclide cystography. Eur J Nucl Med. 2001;28(3):16–20.

51. Mandell GA, et al. Procedure guideline for radionuclide cystography in children. Society of Nuclear Medicine. J Nucl Med. 1997;38(10):1650–4.

52. De Sadeleer C, et al. How good is technetium-99m mercaptoacetyltriglycine indirect cystography? Eur J Nucl Med. 1994;21(3):223–7.

53. Corso A, Ostinelli A, Trombetta MA. "Indirect" radioisotope cystography after the furosemide test: its diagnostic efficacy compared to "direct" study. Radiol Med (Torino). 1989;78(6):645–8.

54. Vlajkovic M, et al. Radionuclide voiding patterns in children with vesicoureteral reflux. Eur J Nucl Med Mol Imaging. 2003;30(4):532–7.

55. Hoberman A, et al. Imaging studies after a first febrile urinary tract infection in young children. N Engl J Med. 2003;348(3):195–202.

56. Stokland E, et al. Imaging of renal scarring. Acta Paediatr Suppl. 1999;88(431):13–21.
57. Goldraich NP, Goldraich LH. Update on dimercapto-succinic acid renal scanning in children with urinary tract infection. Pediatr Nephrol. 1995;9(2):221–6; discussion 227.
58. Mastin ST, Drane WE, Iravani A. Tc-99m DMSA SPECT imaging in patients with acute symptoms or history of UTI. Comparison with ultrasonography. Clin Nucl Med. 1995;20(5):407–12.
59. Majd M, et al. Acute pyelonephritis: comparison of diagnosis with 99mTc-DMSA, SPECT, spiral CT, MR imaging, and power Doppler US in an experimental pig model. Radiology. 2001;218(1):101–8.
60. Applegate KE, et al. A prospective comparison of high-resolution planar, pinhole, and triple-detector SPECT for the detection of renal cortical defects. Clin Nucl Med. 1997;22(10):673–8.
61. Cook GJ, Lewis MK, Clarke SE. An evaluation of 99Tcm-DMSA SPET with three-dimensional reconstruction in 68 patients with varied renal pathology. Nucl Med Commun. 1995;16(11):958–67.
62. Yen TC, et al. A comparative study of evaluating renal scars by 99mTc-DMSA planar and SPECT renal scans, intravenous urography, and ultrasonography. Ann Nucl Med. 1994;8(2):147–52.
63. Takeda M, et al. Value of dimercaptosuccinic acid single photon emission computed tomography and magnetic resonance imaging in detecting renal injury in pediatric patients with vesicoureteral reflux. Comparison with dimercaptosuccinic acid planar scintigraphy and intravenous pyelography. Eur Urol. 1994;25(4):320–5.
64. Mouratidis B, Ash JM, Gilday DL. Comparison of planar and SPECT 99Tcm-DMSA scintigraphy for the detection of renal cortical defects in children. Nucl Med Commun. 1993;14(2):82–6.
65. Sheehy N, et al. Pediatric 99mTc-DMSA SPECT performed by using iterative reconstruction with isotropic resolution recovery: improved image quality and reduced radiopharmaceutical activity. Radiology. 2009;251(2):511–6.
66. Piepsz A, et al. Consensus on renal cortical scintigraphy in children with urinary tract infection. Scientific Committee of Radionuclides in Nephrourology. Semin Nucl Med. 1999;29(2):160–74.
67. Itoh K, et al. Qualitative and quantitative evaluation of renal parenchymal damage by 99mTc-DMSA planar and SPECT scintigraphy. Ann Nucl Med. 1995;9(1):23–8.
68. Craig JC, et al. How accurate is dimercaptosuccinic acid scintigraphy for the diagnosis of acute pyelonephritis? A meta-analysis of experimental studies. J Nucl Med. 2000;41(6):986–93.
69. Chiou YY, et al. Renal fibrosis: prediction from acute pyelonephritis focus volume measured at 99mTc dimercaptosuccinic acid SPECT. Radiology. 2001;221(2):366–70.
70. Yen TC, et al. Identification of new renal scarring in repeated episodes of acute pyelonephritis using Tc-99m DMSA renal SPECT. Clin Nucl Med. 1998;23(12):828–31.
71. Yen TC, et al. Technetium-99m-DMSA renal SPECT in diagnosing and monitoring pediatric acute pyelonephritis. J Nucl Med. 1996;37(8):1349–53.
72. Ell PJ, Gambhir SS. Nuclear medicine in clinical diagnosis and treatment. 3rd ed. Edinburgh: Chuchill Livingstone; 2004.
73. Mandell GA, et al. Procedure guideline for diuretic renography in children. Society of Nuclear Medicine. J Nucl Med. 1997;38(10):1647–50.
74. Rossleigh MA. Renal cortical scintigraphy and diuresis renography in infants and children. J Nucl Med. 2001;42(1):91–5.
75. McCarthy CS, et al. Pitfalls and limitations of diuretic renography. Abdom Imaging. 1994;19(1):78–81.
76. Conway JJ, Maizels M. The "well tempered" diuretic renogram: a standard method to examine the asymptomatic neonate with hydronephrosis or hydrouretero-nephrosis. A report from combined meetings of The Society for Fetal Urology and members of The Pediatric Nuclear Medicine Council – The Society of Nuclear Medicine. J Nucl Med. 1992;33(11):2047–51.
77. Donoso G, et al. 99mTc-MAG3 diuretic renography in children: a comparison between F0 and F+20. Nucl Med Commun. 2003;24(11):1189–93.
78. Wong DC, Rossleigh MA, Farnsworth RH. F+0 diuresis renography in infants and children. J Nucl Med. 1999;40(11):1805–11.
79. Lowe LH, et al. Pediatric renal masses: Wilms tumor and beyond. Radiographics. 2000;20(6):1585–603.
80. Buckley JC, McAninch JW. The diagnosis, management, and outcomes of pediatric renal injuries. Urol Clin North Am. 2006;33(1):33–40, vi.
81. McAleer IM, Kaplan JW. Pediatric genitourinary trauma. Urol Clin North Am. 1995;22(1):177–88.
82. Dacher JN, et al. Rational use of CT in acute pyelonephritis: findings and relationships with reflux. Pediatr Radiol. 1993;23(4):281–5.
83. Tunaci A, Yekeler E. Multidetector row CT of the kidneys. Eur J Radiol. 2004;52(1):56–66.
84. Benko A, et al. Canadian Association of Radiologists: consensus guidelines for the prevention of contrast-induced nephropathy. Can Assoc Radiol J. 2007;58(2):79–87.
85. Slovis TL. Children, computed tomography radiation dose, and the As Low As Reasonably Achievable (ALARA) concept. Pediatrics. 2003;112(4):971–2.
86. Volle E, Park W, Kaufmann HJ. MRI examination and monitoring of pediatric patients under sedation. Pediatr Radiol. 1996;26(4):280–1.
87. Li A, et al. Acute adverse reactions to magnetic resonance contrast media – gadolinium chelates. Br J Radiol. 2006;79(941):368–71.
88. Akgun H, et al. Are gadolinium-based contrast media nephrotoxic? A renal biopsy study. Arch Pathol Lab Med. 2006;130(9):1354–7.

89. Sadowski EA, et al. Nephrogenic systemic fibrosis: risk factors and incidence estimation. Radiology. 2007;243(1):148–57.
90. Thomsen HS, et al. Nephrogenic systemic fibrosis and gadolinium-based contrast media: updated ESUR Contrast Medium Safety Committee guidelines. Eur Radiol. 2013;23(2):307–18.
91. Hoffer FA. Magnetic resonance imaging of abdominal masses in the pediatric patient. Semin Ultrasound CT MR. 2005;26(4):212–23.
92. Rohrschneider WK, et al. US, CT and MR imaging characteristics of nephroblastomatosis. Pediatr Radiol. 1998;28(6):435–43.
93. Israel GM, et al. The use of opposed-phase chemical shift MRI in the diagnosis of renal angiomyolipomas. AJR Am J Roentgenol. 2005;184(6):1868–72.
94. Pretorius ES, Wickstrom ML, Siegelman ES. MR imaging of renal neoplasms. Magn Reson Imaging Clin N Am. 2000;8(4):813–36.
95. Ramchandani P, et al. Impact of magnetic resonance on staging of renal carcinoma. Urology. 1986;27(6): 564–8.
96. Hallscheidt PJ, et al. Preoperative staging of renal cell carcinoma with inferior vena cava thrombus using multidetector CT and MRI: prospective study with histopathological correlation. J Comput Assist Tomogr. 2005;29(1):64–8.
97. Kim D, et al. Abdominal aorta and renal artery stenosis: evaluation with MR angiography. Radiology. 1990;174(3 Pt 1):727–31.
98. Zhang H, Prince MR. Renal MR angiography. Magn Reson Imaging Clin N Am. 2004;12(3):487–503, vi.
99. Schoenberg SO, et al. Renal MR angiography: current debates and developments in imaging of renal artery stenosis. Semin Ultrasound CT MR. 2003; 24(4):255–67.
100. Marcos HB, Choyke PL. Magnetic resonance angiography of the kidney. Semin Nephrol. 2000;20(5): 450–5.
101. Vasbinder GB, et al. Accuracy of computed tomographic angiography and magnetic resonance angiography for diagnosing renal artery stenosis. Ann Intern Med. 2004;141(9):674–82; discussion 682.
102. Kovanlikaya A, et al. Comparison of MRI and renal cortical scintigraphy findings in childhood acute pyelonephritis: preliminary experience. Eur J Radiol. 2004;49(1):76–80.
103. Weiser AC, et al. The role of gadolinium enhanced magnetic resonance imaging for children with suspected acute pyelonephritis. J Urol. 2003;169(6): 2308–11.
104. Leonidas JC, Berdon WE. MR imaging of urinary tract infections in children. Radiology. 1999;210(2):582–4.
105. Ku JH, et al. Is there a role for magnetic resonance imaging in renal trauma? Int J Urol. 2001;8(6): 261–7.
106. Marcos HB, Noone TC, Semelka RC. MRI evaluation of acute renal trauma. J Magn Reson Imaging. 1998;8(4):989–90.
107. Cohen HL, et al. Congenital abnormalities of the genitourinary system. Semin Roentgenol. 2004; 39(2):282–303.
108. Rohrschneider WK, et al. Functional and morphologic evaluation of congenital urinary tract dilatation by using combined static-dynamic MR urography: findings in kidneys with a single collecting system. Radiology. 2002;224(3):683–94.
109. Nolte-Ernsting CC, Adam GB, Gunther RW. MR urography: examination techniques and clinical applications. Eur Radiol. 2001;11(3):355–72.
110. Karabacakoglu A, et al. Diagnostic value of diuretic-enhanced excretory MR urography in patients with obstructive uropathy. Eur J Radiol. 2004;52(3): 320–7.
111. Grattan-Smith JD, Jones RA. MR urography in children. Pediatr Radio. 2006;36:1119–32.
112. Arlen AM, et al. Magnetic resonance urography for diagnosis of pediatric ureteral stricture. J Pediatr Urol. 2014;10(5):792–8.
113. Jones RA, Grattan-Smith JD, Little S. Pediatric magnetic resonance urography. J Magn Reson Imaging. 2011;33(3):510–26.
114. Schmid-Tannwald C, et al. Diffusion-weighted MRI of the abdomen: current value in clinical routine. J Magn Reson Imaging. 2013;37(1):35–47.
115. Lee CU, et al. MR elastography in renal transplant patients and correlation with renal allograft biopsy: a feasibility study. Acad Radiol. 2012;19(7):834–41.
116. Paulson DF, et al. Pediatric urolithiasis. J Urol. 1972;108(5):811–4.
117. Breatnach E, Smith SE. The radiology of renal stones in children. Clin Radiol. 1983;34(1):59–64.
118. Day DL, Scheinman JI, Mahan J. Radiological aspects of primary hyperoxaluria. AJR Am J Roentgenol. 1986;146(2):395–401.
119. Patriquin H, Robitaille P. Renal calcium deposition in children: sonographic demonstration of the Anderson-Carr progression. AJR Am J Roentgenol. 1986;146(6):1253–6.
120. Jevtic V. Imaging of renal osteodystrophy. Eur J Radiol. 2003;46(2):85–95.
121. Lebowitz RL. Urography in children: when should it be done? 1. Infection. Postgrad Med. 1978;64(4):63–72.
122. Lebowitz RL. Urography in children: when should it be done? 2. Conditions other than infection. Postgrad Med. 1978;64(5):61–70.
123. American Academy of Pediatrics: Committee on Radiology. Excretory urography for evaluation of enuresis. Pediatrics. 1980;65(1):A49–50.
124. Lebowitz RL. Excretory urography in children. AJR Am J Roentgenol. 1994;163(4):990.
125. Sourtzis S, et al. Radiologic investigation of renal colic: unenhanced helical CT compared with excretory urography. AJR Am J Roentgenol. 1999; 172(6):1491–4.
126. McNicholas MM, et al. Excretory phase CT urography for opacification of the urinary collecting system. AJR Am J Roentgenol. 1998;170(5):1261–7.

127. O'Malley ME, et al. Comparison of excretory phase, helical computed tomography with intravenous urography in patients with painless haematuria. Clin Radiol. 2003;58(4):294–300.

128. Borthne AS, et al. Pediatric excretory MR urography: comparative study of enhanced and non-enhanced techniques. Eur Radiol. 2003;13(6): 1423–7.

129. Pollack HM, Banner MP. Current status of excretory urography. A premature epitaph? Urol Clin North Am. 1985;12(4):585–601.

130. Carrico C, Lebowitz RL. Incontinence due to an infrasphincteric ectopic ureter: why the delay in diagnosis and what the radiologist can do about it. Pediatr Radiol. 1998;28(12):942–9.

131. Smith H, et al. Routine excretory urography in follow-up of superficial transitional cell carcinoma of bladder. Urology. 1989;34(4):193–6.

132. Kawashima A, et al. Imaging of urethral disease: a pictorial review. Radiographics. 2004;24 Suppl 1:S195–216.

133. Yoder IC, Papanicolaou N. Imaging the urethra in men and women. Urol Radiol. 1992;14(1):24–8.

134. Pavlica P, Barozzi L, Menchi I. Imaging of male urethra. Eur Radiol. 2003;13(7):1583–96.

135. Sclafani SJ, Becker JA. Radiologic diagnosis of extrarenal genitourinary trauma. Urol Radiol. 1985;7(4):201–10.

136. Grignon A, et al. Ureteropelvic junction stenosis: antenatal ultrasonographic diagnosis, postnatal investigation, and follow-up. Radiology. 1986; 160(3):649–51.

137. Wood BP, et al. Ureterovesical obstruction and megaloureter: diagnosis by real-time US. Radiology. 1985;156(1):79–81.

138. Gilsanz V, Miller JH, Reid BS. Ultrasonic characteristics of posterior urethral valves. Radiology. 1982;145(1):143–5.

139. Mascatello VJ, et al. Ultrasonic evaluation of the obstructed duplex kidney. AJR Am J Roentgenol. 1977;129(1):113–20.

140. Nussbaum AR, et al. Ectopic ureter and ureterocele: their varied sonographic manifestations. Radiology. 1986;159(1):227–35.

141. Griffin J, Jennings C, MacErlean D. Ultrasonic evaluation of simple and ectopic ureteroceles. Clin Radiol. 1983;34(1):55–7.

142. Strife JL, et al. Multicystic dysplastic kidney in children: US follow-up. Radiology. 1993;186(3):785–8.

143. Hains DS, et al. Management and etiology of the unilateral multicystic dysplastic kidney: a review. Pediatr Nephrol. 2009;24(2):233–41.

144. Edell SL, Bonavita JA. The sonographic appearance of acute pyelonephritis. Radiology. 1979;132(3):683–5.

145. Rosenfield AT, et al. Acute focal bacterial nephritis (acute lobar nephronia). Radiology. 1979;132(3): 553–61.

146. Bjorgvinsson E, Majd M, Eggli KD. Diagnosis of acute pyelonephritis in children: comparison of sonography and 99mTc-DMSA scintigraphy. AJR Am J Roentgenol. 1991;157(3):539–43.

147. Farmer KD, Gellett LR, Dubbins PA. The sonographic appearance of acute focal pyelonephritis 8 years experience. Clin Radiol. 2002;57(6):483–7.

148. Dacher JN, et al. Renal sinus hyperechogenicity in acute pyelonephritis: description and pathological correlation. Pediatr Radiol. 1999;29(3):179–82.

149. Khanna G, et al. Detection of preoperative wilms tumor rupture with CT: a report from the Children's Oncology Group. Radiology. 2013;266(2):610–7.

150. Khanna G, et al. Evaluation of diagnostic performance of CT for detection of tumor thrombus in children with Wilms tumor: a report from the Children's Oncology Group. Pediatr Blood Cancer. 2012;58(4):551–5.

151. McDonald K, et al. Added value of abdominal cross-sectional imaging (CT or MRI) in staging of Wilms' tumours. Clin Radiol. 2013;68(1):16–20.

152. Stein JP, et al. Blunt renal trauma in the pediatric population: indications for radiographic evaluation. Urology. 1994;44(3):406–10.

153. John SD. Trends in pediatric emergency imaging. Radiol Clin North Am. 1999;37(5):995–1034, vi.

154. Rose JS. Ultrasound in abdominal trauma. Emerg Med Clin North Am. 2004;22(3):581–99, vii.

155. Soudack M, et al. Experience with focused abdominal sonography for trauma (FAST) in 313 pediatric patients. J Clin Ultrasound. 2004;32(2):53–61.

156. Taylor GA, Sivit CJ. Posttraumatic peritoneal fluid: is it a reliable indicator of intraabdominal injury in children? J Pediatr Surg. 1995;30(12):1644–8.

157. Pieretti R, Gilday D, Jeffs R. Differential kidney scan in pediatric urology. Urology. 1974;4(6):665–8.

158. Mandell GA, et al. Procedure guideline for renal cortical scintigraphy in children. Society of Nuclear Medicine. J Nucl Med. 1997;38(10):1644–6.

159. Clausen TD, Kanstrup IL, Iversen J. Reference values for 99mTc-MAG3 renography determined in healthy, potential renal donors. Clin Physiol Funct Imaging. 2002;22(5):356–60.

160. Schofer O, et al. Technetium-99m mercaptoacetyltriglycine clearance: reference values for infants and children. Eur J Nucl Med. 1995;22(11):1278–81.

161. Tsukamoto E, et al. Validity of 99mTc-DMSA renal uptake by planar posterior-view method in children. Ann Nucl Med. 1999;13(6):383–7.

162. Gainza FJ, et al. Evaluation of complications due to percutaneous renal biopsy in allografts and native kidneys with color-coded Doppler sonography. Clin Nephrol. 1995;43(5):303–8.

163. Morin F, Cote I. Tc-99m MAG3 evaluation of recipients with En bloc renal grafts from pediatric cadavers. Clin Nucl Med. 2000;25(8):579–84.

164. Tulchinsky M, Malpani AR, Eggli DF. Diagnosis of urinoma by MAG3 scintigraphy in a renal transplant patient. Clin Nucl Med. 1995;20(1):80–1.

165. Carmody E, et al. Sequential Tc 99m mercaptoacetyltriglycine (MAG3) renography as an evaluator of

early renal transplant function. Clin Transplant. 1993;7(3):245–9.

166. Cohn DA, Gruenewald S. Postural renal transplant obstruction: a case report and review of the literature. Clin Nucl Med. 2001;26(8):673–6.

167. Goodear M, Barratt L, Wycherley A. Intraperitoneal urine leak in a patient with a renal transplant on Tc-99m MAG3 imaging. Clin Nucl Med. 1998; 23(11):789–90.

168. Mange KC, et al. Focal acute tubular necrosis in a renal allograft. Transplantation. 1997;64(10):1490–2.

169. Dubovsky EV, Russell CD, Erbas B. Radionuclide evaluation of renal transplants. Semin Nucl Med. 1995;25(1):49–59.

170. Dubovsky EV, Russell CD. Radionuclide evaluation of renal transplants. Semin Nucl Med. 1988;18(3): 181–98.

171. Nankivell BJ, et al. Diagnosis of kidney transplant obstruction using Mag3 diuretic renography. Clin Transplant. 2001;15(1):11–8.

172. Riccabona M, et al. ESPR Uroradiology Task Force and ESUR Paediatric Working Group – Imaging recommendations in paediatric uroradiology, part V: childhood cystic kidney disease, childhood renal transplantation and contrast-enhanced ultrasonography in children. Pediatr Radiol. 2012;42(10):1275–83.

173. McHugh K, et al. Simple renal cysts in children: diagnosis and follow-up with US. Radiology. 1991;178(2):383–5.

174. Stuck KJ, Koff SA, Silver TM. Ultrasonic features of multicystic dysplastic kidney: expanded diagnostic criteria. Radiology. 1982;143(1):217–21.

175. Patriquin HB, O'Regan S. Medullary sponge kidney in childhood. AJR Am J Roentgenol. 1985;145(2): 315–9.

176. Pretorius DH, et al. Diagnosis of autosomal dominant polycystic kidney disease in utero and in the young infant. J Ultrasound Med. 1987;6(5):249–55.

177. Traubici J, Daneman A. High-resolution renal sonography in children with autosomal recessive polycystic kidney disease. AJR Am J Roentgenol. 2005;184(5):1630–3.

178. Garel LA, et al. Juvenile nephronophthisis: sonographic appearance in children with severe uremia. Radiology. 1984;151(1):93–5.

179. Fredericks BJ, et al. Glomerulocystic renal disease: ultrasound appearances. Pediatr Radiol. 1989;19(3): 184–6.

180. Srinath A, Shneider BL. Congenital hepatic fibrosis and autosomal recessive polycystic kidney disease. J Pediatr Gastroenterol Nutr. 2012;54(5):580–7.

181. El-Assmy A, et al. Kidney stone size and hounsfield units predict successful shockwave lithotripsy in children. Urology. 2013;81(4):880–4.

182. Wilson DA, Wenzl JE, Altshuler GP. Ultrasound demonstration of diffuse cortical nephrocalcinosis in a case of primary hyperoxaluria. AJR Am J Roentgenol. 1979;132(4):659–61.

Antenatal Assessment of Kidney Morphology and Function

2

Khalid Ismaili, Marie Cassart, Fred E. Avni, and Michelle Hall

Introduction

Today, obstetrical two-dimensional (2D) ultrasound (US) is part of routine antenatal care in most western countries. In Europe, three sonographic examinations are performed, one in each trimester [1]. In other countries, including the United States and Canada, only a second-midtrimester examination is performed routinely; with first-trimester or third-trimester examinations performed in case of specific indication [2]. The more systematic use of obstetrical US has led to the discovery of many fetal abnormalities. Congenital abnormalities of the kidney and urinary tract (CAKUT) make up one of the largest groups of congenital anomalies amenable to neonatal care,

representing 0.2–2 % of all newborns [1]. Moreover, dramatic changes have occurred in the management of these children, and nowadays, CAKUTs are mostly found in asymptomatic patients and the treatment applied is mainly preventive. Also the antenatal detection and postnatal follow-up have brought new insights into the natural history of many CAKUTs [3, 4].

Fetal Imaging Methods

Ultrasound is the first line imaging technique used in antenatal diagnosis. It has now been nearly four decades since its first use to evaluate the fetus and it is presently accepted as a safe and noninvasive imaging modality. The most common transducers used are curvilinear sector transducers (3–5 Mhz), which have good penetration of the sound beam and allow visualization of the whole fetus. Higher frequency linear transducers (5–10 Mhz) or transvaginal probes are used for achieving high resolution scans in near fields. The transducers used in clinical daily practice are mostly multifrequency probes allowing harmonic, three-dimensional and Doppler flow imaging. *3D imaging* is mostly used for the study of the face and vertebral column [5], the other organs are well depicted by C imaging. Hence, 3D imaging is currently not routinely performed for urinary tract and kidney diseases. *Doppler*

K. Ismaili (✉) • M. Hall
Departmet of Pediatric Nephrology, Hopital Universitaire des Enfants--Reine Fabiola, 15 Avenue Jean Joseph Crocq, Brussels 1020, Belgium
e-mail: khalid.ismaili@huderf.be; michele.hall@huderf.be

M. Cassart
Department of Pediatric Radiology, Etterbeek-Ixelles Hospital, Rue J. Paquot 63, Brussels 1050, Belgium
e-mail: mcassart@his-izz.be

F.E. Avni
Department of Pediatric Imaging, Jeanne de Flandre Lille University Hospital, Av Eugene Avinee, Lille 59037, France
e-mail: favni@skynet.be

© Springer-Verlag Berlin Heidelberg 2016
D.F. Geary, F. Schaefer (eds.), *Pediatric Kidney Disease*, DOI 10.1007/978-3-662-52972-0_2

imaging is useful to evaluate the vascularization of the organs and fetal well being [2].

MR Imaging is a more recent technique applied to the fetus. The examinations are performed on 1.5–3 Tesla magnets. Although no deleterious effects on the fetus have been identified to date [6], MR imaging is generally avoided during organogenesis in the first trimester. MR is mostly performed in order to establish a more precise diagnosis in cases for which ultrasound cannot completely depict the suspected malformation or anomaly. The advantages of MR are the larger field of view and the better contrast resolution that allow a better characterization of the anatomy of the organs. The indications mostly concern the brain but it is presently extended to the fetal digestive and urinary tracts in specific indications well known by the radiologists in charge. Practically, depending on local habits, sedation can be given to the mother before the examination to reduce fetal movement. No contrast media is injected because at the current time, there is no accepted indication and no sufficient studies determining the potential harmful effects in pregnant women. Fast sequences (20 s) are performed in different planes and can be repeated in case of fetal movements. In urinary tract and kidney diseases the indications of fetal MR imaging are closely circumscribed; they will be illustrated in the next paragraphs.

The Normal Urinary Tract

Bladder

Urine starts to be produced during the ninth week of fetal life. At that time, the urine is collected in the bladder, which can be visualized as a fluid-filled structure within the fetal pelvis. During the second and third trimester, the fetus normally fills and partially or completely empties the bladder approximately every 25 min and the cycle can be monitored during the sonographic examination [7]. The bladder can easily be located by its outline of umbilical arteries, which are identifiable on color Doppler.

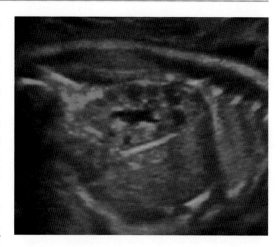

Fig. 2.1 Normal fetal kidney at 32 weeks of GA. Sagittal US scan of the kidney with clear visibility of the cortico-medullary differentiation

Kidneys

Endovaginal probes can be used to visualize fetal anatomic structures earlier than with transabdominal US. Thus, the fetal kidneys can be demonstrated at around 11 weeks endovaginally and around 12–15 weeks with transabdominal probes. During the first trimester, the kidneys appear as hyperechoic oval structures at both sides of the spine (their hyperechogenicity can be compared with that of the liver or spleen) [8]. This echogenicity will progressively decrease and during the third trimester the cortical echogenicity will always be less than that of the liver or spleen. In parallel with the decrease of echogenicity, corticomedullary differentiation will appear at about 14–15 weeks. It should always be visible in fetuses older than 18 weeks (Fig. 2.1). Prominent pyramids should not be misinterpreted as calyceal dilatation.

Growth of the fetal kidneys can be evaluated throughout pregnancy. As a rule, a normal kidney grows at about 1.1 mm per week of gestation.

Evidence of Normally Functioning Urinary Tract

Besides visualization of the bladder and normal kidneys, assessment of the urinary tract should include an evaluation of the amniotic fluid volume. After 14–15 weeks, two thirds of the amniotic fluid is produced by fetal urination and one third by pulmonary fluid. A normal volume of amniotic fluid is mandatory for the proper development of the fetal lungs. This can be confirmed by measuring thoracic diameters or thoracic circumference [9].

Ultrasound Findings as Evidence of Abnormal Fetal Kidney and Urinary Tract

Abnormal US appearance of the kidneys as a pathophysiological base of CAKUT has been described extensively [10, 11]. Anomalies of the urinary system detected in utero are numerous; they can include anomalies of the kidney itself, of the collecting system, of the bladder and of the urethra. In addition, they can be isolated or in association with other systems. Therefore, the sonographic examination should be as meticulous as possible in order to visualize the associated features. These findings, among others, will determine the prognosis.

Abnormal Renal Number

Bilateral renal agenesis is part of Potter's syndrome and is incompatible with extrauterine life. The diagnosis is based on the absence of renal structure and the presence of oligohydramnios after 15 weeks of gestation. Pulmonary hypoplasia is invariably associated and leads to death from respiratory failure soon after birth. In this context, enlarged globular adrenals should not be mistaken for kidneys [12]. The use of color Doppler may help demonstrate the absence of renal arteries and subsequently confirm the diagnosis [13].

Unilateral renal agenesis is more common (1 in 500 pregnancies) and usually has no significant consequence on postnatal life. The pathogenesis of renal agenesis is mostly failure of formation of the metanephros. In addition, interruption in vascular supply and regression of a multicystic dysplastic kidney (MCDK) may also lead to renal agenesis in the fetal period [14]. An investigation after birth is necessary to confirm the status of the remnant kidney and to look for possible associated anomalies [15]. These anomalies can occur both in contiguous structures (such as vertebrae, genital organs, intestines, and anus) and also in noncontiguous structures (such as limbs, heart, trachea, ear, and central nervous system). On the long term, children having ipsilateral uronephropathy are at higher risk of adverse outcome, with a median time to chronic kidney disease of 14.8 years [16].

Abnormal Renal Location

Ectopic kidney, especially in the pelvic area, is part of the differential diagnosis of the "empty renal fossa" in the fetus and may represent 42 % of these cases [15]. The diagnosis of horseshoe or crossed fused kidneys can also be assessed in utero through the demonstration of a typical corticomedullary differentiation [17]. An ectopic kidney is usually small and somewhat malrotated with numerous small blood vessels and associated ureteric anomalies. Ectopic kidneys may be asymptomatic, but complications such as ureteral obstruction, infection, and calculi are common. Therefore, at birth, the anomaly has to be confirmed by US or by MRI and voiding cystourethrography (VCUG) in complex cases.

Abnormal Renal Echogenicity

Hyperechogenicity of the fetal kidney is defined by comparison with the adjacent liver or spleen. This is difficult to assess in the first and second trimester as the kidney is "physiologically" hyperechoic (or isoechoic at the end of the second trimester) to the liver. It is easier to characterize after 28–32 weeks as the renal cortex by that time should be hypoechoic compared to the liver and spleen [8]. Increased echogenicity of the renal parenchyma is nonspecific and occurs as a response to different changes in renal tissue [18]. Interstitial infiltration, sclerosis and multiple microscopic cortical and medullary cysts may account for hyperechogenicity even in the absence of macrocysts. The detection of hyperechoic kidneys represents a difficult diagnostic challenge [19]. The differential diagnosis must be based on kidney size, corticomedullary differentiation, the presence of macrocysts, the degree of dilatation of the collecting system and the amount of amniotic fluid [20]. The diagnosis must also take into account the familial history and the presence of associated anomalies. Metabolic disorders should be added to the long list of causes of hyperechoic kidneys in children. Tyrosinemia, galactosemia, fructosemia, mitochondrial disorders, glutaric aciduria, carnitine palmitoyltransferase II deficiency, congenital disorders of glycosylation, and peroxisomal disorders can all be accompanied by hyperechoic kidneys [21].

So far, the outcome of fetal hyperechoic kidneys can only be accurately predicted in severe cases with significant oligohydramnios [19, 20]. For some patients, the characteristic US patterns will appear after birth or even later. A follow-up is therefore mandatory. It should be stressed that some cases remain unsolved and have to be considered as normal variants [20]. Table 2.1 provides information on the spectrum of renal disorders associated with fetal hyperechoic kidneys.

Abnormal Renal Size

Measurements of the kidneys must be systematic whenever an anomaly of the urinary tract or amniotic fluid volume is suspected. It is therefore important to have standards for renal size and volume measurements covering the complete gestational age range, because renal pathology often presents late in pregnancy [22]. Small kidneys most often correspond to hypodysplasia or damaged kidneys from obstructive uropathy or high-grade vesicoureteral reflux (VUR) [23, 24]. Enlarged kidneys may be related to urinary tract dilatation, renal cystic diseases or tumoral involvement.

Urinary Tract Dilatation

Fetal renal pelvis dilatation is a frequent abnormality that has been observed in 4.5 % of pregnancies [25]. Pyelectasis is defined as dilatation of the renal pelvis whereas pelvicaliectasis and hydronephrosis include dilatation of calyces. In practice, these terms are interchanged and used as descriptions of a dilated renal collecting system regardless of the etiology [26].

The third-trimester threshold value for the anteroposterior (AP) renal pelvis diameter of 7 mm is certainly the best prenatal criterion both for the screening of urinary tract dilatation and for the selection of patients needing postnatal investigation [22, 25].

There are several theories that account for the visibility of the renal pelvis during pregnancy. The distension of the urinary collecting system may be simply a dynamic and physiologic process [27]. Persutte et al. found the size of the fetal renal collecting system to be highly variable over a 2-h period [28]. The tendency of renal pelvis dilatation to resolve spontaneously is supported by normal postnatal renal appearances reported in 36–80 % of cases followed up after birth [29, 30]. However, prenatally detected renal pelvis dilatation may be an indicator of significant urinary tract pathologies [31]. The likelihood of having a clinically significant uropathy is directly proportional to the severity of the hydronephrosis [26]. A summary of the literature describing the postnatal uronephropathies found in neonates who presented with fetal renal pelvis dilatation is given in Table 2.2. The incidence and type of pathology varies considerably between studies, reflecting the differences in prenatal criteria and the variability in postnatal assessment. The two main pathologies found are pelviureteric junction stenosis and VUR. US is the first examination to perform after birth [35]. In babies diagnosed in utero with renal pelvis dilatation, the presence of persistent renal pelvis dilatation or other ultrasonographic abnormalities (such as calyceal or ureteral dilatation, pelvic or ureteral wall thickening and absence of the corticomedullary differentiation) and signs of renal dysplasia (such as small kidney, thinned or hyperechoic cortex or cortical cysts) should determine the need for further investigations [36, 37]. In cases when the

Table 2.1 Conditions associated with hyperechoic kidneys on prenatal ultrasound

	Kidney size	Amniotic fluid volume	Renal cysts	Collecting system	Associated abnormalities	Inheritance	Alternative prenatal diagnosis
Obstruction	−2 to 0 SD	Normal or reduced	Cortical <1 cm	Dilated	No	Sporadic	MRI
Bilateral MCDK	Variable	Reduced	Variable sizes, mostly large	Not seen	Variable if syndromic	Sporadic	MRI
Renal vein thrombosis	0–2 SD	Normal	No	Not seen	Thrombus in the inferior vena cava	Sporadic	Doppler
ARPKD	2–4 SD	Reduced	Small medullary	Not seen	Lung hypoplasia	AR	Genetics
ADPKD	0–2 SD	Normal or reduced	Subcapsular and medullar	Not seen	No	AD	Genetics
Glomerulocystic dysplasia	0–2 SD	Variable	Small cortical	Not seen	Variable if syndromic	Variable	Genetics (HNF1B/TCF2)
Bardet-Biedl syndrome	2–4 SD	Variable	No or medullary	Not seen	Polydactyly	AR	Genetics
Beckwith-Wiedeman syndrome	2 SD	Normal or increased	No or medullary	±	Macrosome, omphalocele	AD or dysomy	Genetics
Perlman syndrome	2 SD	Normal or reduced	No	±	Macrosome	AR	–
Normal variant	0–2 SD	Normal or increased	No	±	No	Sporadic	–

ARPKD Autosomal recessive polycystic kidney disease *ADPKD* Autosomal dominant polycystic kidney disease, *MCDK* Multicystic dysplastic kidney, *AD* Autosomal dominant, *AR* Autosomal recessive, *MRI* Magnetic resonance imaging, *HNF-1β* Hepatocyte nuclear factor-1β

Table 2.2 Incidence of uro-nephropathies in neonates with antenatally diagnosed renal pelvis dilatation

Authors	Year	Threshold value of renal pelvis (mm)	Total	Abnormal (%)	UPJS (%)	VUR (%)	Megaureter (%)	Mild dilatation (%)	Duplex kidney (%)	Other (%)	(%) undergoing surgery
Stocks et al. [33]	1996	4–7	27	70	22	22		26			11
Dudley et al. [32]	1997	5	100	64	3	12	3	43	4	7	3
Jaswon et al. [34]	1999	5	104	45	4	22		8		4	1
Ismaili et al. [29]	2004	4–7	213	39	13	11	7	18[a]	5	3	3

UPJS uretero-pelvic junction stenosis, *VUR* vesicoureteral reflux
[a]In this study mild and transient dilatations were considered as non-significant findings

urinary tract appears normal on neonatal US examinations, no further evaluation is needed [29]. Based on our own experience [29, 36, 38], we propose an algorithm for a rational postnatal imaging strategy (Fig. 2.2). Using this algorithm, we found that very few abnormal cases escaped the work up and that the risk of complications was very low.

Renal Cysts

Renal cystic diseases should be suspected not only in the case of obvious macrocysts but also in the case of hyperechoic kidneys [24]. Cysts may be present in one or both kidneys. Their origin may be genetic, and they may occur as an isolated anomaly or part of a syndrome. Familial history is of a great importance for the diagnosis [39].

Obstructive renal dysplasia and MCDK are the most common entities in which macrocysts can be detected. Obstructive renal dysplasia is associated with urinary tract obstruction that may have resolved at the time of diagnosis, leaving the cystic sequelae behind as the unique evidence that a urinary flow impairment ever existed [8]. In this condition, the cysts measure less than 1 cm and are located within the hyperechoic cortex [20]. MCDK is discussed further under Renal Causes of Fetal Renal Abnormalities in this chapter. Although rare, isolated cortical cysts may be seen in utero. They may persist after birth or regress spontaneously [40].

The most frequent genetically transmitted cystic renal diseases are the autosomal dominant polycystic kidney diseases and abnormalities of the hepatocyte nuclear factor-1β (HNF1B) encoded by the

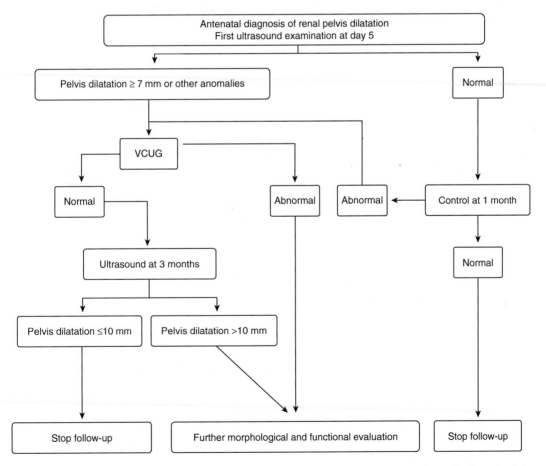

Fig. 2.2 Algorithm of a rational postnatal imaging strategy in infants with mild to moderate fetal renal pelvis dilatation

TCF2 gene [41]. HNF1B diseases are typically associated with bilateral cortical renal microcysts as well as other renal parenchymal abnormalities including MCDK and renal dysplasia [41]. HNF1B plays an important role in the early phases of kidney development [42]. Both the type and the severity of the renal disease are variable in children with HNF1B mutations: from severe prenatal renal failure to normal renal function in adulthood, and there is no obvious correlation between the type of mutation and the type and/or severity of renal disease. Furthermore, the inter- and intrafamilial variability of the phenotype in patients who harbor the same mutation is high, making the genetic counseling particularly difficult in these families [43]. Cystic kidneys are also part of many syndromes (Tables 2.1 and 2.3) with many associated anomalies that are sometimes typical of the underlying pathology.

Renal Tumors

Fetal renal tumors occur only rarely. Mesoblastic nephroma represents the most common congenital renal neoplasm [52]. It is a solitary hamartoma with a usually benign course. Mesoblastic nephroma appears as a large, solitary, predominantly solid, retroperitoneal mass arising and not separable from the adjacent kidney. It does not have a well-defined capsule and may sometimes appear as a partially cystic tumor [8]. In case of a tumor with multiple cysts, a MCDK should be considered first. Mesoblastic nephroma frequently coexists with polyhydramnios although the reason for this association remains unclear [52]. Fetal Wilm's tumor is exceptionally rare and may be indistinguishable from mesoblastic nephroma on imaging [53]. Another differential diagnosis is nephroblastomatosis, which appears either as hyperechoic nodule(s) or as a diffusely enlarged hyperechoic kidney [54]. Renal tumors have to be differentiated from adrenal tumors and intra-abdominal sequestrations [55].

Bladder Abnormalities

On fetal US examinations, the bladder should always be seen from the tenth week of gestation.

Nonvisualization of the bladder in the setting of oligohydramnios is highly suspicious of a bilateral severe renal abnormality with decreased urine production. It is important to carefully analyze the kidneys in order to exclude agenesis or dysplasia associated with poor outcome.

Nonvisualization of the bladder with an otherwise normal sonogram (kidneys and amniotic fluid) may be due to physiologic bladder emptying cycle in the fetus. Normal repletion should be checked within the following 20 min. Persistent non visualized bladder can be due to its inability to store urine, for example in cases of bladder or cloacal extrophy [56]. In this context, no bladder is seen between the two umbilical arteries. Bladder extrophy or cloacal malformations represent a diagnostic challenge on US, and MRI may help to define the pelvic anatomy of the fetus [57].

Enlarged bladder in the first trimester has a poor prognosis. Most of the cases are secondary to urethral atresia or stenosis, some are part of a syndrome (such as Prune Belly), or associated with chromosomal anomalies. Later in pregnancy, megabladder is defined as a cephalo-caudal diameter superior to 3 cm in the second trimester and to 5 cm in the third trimester. Megabladders are mainly due to outflow obstruction or to a major bilateral reflux [58]. It is often difficult to make a clear distinction between both abnormalities, as they may be associated. An irregular and thickened bladder wall is suggestive of an outflow obstruction. Megacystis-microcolon hypoperistalsis (MMH) syndrome is another differential diagnoses that carries a very poor prognosis [59]. It can be excluded by MRI during the third trimester because the colon is well visualized at that time.

Assessment of Fetal Renal Function

In utero, excretion of nitrogenous waste products and regulation of fetal fluid and electrolytes balance as well as acid-base homeostasis are maintained by the interaction of the placenta and maternal blood [60]. Thus, the placenta functions as an in vivo dialysis unit. Several

Table 2.3 Syndromes with cystic renal disease

	Renal cysts	Associated abnormalities	Inheritance	Reference
Meckel-Gruber syndrome	Medullary	Encephalocele, brain/cardiac anomalies, hepatic ductal dysplasia, cleft lip/palate, polydactyly	AR	[44]
Trisomy 9	Medullary	Mental retardation, intrauterine growth retardation, cardiac anomalies, joint contractures, prominent nose, sloping forehead	Chromosomal	[45]
Trisomy 13	Medullary	Mental retardation, intrauterine growth retardation, cardiac anomalies, cleft lip/palate, polydactyly	Chromosomal	[45]
Trisomy 18	Medullary	Mental retardation, intrauterine growth retardation, cardiac anomalies, small face, micrognathia, overlapping digits	Chromosomal	[45]
Bardet-Biedl syndrome	No or medullary	Polysyndactyly, obesity, mental retardation, pigmented retinopathy, hypogonadism	AR	[46]
Zellweger syndrome	Medullary	Hypotonia, seizures, failure to thrive, distinctive face, hepatosplenomegaly	AR	[47]
Ivemark syndrome	No or medullary	Polysplenia, complex heart disease, midline anomalies, situs inversus	Sporadic, AR	[48]
Beckwith-Wiedeman syndrome	Medullary	Overgrowth, macroglossia, omphalocele, hepatoblastoma, Wilm's tumor	Sporadic, AD	[49]
Jeune's syndrome	Medullary	Narrow chest, short limbs, polydactyly, periglomerular fibrosis	AR	[50]
Tuberous sclerosis	Medullary	Mental retardation, seizures, facial angiofibroma, angiomyolipoma, hypopigmented spots, cardiac rhabdomyomas, cerebral hamartomas	AD	[51]

AD Autosomal dominant, *AR* Autosomal recessive

parameters have been used in the evaluation of fetal renal function in fetal life. However, since fetal homeostasis depends on the integrity of the placenta, it is very difficult to assess the functional status of the fetal kidney. Furthermore, changes in the volume or composition of fetal urine may in many instances reflect the condition of the placenta rather than the condition of the fetal kidney [61]. However, exact diagnosis of the renal abnormalities and accurate prediction of the renal function after birth are important tasks, because different renal diseases may require different approaches and therapies. Therefore, in addition to using fetal renal sonography to determine potential fetal renal anatomical abnormalities, it is important to assess function as accurately as possible.

Amniotic Fluid Volume

During the first trimester of gestation the placenta (chorion and amniotic membrane) is the principal source of amniotic fluid, while after 15 weeks fetal kidneys produce the majority of amniotic fluid. Therefore, the assessment of the quantity of amniotic fluid after 15 weeks constitutes the initial step in the evaluation of the fetal urinary tract. Abnormal amounts of amniotic fluid must alert the sonographer to search meticulously for renal and urinary tract anomalies [62]. Assessing amniotic fluid volume is difficult and mostly subjective. However, the four-quadrant sum of amniotic fluid pockets (amniotic fluid index) provides a reproducible method for assessing amniotic fluid volume with interobserver and intraobserver variation of 3–7 % [63].

Various cut-off criteria have been suggested for definition of oligohydramnios by amniotic fluid index, including less than 1st percentile [64], or 5th percentile for gestational age [63]. Oligohydramnios of any cause typically compresses and twists the fetus, thus leading to a recurrent pattern of abnormalities that has been called the oligohydramnios sequence [16]. Oligohydramnios may be caused by decreased production of fetal urine from bilateral renal agenesis or dysplasia, or by reduced egress of urine into the amniotic fluid due to urinary obstruction. Other causes may be fetal death, growth retardation, rupture of the membranes, or post-term gestation (Table 2.4).

In cases of bilateral obstructive uropathy, a recent study found the evaluation of amniotic fluid by the amniotic fluid index to be the most reproducible and inexpensive method to predict renal function after birth [65]. The study also showed that an amniotic fluid index less than the 5th percentile was generally associated with an adverse perinatal outcome. Yet, an amniotic fluid index between the 5th and 25th percentiles should be considered as a warning sign since it may be a subtle indication of renal impairment, especially early in gestation when ultrasonographic signs of renal dysplasia may not be present and when fetal urinanalysis is not available [65].

Finally, one of the most devastating consequences of oligohydramnios, especially before 24 weeks gestation, is pulmonary hypoplasia [9]. Traditional explanations suggest that oligohydramnios causes pulmonary hypoplasia either by compression of the fetal thorax [66] or by encouraging lung liquid loss via the trachea [67]. However, since several morphogenetic pathways governing renal development are shared with lung organogenesis, this sequence is put into question. Some reports suggest that abnormal lung dysplasia may precede the advent of oligohydramnios in fetuses with intrinsic defects of renal parenchymal development [68].

Polyhydramnios, also referred to as hydramnios, is defined as a high level of amniotic fluid. Because the normal values for amniotic fluid volumes increase during pregnancy, this definition will depend on the gestational age of the fetus. During the last 2 months of pregnancy, polyhydramnios usually refers to amniotic fluid volumes greater than 1700–1900 ml. Severe cases are associated with much greater fluid volume excesses. The two major causes of polyhydramnios are reduced fetal swallowing or absorption of amniotic fluid and increased fetal urination (Table 2.4). Increased fetal urination is typically observed in maternal diabetes mellitus, but it may be associated with fetal renal diseases as mesoblastic nephroma [52], Bartter syndrome [69], congenital nephrotic syndrome [70] and alloimmune glomerulonephritis [71].

Fetal Urine Biochemical Markers

Fetal urine biochemistry was first introduced three decades ago as an additional test to improve prediction of renal function after birth [72]. Thereafter, investigators started to establish gestational age-dependent reference ranges for various biochemical parameters of fetal urine [73]. Rapidly, two important pitfalls emerged in this area of research. Initially, biochemical markers were analyzed either from amniotic fluid or bladder sampling based on the debatable assumption that both liquids have nearly identical composition. Subsequently, a practice has emerged whereby reference ranges are only taken from bladder or fetal urinary tract sampling. The second pitfall concerned the pertinence of the use of urinary solutes that are filtered by the glomerulus and reabsorbed by the tubules. These solutes express a tubular damage rather than a compromised GFR and it is therefore questionable if they can accurately predict renal function.

Fetal urine biochemistry is currently used especially in dilated uropathies because of technical difficulties of sampling fetal urines from a nondilated urinary tract, as seen in the majority of nephropathies. β2-microglobulin is the most widely used fetal urinary marker, although other compounds such as calcium, chloride and sodium may also be of interest. Prognostic values of these markers are outlined in Table 2.5. Most fetal urine

Table 2.4 Causes of oligohydramnios and polyhydramnios

	Origin	Pathologies
Oligohydramnios	Uronephropathy	Bilateral renal agenesis
		Bilateral renal dysplasia
		Autosomal recessive polycystic kidney disease
		Bilateral obstructive uropathy
		Bilateral high-grade reflux
		Bladder outlet obstruction
	Other	Premature rupture of membranes
		Placental insufficiency
		Fetal death
		Fetal growth retardation
		Twin-to-twin transfusion (twin donor)
		Maternal drug intake: prostaglandin synthase inhibitors, angiotensin-converting enzyme inhibitors, cocaine
		Postmaturity syndrome
Polyhydramnios	Uronephropathy	Renal tumors, especially mesoblastic nephroma
		Bartter syndrome
		Congenital nephrotic syndrome
		Alloimmune glomerulonephritis
	Other	Maternal diabetes
		Maternal drug intake: lithium,
		Multiple gestations
		Twin-to-twin transfusion (twin recipient)
		Fetal infections: Rubella, Cytomegalovirus, Toxoplasmosis
		Fetal gastrointestinal obstructions: esophageal atresia, duodenal atresia, gastroschisis
		Fetal compressive pulmonary disorders: diaphragmatic hernia, pleural effusions, cystic adenomatoid malformations, narrow thoracic cage
		Neuro-muscular conditions: anencephaly, myotonic dystrophy
		Cardiac anomalies
		Hematologic anomalies (fetal anemia)
		Hydrops fetalis
		Fetal chromosome abnormalities: trisomy 21, trisomy 18, trisomy 13
		Syndromic conditions: Beckwith-Wiedeman syndrome, achondroplasia
		No evident cause

studies agree on the following [74]: (1) fetuses with renal damage (dysplasia) show increased urinary solute concentrations; (2) urinary sodium and calcium yield the best accuracy among measurable electrolytes; (3) β2-microglobulin and cystatin C exhibit better accuracy than the measurement of any single electrolyte; (4) the accuracy of the proposed parameters are, however, far from perfect.

Recent novel approaches to fetal urine biochemistry such as proteomics and metabolomics may yield novel markers that may improve the usefulness of this technique in the near future. Recently, the urinary proteome was analyzed in fetuses with posterior urethral valves [79]. Among 4000 candidate compounds, 26 peptides were strongly associated with early end-stage renal disease.

Table 2.5 Fetal urine biochemical markers of postnatal prognosis

	Normal limits [75]	Good prognosis [76, 77]	Moderate renal failure at age 1 year [78]	Poor prognosis (Neonatal death or termination of pregnancy) [77, 78]
Na+	75–100 mmol/L	<100 mmol/L	59 mmol/L (54–65)	121 mmol/L (100–140)
Ca++	2 mmol/L		2 mmol/L (1.5–2.5)	2 mmol/L (1.5–2.5)
Cl–		<90 mmol/L	57 mmol/L (52–62)	98 mmol/L (85–111)
β2 microglobulin	<4 mg/L	<6 mg/L	6.8 mg/L (4.2–9.4)	19.5 mg/L (11–28)
Cystatin C		<1 mg/L	0.47 mg/L (0.05–4.75)	4.1 mg/L (0.45–13.1)
Osmolarity	<200 mOsm/L	<210 mOsm/L		

Table 2.6 Fetal serum biochemical markers of postnatal prognosis

	Controls [80]	Bilateral hypoplasia and dysplasia [81]	Bilateral uropathies [82]
Outcome:		Good prognosis	Postnatal renal failure
β2-microglobulin	4.28 mg/L (2.95–6.61)	3.2 mg/L (1.5–3.7)	5.3 mg/L (3.5–7.2)
Cystatin C	1.67 mg/L (1.12–2.06)	1.43 mg/L (1.09–1.86)	1.95 mg/L (1.56–4.60)
α1-microglobulin			60.5 mg/L (31.8–90.1)

Fetal Blood Sampling

Fetal blood sampling poses probably greater risks than urine sampling, but it allows a more accurate evaluation of fetal glomerular filtration rate (GFR) [78, 80, 81]. In the fetus, creatinine cannot be used as a marker of GFR because it crosses the placenta and is cleared by the mother. This is not the case for α1-microglobulin, β2-microglobulin and cystatin C, which have been used to predict renal function in uropathies and nephropathies (Table 2.6). This technique may be helpful, especially in cases where fetal urine is difficult to sample. It is, however, unlikely that fetal serum α1-microglobulin, β2-microglobulin and cystatin C will overcome the limitations associated with fetal urinalysis [80]. The only clinically useful information emerging from the studies performed to date is that fetal serum β2-microglobulin remains the best marker of renal function; however, its helpfulness is questionable outside extreme values (less than 3.5 mg/L good outcome; more than 5 mg/L poor outcome) [82].

Ultrasound-Guided Renal Biopsies

Ultrasound-guided renal biopsy would theoretically allow precise definition of the extent of renal damage in obstructed and primarily dysplastic kidneys [83]. However, this is an invasive procedure with a high rate of failure in obtaining an adequate sample [78]. Furthermore, a focal needle aspiration is not representative of the whole kidney parenchyma since renal dysplasia is patchily distributed.

Specific Renal and Urinary Tract Pathologies

Causes of fetal abnormalities of the kidney and urinary tract may be considered as prerenal, renal and postrenal.

Pre-Renal Causes of Fetal Renal Abnormalities

Intrauterine Growth Restriction (IUGR)

Intrauterine growth restriction (IUGR) complicates up to 10% of all pregnancies. It is associated with a perinatal mortality rate that is six to ten times higher when compared to normally grown fetuses and is the second most important cause of perinatal death after preterm delivery. The cause of IUGR is multifactorial. Worldwide, maternal nutritional deficiencies and inadequate utero-placental perfusion are among the most common causes of IUGR.

IUGR caused by placental insufficiency is often associated with oligohydramnios due to reduced urine production rate in these fetuses. This phenomenon is probably due to chronic hypoxemia that leads to the brain-sparing redistribution of oxygenated blood away from nonvital peripheral organs such as the kidneys [60]. As a consequence, fetal renal medullary hyperechogenicity may develop between the 24th and the 37th weeks of gestation due to tubular blockage caused by Tamm-Horsfall protein precipitation, and may be a sign of hypoxic renal insufficiency [84]. IUGR complicated by renal medullary hyperechogenicity suggests a more serious state, because these fetuses have a higher risk of pathological postnatal clinical outcome, such as neonatal mortality (8%), fetal distress leading to cesarean section (36%), transfer to intensive care unit (64%), and perinatal infection (24%) [84]. IUGR not only leads to a low birth weight but it might also reprogram nephrogenesis, which results in a low nephron endowment. According to the hyperfiltration hypothesis, this reduction in renal mass is supposed to lead to glomerular hyperfiltration and hypertension in remnant nephrons with subsequent glomerular injury with proteinuria, systemic hypertension and glomerulosclerosis in adult age [85].

Renal Vein Thrombosis

Renal vein thrombosis is the most common vascular condition in the newborn kidney and represents 0.5/1000 of admissions to neonatal intensive care units [86]. Factors predisposing a neonate to renal vein thrombosis include dehydration, sepsis, birth asphyxia, maternal diabetes, polycythemia and the presence of indwelling umbilical venous catheter [86]. In addition, prothrombotic abnormalities may be present in more than 40% of these babies, such as Protein C or S deficiency,

Factor V Leiden mutation, Lupus anticoagulant and Antithrombin III deficiency [87]. Renal vein thrombosis may also occur in utero. However, the origin of the thrombosis is not always obvious. Sonographically, the fetal kidney appears somewhat enlarged; the cortex may appear hyperechoic and without corticomedullary differentiation. Pathognomonic vascular streaks may be visible in the interlobar areas. Thrombus in the inferior vena cava is a common association [8]. Color Doppler US may be used in addition to grey-scale examination in the assessment of renal vein thrombosis (Fig. 2.3a-c). In the early stages of renal vein thrombosis, intrarenal and renal venous flow and pulsatility may be absent and renal arterial diastolic flow may be decreased, with a raised resistive index. Collateral vessels develop very rapidly and in most cases there are no consequences on further renal development [88]. After birth, the hyperechoic streaks and the thrombus are calcified. This feature helps differentiate antenatal from postnatal onset of the renal vein thrombosis [88].

The Twin-To-Twin Transfusion Syndrome

The twin-to-twin transfusion syndrome complicates 10–15% of monochorionic twin pregnancies [89]. The etiology of this condition is not completely understood but is thought to result from an unbalanced fetal blood supply through the placental vascular shunts, with the larger twin being the recipient and the smaller twin the donor [90]. The twin-to-twin transfusion syndrome is defined by the existence of a oligo-polyhydramnios sequence (that is, the deepest vertical pool being 2 cm or less in the donor's sac and 8 cm or more in the recipient's sac) [89]. Additional phenotypic features in the donor include a small or nonvisible bladder and abnormal umbilical artery Doppler with absent or reverse end-diastolic frequencies. In addition to the neonatal complications of growth restriction, up to 30% of donors have renal failure and/or renal tubular dysgenesis due to the chronic renal hypoperfusion state in utero [89]. In the recipient, confirmatory features include large bladder, cardiac hypertrophy and eventually hydrops. Risk of renal failure in the recipient twin is considerably smaller than in the donor twin. This can be seen as one fetus dying and vascular resistance dropping significantly to cause reversed blood transfusion from the recipient twin to the dead fetus, resulting in hypovolemia and anemia in the live fetus [91].

Maternal Drug Intake

Mother drugs consumption can in certain cases impair fetal renal function or produce congenital renal anomalies.

Renin-Angiotensin System (RAS) Antagonists

Administration of angiotensin converting enzyme inhibitors (ACEIs) and angiotensin type I receptor blockers (ARBs) can severely affect renal development and function at any gestational age. RAS inhibitors lead to tubular dysgenesis, oligohydramnios, growth restriction, neonatal anuria and stillbirth [92–95]. In one study almost 9 % of children exposed to ACEIs during the first trimester (but not later in pregnancy) showed major congenital anomalies (cardiovascular, central nervous system and renal malformations) at a rate 2.7 times that among unexposed infants [93]. The renal anomalies are thought to be caused both directly by antagonism of the fetal intrarenal renin-angiotensin system and indirectly by fetoplacental ischemia resulting from maternal hypotension and a drop of fetal-placental blood flow [60]. Pregnancies exposed to RAS blockers and complicated by oligohydramnios are associated with the highest rate of adverse pregnancy outcomes. Combined monitoring of amniotic fluid volume evaluation and fetal serum β2-microglobulin may be helpful in the management of these pregnancies [96].

Nonsteroidal Antiinflammatory Drugs (NSAID)

Cyclooxygenase type 1 (COX-1) inhibitors such as indomethacin, the most common NSAID used as a tocolytic, definitely reduce urine out-

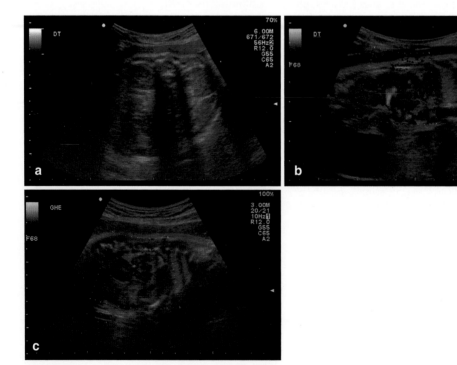

Fig. 2.3 Left renal vein thrombosis (third trimester). (**a**) Axial US scan showing differences of size and echogenicity of both kidneys, The left kidney is enlarged and hyperechoic. (**b**) Coronal US scan showing normal renal venous flow on the right kidney. (**c**) Parasagittal US scan of the left kidney. Renal venous flow is almost absent in comparison with the normal right kidney

put and may lead to oligohydramnios and renal dysfunction [60]. It was hoped that cyclooxygenase type 2 (COX-2) inhibitors would target COX-2 activity and potentially spare COX-1-specific fetal side effects. However, COX-2 expression is higher in fetal as compared to adult kidneys and may even occur constitutively in fetal kidney tissue [60]. Sulindac and nimesulide administration has therefore been linked both to constriction of the ductus arteriosus and oligohydramnios [97].

Cocaine

Maternal cocaine use adversely influences fetal renal function by hypoperfusion and thus influences the fetal renin-angiotensin system. It is also associated with oligohydramnios as well as other fetal vascular complications leading to higher renal artery resistance index and a significant decrease in urine output [98]. However, and contradicting a widely held belief [99], a prospective, large-scale, blinded, systematic evaluation for congenital anomalies in prenatally cocaine-exposed children did not identify any increase in the number or consistent pattern of genitourinary tract malformations [100].

Immunosuppressive Medications During Pregnancy

In the early days of transplantation, physicians worried about the potential effects of immunosuppressive medications on the child-to-be and considered pregnancy ill-advised for patients taking these medications [101]. Despite these concerns, a large number of women with transplanted organs have completed pregnancies [102]. Although some immunosuppressants such as azathioprine and cyclosporine are teratogenic in animals, case reports and registry records have not substantiated any consistent malformation patterns in children of allograft recipients [103]. However, the use of mycophenolate mofetil (MMF) during pregnancy has been associated with teratogenicity in humans [104]. Therefore, European best practice guidelines recommend that women receiving MMF switch to another agent and wait six weeks before they attempt to conceive [105].

Renal Causes of Congenital Abnormalities of the Kidney and Urinary Tract (CAKUT)

CAKUTs are the most common cause of pediatric kidney failure. These disorders are highly heterogeneous, and the etiologic factors are not completely understood. These conditions are genetically variable and encompass a wide range of anatomical defects, such as renal agenesis, renal hypodysplasia, pelviureteric junction stenosis, and VUR. Mutations in genes causing syndromic disorders, such as *HNF1B* and *PAX2* mutations, are detected in only 5–10% of cases [106]. Familial forms of nonsyndromic disease have also been reported, further supporting a genetic determination (such as *DSTYK* gene [107], *CHRM3* gene in Prune belly syndrome [108], *HPSE2* and *LRIG2* genes in Ochoa syndrome [109, 110]. However, owing to locus heterogeneity and small pedigree size, the genetic cause of most familial or sporadic cases remains unknown.

Multicystic Dysplastic Kidney (MCDK)

These kidneys contain bizarrely shaped tubules surrounded by a stroma that includes undifferentiated and metaplastic cells (for example, smooth muscle and cartilage). According to Liebeschuetz [111] the prevalence of MCDK is about 1 in 2400 live births, which is higher than other reports [112]. MCDK is usually unilateral and presents a typical US pattern: multiple noncommunicating cysts of varying size and nonmedial location of the largest cyst, absence of normal renal sinus echoes, and absence of normal renal parenchyma [113]. MCDK may also develop in the upper part of a duplex system or be located in an ectopic position. Unilateral isolated MCDK carries a good prognosis but careful examination of the contralateral kidney is essential because there is a high incidence of associated pathologies, many of which may not be detected until birth [4, 114]. The distinction between MCDK and cystic renal dysplasia associated with urinary tract obstruction may be difficult, especially in the absence of hydronephrosis. This distinction, although helpful in terms of diagnosis, may be somewhat artificial in terms of prognosis, since in either case, the affected kidney has no or minimal functional capacity.

Autosomal Recessive Polycystic Kidney Disease (ARPKD)

ARPKD belongs to the family of cilia-related disorders, has an incidence of 1 in 20,000 live births and may cause fetal and neonatal death in severe cases. Mutations in the *PKHD1* fibrocystin gene are usually demonstrated in this disease [115]. Yet, since some patients survive the neonatal period with few or slight symptoms, different combinations of *PKHD1* gene mutations and its resulting changes in the fibrocystin/polyductin protein structure may at least partially explain the phenotypic variance [116]. The disease is characterized by marked elongation of the collecting tubules that expand into multiple small cysts. The cystic dilatation of the tubules is variable and predominates in the medulla. The outer cortex is spared since it contains no tubules. The classical in utero pattern of ARPKD includes markedly enlarged (+4 SD) hyperechoic kidneys without corticomedullary differentiation. This appearance can be observed in the second trimester. The patterns may evolve and the size of the kidneys may continuously increase during the third trimester. Oligohydramnios and lung hypoplasia may be present, and therefore the prognosis is extremely poor.

Another presentation of ARPKD is of reversed corticomedullary differentiation with large kidneys (+2 to +4 SD) (Fig. 2.4). This finding is probably related to increased interfaces within the medullae and to the presence of material within the dilated tubules [117]. It is an important observation since there are few other causes of reversed corticomedullary differentiation. Liver involvement, typical of the condition, is usually impossible to demonstrate in utero. The differential diagnosis includes the glomerulocystic type of autosomal dominant polycystic kidney disease, Bardet-Biedl syndrome in which polydactyly is present [46] and other rare entities such as bilateral renal tumors, medullary sponge kidney, bilateral nephroblastomatosis, Finnish-type congenital nephrotic syndrome, medullary cystic disease, or congenital metabolic diseases (that is,

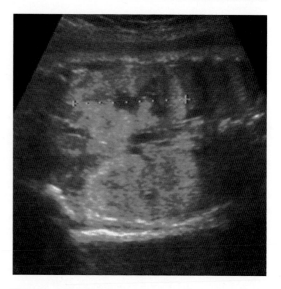

Fig. 2.4 Autosomal recessive polycystic kidney disease. Third trimester-coronal scan through the kidneys that appear large (+3 SD), and hyperechoic

glycogen storage disease or tyrosinosis). Oligohydramnios and absence of urine within the bladder would suggest ARPKD over all these rare entities.

Autosomal Dominant Polycystic Kidney Disease (ADPKD)

ADPKD is a common hereditary kidney disease, with 1/1000 people carrying the mutation. The pathological abnormality consists of a cystic dilatation of all parts of the nephron, which causes the kidneys to enlarge while the cortex and medulla become replaced by cysts, thus leading to end-stage renal failure [117, 118].

There are two major types of ADPKD: type I is caused by mutations in the *PKD1* gene on chromosome 16p13.3 and accounts for 85–90 % of cases [117], and type II is caused by mutations in the *PKD2* gene on chromosome 4q21-22 and accounts for 10–15 % of cases [118]. One or more other genes (type III) are likely to be involved since some obvious cases have none of these mutations. Although the age of clinical onset of this disorder is typically in the third to fifth decade of life, early manifestations during childhood or during the prenatal period have also been reported [119, 120].

There may be two different presentations in utero. In most cases, the kidneys are not grossly enlarged, but the corticomedullary differentiation is increased due to cortical hyperechogenicity. In this type of ADPKD, cysts are unusual in utero; they will develop after birth. Markedly enlarged kidneys resembling ARPKD are another pattern that can be encountered in utero and suggests the glomerulocystic type of ADPKD. In this presentation of the disease, some subcortical cysts may be present in utero and renal failure may be already present at birth [116].

Renal Hypoplasia and Dysplasia

Renal dysplasia refers to abnormal differentiation or organization of cells in the renal parenchyma and is characterized histologically by the presence of primitive ducts and nests of metaplastic cartilage [23, 24]. Hypoplasia is a reduction of the number of nephrons in small kidneys (below -2 SD) [23]. Hypoplasia may coexist with dysplasia and the diagnosis is inferred from the hyperechoic appearance on US caused by the lack of normal renal parenchyma and structurally abnormal small kidneys (Fig. 2.5) [23, 24]. As in most cases the diagnosis is made by US examination, the spectrum of renal dysplasia includes inherited or congenital causes of renal hypoplasia, renal adysplasia, cystic dysplasia, oligomeganephronic hypoplasia, reflux nephropathy and obstructive renal dysplasia [23]. Cases with oligohydramnios have the poorest outcome [121].

A number of developmental genes have been implicated in the pathogenesis of hypodysplastic kidneys [106]: *EYA1* and *SIX1* causing autosomal dominant branchio-oto-renal syndrome [122], *HNF1B/TCF2* associated with autosomal dominant renal cysts and diabetes syndrome [123], and *PAX2* causing autosomal dominant renal-coloboma syndrome [124].

After birth, the prognosis depends on the residual renal function at 6 months of age. Infants with a GFR below 15 ml/min per 1.73 m^2 are at higher risk for early renal replacement therapy [23].

Congenital Nephrotic Syndrome

Congenital nephrotic syndrome is defined as proteinuria leading to clinical symptoms within the 3 first months after birth. Infantile nephrotic syndrome manifests later, in the first year of life. However, these classifications are arbitrary as the majority of early-onset nephrotic syndrome diseases range from fetal life to several years of age [125].

Congenital nephrotic syndrome of the Finnish type (CNF) is characterized by autosomal recessive inheritance and is caused by mutations in the nephrin gene (*NPHS1*) [126]. Most infants are born prematurely, with low birth weight for gestational age. The placenta is enlarged, weighing more than 25 % of the birth weight. Edema is present at birth or appears within a few days due to severe nephrotic syndrome. In utero, the possible development of hydrops fetalis and increased nuchal translucency reflects massive proteinuria accompanied by a relatively high urine output [127, 128]. Because the main part of amniotic fluid α-fetoprotein is derived from fetal urine, high values reflect intrauterine proteinuria [129]. If the α-fetoprotein concentration is 250,000–500,000 µg/L, and especially if there is another child with CNF in the family, it is highly suggestive of CNF.

Other cases of prenatally diagnosed congenital nephrotic syndrome have been reported including Podocin gene (*NPHS2*) mutations [130], Pierson syndrome [131, 132], *PLCE1*

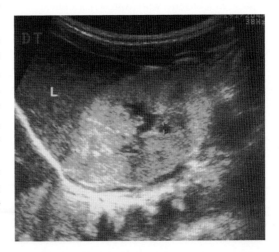

Fig. 2.5 Renal hypodysplasia (third trimester). Sagittal US scan through a hyperechoic small-sized right kidney. A medullar cyst is present (between crosses). *L* liver

gene mutations [133], secondary nephrotic syndrome due to CMV or other intrauterine infections [134] and massive proteinuria in off-springs of mothers with homozygous deficiency for the metallomembrane endopeptidase [71].

Postrenal Causes of Fetal Renal Abnormalities

Dilatations of the renal pelvis, calyces and ureters are the principal signs of impaired urinary flow on antenatal ultrasound scanning.

Pelviureteric Junction Stenosis

Pelviureteric junction stenosis occurs in 13 % of children with antenatally diagnosed renal pelvis dilatation [29] and is characterized by obstruction at the level of the junction between the renal pelvis and the ureter. The anatomical basis for obstruction includes intrinsic stenosis/valves, peripelvic fibrosis, or crossing vessels. Sonographic diagnosis depends on the demonstration of a dilated renal pelvis in the absence of any dilatation of ureter or bladder. It should be particularly suspected when moderate (10–15 mm) or severe (greater than 15 mm) dilatation is seen, when the cavities appear round shaped and in the presence of a perirenal urinoma [26] (Fig. 2.6). Prognosis may be poor in bilateral cases associated with oligohydramnios and hyperechoic parenchyma although individual prognostic predictions are difficult to make. Postnatal management is based on close monitoring of both sonomorphological and functional criteria assessed by radionuclide renogram including renal transit limited to the cortical area, differential function and output function (drainage pattern) [135–137].

Vesicoureteric Reflux (VUR)

VUR is defined as the retrograde flow of urine from the bladder upward within the ureter, sometimes extending into the renal pelvis, calyces and collecting ducts. Fetal renal pelvis dilatation can signal the presence of VUR in 11 % [29] to 30 % [138] of cases with the lower figure being more realistic. Making a precise diagnosis of VUR in

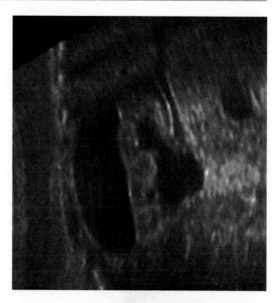

Fig. 2.6 Pelvicaliceal dilatation and perirenal urinoma in a fetus with pelviureteric junction stenosis. Coronal US scan through the right fetal kidney

utero is difficult. However, intermittent renal collecting system dilatation during real-time scanning (Fig. 2.7a, b) or pelvicaliceal wall thickening are sonographic criteria highly suggestive of this diagnosis [139]. Although some children with high-grade, prenatally diagnosed VUR may have associated renal dysplasia [140], VUR related to fetal renal pelvis dilatation was found in a large and prospective study to be of low-grade in 74 % of cases with a high rate of 2-year spontaneous resolution (91 %) [6].

Uretero-Vesical Junction Obstruction (Megaureter)

In utero, under normal conditions, the ureters are not visualized. Megaureter should be suspected in the presence of a serpentine fluid-filled structure with or without dilatation of the renal pelvis and calices (Fig. 2.8) The ureter may be dilated because of obstruction at the level of the junction between the ureter and the bladder or as a result of nonobstructive causes including high-grade reflux. The differential diagnosis relies on VCUG. Megaureter could also be encountered in fetuses and/or newborns with neurogenic bladder or posterior urethral valves. In those cases, specific treatment strategies should be directed

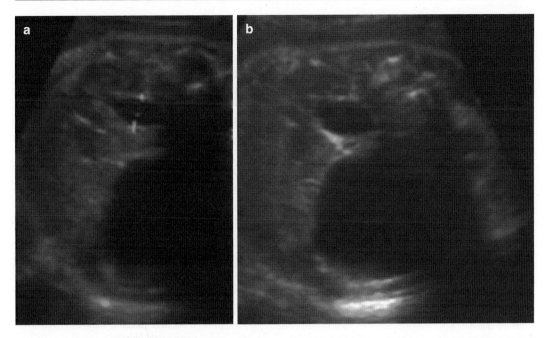

Fig. 2.7 (**a, b**) Fetal vesicoureteral reflux. Transverse scans of the fetal abdomen. Intermittent renal collecting system dilatation during the same antenatal ultrasound examination due to vesicoureteral reflux

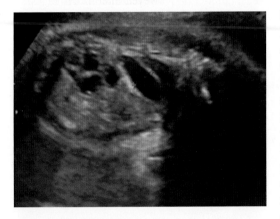

Fig. 2.8 Megaureter. In utero (third trimester) dilatation of the right ureter. Parasagittal scan of the fetal abdomen showing a serpentine fluid-filled structure (between the crosses)

toward the underlying condition. Prognosis of primary megaureter is generally good with most cases resolving spontaneously between ages 12 and 36 months [141]. However, in children with high-grade hydronephrosis, or a retrovesical ureteral diameter of greater than 1 cm, the condition may resolve slowly and in rare cases may require surgery [141].

Duplex Kidneys

Duplication of the renal collecting system is characterized by the presence of a kidney having two pelvic structures with two ureters that may be completely or partially separated [142]. Most cases with non-dilated cavities have no renal impairment and should be considered as normal variants [29]. However, a proportion of duplex kidneys may be associated with significant pathology, usually due to the presence of VUR or obstruction. Fetal urinary tract dilatations are related to complicated renal duplication in 4.7 % of cases [29]. VUR usually involves only the lower pole ureter in 90 % of cases. Compared to single-system reflux, duplex system VUR tends to be of a higher grade with a high incidence of lower pole dysplasia [5, 143]. Obstructive ureteroceles are associated with the upper pole ureter in 80 % of cases, although obstruction of the upper pole may also occur secondary to an ectopic insertion or an isolated vesicoureteric junction obstruction (Fig. 2.9a) [142]. In utero, duplex kidneys are highly suspected in the presence of two separate noncommunicating renal pelves, dilated ureters, cystic structures within one pole, and echogenic cyst in the bladder, representing ureterocele (Fig. 2.9b) [144]. After birth, the classical radiological workup of abnormal duplex kidneys is based on US and VCUG [145]. Most people agree that the surgical approach to complicated duplex systems is largely predicated on the function of the affected renal moiety and the presence or absence of function [145].

Bladder Outlet Obstruction

When bladder obstruction is suspected in the first trimester, the most common causes are Prune Belly syndrome or fibrourethral stenosis, which is mainly associated with chromosomal and multiple congenital anomalies and carries a very poor prognosis [146]. In the second trimester, the most common cause of lower urinary tract obstruction in male fetuses is posterior urethral valves, which are tissue leaflets fanning distally from the prostatic urethra to the external urinary sphincter. The failure of the bladder to empty during an extended examination and the presence of abnormal kidneys and oligohydramnios must raise suspicion of posterior urethral valves. On occasion a megabladder with a thickened wall may be seen

(Fig. 2.10a), and the dilated posterior urethra may take the aspect of a keyhole (Fig. 2.10b). In extreme cases in utero bladder rupture may be observed with extravasation of urine resulting in urinary ascites. This phenomenon was thought to be a protective pop-off mechanism, although recent reports provided evidence against this hypothesis [147].

In many cases there is only a partial obstruction, and amniotic fluid volume can be maintained throughout pregnancy. In some cases, spontaneous rupture of valves appears to occur in utero with the reappearance of cyclical emptying of the bladder. The most reliable prognostic indicators of poor renal functional status are presentation before 24 weeks, oligohydramnios, increased cortical echogenicity, and the absence of corticomedullary differentiation [148].

The prognosis in severe cases is often relatively easy to predict, and perinatal death will occur secondary to pulmonary hypoplasia and renal failure [149]. The renal parenchymal lesions may be secondary to the obstruction but also to associated high-grade reflux. In partial obstruction,

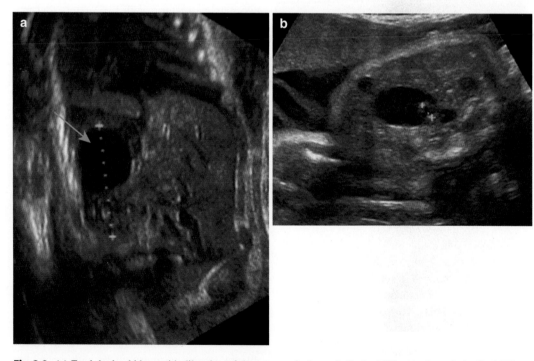

Fig. 2.9 (a) Fetal duplex kidney with dilatation of the upper pole (*arrow*). Sagittal US scan through the fetal kidney. (b) Fetal bladder with ureterocele (between crosses). Axial US scan through the fetal bladder

however, the outcome is less predictable, and late morbidity most commonly takes the form of end-stage renal failure, which affects 15–30 % of individuals some time in childhood [150]. Once the prognosis has been determined as accurately as possible, management of these cases should be performed in a fetal medicine and pediatric surgery reference center. In each new case, the great variability of presentation makes participation of different specialists necessary in the difficult decision-making process. Various options should be discussed, including in utero follow-up with planned postnatal management, termination of pregnancy, and occasionally, in utero therapy.

Fetal Intervention for Lower Urinary Tract Obstruction

One could imagine that an antenatal intervention to relieve the obstruction after diagnosis may restore amniotic fluid levels and that such intervention would allow for normal pulmonary maturation. However, whether an early intervention really prevents progressive renal deterioration and/or improves long-term renal outcomes remains to be demonstrated. A variety of in utero therapeutic approaches to bladder outflow obstruction have been tried. The open surgical technique of fetal vesicostomy has now been abandoned due to significant fetal loss, premature uterine contractions and maternal morbidity [151].

Direct endoscopic ablation of the valves is a more recent technique which requires the introduction of an endoscope into the fetal bladder, leading to ablation of the valves either by laser, saline irrigation or mechanical disruption using guide wire [152, 153]. Direct visualization of the valves, however, is difficult, and it can be difficult to avoid damage to surrounding tissue.

Vesicoamniotic shunting is performed with US guidance using a pigtail shunt, which when inserted leaves one end in the fetal bladder and the other in the amniotic space. This technique,

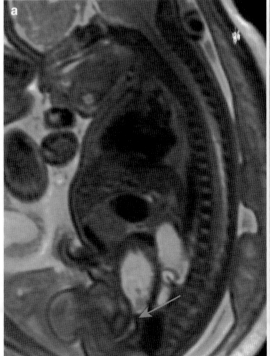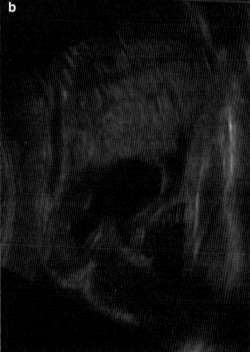

Fig. 2.10 (a) Fetal urethral valve with thickened bladder wall. Posterior urethral dilatation (*arrow*). Sagittal MR image on the fetal pelvis. (b) Megabladder. Third trimester scan. Huge enlargement of the fetal bladder due to posterior urethral valves. The key-hole sign is present

which was first reported in 1982 [154], is preferred to bladder drainage by serial vesico-centesis. A previous systematic review to assess the effectiveness of bladder drainage (vesico amniotic shunting or vesicocentesis) showed that fetal bladder drainage increased fetal survival [155]. However, the studies identified in this systematic review were small, heterogeneous, observational, and nonrandomized trials. Consequently, the potential for bias in the results was substantial. In addition, using survival alone as a marker of efficacy in these patients was misleading, since most of the survivors were left with significant renal morbidity. End-stage renal failure was present in 40 % of those children who survived [75]. Recently, Rachel Morris et al. [156] presented the results of the long-awaited PLUTO (Percutaneous vesicoamniotic shunting in Lower Urinary Tract Obstruction) trial, in which fetuses with fetal lower urinary tract obstruction were randomly assigned to either vesicoamniotic shunting or conservative management. Thirty-one women with singleton pregnancies complicated by lower urinary tract obstruction were included in the trial, with 16 allocated to the vesicoamniotic shunt group and 15 to the conservative management group. Unfortunately, the trial was stopped early because of poor recruitment after only about 20 % of the planned 150 pregnancies were randomly assigned during a 4-year period. Although PLUTO's results have to be interpreted with caution due to the premature termination of the study and the small number of patients [157], postnatal survival was three-times higher in the fetuses receiving vesicoamniotic shunting. However, only two of seven shunted survivors had normal renal function at age 1 year. These results suggest that the chance of newborn babies surviving with normal renal function is very low irrespective of whether or not vesicoamniotic shunting is done. These findings are in line with results from studies in animals, which have shown that renal damage occurs rapidly after the onset of obstruction and might be only partly reversible [158].

In conclusion, the experience with intrauterine shunting techniques as practiced to date suggests that postnatal survival may be improved but little if any improvement of postnatal renal function can be achieved.

References

1. Wiesel A, Queisser-Luft A, Clementi M, Bianca S, Stoll C, the EUROSCAN Study Group. Prenatal detection of congenital renal malformation by fetal ultrasonographic examination: an analysis of 709 030 births in 12 European countries. Eur J Med Genet. 2005;48:131–44.
2. Gagnon A, Wilson RD, Allen VM, Audibert F, Blight C, Brock JA, Désilets VA, Johnson JA, Langlois S, Murphy-Kaulbeck L, Wyatt P. Society of obstetricians and gynaecologists of Canada. Evaluation of prenatally diagnosed structural congenital anomalies. J Obstet Gynaecol Can. 2009;31:875–81.
3. Ismaili K, Hall M, Ham H, Piepsz A. Evolution of individual renal function in children with unilateral complex renal duplication. J Pediatr. 2005;147:208–12.
4. Ismaili K, Hall M, Piepsz A, Wissing KM, Collier F, Schulman C, Avni FE. Primary vesicoureteral reflux detected among neonates with a history of fetal renal pelvis dilatation: a prospective clinical and imaging study. J Pediatr. 2006;148:222–7.
5. Gonçalves L, Espinoza J, Kusanovic JP, Lee W, Nien JK, Joaquin Santolaya-Forgas J, Mari G, Treadwell MC, Romero R. Applications of 2D matrix array for 3D and 4D examination of the fetus: a pictorial essay. J Ultrasound Med. 2006;25:745–55.
6. Michel SC, Rake A, Keller TM, Huch R, König V, Seifert B, Marincek B, Kubik-Huch RA. Fetal cardiographic monitoring in 1.5 T MR imaging. Am J Roentgenol. 2003;180:1159–64.
7. Lee SM, Jun JK, Lee EJ, Lee JH, Park CW, Park JS, Syn HC. Measurement of fetal urine production to differentiate causes of increased amniotic fluid volume. Ultrasound Obstet Gynecol. 2010;36:191–5.
8. Avni FE, Garel L, Hall M, Rypens F. Perinatal approach in anomalies of the urinary tract, adrenals and genital system. In: Avni FE, editor. Perinatal imaging. From ultrasound to MR imaging. New York: Springer; 2002. p. 153–96.
9. Thomas IF, Smith DW. Oligohydramnios: cause of the non renal features of Potter's syndrome including pulmonary hypoplasia. J Pediatr. 1974;84:811–5.
10. Cuckow PM, Nyirady P, Winyard PJ. Normal and abnormal development of the urogenital tract. Prenat Diagn. 2001;21:908–16.
11. Avni FE, Cos T, Cassart M, Massez A, Donner C, Ismaili K, Hall M. Evolution of fetal ultrasonography. Eur Radiol. 2007;17:419–31.
12. Oh KY, Holznagel DE, Ameli JR, Sohaey R. Prenatal diagnosis of renal developmental anomalies associated with an empty renal fossa. Ultrasound Q. 2010;26:233–40.

13. Sepulveda W, Staggianis KD, Flack NJ, Fisk NM. Accuracy of prenatal diagnosis of renal agenesis with color flow imaging in severe second-trimester oligohydramnios. Am J Obstet Gynecol. 1995;173:1788–92.

14. Mesrobian HG, Rushton HG, Bulas D. Unilateral renal agenesis may result from in utero regression of multicystic renal dysplasia. J Urol. 1993;150:793–4.

15. Chow JS, Benson CB, Lebowitz RL. The clinical significance of an empty renal fossa on prenatal sonography. J Ultrasound Med. 2005;24:1049–54.

16. Westland R, Kurvers RA, van Wijk JA, Schreuder MF. Risk factors for renal injury in children with a solitary functioning kidney. Pediatrics. 2013;131:e478–85.

17. Jeanty P, Romero R, Kepple D, Stoney D, Coggins T, Fleischer AC. Prenatal diagnoses in unilateral empty renal fossa. J Ultrasound Med. 1990;9:651–4.

18. Chaumoitre K, Brun M, Cassart M, Maugey-Laulom B, Eurin D, Didier F, Avni EF. Differential diagnosis of fetal hyperechogenic cystic kidneys unrelated to renal tract anomalies: A multicenter study. Ultrasound Obstet Gynecol. 2006;28:911–7.

19. Tsatsaris V, Gagnadoux MF, Aubry MC, Gubler MC, Dumez Y, Dommergues M. Prenatal diagnosis of bilateral isolated fetal hyperechogenic kidneys. Is it possible to predict long term outcome? BJOG. 2002;109:1388–93.

20. Mashiach R, Davidovits M, Eisenstein B, Kidron D, Kovo M, Shalev J, Merlob P, Verdimon D, Efrat Z, Meizner I. Fetal hyperechogenic kidney with normal amniotic fluid volume: a diagnostic dilemma. Prenat Diagn. 2005;25:553–8.

21. Hertz-Pannier L, Déchaux M, Sinico M, Emond S, Cormier-Daire V, Saudubray JM, Brunelle F, Niaudet P, Seta N, de Lonlay P. Congenital disorders of glycosylation type I: a rare but new cause of hyperechoic kidneys in infants and children due to early microcystic changes. Pediatr Radiol. 2006;36:108–14.

22. van Vuuren SH, Damen-Elias HA, Stigter RH, van der Doef R, Goldschmeding R, de Jong TP, Westers P, Visser GH, Pistorius LR. Size and volume charts of fetal kidney, renal pelvis and adrenal gland. Ultrasound Obstet Gynecol. 2012;40:659–64.

23. Ismaili K, Schurmans T, Wissing M, Hall M, Van Aelst C, Janssen F. Early prognostic factors of infants with chronic renal failure caused by renal dysplasia. Pediatr Nephrol. 2001;16:260–4.

24. Winyard P, Chitty L. Dysplastic and polycystic kidneys: diagnosis, associations and management. Prenat Diagn. 2001;21:924–35.

25. Ismaili K, Hall M, Donner C, Thomas D, Vermeylen D, Avni FE. Results of systematic screening for minor degrees of fetal renal pelvis dilatation in an unselected population. Am J Obstet Gynecol. 2003;188:242–6.

26. Ismaili K, Hall M, Piepsz A, Alexander M, Schulman C, Avni FE. Insights into the pathogenesis and natural history of fetuses with renal pelvis dilatation. Eur Urol. 2005;48:207–14.

27. Sherer DM. Is fetal hydronephrosis overdiagnosed? Ultrasound Obstet Gynecol. 2000;16:601–6.

28. Persutte WH, Hussey M, Chyu J, Hobbins JC. Striking findings concerning the variability in the measurement of the fetal renal collecting system. Ultrasound Obstet Gynecol. 2000;15:186–90.

29. Ismaili K, Avni FE, Wissing KM, Hall M. Long-term clinical outcome of infants with mild and moderate fetal pyelectasis: validation of neonatal ultrasound as a screening tool to detect significant nephro-uropathies. J Pediatr. 2004;144:759–65.

30. Sairam S, Al-Habib A, Sasson S, Thilaganathan B. Natural history of fetal hydronephrosis diagnosed on mid-trimester ultrasound. Ultrasound Obstet Gynecol. 2001;17:191–6.

31. Chudleigh T. Mild pyelectasis. Prenat Diagn. 2001;21:936–41.

32. Dudley JA, Haworth JM, McGraw ME, Frank JD, Tizzard EJ. Clinical relevance and implications of antenatal hydronephrosis. Arch Dis Child. 1997;76:F31–4.

33. Stocks A, Richards D, Frentzen B, Richard G. Correlation of prenatal renal pelvic anteroposterior diameter with outcome in infancy. J Urol. 1996;155:1050–2.

34. Jaswon MS, Dibble L, Puri S, Davis J, Young J, Dave R, Morgan H. Prospective study of outcome in antenatally diagnosed renal pelvis dilatation. Arch Dis Child. 1999;80:F135–8.

35. De Bruyn R, Gordon I. Postnatal investigation of fetal renal disease. Prenat Diagn. 2001;21:984–91.

36. Ismaili K, Avni FE, Hall M. Results of systematic voiding cystourethrography in infants with antenatally diagnosed renal pelvis dilation. J Pediatr. 2002;141:21–4.

37. Moorthy I, Joshi N, Cook JV, Warren M. Antenatal hydronephrosis: negative predictive value of normal postnatal ultrasound, a 5-year study. Clin Radiol. 2003;58:964–70.

38. Avni EF, Ayadi K, Rypens F, Hall M, Schulman CC. Can careful ultrasound examination of the urinary tract exclude vesicoureteric reflux in the neonate? Br J Radiol. 1997;70:977–82.

39. Friedman W, Vogel M, Dimer JS, Luttkus A, Buscher U, Dudenhausen JW. Prenatal differential diagnosis of cystic renal disease and urinary tract obstruction: anatomic pathologic, ultrasonographic and genetic findings. Eur J Obstet Gynecol Reprod Biol. 2000;89:127–33.

40. Blazer S, Zimmer EZ, Blumenfeld Z, Zelikovic I, Bronshtein M. Natural history of fetal simple cysts detected early in pregnancy. J Urol. 1999;162:812–4.

41. Decramer S, Parant O, Beaufils S, Clauin S, Guillou C, Kessler S, Aziza J, Bandin F, Schanstra JP, Bellanné-Chantelot C. Nomalies of the TCF2 gene are the main cause of fetal bilateral hyperechogenic kidneys. J Am Soc Nephrol. 2007;18(3):923–33.

42. Coffinier C, Thepot D, Babinet C, Yaniv M, Barra J. Essential role for the hemeoprotein vHNF1/

HNF1beta in visceral endoderm differentiation. Development. 1999;126:4785–94.

43. Heidet L, Decramer S, Pawtowski A, Morinière V, Bandin F, Knebelmann B, Lebre AS, Faguer S, Guigonis V, Antignac C, Salomon R. Spectrum of HNF1B mutations in a large cohort of patients who harbor renal diseases. Clin J Am Soc Nephrol. 2010;5:1079–90.

44. Logan CV, Abdel-Hamed Z, Johnson CA. Molecular genetics and pathogenic mechanisms for the severe ciliopathies: insights into neurodevelopment and pathogenesis of neural tube defects. Mol Neurobiol. 2011;43:12–26.

45. Jones KL. Smith's recognizable patterns of human malformation. 5th ed. Philadelphia: WB Saunders; 1997.

46. Cassart M, Eurin D, Didier F, Guibaud L, Avni EF. Antenatal renal sonographic anomalies and postnatal follow-up of renal involvement in Bardet-Biedl syndrome. Ultrasound Obstet Gynecol. 2004;24:51–4.

47. Waterham HR, Ebberink MS. Genetics and molecular basis of human peroxisome biogenesis disorders. Biochim Biophys Acta. 2012;1822:1430–41.

48. Larson RS, Rudolff MA, Liapis H, Manes JL, Davila R, Kissane J. The Ivemark syndrome: prenatal diagnosis of an uncommon cystic renal lesion with heterogeneous associations. Pediatr Nephrol. 1995;9:594–8.

49. Soejima H, Higashimoto K. Epigenetic and genetic alterations of the imprinting disorder Beckwith-Wiedemann syndrome and related disorders. J Hum Genet. 2013;58:402–9.

50. Baujat G, Huber C, El Hokayem J, Caumes R, Do Ngoc Thanh C, David A, Delezoide AL, Dieux-Coeslier A, Estournet B, Francannet C, Kayirangwa H, Lacaille F, Le Bourgeois M, Martinovic J, Salomon R, Sigaudy S, Malan V, Munnich A, Le Merrer M, Le Quan Sang KH, Cormier-Daire V. Asphyxiating thoracic dysplasia: clinical and molecular review of 39 families. J Med Genet. 2013;50:91–8.

51. Dabora SL, Jozwiak S, Franz DN, Roberts PS, Nieto A, Chung J, Choy YS, Reeve MP, Thiele E, Egelhoff JC, Kasprzyk-Obara J, Domanska-Pakiela D, Kwiatkowski DJ. Mutational analysis in a cohort of 224 tuberous sclerosis patients indicates increased severity of TSC2, compared with TSC1, disease in multiple organs. Am J Hum Genet. 2001;68:64–80.

52. Leclair MD, El-Ghoneimi A, Audry G, Ravasse P, Moscovici J, Heloury Y, French Pediatric Urology Study Group. The outcome of prenatally diagnosed renal tumors. J Urol. 2005;173:186–9.

53. Powis M. Neonatal renal tumours. Early Hum Dev. 2010;86:607–12.

54. Ambrosino MM, Hernanz-Schulman M, Horii SC, Raghavendra BN, Genieser NB. Prenatal diagnosis of nephroblastomatosis in two siblings. J Ultrasound Med. 1990;9:49–51.

55. Daneman A, Baunin C, Lobo E, Pracros JP, Avni F, Toi A, Metreweli C, Ho SS, Moore L. Disappearing suprarenal masses in fetuses and infants. Pediatr Radiol. 1997;27:675–81.

56. Wilcox DT, Chitty LS. Non visualisations of fetal bladder: aetiology and management. Prenat Diagn. 2001;21:977–83.

57. Martin C, Darnell A, Duran C, Bermudez P, Mellado F, Rigol S. Magnetic resonance imaging of the intra uterine fetal genito-urinary tract. Abdominal imaging. New York: Springer; 2004.

58. Pinette M, Blackstone J, Wax J, Cartin A. Enlarged fetal bladder: differential diagnosis and outcomes. J Clin Ultrasound. 2003;31:328–34.

59. Muller F, Dreux S, Vaast P, Dumez Y, Nisand I, Ville Y, Boulot P, Guibourdenche J, the Study Group of the French Fetal Medicine Society. Prenatal diagnosis of Megacystis-Microcolon-Intestinal hypoperistalsis syndrome: contribution of amniotic fluid digestive enzyme essay and fetal urinalysis. Prenat Diagn. 2005;25:203–9.

60. Vanderheyden T, Kumar S, Fisk NM. Fetal renal impairment. Semin Neonatol. 2003;8:279–89.

61. Spitzer A. The current approach to the assessment of fetal renal function: fact or fiction? Pediatr Nephrol. 1996;10:230–5.

62. Hobbins JC, Romero R, Grannum P, Berkovitz RL, Cullen M, Mahony M. Antenatal diagnosis of renal anomalies with ultrasound. I. Obstructive uropathy. Am J Obstet Gynecol. 1984;148:868–77.

63. Moore TR, Cayle JE. The amniotic fluid index in normal human pregnancy. Am J Obstet Gynecol. 1990;162:1168–73.

64. Phelan JP, Smith CV, Broussard A, Small M. Amniotic fluid volume assessment by four-quadrant technique at 32–42 weeks' gestation. J Reprod Med. 1987;32:540–2.

65. Zaccara A, Giorlandino C, Mobili L, Brizzi C, Bilancioni E, Capolupo I, Capitanucci ML, De Genaro M. Amniotic fluid index and fetal bladder outlet obstruction. Do we really need more? J Urol. 2005;174:1657–60.

66. Peters CA, Reid LM, Docimo S, Luetic T, Carr M, Retik AB, Mandell J. The role of the kidney in lung growth and maturation in the setting of obstructive uropathy and oligohydramnios. J Urol. 1991;146:597–600.

67. Laudy JA, Wladimiroff JW. The fetal lung. 1: developmental aspects. Ultrasound Obstet Gynecol. 2000;16:284–90.

68. Smith NP, Losty PD, Connell MG, Meyer U, Jesudason EC. Abnormal lung development precedes oligohydramnios in transgenic murine model of renal dysgenesis. J Urol. 2006;175:783–6.

69. Brochard K, Boyer O, Blanchard A, Loirat C, Niaudet P, Macher MA, Deschenes G, Bensman A, Decramer S, Cochat P, Morin D, Broux F, Caillez M, Guyot C, Novo R, Jeunemaître X, Vargas-Poussou R. Phenotype-genotype correlation in antenatal and neonatal variants of Bartter syndrome. Nephrol Dial Transplant. 2009;24:1455–64.

70. Männikkö M, Kestilä M, Lenkkeri U, Alakurtti H, Holmberg C, Leisti J, Salonen R, Aula P, Mustonen A, Peltonen L, Tryggvason K. Improved prenatal diagnosis of the congenital nephrotic syndrome of the Finnish type based on DNA analysis. Kidney Int. 1997;51:868–72.

71. Nortier J, Debiec H, Tournay Y, Mougenot B, Noel JC, Deschodt-Lackman MM, Janssen F, Ronco P. Neonatal disease in neutral endopeptidase alloimmunization: lessons for immunological monitoring. Pediatr Nephrol. 2005;21:1399–405.

72. Glick PL, Harrisson MR, Golbus MS, Adzick NS, Filly RA, Callen PW, Mahony PS. Management of the fetus with congenital hydronephrosis. II: prognosis criteria and selection for treatment. J Pediatr Surg. 1985;20:376–87.

73. Burghard R, Pallacks R, Gordjani N, Leititis JU, Hackeloer BJ, Brandis M. Microproteins in amniotic fluid as an index of changes in fetal renal function during development. Pediatr Nephrol. 1997;1:574–80.

74. Nicolini U, Spelzini F. Invasive assessment of fetal renal abnormalities: urinalysis, fetal blood sampling and biopsy. Prenat Diagn. 2001;21:964–9.

75. Coplen DE. Prenatal intervention for hydronephrosis. J Urol. 1997;157:2270–7.

76. Crombleholme TM, Harrisson MR, Golbus MS, Longaker MT, Langer JC, Callen PW, Anderson RL, Goldstein RB, Filly RA. Fetal intervention in obstructive uropathy: prognostic indicators and efficacy of intervention. Am J Obstet Gynecol. 1990;162:1239–44.

77. Muller F, Bernard MA, Benkirane A, Ngo S, Lortat-Jacob S, Oury JF, Dommergues M. Fetal urine Cystatine C as a predictor of postnatal renal function in bilateral uropathies. Clin Chem. 1999;45:2292–3.

78. Muller F, Dommergues M, Mandelbrot L, Aubry MC, Nihoul-Fékété C, Dumez Y. Fetal urinary biochemistry predicts postnatal renal function in children with bilateral obstructive uropathies. Obstet Gynecol. 1993;82:813–20.

79. Klein J, Lacroix C, Caubet C, Siwy J, Zürbig P, Dakna M, Muller F, Breuil B, Stalmach A, Mullen W, Mischak H, Bandin F, Monsarrat B, Bascands JL, Decramer S, Schanstra JP. Fetal urinary peptides to predict postnatal outcome of renal disease in fetuses with posterior urethral valves (PUV). Sci Transl Med. 2013;5:198ra106.

80. Bökenkamp A, Dieterich C, Dressler F, Mühlhaus K, Gembruch U, Bald R, Kirschstein M. Fetal serum concentrations of cystatin C and β2-microglobulin as predictors of postnatal kidney function. Am J Obstet Gynecol. 2001;185:468–75.

81. Muller F, Dreux S, Audibert F, Chabaud JJ, Rousseau T, D'Hervé D, Dumez Y, Ngo S, Gubler MC, Dommergues M. Fetal serum β2-microglobulin and cystatin C in the prediction of post-natal renal function in bilateral hypoplasia and hyperechogenic enlarged kidneys. Prenat Diagn. 2004;24:327–32.

82. Nguyen C, Dreux S, Heidet L, Czerkiewicz I, Salomon LJ, Guimiot F, Schmitz T, Tsatsaris V, Boulot P, Rousseau T, Muller F. Fetal serum α-1 microglobulin for renal function assessment: comparison with β2-microglobulin and cystatin C. Prenat Diagn. 2013;33:775–81.

83. Bunduki V, Saldanha LB, Sadek L, Miguelez J, Myiyadahira S, Zugaib M. Fetal renal biopsies in obstructive uropathy: feasibility and clinical correlations – preliminary results. Prenat Diagn. 1998;18:101–9.

84. Suranyi A, Retz C, Rigo J, Schaaps JP, Foidart JM. Fetal renal hyperechogenicity in intrauterine growth retardation: importance and outcome. Pediatr Nephrol. 2001;16:575–80.

85. Schreuder MF, Nauta J. Prenatal programming of nephron number and blood pressure. Kidney Int. 2007;72:265–8.

86. Schmidt B, Andrew M. Neonatal thrombosis: report of a prospective canadian and international registry. Pediatrics. 1995;96:939–43.

87. Marks SD, Massicotte P, Steele BT, Matsell DG, Filler G, Shah PS, Perlman M, Rosenblum ND, Shah VS. Neonatal renal venous thrombosis: clinical outcomes and prevalence of prothrombotic disorders. J Pediatr. 2005;146:811–6.

88. Lalmand B, Avni EF, Nasr A, Katelbant P, Struyven J. Perinatal renal vein thrombosis: US demonstration. J Ultrasound Med. 1990;9:437–42.

89. Wee LY, Fisk NM. The twin-twin transfusion syndrome. Semin Neonatol. 2002;7:187–202.

90. Talbert DG, Bajoria R, Sepulveda W, Bower S, Fisk NM. Hydrostatic and osmotic pressure gradients produce manifestations of fetofetal transfusion syndrome in a computerized model of monochorial twin pregnancy. Am J Obstet Gynecol. 1996;174:598–608.

91. Chiang MC, Lien R, Chao AS, Chou YH, Chen YJ. Clinical consequences of twin-to-twin transfusion. Eur J Pediatr. 2003;162:68–71.

92. Sedman AB, Kershaw DB, Bunchman TE. Recognition and management of angiotensin converting enzyme inhibitor fetopathy. Pediatr Nephrol. 1995;9:382–5.

93. Cooper WO, Hernandez-Diaz S, Arbogast PG, Dudley JA, Dyer S, Gideon PS, Hall K, Ray WA. Major congenital malformations after first-trimester exposure to ACE Inhibitors. N Engl J Med. 2006;354:2443–51.

94. Lambot MA, Vermeylen D, Noel JC. Angiotensin-II-receptor inhibition in pregnancy. Lancet. 2001;357:1619–20.

95. Alwan S, Polifka JE, Friedman JM. Angiotensin II receptor antagonist treatment during pregnancy. Birth Defects Res. 2005;73:123–30.

96. Spaggiari E, Heidet L, Grange G, Guimiot F, Dreux S, Delezoide AL, Renin-Angiotensin System Blockers Study Group, Muller F. Prognosis and outcome of pregnancies exposed to renin-angiotensin system blockers. Prenat Diagn. 2012;32:1071–6.

97. Loudon JA, Groom KM, Bennett PR. Prostaglandin inhibitors in preterm labour. Best Pract Clin Obstet Gynecol. 2003;17:731–44.

98. Mitra SC, Ganesh V, Apuzzio JJ. Effect of maternal cocaine abuse on renal arterial flow and urine output in the fetus. Am J Obstet Gynecol. 1994;171:1556–9.

99. Greenfield SP, Rutigliano E, Steinhardt G, Elder JS. Genitourinary tract malformations and maternal cocaine abuse. Urology. 1991;37:455–9.

100. Behnke M, Eyler FD, Garvan CW, Wobie K. The search for congenital malformations in newborns with fetal cocaine exposure. Pediatrics. 2001;107:E174.

101. No authors listed. Pregnancy and renal disease. Lancet. 1975;2:801–2.

102. McKay DB, Josephson MA. Pregnancy in recipients of solid organs – effects on mother and child. N Engl J Med. 2006;354:1281–93.

103. Ross LF. Ethical considerations related to pregnancy in transplant recipients. N Engl J Med. 2006;354:1313–6.

104. Anderka MT, Lin AE, Abuelo DN, Mitchell AA, Rasmussen SA. Reviewing the evidence for mycophenolate mofetil as a new teratogen: case report and review of the literature. Am J Med Genet A. 2009;149A:1241–8.

105. EBPG Expert Group in Renal Transplantation. European best practice guidelines for renal transplantation. Section IV.10. Long-term management of the transplant recipient – pregnancy in renal transplant recipients. Nephrol Dial Transplant. 2002;17 Suppl 4:50–5.

106. Weber S, Morinière V, Knüppel T, Charbit M, Dusek J, Ghiggeri GM, Jankauskiené A, Mir S, Montini G, Peco-Antic A, Wühl E, Zurowska AM, Mehls O, Antignac C, Schaefer F, Salomon R. Prevalence of mutations in renal developmental genes in children with renal hypodysplasia : results of the ESCAPE study. J Am Soc Nephrol. 2006;17:2864–70.

107. Sanna-Cherchi S, Sampogna RV, Papeta N, Burgess KE, Nees SN, Perry BJ, Choi M, Bodria M, Liu Y, Weng PL, Lozanovski VJ, Verbitsky M, Lugani F, Sterken R, Paragas N, Caridi G, Carrea A, Dagnino M, Materna-Kiryluk A, Santamaria G, Murtas C, Ristoska-Bojkovska N, Izzi C, Kacak N, Bianco B, Giberti S, Gigante M, Piaggio G, Gesualdo L, Kosuljandic Vukic D, Vukojevic K, Saraga-Babic M, Saraga M, Gucev Z, Allegri L, Latos-Bielenska A, Casu D, State M, Scolari F, Ravazzolo R, Kiryluk K, Al-Awqati Q, D'Agati VD, Drummond IA, Tasic V, Lifton RP, Ghiggeri GM, Gharavi AG. Mutations in DSTYK and dominant urinary tract malformations. N Engl J Med. 2013;369:621–9.

108. Weber S, Thiele H, Mir S, Toliat MR, Sozeri B, Reutter H, Draaken M, Ludwig M, Altmüller J, Frommolt P, Stuart HM, Ranjzad P, Hanley NA, Jennings R, Newman WG, Wilcox DT, Thiel U, Schlingmann KP, Beetz R, Hoyer PF, Konrad M, Schaefer F, Nürnberg P, Woolf AS. Muscarinic acetylcholine receptor M3 mutation causes urinary bladder disease and a Prune-Belly-like syndrome. Am J Hum Genet. 2011;89:668–74.

109. Daly SB, Urquhart JE, Hilton E, McKenzie EA, Kammerer RA, Lewis M, Kerr B, Stuart H, Donnai D, Long DA, Burgu B, Aydogdu O, Derbent M, Garcia-Minaur S, Reardon W, Gener B, Shalev S, Smith R, Woolf AS, Black GC, Newman WG. Mutations in HPSE2 cause urofacial syndrome. Am J Hum Genet. 2010;86:963–9.

110. Stuart HM, Roberts NA, Burgu B, Daly SB, Urquhart JE, Bhaskar S, Dickerson JE, Mermerkaya M, Silay MS, Lewis MA, Olondriz MB, Gener B, Beetz C, Varga RE, Gülpınar O, Süer E, Soygür T, Ozçakar ZB, Yalçınkaya F, Kavaz A, Bulum B, Gücük A, Yue WW, Erdogan F, Berry A, Hanley NA, McKenzie EA, Hilton EN, Woolf AS, Newman WG. LRIG2 mutations cause urofacial syndrome. Am J Hum Genet. 2013;92:259–64.

111. Liebeschuetz S, Thomas R. Unilateral multicystic dysplastic kidney (letter). Arch Dis Child. 1997;77:369.

112. James CA, Watson AR, Twining P, Rance CH. Antenatally detected urinary tract abnormalities: changing incidence and management. Eur J Pediatr. 1998;157:508–11.

113. Stuck KJ, Koff SA, Silver TM. Ultrasonic features of multicystic dysplastic kidney: expanded diagnostic criteria. Radiology. 1982;143:217–21.

114. Ismaili K, Avni FE, Alexander M, Schulman C, Collier F, Hall M. Routine voiding cystourethrography is of no value in neonates with unilateral multicystic dysplastic kidney. J Pediatr. 2005;146:759–63.

115. Ward CJ, Hogan MC, Rossetti S, Walker D, Sneddon T, Wang X, Kubly V, Cunningham JM, Bacallao R, Ishibashi M, Milliner DS, Torres VE, Harris PC. The gene mutated in Autosomal recessive polycystic kidney disease encodes a large, receptor-like protein. Nat Genet. 2002;30:259–69.

116. Büscher R, Büscher AK, Weber S, Mohr J, Hegen B, Vester U, Hoyer PF. Clinical manifestations of autosomal recessive polycystic kidney disease (ARPKD): kidney-related and non-kidney-related phenotypes. Pediatr Nephrol. 2014;29(10):1915–25.

117. Wilson PD. Polycystic kidney disease. N Engl J Med. 2004;350:151–64.

118. Mochizuki T, Wu G, Hayashi T, Xenophontos SL, Veldhuisen B, Saris JJ, Reynolds DM, Cai Y, Gabow PA, Pierides A, Kimberling WJ, Breuning MH, Deltas CC, Peters DJ, Somlo S. PKD2, a gene for polycystic kidney disease that encodes an integral membrane protein. Science. 1996;272:1339–42.

119. Brun M, Maugey-Laulom B, Eurin D, Didier F, Avni EF. Prenatal sonographic patterns in autosomal dominant polycystic kidney disease: a multicenter study. Ultrasound Obstet Gynecol. 2004;24:55–61.

120. McDermot KD, Saggar-Malik AK, Economides DL, Jeffrey S. Prenatal diagnosis of autosomal dominant

polycystic kidney disease (PKD1) presenting in utero and prognosis for very early onset disease. J Med Genet. 1998;35:13–6.

121. Avni EF, Thoua Y, Van Gansbeke D, Matos C, Didier F, Droulez P, Schulman CC. The development of hypodysplastic kidney. Radiology. 1985;164:123–5.

122. Ruf RG, Xu PX, Silvius D, Otto EA, Beekmann F, Muerb UT, Kumar S, Neuhaus TJ, Kemper MJ, Raymond Jr RM, Brophy PD, Berkman J, Gattas M, Hyland V, Ruf EM, Schwartz C, Chang EH, Smith RJ, Stratakis CA, Weil D, Petit C, Hildebrandt F. SIX1 mutations cause branchio-oto-renal syndrome by disruption of EYA1-SIX1-DNA complexes. Proc Natl Acad Sci U S A. 2004;101:8090–5.

123. Bingham C, Bulman MP, Ellard S, Allen LI, Lipkin GW, Hoff WG, Woolf AS, Rizzoni G, Novelli G, Nicholls AJ, Hattersley AT. Mutations in the hepatocyte nuclear factor-1beta gene are associated with familial hypoplastic glomerulocystic kidney disease. Am J Hum Genet. 2001;68:219–24.

124. Sanyanusin P, Schimmenti LA, McNoe LA, Ward TA, Pierpont ME, Sullivan MJ, Dobyns WB, Eccles MR. Mutation of the PAX2 gene in a family with optic nerve colobomas, renal anomalies and vesicoureteral reflux. Nat Genet. 1995;9:358–64.

125. Ismaili K, Pawtowski A, Boyer O, Wissing KM, Janssen F, Hall M. Genetic forms of nephrotic syndrome: a single-center experience in Brussels. Pediatr Nephrol. 2009;24:287–94.

126. Kestilä M, Lenkkeri U, Lamerdin J, McCready P, Putaala H, Ruotsalainen V, Morita T, Nissinen M, Herva R, Kashtan CE, Peltonen L, Holmberg C, Olsen A, Tryggvason K. Positionally cloned gene for a novel glomerular protein – nephrin – is mutated in congenital nephrotic syndrome. Mol Cell. 1998;1:575–82.

127. Huttunen NP. Congenital nephrotic syndrome of Finnish type. Study of 75 cases. Arch Dis Child. 1976;51:344–8.

128. Souka AP, Skentou H, Geerts L, Bower S, Nicolaides KH. Congenital nephrotic syndrome presenting with increase nuchal translucency in the first trimester. Prenat Diagn. 2002;22:93–5.

129. Rapola J. Why is congenital nephrotic syndrome associated with a rise in the concentration of alpha-fetoprotein in the amniotic fluid? Pediatr Nephrol. 1990;4:206.

130. Weber S, Gribouval O, Esquivel EL, Morinière V, Tête MJ, Legendre C, Niaudet P, Antignac C. NPHS2 mutation analysis shows genetic heterogeneity of steroid-resistant nephrotic syndrome and low post-transplant recurrence. Kidney Int. 2004;66:571–9.

131. Mark K, Reis A, Zenker M. Prenatal findings in four consecutive pregnancies with fetal pierson syndrome, a newly defined congenital nephrosis syndrome. Prenat Diagn. 2006;26:262–6.

132. Zenker M, Aigner T, Wendler O, Tralau T, Müntefering H, Fenski R, Pitz S, Schumacher V, Royer-Pokora B, Wühl E, Cochat P, Bouvier R, Kraus C, Mark K, Madlon H, Dötch J, Rascher W, Maruniak-Chudek I, Lennert T, Neumann LM, Reis A. Human laminin beta 2 deficiency causes congenital nephrosis with mesangial sclerosis and distinct eye abnormalities. Hum Mol Genet. 2004;13:2625–32.

133. Boyer O, Benoit G, Gribouval O, Nevo F, Pawtowski A, Bilge I, Bircan Z, Deschênes G, Guay-Woodford LM, Hall M, Macher MA, Soulami K, Stefanidis CJ, Weiss R, Loirat C, Gubler MC, Antignac C. Mutational analysis of the PLCE1 gene in steroid resistant nephrotic syndrome. J Med Genet. 2010;47:445–52.

134. Besbas N, Bayrakci US, Kale G, Cengiz AB, Akcoren Z, Akinci D, Kilic I, Bakkaloglu A. Cytomegalovirus-related congenital nephrotic syndrome with diffuse mesangial sclerosis. Pediatr Nephrol. 2006;21:740–2.

135. Ismaili K, Piepsz A. The antenatally detected pelvi-ureteric junction stenosis: advances in renography and stategy of management. Pediatr Radiol. 2013;43:428–35.

136. Ismaili K, Avni FE, Wissing KM, Piepsz A, Aubert D, Cochat P, Hall M. Current management of infants with fetal renal pelvis dilatation: a survey by french-speaking pediatric nephrologists and urologists. Pediatr Nephrol. 2004;19:966–71.

137. Duong HP, Piepsz A, Collier F, Khelif K, Christophe C, Cassart M, Janssen F, Hall M, Ismaili K. Predicting the clinical outcome of antenatally detected unilateral pelviureteric junction stenosis. Urology. 2013;82:691–6.

138. Marra G, Barbieri G, Moioli C, Assael BM, Grumieri G, Caccamo ML. Mild fetal hydronephrosis indicating vesicoureteric reflux. Arch Dis Child. 1994;70:F147–50.

139. Grazioli S, Parvex P, Merlini L, Combescure C, Girardin E. Antenatal and postnatal ultrasound in the evaluation of the risk of vesicoureteral reflux. Pediatr Nephrol. 2010;25:1687–92.

140. Garin EH, Campos A, Homsy Y. Primary vesicoureteral reflux: review of current concepts. Pediatr Nephrol. 1998;12:249–56.

141. McLellan DL, Retik AB, Bauer SB, Diamond DA, Atala A, Mandell J, Lebowitz RL, Borer JG, Peters CA. Rate and predictors of spontaneous resolution of prenatally diagnosed nonrefluxing megaureter. J Urol. 2002;168:2177–80.

142. Whitten SM, Wilcox DT. Duplex systems. Prenat Diagn. 2001;21:952–7.

143. Peppas DS, Skoog SJ, Canning DA, Belman AB. Nonsurgical management of primary vesicoureteric reflux in complete ureteral duplication. Is it justified? J Urol. 1991;146:1594–5.

144. Avni FE, Dacher JN, Stallenberg B, Collier F, Hall M, Schulman CC. Renal duplications: the impact of perinatal US on diagnosis and management. Eur Urol. 1991;20:43–8.

145. Decter RM. Renal duplication and fusion anomalies. Pediatr Clin North Am. 1997;44:1323–41.

146. Jouannic JM, Hyett JA, Pandya PP, Gulbis B, Rodeck CH, Jauniaux E. Perinatal outcome in foetuses with megacystis in the first half of pregnancy. Prenat Diag. 2003;23:340–4.

147. Spaggiari E, Dreux S, Czerkiewicz I, Favre R, Schmitz T, Guimiot F, Laurichesse Delmas H, Verspyck E, Oury JF, Ville Y, Muller F. Fetal obstructive uropathy complicated by urinary ascites: outcome and prognostic value of fetal serum β-2-microglobulin. Ultrasound Obstet Gynecol. 2013;41:185–9.

148. Morris RK, Malin GL, Khan KS, Kilby MD. Antenatal ultrasound to predict postnatal renal function in congenital lower urinary tract obstruction: systematic review of test accuracy. BJOG. 2009;116:1290–9.

149. Housley HT, Harrisson MR. Fetal urinary tract abnormalities. Natural history, pathophysiology, and treatment. Urol Clin North Am. 1998;25:63–73.

150. Dinneen MD, Duffy PG. Posterior urethral valves. Br J Urol. 1996;78:275–81.

151. Holmes N, Harrison MR, Baskin LS. Fetal surgery for posterior urethral valves: long term postnatal outcomes. Pediatrics. 2001;108:36–42.

152. Quintero RA, Hume R, Smith C, Johnson MP, Cotton DB, Romero R, Evans M. Percutaneous fetal cystoscopy and endoscopic fulguration of posterior urethral valves. Am J Obstet Gynecol. 1995;172:206–9.

153. Agarwal SK, Fisk NM. In utero therapy for lower urinary tract obstruction. Prenat Diagn. 2001;21:970–6.

154. Golbus MS, Harrison MR, Filly RA. In utero treatment of urinary tract obstruction. Am J Obstet Gynecol. 1982;142:383–8.

155. Clark TJ, Martin WL, Divakaran TG, Whittle MJ, Kilby MD, Khan KS. Prenatal bladder drainage in the management of fetal lower urinary tract obstruction: a systematic review and metaanalysis. Obstet Gynecol. 2003;102:367–82.

156. Morris RK, Malin GL, Quinlan-Jones E, Middleton LJ, Hemming K, Burke D, Daniels JP, Khan KS, Deeks J, Kilby MD. Percutaneous vesicoamniotic shunting in lower urinary tract obstruction (PLUTO) Collaborative Group. Percutaneous vesicoamniotic shunting versus conservative management for fetal lower urinary tract obstruction (PLUTO): a randomised trial. Lancet. 2013;382:1496–506.

157. Van Mieghem T, Ryan G. The PLUTO trial: a missed opportunity (comment). Lancet. 2013;382:1471–3.

158. Kitagawa H, Pringle KC, Koike J. Vesicoamniotic shunt for complete urinary tract obstruction is partially effective. J Pediatr Surg. 2006;41:394–402.

Damien Noone and Valérie Langlois

Assessment of the Urine

Urine Analysis

The American Academy of Pediatrics does not recommend routine urinalysis as a screening tool for chronic kidney disease in otherwise healthy school aged children [1]. Nonetheless, the value of urine analysis in the evaluation of kidney disease should not be underestimated. Important information can be learned from this simple, quick, and inexpensive test when used in the appropriate setting. Commercially available reagent strips can be used to screen the urine for pH, specific gravity, protein, blood, glucose, ketones, leukocytes, and nitrates. The urine specimen should be fresh and ideally a clean-voided midstream in older children.

Depending on urine concentration, the urine color varies from pale yellow to amber. Red or tea colored urine suggests the presence of blood, hemoglobin, myoglobin, porphyrin, non-pathologic pigments (beets, food color) or medication. Blue to green suggests the presence of biliverdin or pseudomonas infection.

The urine is normally clear but can be cloudy in the presence of leukocytes, epithelial cells, bacteria, or precipitation of amorphous phosphate or amorphous urate. Unusual urine odor can lead to the diagnosis of rare metabolic disorders such as maple syrup urine disease (maple syrup odor), phenylketonuria (musty odor) or hypermethioninemia (fishy odor).

Specific gravity reflects the urinary concentrating and diluting capability of the kidney. In normal conditions, it reflects the hydration status of a person. However, with abnormal kidneys, a very low SG may represent a concentrating defect. It may be useful in distinguishing prerenal states from intrinsic renal disease. Specific gravity usually ranges from 1:001 to 1:035 and can be measured using a urinometer or refractometer, but more commonly using the reagent strips. The reagent strip test is based on pKa change of certain polyelectrolytes in relation to ionic concentration [2].

Urinary pH usually ranges from 5.0 to 8.0 depending on the acid-base balance of the body and can be estimated using the reagent test strip. However, precise measurements need to be obtained using a pH meter with a glass electrode. Urinary pH is important in the diagnosis of renal tubular acidosis and monitoring in the treatment or prevention of urinary stones.

Glucose is not usually present in the urine. Glucose is freely filtered at the level of the glomerulus and reabsorbed in the proximal tubule via a sodium-coupled active transport mechanism.

D. Noone (✉) • V. Langlois
Department of Pediatrics, Division of Nephrology,
The Hospital for Sick Children,
555 University Avenue, Toronto M5G 1X8, Canada
e-mail: damien.noone@sickkids.ca;
valerie.langlois@sickkids.ca

© Springer-Verlag Berlin Heidelberg 2016
D.F. Geary, F. Schaefer (eds.), *Pediatric Kidney Disease*, DOI 10.1007/978-3-662-52972-0_3

Glucosuria can be seen when the serum glucose is above the renal threshold or due to isolated renal glucosuria or proximal tubular disorder such as Fanconi syndrome. Normal values for maximal tubular glucose reabsorption (TmG) in children vary from 254 to 401 mg/min/1.73 m^2 [3]. Reagent test strips are usually impregnated with the enzyme glucose oxidase and only detect glucose. Other sugars can be detected by the copper reduction test such as Clinitest® Tablet (Bayer, Whippany, NJ, USA).

Ketone bodies are formed during the catabolism of fatty acids and include acetoacetic acid, beta hydroxybutyric acid, and acetone. Most reagent strips for ketones are based on a color reaction with sodium nitroprusside and are sensitive for acetoacetic acid but will not detect beta-hydroxybutyric acid and acetone.

Strip tests detect leukocyte esterase, an enzyme found in neutrophils. Nitrites indicate the presence of bacteria capable of reducing dietary nitrate such as *Escherichia coli*, *Enterobacter*, *Citrobacter*, *Klebsiella*, and *Proteus* species. A positive urinalysis for both leucocytes and nitrites is suggestive of bacteriuria or urinary tract infection (UTI), and if both are negative then a UTI is unlikely. If either/or are positive then a further confirmatory urine culture is required [4, 5]. Samples should be processed rapidly to avoid degradation of esterases and false negative results [6]. For children under the age of 2 urinalysis is less reliable for the diagnosis of UTI [5]. For infants less than 1 year of age, microscopic presence of moderate bacteria and >10 white cells/high powered field is more accurate in diagnosing a UTI [5].

Hematuria is defined as the presence of >5 red blood cells (RBC) per high power field in centrifuged urine. Presence of RBCs can only be confirmed by microscopic evaluation of fresh urine. Reagent strips detect RBC, myoglobin, and hemoglobin. The supernatant of a centrifuged urine containing red blood cells will be clear yellow as opposed to being pink if the urine contains hemoglobin or myoglobin. The morphology of the cells can help determine their origin. Presence of dysmorphic red blood cells suggests glomerular hematuria.

Urine Microscopy

> ...the ghosts of dead patients that haunt us do not ask why we did not employ the latest fad of clinical investigation. They ask us, why did you not test my urine?—Sir Robert Grieve Hutchison (1871–1960) [7]

Microscopic evaluation of fresh urine is extremely valuable in the evaluation of renal disease. The presence of casts, cells, and crystals should be sought. Although hyaline and granular casts can be seen in normal states, cellular casts are pathologic. Red blood cell casts are pathognomonic of glomerular disease and white blood cell casts can be seen with pyelonephritis or post-infectious glomerulonephritis.

Crystals are rarely seen in fresh urine but appear after the urine stands for a period of time. Uric acid, calcium oxalate, amorphous urate, cystine, tyrosine, leucine, and cholesterol are usually found in acid urine. Uric acid and calcium oxalate can be seen in normal and pathological conditions. Amorphous urates are of no clinical significance. Cystine, tyrosine, leucine, and cholesterol crystals are always relevant. Cystine crystals are related to cystinuria, leucine crystals can be associated with maple syrup urine disease, methionine malabsorption syndrome and serious liver disease. Tyrosine crystals also occur in serious liver disease, tyrosinosis, and methionine malabsorption syndrome. The presence of cholesterol crystals can indicate excessive tissue breakdown, nephritic or nephrotic conditions [2]. Triple phosphate, calcium carbonate, ammonium biurate, amorphous phosphates and calcium phosphate crystals are usually found in alkaline urine. Calcium carbonate and amorphous phosphate are of no clinical significance.

Detection of urinary eosinophils and its association with acute interstitial nephritis (AIN) was first reported by Galpin et al. [8] and became widely accepted as supportive of a diagnosis of AIN [9]. Hansel's stain replaced Wright's stain, the latter being ineffective when urine pH was <7 and the former revealing the bright red granules of eosinophils. However, eosinophiluria may be seen in prostatitis, cystitis, and glomerulonephritis also, limiting the sensitivity and positive predictive value (PPV) of the test [10]. Compared to kidney biopsy, the gold standard of AIN diagnosis, eosinophiluria lacks sensitivity and specificity and cannot distinguish AIN from acute tubular necrosis [11].

Urinary Protein Excretion

In the normal state, most of the filtered low molecular weight proteins (MW <40,000 Da) are reabsorbed in the proximal tubules. Protein of higher molecular weight such as albumin (MW = 60,000 Da) are not usually filtered. Tamm Horsfall proteins are secreted by the tubular cells in the ascending thick limb of the loop of Henle and are the main protein found in normal urine.

In disease states, increased amount of protein can be found in the urine and may reflect damage in the glomerular barrier (glomerular proteinuria) or impaired tubular reabsorption (tubular proteinuria). In glomerular proteinuria, albumin which is not usually present will be found predominantly. Beta 2 microglobulin, alpha 1 microglobulin, and retinol-binding protein are used as markers of tubular proteinuria.

Proteinuria can vary by age, sex, ethnicity and BMI [12, 13]. In the first month of life proteinuria is four to five times higher than older infants, perhaps reflecting the evolving maturity of the tubules, and the 90th percentile for urinary albumin/creatinine ratio in the neonatal period was reported as 17.5 (90 % Confidence Interval 7.1–79.7) mg/mmol in one study [14]. Normative ranges for urinary albumin/creatinine ratios at different ages are presented in Table 3.1 [15].

The Clinical Practice Guidelines for Chronic Kidney Disease in Children and Adolescents published by the National Kidney Foundation's Kidney Disease Outcomes Quality initiative (KDOQI) [16] recommends that untimed "spot" urine samples should be used to detect and monitor proteinuria in children and adolescents. It is not usually necessary to obtain a timed urine collection. Standard urine dipstick can be used to detect increased total urine proteins and albumin-specific dipsticks are acceptable to detect microalbuminuria. "Microalbuminuria" refers to

Table 3.1 Mean urinary albumin excretion, expressed as an albumin/creatinine ratio

Age	Spot urine mg/mmol
Neonates	5.24
1–3 months	5.01
4–6 months	4.06
7–23 months	1.76
2–4 years old	1.34
3–19 years old	3

Data from Davies et al. [15]

albumin excretion above the normal range but below the level of detection of the standard urine dipstick. Urine protein-to-creatinine or urine albumin-to-creatinine ratio should be done within 3 months of a positive dipstick to confirm proteinuria or albuminuria. Postpubertal children with diabetes of 5 or more year's duration should have urine albumin measured by albumin-specific dipstick or albumin-to-creatinine ratio and this should be performed annually [16, 17].

False positive dipstick can be the result of prolonged immersion of the reagent strip, alkaline urine, presence of pyuria, bacteriuria or mucoprotein [18].

Twenty four hour urine collections have long been the gold standard for quantification of urine protein excretion. However, collection in young children often requires catheterization and is not practical. First morning urine for spot protein-to-creatinine is generally accepted as being valid in the assessment of proteinuria in children [19–21].

Twenty-four hour urine protein excretion of 4 mg/m^2/h and 40 mg/m^2/h is considered in the normal and nephrotic range respectively. Normal urinary albumin excretion is between 30 and 300 mg/day on a 24 h collection, 20–200 µg/min in an overnight collection and 3–30 mg/mmol as measured on a first morning urine sample (Table 3.2) [22]. There can be significant diurnal variation in proteinuria in children and adolescents that is generally not considered pathological and resolves by adulthood. Orthostatic proteinuria is defined as having an elevated protein excretion observed in the upright position but normal excretion in the recumbent position

Table 3.2 Reference values for urinary protein excretion

	24 h collection (mg/m²/h)	24 h collection (mg/m²/day)	Spot urine prot/creat (mg/mg)	Spot urine prot/creat (mg/mmol)
Normal range				
6–24 months		<150	<0.5	<50
>24 months	<4	<150	<0.2	<20
Nephrotic	>40	>3 g/1.73 m²/day		>200

Data from Hogg et al. [16]

and can be assessed on a split 24 h urinary protein assessment [23]. Previous studies reported an incidence of 2–5 % [23]; however, a recent study using 24 h total urinary protein excretion found a much higher incidence of 19.8 % in a cohort of 91 children [20]. Previous studies had used dipstick analysis [23], spot urinary protein to creatinine ratios [24] or timed collections of less than 24 h [20, 25].

In 2006, Mori et al. [26] measured the urine protein-to-creatinine ratio in a cohort of Japanese children with urinary tract abnormalities or glomerular disorders and found that it varies according to body size and composition, reflecting muscle mass. They suggested that evaluation of urine protein-to-creatinine ratio should also consider body height, because, as height and therefore muscle mass (denominator) increases, the ratio will actually decrease. A normative range for urinary protein excretion for the different sexes and as height and body surface area increases remains to be defined [26]. Kim et al. [27] proposed urine protein-to-osmolality ratio as an alternative test to 24 h urinary protein excretion. Urinary protein-to-osmolality corrects for hydration status, can be used in children with decreased muscle mass, and has now been validated in two further pediatric populations against both spot urinary protein-to-creatinine ratio and 24 h urinary protein excretion [28, 29]. A spot urinary protein-to-osmolality above 0.33 mg/L/mosm/kg and 1.75 mg/L/mosm/kg represents abnormal proteinuria in children and nephrotic range proteinuria respectively [29].

Standard urine dipstick test are primarily sensitive to detect albumin. Screening for low molecular weight protein can be done by the sulfosalicylic acid test. The addition of acid to the supernatant of centrifuged urine will cause cloudiness in the presence of any protein in the urine. A negative reagent strip test with a positive sulfosalicylic test is suggestive of low molecular weight proteinuria. Urine protein electrophoresis can confirm the diagnosis. False positive sulfosalicylic test can be produced by large dose of contrast material, penicillin, cephalosporin, sulfonamides metabolites and high uric acid concentration [18].

Assessment of Renal Function

Glomerular Filtration

Glomerular filtration rate (GFR) is the most commonly used measure of kidney function and is used to classify children into the various stages of chronic kidney disease (CKD) as can be seen in Table 3.3 [16]. It can be quantified by measuring the clearance rate of a substance from the plasma. The substance can be endogenous or exogenous. It is often referred to as the "marker". Different markers such as inulin, creatinine, iothalamate, iohexol, EDTA and DTPA are available. The ideal marker must have a stable plasma concentration, should be filtered, not reabsorbed, secreted, synthesized or metabolized by the kidney so that the filtered substance x = the excreted substance x.

The renal clearance of the substance x (Cx) can be obtained by multiplying the urinary concentration of substance x (Ux) times the urinary flow rate in ml/min (V) divided by the plasma concentration of substance x (Px):

$$Cx = Ux * V / Px$$

Table 3.3 NKF-K/DOQI classification of the stages of chronic kidney disease

Stage	Description	GFR (ml/min/1.73 m²)
1	Kidney damage with normal or increased GFR	>90
2	Kidney damage with mild reduction of GFR	60–89
3	Moderate reduction of GFR	30–59
4	Severe reduction of GFR	15–29
5	Kidney failure	<15

Data from Hogg et al. [16]

Inulin

Determination of urinary inulin clearance during a continuous intravenous infusion is considered the "gold standard" method for measurement of GFR. Inulin has all the properties of an ideal marker. Inulin is inert and not synthesized or metabolized by the kidney. It is freely filtered by the glomerulus, and not secreted or reabsorbed in the tubules [30].

The measurement of urinary inulin clearance requires a constant intravenous infusion to maintain a constant level of inulin over a period of 3–4 h. After an equilibration period, timed urinary specimens and plasma are collected every 30 min and urinary and plasma inulin is measured to calculate urinary inulin clearance. The mean clearance of the four to five measurements determines the individual's GFR [31]. Urinary catheterization in young children is often required. To avoid this cumbersome procedure, two methods of plasma inulin clearance have been developed: the continuous infusion method and the single bolus method [32, 33]. The continuous infusion method is based on the concept that once a marker has reached steady state in the plasma and the volume of distribution is saturated, the rate of elimination of the marker will equal the rate of infusion (RI). The clearance of the marker can then be measured [32]:

$$Cx = RI \ x \ / \ Px$$

The equilibration period can take more than 12 h in certain situations. To avoid this long period, a bolus can be given prior to the infusion to reach steady state more rapidly. After a single bolus injection, 10–12 blood samples are collected up to 240 min after injection and the inulin concentration measurements are used to construct a plasma concentration versus time curve (plasma disappearance curve). Plasma clearance of inulin can be calculated by dividing the dose by the area under the plasma concentration-time curve. This method has been shown to give accurate results in adult [34]. van Rossum et al. developed and validated sampling strategies to minimize the number of blood samples making it more acceptable for children [35]. He concluded that two (at 90 and 240 min) to four samples (at 10, 30, 90, 240 min), allow accurate prediction of inulin clearance in pediatric patients with a non significant bias and good imprecision (<15 %) [35]. The single bolus injection method tends to overestimate GFR (average 9.7 ml/min 1.73 m²), but the difference between the two methods becomes smaller at lower GFR (less than 50 ml/min/1.73 m²) [35].

Although measurement of inulin clearance remains the gold standard for assessment of GFR, most laboratories cannot routinely measure inulin which makes this test unpractical. Furthermore, simple and rapid determination of GFR is often needed in clinical practice.

The KDIGO 2012 Clinical Practice Guideline for the Evaluation and Management of Chronic Kidney Disease recommends the use of serum creatinine and a recently derived pediatric specific GFR estimating equation which incorporates a height term, in the initial assessment of pediatric renal function [21].

Serum Creatinine

Creatinine is an amino acid derivative produced in muscle cells. Its production increases in proportion to muscle mass, it is freely filtered, and about 10 % of the creatinine found in urine is secreted by the proximal tubules. Tubular secretion varies among and within individual persons

[36]. Creatinine is used as a measure of renal function. In the past laboratories were using different measurement methods and the lack of standardization was clinically significant. In 2006, the National Kidney Disease Education Program (NKDEP) published recommendations to improve creatinine measurement [37]. KDIGO recommends now that creatinine measurements in all infants and children be derived from methods that minimize confounders and that are calibrated against an international standard [21].

Creatinine Clearance (Ccr)

Creatinine clearance measurement has been widely used and correlates well with inulin clearance within the normal range of GFR [38]. Creatinine has the advantage of being an endogenous marker which precludes the need to use injection. However, as GFR declines the percentage of secreted creatinine in the tubules increases, therefore, Ccr at low GFR will significantly overestimate true GFR [39]. In order to decrease tubular secretion of creatinine and obtain a creatinine clearance more reflective of the true GFR, cimetidine can be given in patients with renal disease [40, 41]. The cimetidine protocol involves the administration of cimetidine (20 mg/kg to a maximum of 1600 mg divided twice daily for a total of five doses) prior to assessment of urinary creatinine clearance. For 24 h prior to the test, a meat-free diet was instigated. Note dose adjustments in cimetidine according to renal function are advised and the complete protocol is reported [42].

Equations to Predict GFR

Schwartz [43] and Counahan [44] first developed equations to predict GFR. In the clearance formula, the numerator $Ucr \times V$ is the excretion rate of creatinine; in steady state this must equal the rate of production. Since the rate of production is a function of muscle mass, Schwartz tested different variables of body size to provide the best correlation with GFR measured by creatinine clearance. The body length appeared to have the best correlation. The GFR can be estimated using the equation known as the Schwartz formula:

$$GFR \left(ml/min/1.73 m^2 \right) = K * Ht/Pcr$$

where K is a constant determined by regression analysis for different ages, Ht = height in cm and Pcr = plasma creatinine.

Kidney disease in children showed that the Schwartz formula overestimates GFR when compared to measured iohexol [45]. This was attributed to the fact that creatinine values determined by enzymatic creatinine assays tend to be lower than those determined by Jaffe method [46].

Subsequently, a number of new equations have been developed and validated. Many of these new equations were developed using a "gold standard" other than inulin and may overestimate GFR. Furthermore, the precision and accuracy of each equation may not be the same at all GFR levels, depending on which populations they were validated against. As per KDIGO, currently the most robust pediatric eGFR formula derived using iohexol disappearance and creatinine measurements which were measured centrally and calibrated and traceable to international standards comes from the CKiD study [21, 47, 48].

The two most common creatinine-based formulas recommended for use in clinical practice (KDIGO) include:

The updated Bedside Schwartz formula [47]

$$eGFR \left(ml/min/1.73 m^2 \right) = 41.3 \times \left(height/Scr \right)$$

where height is in meters and Scr is in mg/dl Schwartz equation that includes BUN [21, 47]:

$$eGFR \left(ml/min/1.73 m^2 \right) = 40.7 \times \left(height/SCr \right)^{0.64} \times \left(30/BUN \right)^{0.202},$$

where height is in meters, Scr and BUN are in mg/dl.

Cystatin C

In order to improve the accuracy of creatinine-based equations, a number of investigators have looked at the use of cystatin C to predict GFR. Cystatin C is a low molecular weight protein (13.36 KD) member of the cystatin superfamily of cysteine protease inhibitors. It is produced by all nucleated cells and exhibits a stable production rate. Cystatin C is freely filtered by the glomerulus and metabolized after tubular reabsorption [49]. Since it is not excreted in urine, its clearance cannot be calculated.

Cystatin C is less influenced by age, gender and muscle mass than creatinine [50]. Levels decline from birth to 1 year of age then remain stable until about 50 years of age. However, Cystatin C levels may be influenced by cigarette smoking, high C reactive protein, steroid use and thyroid disorders [51–53]. One pediatric study showed that for children with CKD stage 3–5 the intrapatient coefficient of variation of cystatin C was significantly lower than that of serum creatinine and proposed that cystatin C is a better tool for longitudinally monitoring patients with advanced CKD [54].

Equations based on cystatin C and/or creatinine using different variables can be found in Table 3.4 [47, 48, 55–59].

Some of the equations were developed using height as one of the variables whereas some are height independent to allow quick estimation of GFR when patient height is not available [56, 57]. These equations were externally validated against the gold standard single injection inulin clearance. The eGFR Pottell was superior to the eGFR-BCCH and comparable to the eGFR Schwartz [60]. Pottel recently developed a new equation to be used in children, adolescents and young adults since none of the previous equations were validated for adolescent and young adults [59]. KDIGO suggest that measuring cystatin C based eGFR (not serum cystatin C) could be undertaken in adults with a creatinine-based eGFR of 45–59 mL/min/1.73 m^2 who do not have markers of kidney damage, such as proteinuria, in an attempt to confirm CKD. No specific recommendation for paediatrics or equation was made [21].

Equations based on multivariates appear to be superior to those using univariate. However, in some situations, a univariate equation might be preferred. For example, since creatinine is highly dependent on muscle mass, a cystatin C based equation may be preferable in patients with reduced muscle mass.

Other Methods

KDIGO suggests measuring GFR using an exogenous filtration marker when more accurate GFR will impact the treatment decision. Since inulin is not widely available, other markers can be used.

Iohexol and Iothalamate
Iohexol is a safe non ionic low osmolar contrast agent (molecular weight MW 821 Da). It is eliminated exclusively by the kidneys, where it is filtered but not secreted, metabolized or reabsorbed. It has less than 2 % binding to protein. Therefore, it makes it an ideal marker of GFR and a good alternative to the use of radiotracers that are not suitable for some patients and require special handling, storage and disposal. Iohexol and Iothalamate have similar kinetic profile but Iohexol has a lower allergic potential [61].

Clearance of iohexol correlates well with measured inulin clearance [45, 61–63]. Gaspari et al. [64] showed a highly significant correlation between GFR measured by the plasma clearance of iohexol (using a two-compartment open–model) and the GFR measured by urinary inulin clearance.

EDTA, DTPA Nuclear GFR
GFR can be accurately measured using a radioactive tracer such as Chromium 51 (51Cr) EDTA or technetium 99m (^{99m}Tc) Diethylenetriaminepentaacetate (DTPA) in children. The most accurate method is based on the plasma disappearance curve after a single bolus injection, fitted by a double exponential curve. The clearance of the radiotracer is calculated as the injected dose divided by the area under the curve [65]. The initial "fast curve" represents the diffusion of the radiotracer in its distribution volume whereas the late slow exponential curve represents its renal clearance. The two-compartment model requires serial blood sampling to obtain an accurate

Table 3.4 Equations to estimate GFR

Name	Equation to estimate GFR	Reference method used to devise
Height dependent		
Updated bedside Schwartz [47]	$eGFR\left(ml/min per 1.73m^2\right) = 41.3\left[Height(m)/Scr mg/dl\right]$	Iohexol
Updated Schwartz '1B' equation [47]	$eGFR\left(ml/min per 1.73m^2\right) = \left[40.7\times Height(m)/Scr mg/dl\right]^{0.64}\times\left[30/BUN\right]^{0.202}$	Iohexol
CKID [47]	$eGFR\left(ml/min per 1.73m^2\right) = 39.1\left[height(m)/Scr(mg/dl)\right]^{0.516}\times\left[1.8/cystatin C(mg/L)\right]^{0.294}$ $\left[30/BUN(mg/dl)\right]^{0.169}\left[1.099\right]if^{male}\left[height(m)/1.4\right]^{0.188}$	Iohexol
Zappiteli [55]	$eGFR\left(ml/min per 1.73m^2\right) = 43.82\left[1/cystatin C\right]0.635\times\left[1/creatinine\right]0.547\times1.35 height$	Iothalamate
Updated CKID [48]	$eGFR\left(ml/min per 1.73m^2\right) = 39.8\left[ht(m)/Scr(mg/dl)\right]^{0.456}\left[1.8/CysC(mg/l)\right]^{0.418}\left[30/BUN(mg/dl)\right]^{0.079}$ $\left[1.076^{male}\right]\left[ht(m)/1.4\right]^{0.179}$	Iohexol
Height independent		
Pottel [56]	$eGFR\left(ml/min per 1.73m^2\right) = 107.3/\left[Scr/(mg/dL)/Q\right]$	Inulin
	Where Q is the median serum creatinine concentration for children based on age and sex	
	Median serum creatinine $(mg/dL) = 0.0270\times age + 0.2329$	
	To express serum creatinine concentration in µmol/L, multiply by 88.4	
Modified BCCH equation [57]	$eGFR\left(ml/min per 1.73m^2\right) = $ Inverse ln of $:8.067+\left(1.034\times ln\left[1/SCr(\mu mol/L)\right]\right)+\left(0.305\times ln\left[age(years)\right]\right)+0.064$ if male	Iothalamate
Filler [58]	$eGFR\left(ml/min per 1.73m^2\right) = 91.62\left[1/CysC\right]1.123$	TcDTPA

plasma disappearance curve. In general, the more numerous blood samples that are acquired over-time, the more accurate the calculated GFR value will be. However, to avoid overly-numerous blood samplings, two simplified methods have been proposed for routine clinical used in children [66].

The Slope-Intercept Method

The slope intercept method requires two blood samples acquired 2 and 4 h post injection and is based on the determination of the late exponential curve. An algorithm must be used to correct for overestimation of the clearance because this method neglects the early exponential curve. Late blood sampling (between 5 and 24 h) is recommended for accuracy in patients with renal clearance below 10–15 ml/min/1.73 m^2.

The Distribution Volume Method

This method only requires one blood sample acquired at 2 h post injection. It appears to be valid for children of any age except for those with very poor renal function (GFR <30 ml/min/1.73 m^2) [65].

One major limitation of these methods is the presence of significant edema. In such a situation the disappearance of the tracer will be influenced by its diffusion into an expanded extracellular volume, and artifactually elevating the calculated GFR. Infiltration of the radiotracer at the injection site can also cause artifactual elevation of GFR.

The effective dose of radiation is approximately 0.011 mSv/examination regardless of the age of the child for Cr-EDTA and twice as high with low GFR (<10 min/1.73 m^2) and 0.1 mSV/examination for Tc-DTPA [65].

Assessment of Tubular Function

Fluid filtered by the glomerulus (plasma ultra-filtrate) enters the proximal tubule where 60–65 % of the filtrate will be reabsorbed [67]. In disorders of the proximal tubule excessive amount of the solutes will be found in the urine. The fractional excretion of sodium and tubular reabsorption of phosphate can be used to assess the integrity of the proximal tubules. Detection of glucosuria and aminoaciduria can also be indicative of proximal tubular disorder in certain situations.

Fractional Excretion of Sodium (FeNa)

This is one of the most commonly used tests of tubular integrity. There is no "normal" for fractional excretion of salt. It has to be interpreted in the context of each patient's sodium and volume status.

In the face of hyponatremic dehydration the appropriate response will be conservation of sodium and water. Therefore, the fractional excretion of salt will be low, usually with a FeNa <1 % in children and less than 2.5 % in neonates. The urinary sodium concentration will be <20 meq/L in children and <30 meq/L in neonates. If tubular damage has occurred such as in acute tubular necrosis, the fractional excretion of salt will be inappropriately elevated. The FeNa will be >2 % in children and >2.5 % in neonates. Urinary sodium will generally be more than 30 meq/L.

However, in certain situations such as when patients are on diuretic therapy, receiving intravenous saline or in patients with salt losing tubulopathies or chronic kidney disease FeNa is unreliable [68, 69]. The FeNa may be substituted by FeUrea, as urea is unaffected by diuretics. A FeUrea <35 % implies pre renal AKI and >50 % intrinsic AKI. High FeNa combined with FeUrea >35 % has a 95 % negative predictive value for intrinsic AKI [70]. The FENa can be calculated as below:

$$Fe\ Na = \frac{U\,Na * PCr * 100}{P\,Na * UCr}$$

U Na = urinary concentration of sodium
P Cr = plasma creatinine
P Na = plasma sodium
U Cr = urinary creatinine

Tubular Reabsorption of Phosphate (TRP)

Eighty five to 95 % of phosphate is usually reabsorbed in the proximal tubule [67]. Phosphate transport is primarily regulated by the plasma phosphate concentration and parathyroid hormone, which alter the Na^+- phosphate carrier activity.

The normal tubular reabsorption of phosphate (TRP) is greater than 85 % and can be calculated:

$$TRP\% = 1 - \frac{(UPO_4 * PCr)}{(PPO_4 * UCr)} * 100$$

U PO_4 = urinary concentration of phosphate
P Cr = plasma creatinine
P PO_4 = plasma concentration of phosphate
U Cr = urinary concentration of creatinine

The renal tubular maximum reabsorption rate of phosphate to glomerular filtration rate (TmP/GFR) was initially described by Bijvoet using phosphate infusion [71]. Its initial use was for diagnosis of hypercalcemia, parathyroid disorders and renal handling of phosphate. Although it is no longer used for evaluation of hypercalcemia, it can still be helpful for evaluation of hypophosphatemia. A nomogram [72] and algorithm [73] were derived from the initial infusion data of Bijvoet and can be used to calculate the TmP/GFR ratio from the TRP. The algorithm is less prone to error and therefore recommended instead of the nomogram [74]. Basically, if the TRP is ≤ 0.86, then $TmP / GFR = TRP \times P_p$ (where P_p = plasma phosphate) and if >0.86 then $TmP / GFR = 0.3 \times TRP / \{1 - (0.8 \times TRP)\} \times P_p$ [73, 74].

Glucosuria

Filtered glucose is usually almost completely reabsorbed in the three segments of the proximal tubule. Glucose is transported across the apical membrane by secondary active transport dependent on the sodium electrochemical gradient generated by the Na-K ATPase. Two sodium-glucose transporters are found in the proximal tubule. The SGLT2 in the early proximal tubule has high capacity and low affinity for glucose and the SGLT1 found in segment 2 and 3 have high affinity and low capacity [75].

The plasma glucose at which glucose reabsorption is maximal is defined as the *threshold for glucose* and the transport capacity when the threshold is reached is called the maximal tubular glucose reabsorption (TmG).

In presence of glucosuria, it is important to determine the serum glucose concentration. The presence of isolated glucosuria with normal serum glucose concentration is usually a result of familial renal glucosuria. Mutations of the SGLT2 coding gene were first described by Santer R et al. in this disorder [76]. Isolated glucosuria with elevated serum glucose is suggestive of diabetes.

Transtubular Potassium Gradient (TTKG)

Potassium is secreted in the late distal and cortical collecting tubules in response to aldosterone. The transtubular potassium gradient is an indirect index of the activity of the potassium secretory process in the cortical distal nephron and reflects the action of aldosterone. It is an important component of the evaluation of hyper and hypokalemia. It can be calculated using the formula proposed by West [77]:

$$TTKG = \frac{UK \div (U\,osm / P\,osm)}{P\,potassium}$$

U K = urinary potassium concentration
U osm = urinary osmolality
P osm = plasma osmolality

The urinary sodium concentration should exceed 25 mmol/L. This ensures sodium reabsorption is not limiting potassium secretion, and urine osmolality should exceed plasma osmolality.

The luminal potassium of the terminal cortical collecting duct is estimated by dividing the urinary potassium by the urine/plasma osmolality since the luminal K concentration is influenced by removal of water in the medullary segments. The serum potassium is an estimate of the peritubular potassium concentration.

TTKG appears to be a good indicator of aldosterone activity in both normal children and in children with hypoaldosteronism and pseudohypoaldosteronism. A TTKG below 4.1 in children or 4.9 in infants is indicative of a state of hypo or pseudohypoaldoserosnism [78]. Ethier et al. define expected values of TTKG under stimuli that are known to modulate excretion of potassium. The expected value during hypokalemia induced from a low potassium diet is less than 2.5 and during acute potassium loading is greater than 10.0 [79]. It may also be useful in distinguishing aldosterone deficiency from resistance by repeating the calculation after initiation of mineralocorticoid therapy [80]. Kamel and Halperin have recently questioned the validity of the TTKG because one of the principle assumptions involved in calculating the TTKG, that the majority of osmoles in the medullary collecting ducts are not reabsorbed, is incorrect, as this is where urea recycling occurs. If more urea is reabsorbed, then the TTKG may overestimate the potassium excretion. As the amount of urea being recycled and excreted in the cortical collecting duct cannot be measured to provide a correction for the formula, the TTKG is no longer considered a valid test [81]. Instead the urinary potassium to creatinine ratio calculated on spot urine can be used. The expected UK/UCr ratio in a patient with hypokalemia should be less than <1.5 mmol K/mmol creatinine), whereas the appropriate renal response to hyperkalemia would be reflected in a UK/UCr ratio >20 mmol K/mmol creatinine [81].

Aminoaciduria

In the normal state, most of the amino acids are reabsorbed in the proximal tubule. Sodium dependant cotransporters are responsible for the transport of glycine and glutamine whereas sodium independents carriers are responsible for the transport of neutral amino acids (leucine, isoleucine and phenylalanine), cystine and dibasic aminoacids (ornithine, arginine and lysine). Mutation in the gene SLC3A1 which encodes a protein responsible for the transport of cystine and the dibasic aminoacids is the cause of the classic form of cystinuria (type I/I) [82, 83].

The cyanide-nitroprusside test is an easy way to detect urinary aminoacids which contain a free sulfhydryl group or disulfide bond such as cystine, cysteine, homocystine and homocysteine and can be performed in the evaluation of nephrolithiasis [2]. Generalized aminoaciduria is usually associated with Fanconi syndrome.

Assessment of Acid Base Status

Total Carbon Dioxide (Total CO_2) and Bicarbonate (HCO_3^-)

Total CO_2 content of blood, plasma or serum consists of an ionized (bicarbonate and carbonate) and a non-ionized (carbonic acid) fraction. The ionized fraction includes HCO_3^-, CO_3^{2-} and carbamino compounds. The non-ionized fraction contains H_2CO_3 and physically dissolved (anhydrous) carbon dioxide. Total CO_2 measurement typically includes both of these fractions.

HCO_3^- results obtained from blood gas analyzer is a calculated parameter. First, pH and pCO_2 are measured and then HCO_3 is calculated using the Henderson-Hasselbach equation:

$$pH = pK1 + \log\left[\left(HCO_3^-\right) \div \left(0.03 * pCO_2\right)\right]$$

pK1 is usually equal to 6.1.

Discrepant values from calculated arterial bicarbonate and measured venous total CO_2 can be seen especially in acutely ill pediatric patients who are prone to large fluctuations in pK1 [84].

Reference range for total CO_2 varies between 17 and 31 mEq/L depending on age. Total CO_2 (tCO_2) and bicarbonate are reduced in the presence of acidosis. K/DOQI clinical practice guidelines for Bone metabolism and Disease in children with CKD [85] recommends that serum level of total CO_2 be measured. Serum levels of total CO_2 should be maintained at ≥ 22 mmol/L in children over 2 years of age, and ≥ 20 mmol/L in neonates and young infants below age 2. Maintaining the serum tCO_2 in the normal range, as suggested by K/DOQI, may also be desirable for better growth in children with CKD [86].

Serum Anion Gap (SAG)

The serum anion gap (SAG) is used in the interpretation of metabolic acidosis in order to determine if there are additional unmeasured anions contributing to the acidosis. It is the difference between the most abundant cations and anions measured in the blood. The serum anion gap is calculated as follows:

$$SAG = Na^+ - \left[Cl^- + HCO3^- \right]$$

Potassium is generally not included in most references. However, if the serum K is significantly high or low, then it will alter the SAG. Reference values reported vary and depend on the method of quantification of the electrolytes by individual laboratories. A typical normal range is 8–16 with a mean of 12 ± 2 as proposed by Halperin et al. [87]. Correction for the serum albumin, a major anion, is advisable as the SAG changes by 2.5 mEq/L for every gram/L change in serum albumin. Corrected SAG can be calculated by using the Figge equation as follows:

$$Corrected\,SAG = SAG + 0.25$$
$$\times \left(normal\,albumin - measured\,albumin\,\left[g/L \right] \right)$$
OR
$$Corrected\,SAG = SAG + 2.5 \times$$
$$\left(normal\,albumin - measured\,albumin\,\left[g/dL \right] \right)$$
[88].

Not correcting for albumin, especially when it is low, may lead to an increased anion gap metabolic acidosis being missed in a significant number of cases [89].

Urine Anion Gap

The urine anion gap is an indirect measurement of ammonium production by the distal nephron. Because ammonium is not routinely measured in most laboratories clinicians need an index of ammonium secretion to use in the evaluation of normal anion gap metabolic acidosis. This was initially proposed by Goldstein et al. [90] and its clinical usefulness was also shown later by Batlle et al. [91].

If ammonium is present, the sum of sodium and potassium will be less than the chloride since ammonium is an unmeasured cation. This test presupposed that the chloride is the predominant anion in the urine balancing the positive charge in urine NH_4^+. Therefore, the urine anion gap can be calculated by the equation:

$$Urine\,anion\,gap = \left(Na + K \right) - Cl$$

A negative urine anion gap suggests gastrointestinal loss of bicarbonate or renal bicarbonate loss whereas a positive urine anion gap suggests the presence of an altered distal urinary acidification [91].

The urine anion gap cannot be used in volume depletion with a urine sodium concentration of less than 25 mmol/L, when there is increased excretion of unmeasured anions such as ketoacid or hippurate, nor in neonates.

Urine Osmolar Gap

Halperin et al. [92] proposed the urine osmolar gap in addition to urine anion gap to ascertain the etiology of normal or increased anion gap metabolic acidosis as well as mixed metabolic acidosis. The urine osmolar gap was defined as the difference between the measured urine osmolality and the sum of the concentration of sodium, potassium, chloride, bicarbonate, urea and glucose. Normally this gap is 80–100 mosm/kgH_2O. Dyck et al. proposed a modification to the urine osmolar gap proposed by Halperin as a better estimate [93]:

$$Osmolar\ gap = 0.5 * \left(\begin{array}{l} Measured\ osmolality - \\ \left(2\left(Na+K\right)+urea+glucose\right) \end{array}\right)$$

Where Na, K, urea and glucose are expressed in mmol/L.

Calculation of the urine osmolar gap will be helpful in excluding glue sniffing, which causes a normal anion gap metabolic acidosis. High concentration of the unmeasured ions ammonium and benzoate will increase the osmolar gap falsely excluding RTA as the cause of acidosis.

Urine: Blood pCO₂ (U-B pCO₂)

Urine-blood pCO_2 can be used for the evaluation of normal anion gap metabolic acidosis with a positive urine net charge to differentiate between deficient ammonium production versus poor hydrogen secretion [94, 95]. The pCO_2 should be measured in alkaline urine. With adequate hydrogen secretion in the distal tubule, the hydrogen will couple with HCO_3 to form H_2CO_3 and then dissociate into CO_2 and H_2O.

Kim et al. [96] evaluated the diagnostic value of the urine-blood pCO_2 in patients diagnosed as having H+-ATPase defect dRTA based on reduced urinary NH4+ and absolute decrease in H+ ATPase immunostaining in intercalated cells. U-B P CO_2 during sodium bicarbonate loading was less than 30 mmHg in all patients with H+ ATPase defect dRTA.

General Biochemistry

Serum Sodium

The reference range for plasma sodium varies with age and method of measurement used. The following reference range for serum sodium is recommended by the Canadian Laboratory Initiative in Pediatric Reference Intervals (CALIPER) database group and the Australasian Association of Clinical Biochemists (AACB); birth – <7 days 132–147 mmol/L, ≥7 days – <2 years 133–145 mmol/L, ≥2 – <12 years 134–145 mmol/L,

and ≥12 – adult 135–145 mmol/L [97, 98]. Serum sodium outside that range can have serious consequences.

Hyponatremia is the results of excess free water or sodium loss. The former is usually associated with expended extracellular fluid where the latter is often seen with volume contraction. Hyponatremia with normal serum osmolality is usually the result of hyperlipidemia, hyperproteinemia or hyperglycemia. Most laboratories now measure serum sodium with ion-specific electrodes and the measurement will not be affected by hyperlipidemia and hyperproteinemia. In the presence of hyperglycemia every 3.4 mmol/l increment in glucose will reduce serum sodium by 1 mmol/l because of water shift from the intracellular space to the extracellular space.

Hypernatremia is usually secondary to water deficit either because of poor intake or increased water loss such as in diabetes insipidus or mellitus. Salt intoxication is a less common cause of hypernatremia.

Serum Potassium

Potassium is an intracellular cation with 98% of body potassium located intracellularly. Cell potassium concentration is about 140 mmol/L, whereas normal range for serum potassium varies between 3.2 and 6.2 mmol/L depending on age. Reference range varies with the method used and age of the child. In infants the upper limit of normal can be as high as 6.2. The upper limit then progressively comes down to about 5.0 to reach the "adult" level. Reference ranges for different methods can be found in reference [99].

Hyperkalemia can be the result of intracellular to extracellular shift in the presence of acidosis, beta blockers, cellular breakdown, and decreased excretion in renal failure, hypoaldosteronism or pseudohypoaldosteronism, and less commonly with increased potassium intake. Pseudohyperkalemia is defined as a serum K+ that exceeds plasma K+ by 0.4 mmol/L on a sample processed within 1 h of venipuncture (delay results in glucose depletion, less ATP generation – the energy source of the sodium-potassium pump) and maintained at room temperature (lower temperatures inhibit the pump leading to potassium leak out of cells). It can occur with prolonged tourniquet use, mechanical factors, excessive crying and respiratory alkalosis, potassium EDTA contamination (associated also with hypocalcemia), leucocytosis, erythrocytosis and thrombocytosis. Platelets release potassium during the clotting process of serum attainment and activated platelets degranulate and release potassium [100, 101]. The benign, dominantly inherited familial pseudohyperkalemia presents as hyperkalemia when the potassium is measured at or below room temperature, but patients do not manifest hyperkalemia at body temperature [102]. It has recently been linked to a mutation in an erythrocyte porphyrin transporter, ABCB6 on chromosome 2 [103]. Hypokalemia is mostly seen in renal tubular disorders such as Fanconi's, Bartter's, Gitelman's syndrome and in hyperaldosteronism.

Serum Calcium, Phosphorus and Calcium-Phosphorus Product

Evaluation of calcium, phosphorus and calcium phosphorus product is reviewed in detail in the guidelines published by K/DOQI [85, 104]. Representative normal values for serum phosphorus, ionized calcium and total calcium can be found in Table 3.5. Pseudohypocalcemia may be seen with gadolinium based contrast agents or in thrombocytosis [105]. The serum phosphate may appear falsely low after mannitol infusion and falsely elevated with hyperbilirubinemia, hyperlipidemia, secondary to amphotericin or if the sample is taken from a central line that has been treated with tissue plasminogen activator [105].

In CKD serum levels of phosphorus should be maintained at or above the age-appropriate lower limits and no higher than the age-appropriate upper limits. For children with CKD stage 5 the serum level of phosphorus should be maintained between 3.5 and 5.5 mg/dL (1.13–1.78 mmol/L) during adolescence and between 4 and 6 mg/dL (1.29–1.94 mmol/L) for children between the ages of 1 and 12 years.

Calcium in blood exists in three fractions: protein-bound calcium, free (ionized) calcium and calcium complexes. Total measured calcium should be corrected if serum albumin is abnormal to better reflect the ionized calcium. The following formula can be used:

$$Corrected\,calcium\,(mg\,/\,dL) = \\ total\,calcium\,(mg\,/\,dL) + 0.8 \times \\ \left[4 - serum\,albumin\,(g\,/\,dL)\right]$$

Ionized calcium is affected by pH since hydrogen ion displaces calcium from albumin. A fall of 0.1 unit in pH will cause approximately a 0.1 meq/L rise in the concentration of ionized calcium. As serum ionized calcium is not routinely measured in most places, K/DOQI guidelines are based on corrected total calcium. Levels should be maintained within normal range for the laboratory used and preferably toward the lower end in CKD stage 5. The serum calcium-phosphorus product should be maintained at <55 mg^2/dl^2 (4.4 mmol^2/L^2) in adolescents greater

Table 3.5 Normal values for serum phosphorus, blood ionized calcium concentrations

Age	Serum phosphorus		Blood ionized calcium (mM)	Total calcium	
	mg/dL	mmol/L[a]		mg/dL	mmol/L[b]
0–3 months	4.8–7.4	1.55–2.39	1.22–1.40	8.8–11.3	2.20–2.83
1–5 years	4.5–6.5	1.45–2.10	1.22–1.32	9.4–10.8	2.35–2.70
6–12 years	3.6–5.8	1.16–1.87	1.15–1.32	9.4–10.3	2.35–2.57
13–20 years	2.3–4.5	0.74–1.45	1.12–1.30	8.8–10.2	2.20–2.55

Data from K/DOQI Clinical practice guidelines for bone metabolism and disease in children with chronic kidney disease [85]

[a]Serum phosphorus converted from mg/dL to mmol/L using a factor of 0.3229

[b]Serum calcium converted from mg/dL to mmol/L using a factor of 0.250

than 12 years and <65 mg^2/dl^2 (5.2 mmol^2/L^2) in younger children [85].

Serum Albumin

Serum albumin is used extensively to assess the nutritional status in children with or without renal disease. Although it is used as a measure of the nutritional state of an individual it can be affected by non-nutritional factor especially in children with chronic kidney disease such as infection, inflammation, hydration status, peritoneal or urinary losses [106]. Children with low serum albumin should be assessed for protein-energy malnutrition if not losing protein.

Serum Uric Acid

Serum uric acid varies with both age and gender and reference intervals have been published [107, 108]. An elevated serum uric acid is rare in childhood as compared to adulthood, and in contrast to adults where gout is the primary cause, hereditary disorders of purine biosynthesis account for the majority of cases in children. These include a deficiency of the enzyme hypoxanthine-guanine phosphoribosyltransferase (Lesch-Nyhan syndrome) and hereditary xanthinuria [109]. Hyperuricemia is also found in familial juvenile hyperuricemic nephropathy in association with mutations in the uromodulin gene [110]. The combination of hyperuricemia, anemia, early onset kidney failure and hypotensive or presyncopal episodes should raise suspicion of the recently described disorder associated with a mutation in the renin gene [111]. The renal cysts and diabetes syndrome caused by mutations in the hepatocyte nuclear factor – 1β (HNF1β) is also associated with hyperuricemia [112]. Patients with HNF1β mutations may also present hypomagnesemia [113].

The kidney is the primary site of excretion of uric acid and hyperuricemia is seen in acute kidney injury, tumor lysis syndrome, and secondary to certain drugs such as thiazides, salycylates and cyclosporine [108]. A pediatric study of over 100 patients with CKD found that 70% of children with an eGFR <60 ml/min/1.73 m^2 had uric acid levels above the normal range [114]. This may become pertinent considering the growing evidence to suggest that hyperuricemia has a causal link with hypertension and possibly also with chronic kidney disease progression [115, 116]. Uric acid might even be a clinically useful marker in the management of essential hypertension in adolescents [117]. Drugs that lower serum uric acid include allopurinol and rasburicase. Also the angiotensin receptor blocker losartan is uricosuric [118] and could be beneficial in hypertensive patients with hyperuricemia while further studies to evaluate the utility and safety of allopurinol are conducted [119]. Allopurinol can increase xanthine and hypoxanthine levels leading to xanthinuria and stones and has been associated with severe dermatological reactions in children [120, 121].

Urinary Calcium

Measurement of calcium excretion should be part of the evaluation of patients with hematuria, nephrocalcinosis and renal stones and can often be useful in the assessment of children with frequency, dysuria, urgency and recurrent UTI [122]. Urinary calcium excretion varies with age being highest in infancy and reaching its nadir during puberty.

Hypercalciuria is usually defined as a urinary calcium excretion of more than 4 mg/kg/day based on the study of Ghazali and Barratt [123]. However, several authors have studied urinary calcium excretion and published reference ranges in their study population [124–128].

Spot urinary calcium/creatinine ratio (usually collected on the second morning fasting urine specimen) correlates well with 24 h calcium excretion, especially for children with normal muscle mass. They can be used for clinical purpose; however, they are more likely to be affected to a greater degree by factors such as recent dietary calcium intake [129]. Sodium, protein, phosphorus, potassium and glucose intake can influence calcium excretion. There is no apparent seasonal variation of urinary calcium/creatinine ratio in children as seen in adults [130].

For those who have reduced muscle mass, urinary calcium/osmolality ratio predicts hypercalciuria with better sensitivity and specificity than urine calcium/creatinine ratio [131, 132].

Urinary Sodium

Measurement of urinary sodium excretion is a valuable part of the evaluation of children with hypercalciuria. Polito et al. found that urinary sodium excretion and 24 h urinary sodium/potassium (U Na/K) excretion was higher in children with hypercalciuria [133]. Urinary sodium excretion was 4 ± 2.4 mmol/kg/day in hypercalciuric children compared to 2.7 mmol/kg/day in ex-hypercalciuric children. Fasting U Na/ K was 3 ± 1.6 versus 2.1 ± 1 mmol/mmol and 24 h UNa/ K 4.2 ± 3.9 versus 2.8 ± 1.5 mmol/mmol in hypercalciuric versus ex-hypercalciuric.

Twenty-four hour urinary sodium can also be used to assess dietary sodium intake in adults on a low sodium diet for the treatment of hypertension where a target 24 h intake of 50–100 mmol/day is recommended [134].

Urinary Magnesium

Magnesium is a known stone inhibitor as it forms complexes with oxalate and reduces supersaturation. Thirty nine percent of children with calcium – oxalate stones in one series had hypomagnesuria defined as magnesium excretion less than 1.2 mg/kg/24 h [135]. Urinary reference limits for Mg/Cr can be found in Table 3.6.

Urinary Citrate

Citrate inhibits calcium-oxalate and calcium-phosphate crystal nucleation, growth and aggregation. In normal circumstances, citrate is freely filtered at the glomerulus with a

Table 3.6 Urinary reference limits for urinary magnesium/creatinine

Age in year	Urinary Mg/Cr Mol/mol (mg/mg)	
	5th percentile	95th percentile
1/12–1	0.4 (0.10)	2.2 (0.48)
1–2	0.4 (0.09)	1.7 (0.37)
2–3	0.3 (0.07)	1.6 (0.34)
3–5	0.3 (0.07)	1.3 (0.29)
5–7	0.3 (0.06)	1.0 (0.21)
7–10	0.3 (0.05)	0.9 (0.18)
10–14	0.2 (0.05)	0.7 (0.15)
14–17	0.2 (0.05)	0.6 (0.13)

Used with permission of Elsevier from Matos et al. [136]

Table 3.7 Mean molar citrate/creatinine ratio

Urinary citrate/creatinine	Girls	Boys
Infants	1.9	0.63
Childhood	0.27	0.33
Adolescence	0.32	0.28

Data from Hoppe and Langman [137]

65–90 % reabsorption rate. Systemic acidosis, potassium depletion, starvation and acetazolamide therapy are all known to decrease urinary citrate. Citrate excretion is age and sex related. Mean molar excretion of citrate is higher in infants than in older age groups, and in infants is higher in females mmol/mmol [137] and can be found in Table 3.7. Citrate excretion of more than 1.6 mmol/1.73 m² in girls and more than 1.9 in boys is considered normal [138].

Hypocitraturia either alone or in association with hypercalciuria is an important risk factor for nephrolithiasis in children [139, 140]. In one study, hypocitraturia defined as citrate excretion <320 mg/1.73 m²/24 h [1.66 mmol/1.73 m²/24 h] was observed in 60.6 % of children with calcium-oxalate stone [135]. A recent study in a stone-forming adult population suggests that urinary calcium to citrate ratio >0.25 mg/mg is predictive of lithogenesis; however, this will need validation in children [141]. Hypocitraturia is a major risk factor for nephrocalcinosis in very low birth weight infants [142] and after kidney transplantation [143].

Urinary Oxalate

Urinary oxalate excretion is significantly increased in primary hyperoxaluria type I (PH I), PH II and PH III and in secondary hyperoxaluria. In PH I, there is excessive endogenous production of oxalate caused by a deficiency of hepatic AGT which catalyzes the peroxisomal conversion of glyoxylate to glycine and in PH II, a deficiency of cytosolic glyoxylate reductase – hydroxypyruvate reductase (GRHPR), an enzyme that catalyzes the reduction of glyoxylate and hydroxypyruvate as well as the dehydrogenation of glycerate [144, 145]. The recently defined PH III is due to a defect in a hepatocyte specific mitochondrial enzyme, 4-hydroxy-2-oxoglutarate aldolase (HOGA) [146].

The secondary forms are due to increased intestinal absorption of oxalate secondary to malabsorptive states or impaired vitamin status. Reference values for oxalate/creatinine can be found in Table 3.8.

Patients suspected of having abnormalities in oxalate metabolism should have more extensive studies including measurement of oxalate, glycolate and l-glycerate and in some cases liver biopsy to assess the activity of alaninine:glyoxylate aminotransferase (AGT) and glyoxylatereductase enzyme.

Elevated oxalate and glycolate are associated with primary hyperoxaluria type I (PH1); however, normal glycolate is found in 25 % of subject with PHI. Elevated urinary oxalate and L-glycerate is the typical finding of hyperoxaluria type II, but likewise L-glycerate is not always detected. Genetic analysis is now considered the gold standard for diagnosis and liver biopsy, to measure intrahepatic enzyme levels, is generally reserved for patients in whom no mutation can be found [144, 145].

Urinary Uric Acid

Increased urinary uric acid excretion can present with microscopic hematuria, abdominal and/or flank pain, dysuria, gravel and macroscopic hematuria. About half of patients with hyperuricosuria will have microlithiasis on ultrasonography [148]. Hyperuricosuria (HU) may be defined by urine uric acid concentration corrected for creatinine clearance >0.53 mg/dL/GFR [149]. The excretion varies with age being highest in infants. However, a simpler estimate of urinary urate excretion can be calculated from the urine urate/creatinine ratio. Reference values for urine urate/creatinine can be found in Table 3.8.

Assessment of the Renin-Angiotensin-Aldosterone System

Renin is a proteolytic enzyme predominantly formed and stored in the juxtaglomerular cells of the kidney. Renal hypoperfusion and increased sympathetic activity are the major physiologic stimuli to renin secretion [67]. When released in

Table 3.8 Urinary reference limits for calcium/creatinine, oxalate/creatinine, urate/creatinine

Age	Urinary calcium/creatinine Mol/mol (mg/mg)*		Urinary oxalate/creatinine Mol/mol (mg/mg)*		Urinary urate/creatinine Mol/mol (mg/mg)*	
	5th	95th	5th	95th	5th	95th
1–6 months	0.09 (0.03)	2.2 (0.81)	0.07 (0.0560)	0.22 (0.175)	0.80 (1/189)	1.60 (2.378)
6 months–1 year	0.09 (0.03)	2.2 (0.81)	0.06 (0.0480)	0.17 (0.139)	0.70 (1.040)	1.50 (2.299)
1–2	0.07 (0.03)	1.5 (0.500)	0.05 (0.04)	0.13 (0.103)	0.50 (0.743)	1.40 (2.080)
2–3	0.06 (0.02)	1.4 (0.41)	0.04 (0.032)	0.10 (0.080)	0.47 (0.698)	1.30 (1.932)
3–5	0.05 (0.02)	1.1 (0.30)	0.03 (0.024)	0.08 (0.064)	0/40 (0.594)	1.1(1.635)
5–7	0.04 (0.01)	0.8 (0.25)	0.03 (0.024)	0.07 (0.056)	0.30 (0.446)	0.80 (1.189)
7–10	0.04 (0.01)	0.7 (0.24)	0.02 (0.016)	0.06 (0.048)	0.26 (0.386)	0.56 (0.832)
10–14	0.04 (0.01)	0.7 (0.24)	0.02 (0.016)	0.06 (0.048)	0.20 (0.297)	0.44 (0.654)
14–17	0.04 (0.01)	0.7 (0.24)	0.02 (0.016)	0.06 (0.048)	0.20(0.297)	0.40 (0.594)

Data from Matos et al. [136]; and from Matos et al. [147]

*Conversions have been performed with higher precision, then rounded for this presentation

the circulation renin cleaves angiotensinogen to produce a decapeptide angiotensin I. Angiotensin I is then converted to an octapeptide, angiotensin II by the angiotensin I-converting enzyme. Angiotensin II is a potent vasoconstrictor and promotes salt and water retention. The converting enzyme is mainly located in the lung but angiotensin II can be synthesized at a variety of sites including the kidney, luminal membrane of vascular endothelial cells, adrenal gland and brain. Angiotensin II promotes renal salt and water reabsorption by stimulation of sodium reabsorption in the early proximal tubule and by indirectly activating aldosterone biosynthesis in the zona glomerulosa of the adrenal cortex.

Measurement of plasma renin activity may not reflect the tissue activity of the local renin-angiotensin system.

Assessment of the renin-angiotensin-aldosterone system may be required in the evaluation of hypokalemia/hyperkalemia, adrenal insufficiency and hypertension, see Table 3.9.

Renin

Renin release is dependent on renal tubular sodium concentration, renal perfusion pressure and beta adrenergic vascular tone. The enzymatic activity of renin can be measured. It is expressed as the amount of angiotensin I generated per unit of time and is expressed in pmol or ng of generated angiotensin I per ml of plasma.

The "normal values" for plasma renin activity (PRA) are highly dependent on sodium intake, time of day, posture, age and method used [150]. PRA varies inversely with age in infants and children. Reference values derived from measurement of PRA in 79 children age 1 month to 15 years in supine position were published in 1975 [151].

PRA can be useful in the management of hypertension to distinguish between a volume dependent hypertension where renin is suppressed and hypertension mediated by excess renin secretion. A value less than 0.65 ng/ml/h suggests renin suppression, while a value above 6.5 ng/ml/h implies high renin activity. This can help guide appropriate therapy [152].

During renal angiography, renal-vein renin sampling may be done to predict feasibility of correcting hypertension or to identify which kidney contributes to the hypertension. When the ratio of renal vein renin from the diseased kidney (R) to renal vein renin from the normal or less diseased contralateral kidney (RC) is above 1.5 (R/RC >1.5) this is considered significant and there is greater probability that blood pressure would be improved after surgery. A ratio between the RC and the infrarenal inferior vena cava of less than 1.3 further supports the finding. Segmental veins within a kidney may also be sampled [153–157].

Aldosterone

Aldosterone is synthesized in the zona glomerulosa of the adrenal gland. It regulates electrolyte excretion and intravascular volume mainly through its effects on the distal tubules and

Table 3.9 Assessment of the renin-angiotensin-aldosterone system

	PRA	PAC	PAC/PRA	BP	Potassium
Primary hyperaldosteronism	Decrease	Increase	Very high >20–50	High	Low
GRA	Decrease	Increase	High	High	N or low
Renin-secreting tumor	Increase	Increase		High	Low
Bartter' syndrome	Increased	Increased		Normal	Low
Renovascular disease	Increased	Increased	<10		
Apparent mineralocorticoid excess, Cushing, licorice ingestion	Low	Low		High	Low

PRA plasma renin activity, *PAC* plasma aldosterone concentration, *BP* blood pressure, *GRA* glucocorticoid remediable hypertension

cortical collecting ducts of the kidneys in which it acts to increase sodium reabsorption and potassium excretion [158].

Aldosterone is measured by radioimmunoassay. As for renin, it is dependent on sodium intake, posture and time of the day. Serum aldosterone concentration will be highest at the time of awakening and lowest shortly after sleep.

Hyperaldosteronism should be sought for in children with hypertension, hypokalemia and metabolic alkalosis [159].

Plasma Aldosterone Concentration (PAC) to Plasma Renin Activity Ratio (PRA)

The plasma aldosterone to plasma renin ratio has been used as a screening tool for diagnosis of hyperaldosteronism prior to confirmation with a suppression test. Both random PAC and PRA should be measured midmorning. Patients should be off aldosterone receptor antagonist, ACE inhibitor and angiotensin receptor blockers for 3–6 weeks and hypokalemia needs to be corrected prior to the test. Any medication that stimulates renin production, such as diuretics, will lead to a false negative result. False positives can be expected with the reduced renin and increased salt and water retention of renal impairment. The patient needs to be in the seated position for 10–15 min after being ambulant for at least 2 h, and midmorning is considered the best time to perform the test [160]. The mean normal value is 4–10 compared to more than 30–50 in patients with primary hyperaldosteronism [161].

Complement Pathway Assessment

The complement system consists of at least 30 plasma membrane proteins that provide an innate defense against microbes and an adjunct or complement to humoral immunity [162, 163]. The complement system is divided in three major pathways: the classical, the lectin and the alternative pathway. The lectin pathway is activated by the binding of lectin (which as a similar structure to C1q) to sugar residues on the surface of a pathogen and the alternative pathway which is an amplification loop for C3 activation is activated by polysaccharide antigens, aggregated IgA, injured cells or endotoxins. The classical pathway is activated by the binding of C1q to the Fc portion of antibody. The alternative pathway is a constitutively active and amplifiable system. Plasma Factor H and Factor I are important fluid phase complement regulators of the alternative pathway, while CD46/Membrane Cofactor Protein, CD55/Decay Accelerating Factor and CD59/Protectin are the principal surface bound regulators. Each of these three pathways of complement activation will lead to the deposition of an activated C3 fragment (C3b) inducing the final steps of the complement cascades which include opsonisation, phagocytosis, induction of inflammation, and formation of the membrane attack complex (MAC) and cytolysis [162–164]. A fourth pathway by which thrombin can directly activate C5 and thus the terminal complement cascade was recently identified [165]. However, the significance of this pathway in the pathogenesis of disease is still unclear. There is an evolving spectrum of kidney diseases now recognized as being either complement-mediated or having complement dysregulation as part of their pathogenesis, and these will be discussed in a later chapter [166].

Evaluation of the complement system will help in the diagnosis of glomerulonephritis. Complement concentrations of the C3 and C4 protein can be measured by immunological methods. CH50 is a functional assay of the classical pathway. All nine components (C1 through C9) are required to have a normal CH50 which assess the ability of the patient's serum to lyse sheep erythrocyte optimally sensitized with rabbit antibody. The CH50 is useful to diagnose hypocomplementemic states (for example congenital C2 deficiency) that would be missed if only C3 and C4 were done. The normal range for serum C3 varies considerably from laboratory to laboratory [167], therefore no normal values are provided in this chapter.

Glomerular disease associated with activation of the classical pathway will typically have a low C4 and C3 whereas disease associated with

Table 3.10 Evaluation of complement activity for the differential diagnosis of glomerulonephritis

	C3	C4	CH50	Associated disease
Activation of classical pathway	Low	Low	Low	SLE, MPGN type I cryoglobulinemia
				Chronic infections
Activation of alternative pathway	Low	Normal		MPGN type II, post infectious GN
Activation of leptin pathway	Normal	Normal		IgA

activation of the alternative pathway will have a low C3 and normal C4 (Table 3.10). Serial assessment of complements can also be helpful in monitoring disease activity in immune complexes mediated disease such as lupus. C4 is less likely to change because one or more C4 null genes are common in SLE therefore patients in remission can continue to have low C4. However, changes in C3 is sensitive to change in disease activity [167].

When a complement-mediated disease is suspected, more in-depth analysis of the complement system can be performed. The principle steps involved in assessing the complement system includes; (i) functional activity assays of global complement pathway function, with the CH50 or AH50, (ii) analysis of individual complement components, (iii) detection of complement activation or split products, typically by ELISA, (iv) measuring complement products such as SC5b-9 in the serum, urine or tissues, (iv) measuring auto-antibodies to various complement components, to the C3 convertase (C3 nephritic factor), or to the alternative pathway regulator CFH and (v), genetic analysis for mutations in C3, CFB, CFH, CFI, CD46/MCP, now linked to various diseases including atypical hemolytic uremic syndrome, membranoproliferative glomerulonephritis and antibody-mediated rejection [168–172].

Laboratory Assessment of Various Glomerulopathies

Antineutrophil Cytoplasmic Antibodies (ANCA)

Antineutrophil cystoplasmic antibodies (ANCA) are IgG autoantibodies directed against constituents of primary granules of neutrophil and monocyte lysosomes. They were first described in 1982 in patients with pauci-immune glomerulonephritis [173]. Indirect immunofluorescence (IIF) and enzyme-linked immunosorbent assay (ELISA) are the most widely used techniques to detect ANCA. By IIF, two major immunostaining patterns can be seen: the diffuse granular cytoplasmic pattern with central accentuation known as C-ANCA and the perinuclear pattern which is defined as perinuclear fluorescence with nuclear extension known as P-ANCA. Diffuse flat cytoplasmic staining without interlobular accentuation can also be seen and is termed atypical C-ANCA. Atypical ANCA includes all other neutrophil-specific or monocyte-specific IIF reactivity, most commonly a combination of cytoplasmic and perinuclear fluorescence. Proteinase 3 and myeloperoxidase are two antigenic targets known to be associated with vasculitis. The cytoplasmic pattern usually suggests the presence of serum proteinase 3 ANCA (PR3-ANCA), whereas perinuclear pattern with nuclear extension will usually be associated with myeloperoxidase ANCA (MPO-ANCA). ELISA is used to prove the presence of myeoloperoxidase and proteinase 3 ANCA [174]. In order to enhance specificity to rule in a diagnosis, both IIF and ELISA are recommended. Occasionally antinuclear antibodies can give a false positive P-ANCA and this can be avoided by fixing the neutrophils with formalin rather than ethanol [175].

More novel assays for ANCA confirmation include capture ELISAs, high sensitivity or anchor ELISAs and automated immunoassays, the latter able to provide a result in under an hour may become more widespread and have a value in deciding when to initiate treatment in difficult cases [175, 176].

Antibodies to a number of azurophilic granule proteins (lactoferrin, elastase, cathepsin G, bactericidal permeability inhibitor, catalase, lysozyme and more) can cause a P-ANCA staining pattern. The ELISA will determine the specific antibody responsible. Only anti-PR3 or anti-MPO antibodies, however, are clinically relevant [177].

ANCA measurement should only be done for patients who are strongly suspected of having vasculitis. Clinical indications for ANCA testing can be found in the International Consensus statement on Testing and reporting of antineutrophil cytoplasmic antibodies [174]. Compliance with guidelines for ANCA testing would decrease the number of false positives which may lead to misdiagnosis and potentially harmful treatments [178].

Granulomatosis with polyangiitis (GPA), microscopic polyangiitis, Churg-Strauss syndrome, renal limited vasculitis and drug induced ANCA-associated vasculitis are associated with positive ANCA. C-ANCA anti-PR3 ANCA typically suggests a diagnosis of GPA whereas P-ANCA anti-MPO associates more with MPA and Churg Strauss syndrome. ANCA are positive in 70–95 % of patients with GPA and MPA but only about 40 % of patients with a diagnosis of Churg Strauss syndrome will be positive [177].

ANCA can also be positive in non vasculitic disease such as antiglomerular basement membrane disease, inflammatory bowel disease and autoimmune disorders.

Both PR3 and MPO ANCA may be found with infectious conditions such as tuberculosis and subacute bacterial endocarditis. Various drugs can also be associated with ANCA positivity. These include propylthiouracil, hydralazine, penicillins, sulfonamides, quinolones, thiazides and allopurinol [177].

Correlation with disease activity was first recognized by van der Woude et al. in 1985 [179]. Although the diagnostic value of ANCA is not disputed, the utility of measuring serial ANCA to monitor disease course, response to treatment or relapse prediction has overall been disappointing [177, 180]. A systematic review on the value of serial ANCA determination for monitoring of patients was inconclusive [181]. Although it is not generally recommended to treat prophylactically, a patient in clinical remission whose titers are elevated should be followed very closely [182]. A rise in ANCA may be predictive of an imminent relapse but this is not universal [183]. MPO-ANCA carries worse renal and adult patient survival [184, 185]. Relapse is more common with PR3-ANCA, especially if there is persistence of PR3 positivity after induction therapy [186–188].

Some progress in terms of the so called ANCA negative vasculitides has been made recently with the discovery of pathogenic versus naturally occurring MPO epitopes, previously undetectable by conventional testing [189]. In the future, epitope specificities may prove useful in distinguishing varying disease characteristics in ANCA associated vasculitides [190].

More recently, Kain et al. detected antibodies against human lysosome-associated membrane protein-2 (LAMP-2), a protein localized to the same neutrophil granules as PR3 and MPO, in over 90 % of patients with ANCA associated vasculitis and glomerulonephritis [191], 17 years after the same authors suspected their involvement in the pauci-immune necrotizing glomerulonephritis [192]. These autoantibodies may only be present early post diagnosis and disappear with the initiation of immunosuppressive therapies and disease remission; however, their relevance as a pathological or serological marker is yet to be determined [193–195].

Anti Nuclear Antibodies (ANA) and Anti-doubled Stranded DNA (Anti dsDNA)

The ANAs are auto-antibodies directed against chromatin and its individual components including double-stranded DNA and histones and some ribonucleoproteins [196]. Although ANAs are frequently found in children without a rheumatic disease [197], they have been associated with several systemic autoimmune disease including systemic lupus erythematosous, scleroderma, mixed connective tissue disease, polymyositis, dermatomyositis, rheumatoid arthritis, Sjögren's syndrome, drug induced lupus, discoid lupus, pauciarticular juvenile chronic arthritis. They are also occasionally seen in autoimmune disease of the thyroid, liver and lungs as well as chronic infectious disease such as mononucleosis, hepatitis C infection, subacute bacterial endocarditis, tuberculosis and HIV and some lymphoproliferative disorders. They do not always signify disease and 13.8 % of the population over age 12 have detectable ANAs, with ANA positivity increasing with age and more common in females [198].

Different types of ANA are known and classified based on their target antigens. Antibodies can be directed against double stranded DNA, individual nuclear histones, nuclear proteins and RNA-protein complexes. As some of these antibodies are more specific for a particular disease they are helpful tests for diagnosis. They are also used for monitoring disease activity. ANA may also precede disease onset [199].

In most laboratories, antinuclear antibodies are measured by an indirect immunofluorescence assay using the human epithelial cell tumor line (Hep2 cells) as the antigenic substrate. Different staining patterns can be seen reflecting the presence of antibodies to one or a combination of nuclear antigens. Those patterns are neither sensitive nor specific for a single disease. In general, a homogenous or chromosomal pattern is more likely in healthy individuals and in those with SLE, whereas a speckled or extrachromosomal pattern implies antibodies against extractable nuclear antigens (ENA) such as Smith antigen. A nucleolar pattern may suggest systemic sclerosis. It is important to emphasize that anti DNA antibodies associated with SLE may also present a speckled or nucleolar pattern [200]. These different immunofluorescent staining patterns may correlate with disease manifestations in SLE. For instance, proliferative lupus nephritis is more commonly associated with a homogenous pattern and organ damage may be less likely with the speckled pattern in SLE [201]. A nuclear, coarse speckled, rather than a dense fine speckled pattern on immunofluorescence, may signify an autoimmune rheumatic disease [202]. This will need further validation before being employed in more widespread clinical practice [203].

The titer of antinuclear antibodies can be helpful clinically. A negative ANA makes a diagnosis of SLE or mixed connective tissue disease very unlikely. ANAs in the sera of a normal healthy childhood population using Hep-2 cells as substrate is reported as 6 % [204], and 16 % at screening dilutions of 1:20 [205]. In healthy individuals ANA titers above 1:40 is found in 32 % above 1:80 in 13 % and above 1:320 in 3 % [206].

The presence of very high titer >1:640 should raise the suspicion of an autoimmune disease. If no diagnosis is made the patients should be followed closely. Lower titers with no clinical sign or symptoms of disease are much less worrisome. In one study, no rheumatic disease was diagnosed in a patient with ANA titres <1:160 and unless there is a high pretest likelihood of a rheumatic disease then ANA has a very low positive predictive value [207].

Anti-ds DNA are relatively specific for SLE and fluctuate with disease activity [208].

Antinucleosome antibody is the earliest marker for the diagnosis of SLE. It is also a superior marker of lupus nephritis [196]. Among those with SLE, the prevalence of antinucleosome antibodies was higher in those with renal disease (58 %) compared to those without nephritis (29 %) [209]. Antibodies to the Smith antigen which is a nuclear non histone protein are very specific for SLE but insensitive.

In SLE, autoantibodies to the complement component C1q are strongly associated with proliferative lupus nephritis, correlate with disease severity, can herald the onset of nephritis and be used to monitor response to therapy [208, 210]. Anti-dsDNA are also strongly associated with nephritis in SLE [208].

References

1. Sekhar DL, Wang L, Hollenbeak CS, Widome MD, Paul IM. A cost-effectiveness analysis of screening urine dipsticks in well-child care. Pediatrics. 2010;125(4):660–3.
2. Graff SL. In: Biello LA, editor. A handbook of routine urinalysis. Philadelphia: Lippincott Williams & Wilkins; 1983.
3. Brodehl J, Franken A, Gellissen K. Maximal tubular reabsorption of glucose in infants and children. Acta Paediatr Scand. 1972;61(4):413–20.

4. Whiting P, Westwood M, Bojke L, Palmer S, Richardson G, Cooper J. Clinical effectiveness and cost-effectiveness of tests for the diagnosis and investigation of urinary tract infection in children: a systematic review and economic model. Health Technol Assess. 2006;10(36):1–154.

5. Mori R, Yonemoto N, Fitzgerald A, Tullus K, Verrier-Jones K, Lakhanpaul M. Diagnostic performance of urine dipstick testing in children with suspected UTI: a systematic review of relationship with age and comparison with microscopy. Acta Paediatr. 2010;99(4):581–4.

6. Kazi BA, Buffone GJ, Revell PA, Chandramohan L, Dowlin MD, Cruz AT. Performance characteristics of urinalyses for the diagnosis of pediatric urinary tract infection. Am J Emerg Med. 2013;31(9): 1405–7.

7. Perazella MA, Coca SG. Traditional urinary biomarkers in the assessment of hospital-acquired AKI. Clin J Am Soc Nephrol. 2012;7(1):167–74.

8. Galpin JE, Shinaberger JH, Stanley TM, Blumenkrantz MJ, Bayer AS, Friedman GS, et al. Acute interstitial nephritis due to methicillin. Am J Med. 1978;65(5):756–65.

9. Sutton JM. Urinary eosinophils. Arch Intern Med. 1986;146(11):2243–4.

10. Nolan 3rd CR, Anger MS, Kelleher SP. Eosinophiluria – a new method of detection and definition of the clinical spectrum. N Engl J Med. 1986;315(24):1516–19.

11. Muriithi AK, Nasr SH, Leung N. Utility of urine eosinophils in the diagnosis of acute interstitial nephritis. Clin J Am Soc Nephrol. 2013;8(11): 1857–62.

12. Trachtenberg F, Barregard L. The effect of age, sex, and race on urinary markers of kidney damage in children. Am J Kidney Dis. 2007;50(6):938–45.

13. Csernus K, Lanyi E, Erhardt E, Molnar D. Effect of childhood obesity and obesity-related cardiovascular risk factors on glomerular and tubular protein excretion. Eur J Pediatr. 2005;164(1):44–9.

14. Hjorth L, Helin I, Grubb A. Age-related reference limits for urine levels of albumin, orosomucoid, immunoglobulin G and protein HC in children. Scand J Clin Lab Invest. 2000;60(1):65–73.

15. Davies AG, Postlethwaite RJ, Price DA, Burn JL, Houlton CA, Fielding BA. Urinary albumin excretion in school children. Arch Dis Child. 1984; 59(7):625–30.

16. Hogg RJ, Furth S, Lemley KV, Portman R, Schwartz GJ, Coresh J, et al. National Kidney Foundation's Kidney Disease Outcomes Quality Initiative clinical practice guidelines for chronic kidney disease in children and adolescents: evaluation, classification, and stratification. Pediatrics. 2003;111(6 Pt 1): 1416–21.

17. Executive summary: standards of medical care in diabetes – 2013. Diabetes Care. 2013;36(Suppl 1): S4–10.

18. Ettenger RB. The evaluation of the child with proteinuria. Pediatr Ann. 1994;23(9):486–94.

19. The CARI Guidelines. Urine protein as diagnostic test: evaluation of proteinuria in children. Nephrology (Carlton). 2004;9 Suppl 3:S15–19.

20. Brandt JR, Jacobs A, Raissy HH, Kelly FM, Staples AO, Kaufman E, et al. Orthostatic proteinuria and the spectrum of diurnal variability of urinary protein excretion in healthy children. Pediatr Nephrol. 2010;25(6):1131–7.

21. Kidney Disease: Improving Global Outcomes (KDIGO) CKD Work Group. KDIGO 2012 clinical practice guideline for the evaluation and management of chronic kidney disease. Kidney Int Suppl. 2013;3:1–150.

22. Jones CA, Francis ME, Eberhardt MS, Chavers B, Coresh J, Engelgau M, et al. Microalbuminuria in the US population: Third National Health and Nutrition Examination Survey. Am J Kidney Dis. 2002;39(3):445–59.

23. Hogg RJ, Portman RJ, Milliner D, Lemley KV, Eddy A, Ingelfinger J. Evaluation and management of proteinuria and nephrotic syndrome in children: recommendations from a pediatric nephrology panel established at the National Kidney Foundation conference on proteinuria, albuminuria, risk, assessment, detection, and elimination (PARADE). Pediatrics. 2000;105(6):1242–9.

24. Park YH, Choi JY, Chung HS, Koo JW, Kim SY, Namgoong MK, et al. Hematuria and proteinuria in a mass school urine screening test. Pediatr Nephrol. 2005;20(8):1126–30.

25. Vehaskari VM, Rapola J. Isolated proteinuria: analysis of a school-age population. J Pediatr. 1982; 101(5):661–8.

26. Mori Y, Hiraoka M, Suganuma N, Tsukahara H, Yoshida H, Mayumi M. Urinary creatinine excretion and protein/creatinine ratios vary by body size and gender in children. Pediatr Nephrol. 2006;21(5): 683–7.

27. Kim HS, Cheon HW, Choe JH, Yoo KH, Hong YS, Lee JW, et al. Quantification of proteinuria in children using the urinary protein-osmolality ratio. Pediatr Nephrol. 2001;16(1):73–6.

28. Serdaroglu E, Mir S. Protein-osmolality ratio for quantification of proteinuria in children. Clin Exp Nephrol. 2008;12(5):354–7.

29. Hooman N, Otoukesh H, Safaii H, Mehrazma M, Shokrolah Y. Quantification of proteinuria with urinary protein to osmolality ratios in children with and without renal insufficiency. Ann Saudi Med. 2005; 25(3):215–18.

30. Smith HS. The kidney structure and function in health and disease. New York: Oxford Univ. Press; 1951.

31. Arant Jr BS, Edelmann Jr CM, Spitzer A. The congruence of creatinine and inulin clearances in children: use of the Technicon AutoAnalyzer. J Pediatr. 1972;81(3):559–61.

32. Cole BR, Giangiacomo J, Ingelfinger JR, Robson AM. Measurement of renal function without urine collection. A critical evaluation of the constant-infusion technic for determination of inulin and para-aminohippurate. N Engl J Med. 1972;287(22):1109–14.

33. Swinkels DW, Hendriks JC, Nauta J, de Jong MC. Glomerular filtration rate by single-injection inulin clearance: definition of a workable protocol for children. Ann Clin Biochem. 2000;37(Pt 1):60–6.

34. Florijn KW, Barendregt JN, Lentjes EG, van Dam W, Prodjosudjadi W, van Saase JL, et al. Glomerular filtration rate measurement by "single-shot" injection of inulin. Kidney Int. 1994;46(1):252–9.

35. van Rossum LK, Cransberg K, de Rijke YB, Zietse R, Lindemans J, Vulto AG. Determination of inulin clearance by single injection or infusion in children. Pediatr Nephrol. 2005;20(6):777–81.

36. Levey AS. Measurement of renal function in chronic renal disease. Kidney Int. 1990;38(1):167–84.

37. Myers GL, Miller WG, Coresh J, Fleming J, Greenberg N, Greene T, et al. Recommendations for improving serum creatinine measurement: a report from the Laboratory Working Group of the National Kidney Disease Education Program. Clin Chem. 2006;52(1):5–18.

38. Schwartz GJ, Brion LP, Spitzer A. The use of plasma creatinine concentration for estimating glomerular filtration rate in infants, children, and adolescents. Pediatr Clin North Am. 1987;34(3):571–90.

39. Atiyeh BA, Dabbagh SS, Gruskin AB. Evaluation of renal function during childhood. Pediatr Rev. 1996;17(5):175–80.

40. Hellerstein S, Berenbom M, Alon US, Warady BA. Creatinine clearance following cimetidine for estimation of glomerular filtration rate. Pediatr Nephrol. 1998;12(1):49–54.

41. van Acker BA, Koomen GC, Koopman MG, de Waart DR, Arisz L. Creatinine clearance during cimetidine administration for measurement of glomerular filtration rate. Lancet. 1992;340(8831):1326–9.

42. Hellerstein S, Berenbom M, DiMaggio S, Erwin P, Simon SD, Wilson N. Comparison of two formulae for estimation of glomerular filtration rate in children. Pediatr Nephrol. 2004;19(7):780–4.

43. Schwartz GJ, Haycock GB, Edelmann Jr CM, Spitzer A. A simple estimate of glomerular filtration rate in children derived from body length and plasma creatinine. Pediatrics. 1976;58(2):259–63.

44. Counahan R, Chantler C, Ghazali S, Kirkwood B, Rose F, Barratt TM. Estimation of glomerular filtration rate from plasma creatinine concentration in children. Arch Dis Child. 1976;51(11):875–8.

45. Schwartz GJ, Furth S, Cole SR, Warady B, Munoz A. Glomerular filtration rate via plasma iohexol disappearance: pilot study for chronic kidney disease in children. Kidney Int. 2006;69(11):2070–7.

46. Schwartz GJ, Work DF. Measurement and estimation of GFR in children and adolescents. Clin J Am Soc Nephrol. 2009;4(11):1832–43.

47. Schwartz GJ, Munoz A, Schneider MF, Mak RH, Kaskel F, Warady BA, et al. New equations to estimate GFR in children with CKD. J Am Soc Nephrol. 2009;20(3):629–37.

48. Schwartz GJ, Schneider MF, Maier PS, Moxey-Mims M, Dharnidharka VR, Warady BA, et al. Improved equations estimating GFR in children with chronic kidney disease using an immunonephelometric determination of cystatin C. Kidney Int. 2012;82(4):445–53.

49. Rule AD, Bergstralh EJ, Slezak JM, Bergert J, Larson TS. Glomerular filtration rate estimated by cystatin C among different clinical presentations. Kidney Int. 2006;69(2):399–405.

50. Finney H, Newman DJ, Price CP. Adult reference ranges for serum cystatin C, creatinine and predicted creatinine clearance. Ann Clin Biochem. 2000;37(Pt 1):49–59.

51. Knight EL, Verhave JC, Spiegelman D, Hillege HL, de Zeeuw D, Curhan GC, et al. Factors influencing serum cystatin C levels other than renal function and the impact on renal function measurement. Kidney Int. 2004;65(4):1416–21.

52. Cimerman N, Brguljan PM, Krasovec M, Suskovic S, Kos J. Serum cystatin C, a potent inhibitor of cysteine proteinases, is elevated in asthmatic patients. Clin Chim Acta. 2000;300(1–2):83–95.

53. Wiesli P, Schwegler B, Spinas GA, Schmid C. Serum cystatin C is sensitive to small changes in thyroid function. Clin Chim Acta. 2003;338(1–2):87–90.

54. Sambasivan AS, Lepage N, Filler G. Cystatin C intrapatient variability in children with chronic kidney disease is less than serum creatinine. Clin Chem. 2005;51(11):2215–16.

55. Zappitelli M, Parvex P, Joseph L, Paradis G, Grey V, Lau S, et al. Derivation and validation of cystatin C-based prediction equations for GFR in children. Am J Kidney Dis. 2006;48(2):221–30.

56. Pottel H, Hoste L, Martens F. A simple height-independent equation for estimating glomerular filtration rate in children. Pediatr Nephrol. 2012;27(6):973–9.

57. Zappitelli M, Zhang X, Foster BJ. Estimating glomerular filtration rate in children at serial follow-up when height is unknown. Clin J Am Soc Nephrol. 2010;5(10):1763–9.

58. Filler G, Priem F, Vollmer I, Gellermann J, Jung K. Diagnostic sensitivity of serum cystatin for impaired glomerular filtration rate. Pediatr Nephrol. 1999;13(6):501–5.

59. Hoste L, Dubourg L, Selistre L, De Souza VC, Ranchin B, Hadj-Aissa A, et al. A new equation to estimate the glomerular filtration rate in children, adolescents and young adults. Nephrol Dial Transplant. 2014;29:1082–91.

60. Blufpand HN, Westland R, van Wijk JA, Roelandse-Koop EA, Kaspers GJ, Bokenkamp A. Height-independent estimation of glomerular filtration rate in children: an alternative to the schwartz equation. J Pediatr. 2013;163(6):1722–7.

61. Gaspari F, Perico N, Ruggenenti P, Mosconi L, Amuchastegui CS, Guerini E, et al. Plasma clearance of nonradioactive iohexol as a measure of glomerular filtration rate. J Am Soc Nephrol. 1995; 6(2):257–63.

62. Stake G, Monn E, Rootwelt K, Monclair T. The clearance of iohexol as a measure of the glomerular filtration rate in children with chronic renal failure. Scand J Clin Lab Invest. 1991;51(8):729–34.

63. Berg UB, Back R, Celsi G, Halling SE, Homberg I, Krmar RT, et al. Comparison of plasma clearance of iohexol and urinary clearance of inulin for measurement of GFR in children. Am J Kidney Dis. 2011;57(1):55–61.

64. Gaspari F, Guerini E, Perico N, Mosconi L, Ruggenenti P, Remuzzi G. Glomerular filtration rate determined from a single plasma sample after intravenous iohexol injection: is it reliable? J Am Soc Nephrol. 1996;7(12):2689–93.

65. Piepsz A, Colarinha P, Gordon I, Hahn K, Olivier P, Sixt R, et al. Guidelines for glomerular filtration rate determination in children. Eur J Nucl Med. 2001;28(3):31–6.

66. Blaufox MD, Aurell M, Bubeck B, Fommei E, Piepsz A, Russell C, et al. Report of the Radionuclides in Nephrourology Committee on renal clearance. J Nucl Med. 1996;37(11):1883–90.

67. Rose B. In: Dereck J, Muza N, editors. Clinical physiology of acid-base and electrolyte disorders. 4th ed. New York: McGraw-Hill; 1994. p. 66–103.

68. Perazella MA, Bomback AS. Urinary eosinophils in AIN: farewell to an old biomarker? Clin J Am Soc Nephrol. 2013;8(11):1841–3.

69. Pepin MN, Bouchard J, Legault L, Ethier J. Diagnostic performance of fractional excretion of urea and fractional excretion of sodium in the evaluations of patients with acute kidney injury with or without diuretic treatment. Am J Kidney Dis. 2007;50(4):566–73.

70. Vanmassenhove J, Glorieux G, Hoste E, Dhondt A, Vanholder R, Van Biesen W. Urinary output and fractional excretion of sodium and urea as indicators of transient versus intrinsic acute kidney injury during early sepsis. Crit Care. 2013;17(5):R234.

71. Bijvoet OL. Relation of plasma phosphate concentration to renal tubular reabsorption of phosphate. Clin Sci. 1969;37(1):23–36.

72. Walton RJ, Bijvoet OL. Nomogram for derivation of renal threshold phosphate concentration. Lancet. 1975;2(7929):309–10.

73. Kenny AP, Glen AC. Tests of phosphate reabsorption. Lancet. 1973;2(7821):158.

74. Barth JH, Jones RG, Payne RB. Calculation of renal tubular reabsorption of phosphate: the algorithm performs better than the nomogram. Ann Clin Biochem. 2000;37(Pt 1):79–81.

75. Hummel CS, Lu C, Loo DD, Hirayama BA, Voss AA, Wright EM. Glucose transport by human renal Na+/D-glucose cotransporters SGLT1 and SGLT2. Am J Physiol Cell Physiol. 2011;300(1):C14–21.

76. Santer R, Kinner M, Schneppenheim R, Hillebrand G, Kemper M, Ehrich J, et al. The molecular basis of renal glucosuria: mutations in the gene for a renal glucose transporter (SGLT2). J Inherit Metab Dis. 2000;23 Suppl 1:178.

77. West ML, Bendz O, Chen CB, Singer GG, Richardson RM, Sonnenberg H, et al. Development of a test to evaluate the transtubular potassium concentration gradient in the cortical collecting duct in vivo. Miner Electrolyte Metab. 1986;12(4):226–33.

78. Rodriguez-Soriano J, Ubetagoyena M, Vallo A. Transtubular potassium concentration gradient: a useful test to estimate renal aldosterone bio-activity in infants and children. Pediatr Nephrol. 1990; 4(2):105–10.

79. Ethier JH, Kamel KS, Magner PO, Lemann Jr J, Halperin ML. The transtubular potassium concentration in patients with hypokalemia and hyperkalemia. Am J Kidney Dis. 1990;15(4):309–15.

80. Choi MJ, Ziyadeh FN. The utility of the transtubular potassium gradient in the evaluation of hyperkalemia. J Am Soc Nephrol. 2008;19(3):424–6.

81. Kamel KS, Halperin ML. Intrarenal urea recycling leads to a higher rate of renal excretion of potassium: an hypothesis with clinical implications. Curr Opin Nephrol Hypertens. 2011;20(5):547–54.

82. Calonge MJ, Gasparini P, Chillaron J, Chillon M, Gallucci M, Rousaud F, et al. Cystinuria caused by mutations in rBAT, a gene involved in the transport of cystine. Nat Genet. 1994;6(4):420–5.

83. Saadi I, Chen XZ, Hediger M, Ong P, Pereira P, Goodyer P, et al. Molecular genetics of cystinuria: mutation analysis of SLC3A1 and evidence for another gene in type I (silent) phenotype. Kidney Int. 1998;54(1):48–55.

84. Kost GJ, Trent JK, Saeed D. Indications for measurement of total carbon dioxide in arterial blood. Clin Chem. 1988;34(8):1650–2.

85. K/DOQI Working Group. K/DOQI Clinical practice guidelines for bone metabolism and disease in children with chronic kidney disease. Am J Kidney Dis. 2005;46(4):12–100.

86. Rees L, Jones H. Nutritional management and growth in children with chronic kidney disease. Pediatr Nephrol. 2013;28(4):527–36.

87. Halperin ML, Kamel KS, Goldstein MB. Fluid, electrolyte, and acid-base physiology : a problem-based approach. 3rd ed. Philadelphia: W.B. Saunders; 2010.

88. Figge J, Jabor A, Kazda A, Fencl V. Anion gap and hypoalbuminemia. Crit Care Med. 1998;26(11): 1807–10.

89. Srivastava T, Garg U, Chan YR, Alon US. Essentials of laboratory medicine for the nephrology clinician. Pediatr Nephrol. 2007;22(2):170–82.

90. Goldstein MB, Bear R, Richardson RM, Marsden PA, Halperin ML. The urine anion gap: a clinically useful index of ammonium excretion. Am J Med Sci. 1986;292(4):198–202.

91. Batlle DC, Hizon M, Cohen E, Gutterman C, Gupta R. The use of the urinary anion gap in the diagnosis

of hyperchloremic metabolic acidosis. N Engl J Med. 1988;318(10):594–9.

92. Halperin ML, Margolis BL, Robinson LA, Halperin RM, West ML, Bear RA. The urine osmolal gap: a clue to estimate urine ammonium in "hybrid" types of metabolic acidosis. Clin Invest Med. 1988;11(3): 198–202.

93. Dyck RF, Asthana S, Kalra J, West ML, Massey KL. A modification of the urine osmolal gap: an improved method for estimating urine ammonium. Am J Nephrol. 1990;10(5):359–62.

94. Halperin ML, Goldstein MB, Haig A, Johnson MD, Stinebaugh BJ. Studies on the pathogenesis of type I (distal) renal tubular acidosis as revealed by the urinary PCO2 tensions. J Clin Invest. 1974;53(3): 669–77.

95. DuBose Jr TD, Caflisch CR. Validation of the difference in urine and blood carbon dioxide tension during bicarbonate loading as an index of distal nephron acidification in experimental models of distal renal tubular acidosis. J Clin Invest. 1985;75(4):1116–23.

96. Kim S, Lee JW, Park J, Na KY, Joo KW, Ahn C, et al. The urine-blood PCO gradient as a diagnostic index of H(+)-ATPase defect distal renal tubular acidosis. Kidney Int. 2004;66(2):761–7.

97. Southcott EK, Kerrigan JL, Potter JM, Telford RD, Waring P, Reynolds GJ, et al. Establishment of pediatric reference intervals on a large cohort of healthy children. Clin Chim Acta. 2010;411(19-20):1421–7.

98. Colantonio DA, Kyriakopoulou L, Chan MK, Daly CH, Brinc D, Venner AA, et al. Closing the gaps in pediatric laboratory reference intervals: a CALIPER database of 40 biochemical markers in a healthy and multiethnic population of children. Clin Chem. 2012;58(5):854–68.

99. Soldin SJ, Brugnara C, Wong EC, editors. Pediatric reference ranges. 4th ed. Washington, DC: AACC Press; 2003.

100. Sevastos N, Theodossiades G, Archimandritis AJ. Pseudohyperkalemia in serum: a new insight into an old phenomenon. Clin Med Res. 2008;6(1):30–2.

101. Asirvatham JR, Moses V, Bjornson L. Errors in potassium measurement: a laboratory perspective for the clinician. N Am J Med Sci. 2013;5(4):255–9.

102. Stewart GW, Corrall RJ, Fyffe JA, Stockdill G, Strong JA. Familial pseudohyperkalaemiaa new syndrome. Lancet. 1979;2(8135):175–7. Epub 1979/07/28.

103. Andolfo I, Alper SL, Delaunay J, Auriemma C, Russo R, Asci R, et al. Missense mutations in the ABCB6 transporter cause dominant familial pseudohyperkalemia. Am J Hematol. 2013;88(1):66–72.

104. Kidney Disease: Improving Global Outcomes (KDIGO) CKD-MBD Work Group. KDIGO clinical practice guideline for the diagnosis, evaluation, prevention, and treatment of chronic kidney disease-mineral and bone disorder (CKD-MBD). Kidney Int Suppl. 2009;76(113):S1–130.

105. Liamis G, Liberopoulos E, Barkas F, Elisaf M. Spurious electrolyte disorders: a diagnostic chal-

lenge for clinicians. Am J Nephrol. 2013;38(1): 50–7.

106. Clinical practice guidelines for nutrition in chronic renal failure. K/DOQI, National Kidney Foundation. Am J Kidney Dis. 2000;35(6 Suppl 2):S1–140.

107. Clifford SM, Bunker AM, Jacobsen JR, Roberts WL. Age and gender specific pediatric reference intervals for aldolase, amylase, ceruloplasmin, creatine kinase, pancreatic amylase, prealbumin, and uric acid. Clin Chim Acta. 2011;412(9-10): 788–90.

108. Fathallah-Shaykh SA, Cramer MT. Uric acid and the kidney. Pediatr Nephrol. 2013;29:999–1008.

109. Cameron JS, Moro F, Simmonds HA. Gout, uric acid and purine metabolism in paediatric nephrology. Pediatr Nephrol. 1993;7(1):105–8.

110. Dahan K, Devuyst O, Smaers M, Vertommen D, Loute G, Poux JM, et al. A cluster of mutations in the UMOD gene causes familial juvenile hyperuricemic nephropathy with abnormal expression of uromodulin. J Am Soc Nephrol. 2003;14(11):2883–93.

111. Zivna M, Hulkova H, Matignon M, Hodanova K, Vylet'al P, Kalbacova M, et al. Dominant renin gene mutations associated with early-onset hyperuricemia, anemia, and chronic kidney failure. Am J Hum Genet. 2009;85(2):204–13.

112. Bingham C, Ellard S, van't Hoff WG, Simmonds HA, Marinaki AM, Badman MK, et al. Atypical familial juvenile hyperuricemic nephropathy associated with a hepatocyte nuclear factor-1beta gene mutation. Kidney Int. 2003;63(5):1645–51.

113. Adalat S, Woolf AS, Johnstone KA, Wirsing A, Harries LW, Long DA, et al. HNF1B mutations associate with hypomagnesemia and renal magnesium wasting. J Am Soc Nephrol. 2009;20(5):1123–31.

114. Noone DG, Marks SD. Hyperuricemia is associated with hypertension, obesity, and albuminuria in children with chronic kidney disease. J Pediatr. 2013;162(1):128–32.

115. Ruilope LM, Pontremoli R. Serum uric acid and cardio-renal diseases. Curr Med Res Opin. 2013;29 Suppl 3:25–31.

116. Feig DI, Johnson RJ. Hyperuricemia in childhood primary hypertension. Hypertension. 2003;42(3):247–52.

117. Yanik M, Feig DI. Serum urate: a biomarker or treatment target in pediatric hypertension? Curr Opin Cardiol. 2013;28(4):433–8.

118. Hamada T, Ichida K, Hosoyamada M, Mizuta E, Yanagihara K, Sonoyama K, et al. Uricosuric action of losartan via the inhibition of urate transporter 1 (URAT 1) in hypertensive patients. Am J Hypertens. 2008;21(10):1157–62.

119. Feig DI, Soletsky B, Johnson RJ. Effect of allopurinol on blood pressure of adolescents with newly diagnosed essential hypertension: a randomized trial. JAMA. 2008;300(8):924–32.

120. Sikora P, Pijanowska M, Majewski M, Bienias B, Borzecka H, Zajczkowska M. Acute renal failure due to bilateral xanthine urolithiasis in a boy with Lesch-Nyhan syndrome. Pediatr Nephrol. 2006;21(7):1045–7.

121. Chao J, Terkeltaub R. A critical reappraisal of allopurinol dosing, safety, and efficacy for hyperuricemia in gout. Curr Rheumatol Rep. 2009;11(2):135–40.

122. Biyikli NK, Alpay H, Guran T. Hypercalciuria and recurrent urinary tract infections: incidence and symptoms in children over 5 years of age. Pediatr Nephrol. 2005;20(10):1435–8.

123. Ghazali S, Barratt TM. Urinary excretion of calcium and magnesium in children. Arch Dis Child. 1974;49(2):97–101.

124. Moore E, Coe F, McMann B, Favus M. Idiopathic hypercalciuria in children: prevalence and metabolic characteristics. J Pediatr. 1978;92(6):906–10.

125. Sorkhi H, Haji Aahmadi M. Urinary calcium to creatinin ratio in children. Indian J Pediatr. 2005; 72(12):1055–6.

126. De Santo NG, Di Iorio B, Capasso G, Paduano C, Stamler R, Langman CB, et al. Population based data on urinary excretion of calcium, magnesium, oxalate, phosphate and uric acid in children from Cimitile (southern Italy). Pediatr Nephrol. 1992;6(2): 149–57.

127. So NP, Osorio AV, Simon SD, Alon US. Normal urinary calcium/creatinine ratios in African-American and Caucasian children. Pediatr Nephrol. 2001;16(2): 133–9.

128. Vachvanichsanong P, Lebel L, Moore ES. Urinary calcium excretion in healthy Thai children. Pediatr Nephrol. 2000;14(8–9):847–50.

129. Butani L, Kalia A. Idiopathic hypercalciuria in children – how valid are the existing diagnostic criteria? Pediatr Nephrol. 2004;19(6):577–82.

130. Hilgenfeld MS, Simon S, Blowey D, Richmond W, Alon US. Lack of seasonal variations in urinary calcium/creatinine ratio in school-age children. Pediatr Nephrol. 2004;19(10):1153–5.

131. Richmond W, Colgan G, Simon S, Stuart-Hilgenfeld M, Wilson N, Alon US. Random urine calcium/osmolality in the assessment of calciuria in children with decreased muscle mass. Clin Nephrol. 2005;64(4):264–70.

132. Mir S, Serdaroglu E. Quantification of hypercalciuria with the urine calcium osmolality ratio in children. Pediatr Nephrol. 2005;20(11):1562–5.

133. Polito C, La Manna A, Maiello R, Nappi B, Siciliano MC, Di Domenico MR, et al. Urinary sodium and potassium excretion in idiopathic hypercalciuria of children. Nephron. 2002;91(1):7–12.

134. Bray GA, Vollmer WM, Sacks FM, Obarzanek E, Svetkey LP, Appel LJ. A further subgroup analysis of the effects of the DASH diet and three dietary sodium levels on blood pressure: results of the DASH-Sodium trial. Am J Cardiol. 2004;94(2): 222–7.

135. Tefekli A, Esen T, Ziylan O, Erol B, Armagan A, Ander H, et al. Metabolic risk factors in pediatric and adult calcium oxalate urinary stone formers: is there any difference? Urol Int. 2003;70(4):273–7.

136. Matos V, van Melle G, Boulat O, Markert M, Bachmann C, Guignard JP. Urinary phosphate/creatinine, calcium/creatinine, and magnesium/creatinine ratios in a healthy pediatric population. J Pediatr. 1997;131(2):252–7.

137. Hoppe B, Langman CB. Hypocitraturia in patients with urolithiasis. Arch Dis Child. 1997;76(2): 174–5.

138. Hoppe B, Jahnen A, Bach D, Hesse A. Urinary calcium oxalate saturation in healthy infants and children. J Urol. 1997;158(2):557–9.

139. Karabacak OR, Ipek B, Ozturk U, Demirel F, Saltas H, Altug U. Metabolic evaluation in stone disease metabolic differences between the pediatric and adult patients with stone disease. Urology. 2010; 76(1):238–41.

140. DeFoor WR, Jackson E, Minevich E, Caillat A, Reddy P, Sheldon C, et al. The risk of recurrent urolithiasis in children is dependent on urinary calcium and citrate. Urology. 2010;76(1):242–5.

141. Arrabal-Polo MA, Arrabal-Martin M, Arias-Santiago S, Garrido-Gomez J, Poyatos-Andujar A, Zuluaga-Gomez A. Importance of citrate and the calcium : citrate ratio in patients with calcium renal lithiasis and severe lithogenesis. BJU Int. 2013; 111(4):622–7.

142. Sikora P, Roth B, Kribs A, Michalk DV, Hesse A, Hoppe B. Hypocitraturia is one of the major risk factors for nephrocalcinosis in very low birth weight (VLBW) infants. Kidney Int. 2003;63(6):2194–9.

143. Stapenhorst L, Sassen R, Beck B, Laube N, Hesse A, Hoppe B. Hypocitraturia as a risk factor for nephrocalcinosis after kidney transplantation. Pediatr Nephrol. 2005;20(5):652–6.

144. Hoppe B. An update on primary hyperoxaluria. Nat Rev Nephrol. 2012;8(8):467–75.

145. Cochat P, Rumsby G. Primary hyperoxaluria. N Engl J Med. 2013;369(7):649–58.

146. Belostotsky R, Seboun E, Idelson GH, Milliner DS, Becker-Cohen R, Rinat C, et al. Mutations in DHDPSL are responsible for primary hyperoxaluria type III. Am J Hum Genet. 2010;87(3):392–9.

147. Matos V, Van Melle G, Werner D, Bardy D, Guignard JP. Urinary oxalate and urate to creatinine ratios in a healthy pediatric population. Am J Kidney Dis. 1999;34(2):e1.

148. La Manna A, Polito C, Marte A, Iovene A, Di Toro R. Hyperuricosuria in children: clinical presentation and natural history. Pediatrics. 2001;107(1):86–90.

149. Stapleton FB, Nash DA. A screening test for hyperuricosuria. J Pediatr. 1983;102(1):88–90.

150. Azizi M, Menard J. Review: measurement of plasma renin: a critical review of methodology. J Renin Angiotensin Aldosterone Syst JRAAS. 2010;11(2):89–90.

151. Dillon MJ, Ryness JM. Plasma renin activity and aldosterone concentration in children. Br Med J. 1975;4(5992):316–19.

152. Olson N, DeJongh B, Hough A, Parra D. Plasma renin activity-guided strategy for the management of hypertension. Pharmacotherapy. 2012;32(5):446–55.

153. Dillon MJ. The diagnosis of renovascular disease. Pediatr Nephrol. 1997;11(3):366–72.

154. Tash JA, Stock JA, Hanna MK. The role of partial nephrectomy in the treatment of pediatric renal hypertension. J Urol. 2003;169(2):625–8.

155. Goonasekera CD, Shah V, Wade AM, Dillon MJ. The usefulness of renal vein renin studies in hypertensive children: a 25-year experience. Pediatr Nephrol. 2002;17(11):943–9.

156. McLaren CA, Roebuck DJ. Interventional radiology for renovascular hypertension in children. Tech Vasc Interv Radiol. 2003;6(4):150–7.

157. Dillon MJ, Shah V, Barratt TM. Renal vein renin measurements in children with hypertension. Br Med J. 1978;2(6131):168–70.

158. White PC. Disorders of aldosterone biosynthesis and action. N Engl J Med. 1994;331(4):250–8.

159. Whitworth JA. Mechanisms of glucocorticoid-induced hypertension. Kidney Int. 1987;31(5):1213–24.

160. Stowasser M, Ahmed AH, Pimenta E, Taylor PJ, Gordon RD. Factors affecting the aldosterone/renin ratio. Hormone and metabolic research = Hormon- und Stoffwechselforschung = Hormones et metabolisme. Horm Metab Res. 2012;44(3):170–6.

161. Blumenfeld JD, Sealey JE, Schlussel Y, Vaughan Jr ED, Sos TA, Atlas SA, et al. Diagnosis and treatment of primary hyperaldosteronism. Ann Intern Med. 1994;121(11):877–85.

162. Walport MJ. Complement. First of two parts. N Engl J Med. 2001;344(14):1058–66.

163. Walport MJ. Complement. Second of two parts. N Engl J Med. 2001;344(15):1140–4.

164. Thurman JM, Holers VM. The central role of the alternative complement pathway in human disease. J Immunol. 2006;176(3):1305–10.

165. Huber-Lang M, Sarma JV, Zetoune FS, Rittirsch D, Neff TA, McGuire SR, et al. Generation of C5a in the absence of C3: a new complement activation pathway. Nat Med. 2006;12(6):682–7.

166. Vernon KA, Cook HT. Complement in glomerular disease. Adv Chronic Kidney Dis. 2012;19(2): 84–92.

167. Hebert LA, Cosio FG, Neff JC. Diagnostic significance of hypocomplementemia. Kidney Int. 1991; 39(5):811–21.

168. Harboe M, Thorgersen EB, Mollnes TE. Advances in assay of complement function and activation. Adv Drug Deliv Rev. 2011;63(12):976–87.

169. Mollnes TE, Jokiranta TS, Truedsson L, Nilsson B, Rodriguez de Cordoba S, Kirschfink M. Complement analysis in the 21st century. Mol Immunol. 2007;44(16):3838–49.

170. Dragon-Durey MA, Blanc C, Marinozzi MC, van Schaarenburg RA, Trouw LA. Autoantibodies against complement components and functional consequences. Mol Immunol. 2013;56(3):213–21.

171. Botto M, Kirschfink M, Macor P, Pickering MC, Wurzner R, Tedesco F. Complement in human diseases: lessons from complement deficiencies. Mol Immunol. 2009;46(14):2774–83.

172. Malina M, Roumenina LT, Seeman T, Le Quintrec M, Dragon-Durey MA, Schaefer F, et al. Genetics of hemolytic uremic syndromes. Presse Med. 2012; 41(3 Pt 2):e105–14.

173. Davies DJ, Moran JE, Niall JF, Ryan GB. Segmental necrotising glomerulonephritis with antineutrophil antibody: possible arbovirus aetiology? Br Med J (Clin Res Ed). 1982;285(6342):606.

174. Savige J, Gillis D, Benson E, Davies D, Esnault V, Falk RJ, et al. International consensus statement on testing and reporting of antineutrophil cytoplasmic antibodies (ANCA). Am J Clin Pathol. 1999;111(4): 507–13.

175. Elena C. L28. Relevance of detection techniques for ANCA testing. Presse Med. 2013;42(4 Pt 2):582–4.

176. Csernok E. ANCA testing: the current stage and perspectives. Clin Exp Nephrol. 2013;17(5):615–18.

177. Radice A, Bianchi L, Sinico RA. Anti-neutrophil cytoplasmic autoantibodies: methodological aspects and clinical significance in systemic vasculitis. Autoimmun Rev. 2013;12(4):487–95.

178. Mandl LA, Solomon DH, Smith EL, Lew RA, Katz JN, Shmerling RH. Using antineutrophil cytoplasmic antibody testing to diagnose vasculitis: can test-ordering guidelines improve diagnostic accuracy? Arch Intern Med. 2002;162(13):1509–14.

179. van der Woude FJ, Rasmussen N, Lobatto S, Wiik A, Permin H, van Es LA, et al. Autoantibodies against neutrophils and monocytes: tool for diagnosis and marker of disease activity in Wegener's granulomatosis. Lancet. 1985;1(8426):425–9.

180. Sinclair D, Stevens JM. Role of antineutrophil cytoplasmic antibodies and glomerular basement membrane antibodies in the diagnosis and monitoring of systemic vasculitides. Ann Clin Biochem. 2007;44(Pt 5):432–42.

181. Birck R, Schmitt WH, Kaelsch IA, van der Woude FJ. Serial ANCA determinations for monitoring disease activity in patients with ANCA-associated vasculitis: systematic review. Am J Kidney Dis. 2006;47(1):15–23.

182. Bosch X, Guilabert A, Font J. Antineutrophil cytoplasmic antibodies. Lancet. 2006;368(9533): 404–18.

183. Tomasson G, Grayson PC, Mahr AD, Lavalley M, Merkel PA. Value of ANCA measurements during remission to predict a relapse of ANCA-associated vasculitis – a meta-analysis. Rheumatology (Oxford). 2012;51(1):100–9.

184. Flossmann O, Berden A, de Groot K, Hagen C, Harper L, Heijl C, et al. Long-term patient survival in ANCA-associated vasculitis. Ann Rheum Dis. 2011;70(3):488–94.

185. Sinico RA, Di Toma L, Radice A. Renal involvement in anti-neutrophil cytoplasmic autoantibody associated vasculitis. Autoimmun Rev. 2013;12(4):477–82.

186. Walsh M, Flossmann O, Berden A, Westman K, Hoglund P, Stegeman C, et al. Risk factors for relapse

of antineutrophil cytoplasmic antibody-associated vasculitis. Arthritis Rheum. 2012;64(2):542–8.

187. Sanders JS, Stassen PM, van Rossum AP, Kallenberg CG, Stegeman CA. Risk factors for relapse in antineutrophil cytoplasmic antibody (ANCA)-associated vasculitis: tools for treatment decisions? Clin Exp Rheumatol. 2004;22(6 Suppl 36):S94–101.

188. Sanders JS, Huitma MG, Kallenberg CG, Stegeman CA. Prediction of relapses in PR3-ANCA-associated vasculitis by assessing responses of ANCA titres to treatment. Rheumatology (Oxford). 2006;45(6):724–9.

189. Roth AJ, Ooi JD, Hess JJ, van Timmeren MM, Berg EA, Poulton CE, et al. Epitope specificity determines pathogenicity and detectability in ANCA-associated vasculitis. J Clin Invest. 2013;123(4):1773–83.

190. Gou SJ, Xu PC, Chen M, Zhao MH. Epitope analysis of anti-myeloperoxidase antibodies in patients with ANCA-associated vasculitis. PLoS One. 2013;8(4):e60530.

191. Kain R, Exner M, Brandes R, Ziebermayr R, Cunningham D, Alderson CA, et al. Molecular mimicry in pauci-immune focal necrotizing glomerulonephritis. Nat Med. 2008;14(10):1088–96.

192. Kain R, Matsui K, Exner M, Binder S, Schaffner G, Sommer EM, et al. A novel class of autoantigens of anti-neutrophil cytoplasmic antibodies in necrotizing and crescentic glomerulonephritis: the lysosomal membrane glycoprotein h-lamp-2 in neutrophil granulocytes and a related membrane protein in glomerular endothelial cells. J Exp Med. 1995;181(2):585–97.

193. Kain R, Tadema H, McKinney EF, Benharkou A, Brandes R, Peschel A, et al. High prevalence of autoantibodies to hLAMP-2 in anti-neutrophil cytoplasmic antibody-associated vasculitis. J Am Soc Nephrol. 2012;23(3):556–66.

194. Roth AJ, Brown MC, Smith RN, Badhwar AK, Parente O, Chung H, et al. Anti-LAMP-2 antibodies are not prevalent in patients with antineutrophil cytoplasmic autoantibody glomerulonephritis. J Am Soc Nephrol. 2012;23(3):545–55.

195. Kain R. L29. Relevance of anti-LAMP-2 in vasculitis: why the controversy. Presse Med. 2013;42(4 Pt 2):584–8.

196. Saisoong S, Eiam-Ong S, Hanvivatvong O. Correlations between antinucleosome antibodies and anti-double-stranded DNA antibodies, C3, C4, and clinical activity in lupus patients. Clin Exp Rheumatol. 2006;24(1):51–8.

197. Malleson PN, Sailer M, Mackinnon MJ. Usefulness of antinuclear antibody testing to screen for rheumatic diseases. Arch Dis Child. 1997;77(4):299–304.

198. Satoh M, Chan EK, Ho LA, Rose KM, Parks CG, Cohn RD, et al. Prevalence and sociodemographic correlates of antinuclear antibodies in the United States. Arthritis Rheum. 2012;64(7):2319–27.

199. Pisetsky DS. Antinuclear antibodies in rheumatic disease: a proposal for a function-based classification. Scand J Immunol. 2012;76(3):223–8.

200. Servais G, Karmali R, Guillaume MP, Badot V, Duchateau J, Corazza F. Anti DNA antibodies are not restricted to a specific pattern of fluorescence on HEp2 cells. Clin Chem Lab Med. 2009;47(5):543–9.

201. Frodlund M, Dahlstrom O, Kastbom A, Skogh T, Sjowall C. Associations between antinuclear antibody staining patterns and clinical features of systemic lupus erythematosus: analysis of a regional Swedish register. BMJ Open. 2013;3(10): e003608.

202. Mariz HA, Sato EI, Barbosa SH, Rodrigues SH, Dellavance A, Andrade LE. Pattern on the antinuclear antibody-HEp-2 test is a critical parameter for discriminating antinuclear antibody-positive healthy individuals and patients with autoimmune rheumatic diseases. Arthritis Rheum. 2011;63(1):191–200.

203. Fritzler MJ. The antinuclear antibody test: last or lasting gasp? Arthritis Rheum. 2011;63(1):19–22.

204. Haynes DC, Gershwin ME, Robbins DL, Miller 3rd JJ, Cosca D. Autoantibody profiles in juvenile arthritis. J Rheumatol. 1986;13(2):358–63.

205. Cabral DA, Petty RE, Fung M, Malleson PN. Persistent antinuclear antibodies in children without identifiable inflammatory rheumatic or autoimmune disease. Pediatrics. 1992;89(3):441–4.

206. Tan EM, Feltkamp TE, Smolen JS, Butcher B, Dawkins R, Fritzler MJ, et al. Range of antinuclear antibodies in "healthy" individuals. Arthritis Rheum. 1997;40(9):1601–11.

207. Abeles AM, Abeles M. The clinical utility of a positive antinuclear antibody test result. Am J Med. 2013;126(4):342–8.

208. Marks SD, Tullus K. Autoantibodies in systemic lupus erythematosus. Pediatr Nephrol. 2012;27(10): 1855–68.

209. Cervera R, Vinas O, Ramos-Casals M, Font J, Garcia-Carrasco M, Siso A, et al. Anti-chromatin antibodies in systemic lupus erythematosus: a useful marker for lupus nephropathy. Ann Rheum Dis. 2003;62(5):431–4.

210. Pickering MC, Botto M. Are anti-C1q antibodies different from other SLE autoantibodies? Nat Rev Rheumatol. 2010;6(8):490–3.

Genetic Diagnosis of Renal Diseases: Basic Concepts and Testing

4

Aoife Waters and Mathieu Lemaire

In an age of competing medical priorities why should health-care professionals who are already overloaded with information develop core competencies in genetics and genomics? [1]

Introduction

Over the past decade, remarkable advances have been made in our understanding of the human genome through the development of genotyping arrays and next-generation sequencing techniques. These technological advances have allowed us to examine the consequences of various types of genomic variations on the phenotype of patients in an unparalleled manner. Identification of mutations in novel genes associated with rare renal diseases has forced dramatic pathophysiologic revisions owing to discovery of links to unexpected biochemical pathways or structural scaffolds. These provide not only a firm molecular diagnosis for hitherto "idiopathic" conditions, but also offer hope for

new therapeutic strategies for diseases that would otherwise have an unfavorable prognosis. The last few years have have witnessed great improvements in our understanding of the role of common genetic variation in the pathogenesis of complex renal diseases, although the promises of clinical utility are far from reality [2]. In this chapter, we will outline recent developments made in various fields related to genomic medicine, with a particular emphasis on how these will translate into the daily clinical practice of pediatric nephrologists.

General Genetic/Genomic Concepts

Deoxyribonucleic Acid (DNA)

In 1962, the Nobel Prize in Medicine was awarded to Watson and Crick together with Maurice Wilkins for their discovery of the structure of deoxyribonucleic acid (DNA). DNA is a critical participant in the execution and regulation of biological processes that are critical for living organisms to develop and survive. Constituting the double helix structure of DNA are two twisting, paired strands which are packed full with information via the systematic arrangement of four nucleotide bases – adenine (A), thymine (T), guanine (G), and cytosine (C) – the "genetic alphabet" [3]. Opposite strands anneal together in a very specific way, via the pairing of bases: A binds to T, and C to G. If one strand's

A. Waters (✉)
Department of Nephrology, Hospital NHS
Foundation Trust, Great Ormond Street,
London WC1N 3JH, UK
e-mail: aoife.waters@ucl.ac.uk

M. Lemaire (✉)
Division of Nephrology, The Hospital for
Sick Children Scientist-track Investigator,
Sick Kids Research Institute, 686 BAy street,
Toronto M5G0A4, Canada
e-mail: mathieu.lemaire@sickkids.ca

© Springer-Verlag Berlin Heidelberg 2016
D.F. Geary, F. Schaefer (eds.), *Pediatric Kidney Disease*, DOI 10.1007/978-3-662-52972-0_4

nucleotide sequence reads ATTCGG, the other strand will read TAAGCC; these are referred to as the positive and negative strands, respectively.

Gene

A gene refers to segments of DNA that carries the sequencing code for all the building blocks necessary for cells to thrive. Two sequential processes are key: transcription and translation. Transcription is the process by which a ribonucleic acid (RNA) strand is made to match exactly all nucleotides that make up a particular gene. It is critical to preserve both nucleotide identity and order because it is a key determinant of the function of RNAs. The most well-known RNA molecules made this way are messenger RNA (mRNA), which are the key players in the translation (or encoding) of proteins. During this process, which occurs in ribosomes, the sequence of mRNA molecules is read in triplets of nucleotides, known as codons, and this specifies which amino acid is added next during protein synthesis (Fig. 4.1). The recent discoveries of a dizzying array of non-coding RNA

molecules have added an unexpected level of complexity: the RNA world is much more than mRNAs. We are only starting to understand how these non-coding RNAs carry cellular functions by themselves, without requiring translation into proteins.

Genome

A genome represents an organism's complete DNA sequence. The Human Genome Project, an international effort to sequence the entire human genome (six billion nucleotides), was completed in 2001 after more than 10 years of work and billions in research funding [4]. DNA from 13 anonymous individuals of European descent was used to build what is now referred to as the human reference genome. In principle, the human reference genome should be a repository containing a representative whole genome sequence for a prototypical human. Following publication of the draft sequence in 2001, a high-quality reference sequence followed in 2004 and has been succeeded by ongoing efforts through the Genome Reference Consortium to improve the quality and

1st base	2nd base					3rd base
	T	C	A	G		
T	TTT (Phe/F) Phenylalanine	TCT	TAT (Tyr/Y) Tyrosine	TGT (Cys/C) Cysteine		T
	TTC	TCC	TAC	TGC		C
	TTA	TCA (Ser/S) Serine	TAA (X) stop	TGA (X) stop		A
	TTG	TCG	TAG (X) stop	TGG (Trp/W) Tryptophan		G
C	CTT (Leu/L) Leucine	CCT	CAT (His/H) Histidine	CGT (Arg/R) Arginine		T
	CTC	CCC (Pro/P) Proline	CAC	CGC		C
	CTA	CCA	CAA (Gln/Q) Glutamine	CGA		A
	CTG	CCG	CAG	CGG		G
A	ATT (Ile/I) Isoleucine	ACT	AAT (Asn/N) Aspargine	AGT (Ser/S) Serine		T
	ATC	ACC (Thr/T) Threonine	AAC	AGC		C
	ATA	ACA	AAA (Lys/K) Lysine	AGA (Arg/R) Arginine		A
	ATG (Met/M) Methionine	ACG	AAG	AGG		G
G	GTT (Val/V) Valine	GCT	GAT (Asp/D) Aspartic acid	GGT (Gly/G) Glycine		T
	GTC	GCC (Ala/A) Alanine	GAC	GGC		C
	GTA	GCA	GAA (Glu/E) Glumatic acid	GGA		A
	GTG	GCG	GAG	GGG		G

Amino acid properties
■ Nonpolar
  Polar
■ Basic
■ Acidic
■ Nonsense

Fig. 4.1 DNA codons and associated amino acids. The three nucleotides (codons) that make up the 20 different amino acids (and stop signal) are presented, along with the single-letter data-base codes. To obtain the various codons, one simply needs to integrate the value of the first (*left*), second (*top*) and third (*right*) bases. To obtain the RNA codons, Key properties of amino acids are indicated in the *color* legend at the *right* (Source: Modified from Wikipedia, http://en.wikipedia.org/wiki/DNA_codon_table. Creative Commons Attribution-ShareAlike 3.0 Unported License)

coverage of low-complexity, repetitive, and hard to resolve regions.

Whilst the exact number of genes remains unknown, current estimates yield approximately ~20,000 protein-coding genes that reside in only about 1 % of the human genome. Further constituents of the genome include RNA genes, regulatory sequences, and repetitive DNA sequences. Ongoing research by the Encyclopedia of DNA Elements (ENCODE) project suggests that ~80 % of the human genome is functionally active: non-protein coding DNA must be implicated in a significant number of regulatory processes including gene-gene regulation, gene-protein interaction and the transcription of non-translated RNA.

Genetic vs. Genomic

It is now common, but incorrect, to use the terms "Genetic" and "Genomic" as synonyms. The former refers to investigations restricted to a small number of genes at once, while the latter applies to tests that involve genome-wide interrogations.

Other Omics

There is now an increasing number of other "omics" sciences being actively developed in parallel to and in conjunction with genomics, such as proteomics, transcriptomics and metabolomics. It is, however, beyond the scope of this chapter to cover these in any details. These topics are expertly covered in Chap. 6.

Online Resources
Human Genetics: http://goo.gl/mTvVJt;
Pedigree: http://goo.gl/mTvVJt;
Broad Institute videos: http://goo.gl/rkpCBv

Variations in the Genome

Several different classes of DNA sequence variations are observed when comparing the genomes of different individuals. A variation may also be classified as a mutation which is defined as a change of the nucleotide sequence when compared to the Human reference genome; a mutation is not necessarily pathogenic. These alterations may be caused by a number of mechanisms, including unrepaired DNA damage (caused by mutagens such as radiation or chemicals), DNA polymerase errors during replication, or insertion or deletion of DNA segments by mobile genetic elements. Below, we will describe the different kinds of mutations after a short discussion on their key characteristics. Implicit to these discussions is that these mutations are all germline, which means that all cells of an individual carry the mutation, and this mutation is passed on to subsequent generations according to Mendel's law of allele segregation. This is in contrast to somatic mutations that are only present in a restricted subset of cells. This topic, which is most relevant to cancer genetics, will not be covered further here; interested readers are directed to a recent review [5].

How to Assess Genomic Variations

One of the key features that will allow genomic medicine to flourish in the clinic is the ability to reliably assess whether a given mutation is likely to affect protein function or not. When appraising a particular mutation, there are a number of important characteristics to consider. Below, we will briefly describe four such characteristics, including frequency, location, mutation type and conservation. This section introduces many key concepts that will be used frequently throughout this chapter. Please refer to Fig. 4.2 for an illustration of the various concepts.

Is the Allele Common or Rare?
The first consideration is to assess how frequent is the mutation observed in the general population. The most useful piece of information to do this is the minor allele frequency (MAF), which is calculated by dividing the number of mutant alleles in a sample by the number of wild type alleles (each individuals has two alleles since human are diploid organisms). MAF data for common variants are easily retrieved from online databases such as dbSNP [6]. A common variant

Fig. 4.2 An approach to assess a mutation. We present a simple workflow to assess mutations that include four steps. These are based on allele frequency, mutation location and type and degree of conservation. *Underlined terminal nodes* indicate the mutations most likely to cause human diseases

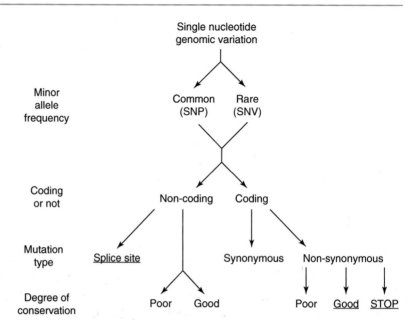

is distinguished from rare ones when the MAF is between 1 and 49 % (the major allele frequency is always >50 %). This concept is important because common mutations are expected to have low probability to cause untoward effects when compared to rare ones. Indeed, natural selection should eventually lead to the gradual elimination of all deleterious alleles that affect reproductive fitness (i.e., the ability to procreate).

Coding vs. Non-coding

The second distinction relates to the location of the mutation in the genome: is it in a region that is involved in protein coding or not? Because we have rich knowledge about protein-coding DNA (exons) and their functions, most studies and clinical tests tend to focus on these regions of the genome, collectively known as the exome. "Non-coding" DNA, which is comprised of intronic and intergenic segments, does not contain only "junk" DNA as this is where one finds a host of regulatory elements such as promoters, enhancers, silencers and insulators, as well as microRNAs. There is mounting evidence that there is in fact no such thing as junk DNA as 80 % of the entire genome plays an important role one way or another [7].

There is one type of intronic mutations that have a special status in clinical genetics: splice site mutations that change key nucleotides in one of the specific sites that are critical for splicing introns during the processing of precursor mRNA into mature mRNA. Abolishment of a splicing site results in retention of introns in mature mRNA molecules and lead to the production of aberrant proteins.

Mutation Type

Third, it is important to determine if an exonic mutation will result in the insertion of different amino acid in the encoded protein, in which case it is referred to as a non-synonymous substitution (Fig. 4.3). These changes are important in clinical genetics because they are most likely to alter the function of the encoded protein. To determine if a non-synonymous mutation may be pathologic, one needs to assess if the physicochemical properties of the original amino acid are preserved (size, charge, and polarity) and also the degree of amino acid conservation (see next section).

There are three instances where a substitution will be expected to be deleterious without requiring these analyses. First, changing any amino acids to a nonsense (or stop) codon will result in

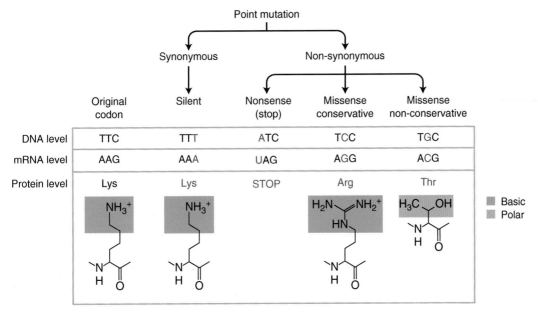

Fig. 4.3 Different types of point mutations. This figure illustrates how a single point mutation in a given codon can change the encoded amino acid in many ways. A conservative missense mutation is one that keep some or all of the original amino acid properties intact (Source: Modified from Wikipedia: http://goo.gl/cTHdD9. GNU Free Documentation License, Version 1.2)

the production of a truncated protein. Second, substituting a start codon (which is always a methionine) for any other amino acid will cause problems because protein translation cannot be initiated properly: no protein is produced. Third, any mutations at a stop codon will also cause problems because the protein made will be longer than the wild type, and as a result will include extra amino acids that may interfere with the proper function of the protein.

Mutations that do not result in an amino acid change are referred to as a synonymous variants; this is possible because many amino acids are generated from different codons (Fig. 4.1). They are also known as silent mutations since in most instances (but not always [8]), they have little to no effect on the function of the encoded proteins.

Degree of Conservation

Finally, one needs to determine if the mutation occurs at a genomic position that is highly conserved when compared to the genomes of other species. It is possible to do this comparison rapidly since we have the entire genomic sequences of many different species (e.g., from humans to mice, frog, and fruit fly). This analysis is most meaningful for coding segments because one can directly compare the amino acid sequences of the same protein made by different organisms (orthologs).

Such comparisons support the notion that the degree of interspecies amino acid variation is indirectly proportional to the functional importance of the amino acid. For example, key residues within the catalytic domain of protein kinases are conserved as a functional unit amongst all kinases of any species [9]. Kinases are enzymes that transfer a phosphate group from ATP to tyrosine, serine or threonine residues on target proteins. It is also possible to assess the degree of conservation for mutations occurring in non-coding regions, but it is a much more challenging exercise because nearly all positions are poorly conserved across species (the exceptions are the small regulatory elements) [10].

Single Nucleotide Polymorphisms

Strictly speaking, a SNP is single base substitution at a specific genomic locus which makes this position different from that of the Human Reference Genome. However, common usage has SNP also defined as a "common variant" on the basis on a population minor allele frequency of >1%. Single nucleotide mutations may occur anywhere in the genome. That the bulk of SNPs are located in non-coding segments is hardly surprising since they constitute ~99% of the genome. As discussed above, the vast majority of SNPs have long been thought to be benign because they are so common. However, lack of clear clinical significance does not mean that SNPs are useless, far from it.

Over the years, geneticists have long used a variety of genetic markers to study human genetic variation with greater depth and accuracy. SNPs emerged as the genetic marker of choice around 2000. It was preceded by three other "generations" of markers: restriction length fragment polymorphisms (~1980), variable number of tandem repeat (~1985), and short tandem repeat polymorphism (~1989) [11]. The rise of SNPs as markers is in large part due to the momentum created by the HapMap project, which aimed to catalogue millions of SNPs in hundreds of subjects from many ethnicities [12]. This resulted in marked improvements in the reliability, efficiency and costs of high throughput SNP genotyping (see section below).

SNPs proved to be invaluable to study haplotype patterns in humans. Haplotypes are genomic segments on a chromosome that are defined by a combination of alleles that are consistently inherited together [13]. This phenomenon is termed linkage disequilibrium (LD) since these alleles are linked to each other more often than not because recombination events occur outside of the LD block. Because of the low diversity of genetic variation within LD blocks, genotyping a subset of SNPs provides a fingerprint of the underlying haplotype without having to genotype all alleles: these are known as "tag SNPs" [12]. The concepts described here will be useful for the sections on linkage analysis, homozygosity mapping and genome-wide associations.

Online Resources
dbSNP: http://www.ncbi.nlm.nih.gov/SNP/;
HapMap: http://hapmap.ncbi.nlm.nih.gov

Single Nucleotide Variants

Single nucleotide variants (SNV) are rare mutations, defined as minor allele frequency of <1% in the general population. As a whole, SNVs are scattered throughout the genome and include both synonymous and non-synonymous variants. When comparing non-synonymous SNPs and SNVs, the latter are much more likely to be at well-conserved positions (or damaging) than their counterpart. As a result, it is not surprising that highly penetrant disease-causing variants for monogenic conditions are overwhelmingly non-synonymous SNVs. More in-depth discussion of SNVs will be provided below in the section of Mendelian conditions.

When dealing with a rare condition, one needs to determine whether the mutation is truly rare (or novel) by interrogating a variety of publicly available variant databases such as dbSNP [6]. Most of these resources have been generated using samples from subjects of European descent. As a result, interpretation of variants from patients that are not "European" is problematic because usually one does not have access to the optimal control group. This phenomenon, called population stratification, makes the search for pathogenic mutations more challenging because variants that are common in one population may be rare (or even absent) in another. Hence, the validity of the interpretation of pathogenicity for a given variant is deeply impacted by the patient's ethnic background. The magnitude of this problem will be lessened as more non-European subjects are sequenced through various efforts worldwide (such as the 1000 Genomes Project [14]).

An additional layer of complexity comes from the fact that reported ethnicity is notoriously unreliable. This is particularly true in localities where multiethnic families are common: the genetic make-up of your patient may be much more complex than being "European" (a concept often referred to as genomic admixture) [15]. To circumvent this problem, researchers use unbiased measures of ethnicity that relies on the SNP genotyping data (such as principal components analysis) [16]; this approach is, however, not routinely used by clinical diagnostic laboratories.

Structural Variations

Structural variation is defined as any genomic change that does not implicate a single base substitution. Recent data show that at least 5000–10,000 structural differences will be found when comparing the genomes of two unrelated individuals [17]. dbVar is a database equivalent to dbSNP, but for variants >50 bp in length [18]. Below, we will briefly describe the most common types of structural variations while also providing, whenever possible, examples from the renal literature. While we are only starting to grasp the magnitude, complexity and ramifications of structural variations on human biology and disease, we believe it worthwhile for pediatricians to familiarize themselves with these topics since these will undoubtedly become "household" terminology in the clinic in the near future.

Small Insertions and Deletions

There are three types of structural variations that involve short genomic segments (typically, from a few to thousands of base pairs). These include situations where nucleotides are either added or removed, which are respectively known as insertions and deletions. A duplication is a special type of insertion because it involves the addition of specific nucleotide sequence that already exists in the vicinity. The distinction between small and large structural events (discussed in the next section) is somewhat arbitrary.

For events involving very short segments that are located within an exon, whether such an alteration is deleterious or not for proteins depends largely on the number of nucleotides involved. If it is a multiple of 3 (for example, insertion of AGGACG), it simply adds a few extra amino acids to the protein (in this case, arginine "AGG" and threonine "ACG") since codons are made of three nucleotides. This type of alteration is usually benign because it does not alter the way the mRNA sequence is "read" after the insertion (i.e., the amino acid sequence of rest of the protein is unchanged). If it is not a multiple of 3 (for example, insertion of a single A), it dramatically changes the way the mRNA sequence is interpreted: this shifts the reading frame of the mRNA, resulting in early termination of translation, and production of a truncated protein (Fig. 4.4a) [19].

Frameshift mutations are commonly found in genes known to cause Mendelian conditions affecting the kidney. Insertion of a single cystine residue in the gene mucin1 (MUC1) was recently found in multiple unrelated families with medullary cystic kidney disease type 1 using a unique combination of sequencing and bioinformatic techniques [19]. What is fascinating about this story is that while multiple linkage studies pointed to a small genomic segment on chromosome 1 (where MUC1 is located) [21], the disease-causing mutations remained elusive even to next-generation sequencing approaches. Indeed, for all families, the C insertion lies in an exon that is enriched in C residues, thereby making it very difficult to tease out bone fide mutations from sequencing errors (Fig. 4.4b).

For events involving slightly larger segments (for example, deletion of exons 6 and 7), the functional consequences are related to either absence of an important domain (these exons contain a kinase domain) or to aberrant tertiary protein structure (direct linking of exons 5 and 8 results in a misfolded protein). Small deletions have been described in patients with Alport syndrome [22]. A large duplication of complement factor H-related protein 5 gene (CFHR5) genes have been described in patients with C3 glomerulopathy [23, 24].

Copy Number Variations

Large-scale insertions, duplication or deletions are collectively referred to as copy number variants (CNV; Fig. 4.4c). They are detected using the same microarray-based technologies used for GWAS studies [25]. Most CNVs are predicted to be benign since the majority are common in the

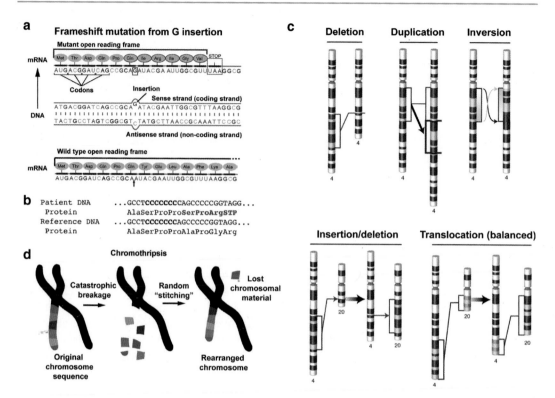

Fig. 4.4 Structural variations. (TIF). Illustration of various types of structural variations. (**a**) Illustration of the impact of insertion of a single base in a coding exon. The shift in the reading frame causes a major change in the amino acid sequence. The encoded protein is truncated because a new stop codon is created by the frameshift. (**b**) Example of a C insertion (*red*) in a genomic segment that is highly enriched in cystine (*bold*). The impact on the amino acid sequence is presented below the DNA sequences. (**c**) Examples of large-scale structural changes. (**d**) This schematic presents the model by which the process of chromothripsis is explained (Sources: **a, c**: Modified from NHGRI digital image database https:// www.genome.gov/dmd/. Public Domain; **b**: Modified with permission from Kirby et al. [19]; **d** Inspired from Fig. 1 from Tubio and Estivill [20])

general population. Large hemizygous or homozygous deletions, especially when rare and leading to abrogation of a single gene, are the simplest CNVs to interpret phenotypically: this copy number loss is equivalent to a gene knockout. For example, studies on patients with large deletions led to the discovery of the first genes causing Dent's disease (CLCN5, on chromosome X) [26], Alport syndrome (COL4A5, on chromosome X) [27], and nephronophthisis (NPHP1, on chromosome 2) [28].

It is not straightforward to predict the functional impact of other types of CNVs, even those strongly associated with human diseases. In most instances, gene dosage is thought to be reflected proportionally in the levels of gene expression [29]. For example, a copy number gain/loss may result in higher/lower expression of a given protein; the amino acid sequence of this protein is unchanged. The most prominent example of this in the renal literature comes from studies on the genetic basis of lupus nephritis: SLE patients with low copy numbers (0 or 1 per chromosome) of the gene encoding Fc receptor for IgG (FCGR3B) were more likely to develop renal disease than those who had more than 1 [30]. It was recently shown that patients with congenital kidney malformation are much more likely to harbor large and rare heterozygous CNVs in any region of the genome when compared to unaffected controls [31]. Tumor-specific copy number gains and losses have been observed in clear cell renal cell carcinoma, particularly when there is no germline mutation in the gene VHL [32, 33].

Copy Neutral Variations

Copy neutral variation, defined as genomic alterations that do not affect the overall number of copies of genes, includes inversion and translocation (Fig. 4.4c). These may cause disease in several ways. The function of genes may be abnormal if the inversion/translocation is accompanied by random loss of parts of the rearranged genomic segment that play an important role (i.e., it is "unbalanced"). Balanced copy neutral variations can also be pathogenic. Indeed, if the boundaries of the structural change occur in the middle of a gene, it may disrupt normal transcription of that gene (since contiguous exons are now far apart). Even if gene integrity is preserved, aberrant gene expression may be observed because of interference with the function of regulatory elements such as promoters, enhancers, silencers, insulators [34].

There are only few examples of patients with renal conditions caused by balanced copy neutral variations [35-37]. One explanation for this is that commonly used genomic techniques are unable to detect these types of rearrangements. Thus clinicians who have patients with a clear phenotype but without mutations in the known gene(s) should consider asking for copy neutral variations testing.

Chromothripsis

Recent advances in DNA sequencing and bioinformatics now allow interrogation of genomes at an unprecedented resolution: it was instrumental in the discovery of yet another type of structural variation, namely chromothripsis (which means chromosomes shattered to pieces). Chromothripsis is suspected when a chromosome is found to harbor two or more complex structural rearrangements (Fig. 4.4d). This phenomenon was first described as a type of somatic structural variation present only in cancer cells [38]. Many similar reports followed shortly thereafter, suggesting that this mechanism is common in tumors [39]. The current working model states that chromothripsis arises from a single catastrophic event causing shattering of one or more chromosomes followed by formation of a chromosome-like structure via random stitching of the fragments [40].

Of utmost interest for pediatricians is the fact that a chromothripsis-like phenomenon has been reported as de novo germline variation in patients with congenital diseases [41, 42]. Recent evidence suggests that the underlying mechanism is analogous to that described for cancer cells; the main difference being that the shattering process is much more circumscribed in so-called "constitutional chromothripsis" [43].

Online Resources

dbVar: http://www.ncbi.nlm.nih.gov/dbvar/

Modes of Inheritance

An allele is one of a number of copies of the same gene or locus. Every person has two copies of every gene on autosomal chromosomes, one inherited from the mother and one inherited from the father. The occurrence of two copies of the same allele results in a homozygous genotype for that allele whereas the presence of two different alleles results in a heterozygous genotype for each allele. How recessive or dominant genotypic interactions can influence the expression of the characteristic traits of the underlying genetic variation is described in the following sections. Please see Fig. 4.5 for pedigrees displaying the typical inheritance patterns, and Table 4.1 for clinical examples.

Dominant Genotypes

Dominant genotypes are seen when the heterozygous genotype are associated with phenotypic expression. Dominant genotypes arise when one allele dominates by masking the phenotypic expression of the other allele at the same genetic locus. For example, where a gene exists in two allelic forms (designated A and B), a combination of three different genotypes is possible: AA, AB, and BB. If AA and BB individuals (homozygotes) show different forms of some trait (phenotypes), and AB individuals

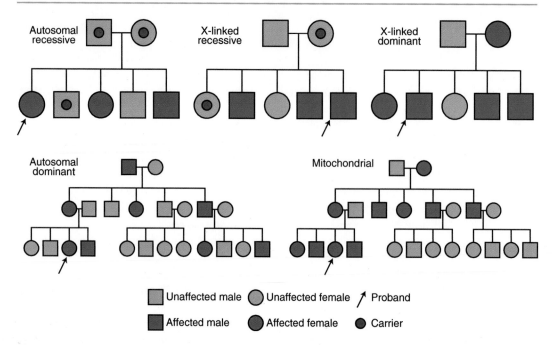

Fig. 4.5 Examples of pedigrees for most common types of inheritance. Examples of classic pedigrees for kindreds with patterns of inheritance consistent with autosomal recessive, autosomal dominant, X-linked recessive, X-linked dominant and mitochondrial

Table 4.1 Examples of renal diseases for the main types of inheritance

Inheritance patterns	Diseases	Genes	OMIM #
Autosomal recessive	Congenital nephrotic syndrome	NPHS1 [44]	256300
Autosomal dominant	Polycystic kidney disease	PKD1 [45]	173900
X-linked recessive	Dent's disease	CLCN5 [46]	300009
X-linked dominant	X-linked hypophosphatemic rickets	PHEX [47]	307800
Mitochondrial	Hypomagnesemia, hypertension, and hypercholesterolemia	Mitochondrial tRNA(Ile) [48]	500005

(heterozygotes) show the same phenotype as AA individuals, then allele A is said to dominate or be dominant to or show dominance to allele B, and B is said to be recessive to A. If instead AB has the same phenotype as BB, B is said to be dominant to A.

Recessive Genotypes

Recessive genotypes are seen when the homozygous genotype and not the heterozygous genotype are associated with phenotypic expression. Thus, both parents have to be carriers of a recessive trait in order for a child to express that trait.

If both parents are carriers, there is a 25 % chance for each child to show the recessive trait in the phenotype. Thus if the parents are closely related (consanguineous) the probability of both having inherited the same allele is increased and as a result the probability of the children showing the recessive trait is increased as well.

X-Linked

X-linked inheritance means that the gene causing the trait or the disorder is located on the X chromosome. Females have two X chromosomes, while males have one X and one Y chromosome.

X-Linked Recessive

X-linked recessive (XLR) inheritance is a mode of inheritance in which a mutation in a gene on the X chromosome causes the phenotype to be expressed (1) in males (who are necessarily hemizygous for the gene mutation because they have only one X chromosome) and (2) in females who are homozygous for the gene mutation (i.e., they have a copy of the gene mutation on each of their two X chromosomes).

Carrier females who have only one copy of the mutation do not usually express the phenotype, although differences in X chromosome inactivation can lead to varying degrees of clinical expression in carrier females since some cells will express one X allele and some will express the other.

X-Linked Dominant

X-linked dominance (XLD), is when the dominant gene is carried on the X chromosome and is responsible for manifestation of the disorder. It is less common than the X-linked recessive type. In XLD, only one copy of the allele is sufficient to cause the disorder when inherited from a parent who has the disorder.

X-linked dominant traits do not necessarily affect males more than females (unlike X-linked recessive traits). The exact pattern of inheritance varies, depending on whether the father or the mother has the trait of interest. All daughters of an affected father will also be affected but none of his sons will be affected (unless the mother is also affected). In addition, the mother of an affected son is also affected (but not necessarily the other way round).

Mitochondrial

Inheritance from a single parent can give rise to disease (uniparental isodisomy). Some renal phenotypes arise solely by maternal inheritance and are characterized by mitochondrial dysfunction. Mitochondrial DNA (mtDNA) is derived from the mother because it exists in much higher concentrations in ova compared to sperm. Furthermore, sperm mtDNA tends to get degraded in fertilized ova and sperm mtDNA fails to enter the ovum in several organisms.

Genetic/Genomic Methods

SNP Genotyping

Because of the unique properties of SNPs, there has been considerable interest in developing high-throughput technologies that would allow simultaneous testing of a large number of SNPs cheaply and reliably. The starting point is always a solution containing the patient's fragmented DNA. The two most successful approaches apply this solution onto a microarray seeded with specific oligonucleotide probes directed against the sequence surrounding the target common variants (with minor allele frequencies of at least 1 %).

The first method relies on non-enzymatic hybridization of single-stranded DNA to probes: a perfect match generates a light signal, but a fragment harboring a variant does not. The second uses DNA polymerase to add one of four fluorescent-labeled nucleotide (A, C, T, or G), thus extending the probe by one base specifically at the SNP locus. SNP genotyping was rapidly adopted by investigators as the method of choice to investigate the links between common genetic variants and human disease [49].

Current estimate show that a typical Human genome (three billion base pairs in total) harbors five million SNPs: this corresponds to roughly 1 SNP every ~1000 bases. While early versions of these arrays contained <100,000 SNPs scattered throughout the genome, current platforms routinely interrogate one to two million SNPs at once (1 SNP every 1500–2000 bases). This means that we currently have unprecedented precision in our assessment of common genetic variation. As described below, SNP genotyping has proved useful for many types of investigations, such as for example assessment of linkage, genome-wide association, ancestral heritage, and copy-number variations.

Linkage Analysis

For decades, genetic linkage analysis has proved to be a powerful method to uncover short genomic segments that harbor disease-causing genes for Mendelian conditions. The concepts of co-segregation, phase, linkage disequilibrium and haplotype, which were described above, are central to this analysis (Fig. 4.6a, b). The goal is to identify "non-random segregation of disease phenotypes with discrete chromosomal segments" [50]. When performed with current technologies, the first step is to obtain dense SNP genotyping data for all individuals in the family that provided a blood sample. The genotyping platforms typically record genotypes for millions of common variants (minor allele frequency >1 % in the general population) that are scattered throughout the genome. On that basis, this approach is often referred to as a "genome-wide linkage scan."

Next is the identification of all series of contiguous SNPs that travel together (haplotypes) in all affected individuals, but not in healthy relatives (Fig. 4.6a, b). Using this approach, one can confidently exclude most of the genome and focus efforts on the incriminated genomic segments, which may contain any number of candidate genes (from zero to many). One key concept to understand is that the SNPs used for linkage analysis almost never turn out to be the disease-causing variant per se since the common variants on the SNP genotyping platform cannot be the

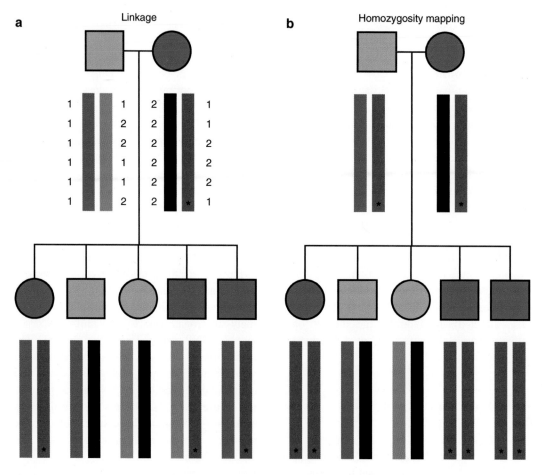

Fig. 4.6 Linkage analysis and homozygosity mapping. (**a**) Illustration of linkage analysis, with the disease haplotype (genomic segment harboring the disease-causing mutation) in *red*. If an autosomal dominant pattern of inheritance with complete penetrance is suspected, all (and only) affected individuals should share the pathogenic heterozygous haplotype. Each colored segments represent different haplotypes because they harbor differ-

ent sequences of alleles at similar genomic positions (in this case, six loci are shown, each with two possible alleles, 1 or 2). (**b**) Homozygosity mapping seeks to identify homozygous segments that are present only in affected individuals (*red*). While a consanguineous union increases the probability of an autosomal recessive condition, outbred parents may share short genomic segments because of very distant common ancestors

primary cause for a rare Mendelian condition. These SNPs are called tag SNPs because they effectively flag specific genomic segments (haplotype) that contain the rare disease-causing variant.

The larger the number of samples from affected and unaffected individuals, the higher the precision of linkage analysis. This approach is thus most fruitful when dealing with large kindreds with multiple affected individuals, and it is not useful when dealing with families with a single affected individual. Obtaining a large number of blood samples from unaffected first degree relatives is also key as one can exclude a larger number of "healthy" haplotypes. Combining linkage analysis performed on two or more unrelated kindreds with similar phenotypes allows for narrowing down the number and length of the target genomic segments since the disease-causing gene must lie within the segment that is shared between kindreds (if caused by mutations in the same gene).

Up until recently, most genes associated with Mendelian conditions were discovered using linkage analysis. This is true for renal conditions as well. Nowadays, gene discovery projects are done with whole-genome and whole-exome sequencing using analytic procedures that are closely related to that of linkage analysis (see below). Instead of using common variants as genomic markers for the disease locus, one can directly find the disease-causing mutation (which is expected to be rare or novel since the disease under scrutiny is rare).

Homozygosity Mapping

Genetic analysis of consanguineous families with multiple individuals exhibiting a similar disease phenotype is in theory simpler than for outbred kindreds because of a much higher prior probability that the disease follows an autosomal recessive pattern of inheritance (Fig. 4.6a, b) [51]. Homozygosity mapping [52], which is the method of choice in this context, is a version of linkage analysis that is streamlined by restricting the playing field to genomic segments that are homozygous only in affected individuals [53]. The entire set of homozygous segments has been termed the "autozygome" because autozygosity refers to homozygosity in the context of consanguinity [54]. This method relies on identity-by-descent because one would expect to find a single founder mutation that originated from a common ancestor. As in traditional linkage analyses, testing of unaffected parents and siblings is critical to make sure that only affected individuals carry the recessive genotypes (monogenic disorders typically have complete penetrance).

Ideally, homozygosity mapping points to a single homozygous genomic segment. Interestingly, homozygosity mapping is at times problematic when investigating highly inbred families because there may be many shared homozygous segments [55]. Alternatively, there are many examples of closed communities that have over time accumulated two distinct pathogenic mutations in the same gene (from two different ancestors): this was found because affected subjects from highly consanguineous families were unexpected compound heterozygotes [56, 57]. There is evidence from the renal literature that homozygosity mapping may also be useful to investigate a subject from an outbred family for whom a recessive pattern of inheritance is suspected [58].

Since most of these conditions are first diagnosed clinically during childhood, pediatricians should know about this approach. The history of kidney disease genetics is replete with examples of successful applications of identity-by-descent methodology to identify novel disease-causing genes. While homozygosity mapping is better known as a research tool for gene discovery, it is emerging as a critical tool for clinical genetics as well, particularly when dealing with patients from consanguineous unions that have a condition with many possible genetic causes [59]. For examples, this approach reduced diagnostic costs and streamlined patient care when applied to a large number of patients with a clinical diagnosis of Bardet-Biedl syndrome [60].

Genome-Wide Association Study

In many ways, a genome-wide association study (GWAS) is very similar to a linkage study. Indeed, both test to see if there is a statistical association between any of one to two millions SNPs and a particular trait that may be recorded as a variable that is either continuous (systolic blood pressure, in mmHg) or a dichotomous (hypertension: yes or no). There are two major differences between these study designs. First, while the focus of linkage studies is on families with affected and unaffected individuals, GWAS methodology actively prohibits inclusion of close relatives in the same study to avoid bias. Second, linkage and GWAS studies use the same set of tag SNPs to flag haplotypes harboring rare disease-causing mutations or common risk alleles, respectively.

Anyone reading an article reporting on the results of a GWAS for the first time is usually struck by the extremely low p-values required to identify valid associations: the typical genome-wide significance threshold for GWAS studies is 5×10^{-8}. Such low p-values are necessary to minimize the chances of reporting false positive associations, which become increasingly common as the number of tests performed increases. While on a different scale, this concept should be familiar to physicians ordering lab tests. The new p-value threshold is simple to calculate: 0.05 divided by the number of tests performed (in this case 1×10^{-6} SNPs). When reading any article, it is good practice for physicians to systematically calculate the number of tests performed and independently calculate the corrected p-value threshold, if applicable.

Flag SNPs with p-values below the set threshold identify target haplotypes, each of which usually contain many genes. It is important to realize that GWAS does not make it possible to pinpoint which of these genes is the culprit. This is critical because it influences the way GWAS results are reported in the literature. The tradition is to name an incriminated haplotype after the gene within that haplotype that is the authors' best guess based on available evidence. This approach does not convey the inherent uncertainty behind such statements (see Box 4.1).

Box 4.1: The MYH9 vs. APOL1 Story One of the best examples of an educated guess that misfired is from the Nephrology literature.

Simultaneous reports from two independent teams found a very strong association between the gene encoding myosin heavy-chain 9 (MYH9) and glomerular disease in African-American adult patients [61, 62]. This was a reasonable guess given that many associated SNPs were clustered near or within MYH9, and given that autosomal dominant mutations in MYH9 cause diseases with a complex, multi-systemic phenotype that include an Alport-like glomerulonephritis that often leads to end-stage renal disease [63, 64]. However, sequencing of all MYH9 exons did not reveal the underlying risk allele(s).

Taking a deeper look at similar cohorts, a third team finally solved the riddle: the associated risk alleles were in a distinct gene named APOL1, located on the same haplotype [65]. These renal risk alleles are common in African-Americans because they also confer a positive advantage via more efficient APOL1-dependent killing of trypanosome parasites. A recent review provides more details about this remarkable story [66]. A prospective study confirmed that African-American individuals harboring the APOL1 alleles have higher risk of progression to ESRD or CKD over time [67].

Online Resources
Single base primer extension genotyping: http://goo.gl/lt133E; Linkage: http://goo.gl/PPK5hZ

Polymerase Chain Reaction

Polymerase Chain Reaction (PCR) is the method of choice to amplify specific DNA segments. Most current DNA sequencing technologies are dependent on PCR amplification to generate a reliable signal that is translated into the DNA sequence itself through various ingenious means (Fig. 4.7). PCR takes advantage of a DNA polymerase enzyme that is highly resistant to heat such that it is still functional following multiple rounds of heating/cooling. Heat is necessary to break the double stranded DNA into single strands that can then be copied by the DNA polymerase using the supplied deoxy nucleotide (dNTPs). The reaction also requires primers pairs

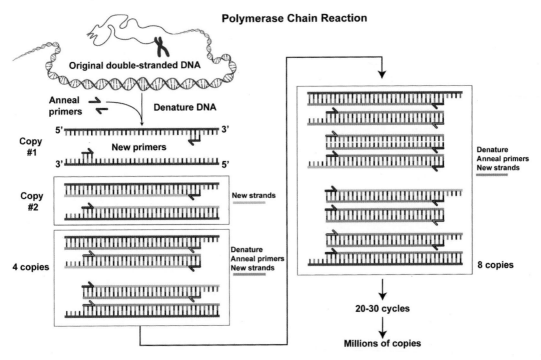

Fig. 4.7 Polymerase chain reaction. Illustration of the amplification process that occurs when DNA is subjected to PCR. Specific oligonucleotide primers, heat-resistant DNA polymerase and unlabeled nucleotides are added to the solution containing the starting DNA. The mix i subjected to heat to denature DNA. Once temperature is reduced, the primers anneal to single-stranded DNA segments and new strands are synthesized by DNA polymerase enzyme. The first cycle generates two new strands, the second cycle four new strands. Ultimately, millions of copies of this segment are generated after 20–30 cycles (Sources: Modified from NHGRI digital image database. www.genome.gov. Public Domain)

that are synthesized in the laboratory: these are made out of a series of ~20 nucleotides that match a very specific region of the genome. Now that the human reference genome is well established, it is simple to design primers pairs located around the target genomic segment of interest that is no more than 1000 base pairs in length.

The main drawback of PCR-based methods is that the DNA polymerase sometimes inserts the wrong nucleotide at a given position during the copying process. When one such amplified segment is subjected to DNA sequencing, one could be mistaken to think that it is a mutation when in fact there is none in the original DNA. It is thus important to validate all mutations deemed "pathologic" via PCR re-amplification a fresh sample of DNA followed by Sanger sequencing (method discussed below). The reason why this step is useful is that most of these errors occur at random, which means that the same mistake is very unlikely to be observed at the same locus in a separate experiment.

Online Resources

PCR: http://goo.gl/0ZMv70

DNA Sequencing Technologies

DNA sequencing determines the precise order of the four bases adenine, guanine, cytosine and thymidine in a single strand of DNA. Sequences of individual genes, or clusters of genes, full chromosomes or the whole genome has greatly facilitated our understanding of the basic biological mechanisms of human disease. DNA sequencing was first developed in the 1970s [68] and rapid sequencing methods using the 'chain termination method' was developed by Sanger in 1977 [69].

Sanger Method

DNA replication requires the presence of a single strand of DNA template, dNTPs, DNA polymerase and DNA primers. Under normal conditions, the 3'-OH terminus of the dNTPs facilitates the formation of a phosphodiesterase bond between two nucleotides catalyzed by the enzyme, DNA polymerase. The 'chain termination method' relies on the incorporation of dideoxy NTPs (ddNTPs) lacking a 3'-OH terminus such that extension of DNA thereby ceases during the replication process (Fig. 4.8a–d). Fluorescent-labeled ddNTPs are employed in the automated sequencing methods which rely on wavelength determination to identify the different ddNTPs in a given sequence [70].

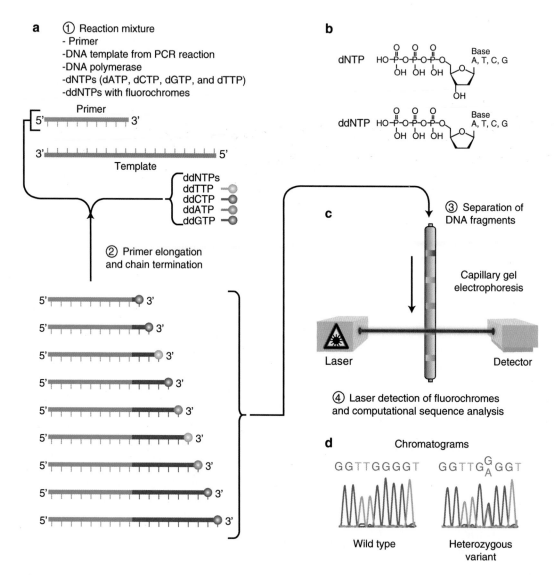

Fig. 4.8 Sanger sequencing with fluorescent-labelled ddNTPs. (**a**) Reagents necessary for Sanger sequencing. (**b**) Illustration of the structural difference between dNTP and ddNTP. (**c**) Capillary gel electrophoresis of elongated fragments and detection of added fluorochrome-labeled base with laser detection. (**d**) Example of the output in the form of a chromatogram; the same sequence is presented from a subject who is wild type and another that harbor a heterozygous G to A substitution (Source: Modified from Wikipedia, http://goo.gl/jF2LWo. Creative Commons Attribution-ShareAlike 3.0 Unported License. Author of original figure is User Estevezj)

Online Resources
Sanger sequencing: http://goo.gl/dUkRuv

Next Generation Sequencing Methods

Sanger sequencing can be laborious and expensive. A number of new sequencing technologies called next-generation sequencing (NGS) technologies have been developed that have significantly reduced the cost and time required for sequencing [71]. Unlike the Sanger method where a single predefined target is required for each sequencing reaction, NGS platforms allow for the sequencing of many millions of target molecules in parallel (Fig. 4.9a–c). DNA molecules are immobilized on a solid surface and are sequenced in situ by a stepwise incorporation of fluorescent-labeled nucleotides or oligonucleotides. "Clusters" of identical DNA are generated by the clonal amplification of template DNA, hence the term 'massive parallel deep sequencing' used to describe NGS. Platforms vary, with some covering fewer genomic regions than others, some are able to detect a greater total number of variants with additional sequencing while others capture untranslated regions, which are not targeted by other platforms [72].

Massive parallel sequencing has greatly facilitated investigations of variations within the human genome. In January 2008, the 1000 Genomes Project was launched with the objective of establishing a detailed catalogue of human genetic variation [73]. Utilizing the genomic sequences of 2500 anonymous participants from a number of different ethnic groups worldwide and using a combination of methods including low-coverage genome sequencing and targeted re-sequencing of coding regions, the primary goals of this project were to discover SNPs at frequencies of 1 % or higher in diverse populations; to uncover rare SNPs with frequencies of 0.1–0.5 % in functional gene regions; and to reveal structural variants, such as copy number variants, insertions, and deletions. The results of a pilot project involving more than 1000 genomes was completed in May 2011 [74]. This resource is publicly available and can be used by researchers to identify variants in regions that are suspected of being associated with disease. By identifying and cataloguing most of the common genetic variants in the populations studied, this project has generated data that will serve as an invaluable reference for clinical interpretation of genomic variation.

Third Generation Sequencing Methods

Newer or 'third generation' approaches have emerged that aim to sequence the single DNA molecule in real time without prior amplification. The potential benefits of using single-molecule sequencing are minimal input DNA requirements, elimination of amplification bias, faster turnaround times, and longer read lengths that allow for some haplotyping of sequence information.

Online Resources
PacBio: http://goo.gl/SUaIls; IonTorrent: http://goo.gl/552MKe

Whole-Exome Sequencing

Owing to the fact that about 85 % of all disease-causing mutations in Mendelian disorders are within coding exons, the recent application of massive parallel deep-sequencing with exon capture has shown the efficacy of this technique for the rapid identification of mutations in single-gene disorders [75, 76]. Almost 7 years has passed since targeted enrichment of an exome by hybridization of shotgun libraries was first described [77]. Two years later, the targeted capture and massive parallel sequencing of the exomes of 12 humans was published [78]. The following year, the first reports emerged on the use of whole exome sequencing in gene identification [79]. Since then, the genetic etiology of over 300 Mendelian diseases has been discovered in no less than 4 years.

Exome sequencing involves the targeted re-sequencing of all protein-coding sequences, which requires 5 % as much sequencing as a whole human genome (Fig. 4.10a–d) [78]. As the majority of Mendelian disorders are due to mutations that disrupt protein-coding sequences,

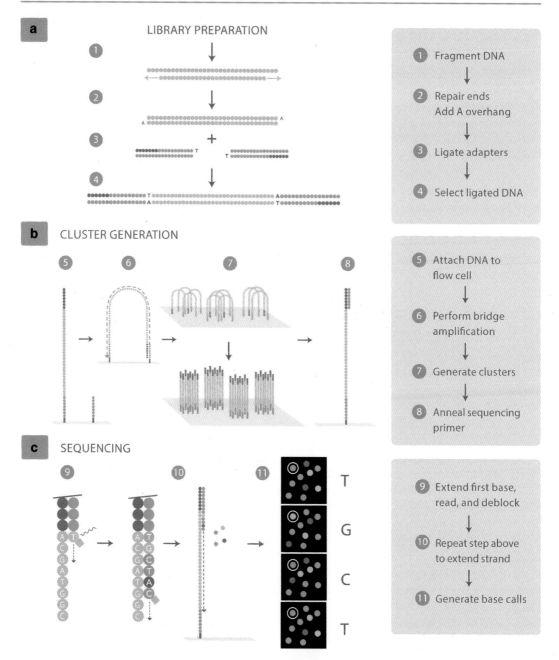

Fig. 4.9 Illumina® sequencing technology overview. This figure illustrates the steps necessary to sequence genomic DNA fragments using the Illumina® sequencing technology. These include (**a**) library preparation, (**b**) cluster generation and (**c**) sequencing. Additional details are provided in the *gray boxes* (All images courtesy of Illumina, Inc., Dan Diego, CA, USA. All rights reserved)

the use of exome capture to identify allelic variants in rare monogenic disorders is well justified. Furthermore, highly functional variations can also be accounted for by changes in splice acceptor and donor sites, sequences of which will also be targeted by exome capture.

The major advantage of whole exome sequencing is that virtually all variants within an

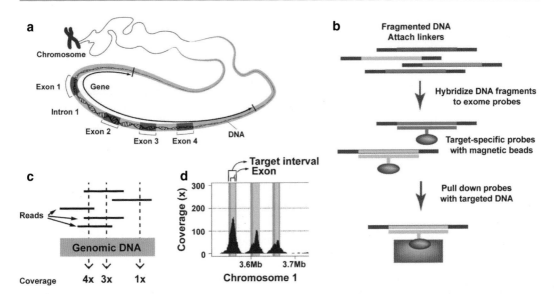

Fig. 4.10 Whole-exome capture and sequencing. (**a**) Representation of a gene and its exons and introns. (**b**) Illustration of the exome capture process. In this case, the oligonucleotide probes designed to specifically anneal to all exons in the the genomes are in solution. They are easily pulled out from the solution the probes are linked to magnetic beads. Another exome capture system has probes attached to a microarray. (**c**) Illustration of the concept of reads and coverage for a small genomic segment. These are key concepts in genomics. (**d**) Illustration of the skewed distribution of read coverage with exome capture to the exonic segments (Sources: **a**: Modified from NHGRI digital image database. www.genome.gov. Public Domain; **b**: Modified from Wikipedia. http://goo.gl/OZBw4z. Creative Commons Attribution-ShareAlike 3.0 Unported License. Author of original figure is SarahKusala; **d** Courtesy of Murim Choi.)

individual's genome are uncovered simultaneously. This allows for direct examination of the list of variants and candidate gene selection in the presence or absence of mapping studies. Variant listing is dependent on several factors that are dependent on the technology used. For example, the type of capture kit, the sequencing platform and sequencing depth can influence the variant listing. Additionally, the lists produced will depend on the alignment algorithms and the stringency settings of the bioinformatics tools employed for identifying variants. Capture kits are continuously improving, initially having covered 27 Mb and 180,000 coding exons to now up to 62 Mb of the human genome and over 201,121 coding exons. Each platform uses biotinylated oligonucleotide baits complementary to the exome targets to hybridize sequencing libraries prepared from fragmented genomic DNA. These bound libraries are enriched for targeted regions by pull-down with magnetic streptavidin beads and then sequenced.

Online Resources
NHGRI TV: http://goo.gl/U0Uu1O

Whole-Genome Sequencing

Whole-genome sequencing (WGS) involves sequencing the complete DNA sequence encompassing all six billion nucleotide bases in the 23 chromosome pairs of a diploid human genome [80]. The main difference between WGS and WES is that WGS covers the entire genome, including all exons [81]. As a result, it includes the exome and allows detection of mutations in non-coding DNA elements that are missed by WES. While we cannot efficiently analyzed such mutations right now, it is fair to assume that we will be in a good position to do so in a few years. Once the tools exist to assess non-coding variants, re-analysis of "negative" WGS datasets would be very simple. On the other hand, patients who underwent WES studies that proved uninformative (i.e., no causative coding variant was identified) would have to be studied again with WGS.

Yet another significant advantage over WES is the much improved ability to uncover various types of CNVs, such as insertions, duplications and deletions [82]. This is possible because of the introduction of paired-end mapping of sequence reads: a CNV is flagged when the 75 bp reads generated from both ends of genomic fragments of known length (~300 bp) are aligned farther (or closer) than anticipated (Fig. 4.11a–g) [83]. The earliest example of genome-wide CNV interrogation using WGS data revealed 1000 large structural variations per genome, which is much more than anticipated [84]. However, the gold standard for thorough investigation of structural variations remains comparative genomic hybridization (CGH) microarray techniques.

We will use one of the first published WGS study (based on James Watson's DNA) to illustrate how comprehensive is the dataset created [85]. More than 100 million high quality short-read sequences were produced, containing a total of 24.5 billion DNA bases. This allowed the investigators to "read" every base of Watson's genomes on average seven-times – this is the referred to as the "coverage," and the higher it is, the more confident you are that the mutations identified are true. After processing the data with various bioinformatics tools, a total of three million high quality variants were ultimately identified, of which ~10,000 were non-synonymous mutations (0.3%). More than 65,000 insertions and twice as many deletions were also found with these data.

When compared to WES, one of the biggest challenges of WGS is the substantially larger volume of data generated (estimated to be over 1 terabyte per genome). This has significant implications because the raw aligned data will typically be stored long-term. The issue is that sequencing costs have decreased much more rapidly than the costs associated with the infrastructure necessary to store and process these data [86]. For example, even when Watson's team was done processing his data back in 2008 [85], they would have to keep the data indefinitely in case re-analysis was deemed necessary. Consequently,

teams interested to implement WGS as opposed to WES have to be ready to face significant challenges with regards to storing data.

Another big challenge is the much higher number of variants identified in a WGS dataset. Indeed, it is not easy to pinpoint the disease-causing variant from the many hundreds of variants that remain after various bioinformatics filters. In comparison, one has to investigate ~50–100 coding variants after filtering WES data.

Furthermore, it will be essential for accurate and comprehensive characterization of disease phenotypes to greatly assist the analysis of an individual's phenotype. It has been shown that the presence of bi-allelic variants can greatly influence a disease phenotype and data generated by WGS will likely increase our understanding of the molecular intersection of biologically relevant pathways.

As the cost of a whole genome is still expensive, currently over £2000 per genome, whole exome sequencing remains the preferred strategy for molecular genetic diagnosis as this remains a more cost effective strategy than Sanger sequencing in genetically heterogeneous conditions. However, limitations exist with both technologies and the major challenges posed by both strategies will involve the logistics of delivering genome sequence information to clinicians and, how, we, as clinicians use the data, and how patients and their families deal with the incidental findings.

Clinical Implementation in Nephrology

Finding Pathogenic Mutations for Mendelian Disease

Nowadays, most pediatric nephrologists will send blood samples for genetic testing a few times a year for patients with a wide range of conditions. This may be done to establish a firm molecular diagnosis for a patient, to verify if relatives are carriers. New non-invasive techniques are also emerging to obtain antenatal molecular diagnosis from maternal blood [87]. The interested reader is

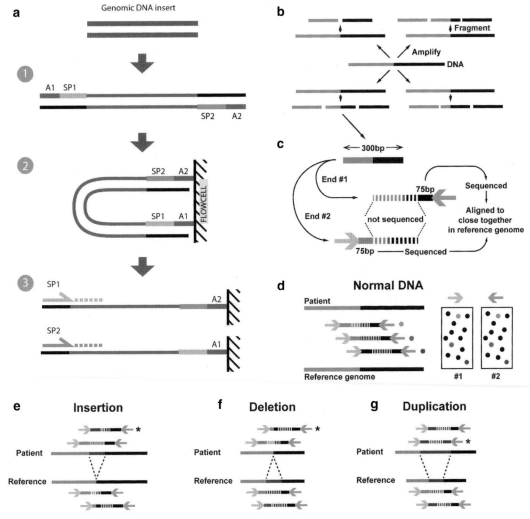

Fig. 4.11 Paired-end sequencing to detect structural variations. (a) Preparation DNA sample for standard next-generation sequencing using paired-end. Genomic DNA from the patient is amplified, and then fragmented into small pieces. Only fragments with lengths ~200–250 base pairs are selected for sequencing (genomic DNA inserts). The steps described are as follows: (1) Adapter (*A1* and *A2*) with sequencing primer sites (*SP1* and *SP2*) are ligated onto DNA fragments; (2) Template clusters are formed on the flow cell by bridge amplification; (3) Clusters are then sequenced by synthesis from the paired primers sequentially. (b) Illustration of amplification of DNA, random fragmentation of amplified segments; in this case, fragments of similar sizes are illustrated. (c) Illustration of the two-step process leading to paired-end sequencing. The fragment size selected for is 300 base pairs, and 75 base pairs are sequenced at each end. The *dotted lines* represent segments that are not directly sequenced in that fragment. (d) Schematic showing how paired-end reads from a small genomic region from a patient with normal DNA align to the reference genome. The right-hand side shows the position of the clusters from which the data for each reads come from. Each DNA fragment is linked to a specific cluster on the flow cell thus linking the first and second sequencing data. Also shown are examples of how paired-end sequencing is useful to identify for insertions (e), deletion (f) or duplications (g). (a: Figure modified from original Illumina® paired-end sequencing workflow. Illumina, San Diego, CA, USA. All rights reserved)

directed to recent reviews on the topic of genetic testing applied to Nephrology [88, 89].

The first set of investigations is usually to sequence genes known to cause a particular condition to uncover possible pathogenic mutations. Up until recently, this was done using PCR amplification and Sanger sequencing of all exons of these genes. However, it appears inevitable that very soon the same diagnostic procedures will be achieved using whole exome or whole-genome sequencing because of decreasing prices and widespread availability. There are already early reports describing the successes and challenges of this approach in the clinical realm: a confident molecular diagnosis was confirmed in ~25% of cases tested within ~10–15 weeks [90-92]. In theory, a molecular diagnosis may be obtained within 2–3 days (and probably faster as the technology improves): this would be particularly useful for patients in the neonatal intensive care unit [93]. A clear advantage and yet another challenge of this approach is the ability to interrogate all of the other genes if no mutation in known genes is found.

The simplest scenario is when the mutation identified has already been described in other patients with a similar phenotype. Unfortunately, an alternative scenario is much more common: the report states that there is a variant of "unknown significance" in a gene known to cause this disease (i.e., it has not been described beforehand). While this may be frustrating since it does not provide a firm answer to the family, we provide a case that illustrates what a pediatric nephrologist can do to evaluate such a report (see clinical vignette). It emphasizes the usefulness of simple concepts that were discussed earlier in this chapter, such as co-segregation, allele frequency, and amino acid conservation.

Physicians need to be prepared to revisit the diagnosis since databases are evolving, and should make this clear with the patient and his/her parents. Current protocols used by leaders in the field stipulate systematic rechecks of all data-sets every 6 months, with automatic reporting to the ordering physician if new findings emerge [91, 92]. This is critical because as public data-base are populated with an increasing number of pathogenic variants over time, or novel disease-causing genes, the output of bioinformatic analyses performed changes. Thus, an initial negative report from next generation sequencing testing may very well yield a confident molecular diagnosis in the near future. Since the criteria for a mutation to be deemed pathogenic are very stringent, it is, however, unlikely that the interpreta-

tion of such a mutation will be overturned. A recent study showed that the curation of mutation databases is surprisingly unreliable: sequencing of ~438 target genes in 52 parent-child trios revealed that ~25% of mutations flagged as "likely pathogenic" in healthy parents were likely to be benign [94].

Clinical Vignette

A young patient with a clinical diagnosis of congenital nephrotic syndrome spent many months as in-patient. Since the parents are first cousins, an autosomal recessive form of CNS was expected; the patient has a 2-year old female sibling that is apparently healthy (Fig. 4.12). There is no prior family history of CNS. A few months back, your colleagues made sure to send blood samples from all first-degree relatives for genetic testing of the usual CNS gene panel, which includes Sanger sequencing of the genes NPHS1 and NPHS2. You are seeing the patient and his parents today in the clinic to discuss the report issued by the diagnostic laboratory.

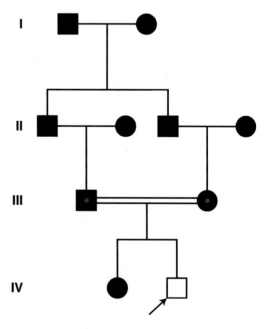

Fig. 4.12 Pedigree for patient with CNS. *Black* and *white* symbols represent affected and unaffected subjects, respectively. *Red dots* and *double lines* denote heterozygous carriers and consanguineous unions, respectively. *Black arrowhead* identifies the proband

The report highlights potentially relevant alterations. The homozygous mutation in NPHS1 (p.I759T) is considered a "variant of unknown significance" because it has not been described before in other patients with CNS. Furthermore, there are no in vitro studies that have tested whether NPHS1 harboring this specific mutation is dysfunctional. The two parents and the unaffected sibling are all confirmed heterozygous for NPHS1 p.I759T – thus the pattern of cosegregation is consistent with this mutation being potentially pathogenic. In preparation for your meeting with the family, you decide to further investigate to see if this mutation could be pathogenic. Indeed, finding a convincing mutation in a gene known to be associated with a particular disease subtype (in this case, CNS) is one situation in contemporary medicine where diagnostic parsimony may be exercised with confidence, a principle often referred to as Occam's Razor.

First, you check on the public version of the Human Gene Mutation Database (HGMD) to make sure that this mutation was indeed never reported (free registration required for access); an alternative resource is ClinVar. These resources present a comprehensive list of mutations causing Mendelian condition that are curated by experts that are freely available to users from academic institutions. As shown in Fig. 4.13a, b, you confirm that this mutation has not been reported; it would be worthwhile to consider checking this database yearly as more mutations are continuously added to the database. Indeed, if another unrelated patient with CNS is reported to have the exact same homozygous mutation, you could consider this as virtual proof of pathogenicity because the probability of seeing this by chance alone is very low.

Second, you decide to take advantage of bioinformatic tools available online to predict how likely your patient's mutation is to affect protein function. You decide to use the software Condel because it is easy to use, the interpretation of the output is simple, and its predictions outperform that of three other leading software: Polyphen2, SIFT and MutationAssessor (Fig. 4.14a–d). That Condel is the best prediction tools is not surprising because it actually integrates the outputs of these

three leading softwares, which are sometimes contradictory. All determine the pathogenic potential of missense mutations by using information about the degree of amino acid conservation between various species, the predicted impact of the specific amino acid change (based on physicochemical properties of amino acids, such as size, charge, and polarity) compounded to some advanced computing methodologies (machine learning). In this case, an isoleucine to threonine substitution is deemed neutral despite excellent conservation because this change is known to be well tolerated by proteins. It is thus very unlikely (but not 100% certain) that this mutation is pathogenic.

Online Resources

HGMD: http://www.hgmd.cf.ac.uk/; ClinVar: http://www.ncbi.nlm.nih.gov/clinvar/; CONDEL: http://bg.upf.edu/condel/analysis; SIFT: http://goo.gl/7eKRfY; Polyphen2: http://goo.gl/EZK28; MutationAssessor: http://mutationassessor.org/; BLAST: http://blast.ncbi.nlm.nih.gov/

Genetic Heterogeneity

Genetic (or locus) heterogeneity is recognized when a particular phenotype may be caused by mutations in different genes. Nephronophthisis is one of the best examples of locus heterogeneity from the renal literature, with disease-causing mutations reported in ~30 genes (Table 4.2). Functional studies have shown that the majority of the encoded proteins by these genes are localized and play important roles at the centrosomes, basal bodies and cilia. This led to the proposition that these structures are central in the pathogenesis of nephronopthisis [95]. It is important to note that locus heterogeneity is common amongst many renal monogenic conditions, such atypical hemolytic uremic syndrome [96], nephrotic syndrome [97], distal renal tubular acidosis [98], Dent's disease [99], or primary hyperoxaluria [100].

Pleiotropy is the mirror image of genetic heterogeneity: mutations in the same gene cause different phenotypes. Incidentally, nephronophthisis also provides many well-documented cases of pleiotropy (Table 4.2). For example, the study of

The Human Gene Mutation Database
at the Institute of Medical Genetics in Cardiff

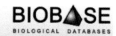

Gene Symbol	Chromosomal location	Gene name	cDNA sequence	Extended cDNA	Mutation viewer
NPHS1	19q13.1	Nephrosis 1, congenital, Finnish type		Not available	BIOBASE Feature available to subscribers

Mutation type	Number of mutations				Mutation data
Missense/nonsense	87	97	113	125	Get mutations
Splicing	14	16	20	22	Get mutations
Regulatory	0	0	0	0	No mutation
Small deletions	20	24	25	28	Get mutations
Small insertions	10	10	10	10	Get mutations
Small indels	2	2	2	2	Get mutations
Gross deletions	0	0	1	0	No mutation
Gross insertions/duplications	0	0	0	0	No mutation
Complex rearrangements	0	0	0	0	No mutation
Repeat variations	0	0	0	0	No mutation
Total	133	149	171	188	
Year	2012	2013	2014	2015	

b

Accession Number	Codon change	Amino acid change	Codon number	Genomic coordinates & HGVS nomenclature	Phenotype	Reference
CM990964	TCT-TGT	Ser-Cys	724	BIOBASE Feature available to subscribers	Congenital nephrotic syndrome, Finnish type	Lenkkeri (1999) Am J Hum Genet **64**, 51
CM011440	GCT-GTT	Ala-Val	739	BIOBASE Feature available to subscribers	Congenital nephrotic syndrome, Finnish type	Beltcheva (2001) Hum Mutat **17**, 368
CM990965	cCGT-TGT	Arg-Cys	743	BIOBASE Feature available to subscribers	Congenital nephrotic syndrome, Finnish type	Lenkkeri (1999) Am J Hum Genet **64**, 51
CM044681	AGC-AAC	Ser-Asn	786	BIOBASE Feature available to subscribers	Minimal change nephrotic syndrome ?	Lahdenkari (2004) Kidney Int **65**, 1856
CM044685	gCGC-TGC	Arg-Cys	800	BIOBASE Feature available to subscribers	Minimal change nephrotic syndrome ?	Lahdenkari (2004) Kidney Int **65**, 1856

Fig. 4.13 HGMD®'s webpage for NPHS1. (**a**) The change in the number of mutations for each category is indicated for 2012 and 2013. (**b**) Pathogenic nonsynonymous mutations in NHPS1 documented in HGMD. After scrolling down to the correct position in the list, it is clear that there is no variant at position isoleucine 759. Description of the phenotype and hyperlinks to the original references are provided for each mutation (Source: http://www.hgmd.cf.ac.uk. Copyright © Cardiff University 2015. All rights reserved. The Human Gene Mutation Database at the Institute of Medical Genetics in Cardiff)

patients with unique phenotypes within the nephronophthisis spectrum using whole-exome sequencing led to the identification of novel candidate genes that were previously associated with completely distinct disorders, such as SLC4A1 or AGXT [101]. The first gene, which encodes the anion exchanger 1 protein, was previously associated with hereditary spherocytosis [102] or distal tubular renal acidosis [98], while the second one is a well-established cause for primary hyperoxaluria: it encodes an enzyme involved in glyoxylate metabolism [100].

Interestingly, a substantial number of patients with nephronophthisis (~40%) remain genetically undefined. The same is true for many other renal conditions. This will proved to be a fertile

a

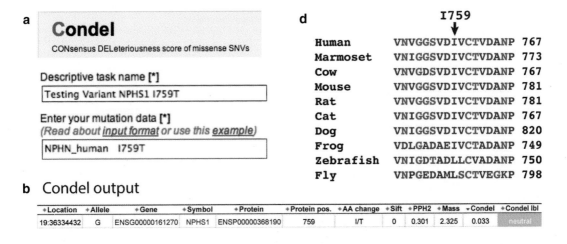

b Condel output

◆Location	◆Allele	◆Gene	◆Symbol	◆Protein	◆Protein pos.	◆AA change	◆Sift	◆PPH2	◆Mass	▾Condel	◆Condel lbl
19:36334432	G	ENSG00000161270	NPHS1	ENSP00000368190	759	I/T	0	0.301	2.325	0.033	neutral

c

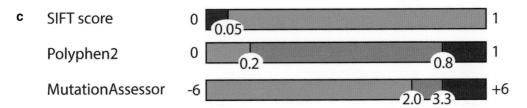

Fig. 4.14 Assessing mutations for pathogenicity. (**a**) The ranges of score for SIFT, Polyphen2 and MutationAssessor. Pathogenic mutations are in the *red* zone. Because they use different approaches to reach this conclusion, their predictions for the same mutation are often different. (**b**) Condel is a new software that extracts and integrate the outputs from all three softwares to reach a conclusion about the pathogenic potential of a particular mutation. For this task, it outperforms the other three softwares. (**c**) Example of Condel output for I759T. The overall conclu-sion is that I759T is predicted to be neutral. While SIFT predicts it to be damaging (0=red), both Polyphen2 (0.3) and MutationAssessor (2.3) are ambivalent (both are in the *"gray"* zone). (**d**) Multiple species protein sequence alignment done using BLAST shows that position I759 is well-conserved down to fly (leucine and isoleucine are interchangeable). Each letter represents an amino acid; the number on the right-hand side indicate the position of the last amino acid of the series presented in a given ortholog

ground to display the utility of whole-exome and/or whole-genome sequencing and will undoubt-edly lead to the identification of many other unexpected candidate genes [103, 104].

Online Resources
Renal gene: http://www.renalgenes.org/

Finding Risk Alleles for Complex Diseases

One of the promises of genomic medicine is for knowledge about a patient's genome to play a central role in the management of complex medical conditions. Classic examples of complex disease include essential hypertension, diabetes mellitus type II, steroid-sensitive nephrotic syn-drome, and congenital malformation of the kid-ney and/or urinary tract. For example, pediatric nephrologists could optimize prevention and/or treatment of steroid-sensitive nephrotic syn-drome, thus realizing the guiding principles of personalized medicine. While this will undoubt-edly change the face of clinical medicine, as described below, we are unfortunately years away from enacting this scenario.

In contrast to Mendelian conditions that are caused by highly penetrant mutations in one gene, complex diseases are not rare and are caused by multiple factors. Detailed epidemiological studies have shown that for

Table 4.2 Genetic heterogeneity among nephronophthisis-associated ciliopathies

Genes	Nephronophthisis syndromes											OMIM #
	BBS	CED	COACH	JATD	JBTS	LCA	MKS	MSS	MORM	NPHP	SLS	
AGXT										■		604285
AH1					■							608894
ANKS6										■		615370
ARL13B					■							608922
CC2D2A			■				■					612013
CEP164						■						614848
CEP290	■				■					■		610142
CEP41					■							610523
GLIS2										■		608539
IFT122		■										606045
IFT140				■				■				614620
IFT43		■										614068
INPP5E					■				■			613037
INVS										■	■	243305
IQCB1										■	■	609237
MRE11											■	600814
NEK8										■		609799
NPHP1					■					■	■	607100
NPHP3							■			■	■	608002
NPHP4										■	■	607215
RPGRIPL1				■			■					610937
SDCCAG8	■									■	■	613524
SLC4A1										■		109270
SLC41A1										■		610801
TMEM138					■							614459
TMEM216					■		■					613277
TMEM67			■		■		■			■		609884
TTC21B				■						■		612014
WDR19			■	■								608151
XPNPEP3										■		613553
ZNF423										■		604557

BBS Bardet-Biedl Syndrome, *CED* Cranioectodermal dysplasia, *COACH* syndrome characterized by cerebellar vermis hypo/aplasia, oligophrenia, congenital ataxia, ocular coloboma, and hepatic fibrosis, *JATD* Jeune asphyxiating thoracic dystrophy, *JBTS* Joubert Syndrome, *LCA* Leber's Congenital Amaurosis, *MKS*, Meckel-Gruber Syndrome, *MMS* Mainzer-Saldino syndrome, *MORM*, syndrome characterized by mental retardation, truncal obesity, retinal dystrophy, and micropenis, *NPHP* nephronopthisis, *SLS* Senior Loken Syndrome

many of these conditions, environmental and genetic factors are major determinants of trait expression. Current models implicate the interaction of multiple low penetrance variants in many genes. These are based on studies of heritability, defined as the fraction of phenotypic variation that is likely explained by genetic variation [105]. Heritability is estimated from the phenotypic correlations among related individuals, using families with multiple affects individuals as well as twin studies. A prime example of a complex trait with high heritability is adult essential hypertension [106].

Finding the genetic basis for complex traits could have significant public health implications. First, it may help identify at-risk individuals early on, thereby perhaps allowing for prevention of long-term, largely preventable health consequences. Second, it may be an important tool to decide the type and dose of medication that is best suited for a given patient, which would be a major advance towards the realization of personalized medicine. Below, we will discuss the two competing theories of complex trait genetics and the methodologies employed to find associations, while providing examples from the renal literature.

Complex Diseases: Associated with Common and/or Rare Variants?

There are two predominant explanatory models of complex disease genetic causation: the complex disease, common variants (CDCV) and the complex disease, rare variants (CDRV) hypotheses (Fig. 4.15) [107]. Both assume that multiple genes are implicated in the pathophysiology of common traits. The first hypothesis states that the genetic landscape of common traits is mostly comprised of common variants (minor allele frequency >1 %), each with a very small contribution to the overall phenotype. The alternative

hypothesis suggests that rare variants (minor allele frequency <1 %) with larger effects are largely responsible. Up until recently, the technology to perform the comprehensive genomic analyses required to unravel the genetic architecture of complex diseases did not exist: the predominant working model was CDRV.

The CDCV hypothesis was first to be tested rigorously owing to technological and methodological developments related to SNP genotyping. This opened the gates for a flurry of genome-wide association scans (GWAS) performed on common SNPs. Reliable investigations of the CDRV hypothesis was beyond reach until the emergence of cheap high-throughput sequencing and the development of exome capture.

Genome-Wide Association Studies

Many GWAS studies focused on renal conditions have now been completed – all include only adult subjects [108]. Some studies were focused on dichotomous disease outcomes, such as hypertension, diabetic nephropathy, IgA nephropathy,

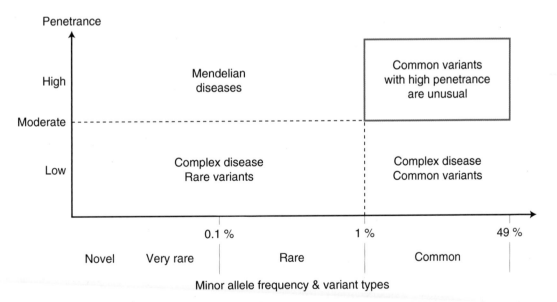

Fig. 4.15 The relationship between minor allele frequency and penetrance to explain the genetic basis of complex diseases. This graph illustrates the relationship between minor allele frequency and penetrance of phenotype. Typically, common variants that have a phenotypic effect have low penetrance. On the other hand, rare variants are expected to results in a much higher penetrance. This is due to the fact that penetrance is one of the main factor driving the selective pressure for/against a particular phenotype. Most variants identified thus far for Mendelian conditions are in the *left upper quadrant* while those associated with complex diseases fit in the *right lower quadrant*

CKD, ESRD/FGSG and kidney stones [108]. Others tested the association with relevant continuous variables like blood pressure, eGFR, serum creatinine, creatinine clearance, albumin-to-creatinine ratio, or serum cystatin C [108, 109]. Unfortunately, there are few variants showing robust association with a given trait that are replicated across distinct studies. These SNPs typically explain very little of the phenotypic variability observed in patients: this phenomenon, which is not unique to nephrology studies, has been termed the "missing heritability" [110]. Many of these studies have, however, provided unique insights in the biological pathways that cause disease that were hitherto immune to detection [111].

There are currently no published GWAS that enrolled children with kidney diseases. As a result of this research lag, children may not benefit from the realization of genomic medicine as rapidly as adult patients [112]. Indeed, it is likely that advances percolating from adult studies will not translate into concrete measures for children for two main reasons. First, the important pediatric public health problems that could be addressed "genomically" are not on the adult medicine "radar" (e.g., nephrotic syndrome). Second, even when diagnoses are congruent (e.g., hypertension), it is unclear how useful results from large adult studies will apply to pediatric care since the underlying pathophysiology is often distinct (due to growth and development) [113, 114]. Thankfully, this situation is likely to change, with projects well underway to perform association studies focused on pediatric nephrotic syndrome [109] or CKD [115], among others. Even then, sample size will remain a big problem unless studies planned include multiple centers from many different countries. Perhaps we should strive to emulate our colleagues from the Children's Oncology Group (COG) who achieved remarkable clinical results by enrolling more than 90 % of all children treated at COG-affiliated centers in a randomized controlled trial [116].

Source of Missing Heritability: Rare Variants?

A substantial proportion of the genetic contribution to complex traits thus remains unexplained.

The next logical step is to determine the impact of rare variants on such phenotypes using whole-genome or – exome sequencing [117]. Unfortunately, because the variants are rare, the sample sizes required to draw conclusions are prohibitively large (10,000–100,000 subjects at a minimum) [118, 119]. As a result, few studies testing the CDRV hypothesis have been published [120]. There is early evidence supporting the importance of rare variants in three genes involved in renal salt transport in modulating hypertension risk [121]. Other aspects that could also play a role in the pathophysiology of complex traits include epigenetic factors [122], gene-gene interactions (epistasis) [123], and/or gene-environment interactions [124]. An alternative explanation recently put forward is that heritability may have been overestimated all along [125]. Finally, the complexity of underlying genetic architecture of these diseases may be such that it is not possible to unravel with our current experimental tools [126].

Pharmacogenetics/Pharmacogenomics

Most current studies attempt to link genetic polymorphisms in a small number of genes with known function in drug metabolism. As such, they establish the pharmacogenetic profiles for patients. Very few studies, particularly when enrolling pediatric subjects, perform pharmacogenomic profiling, which involve genome-wide interrogations. One of the major promises of personalized medicine is that drug prescriptions will be tailored based on a patient's pharmacogenetic profile. This promise is within reach because of extensive knowledge accumulated about two of the key determinants of drugs' pharmacokinetic and pharmacodynamics properties.

First, a group of enzymes add specific chemical groups to the parent compound: this way, drugs are metabolized to their active form, or they are modified to enhance excretion. Cytochrome P-450 oxidases (CYP) and uridine diphosphate-glucuronosyl transferase (UGT) are two of the most prominent family of enzymes of this class. The second class are transporters that mediate the efflux of drugs outside of cells, thereby limiting their therapeutic benefits. Many great examples are provided by transporter proteins that are part of the ATP-binding Cassette (ABC) superfamily. The other key development is the increasing knowledge about the physiological impact of SNPs in genes encoding proteins that play important roles in both of these processes. Below, we will describe issues that relate specifically to the realization of pharmacogenetics for pediatric nephrology patients, while also providing concrete examples from the literature.

Four main issues plague the field of pediatric pharmacogenetics in general. First, the vast majority of pharmacogenetics studies are done exclusively with adult subjects. Unfortunately, these findings can not be directly extrapolated to children because of the impact that growth and development have on pharmacologic parameters. Second, there are currently very few studies reporting specifically on the association of genetic polymorphisms with pharmacologic parameters in pediatric subjects. Third, the predictive power of most pediatric studies is effectively limited by small sample sizes (typically less than 100). Finally, all studies conducted thus far are retrospective and have not been able to test if inclusion of pharmacogenetic data influences outcomes. It is therefore not surprising that there are currently very few tests that are ready for prime time for pediatric patients.

In both adult [127] and pediatric nephrology [128], the most active research in pharmacogenetics relates to key agents used in current renal transplantation cocktails. Calcineurin inhibitors were logical candidates for such studies since they have proved to be valuable as steroid-sparing agents, but are known to cause significant, level-dependent nephrotoxicity. A single study with 104 pediatric kidney transplant recipients treated with cyclosporin showed no evidence that genotyping for polymorphisms in genes from the CYP and ABC families helped optimize patient care [129]; these results largely echo the consensus opinion derived from similar adult studies [127]. In contrast, implementation of pharmacogenetic profiling is probably closer to reality for tacrolimus: testing for polymorphisms in CYP3A5 identified in adult studies [127] was found to be predictive when tested in 30 teenage kidney transplant recipients [130]. There are also data from two small studies on pediatric kidney transplant recipients treated with MMF that report promising associations with UGT polymorphisms that require corroboration [131, 132].

Two additional hurdles will complicate the implementation of pharmacogenetics specifically in renal transplant protocols. First, benefits of genotyping above and beyond current gold standard will be necessary. This may proved a difficult task since therapeutic drug monitoring (TDM) of various immunosuppressive medications allows personalization of doses within days to weeks [127]. There is evidence that at least in adult patients, pharmacogenetics leads to more rapid optimization of drug dosage, but it does not appear to translate into better outcomes [133]. Second, the ability of any predictive indices, including pharmacogenetics, to impact clinical outcomes will always be hampered by the polypharmacy that is inherent to most renal transplant drug cocktails because of complex drug-drug interactions [127].

Warfarin is yet another medication relevant to pediatric nephrologists that has been extensively studied for pharmacogenetic applications. Studies in adult subjects have shown that polymorphisms in the genes encoding the target of warfarin VKORC1 (vitamin K epoxide reductase complex subunit 1) or its main metabolizing CYP (CYP2C9) are helpful to predict warfarin disposition [134]. Data emerging from pediatric studies testing the same polymorphism are unfortunately not as clear [135].

While pharmacogenetics offers the potential of individualized treatment strategies, it is critical to obtain solid evidence of clinical utility before widespread clinical implementation. A great source of information for interested physicians is the Clinical Pharmacogenetics Implementation Consortium (CPIC), a project aimed at addressing "some of the barriers to implementation of pharmacogenetic tests into clinical practice."

Online Resources
CPIC: http://goo.gl/rDw2SQ

Barriers to Implementation in the Clinic

There is a lot of hype and high expectation that remain largely unrealistic. Apart from diagnosis of rare disease and some rare applications in pharmacogenomics, the real-world impact of genomics has yet to impact the clinic. Notwithstanding the knowledge limitations that are inherent in the implementation delays, there are a number of other issues that will hamper this process, some of which are discussed below.

Health Literacy and Numeracy

Patients
Adequate health literacy skills are necessary for patients to understand a discussion about genomic issues and to appropriately consent for testing. Health literacy is defined as "the degree to which individuals can obtain, process, and understand the basic health information and services needed to make appropriate health decisions" [136]. A survey of general US adults demonstrated poor health literacy in ~30–40 % [137]. Not surprisingly, the situation is even worse when these skills are assessed in the context of genomics issues [138]. Apparent familiarity with genetic concepts is common in adults, but physicians should be alert to the fact that understanding of basic genetic concepts is often limited [139].

Health numeracy skills are also critical for patients to grasp the predictive nature of most discussions that relate to genomic health decisions. Indeed, statistics and probabilities are integral part of these discussions. Health numeracy is defined as "the degree to which individuals have the capacity to access, process, interpret, communicate, and act on numerical, quantitative, graphical, biostatistical, probabilistic health information needed to make effective health decisions" [140]. A recent survey revealed that ~50 % of adult sub-

jects have basic or minimal numeracy skills [137]. In contrast to health literacy, this subject has been little studied [138].

While these issues cannot be ignored, they should not jeopardize patient care. Given that time is limited in the clinic, it may not be possible for the treating physician to spend time to explain basic concepts. The critical point is to rapidly assess if the patient (or their caretaker) has at least a basic understanding of the issues at stake, and take measures to try to address perceived inadequacies. If the family has access to Internet and is motivated to learn independently, the physician may provide the address of reputable websites focused on teaching basic genetic concepts to a general audience (see list below).

Resources for Patients
Genetic Science Learning Center:
    http://learn.genetics.utah.edu/
NHGRI educational material:
    http://www.genome.gov/education/
Genetics Home Reference:
    http://ghr.nlm.nih.gov/
NNSGRC Genetics Information for Parents and
    Families: http://goo.gl/1WFa67
Internet-based tool to record details of family
    history (US Surgeon General initiative):
    http://goo.gl/QcFmH

Physicians
Another important issue that is emerging is the gap between what physicians will need to know to implement genomic science in clinical practice, and what they actually know [1, 141]. Given the scarcity of health care professionals with an expertise in genetics and genomics [142], which is unlikely to change in the next few years, it is possible that these inadequacies may hamper the deployment of genomic medicine when it is ready for widespread implementation. There are many resources in the literature [1], in print and online (see list below) that may help bridge that gap for practicing physicians.

While most physicians agree that a good understanding of basic statistical concepts is necessary in contemporary medicine, very few feel confident of their own skills [143]. This is a long-standing problem that has been repeatedly documented in Europe and North America [144-146]. Up until recently, these skills were deemed important by physicians espousing the principles of evidence-based medicine. The advent of genomic medicine will hopefully trigger a renewed interest for physicians to acquire basic quantitative skills. Medical schools are currently adapting curricula to reflect these changes such that current physicians-in-training will be better prepared [147-149].

Resources for Physicians (* Indicates Not Free)

Book from AAP: Robert A Saul, Medical Genetics in Pediatric Practice, 2013, 503 p., American Academy of Pediatrics ISBN:978-1-58110-496-7.
   Mobile Apps:

Talking Glossary of Genetic Terms (NIHGRI); iPhone
Act Sheets (ACMG); iPhone and Android
*PediaGene (free for AAP members; $); iPhone and Android
BioGene; iPhone and Android
GeneticCode; iPhone
Gene Screen; iPhone
Gene tutor; iPhone and Android
*Genetics 4 Medics; iPhone ($5) Android (free)

   Free learning web resource:

Online Mendelian Inheritance in Man (OMIM):
   http://omim.org
CDC – Public Health Genomics:
   http://www.cdc.gov/genomics/
CDC – Pediatric Genetics: http://goo.gl/YV6KIE
European Rare Disease: http://www.orpha.net/
Human Gene Mutation Database:
   http://www.hgmd.cf.ac.uk/
Geneforum: http://www.geneforum.org/
Center for Genomics and Public Health:
   http://goo.gl/XvA7TI

   Genetic Testing:

Gene tests: http://Genetests.org
NCI – Gene testing: http://goo.gl/rZjCXX

Lab tests Online – The Universe of Genetic Testing: http://goo.gl/DzsKVV
NIH Genetic Testing Registry:
   http://www.ncbi.nlm.nih.gov/gtr/

   Online tutorials:

Open Helix: http://www.openhelix.com
OMIM: http://goo.gl/VITq9x
*Genetics Home Reference: http://goo.gl/xLt37E
HGMD: http://goo.gl/hgYqIx
Genetics in Primary Care Institute (AAP):
   http://goo.gl/cxwV6V

Test Costs and Gene Patents

Both governmental programs and insurance companies will usually agree to defray the costs of tests that are ordered by physicians, are relevant to the patient's condition, and may lead to a concrete change in the plan of care. Ideally, the cost of tests would not play a major role in this decision, but up until recently, it did for a few genetic tests that were prohibitively expensive (thousands of dollars). These high prices were driven in large part by strict enforcement of gene patents held by a few companies. For example, the price of BRCA1 and 2 tripled once the company Myriad genetics decided to exercise a strict monopoly for its genes patents [150].

Since ~40% of the human genes have been patented [151], this had the potential to be a major hurdle in the development of personalized medicine based on genomic testing [152]. This situation changed dramatically following the recent US Supreme Court judgment that invalidated the gene patents held by Myriad Genetics [153].

Demonstration of Efficacy and Cost-Effectiveness

With the gene patent barriers now down and the availability of cheap sequencing, the next big obstacle to promised widespread clinical implementation of genomic tests [154] will be demonstration of efficacy and cost-effectiveness for

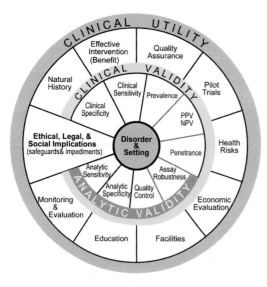

Fig. 4.16 Illustration of the ACCE framework use to evaluate genetic tests. Evaluation of genetic tests with ACCE is based on four criteria: analytic validity, clinical validity, clinical utility and associated ethical, legal and social implications (ELSI). It is meant to be an up-to-date source of information for policy makers to allow informed decision making. This figure illustrates the various components that are studied for each category. Analytic validity is defined as how accurately and reliably the test measures the genotype of interest. Clinical validity is defined as how consistently and accurately the test detects or predicts the intermediate or final outcomes of interest. Clinical utility is defined as how likely the test is to significantly improve patient outcomes. ELSI is defined as the ethical, legal, and social implications that may arise in the context of using the test (Source: http://www.cdc.gov/genomics/gtesting/ACCE/. Public Domain)

common conditions [155]. At the request of the CDC, a committee of experts proposed to use a specific set of criteria to assess whether a particular genetic test ought to be implemented in the clinic. It is referred to as ACCE, an acronym that reflects the four criteria that need to be fulfilled: Analytic validity, Clinical validity, Clinical utility and associated Ethical, legal and social implications.

As seen in Fig. 4.16, this is an ambitious task that requires integration of data from many different spheres of expertise. Genomic tests will also need to be analyzed using the ACCE multifaceted approach: this will likely prove to be a lengthier process since in theory, each gene-

disease combination will undergo similar in-depth examination. The CDC also formed another committee named Evaluation of Genomic Applications in Practice and Prevention (EGAPP) that is aimed at prospective integration of published data within the ACCE framework. Interested physicians should consult the EGAPP website for regular updates on this topic.

It is sobering to review the most up-to-date EGAPP recommendations, which are focused only on common diseases with significant public health burden: there is "insufficient evidence to recommend for or against use" of well-studied genetic tests for breast cancer, cardiovascular disease, depression, diabetes, and prostate cancer; only genetic testing for KRAS mutation in colorectal cancer fulfills all requirements. Children are typically not mentioned in articles on this topic; if they are mentioned, it is as part of the subjects that are excluded [156].

Ethical and Legal Issues

As clinical use of sequencing technologies become increasingly widespread, practicing nephrologists should expect to have to deal with a new set of issues when discussing results with their patients. As the price of whole exome and/or exome sequencing decreases over time, these technologies will supplant current approaches that are more targeted, such as Sanger sequencing. This is a drastic change in practice since clinicians will now have to deal with genome-wide data that are not restricted to genes known to be associated with a given condition. With these changes comes a complex set of issues that every physician is likely to encounter in the near future. These include dealing with misattributed paternity and handling incidental genetic findings. Physicians should also be able to discuss how genomic medicine may affect patient privacy and how these results may lead to genetic discrimination. Below, we provide a brief introduction to these concepts that will provide interested physicians with a good starting point or springboard to learn more about these topics.

Nonpaternity

One important consideration when performing genetic testing is to be cognizant of the fact that misattributed paternity, also referred to as nonpaternity, is observed in ~10% of tested individuals (range 1–30%) [157]. In the clinical arena, this problem will be encountered in two main scenarios: first, in the context of HLA testing when assessing the parents as potential organ donors [158]; the other situation is when diagnosing a genetic condition, particularly if it is a recessive disease and the father does not harbor the mutation [159].

The treating team should strongly consider consulting a medical geneticist or a genetic counsellor since they are trained to handle these situations. In addition, they can help to calculate and interpret the paternity index, the most useful measure of paternity testing [160]. This method relies on genotyping of 10–15 additional loci for each member of the trio, the assumption being that: each parent shares ~50% of variants with their child. Rarely, a paternally-inherited de novo mutation may explain these findings when paternity testing confirms that the father is indeed genetically related to the patient.

In most jurisdictions, there are no guidelines, rules or laws that dictate what a clinical team should do in these circumstances. Proponents of nondisclosure emphasize the importance of nonmaleficence, while those that advocate for disclosure invoke respect for patient autonomy and truth telling [161]. Treating physicians should be aware that nearly all genetic specialists in the US [162] or abroad [163] have consistently favored disclosure, but only to the mother. This was also the recommendation from a report published by the Institute of Medicine in 1994 [164].

Medically-Actionable Variants

Another dilemma that stems from the introduction of genome sequencing in the clinic is how incidental genomic findings, also known as "incidentalomas", should be handled. This dilemma is particularly acute when dealing with so-called "medically-actionable, pathologic mutations". These are defined as variants in genes known to be associated with severe Mendelian diseases for which there is good evidence of benefit from specific preventive measures, or therapies. A debate on whether one has a duty to report such findings has been raging for a few years in the genetic research community: a recent consensus opinion states that such findings should be reported to subjects who have a priori consented to receive information about incidental findings [165]. The debate is now overflowing to the clinical world.

Recently published policy guidelines put forth by the American College of Medical Genetics recommends mandatory reporting of variants found via clinical sequencing and deemed to be likely pathogenic in 57 genes associated with 24 monogenic conditions [166]. In stark contrast to the research guidelines mentioned above, these incidental findings would have to be reported to patients even if they did not consent to receive this information. While providing valuable information to patients and their families, enactment of these guidelines would add extra work that may not be accommodated easily with the current clinical workforce. Interrogation of whole-genome sequencing data from 500 Caucasians and 500 African-American "healthy" adults revealed that ~1–3% of subjects tested harbor at least one mutation in one of these genes [167]. Adjudication of which incidental findings are actionable is not straight forward [168].

Importantly for pediatricians, these recommendations make no exceptions in that regard for children, even for genes that cause adult-onset conditions [166]. This suggestion is based on the fact that it may be critical for the parents themselves to know about these incidental findings. It is predicted that more restricted reporting of such variants will be recommended for children once clinical sequencing becomes more widespread: indeed, this argument will be moot when the parents also have their own sequencing data [166]. Table 4.3 provides a list of genes that are relevant to the practice of pediatric nephrologists: all follow an autosomal dominant pattern of inheritance, and are the primary cause for a variety of cancers [166].

Table 4.3 Conditions and/or syndromes with clinically-actionable mutations that are relevant to pediatric nephrologists

Conditions	Gene	OMIM #	Patients affected	Mode of inheritance	Clinical impact of variants
VHLS	VHL	193300	Child/adult	AD	Known and expected
MEN type 1	MEN1	131100	Child/adult	AD	Known and expected
MEN type 2	RET	171400	Child/adult	AD	Known
		162300			
HPPS type 1	SDHD	168000	Child/adult	AD	Known and expected
HPPS type 2	SDHAF2	601650	Child/adult	AD	Known
HPPS type 3	SDHC	605373	Child/adult	AD	Known and expected
HPPS type 4	SDHB	115310	Child/adult	AD	Unknown
TSC type 1	TSC1	191100	Child	AD	Known and expected
TSC type 2	TSC2	613254	Child	AD	Known and expected
Wilms tumor	WT1	194070	Child	AD	Known and expected
NF type 2	NF2	101100	Child/adult	AD	Known and expected

HPPS Hereditary paraganglioma–pheochromocytoma syndrome, *MEN* Multiple endocrine neoplasia, *NF* Neurofibromatosis, *TSC* Tuberous sclerosis complex, *VHLS* Von Hippel-Lindau syndrome

Privacy

All physicians are keenly aware that patient privacy is paramount. Most are also cognizant of data that could be used as unique identifiers: name, birth date, home address, social security number, etc. When stripped of these data, samples or datasets are deemed de-identified. Like most pediatric sub-specialists, pediatric nephrologists routinely take care of patients with very rare conditions. For such patients, it is unclear how "de-identified" the information really is if the diagnosis is part of the data that may be shared. For example, inclusion of this information in public databases could lead to the de facto identification of a specific patient, particularly if the condition is associated with a visible phenotype. For this reason, some jurisdictions have added rare (UK) or unique (USA) characteristics of patients to the list of unique identifiers [169].

One recent challenge to the privacy of patients stems from the emergence of genomic medicine because genomic data is not considered as a unique identifier per se. This is likely to become even more challenging as the pressures from the research community grow to have as many genomes available publicly as possible [170]. Given the fact that humans differ at ~0.1 % of the 3.2 billion bases of the genome, and given a world population of six billion, current estimates

show that genotyping data from 30 to 80 alleles would be sufficient to provide unique genomic fingerprinting for every individual [171]. This number is amazingly small when compared to the datasets from whole exome and whole-genome sequencing, which provide thousands of such alleles. Thus, re-identification of a de-identified dataset is simple if one can genotype a sample obtained from an individual that may then be used to find a perfect match against all available genomic datasets (or near-perfect match for close relatives).

In a recent tour-de-force, it was shown that it is possible to trace the original subject linked to a particular genomic dataset by combining the analysis with data from publicly available genealogical databases [172]. The "investigators-hackers" were able to do this with the following publicly available information in hand: whole-genome sequencing data, gender (males), age when the samples were provided, and state where the men lived at the time (Utah).

As front-line responders dealing with keen parents who are very likely to use the internet to find health information [173], pediatricians should be prepared to answers questions about the impact of genomic medicine on privacy of their patients. The current status is that there is still considerable uncertainty in the field, but the consensus appears to be that complete de-identification of genomic datasets is far more complex than expected [174].

Genetic Discrimination

The rapid developments in the sequencing and analysis of genomic information have forced a debate about the potential real-life consequences for patients when it is used in the clinic [175]. The reporting of diagnostic and/or incidental findings opens the door to genetic discrimination, which is defined as an "adverse treatment that is based solely on the genotype of asymptomatic individuals" [176].

Knowledge about genetic or familial risks for a variety of diseases has been used to justify health insurers' refusal of at-risk patients [177] or employers' dismissal of potential or current employees [178]. Most Europeans countries have enacted legislation against this type of discrimination since the 1990s [179]. US congress followed suit in 2008 with the passage of Genetic Information Nondiscrimination Act (GINA) [180]. Canada remains the only G8 country without such legislation, and Canadians are routinely refused life and/or disability insurance because of genetic risk factors [181]. Similar problems also occur in other developed nations with national health care systems, such as Japan [182] or Australia [183].

All pediatricians ordering genetic tests for their patients should seek information about the current legal framework in their countries as these may have immediate implications for the family as a whole. These issues should ideally be discussed with the family before ordering the tests.

Direct-to-Consumer Testing of Presymptomatic Minors

The first direct-to-consumer (DTC) genetic testing companies started to operate more than 10 years ago. Up until recently, they existed in a legislative void: because the tests used were developed internally (known as "home brews"), they are exempt from tight regulations that apply to most diagnostic tests [184]. As a result of this, they were able to offer tests of questionable value, without oversight, and without interactions with a health care professional before or after testing [185]. Once it became clear that thousands of people were paying for these services, regulatory bodies in many countries started to pay closer attention to the products offered by these companies [186], but changes in regulation have been slow to come [187]. The interested reader is directed to recent exhaustive reviews for more details on this complex topic [188, 189]. For the purpose of this discussion, we will focus on issues that relate to DTC testing when applied specifically to children.

Many direct-to-consumer (DTC) genetic testing companies, most notably 23andMe, agree to perform pre-symptomatic or predictive genetic testing on children [190]. This is in direct contradiction to professional guidelines promulgated by most professional organizations, which state that such tests should only be performed once the child can provide informed consent for themselves [191]. Additional concerns raised by the behavior of DTC companies is that there is no requirement for these findings to be medically actionable (i.e., at a minimum, a way to prevent or treat the condition must exist to offer such tests to minors) [190]. The FDA has been investigating to determine whether tighter regulations are necessary for these companies.

Pediatrician should expect to be asked for advice with regard to performing DTC genetic testing on their patients, or they may be asked to help interpret the results of such tests [192]. It may also lead to new consultations for asymptomatic children because a number of renal conditions are included in mainstream DTC reports (for example, carrier status for ARPKD, primary hyperoxaluria type 2, and tyrosinemia type 1). Since DTC companies do not spend time to explain the ethical and legal issues that stem from such testing (discussed above), the onus will be on the treating physician to do so. Unless clinically indicated, pediatricians should strongly consider refraining from ordering additional diagnostic tests triggered solely from the results of DTC genetic testing as the clinical validity of many of the findings have yet to be established [193]. In a significant turn of events, the US Federal Drug Administration (FDA) asked 23andme to stop marketing these tests to consumers starting in November, 2013; the FDA will now require DTC genomic companies to undergo regulatory clearances that are typical for genetic tests used in the clinic.

Online Resources
FDA letter to 23andme: http://goo.gl/Xrx48Z; 23andme: https://www.23andme.com/health/

Glossary of Terms

Alleles Alternative forms of a gene at the same locus

Alternative splicing Formation of diverse mRNAs through differential splicing of an mRNA precursor

Autosome Any chromosome (1–22) other than the sex chromosomes X and Y

cDNA, complementary DNA DNA sequence that contains only exonic sequences and was made from an mRNA molecule

Centimorgan Length of DNA that on average has 1 crossover per 100 gametes

Cis Location of two genes/changes on the same chromosome

Codon Three consecutive bases/nucleotides in DNA/RNA that specify an amino acid

Compound heterozygote Individual with two different mutant alleles at a locus

Consanguineous Mating between individuals who share at least one common ancestor

Conservation Sequence similarity for genes present in two distinct organisms or for gene families; can be detected by measuring the sequence similarity at the nucleotide (DNA or RNA) or amino acid (protein) level

Crossover Exchange of genetic material between homologous chromosomes during meiosis

Digenic inheritance Two genes interacting to produce a disease phenotype

Diploid Chromosome number of somatic cells

Domain Segment of a protein associated with a specialized structure or function

Dominant Trait expressed in the heterozygote

Downstream Sequence that is distal or 3′ from the reference point

Empiric risk Recurrence risk based on experience rather than calculation

Epigenetics Term describing nonmutational phenomena (e.g., methylation and acetylation) that modify the expression of a gene

Euchromatin Majority of nuclear DNA that remains relatively unfolded during most of the cell cycle and is therefore accessible to transcriptional machinery

Exon Segment of a gene (usually protein coding) that remains after splicing of the primary RNA transcript

Expressivity Variation in the severity of a genetic trait

Genotype Genetic constitution of the organism; usually refers to a particular pair of alleles the individual carries at a given locus of the genome

Germline Cell lineage resulting in eggs or sperm

Germline mutation Any detectable, heritable variation in the lineage of germ cells transmitted to offspring while those in somatic cells are not

Gonadal (germline) mosaicism Occurrence of more than one genetic constitution in the precursor cells of eggs or sperm

Haplotype Group of nearby, closely linked alleles inherited together as a unit

Heterozygote Person with one normal and one mutant allele at a given locus on a pair of homologous chromosomes

Homozygote Person with identical alleles at a given locus on a pair of homologous chromosomes

Imprinting Parent-specific expression or repression of genes or chromosomes in offspring

Intron Segment of a gene transcribed into the primary RNA transcript but excised during exon splicing, thus does not code for a protein

Isodisomy, uniparental Inheritance of two copies of one homologue of a chromosome from one parent, with loss of the corresponding homologue from the other parent

Karyotype Classified chromosome complement of an individual or a cell

Lyon hypothesis (X inactivation) Principle of inactivation of one of the two X chromosomes in normal female cells (first proposed by Dr. Mary Lyon)

Mendelian Following patterns of inheritance originally proposed by Gregor Mendel

Monogenic disorder Caused by mutations in a single gene

Mosaicism Occurrence of more than one genetic constitution arising in an individual after fertilization

Multifactorial disorder Caused by the interaction of multiple genetic and environmental factors

Mutation Change from the normal to an altered form of a particular gene that has harmful; pathogenic effects

Oligogenic inheritance Character that is determined by a small number of genes acting together

Penetrance Frequency with which a genotype manifests itself in a given phenotype

Phenotype Visible expression of the action of a particular gene; the clinical picture resulting from a genetic disorder

Pleiotropy Multiple effects of a single gene

Polymerase chain reaction (PCR) Amplification of DNA using a specific technique that allows analysis of minute original amounts of DNA

Polymorphism Usually used for any sequence variant present at a frequency greater than 1 % in a population

Recessive A trait expressed only when both alleles at a given genetic locus are altered

Recombination Separation of alleles that are close together on the same chromosome by crossing over of homologous chromosomes at meiosis

SNP (single nucleotide polymorphism) Usually used for any sequence variant present at a frequency greater than 1 % in a population

Somatic Involving the body cells rather than the germline

Syndrome, genetic Nonrandom combination of features

Teratogen Any agent causing congenital malformations

Trans Location of two genes/changes on opposite chromosomes of a pair

Transcription Production of mRNA from the DNA template

Translation The process by which protein is synthesized from an mRNA sequence

References

1. Guttmacher AE, Porteous ME, Mcinerney JD. Educating health-care professionals about genetics and genomics. Nat Rev Genet. 2007;8:151–7.
2. Stanescu HC, Arcos-Burgos M, Medlar A, et al. Risk HLA-DQA1 and PLA(2)R1 alleles in idiopathic membranous nephropathy. N Engl J Med. 2011;364: 616–26.
3. Watson JD, Crick FH. Molecular structure of nucleic acids; a structure for deoxyribose nucleic acid. Nature. 1953;171:737–8.
4. Schmutz J, Wheeler J, Grimwood J, et al. Quality assessment of the human genome sequence. Nature. 2004;429:365–8.
5. Watson IR, Takahashi K, Futreal PA, Chin L. Emerging patterns of somatic mutations in cancer. Nat Rev Genet. 2013;14:703–18.
6. Sherry ST, Ward MH, Kholodov M, et al. dbSNP: the NCBI database of genetic variation. Nucleic Acids Res. 2001;29:308–11.
7. Bernstein BE, Birney E, Dunham I, Green ED, Gunter C, Snyder M. An integrated encyclopedia of DNA elements in the human genome. Nature. 2012;489: 57–74.
8. Sauna ZE, Kimchi-Sarfaty C. Understanding the contribution of synonymous mutations to human disease. Nat Rev Genet. 2011;12:683–91.
9. Izarzugaza JM, Hopcroft LE, Baresic A, Orengo CA, Martin AC, Valencia A. Characterization of pathogenic germline mutations in human protein kinases. BMC Bioinforma. 2011;12 Suppl 4:S1.
10. Spielmann M, Mundlos S. Structural variations, the regulatory landscape of the genome and their alteration in human disease. Bioessays. 2013;35:533–43.
11. Nakamura Y. DNA variations in human and medical genetics: 25 years of my experience. J Hum Genet. 2009;54:1–8.
12. Consortium IH. The International HapMap Project. Nature. 2003;426:789–96.
13. Consortium IH. A haplotype map of the human genome. Nature. 2005;437:1299–320.
14. Pybus M, Dall'Olio GM, Luisi P, et al. 1000 Genomes Selection Browser 1.0: a genome browser dedicated to signatures of natural selection in modern humans. Nucleic Acids Res. 2014;42:D903–9.
15. Alves I, Sramkova Hanulova A, Foll M, Excoffier L. Genomic data reveal a complex making of humans. PLoS Genet. 2012;8:e1002837.
16. Reich D, Price AL, Patterson N. Principal component analysis of genetic data. Nat Genet. 2008;40: 491–2.
17. Mills RE, Walter K, Stewart C, et al. Mapping copy number variation by population-scale genome sequencing. Nature. 2011;470:59–65.

18. Church DM, Lappalainen I, Sneddon TP, et al. Public data archives for genomic structural variation. Nat Genet. 2010;42(10):813–4. [letter].

19. Kirby A, Gnirke A, Jaffe DB, et al. Mutations causing medullary cystic kidney disease type 1 lie in a large VNTR in MUC1 missed by massively parallel sequencing. Nat Genet. 2013;45:299–303.

20. Tubio JM, Estivill X. Cancer: when catastrophe strikes a cell. Nature. 2011;470(7335):476.

21. Christodoulou K, Tsingis M, Stavrou C, et al. Chromosome 1 localization of a gene for autosomal dominant medullary cystic kidney disease. Hum Mol Genet. 1998;7:905–11.

22. Antignac C, Knebelmann B, Drouot L, et al. Deletions in the COL4A5 collagen gene in X-linked Alport syndrome. Characterization of the pathological transcripts in nonrenal cells and correlation with disease expression. J Clin Invest. 1994;93:1195–207.

23. Medjeral-Thomas N, Malik TH, Patel MP, et al. A novel CFHR5 fusion protein causes C3 glomerulopathy in a family without Cypriot ancestry. Kidney Int. 2014;85(4):933–7.

24. Gale DP, de Jorge EG, Cook HT, et al. Identification of a mutation in complement factor H-related protein 5 in patients of Cypriot origin with glomerulonephritis. Lancet. 2010;376:794–801.

25. Barnes MR, Breen G. A short primer on the functional analysis of copy number variation for biomedical scientists. Methods Mol Biol. 2010;628:119–35.

26. Pook MA, Wrong O, Wooding C, Norden AG, Feest TG, Thakker RV. Dent's disease, a renal Fanconi syndrome with nephrocalcinosis and kidney stones, is associated with a microdeletion involving DXS255 and maps to Xp11.22. Hum Mol Genet. 1993;2:2129–34.

27. Barker DF, Hostikka SL, Zhou J, et al. Identification of mutations in the COL4A5 collagen gene in Alport syndrome. Science. 1990;248:1224–7.

28. Hildebrandt F, Otto E, Rensing C, et al. A novel gene encoding an SH3 domain protein is mutated in nephronophthisis type 1. Nat Genet. 1997;17:149–53.

29. Henrichsen CN, Chaignat E, Reymond A. Copy number variants, diseases and gene expression. Hum Mol Genet. 2009;18:R1–8.

30. Aitman TJ, Dong R, Vyse TJ, et al. Copy number polymorphism in Fcgr3 predisposes to glomerulonephritis in rats and humans. Nature. 2006;439:851–5.

31. Sanna-Cherchi S, Kiryluk K, Burgess KE, et al. Copy-number disorders are a common cause of congenital kidney malformations. Am J Hum Genet. 2012;91:987–97.

32. Shuib S, Wei W, Sur H, et al. Copy number profiling in von Hippel-Lindau disease renal cell carcinoma. Genes Chromosomes Cancer. 2011;50:479–88.

33. Girgis AH, Iakovlev VV, Beheshti B, et al. Multilevel whole-genome analysis reveals candidate biomarkers in clear cell renal cell carcinoma. Cancer Res. 2012;72:5273–84.

34. Riethoven JJ. Regulatory regions in DNA: promoters, enhancers, silencers, and insulators. Methods Mol Biol. 2010;674:33–42.

35. Reilly DS, Lewis RA, Ledbetter DH, Nussbaum RL. Tightly linked flanking markers for the Lowe oculocerebrorenal syndrome, with application to carrier assessment. Am J Hum Genet. 1988;42:748–55.

36. Hertz JM, Persson U, Juncker I, Segelmark M. Alport syndrome caused by inversion of a 21 Mb fragment of the long arm of the X-chromosome comprising exon 9 through 51 of the COL4A5 gene. Hum Genet. 2005;118:23–8.

37. Vervoort VS, Smith RJ, O'Brien J, et al. Genomic rearrangements of EYA1 account for a large fraction of families with BOR syndrome. Eur J Hum Genet. 2002;10:757–66.

38. Stephens PJ, Greenman CD, Fu B, et al. Massive genomic rearrangement acquired in a single catastrophic event during cancer development. Cell. 2011;144:27–40.

39. Forment JV, Kaidi A, Jackson SP. Chromothripsis and cancer: causes and consequences of chromosome shattering. Nat Rev Cancer. 2012;12:663–70.

40. Maher CA, Wilson RK. Chromothripsis and human disease: piecing together the shattering process. Cell. 2012;148:29–32.

41. Kloosterman WP, Guryev V, van Roosmalen M, et al. Chromothripsis as a mechanism driving complex de novo structural rearrangements in the germline. Hum Mol Genet. 2011;20:1916–24.

42. Chiang C, Jacobsen JC, Ernst C, et al. Complex reorganization and predominant non-homologous repair following chromosomal breakage in karyotypically balanced germline rearrangements and transgenic integration. Nat Genet. 2012;44:390–7. S1.

43. Kloosterman WP, Tavakoli-Yaraki M, van Roosmalen MJ, et al. Constitutional chromothripsis rearrangements involve clustered double-stranded DNA breaks and nonhomologous repair mechanisms. Cell Rep. 2012;1:648–55.

44. Kestila M, Lenkkeri U, Mannikko M, et al. Positionally cloned gene for a novel glomerular protein – nephrin – is mutated in congenital nephrotic syndrome. Mol Cell. 1998;1:575–82.

45. Consortium TIPKD. Polycystic kidney disease: the complete structure of the PKD1 gene and its protein. The International Polycystic Kidney Disease Consortium. Cell. 1995;81:289–98.

46. Lloyd SE, Pearce SH, Fisher SE, et al. A common molecular basis for three inherited kidney stone diseases. Nature. 1996;379:445–9.

47. Consortium THYP. A gene (PEX) with homologies to endopeptidases is mutated in patients with X-linked hypophosphatemic rickets. The HYP Consortium. Nat Genet. 1995;11:130–6.

48. Wilson FH, Hariri A, Farhi A, et al. A cluster of metabolic defects caused by mutation in a mitochondrial tRNA. Science. 2004;306:1190–4.

49. Ragoussis J. Genotyping technologies for genetic research. Annu Rev Genomics Hum Genet. 2009;10:117–33.

50. Maloy S. Brenner's online encyclopedia of genetics, 2nd edition: vol 1–4. In: Maloy S, Hughes K, editors. Brenner's encyclopedia of genetics. San Diego: Academic; 2013. p. 250–1.

51. Hamamy H, Antonarakis SE, Cavalli-Sforza LL, et al. Consanguineous marriages, pearls and perils: Geneva International Consanguinity Workshop Report. Genet Med. 2011;13:841–7.

52. Lander ES, Botstein D. Homozygosity mapping: a way to map human recessive traits with the DNA of inbred children. Science. 1987;236:1567–70.

53. Alkuraya FS. Unit 6.12: Discovery of rare homozygous mutations from studies of consanguineous pedigrees. Curr Protoc Hum Genet. 2012;75:1–13.

54. Alkuraya FS. Autozygome decoded. Genet Med. 2010;12:765–71.

55. Miano MG, Jacobson SG, Carothers A, et al. Pitfalls in homozygosity mapping. Am J Hum Genet. 2000;67:1348–51.

56. Bolk S, Puffenberger EG, Hudson J, Morton DH, Chakravarti A. Elevated frequency and allelic heterogeneity of congenital nephrotic syndrome, Finnish type, in the old order Mennonites. Am J Hum Genet. 1999;65(6):1785–90.[letter].

57. Frishberg Y, Ben-Neriah Z, Suvanto M, et al. Misleading findings of homozygosity mapping resulting from three novel mutations in NPHS1 encoding nephrin in a highly inbred community. Genet Med. 2007;9:180–4.

58. Hildebrandt F, Heeringa SF, Ruschendorf F, et al. A systematic approach to mapping recessive disease genes in individuals from outbred populations. PLoS Genet. 2009;5:e1000353.

59. Alkuraya FS. Homozygosity mapping: one more tool in the clinical geneticist's toolbox. Genet Med. 2010;12:236–9.

60. Abu Safieh L, Aldahmesh MA, Shamseldin H, et al. Clinical and molecular characterisation of Bardet-Biedl syndrome in consanguineous populations: the power of homozygosity mapping. J Med Genet. 2010;47:236–41.

61. Kao WH, Klag MJ, Meoni LA, et al. MYH9 is associated with nondiabetic end-stage renal disease in African Americans. Nat Genet. 2008;40:1185–92.

62. Kopp JB, Smith MW, Nelson GW, et al. MYH9 is a major-effect risk gene for focal segmental glomerulosclerosis. Nat Genet. 2008;40:1175–84.

63. Peterson LC, Rao KV, Crosson JT, White JG. Fechtner syndrome – a variant of Alport's syndrome with leukocyte inclusions and macrothrombocytopenia. Blood. 1985;65:397–406.

64. Seri M, Pecci A, Di Bari F, et al. MYH9-related disease: May-Hegglin anomaly, Sebastian syndrome, Fechtner syndrome, and Epstein syndrome are not distinct entities but represent a variable expression of a single illness. Medicine (Baltimore). 2003;82:203–15.

65. Genovese G, Friedman DJ, Ross MD, et al. Association of trypanolytic ApoL1 variants with kidney disease in African Americans. Science. 2010;329:841–5.

66. Friedman DJ, Pollak MR. Genetics of kidney failure and the evolving story of APOL1. J Clin Invest. 2011;121:3367–74.

67. Parsa A, Kao WH, Xie D, et al. APOL1 risk variants, race, and progression of chronic kidney disease. N Engl J Med. 2013;369:2183–96.

68. Min Jou W, Haegeman G, Ysebaert M, Fiers W. Nucleotide sequence of the gene coding for the bacteriophage MS2 coat protein. Nature. 1972;237:82–8.

69. Sanger F, Nicklen S, Coulson AR. DNA sequencing with chain-terminating inhibitors. Proc Natl Acad Sci U S A. 1977;74:5463–7.

70. Smith LM, Sanders JZ, Kaiser RJ, et al. Fluorescence detection in automated DNA sequence analysis. Nature. 1986;321:674–9.

71. Metzker ML. Sequencing technologies – the next generation. Nat Rev Genet. 2010;11:31–46.

72. Loman NJ, Misra RV, Dallman TJ, et al. Performance comparison of benchtop high-throughput sequencing platforms. Nat Biotechnol. 2012;30:434–9.

73. Abecasis GR, Altshuler D, Auton A, et al. A map of human genome variation from population-scale sequencing. Nature. 2010;467:1061–73.

74. Buchanan CC, Torstenson ES, Bush WS, Ritchie MD. A comparison of cataloged variation between International HapMap Consortium and 1000 Genomes Project data. J Am Med Inform Assoc. 2012;19:289–94.

75. Ng PC, Levy S, Huang J, et al. Genetic variation in an individual human exome. PLoS Genet. 2008;4:e1000160.

76. Choi M, Scholl UI, Ji W, et al. Genetic diagnosis by whole exome capture and massively parallel DNA sequencing. Proc Natl Acad Sci U S A. 2009;106:19096–101.

77. Hodges E, Xuan Z, Balija V, et al. Genome-wide in situ exon capture for selective resequencing. Nat Genet. 2007;39:1522–7.

78. Ng SB, Turner EH, Robertson PD, et al. Targeted capture and massively parallel sequencing of 12 human exomes. Nature. 2009;461:272–6.

79. Ng SB, Bigham AW, Buckingham KJ, et al. Exome sequencing identifies MLL2 mutations as a cause of Kabuki syndrome. Nat Genet. 2010;42:790–3.

80. Levy S, Sutton G, Ng PC, et al. The diploid genome sequence of an individual human. PLoS Biol. 2007;5:e254.

81. Bick D, Dimmock D. Whole exome and whole genome sequencing. Curr Opin Pediatr. 2011;23:594–600.

82. Stankiewicz P, Lupski JR. Structural variation in the human genome and its role in disease. Annu Rev Med. 2010;61:437–55.

83. Medvedev P, Stanciu M, Brudno M. Computational methods for discovering structural variation with next-generation sequencing. Nat Methods. 2009;6:S13–20.

84. Korbel JO, Urban AE, Affourtit JP, et al. Paired-end mapping reveals extensive structural variation in the human genome. Science. 2007;318:420–6.

85. Wheeler DA, Srinivasan M, Egholm M, et al. The complete genome of an individual by massively parallel DNA sequencing. Nature. 2008;452:872–6.

86. Sboner A, Mu XJ, Greenbaum D, Auerbach RK, Gerstein MB. The real cost of sequencing: higher than you think! Genome Biol. 2011;12:125.

87. Kitzman JO, Snyder MW, Ventura M, et al. Noninvasive whole-genome sequencing of a human fetus. Sci Transl Med. 2012;4:137ra76.

88. Knob AL. Principles of genetic testing and genetic counseling for renal clinicians. Semin Nephrol. 2010;30:431–7.

89. Li Y, Kottgen A. Genetic investigations of kidney disease: core curriculum 2013. Am J Kidney Dis. 2013;61:832–44.

90. Gahl WA, Markello TC, Toro C, et al. The National Institutes of Health Undiagnosed Diseases Program: insights into rare diseases. Genet Med. 2012;14:51–9.

91. Jacob HJ, Abrams K, Bick DP, et al. Genomics in clinical practice: lessons from the front lines. Sci Transl Med. 2013;5:194cm5.

92. Yang Y, Muzny DM, Reid JG, et al. Clinical whole-exome sequencing for the diagnosis of Mendelian disorders. N Engl J Med. 2013;369:1502–11.

93. Saunders CJ, Miller NA, Soden SE, et al. Rapid whole-genome sequencing for genetic disease diagnosis in neonatal intensive care units. Sci Transl Med. 2012;4:154ra135.

94. Bell CJ, Dinwiddie DL, Miller NA, et al. Carrier testing for severe childhood recessive diseases by next-generation sequencing. Sci Transl Med. 2011;3:65ra4.

95. Bettencourt-Dias M, Hildebrandt F, Pellman D, Woods G, Godinho SA. Centrosomes and cilia in human disease. Trends Genet. 2011;27:307–15.

96. Kavanagh D, Goodship TH, Richards A. Atypical hemolytic uremic syndrome. Semin Nephrol. 2013;33:508–30.

97. Joshi S, Andersen R, Jespersen B, Rittig S. Genetics of steroid-resistant nephrotic syndrome: a review of mutation spectrum and suggested approach for genetic testing. Acta Paediatr. 2013;102:844–56.

98. Batlle D, Haque SK. Genetic causes and mechanisms of distal renal tubular acidosis. Nephrol Dial Transplant. 2012;27:3691–704.

99. Devuyst O, Thakker RV. Dent's disease. Orphanet J Rare Dis. 2010;5:28.

100. Hoppe B. An update on primary hyperoxaluria. Nat Rev Nephrol. 2012;8:467–75.

101. Gee HY, Otto EA, Hurd TW, et al. Whole-exome resequencing distinguishes cystic kidney diseases from phenocopies in renal ciliopathies. Kidney Int. 2013;85:880–7.

102. Gallagher PG. Disorders of red cell volume regulation. Curr Opin Hematol. 2013;20:201–7.

103. Chaki M, Airik R, Ghosh AK, et al. Exome capture reveals ZNF423 and CEP164 mutations, linking renal ciliopathies to DNA damage response signaling. Cell. 2012;150:533–48.

104. Hurd TW, Otto EA, Mishima E, et al. Mutation of the Mg2+ transporter SLC41A1 results in a nephronophthisis-like phenotype. J Am Soc Nephrol. 2013;24:967–77.

105. Zaitlen N, Kraft P. Heritability in the genome-wide association era. Hum Genet. 2012;131:1655–64.

106. Ehret GB. Genome-wide association studies: contribution of genomics to understanding blood pressure and essential hypertension. Curr Hypertens Rep. 2010;12:17–25.

107. Schork NJ, Murray SS, Frazer KA, Topol EJ. Common vs. rare allele hypotheses for complex diseases. Curr Opin Genet Dev. 2009;19:212–9.

108. Kottgen A. Genome-wide association studies in nephrology research. Am J Kidney Dis. 2010;56:743–58.

109. Hussain N, Zello JA, Vasilevska-Ristovska J, et al. The rationale and design of Insight into Nephrotic Syndrome: Investigating Genes, Health and Therapeutics (INSIGHT): a prospective cohort study of childhood nephrotic syndrome. BMC Nephrol. 2013;14:25.

110. Eichler EE, Flint J, Gibson G, et al. Missing heritability and strategies for finding the underlying causes of complex disease. Nat Rev Genet. 2010;11:446–50.

111. Hirschhorn JN. Genomewide association studies – illuminating biologic pathways. N Engl J Med. 2009;360:1699–701.

112. Arnold D, Jones BL. Personalized medicine: a pediatric perspective. Curr Allergy Asthma Rep. 2009;9:426–32.

113. Kearns GL, Abdel-Rahman SM, Alander SW, Blowey DL, Leeder JS, Kauffman RE. Developmental pharmacology – drug disposition, action, and therapy in infants and children. N Engl J Med. 2003;349:1157–67.

114. Leeder JS. Translating pharmacogenetics and pharmacogenomics into drug development for clinical pediatrics and beyond. Drug Discov Today. 2004;9:567–73.

115. Staples A, Wong C. Risk factors for progression of chronic kidney disease. Curr Opin Pediatr. 2010;22:161–9.

116. O'Leary M, Krailo M, Anderson JR, Reaman GH. Progress in childhood cancer: 50 years of research collaboration, a report from the Children's Oncology Group. Semin Oncol. 2008;35:484–93.

117. Goldstein DB. Common genetic variation and human traits. N Engl J Med. 2009;360:1696–8.

118. Kryukov GV, Shpunt A, Stamatoyannopoulos JA, Sunyaev SR. Power of deep, all-exon resequencing for discovery of human trait genes. Proc Natl Acad Sci U S A. 2009;106:3871–6.

119. Tennessen JA, Bigham AW, O'Connor TD, et al. Evolution and functional impact of rare coding

variation from deep sequencing of human exomes. Science. 2012;337:64–9.

120. Panoutsopoulou K, Tachmazidou I, Zeggini E. In search of low-frequency and rare variants affecting complex traits. Hum Mol Genet. 2013;22:R16–21.

121. Ji W, Foo JN, O'Roak BJ, et al. Rare independent mutations in renal salt handling genes contribute to blood pressure variation. Nat Genet. 2008;40:592–9.

122. Slatkin M. Epigenetic inheritance and the missing heritability problem. Genetics. 2009;182:845–50.

123. Hemani G, Knott S, Haley C. An evolutionary perspective on epistasis and the missing heritability. PLoS Gene. 2013;9:e1003295.

124. Kaprio J. Twins and the mystery of missing heritability: the contribution of gene-environment interactions. J Intern Med. 2012;272:440–8.

125. Zuk O, Hechter E, Sunyaev SR, Lander ES. The mystery of missing heritability: genetic interactions create phantom heritability. Proc Natl Acad Sci U S A. 2012;109:1193–8.

126. Janssens AC, van Duijn CM. Genome-based prediction of common diseases: advances and prospects. Hum Mol Genet. 2008;17:R166–73.

127. Elens L, Bouamar R, Shuker N, Hesselink DA, van Gelder T, van Schaik RH. Clinical implementation of pharmacogenetics in kidney transplantation: CNIs in the starting blocks. Br J Clin Pharmacol. 2014;77(4):715–28.

128. Zhao W, Fakhoury M, Jacqz-Aigrain E. Developmental pharmacogenetics of immunosuppressants in pediatric organ transplantation. Ther Drug Monit. 2010;32:688–99.

129. Fanta S, Niemi M, Jonsson S, et al. Pharmacogenetics of cyclosporine in children suggests an age-dependent influence of ABCB1 polymorphisms. Pharmacogenet Genomics. 2008;18:77–90.

130. Ferraresso M, Tirelli A, Ghio L, et al. Influence of the CYP3A5 genotype on tacrolimus pharmacokinetics and pharmacodynamics in young kidney transplant recipients. Pediatr Transplant. 2007;11: 296–300.

131. Prausa SE, Fukuda T, Maseck D, et al. UGT genotype may contribute to adverse events following medication with mycophenolate mofetil in pediatric kidney transplant recipients. Clin Pharmacol Ther. 2009;85:495–500.

132. Zhao W, Fakhoury M, Deschenes G, et al. Population pharmacokinetics and pharmacogenetics of mycophenolic acid following administration of mycophenolate mofetil in de novo pediatric renal-transplant patients. J Clin Pharmacol. 2010;50:1280–91.

133. Thervet E, Loriot MA, Barbier S, et al. Optimization of initial tacrolimus dose using pharmacogenetic testing. Clin Pharmacol Ther. 2010;87:721–6.

134. Eby C. Warfarin pharmacogenetics: does more accurate dosing benefit patients? Semin Thromb Hemost. 2012;38:661–6.

135. Vear SI, Stein CM, Ho RH. Warfarin pharmacogenomics in children. Pediatr Blood Cancer. 2013;60: 1402–7.

136. Nielsen-Bohlman L, Panzer AM, Kindig DA. Health literacy: a prescription to end confusion. Washington, DC: National Academies Press; 2004.

137. Kutner M, Greenburg E, Jin Y, Paulsen C. The health literacy of America's adults: results from the 2003 National Assessment of Adult Literacy, NCES 2006-483. Washington, DC: National Center for Education Statistics; 2006.

138. Lea DH, Kaphingst KA, Bowen D, Lipkus I, Hadley DW. Communicating genetic and genomic information: health literacy and numeracy considerations. Public Health Genomics. 2011;14:279–89.

139. Lanie AD, Jayaratne TE, Sheldon JP, et al. Exploring the public understanding of basic genetic concepts. J Genet Couns. 2004;13:305–20.

140. Golbeck AL, Ahlers-Schmidt CR, Paschal AM, Dismuke SE. A definition and operational framework for health numeracy. Am J Prev Med. 2005;29:375–6.

141. Selkirk CG, Weissman SM, Anderson A, Hulick PJ. Physicians' preparedness for integration of genomic and pharmacogenetic testing into practice within a major healthcare system. Genet Test Mol Biomarkers. 2013;17:219–25.

142. Cooksey JA, Forte G, Benkendorf J, Blitzer MG. The state of the medical geneticist workforce: findings of the 2003 survey of American Board of Medical Genetics certified geneticists. Genet Med. 2005;7:439–43.

143. West CP, Ficalora RD. Clinician attitudes toward biostatistics. Mayo Clin Proc. 2007;82:939–43.

144. Weiss ST, Samet JM. An assessment of physician knowledge of epidemiology and biostatistics. J Med Educ. 1980;55:692–7.

145. Wulff HR, Andersen B, Brandenhoff P, Guttler F. What do doctors know about statistics? Stat Med. 1987;6:3–10.

146. Rao G. Physician numeracy: essential skills for practicing evidence-based medicine. Fam Med. 2008;40: 354–8.

147. Rao G, Kanter SL. Physician numeracy as the basis for an evidence-based medicine curriculum. Acad Med. 2010;85:1794–9.

148. Patay BA, Topol EJ. The unmet need of education in genomic medicine. Am J Med. 2012;125:5–6.

149. Dhar SU, Alford RL, Nelson EA, Potocki L. Enhancing exposure to genetics and genomics through an innovative medical school curriculum. Genet Med. 2012;14:163–7.

150. Matloff E, Caplan A. Direct to confusion: lessons learned from marketing BRCA testing. Am J Bioeth. 2008;8:5–8.

151. Rosenfeld J, Mason CE. Pervasive sequence patents cover the entire human genome. Genome Med. 2013;5:27.

152. Klein RD. AMP v Myriad: the supreme court gives a win to personalized medicine. J Mol Diagn. 2013;15:731–2.

153. Graff GD, Phillips D, Lei Z, Oh S, Nottenburg C, Pardey PG. Not quite a myriad of gene patents. Nat Biotechnol. 2013;31:404–10.

154. Guttmacher AE, Collins FS. Realizing the promise of genomics in biomedical research. JAMA. 2005;294:1399–402.

155. Janssens AC. Is the time right for translation research in genomics? Eur J Epidemiol. 2008;23:707–10.

156. Wade CH, McBride CM, Kardia SL, Brody LC. Considerations for designing a prototype genetic test for use in translational research. Public Health Genomics. 2010;13:155–65.

157. Lucassen A, Parker M. Revealing false paternity: some ethical considerations. Lancet. 2001;357:1033–5.

158. Schroder NM. The dilemma of unintentional discovery of misattributed paternity in living kidney donors and recipients. Curr Opin Organ Transplant. 2009;14:196–200.

159. Macintyre S, Sooman A. Non-paternity and prenatal genetic screening. Lancet. 1991;338:869–71.

160. Gjertson DW, Brenner CH, Baur MP, et al. ISFG: recommendations on biostatistics in paternity testing. Forensic Sci Int Genet. 2007;1:223–31.

161. Ross LF. Disclosing misattributed paternity. Bioethics. 1996;10:114–30.

162. Wertz DC, Fletcher JC. Ethics and medical genetics in the United States: a national survey. Am J Med Genet. 1988;29:815–27.

163. Wertz DC, Fletcher JC, Mulvihill JJ. Medical geneticists confront ethical dilemmas: cross-cultural comparisons among 18 nations. Am J Hum Genet. 1990;46:1200–13.

164. Andrews LB, Fullarton JE, Holtzman NA, Motulsky AG, editors. Assessing genetic risks: implications for health and social policy. Washington, DC: National Academies Press; 1994. p. 311.

165. Wolf SM, Crock BN, Van Ness B, et al. Managing incidental findings and research results in genomic research involving biobanks and archived data sets. Genet Med. 2012;14:361–84.

166. Green RC, Berg JS, Grody WW, et al. ACMG recommendations for reporting of incidental findings in clinical exome and genome sequencing. Genet Med. 2013;15:565–74.

167. Dorschner MO, Amendola LM, Turner EH, et al. Actionable, pathogenic incidental findings in 1,000 participants' exomes. Am J Hum Genet. 2013;93:631–40.

168. Hayeems RZ, Miller FA, Li L, Bytautas JP. Not so simple: a quasi-experimental study of how researchers adjudicate genetic research results. Eur J Hum Genet. 2011;19:740–7.

169. Eguale T, Bartlett G, Tamblyn R. Rare visible disorders/diseases as individually identifiable health information. AMIA Annu Symp Proc. 2005:947.

170. Kaye J. The tension between data sharing and the protection of privacy in genomics research. Annu Rev Genomics Hum Genet. 2012;13:415–31.

171. Lin Z, Owen AB, Altman RB. Genetics. Genomic research and human subject privacy. Science. 2004;305:183.

172. Gymrek M, McGuire AL, Golan D, Halperin E, Erlich Y. Identifying personal genomes by surname inference. Science. 2013;339:321–4.

173. Fox S. After Dr Google: peer-to-peer health care. Pediatrics. 2013;131 Suppl 4:S224–5.

174. Rodriguez LL, Brooks LD, Greenberg JH, Green ED. Research ethics. The complexities of genomic identifiability. Science. 2013;339:275–6.

175. Collins FS, Mckusick VA. Implications of the Human Genome Project for medical science. JAMA. 2001;285:540–4.

176. Rothstein MA, Anderlik MR. What is genetic discrimination, and when and how can it be prevented? Genet Med. 2001;3:354–8.

177. Hudson KL, Rothenberg KH, Andrews LB, Kahn MJ, Collins FS. Genetic discrimination and health insurance: an urgent need for reform. Science. 1995;270:391–3.

178. Rothenberg K, Fuller B, Rothstein M, et al. Genetic information and the workplace: legislative approaches and policy changes. Science. 1997;275:1755–7.

179. Van Hoyweghen I, Horstman K. European practices of genetic information and insurance: lessons for the Genetic Information Nondiscrimination Act. JAMA. 2008;300:326–7.

180. Hudson KL, Holohan MK, Collins FS. Keeping pace with the times – the Genetic Information Nondiscrimination Act of 2008. N Engl J Med. 2008;358:2661–3.

181. Bombard Y, Veenstra G, Friedman JM, et al. Perceptions of genetic discrimination among people at risk for Huntington's disease: a cross sectional survey. BMJ. 2009;338:b2175.

182. Murashige N, Tanimoto T, Kusumi E. Fear of genetic discrimination in Japan. Lancet. 2012;380:730.

183. Taylor S, Treloar S, Barlow-Stewart K, Stranger M, Otlowski M. Investigating genetic discrimination in Australia: a large-scale survey of clinical genetics clients. Clin Genet. 2008;74:20–30.

184. Anon. What's brewing in genetic testing. Nat Genet. 2002;32:553–54.

185. Hudson K, Javitt G, Burke W, Byers P. ASHG Statement* on direct-to-consumer genetic testing in the United States. Obstet Gynecol. 2007;110:1392–5.

186. McCarthy M. FDA halts sale of genetic test sold to consumers. BMJ. 2013;347:f7126.

187. Borry P, van Hellemondt RE, Sprumont D, et al. Legislation on direct-to-consumer genetic testing in seven European countries. Eur J Hum Genet. 2012;20:715–21.

188. Bloss CS, Darst BF, Topol EJ, Schork NJ. Direct-to-consumer personalized genomic testing. Hum Mol Genet. 2011;20:R132–41.

189. Caulfield T, McGuire AL. Direct-to-consumer genetic testing: perceptions, problems, and policy responses. Annu Rev Med. 2012;63:23–33.

190. Howard HC, Avard D, Borry P. Are the kids really all right? Direct-to-consumer genetic testing in chil-

dren: are company policies clashing with professional norms? Eur J Hum Genet. 2011;19:1122–6.

191. Borry P, Fryns JP, Schotsmans P, Dierickx K. Carrier testing in minors: a systematic review of guidelines and position papers. Eur J Hum Genet. 2006;14: 133–8.

192. Tracy EE. Are doctors prepared for direct-to-consumer advertising of genetics tests? Obstet Gynecol. 2007;110:1389–91.

193. McGuire AL, Burke W. An unwelcome side effect of direct-to-consumer personal genome testing: raiding the medical commons. JAMA. 2008;300:2669–71.

Anette Melk

Introduction

The gold standard for renal tissue analysis is the renal biopsy. It is routinely performed to allow histological diagnoses of renal diseases and determine the extent of damage in native and allograft kidneys. However, there has been controversy over the use and interpretation of renal biopsies. Issues include sampling errors and reproducibility between different observers. More importantly, histopathological assessment has failed to predict progression or regression of renal diseases reducing the value of renal biopsies as a guide for clinical therapeutic approaches. Because of this, researchers have always tried to use new methods in order to add more validity and prognostication. Needle biopsies were performed already in the 1930s, but renal biopsies as clinical diagnostic tool were introduced in the 1960s when Jones silver stain and the new techniques of electron microscopy (EM) and immunofluorescence (IF) became available. In the 1970s, immunohistological methods were applied to identify, localize and semi-quantify immune deposits, extracellular matrix proteins and cellular infiltrates. The developments in the late 1980s and 1990s have been focused on methods to measure RNA and DNA. With the ongoing advances in renal imaging this non-invasive, indirect technique may become the ultimate way of analyzing renal tissue in the future.

Renal Biopsy

Procedure

In children, renal biopsies were done using open exposure of the kidney until 1962 when White in England and in 1970 Metcoff in the United States described a modified needle biopsy procedure for children including infants [1–3]. Today percutaneous renal biopsies in children are done under ultrasound guidance and have become a routine procedure. A recent report on the 22-year experience on 9288 native kidneys biopsies (715 from children) from the Norwegian Kidney Biopsy Registry came to the conclusion that the percutaneous renal biopsy is a low-risk procedure at all ages [4].

Despite differences in details, the procedures for a renal biopsy are relatively standardized. In preparation for the biopsy the patient and the parents have to be informed about the possible risks of the biopsy and the potential therapeutic consequences. For safety, laboratory values that should be obtained include hemoglobin, platelet count, prothrombin time, partial thromboplastin time and bleeding time if uremic. In addition, serum creatinine, electrolytes and a urine dip stick

A. Melk, MD, PhD
Department of Kidney, Liver and Metabolic Diseases,
Hannover Medical School, Carl-Neuberg-Str. 1,
Hannover 30625, Germany
e-mail: melk.anette@mh-hannover.de

© Springer-Verlag Berlin Heidelberg 2016
D.F. Geary, F. Schaefer (eds.), *Pediatric Kidney Disease*, DOI 10.1007/978-3-662-52972-0_5

analysis are useful as baseline parameters in case of occurring complications. Prior to performing the biopsy the nephrologist should be aware of the patient's renal anatomy. Most commonly ultrasound examination is used to exclude contraindications such as single kidneys, small kidneys, and large cysts.

Small children will receive general anesthesia. In larger children the procedure can safely be performed with mild sedation allowing for cooperation of the patient, but many centers use general anesthesia even in larger children. Briefly, the patient is placed in prone position with a foam roll under the upper part of the abdomen. The kidneys are localized by ultrasound from the back. The kidney, of which the lower pole is easiest to reach, is chosen for biopsy. In most cases this will be the right kidney. The exact position of the kidney during inspiration is determined and after marking the intended entry position of the needle on the skin, the skin is cleaned with an antiseptic solution. If the patient is only sedated, the skin, the subcutaneous tissue and the muscle are infiltrated with a local anesthetic. After a

small incision the needle mounted on the semiautomated spring loaded biopsy gun is carefully introduced under ultrasound guidance until the kidney is almost reached. Manually operated needles have been widely replaced by biopsy guns because of the easier use and lower complication rates. The patient is then advised to take a breath and hold the air. In case of general anesthesia, the anesthesist will hold the patient in deep inspiration. The needle is quickly advanced to the capsule of the kidney and the biopsy is taken (Fig. 5.1a, b). Ideally, the whole procedure is followed on the ultrasound screen to visualize the path of the biopsy needle.

After the procedure the patient usually stays in bed for 24 h with compression of the puncture site. However, during the past several years, renal biopsies have been performed on an outpatient basis, where stable patients are discharged after about 8 h [5]. To assure brisk diuresis the patient receives either a glucose/sodium chloride solution intravenously and/or is asked to drink a lot. Urine is collected in single portions and is examined with urine dip sticks. Hemoglobin levels and

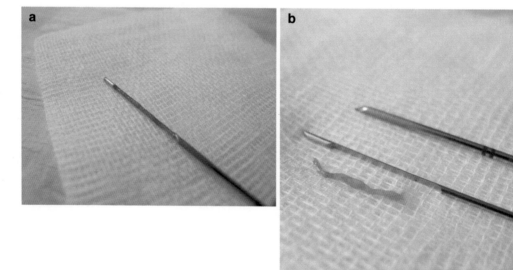

Fig. 5.1 Renal biopsy needle and biopsy specimen. (**a**) Biopsy specimen still captured in the notch of the stylet. (**b**) Biopsy specimen sitting next to the inner needle and outer trocar.

ultrasound controls are performed in most centers after 4–6 h and after 24 h. Hourly controls of blood pressure and heart rate have to be done.

The primary major complication remains macroscopic hematuria that is seen in 0.8–12 % of biopsies performed in pediatric patients. Other complications may include subcapsular or perirenal hematoma, possible need for transfusion, infection, and pain requiring medication. Arteriovenous fistulas are diagnosed more often in recent years because of the improvement in Doppler ultrasound technique. Table 5.1 provides an overview of the efficacy and most frequent complications with regard to different biopsy techniques over a period of three decades [6].

Processing of Biopsy Specimens

As important as accurate performance of the biopsy is adequate processing and interpretation of the specimen [7, 8]. The Renal Pathology Society has therefore published practice guidelines that address specimen handling and processing [9].

Prior to fixation each core should be examined for the presence and number of glomeruli by light microscopy with tenfold magnification. Based on sample size and location this examination should lead to a decision on whether more renal tissue is needed. One should take into account the number of glomeruli as well as the suspected diseases

process. It cannot be emphasized enough that adequacy of sample size is crucial for the validity of a biopsy specimen. In order to diagnose a focal disease process such as focal segmental glomerulosclerosis (FSGS) recognition of a single abnormal glomerulus is required. The probability to make this diagnosis depends on the fraction of affected glomeruli per kidney as well as on the glomeruli present in a given biopsy specimen. The same holds true for the assessment of the extent of a disease with variable pathologic involvement among glomeruli. Corwin et al. have published estimates on the minimum number of abnormal glomeruli required in a biopsy core to infer with 95 % confidence that a disease process involves 20 %, 50 % or 80 % of the kidney (Table 5.2). Glomeruli within the juxtamedullary region are the ones to be involved first with FSGS, highlighting the importance that this area is represented in the sample. Overrepresentation of global sclerosis, however, may result from subcapsular cortical specimens and needs to be considered when dealing with wedge biopsy taken during an open biopsy of the native kidney or at implantation of a renal transplant. For pediatric biopsies it is also of note that the number of glomeruli that are retrieved per centimeter core length decreases with age (Fig. 5.2) [6].

Appropriate fixation of the biopsy should be done as soon as possible because small cores can dry out fast. The choice of fixatives should be discussed with the local renal pathologist. In

Table 5.1 Historical evolution of percutaneous biopsy technology in children. While the efficacy significantly improved over time, the rate of complications did not change

Periods	1969–1974	1974–1985	1985–1990	1990–1992	1992–1996
Needle	Silverman	TrueCut	TrueCut	Biopty	Biopty
Localization of kidney	Radiocontrast imaging	Radiocontrast imaging	Pre-biopsy ultrasound	Pre-biopsy ultrasound	Ultrasound guidance
Efficacy					
No. of passes per session, %	3.04	2.98	2.86	2.60	2.45
Tissue-yielding punctures, %	78	87	90	87	94
No. of glomeruli per session	22.3	24.3	26.4	28.4	33.7
Complications					
Microhematuria, %	21.7	32.5	26.3	47.0	40.3
Macrohematuria, %	2.7	16.7	15.8	8.3	4.4
Perirenal hematoma, %			32.3	46.7	55.8

Used with permission of Karger Publishers from Feneberg et al. [6]

Table 5.2 Minimum number of harvested glomeruli required to allow concluding a minimal fractional involvement (e.g., % sclerotic glomeruli in FSGS, % crescents in extracapillary GN)

Number of harvested glomeruli	Minimal number of abnormal glomeruli (absolute and %) required to reliably estimate extent of involvement		
	≥80%	≥50%	≥20%
8	8 (100)	7 (88)	3 (38)
10	10 (100)	8 (80)	4 (40)
12	12 (100)	9 (75)	5 (42)
15	14 (93)	11 (73)	6 (40)
20	19 (95)	14 (70)	7 (35)
25	23 (92)	17 (68)	9 (36)
30	28 (93)	20 (66)	10 (33)
35	32 (91)	23 (66)	11 (31)
40	36 (90)	26 (65)	12 (30)

Used with permission of Karger Publishers from Corwin et al. [10]

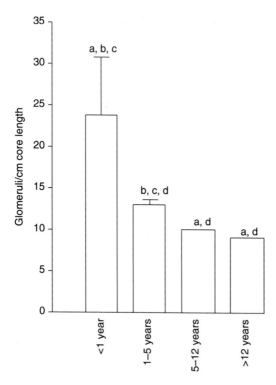

Fig. 5.2 Number of glomeruli per centimeter core length derived from native kidneys shown for different age groups (Used with permission of Karger Publishers from Feneberg et al. [6])

pediatric renal diseases, light microscopy (LM) alone can be insufficient to make a diagnosis. Therefore, specimens for IF and EM should be obtained. Because of the superior morphology, some renal pathologists prefer fixation with Bouin's alcohol picrate solution. This, however, may lead to problems if immunohistochemistry (IHC) staining needs to be performed. Fixation with paraformaldehyde or buffered formalin (4%, pH 7.2–7.4) followed by paraffin embedding is therefore common practice in most pathology departments. For IF, renal tissue should be "snap-frozen" in liquid nitrogen or can be placed in tissue transport media or isotonic sodium chloride solution if transported to the laboratory immediately. Specimens for EM are usually fixed in a solution containing 0.1–3% glutaraldehyde.

LM specimens should be sectioned at a thickness of 2 μm or less by an experienced technician. Subtle pathologic changes are more easily detected in thinner sections and section thickness is an important issue for glomerular pathology, especially when assessing for cellularity.

A variety of histochemical stains are used to evaluate renal biopsies (Fig. 5.3a–f). Typically biopsy specimens are stained with hematoxylin and eosin (H+E), periodic acid-Schiff (PAS) or periodic acid-methenamine silver (Jones silver) and Masson's trichrome. H+E is used for general morphology and reference, whereas the other three stains provide a clear distinction of extracellular matrix from cytoplasm. Depending on indication Congo red stain (amyloid), Kossa stain (calcifications), elastic tissue stain (loss of elasticity in arteries, arterial thickening) and other stains are used. IF uses fluorophore-labelled antibodies to detect and localize immunoglobulins (IgA, IgG, IgM) and their light chains (k, λ), components of the classical or alternative complement pathways (C1q, C3c, C4), albumin and fibrinogen. In transplant biopsies, staining for C4d, a fragment within the complement pathway, has become a major diagnostic tool in antibody-mediated rejection [11]. The pattern of fluorescence positive stain should be noted, such as mesangial versus capillary staining and linear or granular staining. The granular pattern has an

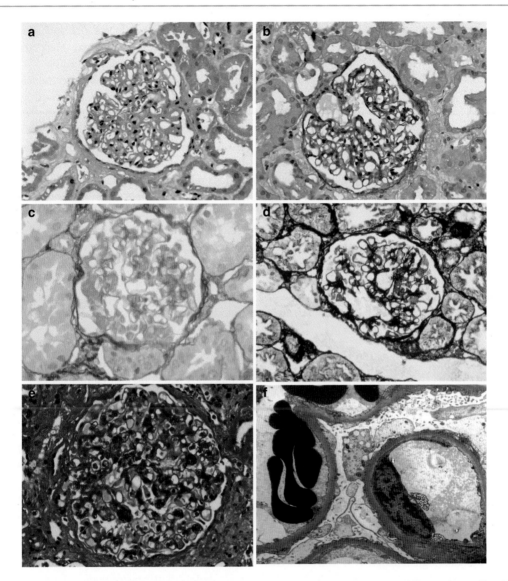

Fig. 5.3 Overview of the different stainings that are used to evaluate a renal biopsy. Representative light (**a-e**) and electron microscopy (**f**) of minimal change glomerulopathy (MCGN) with mild hypercellularity. (**a**) Hematoxylin eosin stain (HE): the HE stain is the work horse of pathology; it is useful to get a first idea about glomerular changes such as proliferation and matrix deposition. In the case of MCGN the glomerulus shows a slightly increased number of mesangial cells, open capillaries, no evidence of intra- or extracapillary proliferation and normal thickness of glomerular basement membrane (GBM). (**b**) Periodic acid-Schiffs (PAS) stain: PAS staining is helpful to analyze changes in glomerular cell number and GBM in more detail. In the case of MCGN mild segmental hypercellularity (*) and normal thickness of GBM without any irregularities is seen. Some podocytes (*arrows*) are slightly enlarged and appear detached from the GBM. (**c**) Sirius red stain (fibrous tissue stain): This fibrous tissue stain is helpful to analyze the amount of fibrous tissue (fibrosis) of glomeruli and most importantly the interstitial tissue (interstitial fibrosis). In the case of MCGN a normal amount of fibrous tissue is found in Bowmans capsule and no increase in mesangial matrix is visible. (**d**) Silver stain: the silver stain is most useful to detect thickening and irregularities of the GBM. In the case of MCGN no thickening and spike formation is seen. (**e**) Acid fuchsin-Orange G stain (SFOG): This stain is helpful to detect protein deposition, i.e., immune complex formation, which appear in bright red within the mesangial matrix or the GBM. In the case of MCGN no immune deposits are present. (**f**) Electron microscopy of a capillary loop shows typical changes in MCGN, i.e., normal thickness of GBM with no evidence immune complex deposition, but with effacement of podocyte foot processes and loss of endothelial fenestration (All: Courtesy of of Dr. Kerstin Amann, Erlangen)

EM counterpart and corresponds to extracellular, electron dense masses.

EM studies do not need to be part of the routine work up of every kidney biopsy. However, EM plays an important diagnostic role in almost half the cases 50 % of cases and is essential for a correct diagnosis in up to 21 % [12, 13]. Even though it is sometimes possible to omit EM after evaluation of LM and IF, specimens for EM studies should always be procured. EM can localize deposits (mesangial, subendothelial, or subepithelial). EM is able to detect changes in cell structure (e.g., fusion of podocyte foot processes, podocyte vacuolization) and alterations of the basement membrane (thickening, thinning, splicing, duplication and other irregularities). The definite diagnosis of, e.g., minimal change nephropathy, Alport's disease or thin basement membrane disease requires EM [14, 15].

Histopathological Assessment

Abnormalities in renal structures can occur in all four compartments of the kidney: glomeruli, tubules, interstitium and vasculature [16, 17]. Numerous consensus classifications have been developed for specific diseases [18–22] and those classifications, as well as the specific pathological changes seen with certain diseases, are discussed in the relevant chapters of this textbook. This chapter provides a general overview on the various histopathological features that can be encountered while reading a biopsy [8, 23, 24].

Glomerular changes are the primary pathological event in many renal diseases. If glomeruli are affected it needs to be decided whether these changes are *diffuse* (defined as ≥50 % of glomeruli involved) or whether the disease process is *focal* (defined as <50 % of glomeruli involved). By assessing single glomeruli a decision has to be made whether the disease process involves only part of the glomerulus, i.e., is *segmental*, or the whole glomerulus, which is considered *global*. *Glomerular sclerosis* refers to an increase in extracellular material (e.g., hyaline) within the mesangium that leads to compression of the capillaries. The capillary basement membrane has a wrinkled appearance and adhesions to Bowman's capsule are found. Depending on the expansion of the sclerotic lesion it can be either segmental or global. *Hypercellularity* is a descriptive term reflecting an increased number of cells (e.g., mesangial cells, endothelial cells, inflammatory cells) in the mesangial space, internal to the glomerular basement membrane or in the Bowman's space, which is called mesangial, endocapillary or extracapillary hypercellularity respectively. Glomerular diseases involving hypercellularity are often called "proliferative". Changes of the basement membrane that can be seen by light microscopy involve *thickening of the basement membrane and basement membrane double layering*. Whereas the first is caused by the accumulation of basement membrane material, the latter is meant to be caused by peripheral interposition of mesangial material. Severe glomerular diseases show the formation of *crescents*. Crescents are located in the urinary space of the glomerulus and consist of cells and extracellular material. The proportion of glomeruli affected by crescents is of enormous prognostic importance in acute glomerulonephritis/vasculitis. The most subtle glomerular damage is *effacement of foot process* and refers to the loss of normal podocyte morphology with an undivided cytoplasmic mass covering the basement membrane. Effacement of foot processes cannot be seen by light microscopy, but is easily found by electron microscopy.

Tubular cells can show various signs of damage. This includes loss of brush border (in proximal tubules), flattening of the tubular epithelium, and detachment of tubular cells from the basement membrane, necrosis and apoptosis. Mitosis of tubular cells is often found after an episode of acute tubular necrosis as a sign of repair. *Tubulitis*, an important feature in acute allograft rejection, refers to the presence of inflammatory cells that have crossed the tubular basement membrane and infiltrate the tubular epithelium. Tubular changes when chronic occur as *tubular atrophy*. Atrophic tubules have a reduced diameter and a thickened basement membrane. Tubular atrophy is often accompanied by interstitial fibrosis. Another type of tubular pathology is the *accumulation of droplets* containing various substances. This for example can occur in patients with heavy proteinuria or with various storage diseases. A foamy appearance of the tubular epithelium is called *vacuolization* and can occur with several conditions. *Intranuclear inclusions* can indicate viral infection (see below), can occur non-specifically with different nephropathies, and can also reflect regeneration after acute tubular necrosis. The occurrence of coagulated proteins or formed elements in the tubular lumen is described as *tubular casts* (e.g., RBC casts).

Interstitial changes are *edema, fibrosis and infiltration by inflammatory cells.* Edema indicates acute diseases whereas fibrosis is the sequelae of chronic renal damage. In both cases tubules are no longer "sitting back to back" but are separated by interstitial material. The degree of interstitial fibrosis is of prognostic importance in chronic kidney diseases. In many instances, the degree of interstitial fibrosis found in a primary glomerular disease is a more powerful predictor of outcome than the glomerular changes themselves. Infiltration of inflammatory cells can be the cause of renal disease such as acute interstitial nephritis or acute transplant rejection, but an interstitial infiltrate can also be a mere accompanying phenomenon, e.g., in fibrosis.

The renal vasculature can also show a range of pathological changes. Inflammation (vasculitis) may affect any vessel. If only the arterial subendothelial space is affected, this subtype is called *endothelialitis,* a finding peculiar to vascular rejection. Direct damage of endothelial cells, e.g., through E.coli toxins in hemolytic uremic syndrome (see Chap. 26), leads to *thrombotic microangiopathy* with endothelial cell swelling and intimal edema that is followed by platelet fibrin thrombi. Hypertension can lead to vascular changes affecting all parts of the arterial wall. This includes *fibrous intimal thickening* and medial hypertrophy. Overall the vessel walls can be thickened and hyalinized, in extreme cases leading to complete obstruction of the vessel lumen. Very high blood pressure can result in *fibrinoid necrosis,* an endpoint also seen in other thrombotic microangiopathies.

Pathologists summarize the findings seen in the different renal compartment based investigating the biopsy with the tools LM, IF, IHC and EM. Recently, a minimum reporting standard for nonneoplastic biopsies has been proposed to facilitate optimal communication between pathologists and nephrologists an eventually to optimize patients care [25].

Protein Analysis

Proteins in renal tissue are classically analyzed by immunostaining, using either IF or IHC for visualization. Both techniques use antibodies or antisera directed against the protein of interest. They can be performed both in native and formalin-fixed tissues. As fixatives can mask protein epitopes, antigen retrieval steps become necessary, particularly for nuclear antigens. Detection and visualization of unlabeled primary antibody that specifically binds the target epitope is achieved by a secondary antibody, which for IF carries a fluorophore or for IHC either peroxidase or alkaline phosphatase. In order to further enhance the signal, especially if the target antigen is rarely expressed, amplification systems such as the streptavidin-biotin-peroxidase system are used for IHC. Direct IF or IHC, for which the primary antibody is linked to a fluorophore or peroxidase, is also possible.

Both IF and IHC have advantages and disadvantages. IF is most often performed on frozen sections. It is a technically easy and fast procedure. Processing, sectioning and staining can be performed within 1–2 h. Even though the cost of the procedure itself is low, storage is difficult as the fluorophores fade over time. A broad range of suitable antibodies is available and background staining is usually not a problem. However, in case of frozen sections an additional sample for assessment of histopathological details may be required to provide good morphology. IHC can be done using the same tissue as for LM. It will provide much better morphological details and causes permanent staining, in contrast to IF. IHC is highly sensitive because of the possibility to enhance the signal by certain amplifiers, but can be technically challenging (e.g., due to higher background staining) and expensive.

Some of the applications of IF and IHC in nonneoplastic renal biopsies have already been described above as they are part of the standard work-up of biopsy specimens. Some pathology centers prefer to use IHC even for the standard workup because of the possibility to store and archive the slides for future comparisons. In addition, IHC is used to detect subtypes of type IV collagen (see Chap. 18, Alport Syndrome and Thin Basement Membrane Nephropathy) and viral antigens, especially in allograft biopsies, although PCR techniques are currently taking over because of their higher sensitivity. A practical example for virus detection with IHC is BK polyoma virus. Demonstration of typical smudgy tubular cells with enlarged nuclei gives direct evidence for viral tissue invasiveness [26]. A pleomorphic infiltrate with lymphocytes, plasma cells and PMNs is highly suspicious of BK virus nephropathy. Diagnostic confirmation can be achieved by IHC using a monoclonal antibody directed against simian virus 40 (SV-40) large T antigen, which is common to all known polyoma viruses [16]. In case expansile/dysplastic plasma cells are found in the interstitium of an allograft biopsy specimen, staining for Epstein-Barr virus (EBV) may be useful to make the diagnosis of post-transplant lymphoproliferative disorder (PTLD) as most but not all PTLDs are EBV positive [27].

While proteomic tools represent a major technological advancement in protein analysis, they have not been included in the routine work-up of renal biopsies to date. Proteomics has been coined the "non-invasive renal biopsy", reflecting that most proteomics approaches nowadays are performed in urine. Proteomic analysis in renal tissue has been used to identify biomarkers enabling diagnosis, disease monitoring, and treatment of renal malignances, especially renal cell carcinoma [28–30]. Proteomic tools may become increasingly interesting to study microdissected structures from biopsies [31, 32] as demonstrated for different glomerular diseases [31–33] and amyloidosis [34–37]. For example, mass spectrometry, by providing the molecular composition of microdissected deposits, is a sensitive and specific technique to accurately diagnose renal amyloidosis [35, 36, 38]. These promising preliminary results and the fact that formalin-fixed tissue even from archived tissue blocks can be used for such analyses will support future use of this approach [39, 40].

RNA Analysis

Methods that measure RNA in small biopsy samples have been applied to analyze diseased native kidneys as well as renal allografts. The sensitivity of RT-PCR exceeds that of Northern blotting and RNA protection assays by 100–1000-fold and cDNA based expression analysis has become the leading tool in recent years [41]. As little as 10 % of a biopsy core is sufficient for molecular analysis [42]. The need to immediately process or freeze tissue samples in liquid nitrogen because of RNA instability has been overcome by new RNase inhibitors that stabilize and protect the integrity of RNA in unfrozen tissue samples. Importantly, it has been shown that renal tissue stored in these agents can still be microdissected and is suitable for immunohistochemical analysis [42]. Hence, RNA expression can also be evaluated from fixed and processed renal biopsy samples, allowing for molecular analysis in combination with routine histology assessments. If frozen sections have been generated, RNA can be isolated using standard protocols, but techniques for RNA isolation from formaldehyde-fixed, paraffin-embedded tissues have also been described [43]. This methodology enables RNA analysis even after years of storage, allowing for a correlation of expression profiles from archived materials with the subsequent clinical disease course.

Even with these sensitive methods of RNA detection, the kidney's different compartments contribute or respond differently to diseases or injury and signals may be underestimated or even missed. Manual dissection, sieving, or laser-assisted microdissection have been used to compare glomeruli with tubulointerstitium or to study rare cells [44]. Using laser-assisted microdissection a defined histological structure can be selected from a given biopsy slide, allowing direct correlation of information from histology and gene expression for the same nephron segments. While the technique has been successfully used in fixed renal tissue [45, 46], the challenge is to retrieve sufficient high-quality material. Several technical reports have been published [43, 47–49]. Laser-assisted microdissection is often used in combination with RNA amplification protocols with 1000-fold linear amplification efficiency to generate gene profiles that are specific for a certain nephron segment. This approach has been used to generate expression profiles of single glomeruli derived from biopsies of lupus nephritis [50]. The study revealed considerable kidney-to-kidney heterogeneity, whereas glomerulus-to-glomerulus variation within a kidney was less marked.

High throughput gene expression technologies emerged in the mid 1990s and a number of different microarray platforms became available. A microarray chip assembles a number of gene-specific probes (clones or oligonucleotides) spotted on a small surface area with high density. The underlying principle of microarray is that after labeling transcripts from a specific sample and hybridizing them to an array, the amount of sample material bound to the specific complementary probe set is measured. As variation across the different platforms is an important issue, a number of studies have compared different platforms. Some claimed a significant divergence across technologies, whereas others found an acceptable level of concordance [51, 52]. Nowadays chips are commercially available from different suppliers and the method is highly standardized, which allows for comparison and exchange of data between different laboratories as long as the same chips are utilized. In contrast to those high density arrays, low density arrays allow for the simultaneous evaluation of a few hundred genes and are based on a reverse transcriptase-polymerase chain reaction (RT-PCR) technique.

Gene expression profiling has been performed investigating large cohorts of patients with native renal diseases or after renal transplantation [53, 54]. The major challenge of any of those

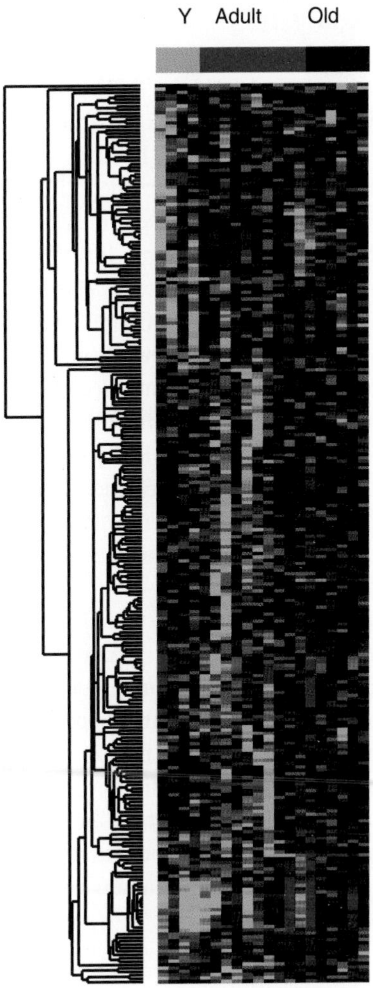

Fig. 5.4 Dendrogram used in gene array analysis. Hierarchical cluster of genes that are differentially expressed based on renal age (*Y* young kidneys, *A* adult kidneys, *O* old kidneys). The color from *green* to *red* reflects increasing gene expression

expression analyses remains the extraction of biological insight from such information. Ideally, one would like to recognize specific patterns or pathways involved in certain diseases (Fig. 5.4). Approaches combining conventional histological assessment with molecular analysis for transplant biopsies, called the virtual microscope, have created a new understanding of transplant disease states and their outcomes [55–57]. Despite strong associations described for certain genes with specific diseases, none of those genes have made it into routine diagnostics to date.

DNA Analysis

Detection of viral DNA by PCR using sequence specific primers has been described for a large panel of viruses such as BK virus, CMV, EBV, other herpes viruses, and hepatitis B virus [58–61], but is hardly used in clinical practice. Measurements of viral load to diagnose and monitor affected patients, especially after transplantation – see also Chap. 70, Prevention and Treatment of Infectious Complications in Pediatric Renal Transplant Recipients – are preferentially performed in blood and urine [62–64]. Pathologists typically combine this information, the histopathological features and the available immunostaining methods to make the diagnosis of a virus-associated process in the kidney.

Molecular cytogenetic techniques such as chromosomal comparative genomic hybridization (CGH) are performed on tumor tissue. These techniques have improved the diagnosis of chromosomal aberrations, e.g., in Wilms' tumor, but have only a limited resolution across the whole genome. The development of genomic arrays allows the assessment of the whole genome at a much higher resolution at a sub-microscopic or sub-band level [65, 66].

Indirect Measurements

Even though the complication rate with renal biopsies is low, taking a biopsy is still an invasive procedure. Therefore methodological progress should aim for indirect and non-invasive methods to assess the status of a kidney *in vivo* in order to minimize the need for renal biopsies.

The kidney is suited well for indirect measurements, as urine represents an easily accessible direct readout of the organ of interest. Indeed, proteinuria has been used for decades as a biomarker of renal disease activity; however, it lacks disease specificity. Ideally, one would like to develop screens for a limited number of markers that are highly sensitive and specific for individual disease entities and can be used as diagnostic tools.

Due to the possibility to extract RNA from cells or exosomes shed into the urine, some of the novel RNA detecting technologies discussed in earlier paragraphs have been applied to urine. Measurements of CD3ε mRNA, IP-10 mRNA, and 18S rRNA levels in urinary cells, have been postulated to detect or predict the outcome of acute rejection in renal allograft recipients [67]. A panel of differentially expressed microRNAs in transplant kidneys prior to histological allograft injury was identified to potentially monitor graft function and anticipate progression to chronic allograft dysfunction [68].

Another approach is the analysis of the urinary proteome [69], which is discussed in Chap. 6.

Imaging methods as indirect tools to evaluate renal tissue have been discussed elsewhere (Chap. 1). It is important to mention that novel functional magnetic resonance imaging (MRI) techniques allow for detailed assessments of both renal stucture and function. While arterial spin labeling measures renal perfusion [70], diffusion-weighted MRI enables the assessment of renal fibrosis and microstructure and blood oxygen level dependent (BOLD) imaging detects renal hypoxia [71, 72]. These methods are not yet widely available and are currently mainly used to inform about renal angioplasty indications. It is conceivable that with further technological progress MRI technology could become applicable to quantitate tubulointerstitial scarring, replacing the need for histopathological assessment in certain clinical settings.

References

1. Morales P, Hamilton K, Brown J, Hotchkiss RS. Open renal biopsy. J Urol. 1961;86:501–3.
2. White RH. Observations on percutaneous renal biopsy in children. Arch Dis Child. 1963;38:260–6.
3. Metcoff J. Needles for percutaneous renal biopsy in infants and children. Pediatrics. 1970;46:788–9.
4. Tondel C, Vikse BE, Bostad L, Svarstad E. Safety and complications of percutaneous kidney biopsies in 715 children and 8573 adults in Norway 1988–2010. Clin J Am Soc Nephrol. 2012;7:1591–7.
5. Sweeney C, Geary DF, Hebert D, Robinson L, Langlois V. Outpatient pediatric renal transplant

biopsy – is it safe? Pediatr Transplant. 2006;10: 159–61.

6. Feneberg R, Schaefer F, Zieger B, et al. Percutaneous renal biopsy in children: a 27-year experience. Nephron. 1998;79:438–46.

7. Amann K, Haas CS. What you should know about the work-up of a renal biopsy. Nephrol Dial Transplant. 2006;21:1157–61.

8. Fogo AB. Approach to renal biopsy. Am J Kidney Dis. 2003;42:826–36.

9. Walker PD, Cavallo T, Bonsib SM. Practice guidelines for the renal biopsy. Mod Pathol. 2004;17: 1555–63.

10. Corwin HL, Schwartz MM, Lewis EJ. The importance of sample size in the interpretation of the renal biopsy. Am J Nephrol. 1988;8:85–9.

11. Racusen LC, Colvin RB, Solez K, et al. Antibody-mediated rejection criteria – an addition to the Banff '97 classification of renal allograft rejection. Am J Transplant. 2003;3:708–14.

12. Haas M. A reevaluation of routine electron microscopy in the examination of native renal biopsies. J Am Soc Nephrol. 1997;8:70–6.

13. Siegel NJ, Spargo BH, Kashgarian M, Hayslett JP. An evaluation of routine electron microscopy in the examination of renal biopsies. Nephron. 1973;10:209–15.

14. Pirson Y. Making the diagnosis of Alport's syndrome. Kidney Int. 1999;56:760–75.

15. Morita M, White RH, Raafat F, Barnes JM, Standring DM. Glomerular basement membrane thickness in children. A morphometric study. Pediatr Nephrol. 1988;2:190–5.

16. Liptak P, Kemeny E, Ivanyi B. Primer: histopathology of polyomavirus-associated nephropathy in renal allografts. Nat Clin Pract Nephrol. 2006;2:631–6.

17. Jennette JC, Olson JL, Schwartz MM, Silva FG. Primer on the pathologic diagnosis of renal disease. In: Jennette JC, Olson JL, Schwartz MM, Silva FG, editors. Heptinstall's pathology of the kidney. Philadelphia: Lippincott Williams & Wilkins; 2007. p. 97–123.

18. D'Agati VD, Fogo AB, Bruijn JA, Jennette JC. Pathologic classification of focal segmental glomerulosclerosis: a working proposal. Am J Kidney Dis. 2004;43:368–82.

19. Weening JJ, D'Agati VD, Schwartz MM, et al. The classification of glomerulonephritis in systemic lupus erythematosus revisited. Kidney Int. 2004;65: 521–30.

20. Coppo R, Troyanov S, Camilla R, et al. The Oxford IgA nephropathy clinicopathological classification is valid for children as well as adults. Kidney Int. 2010;77:921–7.

21. Cattran DC, Coppo R, Cook HT, et al. The Oxford classification of IgA nephropathy: rationale, clinicopathological correlations, and classification. Kidney Int. 2009;76:534–45.

22. Roberts IS, Cook HT, Troyanov S, et al. The Oxford classification of IgA nephropathy: pathology defini-tions, correlations, and reproducibility. Kidney Int. 2009;76:546–56.

23. Camous X, Pera A, Solana R, Larbi A. NK cells in healthy aging and age-associated diseases. J Biomed Biotechnol. 2012;2012:195956.

24. Racusen LC, Solez K, Colvin RB, et al. The Banff 97 working classification of renal allograft pathology. Kidney Int. 1999;55:713–23.

25. Chang A, Gibson IW, Cohen AH, et al. A position paper on standardizing the nonneoplastic kidney biopsy report. Clin J Am Soc Nephrol. 2012;7:1365–8.

26. Drachenberg CB, Papadimitriou JC. Polyomavirus-associated nephropathy: update in diagnosis. Transpl Infect Dis. 2006;8:68–75.

27. Meehan SM, Domer P, Josephson M, et al. The clinical and pathologic implications of plasmacytic infiltrates in percutaneous renal allograft biopsies. Hum Pathol. 2001;32:205–15.

28. Boysen G, Bausch-Fluck D, Thoma CR, et al. Identification and functional characterization of pVHL-dependent cell surface proteins in renal cell carcinoma. Neoplasia. 2012;14:535–46.

29. Kurban G, Gallie BL, Leveridge M, et al. Needle core biopsies provide ample material for genomic and proteomic studies of kidney cancer: observations on DNA, RNA, protein extractions and VHL mutation detection. Pathol Res Pract. 2012;208:22–31.

30. Zacchia M, Vilasi A, Capasso A, et al. Genomic and proteomic approaches to renal cell carcinoma. J Nephrol. 2011;24:155–64.

31. Sethi S, Theis JD, Vrana JA, et al. Laser microdissection and proteomic analysis of amyloidosis, cryoglobulinemic GN, fibrillary GN, and immunotactoid glomerulopathy. Clin J Am Soc Nephrol. 2013;8:915–21.

32. Satoskar AA, Shapiro JP, Bott CN, et al. Characterization of glomerular diseases using proteomic analysis of laser capture microdissected glomeruli. Mod Pathol. 2012;25:709–21.

33. Nakatani S, Wei M, Ishimura E, et al. Proteome analysis of laser microdissected glomeruli from formalin-fixed paraffin-embedded kidneys of autopsies of diabetic patients: nephronectin is associated with the development of diabetic glomerulosclerosis. Nephrol Dial Transplant. 2012;27:1889–97.

34. Brambilla F, Lavatelli F, Merlini G, Mauri P. Clinical proteomics for diagnosis and typing of systemic amyloidoses. Proteomics Clin Appl. 2013;7:136–43.

35. Sethi S, Vrana JA, Theis JD, et al. Laser microdissection and mass spectrometry-based proteomics aids the diagnosis and typing of renal amyloidosis. Kidney Int. 2012;82:226–34.

36. Sethi S, Theis JD, Leung N, et al. Mass spectrometry-based proteomic diagnosis of renal immunoglobulin heavy chain amyloidosis. Clin J Am Soc Nephrol. 2010;5:2180–7.

37. Klein CJ, Vrana JA, Theis JD, et al. Mass spectrometric-based proteomic analysis of amyloid neuropathy type in nerve tissue. Arch Neurol. 2011; 68:195–9.

38. Nasr SH, Said SM, Valeri AM, et al. The diagnosis and characteristics of renal heavy-chain and heavy/light-chain amyloidosis and their comparison with renal light-chain amyloidosis. Kidney Int. 2013;83:463–70.

39. Nasr SH, Fidler ME, Cornell LD, et al. Immunotactoid glomerulopathy: clinicopathologic and proteomic study. Nephrol Dial Transplant. 2012;27:4137–46.

40. Maes E, Broeckx V, Mertens I, et al. Analysis of the formalin-fixed paraffin-embedded tissue proteome: pitfalls, challenges, and future prospectives. Amino Acids. 2013;45:205–18.

41. Kretzler M, Cohen CD, Doran P, et al. Repuncturing the renal biopsy: strategies for molecular diagnosis in nephrology. J Am Soc Nephrol. 2002;13:1961–72.

42. Cohen CD, Frach K, Schlondorff D, Kretzler M. Quantitative gene expression analysis in renal biopsies: a novel protocol for a high-throughput multicenter application. Kidney Int. 2002;61:133–40.

43. Jonigk D, Modde F, Bockmeyer CL, Becker JU, Lehmann U. Optimized RNA extraction from non-deparaffinized, laser-microdissected material. Methods Mol Biol. 2011;755:67–75.

44. Emmert-Buck MR, Bonner RF, Smith PD, et al. Laser capture microdissection. Science. 1996;274:998–1001.

45. Jiang R, Scott RS, Hutt-Fletcher LM. Laser capture microdissection for analysis of gene expression in formalin-fixed paraffin-embedded tissue. Methods Mol Biol. 2011;755:77–84.

46. Cohen CD, Grone HJ, Grone EF, et al. Laser microdissection and gene expression analysis on formaldehyde-fixed archival tissue. Kidney Int. 2002;61:125–32.

47. Woroniecki RP, Bottinger EP. Laser capture microdissection of kidney tissue. Methods Mol Biol. 2009;466:73–82.

48. Noppert SJ, Eder S, Rudnicki M. Laser-capture microdissection of renal tubule cells and linear amplification of RNA for microarray profiling and real-time PCR. Methods Mol Biol. 2011;755:257–66.

49. De SW, Cornillie P, Van PM, et al. Quantitative mRNA expression analysis in kidney glomeruli using microdissection techniques. Histol Histopathol. 2011;26:267–75.

50. Peterson KS, Huang JF, Zhu J, et al. Characterization of heterogeneity in the molecular pathogenesis of lupus nephritis from transcriptional profiles of laser-captured glomeruli. J Clin Invest. 2004;113:1722–33.

51. Sarmah CK, Samarasinghe S. Microarray gene expression: a study of between-platform association of Affymetrix and cDNA arrays. Comput Biol Med. 2011;41:980–6.

52. Carter SL, Eklund AC, Mecham BH, Kohane IS, Szallasi Z. Redefinition of Affymetrix probe sets by sequence overlap with cDNA microarray probes reduces cross-platform inconsistencies in cancer-associated gene expression measurements. BMC Bioinformatics. 2005;6:107.

53. Halloran PF, Pereira AB, Chang J, et al. Microarray diagnosis of antibody-mediated rejection in kidney transplant biopsies: an international prospective study (INTERCOM). Am J Transplant. 2013;13:2865–74.

54. Halloran PF, Reeve JP, Pereira AB, Hidalgo LG, Famulski KS. Antibody-mediated rejection, T cell-mediated rejection, and the injury-repair response: new insights from the Genome Canada studies of kidney transplant biopsies. Kidney Int. 2014;85:258–64.

55. Mengel M, Campbell P, Gebel H, et al. Precision diagnostics in transplantation: from bench to bedside. Am J Transplant. 2013;13:562–8.

56. Ozluk Y, Blanco PL, Mengel M, et al. Superiority of virtual microscopy versus light microscopy in transplantation pathology. Clin Transplant. 2012;26:336–44.

57. Einecke G, Reeve J, Sis B, et al. A molecular classifier for predicting future graft loss in late kidney transplant biopsies. J Clin Invest. 2010;120:1862–72.

58. Liapis H, Storch GA, Hill DA, Rueda J, Brennan DC. CMV infection of the renal allograft is much more common than the pathology indicates: a retrospective analysis of qualitative and quantitative buffy coat CMV-PCR, renal biopsy pathology and tissue CMV-PCR. Nephrol Dial Transplant. 2003;18:397–402.

59. Gupta M, Filler G, Kovesi T, et al. Quantitative tissue polymerase chain reaction for Epstein-Barr virus in pediatric solid organ recipients. Am J Kidney Dis. 2003;41:212–9.

60. Randhawa P, Shapiro R, Vats A. Quantitation of DNA of polyomaviruses BK and JC in human kidneys. J Infect Dis. 2005;192:504–9.

61. Gupta M, Diaz-Mitoma F, Feber J, et al. Tissue HHV6 and 7 determination in pediatric solid organ recipients – a pilot study. Pediatr Transplant. 2003;7:458–63.

62. Bechert CJ, Schnadig VJ, Payne DA, Dong J. Monitoring of BK viral load in renal allograft recipients by real-time PCR assays. Am J Clin Pathol. 2010;133:242–50.

63. Kotton CN, Kumar D, Caliendo AM, et al. Updated international consensus guidelines on the management of cytomegalovirus in solid-organ transplantation. Transplant. 2013;96:333–60.

64. Lautenschlager I, Razonable RR. Human herpesvirus-6 infections in kidney, liver, lung, and heart transplantation: review. Transpl Int. 2012;25:493–502.

65. Rassekh SR, Chan S, Harvard C, et al. Screening for submicroscopic chromosomal rearrangements in Wilms tumor using whole-genome microarrays. Cancer Genet Cytogenet. 2008;182:84–94.

66. Gambin T, Stankiewicz P, Sykulski M, Gambin A. Functional performance of aCGH design for clinical cytogenetics. Comput Biol Med. 2013;43:775–85.

67. Suthanthiran M, Schwartz JE, Ding R, et al. Urinary-cell mRNA profile and acute cellular rejection in kidney allografts. N Engl J Med. 2013;369:20–31.

68. Maluf DG, Dumur CI, Suh JL, et al. The urine microRNA profile may help monitor post-transplant renal graft function. Kidney Int. 2014;85:439–49.

69. Decramer S, Wittke S, Mischak H, et al. Predicting the clinical outcome of congenital unilateral uretero-pelvic junction obstruction in newborn by urinary proteome analysis. Nat Med. 2006;12:398–400.

70. Hueper K, Gutberlet M, Rong S, et al. Acute kidney injury: arterial spin labeling to monitor renal perfusion impairment in mice-comparison with histopathologic results and renal function. Radiology. 2014;270:117–24.

71. Inoue T, Kozawa E, Okada H, et al. Noninvasive evaluation of kidney hypoxia and fibrosis using magnetic resonance imaging. J Am Soc Nephrol. 2011;22:1429–34.

72. Gloviczki ML, Glockner JF, Crane JA, et al. Blood oxygen level-dependent magnetic resonance imaging identifies cortical hypoxia in severe renovascular disease. Hypertension. 2011;58:1066–72.

Omics Tools for Exploration of Renal Disorders

6

Joost P. Schanstra, Bernd Mayer,
and Christoph Aufricht

Abbreviations

12PUV	Fetal urinary proteome based classifier of severe renal disease in PUV
2DE	Two-dimensional electrophoresis
CE	Capillary electrophoresis
CKD	Chronic kidney disease
ECM	Extracellular matrix
ESRD	End stage renal disease
LC	Liquid chromatography
miRNA	microRNA
MRM	Multiple reaction monitoring
MS	Mass spectrometry
MS/MS	Tandem mass spectrometry
MudPIT	Multidimensional protein identification technology
ncRNA	Non coding RNA
PAGE	Polyacrylamide gel electrophoresis
PUV	Posterior urethral valves
SELDI	Surface-enhanced laser desorption/ionization
SNP	Single nucleotide polymorphism
UPJ	Ureteropelvic junction
UUO	Unilateral ureteral obstruction

J.P. Schanstra (✉)
Institute National de la Sante e de la Recherche
Medicale (INSERM), U1048, Institute of
Cardiovascular and Metabolic Disease,
1 Avenue J Poulhes, Toulouse 31432, France

Université Toulouse III Paul-Sabatier, Toulouse, France
e-mail: joost-peter.schanstra@inserm.fr

B. Mayer
Emergentec Biodevelopment GmbH,
Gersthoferstrasse 29-31, Vienna 1180, Austria
e-mail: bernd.mayer@emergentec.com

C. Aufricht
Department of Pediatrics and Adolescent Medicine,
Medical University of Vienna, Waehringer Guertel
18-20, Vienna 1090, Austria
e-mail: christoph.aufricht@meduniwien.ac.at

Omics?

For many pediatric nephrologists, omics is still a buzzword. However, in almost every scientific meeting or clinical symposium omics-based technologies are part of the agenda.

Omics technologies have entered in broad scale translational and applied clinical research in recent years. This is a remarkable development considering the fact that the first publication of the human genetic code laying the foundations for comprehensive analysis of molecular features appeared just about a decade ago. These advancements are to be attributed mainly to advancements on the technology side, be it miniaturization and parallelization involving beads and microarrays, or improvements in separation techniques and resolution on the mass spectrometry side.

On a conceptual side all these improvements have led to the term "Omics revolution" as they provide the opportunity of truly explorative research, departing from classical hypothesis-driven, reductionist approaches [1]. Omics techniques have even contributed to the

© Springer-Verlag Berlin Heidelberg 2016
D.F. Geary, F. Schaefer (eds.), *Pediatric Kidney Disease*, DOI 10.1007/978-3-662-52972-0_6

identification of novel classes of molecular regulators such as the non-coding RNAs as a result of transcriptomics studies initially performed in the ENCODE project [2]. At present an inflation of omics disciplines is seen, *with the major omics tracks in genetics (genomics), transcripts (transcriptomics), proteins (proteomics) and metabolites (metabolomics)* (the "big 4"), but further complemented by dozens of further "Omes" [3].

Important to note, omics in clinical research means in the first place a discovery procedure aimed at identifying novelty with respect to human disease, which in turn may contribute to the development of biomarkers and exploration of novel therapy targets. However, experimental tools utilized in omics as high-throughput sequencing or mass spectroscopy may serve as technology platforms for multiplexed assays, e.g., for determining genetic variants or specific peptide, protein or metabolite patterns, as outlined below for proteomics-based biomarker panels. As for any assays for use in clinical practice also for such more complex platforms technical qualification, next to demonstration of added value in clinical use need to be in place.

For the big 4 in Omics, handling of an experiment, although demanding machinery-specific technical expertise, has essentially become a standard procedure in many clinical research laboratories. Table 6.1 provides an overview of omics research activities in specific areas of nephrology.

If we remember the course of development of established diagnostic parameters and therapeutic interventions, it becomes obvious that the advent of new technologies has always been more or less rapidly followed by the development of new diagnostic and therapeutic tools. Steps

forward on deriving meaningful information out of "big data" resulted in the vision and promise that omics-based tools will improve current standards in medicine. However, are omics based technologies already clinically applicable diagnostic tools? Will they ever be? This chapter aims to provide the clinically orientated pediatric nephrologist with selected insights and a general understanding of the topic by combining a global tutorial with specific scientific discussions in order to allow critical appraisal of the current status of omics based, primarily diagnostic, tools.

Omics for Improved Description of Disease

Complex clinical phenotypes as exhibited by kidney disease can, in general, not be described in detail on the level of single molecular features. It has been repeatedly shown that identification of an association of single molecular characteristics, be it on the genomic mutation level or aberrant abundance of transcripts, proteins or metabolites with a specific disease phenotype, is not sufficient to assess essential elements of pathology and pathophysiology, or to efficiently predict disease outcome [4, 5]. In contrast, a combination of biomarkers – i.e., a panel or profile – covering disease complexity, while being less sensitive to inter-individual variations, appears more suitable to describe or represent a clinical presentation. Tools related to omics are employed with the aim to collectively describe or analyze multiple molecular features.

Genomics aims to cover variations within the genes (of protein- as well as non-protein coding reading frames together with regulatory areas).

Table 6.1 Number of publications in PubMed (As of November 2013) using Omics technologies assigned to general kidney diseases, acute kidney injury and chronic kidney disease

	Genome-wide association studies	Transcriptomics	Proteomics	Metabolomics
Kidney diseases	147	1028	372	65
Acute kidney injury	0	15	28	8
Chronic kidney disease	37	49	39	10

In a growing number of conditions the identification of the underlying genetic abnormality can potentially modify clinical management. Examples include: (i) patients with steroid-resistant nephrotic syndrome harboring mutations in certain mitochondrial genes may benefit from coenzyme Q10 treatment [6], (ii) screening for WT1 in steroid-resistant nephrotic syndrome would allow the identification of patients with risk of rapid progression to ESRD or developing tumors [7], and (iii) screening of patients with atypical hemolytic uremic syndrome for mutations in complement genes may inform on decisions about kidney transplantation [8]. However, in chronic, multifactorial diseases there is still lack of evidence that individual mutations are causally implicated in risk and progression. In kidney disease, mutations in the transcription factor HNF1β are a good example of the lack of correlation between geno- and phenotype. HNF1β mutations (deletions or point mutations) are associated with a large spectrum of renal and extrarenal phenotypes [9, 10] with a highly variable prognosis [11]. Therefore, although genes describe the potential predisposition for a disease or progression, actual disease presentation at present is not (yet) captured by genomic analysis. Significant genetic analysis programs of common genetic variants (single nucleotide polymorphisms (SNPs)) have been conducted and are further ongoing with the aim of unraveling the relevance of genetic background, specifically the combination of SNPs, for diseases of the kidney. As an example, mutations in uromodulin (UMOD) are reported to cause rare, autosomal dominant, primary tubulointerstitial kidney diseases, particularly familial juvenile hyperuricemic nephropathy [12], whereas common SNPs in the same gene induce salt-sensitive hypertension and kidney damage [13].

Transcriptome levels (i.e., mRNA and noncoding(nc)RNA) potentially better describe disease activity, but certainly mRNA expression only serves as an approximation of effective protein concentration and activity [14]. Another practical issue to take care of with mRNA is its inherent instability bearing the risk of inducing artefacts of variation in mRNA levels after isolation. This is especially the case for urinary mRNAs that only can be obtained from freshly collected urine. However, a recent large scale study described the successful use of a urinary-cell mRNA profile to predict acute cellular rejection in kidney allografts [15]. The study was carried out using frozen cellular pellets obtained from freshly collected urine samples. The three-gene signature in this study had 79 % sensitivity and 78 % specificity to discriminate between biopsy specimens showing no rejection and those showing acute cellular rejection. Prospective studies to assess whether this urinary signature and the routine use of urinary–cell mRNA can alter the requirement for allograft biopsies and be used in transplant management will be necessary.

MicroRNAs (miRNAs) are a class of small, non-coding RNAs that act as posttranscriptional regulators by binding and preferentially repressing translation of target mRNAs. Close to a thousand miRNAs have been identified up to now [16] and miRNAs have been predicted to have regulatory impact on >60 % of all protein-coding human genes [17]. miRNAs are excreted into body fluids [18] and -unlike mRNAs- are stable since they are complexed with RNA-binding proteins or packaged in lipid vesicles, shielding them from degradation by ribonucleases [19, 20]. A rapidly increasing body of evidence suggests aberrant in situ miRNA expression in human renal diseases such as diabetic nephropathy [21], IgA nephropathy [22], lupus nephritis [23], allograft rejection [24], and renal tumours [25]. miRNA profiles show distinct expression patterns in different body fluids. The stable, tissue- and fluid-specific expression pattern of extracellular miRNAs and their sensitive detection by PCR/microarray technology makes them promising candidates for molecular disease phenotyping and as biomarkers. Preliminary, but mostly small scale studies showed associations of specific urinary miRNAs to diabetic nephropathy [26], acute kidney injury [27], idiopathic nephrotic syndrome [28], IgA nephropathy [29] and chronic kidney disease [30]. A recent, larger scale study including an independent validation phase showed the association of specific miRNAs present in urinary cell pellets to be predictive of histological allograft injury [31]. These studies show the potential of urinary miRNAs as markers of specific kidney diseases although larger studies are scarce and prospective validation comparing to current gold standards are still absent.

A significant advantage of transcriptomics data is their annotation and coverage level: In single gene array experiments virtually all protein coding transcripts (about 20,000) can be assessed on their concentration level, and also for miRNAs arrays covering the entire set (up to 2000 sequences including predicted miRNA sequences) have become available, and the experimental design provides direct information on the molecular species measured. Additionally, arrays with splice variant-specific probes allow to approximate protein isoform concentrations.

The *proteome* is most likely to be the closest component to study the actual (chronic) disease activity, since long term key changes, for example the development of fibrosis in chronic kidney disease (CKD), is more directly reflected by changes in protein levels of components, e.g., of the extracellular matrix (ECM [32]. Specific examples of the use of proteomics in pediatric nephrology will be presented in detail below.

Although the levels of *metabolites* in body fluids clearly reflects disease activity, they are subject to a large degree of variation: food intake significantly modifies metabolite composition in body fluids [33, 34] and standard protocols for metabolome analysis have only recently been proposed for serum and plasma [35]. In addition due to the "distance" from protein activity generating the respective metabolites, the information extracted from metabolites is frequently far more difficult to interpret, as the metabolite concentration is a result of the regulatory status of many different, protein-driven processes, and equally important metabolites themselves are reactive species forming a reaction network among themselves and the environment. Technically, metabolome analysis is challenging as well. Although nuclear magnetic resonance (NMR) spectros-

copy is highly reproducible, it has low sensitivity only allowing the detection of a few hundred metabolites of the estimated 7800 human metabolites [36]. Chromatography coupled to mass spectrometry (MS) allows the detection of many more metabolites (thousands) but is less reproducible and solutions to deal with this low reproducibility have been proposed only recently [37, 38]. This has resulted in the publication of only a few small scale exploratory studies of the metabolome in human kidney disease. This includes the analysis of the urinary metabolome in the context of autosomal dominant polycystic kidney disease [39] and acute kidney injury after cardiac surgery [40] and plasma metabolome analysis of type 2 diabetic patients progressing to ESRD [41].

Procedural Issues in Omics Research

The first aspect challenging omics research is the mere flood of data generated in short term, leading to the "big data" challenge in clinical research [42]. Whereas transcriptomics may end up in only MB-sized data still allowing analysis on regular desktop machines, genetic and proteome studies generate GB to TB of data, necessitating the development of efficient computational infrastructures.

In addition, having a clinical sample and being able to carry out omics experiments does not necessarily lead to useful biomarkers. This has led to a number of early claims of candidate molecules discovered in, e.g., proteomics approaches that were not substantiated in subsequent studies [5, 43]. This situation has created doubt about the value of clinical proteomics. This is the reason for the appearance of "guidelines of clinical proteomics" [44, 45] and specific submission requirements in journals regularly publishing articles on clinical proteomics. Although initially developed for proteomics studies, these recommendations are straightforward and broadly applicable regardless of the omics technology used, the samples investigated or epidemiological design. The major recommendations are listed below (Fig. 6.1):

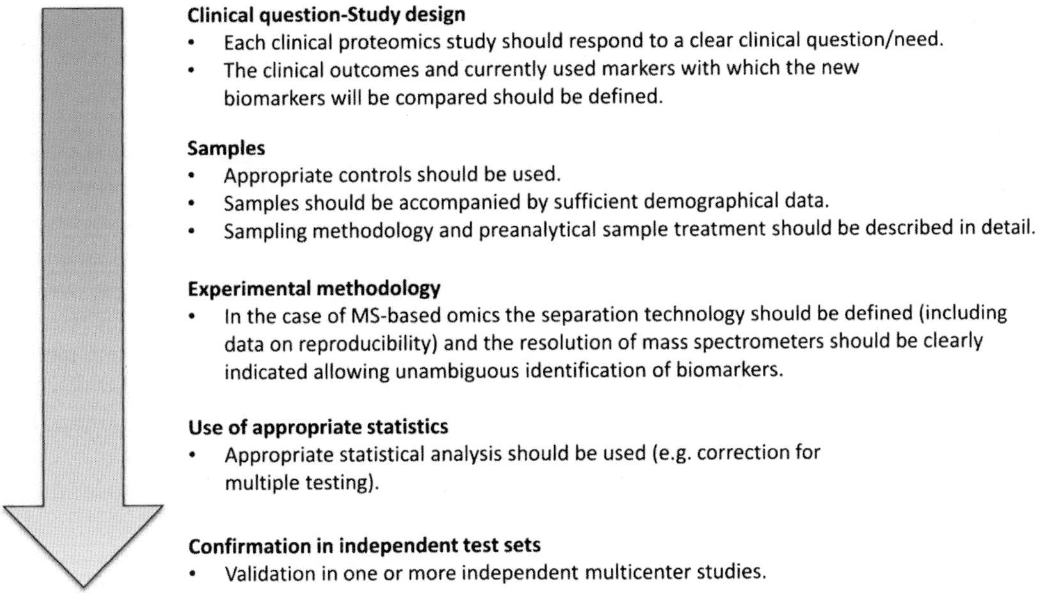

Clinical question-Study design
- Each clinical proteomics study should respond to a clear clinical question/need.
- The clinical outcomes and currently used markers with which the new biomarkers will be compared should be defined.

Samples
- Appropriate controls should be used.
- Samples should be accompanied by sufficient demographical data.
- Sampling methodology and preanalytical sample treatment should be described in detail.

Experimental methodology
- In the case of MS-based omics the separation technology should be defined (including data on reproducibility) and the resolution of mass spectrometers should be clearly indicated allowing unambiguous identification of biomarkers.

Use of appropriate statistics
- Appropriate statistical analysis should be used (e.g. correction for multiple testing).

Confirmation in independent test sets
- Validation in one or more independent multicenter studies.

Fig. 6.1 Roadmap of clinical omics aiming at the identification and validation of clinically useful biomarkers of disease

- Besides these technicalities the key component of any successful (omics) experiment is the choice of an appropriate study design, starting with precisely defined clinical phenotype inclusion criteria [46], supply of sufficient demographic and/or clinical data, a clearly defined clinical question with precise definition of outcomes/end-points, and reference to current clinical tests (if any) to be improved upon.
- Next, appropriate and highly standardized sample procurement is crucial for omics studies. Sufficient information about the sampling methodology including a description of specimen collection, handling and storage (i.e., type of containers, stabilizing solutions) and assurance of having all samples collected in the same manner. A bias can be introduced, e.g., if urine is collected at home or in the clinic. Formalin-embedded tissue may be acceptable for miRNA transcriptomics, but is less appropriate for mRNA profiling where fresh frozen material is preferred. Further constraints apply, e.g., for plasma proteomics (as outlined below, and Table 6.2), or sample freeze-thaw cycle implications on metabolomics results.
- Appropriate positive and negative controls must be defined. A healthy control population does often not reflect the clinical situation encountered and biomarkers identified in such a study will potentially be invalid in follow-up studies. Controls with related or similar diseases are clearly more appropriate. Hence controls for biomarkers of diabetic kidney disease would be diabetic patients, matched for parameters as age, without diabetic kidney disease.
- Sufficient information about the experimental methodology. In proteomics, separation technology (see below) and resolution of mass spectrometers needs to be mentioned. Low resolution mass spectrometers will lead to non-reproducible results and ambiguous attribution of signals. From this follows that protein based markers must be identified unambiguously by tandem MS. With the current state-of-art this is not always possible and in that case a unique identifier based on parameters such as molecular mass, migration/retention time in separation, or interaction

Table 6.2 Advantages and disadvantages of bodily fluids, potential sources of biomarker proteins used in nephrology

	Pros	Cons
Blood	Easily accessible	Highly complex body fluid (plasma)
	In contact with all organs	Proteolytic activity may remain, hence increased variability (serum)
		A few abundant proteins make up the majority of the blood protein content
Urine	Easily accessible	Content varies (daily fluid intake, circadian rhythms and exercise).
	Under physiological conditions 70 % of the proteins are kidney derived	Content is highly diluted
	Stable	
Amniotic fluid	Content closely resembles that of fetal plasma in first half of pregnancy	Is obtained invasively
	Content closely resembles that of fetal urine in second half of the pregnancy (hence expected to be stable)	Content varies during the day
		Low protein content

with an antibody must be provided. Hence the use of high resolution mass spectrometers is preferred.

- Appropriate statistical approaches should be employed. It sometimes appears that the rigor in study design and analysis procedures does not keep up with the data size generated, although specifically in omics experiments the "curse of dimensionality" needs to be taken into consideration: Whereas in conventional clinical research studies the number of samples analyzed by far exceeds the number of parameters tested, omics behaves reciprocally. In

consequence, adequate sample size is pivotal specifically in omics studies. Minimum sample size may range from about 15–30 per group for, e.g., a proteomics (containing a few thousand features) or transcriptomics experiment (20,000 features) assuming less than 100 features as being finally identified as showing differential abundance, to many 1000 samples for a genome-wide association study (several million SNP features). Multiplicity of testing in most cases cannot be addressed any more by strict Bonferroni correction but alternative correction for controlling type I error is used [47].

- Confirmation in independent test-sets. On top of using appropriate statistics, validation of biomarkers in an independent test set (not used for the discovery of the biomarkers) needs to be performed since most statistical approaches used for biomarker evaluation assume (i) an even distribution of features across the data (similar variance in control and disease groups, and the absence of covariates), (ii) that the findings can be generalized, and (iii) that an association exists only with the investigated condition. This is generally not true and as a consequence, most biomarkers with promising results in a first data set will turn out to have less promising results in independent data sets.

Proteomics

As discussed above, since the proteins serve as the effector phase of cellular events, we have chosen to mainly focus on the use of proteome analysis applied to pediatric nephrology.

Biospecimens (Table 6.2)

Blood is a relatively easily accessible body fluid, and consequently many groups have analyzed the blood (serum or plasma) proteome. However, a number of challenges are currently associated to proteome analysis of blood. The most prominent issue is whether plasma or serum should be used [48]. Serum has the advantage of being depleted from abundant coagulation factors, but it is likely that proteolytic activity persists, which can lead to protein degradation upon sample treatment and storage and thus result in alteration of the serum proteome [49]. This contributes to experimental inaccuracy, and hampers comparison of serum proteome or peptidome profiles between individuals. Alternatively, plasma, the most complex body fluid, can be used. This high complexity is mainly due to the dynamic range with which proteins and peptides are found, spanning ten orders of magnitude [48, 50]. The ten most abundant proteins represent >90 % of the total plasma content, with albumin being first, and may interfere with the identification of less abundant proteins. Highly abundant proteins can be removed by employing depletion techniques, but this removal potentially introduces biases and may induce loss of the low abundance proteins and peptides: it has been shown that depletion of albumin induces the additional loss of ~1000 low abundance proteins and increases variability [51]. Thus, although blood analysis has a large potential to provide us with biomarkers of (kidney) disease, both plasma and serum proteomics have their drawbacks that need to be overcome. Targeted proteomics by multiple reaction monitoring might be a solution to this problem. Alternatively, elaborate upfront separation and fractionation techniques may prove beneficial on technical variability.

In contrast to blood, *urine* has evolved as a reliable source of biomarkers for a large variety of diseases [52, 53]. Around 70 % of the urinary proteins are estimated to originate from the kidney and the urinary tract [54]. However, the remainder derives from circulating peptides and small proteins that are transported in blood and filtered or secreted in urine. Therefore, urine contains potential not only biomarkers of kidney disease but also of diseases from more distant sites. For example, urinary biomarkers for cholangiocarcinoma [55], acute graft-versus-host disease [56], coronary artery disease [57] and Kawasaki disease (systemic vasculitis) [58] have been identified. Compared to plasma and serum, urine has the advantage that highly abundant plasma proteins are absent (except in strongly albuminuric

diseases). In addition, the urinary protein and peptide content is particularly stable. Finally, urine is non-invasive to collect and can be obtained in large quantities. On the other hand, urine has the drawbacks of showing variations in the protein and peptides concentration due to differences in the daily fluid intake, circadian rhythms and exercise, and thus potentially varies depending on the point in time when it is obtained. However, this is only a minor shortcoming which can be corrected by a variety of normalizing methods [59].

Besides soluble urinary proteins and peptides, proteins in urine can be contained in so called *exosomes* [60]. Exosomes are 40–100 nm membrane vesicles secreted into the extracellular space (including urine) by numerous cell types. Exosomes contain proteins, mRNAs, miRNAs, and signalling molecules that reflect the physiological state of their cells of origin and consequently provide a rich source of potential biomarker molecules. Normal urine contains exosomes that derive from every epithelial cell type facing the urinary space. Exosome isolation techniques provide a more than 30-fold enrichment of exosomal proteins, allowing proteins that are minor components of whole urine to be readily detectable immunochemically or by proteome analysis techniques [61]. Exosome analysis may be particularly useful for classification of disease processes involving the renal tubule, such as lysosomal storage diseases and transporter mutations [62, 63]. In addition, urinary exosomes contain multiple transcription factors, and their analysis has been proposed as a means of noninvasively detecting and monitoring various glomerular diseases [64].

While the exosome strategy appears intriguing, exosome isolation is not trivial and requires careful standardization of pre-analytical and analytical conditions [61]. Exosome omics studies may therefore be less amendable for routine clinical application.

Amniotic fluid (AF) is a significant contributor to fetal health and growth and protects the fetus physically [65]. Protein concentrations in AF are low, and associated to a relatively high carbohydrate and lipid content. In addition, many of the proteins present in AF are gluco-conjugated, protecting these proteins from degradation [66]. The content of AF fluid changes with gestational age: initially AF is essentially derived from maternal plasma, subsequently in the early fetal period the composition of AF is similar to that of fetal plasma. As of the second half of the pregnancy AF is mostly composed of fetal urine and of secretion of oral, nasal, tracheal and pulmonary fluids after swallowing and expiration [65]. Given the contribution of fetal urine in that period AF is a potential reservoir for developmental renal diseases.

Urinary Proteins Versus Naturally Occurring Peptides

Being a direct "readout" of the organ of interest, urine is the body fluid of choice for the search for biomarkers of kidney disease. Urine contains both proteins and naturally occurring peptides (Fig. 6.2a). To obtain clinically useful biomarkers, the preparation of the sample before proteome analysis needs to be as simple as possible to reduce the chance of selecting biomarkers due to biases introduced by sample handling. This minimal, preanalytical intervention can be achieved for naturally occurring peptides, since the only interventions are desalting and concentration, but is more difficult to establish for proteins. To be analyzed with high mass precision by mass spectrometry, all proteins need to be converted into peptides. Hence, proteins need to be enzymatically digested (usually with trypsin) into peptides. When all samples are processed in parallel (i.e., all samples to be analyzed are treated with the same lot of trypsin at the same time under exactly the same conditions) this will not lead to much experimental variation. However, when additional samples need to be analyzed (e.g., at a different point in time) it is highly unlikely that the proteins contained in these samples will receive exactly the same treatment to generate peptides as in the original samples. This induces experimental variability between these lots of samples and impairs comparability. Hence, currently naturally occurring urinary peptides (not

subjected to these preanalytical steps to produce peptides from proteins) are more amenable to become biomarkers of disease. However, urinary proteins do not need to be put aside since significant information on disease pathophysiology is most likely derived from the trypsin digested urinary proteins. More recently, due to technological improvements, so called "top-down" proteomics allowing to study intact proteins is becoming available, opening the possibility to evaluate the suitability of intact proteins as biomarkers of disease [67].

Tools for Proteome Analysis

Analysis of the proteome, the description or study of the total protein content of a sample, is a complex task given that the total number of proteins and/or its derived peptides easily reaches several tens of thousands (Fig. 6.2a). It is therefore an illusion that in the short term we will be able to analyze all in one experiment. Currently, most proteome analyses cover several thousands of proteins and peptides. Due to the large dynamic range observed in most biological samples including bodily fluids, analysis of a proteome involves some kind of fractionation of the sample. This fractionation step is followed by mass spectrometry (MS) analysis allowing to determine the quantity and exact mass and/or identity (if tandem MS is used) of a specific peptide (Fig. 6.2b).

Fractionation is necessary to reduce the complexity of the sample since the direct injection of a complex biological sample into a mass spectrometer will allow only the detection of a few of the most abundant proteins. Modern fractionation technologies include liquid chromatography (LC) and capillary electrophoresis (CE). Although surface-enhanced laser desorption/ ionization (SELDI)-MS was a very promising technology for both fractionation and MS analysis of proteins and peptides from body fluids [68] it has been largely abandoned due to reproducibility issues [69–74]. Two-dimensional gel electrophoresis (2DE) was until recently the method of choice for the analysis of proteins but, due to gel-to-gel variability and low reproduc-

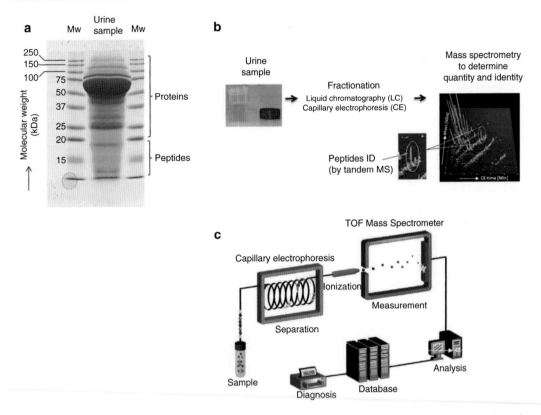

Fig. 6.2 Urinary proteome analysis. (**a**) Unidimensional poly-acrylamide gel analysis of a proteinuric sample showing few major urinary proteins and large dynamic range. Albumin can be clearly distinguished as major 50–75 kDa band. Peptides represent lower molecular weight proteins (<20 kDa). *Mw* molecular weight markers. (**b**) Standard proteome analysis workflow. The complexity of biological samples precludes direct analysis by mass spectrometry and necessitates chromatographic fractionation (liquid chromatography (LC) or capillary electrophoresis (CE)). Resulting fractions are then analyzed by mass spectrometry (MS) to determine protein quantity and identity. Peptides are identi-fied by mass and migration time, with signal intensity reflecting relative abundance. Sequencing of peaks of interest by tandem-MS allows peptide identification. (**c**) Schematic drawing of the on-line coupling of capillary electrophoresis to the mass spectrometer (CE-MS). CE separates polypeptides according to their charge and size. After separation, peptides are ionised on-line by application of high voltage and analysed in the mass spectrometer. CE-MS yields ~ 1000 MS spectra, which are evaluated using appropriate software (**b** Used with permission of Springer Science + Business Media from Mischak and Schanstra [117] **c** Used with permission from Klein et al. [99])

ibility, the difficulty to automate the process and considerable sample processing times, it is now gradually being abandoned as well.

Capillary Electrophoresis (CE)

CE can be used to separate ionic species (such as small proteins and peptides) by their charge, frictional forces and hydrodynamic radius. CE can be coupled on-line to MS. In Fig. 6.2c the main components of CE-MS are shown and their typical characteristics are described. CE-MS is most frequently used in proteome analysis for the

fractionation of peptides and small proteins (<20 kDa). CE-MS allows the reproducible analysis of several thousand polypeptides within a time range of 45–60 min ([24]; the detection of urinary peptides is shown in Fig. 6.2b). It uses inexpensive liquid-filled capillaries that can be cleaned and reconditioned after each run [14]. No elution gradients are required for separation, since the migration of the analyte is controlled by the electric field strength [75], hence limiting the risk of interference with subsequent detection by MS [76]. CE-MS is limited to the detection of small proteins and peptides. In addition, only a small sample volume can be loaded onto the capillary, which decreases somewhat the sensitivity of the detection. Overall, the CE-MS technology has developed into a commonly used proteomic technology, especially in the field of low-molecular weight proteome profiling (i.e., peptidome), and has been successfully applied in several clinical studies [77–79]. A major advantage, owing to the reproducibility of the detection, is that CE-MS can be used for both the discovery and validation phases of studies, since it is not necessary to work in batches. This characteristic potentially allows implementation of this mass spectrometry-based analysis in a routine clinical setting.

Liquid Chromatography (LC)

LC is a frequently used, high-resolution method allowing the separation of significant quantities of small proteins and peptides mostly based on reversed phase, ion exchange, or size exclusion chromatography [80, 81]. The remainder of the steps in LC and on-line coupling to MS is comparable to CE-MS (Fig. 6.2c). In contrast to CE-MS, LC-MS in this configuration cannot be used for the validation of selected biomarkers. However, newer LC-MS/MS technologies ("multiple reaction monitoring," (MRM)) hold promise for potential future use as clinical proteomics platforms.

In addition to providing high sensitivity by virtue of the high loading capacity of LC columns, LC also allows the addition of further separation steps, thus enabling multidimensional fractionation that can generate a large number of data points. For example, in the multidimensional protein identification technology (MudPIT) [82] cation exchange pre-fractionation followed by reversed phase separation is used. The advantages of MudPIT are also its drawbacks: the multiple dimensions make MudPIT time consuming. It is thus nearly impossible to screen hundreds of samples with this technology. Moreover, the multidimensional separations in MudPIT make the comparative analysis of MudPIT-produced data highly challenging [83]. For these reasons the use of LC-MS/MS is currently limited to the initial discovery phase of biomarker research.

In the next section we will give two selected examples of proteome analysis-based studies in the field of pediatric nephrology aiming at the discovery and validation of urinary biomarkers of obstructive nephropathy.

Selected Examples of Clinical Proteomics Studies in Pediatric Nephrology

Ureteropelvic Junction Obstruction

Ureteropelvic junction (UPJ) obstruction is a relatively frequent anomaly (1/1500 births, [84]) characterized by stenosis of the intersection of renal pelvis and ureter, which may induce retention of urine in the kidney and, in severe cases, lead to pressure-induced renal tissue damage. Ultrasound screening detects the majority of cases before birth. Neonates with urodynamically relevant UPJ obstruction need close surveillance with repetitive isotope excretion scans up to the age of 2 years, to identify those in need for surgical removal of the stenosis (Fig. 6.3a).

Several laboratories have searched for urinary markers of UPJ obstruction predicting the eventual need for surgery at an early stage. Targeted searches for urinary protein markers potentially involved in the etiology of obstructive nephropathy (e.g., epidermal growth factor, transforming growth factor beta, monocyte attractant protein 1) did not identify valid predictors of the outcome of UPJ obstruction [53, 85]. In contrast to this candidate protein approach, Decramer et al. analyzed the urinary peptidome using CE-MS of UPJ obstruction patients [78] with the aim to identify outcome biomarkers. The discovery phase of the study included only UPJ obstruction patients representing either mild UPJ obstruction (n = 19, all evolving to spontaneous resolution of the obstruction) or severe UPJ obstruction (n = 19, all scheduled to be operated early in life). An age-matched control group (n = 13) was included as well. This approach yielded a panel of 51 peptide biomarkers with differential urinary abundance between the groups. These were combined in a statistical model that allowed distinguishing between the mild and severe obstruction group in

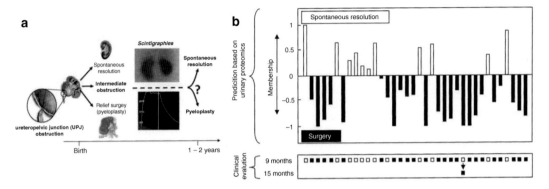

Fig. 6.3 Use of urinary proteomics to predict outcome of UPJ obstruction. (**a**) A subset of newborns with severe UPJ obstruction needs surgical correction while another, larger group with mild obstruction evolves to spontaneous resolution of obstruction. The remaining group with 'intermediate' obstruction needs regular monitoring to determine the evolution of the pathology. (**b**) Urinary protein profiles from 36 patients with 'intermediate' UPJ obstruction were classified using a hierarchic disease model based on polypeptides discriminating between healthy neonates, subjects with spontaneous resolution and individuals with persistent UPJ obstruction requiring surgery. A negative score suggests evolution towards surgery, a positive value evolution towards spontaneous resolution of UPJ obstruction. Prediction was compared with the clinical evolution after 9 and 15 months of follow-up. This resulted in 34 out of 36 correct predictions (94 %) at 9 months and 97 % (35/36) at 15 months as one patient evolved to severe UPJ obstruction at a late stage (*arrow*) (Used with permission from Decramer et al. [52])

the training population. Next, urine was prospectively collected from 36 additional patients with intermediate UPJ obstruction, the patient group in need of close surveillance with the greatest potential benefit from valid biomarkers (Fig. 6.3a). The urinary peptidome of these patients was analyzed with CE-MS and based on the presence of the 51 potential biomarkers it was predicted whether these patients would evolve towards mild or severe obstruction. The prediction was made before 3 months of age and the clinical outcome was assessed after 15 months of follow-up. Prediction was correct in 35 out of 36 patients several months in advance of either surgery or spontaneous resolution of the obstruction (Fig. 6.3b) [78, 86, 87]. The panel of 51 biomarkers was subsequently successfully validated in an independent small scale study [88]. A large scale multicenter validation study including ~300 patients is underway which, if successful, should pave the way towards clinical implementation, reduce treatment costs and be highly cost-effective in terms of quality of life gain [89].

Posterior Urethral Valves-Fetal Urine

Posterior urethral valves (PUV) is a rare developmental disease (incidence: 1:5000–1:8000 live male births [90]) which represents the most common cause of lower urinary tract obstruction in males. PUV induces obstructive nephropathy and renal dysplasia [91]. Approximately 20–30 % of the infants with PUV surviving the neonatal period progress to ESRD in the first decade of life, and the majority progress to CKD [92–94]. Most cases of PUV are diagnosed by antenatal ultrasound and confirmed postnatally by voiding cystourethrography and cystoscopy [95]. An immense clinical challenge upon antenatal detection of PUV is to predict post-natal renal function. Current methods to predict these outcomes in utero are controversial [96, 97]; a considerable fraction of patients with prenatally diagnosed severe renal and urinary tract malformation including PUV for whom termination of pregnancy was proposed but refused had normal serum creatinine at a median age of 29 months [98]. Current methods include ultrasound-based quantitation of amniotic fluid and assessment of the renal parenchyma, and concentration of fetal urine analytes, such as sodium and β2-microglobulin (β2m) (see also Chap. 2). Similarly to postnatal urine, fetal urine potentially contains biomarkers of disease. Klein et al. [99] studied the fetal urinary peptidome with the aim to detect biomarkers that can predict post-natal function in fetuses with PUV. They detected over 4000 peptides in fetal urine. Using a discovery cohort of 28 patients with PUV, 26 fetal urine peptides were identified that were specifically associated with PUV patients with early ESRD. A classifier based on 12 of these fetal urine peptides (12PUV classifier) predicted postnatal renal function with 88 % sensitivity and 95 % specificity in an independent blinded validation cohort of 38 PUV patients. This fetal urinary peptide-based classifier outperformed all conventional clinical parameters, none of which reached the same level of predictive sensitivity and specificity.

Currently, no treatment for PUV exists and even in utero repair of the valves does not improve outcome [100]. However, the failure of prenatal surgery may be due to the absence of appropriate selection criteria [101]. The 12PUV classifier might help selecting fetuses that will benefit from in utero repair. In addition, this fetal urine proteome-based classifier will potentially allow truly informed prenatal counseling, and hopefully will avoid unnecessary termination of pregnancy. Furthermore, prediction of postnatal renal function will be helpful in tailoring clinical follow-up and planning for renal replacement therapy. Most importantly, reliable prediction of postnatal outcomes would greatly reduce the psychological burden of prognostic uncertainty imposed on the affected families.

Implementation

The two examples above show that modern clinical proteomics-based methods can identify new disease markers that will most likely contribute to improved patient management in areas of pediatric nephrology that did not advance substantially for decades. Finally, in addition to this benefit for the patient, incorporation of such a urinary proteome analysis early in the evaluation of UPJ obstruction would significantly reduce costs and be an effective measure in terms of health economics. Incorporating the urinary peptidome analysis in the management of UPJ obstruction increases cost-effectiveness by $8000

per quality adjusted life year (QALY) per patient [89]. An important issue is how to implement these proteome-based results in the clinic.

MS-Based Tools

MS is not yet routinely used in the clinic. However, in contrast to LC-MS and 2DE-MS, CE-MS can be used not only in the discovery and validation phase of clinical proteomics studies but also as a routine proteomics-based clinical platform: analysis of the same samples by CE-MS in different laboratories for both a CKD classifier [102] and the 12PUV classifier [99] showed highly reproducible results. Thus, implementation of an MS-based test to analyze the urinary peptidome using CE-MS in a clinical setting can be foreseen. Urine can be obtained in the clinic, frozen, and then sent to a central laboratory for CE-MS analysis (with a turnaround time of ~2 days once a sample is received).

Other MS-based tools for implementation in a clinical setting are under development. This is mostly based on targeted-MS such as MRM where multiple preselected protein fragments are quantified in body fluids. Proof-of-principle for clinical use is available for this MS-based approach [103–105], but actual clinical studies are still lacking.

Non MS-Based Tools

Whereas in early proteome studies disease signatures included unknown molecular entities (e.g., defined by a specific mass and/or migration time on CE or LC), advances in MS have now identified most of these previously unknown proteins and peptides. This theoretically opens up the possibility to transform MS-based signatures in a multiplex assay more amenable to be implemented in a routine clinical context (e.g., antibody based ELISA analysis). However, although the development of an ELISA for detecting a single protein is rather straightforward, the production of antibodies specific for individual peptide fragments often faces specificity issues. In addition, while it may be feasible to develop an ELISA for a single peptide fragment using a combination of antibodies, it is largely impossible to establish ELISA systems for multiple peptides comprising entire classifiers as described above (e.g., 12 for PUV or 51 for UPJ obstruction).

An emerging multiplex approach involves the use of aptamers. Nucleic acid aptamers are nucleic acid species that have been engineered through repeated rounds of in vitro selection to bind to various molecular targets such as small molecules. Aptamers are useful in biotechnological and therapeutic applications as they offer molecular recognition properties that rival that of the commonly used biomolecule, antibodies. Although their use in peptide-based classifiers still needs to be proven, the use of aptamers-based technology was reported to enable the detection of 60 potential CKD biomarkers from plasma in a cross-sectional study [106].

Omics for Better Insight in Disease Mechanisms

Certainly, the definition of urine proteome-based classifiers for diseases such as unilateral ureteral obstruction (UUO) in the clinical setting also reframes the interpretation of molecular patho-logical changes associated with these diseases in well controlled experimental settings applying omics based tools. For example, Springer et al. recently characterized the renal tissue molecular fingerprint of the cellular responses to severe obstruction in an animal model of fetal complete unilateral ureteral obstruction [107]. Global gene expression analysis provided an open approach for explorative data analysis, and subsequent bio-informatics analysis of the transcript profiles allowed robust identification of concerted molec-ular processes involved in the UUO phenotype. In this first combined transcriptomics and bioin-formatics approach, Springer et al. not only focused on main established pathomechanisms (such as tubular inflammation, tubular apoptosis and renal fibrosis) but also searched for novel molecular mechanisms of potential biological relevance. Transcriptomics analysis was per-formed 2 weeks after the intervention – reflecting the time of the earliest interventions in the human setting. More than 509 gene products were

identified for exhibiting significantly different concentration between biopsies from obstructed versus non-obstructed fetal sheep kidneys. Bioinformatics identified seven biological pro-cesses involved in cellular structural, metabolic and signaling activities that have in large parts not been described before. Aligning these data with the urinary proteome may eventually pro-vide new and clinically relevant insights on the pathophysiologic background of early predictive markers involved in the pathogenesis of fetal uropathy.

Integration of Omics Results

Results of Omics studies may be combined for integrative analysis, either within an omics domain (e.g., transcriptomics meta-analysis) or across domains (e.g., combining transcriptomics and proteomics [108]). Omics integration aims a:t (i) directly contributing to biomarker identifi-cation utilizing Omics-track specific bioinfor-matics (Fig. 6.4a), (ii) evaluating the robustness of identified signatures (Fig. 6.4b), and (iii) to enable molecular (mechanistic) interpretation and plausibility evaluation of molecular signa-tures for rational biomarker selection (Fig. 6.4c).

Testing robustness is straight forward: Components of an omics signature characteriz-ing a specific phenotype should be stable when comparing individual profiling experiments. A multitude of omics profile data have become organized in the public domain (e.g., in Gene Expression Omnibus (www.ncbi.nlm.nih.gov/geo/), ArrayExpress (www.ebi.ac.uk/arrayex-press/), or PRIDE (www.ebi.ac.uk/pride/)), pro-viding highly valuable sources for signature comparison. Also repositories with dedicated focus on kidney diseases have been established, including Nephromine (www.nephromine.org) or KUPKB (www.kupkb.org) [109, 110]. The comparison is performed on the level of indi-vidual molecular features, requiring consolida-tion of signatures on a common denominator which is usually the level of protein coding genes. In practice, such direct comparisons often demonstrate only limited accordance due

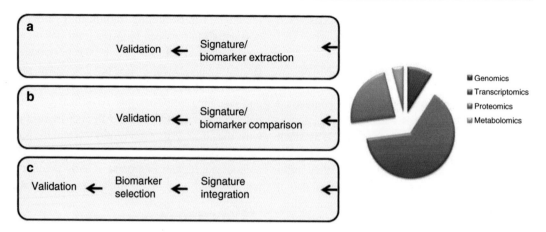

Fig. 6.4 Strategies for Omics profile analysis (Major Omics tracks from Table 6.1) towards biomarker discovery. (**a**) Statistics-based approach for direct delineation of biomarker candidates. (**b**) comparative approach for strengthening robustness of biomarker candidates before forwarding to validation. (**c**) Integrative approach via linking to molecular processes and pathways, from there selecting biomarker candidates

to experimental and biological variability. However, signatures identified in individual studies may show more extensive overlap if interpreted in their mechanistic context. A simple way of accounting for biological background in omics signatures is pathway enrichment analysis [111]. For example, if fibrosis is a histological finding, a respective omics signature might display an enrichment of molecular features involved in the TGF-beta signaling pathway. Analytical tools such as GSEA (www. broadinstitute.org/gsea) or DAVID [112] allow computation of such pathway enrichment using the omics signature as input. Hence, at this stage of analysis the evaluation of reliability and robustness of omics signatures incorporates an analysis of the mechanistic coherence and plausibility of underlying molecular interactions and their functional context. This step bears the additional potential of deriving drug target hypotheses from the molecular signature.

For a diagnostic or prognostic biomarker the association with the clinical phenotype or endpoint of interest is sufficient, and additional validation is achieved by studying therapeutic or preventive measures taken as a consequence of the biomarker test result. Such association of a biomarker and clinical phenotype may exhibit excellent sensitivity, but limited specificity. A biomarker indicative for inflammation may be clearly

linked to inflammatory kidney disease, but various other clinical phenotypes may also be represented by this molecular proxy. For instance, CRP is independently associated with increased rate of kidney function loss in chronic kidney disease [113] but also represents a non-specific marker of inflammation. Integrative Omics analysis aims to identify biomarker candidates with high sensitivity as well as specificity, ideally fulfilled by markers causally afflicted with organ-specific pathophysiology. Substantial efforts have been initiated using integrative Omics in Systems Biology or Systems Medicine approaches, as recently reviewed for kidney diseases by He et al. [114]. These approaches utilize interaction networks for building descriptive models of clinical phenotypes [1, 115]. Integrative molecular modeling has become available for various kidney diseases, traversing omics signatures into molecular process and pathway sets [116].

Conclusion

We hope that the information given in this chapter allows an informed view of the potential value of omics based tools in pediatric nephrology. However, we still owe you a response to the question whether omics based tools can be already regarded as established diagnostics. In pharmaceutical research, novel compounds are mostly derived from pathophysiological and molecular biology data. Following preclinical development, candidate compounds, after careful safety testing in a mostly healthy population, are applied in well selected patient populations in order to demonstrate "proof of concept" in the second phase of clinical development. Only after successful completion of phase 2, large patient populations are involved in phase 3 studies that should reflect "clinical reality." In view of this analogy, omics based diagnostic tools in pediatric nephrology are currently undergoing the transition into the "proof of concept" phase. In adult nephrology the field of urinary biomarkers has advanced faster, mainly due to the larger available population sizes. The urinary proteomics-based, multicentric, interventional PRIORITY trial will assess in more than 3000 patients the prognostic capabilities of a validated urinary proteome based classifier, as well as the benefit of targeted early intervention based on the urinary proteome score. However, as of today the question is still open whether omics based tools will transform routine diagnostics, or whether they will primarily be employed to improve current diagnostic tools by identification of individual new biomarkers, as well as for screening purposes in the development of new drugs.

References

1. Mayer P, Mayer B, Mayer G. Systems biology: building a useful model from multiple markers and profiles. Nephrol Dial Transplant. 2012;27(11):3995–4002.
2. Djebali S, Davis CA, Merkel A, Dobin A, Lassmann T, Mortazavi A, et al. Landscape of transcription in human cells. Nature. 2012;489(7414):101–8.
3. Prohaska SJ, Stadler PF. The use and abuse of -omes. Methods Mol Biol. 2011;719:173–96.
4. Hurst RE. Does the biomarker search paradigm need re-booting? BMC Urol. 2009;9:1.
5. Rifai N, Gillette MA, Carr SA. Protein biomarker discovery and validation: the long and uncertain path to clinical utility. Nat Biotechnol. 2006;24(8):971–83.
6. Ashraf S, Gee HY, Woerner S, Xie LX, Vega-Warner V, Lovric S, et al. ADCK4 mutations promote steroid-resistant nephrotic syndrome through CoQ10 biosynthesis disruption. J Clin Invest. 2013;123(12):5179–89.
7. Lipska BS, Ranchin B, Iatropoulos P, Gellermann J, Melk A, Ozaltin F, et al. Genotype-phenotype associations in WT1 glomerulopathy. Kidney Int. 2014;85(5):1169–78.
8. Bresin E, Rurali E, Caprioli J, Sanchez-Corral P, Fremeaux-Bacchi V, Rodriguez de Cordoba S, et al. Combined complement gene mutations in atypical hemolytic uremic syndrome influence clinical phenotype. J Am Soc Nephrol. 2013;24(3):475–86.
9. Decramer S, Parant O, Beaufils S, Clauin S, Guillou C, Kessler S, et al. Anomalies of the TCF2 gene are the main cause of fetal bilateral hyperechogenic kidneys. J Am Soc Nephrol. 2007;18(3):923–33.
10. Heidet L, Decramer S, Pawtowski A, Moriniere V, Bandin F, Knebelmann B, et al. Spectrum of HNF1B mutations in a large cohort of patients who harbor renal diseases. Clin J Am Soc Nephrol. 2010;5(6):1079–90.
11. Faguer S, Decramer S, Chassaing N, Bellanne-Chantelot C, Calvas P, Beaufils S, et al. Diagnosis, management, and prognosis of HNF1B nephropathy in adulthood. Kidney Int. 2011;80(7):768–76.
12. Sedor JR. Uromodulin and translational medicine: will the SNPs bring zip to clinical practice? J Am Soc Nephrol. 2010;21(2):204–6.
13. Trudu M, Janas S, Lanzani C, Debaix H, Schaeffer C, Ikehata M, et al. Common noncoding UMOD gene variants induce salt-sensitive hypertension and kidney damage by increasing uromodulin expression. Nat Med. 2013;19(12):1655–60.
14. Maier T, Guell M, Serrano L. Correlation of mRNA and protein in complex biological samples. FEBS Lett. 2009;583(24):3966–73.
15. Suthanthiran M, Schwartz JE, Ding R, Abecassis M, Dadhania D, Samstein B, et al. Urinary-cell mRNA profile and acute cellular rejection in kidney allografts. N Engl J Med. 2013;369(1):20–31.
16. Griffiths-Jones S, Saini HK, van Dongen S, Enright AJ. miRBase: tools for microRNA genomics. Nucleic Acids Res. 2008;36(Database issue):D154–8.
17. Friedman RC, Farh KK, Burge CB, Bartel DP. Most mammalian mRNAs are conserved targets of microRNAs. Genome Res. 2009;19(1):92–105.
18. Weber JA, Baxter DH, Zhang S, Huang DY, Huang KH, Lee MJ, et al. The microRNA spectrum in 12 body fluids. Clin Chem. 2010;56(11):1733–41.
19. Wang K, Zhang S, Weber J, Baxter D, Galas DJ. Export of microRNAs and microRNA-protective protein by mammalian cells. Nucleic Acids Res. 2010;38(20):7248–59.
20. Gibbings DJ, Ciaudo C, Erhardt M, Voinnet O. Multivesicular bodies associate with components of miRNA effector complexes and modulate miRNA activity. Nat Cell Biol. 2009;11(9):1143–9.
21. McClelland A, Hagiwara S, Kantharidis P. Where are we in diabetic nephropathy: microRNAs and biomarkers? Curr Opin Nephrol Hypertens. 2014;23(1):80–6.
22. Dai Y, Sui W, Lan H, Yan Q, Huang H, Huang Y. Microarray analysis of micro-ribonucleic acid expression in primary immunoglobulin A nephropathy. Saudi Med J. 2008;29(10):1388–93.

23. Dai Y, Sui W, Lan H, Yan Q, Huang H, Huang Y. Comprehensive analysis of microRNA expression patterns in renal biopsies of lupus nephritis patients. Rheumatol Int. 2009;29(7):749–54.

24. Sui W, Dai Y, Huang Y, Lan H, Yan Q, Huang H. Microarray analysis of MicroRNA expression in acute rejection after renal transplantation. Transpl Immunol. 2008;19(1):81–5.

25. Gottardo F, Liu CG, Ferracin M, Calin GA, Fassan M, Bassi P, et al. Micro-RNA profiling in kidney and bladder cancers. Urol Oncol. 2007;25(5):387–92.

26. Argyropoulos C, Wang K, McClarty S, Huang D, Bernardo J, Ellis D, et al. Urinary microRNA profiling in the nephropathy of type 1 diabetes. PLoS One. 2013;8(1):e54662.

27. Ramachandran K, Saikumar J, Bijol V, Koyner JL, Qian J, Betensky RA, et al. Human miRNome profiling identifies microRNAs differentially present in the urine after kidney injury. Clin Chem. 2013;59(12):1742–52.

28. Luo Y, Wang C, Chen X, Zhong T, Cai X, Chen S, et al. Increased serum and urinary microRNAs in children with idiopathic nephrotic syndrome. Clin Chem. 2013;59(4):658–66.

29. Wang G, Kwan BC, Lai FM, Chow KM, Li PK, Szeto CC. Urinary miR-21, miR-29, and miR-93: novel biomarkers of fibrosis. Am J Nephrol. 2012;36(5):412–8.

30. Szeto CC, Ching-Ha KB, Ka-Bik L, Mac-Moune LF, Cheung-Lung CP, Gang W, et al. Micro-RNA expression in the urinary sediment of patients with chronic kidney diseases. Dis Markers. 2012;33(3):137–44.

31. Maluf DG, Dumur CI, Suh JL, Scian MJ, King AL, Cathro H, et al. The urine microRNA profile may help monitor post-transplant renal graft function. Kidney Int. 2014;85(2):439–49.

32. Rossing K, Mischak H, Rossing P, Schanstra JP, Wiseman A, Maahs DM. The urinary proteome in diabetes and diabetes-associated complications: new ways to assess disease progression and evaluate therapy. Proteomics Clin Appl. 2008;2(7–8):997–1007.

33. Winnike JH, Busby MG, Watkins PB, O'Connell TM. Effects of a prolonged standardized diet on normalizing the human metabolome. Am J Clin Nutr. 2009;90(6):1496–501.

34. Heinzmann SS, Merrifield CA, Rezzi S, Kochhar S, Lindon JC, Holmes E, et al. Stability and robustness of human metabolic phenotypes in response to sequential food challenges. J Proteome Res. 2012;11(2):643–55.

35. Dunn WB, Broadhurst D, Begley P, Zelena E, Francis-McIntyre S, Anderson N, et al. Procedures for large-scale metabolic profiling of serum and plasma using gas chromatography and liquid chromatography coupled to mass spectrometry. Nat Protoc. 2011;6(7):1060–83.

36. Wishart DS, Knox C, Guo AC, Eisner R, Young N, Gautam B, et al. HMDB: a knowledgebase for the human metabolome. Nucleic Acids Res. 2009;37(Database issue):D603–10.

37. Zelena E, Dunn WB, Broadhurst D, Francis-McIntyre S, Carroll KM, Begley P, et al. Development of a robust and repeatable UPLC-MS method for the long-term metabolomic study of human serum. Anal Chem. 2009;81(4):1357–64.

38. Begley P, Francis-McIntyre S, Dunn WB, Broadhurst DI, Halsall A, Tseng A, et al. Development and performance of a gas chromatography-time-of-flight mass spectrometry analysis for large-scale nontargeted metabolomic studies of human serum. Anal Chem. 2009;81(16):7038–46.

39. Gronwald W, Klein MS, Zeltner R, Schulze BD, Reinhold SW, Deutschmann M, et al. Detection of autosomal dominant polycystic kidney disease by NMR spectroscopic fingerprinting of urine. Kidney Int. 2011;79(11):1244–53.

40. Beger RD, Holland RD, Sun J, Schnackenberg LK, Moore PC, Dent CL, et al. Metabonomics of acute kidney injury in children after cardiac surgery. Pediatr Nephrol. 2008;23(6):977–84.

41. Niewczas MA, Sirich TL, Mathew AV, Skupien J, Mohney RP, Warram JH, et al. Uremic solutes and risk of end-stage renal disease in type 2 diabetes: metabolomic study. Kidney Int. 2014;85(5):1214–24.

42. Costa FF. Big data in biomedicine. Drug Discov Today. 2014;19:433–40.

43. Alaiya A, Al-Mohanna M, Linder S. Clinical cancer proteomics: promises and pitfalls. J Proteome Res. 2005;4(4):1213–22.

44. Mischak H, Allmaier G, Apweiler R, Attwood T, Baumann M, Benigni A, et al. Recommendations for biomarker identification and qualification in clinical proteomics. Sci Transl Med. 2010;2(46):46ps2.

45. Mischak H, Ioannidis JP, Argiles A, Attwood TK, Bongcam-Rudloff E, Broenstrup M, et al. Implementation of proteomic biomarkers: making it work. Eur J Clin Invest. 2012;42(9):1027–36.

46. Mayer G, Heinze G, Mischak H, Hellemons ME, Heerspink HJ, Bakker SJ, et al. Omics-bioinformatics in the context of clinical data. Methods Mol Biol. 2011;719:479–97.

47. Dunkler D, Sanchez-Cabo F, Heinze G. Statistical analysis principles for Omics data. Methods Mol Biol. 2011;719:113–31.

48. Avent ND, Plummer ZE, Madgett TE, Maddocks DG, Soothill PW. Post-genomics studies and their application to non-invasive prenatal diagnosis. Semin Fetal Neonatal Med. 2008;13(2):91–8.

49. Kolch W, Neususs C, Pelzing M, Mischak H. Capillary electrophoresis-mass spectrometry as a powerful tool in clinical diagnosis and biomarker discovery. Mass Spectrom Rev. 2005;24(6):959–77.

50. Metzger J, Luppa PB, Good DM, Mischak H. Adapting mass spectrometry-based platforms for clinical proteomics applications: the capillary electrophoresis coupled mass spectrometry paradigm. Crit Rev Clin Lab Sci. 2009;46(3):129–52.

51. Shen Y, Kim J, Strittmatter EF, Jacobs JM, Camp 2nd DG, Fang R, et al. Characterization of the human blood plasma proteome. Proteomics. 2005;5(15):4034–45.

52. Decramer S, Gonzalez de Peredo A, Breuil B, Mischak H, Monsarrat B, Bascands JL, et al. Urine in clinical proteomics. Mol Cell Proteomics. 2008;7(10):1850–62.

53. Caubet C, Lacroix C, Decramer S, Drube J, Ehrich JH, Mischak H, et al. Advances in urinary proteome analysis and biomarker discovery in pediatric renal disease. Pediatr Nephrol. 2010;25(1):27–35.

54. Thongboonkerd V, Malasit P. Renal and urinary proteomics: current applications and challenges. Proteomics. 2005;5(4):1033–42.

55. Metzger J, Negm AA, Plentz RR, Weismuller TJ, Wedemeyer J, Karlsen TH, et al. Urine proteomic analysis differentiates cholangiocarcinoma from primary sclerosing cholangitis and other benign biliary disorders. Gut. 2013;62(1):122–30.

56. Weissinger EM, Metzger J, Dobbelstein C, Wolff D, Schleuning M, Kuzmina Z, et al. Proteomic peptide profiling for preemptive diagnosis of acute graft-versus-host disease after allogeneic stem cell transplantation. Leukemia. 2014;28(4):842–52.

57. Delles C, Schiffer E, von Zur Muhlen C, Peter K, Rossing P, Parving HH, et al. Urinary proteomic diagnosis of coronary artery disease: identification and clinical validation in 623 individuals. J Hypertens. 2010;28(11):2316–22.

58. Kentsis A, Shulman A, Ahmed S, Brennan E, Monuteaux MC, Lee YH, et al. Urine proteomics for discovery of improved diagnostic markers of Kawasaki disease. EMBO Mol Med. 2013;5(2):210–20.

59. Schiffer E, Mischak H, Novak J. High resolution proteome/peptidome analysis of body fluids by capillary electrophoresis coupled with MS. Proteomics. 2006;6(20):5615–27.

60. Pisitkun T, Shen RF, Knepper MA. Identification and proteomic profiling of exosomes in human urine. Proc Natl Acad Sci U S A. 2004;101(36):13368–73.

61. Zhou H, Yuen PS, Pisitkun T, Gonzales PA, Yasuda H, Dear JW, et al. Collection, storage, preservation, and normalization of human urinary exosomes for biomarker discovery. Kidney Int. 2006;69(8):1471–6.

62. Conde-Vancells J, Rodriguez-Suarez E, Gonzalez E, Berisa A, Gil D, Embade N, et al. Candidate biomarkers in exosome-like vesicles purified from rat and mouse urine samples. Proteomics Clin Appl. 2010;4(4):416–25.

63. Esteva-Font C, Wang X, Ars E, Guillen-Gomez E, Sans L, Gonzalez Saavedra I, et al. Are sodium transporters in urinary exosomes reliable markers of tubular sodium reabsorption in hypertensive patients? Nephron Physiol. 2010;114(3):25–34.

64. Zhou H, Cheruvanky A, Hu X, Matsumoto T, Hiramatsu N, Cho ME, et al. Urinary exosomal transcription factors, a new class of biomarkers for renal disease. Kidney Int. 2008;74(5):613–21.

65. Underwood MA, Gilbert WM, Sherman MP. Amniotic fluid: not just fetal urine anymore. J Perinatol. 2005;25(5):341–8.

66. Tsangaris GT, Anagnostopoulos AK, Tounta G, Antsaklis A, Mavrou A, Kolialexi A. Application of proteomics for the identification of biomarkers in amniotic fluid: are we ready to provide a reliable prediction? EPMA J. 2011;2(2):149–55.

67. Yates 3rd JR, Kelleher NL. Top down proteomics. Anal Chem. 2013;85(13):6151.

68. Petricoin EF, Ardekani AM, Hitt BA, Levine PJ, Fusaro VA, Steinberg SM, et al. Use of proteomic patterns in serum to identify ovarian cancer. Lancet. 2002;359(9306):572–7.

69. Check E. Proteomics and cancer: running before we can walk? Nature. 2004;429(6991):496–7.

70. Baggerly KA, Morris JS, Coombes KR. Reproducibility of SELDI-TOF protein patterns in serum: comparing datasets from different experiments. Bioinformatics. 2004;20(5):777–85.

71. Schaub S, Wilkins J, Weiler T, Sangster K, Rush D, Nickerson P. Urine protein profiling with surface-enhanced laser-desorption/ionization time-of-flight mass spectrometry. Kidney Int. 2004;65(1):323–32.

72. Neuhoff N, Kaiser T, Wittke S, Krebs R, Pitt A, Burchard A, et al. Mass spectrometry for the detection of differentially expressed proteins: a comparison of surface-enhanced laser desorption/ionization and capillary electrophoresis/mass spectrometry. Rapid Commun Mass Spectrom. 2004;18(2):149–56.

73. Rogers MA, Clarke P, Noble J, Munro NP, Paul A, Selby PJ, et al. Proteomic profiling of urinary proteins in renal cancer by surface enhanced laser desorption ionization and neural-network analysis: identification of key issues affecting potential clinical utility. Cancer Res. 2003;63(20):6971–83.

74. Albrethsen J, Bogebo R, Olsen J, Raskov H, Gammeltoft S. Preanalytical and analytical variation of surface-enhanced laser desorption-ionization time-of-flight mass spectrometry of human serum. Clin Chem Lab Med. 2006;44(10):1243–52.

75. Gaspar A, Englmann M, Fekete A, Harir M, Schmitt-Kopplin P. Trends in CE-MS 2005–2006. Electrophoresis. 2008;29(1):66–79.

76. Neususs C, Pelzing M, Macht M. A robust approach for the analysis of peptides in the low femtomole range by capillary electrophoresis-tandem mass spectrometry. Electrophoresis. 2002;23(18):3149–59.

77. Theodorescu D, Wittke S, Ross MM, Walden M, Conaway M, Just I, et al. Discovery and validation of new protein biomarkers for urothelial cancer: a prospective analysis. Lancet Oncol. 2006;7(3):230–40.

78. Decramer S, Wittke S, Mischak H, Zurbig P, Walden M, Bouissou F, et al. Predicting the clinical outcome of congenital unilateral ureteropelvic junction obstruction in newborn by urinary proteome analysis. Nat Med. 2006;12(4):398–400.

79. Kaiser T, Kamal H, Rank A, Kolb HJ, Holler E, Ganser A, et al. Proteomics applied to the clinical follow-up of patients after allogeneic hematopoietic stem cell transplantation. Blood. 2004;104(2):340–9.

80. Aebersold R, Mann M. Mass spectrometry-based proteomics. Nature. 2003;422(6928):198–207.

81. Issaq HJ, Conrads TP, Janini GM, Veenstra TD. Methods for fractionation, separation and profiling of proteins and peptides. Electrophoresis. 2002;23(17):3048–61.

82. Delahunty CM, Yates 3rd JR. MudPIT: multidimensional protein identification technology. Biotechniques. 2007;43(5):563, 5, 7 passim.

83. Gaspari M, Verhoeckx KC, Verheij ER, van der Greef J. Integration of two-dimensional LC-MS with multivariate statistics for comparative analysis of proteomic samples. Anal Chem. 2006;78(7):2286–96.

84. Chang CP, McDill BW, Neilson JR, Joist HE, Epstein JA, Crabtree GR, et al. Calcineurin is required in urinary tract mesenchyme for the development of the pyeloureteral peristaltic machinery. J Clin Invest. 2004;113(7):1051–8.

85. Klein J, Gonzalez J, Miravete M, Caubet C, Chaaya R, Decramer S, et al. Congenital ureteropelvic junction obstruction: human disease and animal models. Int J Exp Pathol. 2011;92(3):168–92.

86. Decramer S, Bascands JL, Schanstra JP. Non-invasive markers of ureteropelvic junction obstruction. World J Urol. 2007;25(5):457–65.

87. Decramer S, Zurbig P, Wittke S, Mischak H, Bascands JL, Schanstra JP. Identification of urinary biomarkers by proteomics in newborns: use in obstructive nephropathy. Contrib Nephrol. 2008;160:127–41.

88. Drube J, Zurbig P, Schiffer E, Lau E, Ure B, Gluer S, et al. Urinary proteome analysis identifies infants but not older children requiring pyeloplasty. Pediatr Nephrol. 2010;25(9):1673–8.

89. Mesrobian HG. The value of newborn urinary proteome analysis in the evaluation and management of ureteropelvic junction obstruction: a cost-effectiveness study. World J Urol. 2009;27(3):379–83.

90. Krishnan A, de Souza A, Konijeti R, Baskin LS. The anatomy and embryology of posterior urethral valves. J Urol. 2006;175(4):1214–20.

91. Smith JM, Stablein DM, Munoz R, Hebert D, McDonald RA. Contributions of the transplant registry: the 2006 annual report of the North American Pediatric Renal Trials and Collaborative Studies (NAPRTCS). Pediatr Transplant. 2007;11(4):366–73.

92. Drozdz D, Drozdz M, Gretz N, Mohring K, Mehls O, Scharer K. Progression to end-stage renal disease in children with posterior urethral valves. Pediatr Nephrol. 1998;12(8):630–6.

93. Parkhouse HF, Barratt TM, Dillon MJ, Duffy PG, Fay J, Ransley PG, et al. Long-term outcome of boys with posterior urethral valves. Br J Urol. 1988;62(1):59–62.

94. Lopez Pereira P, Espinosa L, Martinez Urrutina MJ, Lobato R, Navarro M, Jaureguizar E. Posterior urethral valves: prognostic factors. BJU Int. 2003;91(7):687–90.

95. de Bruyn R, Marks SD. Postnatal investigation of fetal renal disease. Semin Fetal Neonatal Med. 2008;13(3):133–41.

96. Morris RK, Quinlan-Jones E, Kilby MD, Khan KS. Systematic review of accuracy of fetal urine analysis to predict poor postnatal renal function in cases of congenital urinary tract obstruction. Prenat Diagn. 2007;27(10):900–11.

97. Morris RK, Malin GL, Khan KS, Kilby MD. Antenatal ultrasound to predict postnatal renal function in congenital lower urinary tract obstruction: systematic review of test accuracy. BJOG. 2009;116(10):1290–9.

98. Hogan J, Dourthe ME, Blondiaux E, Jouannic JM, Garel C, Ulinski T. Renal outcome in children with antenatal diagnosis of severe CAKUT. Pediatr Nephrol. 2012;27(3):497–502.

99. Klein J, Lacroix C, Caubet C, Siwy J, Zurbig P, Dakna M, et al. Fetal urinary peptides to predict postnatal outcome of renal disease in fetuses with Posterior Urethral Valves (PUV). Sci Transl Med. 2013;5(198):198ra06.

100. Lopez Pereira P, Martinez Urrutia MJ, Jaureguizar E. Initial and long-term management of posterior urethral valves. World J Urol. 2004;22(6):418–24.

101. Nasir AA, Ameh EA, Abdur-Rahman LO, Adeniran JO, Abraham MK. Posterior urethral valve. World J Pediatr. 2011;7(3):205–16.

102. Mischak H, Vlahou A, Ioannidis JP. Technical aspects and inter-laboratory variability in native peptide profiling: the CE-MS experience. Clin Biochem. 2013;46(6):432–43.

103. Huttenhain R, Soste M, Selevsek N, Rost H, Sethi A, Carapito C, et al. Reproducible quantification of cancer-associated proteins in body fluids using targeted proteomics. Sci Transl Med. 2012;4(142):142ra94.

104. Addona TA, Abbatiello SE, Schilling B, Skates SJ, Mani DR, Bunk DM, et al. Multi-site assessment of the precision and reproducibility of multiple reaction monitoring-based measurements of proteins in plasma. Nat Biotechnol. 2009;27(7):633–41.

105. Agger SA, Marney LC, Hoofnagle AN. Simultaneous quantification of apolipoprotein A-I and apolipoprotein B by liquid-chromatography-multiple- reaction-monitoring mass spectrometry. Clin Chem. 2010;56(12):1804–13.

106. Gold L, Ayers D, Bertino J, Bock C, Bock A, Brody EN, et al. Aptamer-based multiplexed proteomic technology for biomarker discovery. PLoS One. 2010;5(12):e15004.

107. Springer A, Kratochwill K, Bergmeister H, Csaicsich D, Huber J, Bilban M, et al. A combined transcriptome and bioinformatics approach to

unilateral ureteral obstructive uropathy in the fetal sheep model. J Urol. 2012;187(2):751–6.

108. Perco P, Muhlberger I, Mayer G, Oberbauer R, Lukas A, Mayer B. Linking transcriptomic and proteomic data on the level of protein interaction networks. Electrophoresis. 2010;31(11):1780–9.

109. Klein J, Jupp S, Moulos P, Fernandez M, Buffin-Meyer B, Casemayou A, et al. The KUPKB: a novel Web application to access multiomics data on kidney disease. FASEB J. 2012;26(5):2145–53.

110. Moulos P, Klein J, Jupp S, Stevens R, Bascands JL, Schanstra JP. The KUPNetViz: a biological network viewer for multiple -omics datasets in kidney diseases. BMC Bioinformatics. 2013;14:235.

111. Subramanian A, Tamayo P, Mootha VK, Mukherjee S, Ebert BL, Gillette MA, et al. Gene set enrichment analysis: a knowledge-based approach for interpreting genome-wide expression profiles. Proc Natl Acad Sci U S A. 2005;102(43):15545–50.

112. da Huang W, Sherman BT, Lempicki RA. Systematic and integrative analysis of large gene lists using DAVID bioinformatics resources. Nat Protoc. 2009;4(1):44–57.

113. Tonelli M, Sacks F, Pfeffer M, Jhangri GS, Curhan G, Cholesterol and Recurrent Events (CARE) Trial Investigator, et al. Biomarkers of inflammation and progression of chronic kidney disease. Kidney Int. 2005;68(1):237–45.

114. He JC, Chuang PY, Ma'ayan A, Iyengar R. Systems biology of kidney diseases. Kidney Int. 2012;81(1):22–39.

115. Keller BJ, Martini S, Sedor JR, Kretzler M. A systems view of genetics in chronic kidney disease. Kidney Int. 2012;81(1):14–21.

116. Fechete R, Heinzel A, Perco P, Monks K, Sollner J, Stelzer G, et al. Mapping of molecular pathways, biomarkers and drug targets for diabetic nephropathy. Proteomics Clin Appl. 2011;5(5–6): 354–66.

117. Mischak H, Schanstra JP. CE-MS in biomarker discovery, validation, and clinical application. Proteomics Clin Appl. 2011;5(1–2):9–23.

Approaches to Clinical Research in Pediatric Nephrology

Anja Sander and Scott M. Sutherland

Introduction

"Pediatric nephrology is a discipline in serious need of high-quality clinical research. Despite the fact that many sound clinical studies have been conducted in the pediatric kidney disease population […], our understanding of many childhood kidney diseases remains limited. In addition, many of the treatments offered to children with kidney disease are supported either only by weak evidence in the pediatric population or by evidence of variable quality in adult populations" [1].

In this chapter we will address research opportunities helpful on the way to evidence based medicine and focus on how to conduct meaningful clinical studies, referring especially to problems in this patient population.

A. Sander (✉)
Institute of Medical Biometry
and Informatics,
University of Heidelberg,
Im Neuenheimer Feld 130.3, Heidelberg 69121,
Germany
e-mail: sander@imbi.uni-heidelberg.de

S.M. Sutherland
Department of Pediatrics,
Division of Pediatric Nephrology,
Lucile Packard Children's Hospital, Stanford
University, 300 Pasteur Drive, Rm G-306,
Stanford, CA 94304, USA
e-mail: suthersm@standford.edu

Evidence Based Medicine

Clinical decision-making has undergone dramatic changes in the past few decades. Once considered an "art" based on personal experience and intuition, the inflationary increase of clinical research activities and accessibility of information in the digital age increasingly allows clinicians to make decisions based on scientific evidence. This requires a meaningful filtration and judgment of available information to decide and act on. In this context, "evidence based medicine is the conscientious, explicit, and judicious use of current best evidence in making decisions about the care of individual patients" [2]. This implies to integrate individual clinical expertise with the best available external evidence considering preferences of the patient/patients' choice. External evidence means clinically relevant research for the present question.

Hierarchies of evidence are usually ordered as follows [3, 4]:

- Systematic review of Randomized Controlled Trials (RCTs)
- Individual RCT of high quality
- Systematic review of observational studies
- Individual observational study and low quality RCT
- Systematic review of case-control studies
- Individual case-control study
- Case series (and poor-quality cohort and case-control studies)
- Opinion of experts in the field

© Springer-Verlag Berlin Heidelberg 2016
D.F. Geary, F. Schaefer (eds.), *Pediatric Kidney Disease*, DOI 10.1007/978-3-662-52972-0_7

Well-planned and well-conducted controlled clinical trials, randomized and blinded if possible, are the most reliable way to obtain unbiased estimations of treatment effects. Together with systematic reviews of several such randomized trials they are the *gold standard* for evaluating the effect of treatments. However, evidently some therapeutic issues do not require or justify randomized trials (e.g., successful interventions for otherwise fatal conditions) or cannot wait for the trial to be conducted. In such cases, "we must follow the trial to the next best external evidence and work from there" [2].

In some circumstances the conduct of sufficiently powered clinical studies is challenging, e.g., in rare diseases. Some approaches for improving the power and increasing the feasibility of a study are mentioned in the section "Clinical Trials in pediatric populations."

EBM Approaches in Nephrology

Several approaches have been undertaken to systematically review medical evidence and establish clinical practice guidelines according to EBM principles in nephrology. The Cochrane Consortium comprises a Renal Review Group that has completed an impressive number of 49 systematic reviews under the category "Child health – Kidney disease" (status as of March 2015). The topics include chronic kidney disease (n=17) and end-stage kidney disease (n=7), urinary tract infection (n=8 and urology (n=4), acute kidney injury (n=5), kidney transplant (n=5), and drugs and the kidney (n=3) [5].

In the US, the National Kidney Foundation Kidney Disease Outcomes Quality Initiative (NKF KDOQI) has provided evidence-based guidelines for all stages of chronic kidney disease and related complications since 1997 [6]. EBM criteria were stringently applied in the development of the guidelines, which comprise the following topics: anemia, bone metabolism, diabetes, hypertension and nutrition in chronic kidney disease, hemodialysis and peritoneal dialysis adequacy, vascular access, and cardiovascular disease in dialysis patients. While most guidelines contain pediatric

sections, specific pediatric guidelines were released for nutrition and CKD-associated mineral and bone disease (CKD-MBD).

Encouraged by the wide adoption of the KDOQI guidelines, the International Society of Nephrology launched the "Kidney Disease – Improving global Outcomes (KDIGO)" initiative [7]. The KDIGO Board invites experts from around the globe to develop evidence-based clinical practice guidelines. To date, guidelines on acute kidney injury, CKD evaluation and management, CKD-MBD, anemia, blood pressure, lipids, and hepatitis C in CKD, care of kidney transplant recipients, and glomerulonephritis have been developed and published.

Study Types in Medical Research

Epidemiological Studies

Cross-Sectional Studies
Cross-sectional studies are like snapshots in time. Data on exposure, outcome, and covariates are collected at a defined time point for a specified (patient) population. This study design is suitable for estimation of prevalences and examination of chronic diseases and prolonged exposures. Relative frequencies can be assessed; however, incidence estimation is not possible. While cross-sectional studies can be used to generate research hypotheses, causality inferences with regards to risk factors and treatment effects cannot be made. Cross-sectional studies are not suitable to evaluate rare diseases or rare events.

Cohort Studies
In a cohort study a group of individuals is followed over time with the purpose of observing an outcome of interest and identifying risk factors. This study type is observational and longitudinal. While data on exposures and covariates can be collected prospectively or retrospectively, the follow-up phase, sometimes over years or decades, is always prospective. Cohort studies allow estimation of incidences. This study design is suitable for examination of rare exposures, but not for evaluation of rare outcomes or rare diseases.

Case-Control Studies

In contrast to cohort studies where subjects are observed before an outcome of interest has occurred, in case-control studies individuals with an outcome of interest (cases) are compared with subjects who do not (yet) show this outcome (controls). Exposure data are collected retrospectively. The aim is the identification of risk factors for becoming a "case," i.e., developing an outcome of interest. The selection of cases and controls should be conducted based on pre-specified criteria. To achieve comparable groups, cases and controls are usually matched for important covariates such as age, sex or renal function. Nonetheless, this study design is prone to selection bias.

Case-control studies are especially suitable for research in rare diseases. However, estimation of incidences is not possible and the chronology of exposures and outcomes often remains unclear.

Systematic Reviews and Meta-Analyses

In systematic reviews all literature relevant to a research question is objectively summarized to give an overview of existing evidence. In contrast to a systematic review, a simple review is not based on an exhaustive literature search and can comprise subjective opinions of the authors. In either case results from different studies were summarized only qualitatively. A systematic review can contain a meta-analysis, which quantitatively combines results from similar studies using statistical methods. After a comprehensive literature search data from comparable studies are pooled to get a combined estimate of the treatment effect with improved precision in comparison to the single studies. For this purpose, individual patient data can be used, if available, or summary measures. A distinction is made between systematic reviews based on RCTs and those based on observational studies. The Cochrane Collaboration is a valuable source of high-quality systematic reviews and meta-analyses. An overview of recent Cochrane reviews in the field of pediatric nephrology is given in Table 7.1.

Clinical Trials

Clinical trials are defined as "any form of *planned experiment* which involves patients and is designed to elucidate the most appropriate treatment of future patients with a given medical condition" [8]. In this context the term "trial" is equivalent to "study." This can be both interventional/experimental and non-interventional/observational studies. Based on a sample of patients a generalization for the respective population should be derived.

On the way to drug approval a new drug has to be evaluated in a series of trials. Usually, this process can be divided into four phases. In *phase I* the drug is, after preclinical testing, firstly examined in humans, often using healthy volunteers. Exceptions are oncology trials which often include patients since treatments commonly cause severe side effects. Primary objectives are the pharmacokinetic and pharmacodynamic description of the drug and determination of acceptable dosage through dose escalation. The first description of efficacy and further evaluation of pharmacology, side effects, and dose-effect relationship is undertaken in *phase II* in a limited number of patients. Subsequently, *Phase III* trial programs are aimed to provide definitive proof of efficacy, most relevant for regulatory drug approval. Here, the investigated drug is compared with placebo or standard treatment, if existing, in a rigorous setting including a sufficiently large number of patients to demonstrate efficacy and assess tolerance. An example of a *phase III* trial is the ESCAPE trial, in which the effect of intensified vs. conventional blood pressure control on progression of renal disease in children with chronic kidney disease was assessed [9]. Another example is the randomized, placebo-controlled, double-blind RIVUR trial, which evaluated the effect of antimicrobial metaphylaxis in children with vesicoureteral reflux after urinary tract infection [10].

After *phase III* trials have provided proof of efficacy and global safety with subsequent marketing approval, the clinical experience with newly approved drugs is further monitored to provide more detailed long-term safety informa-

Table 7.1 Overview on recent Cochran reviews in the field of pediatric nephrology

Study title	Year (update)	Number of included studies	Number of patients	Children only	Children and adults
Procalcitonin, C-reactive protein, and erythrocyte sedimentation rate for the diagnosis of acute pyelonephritis in children	2015	24	4622	x	
Antibiotics for acute pyelonephritis in children	2014	27	4452	x	
Interventions for covert bacteriuria in children	2012	3	460	x	
Long-term antibiotics for preventing recurrent urinary tract infection in children	2011	12	1557	x	
Short versus standard duration oral antibiotic therapy for acute urinary tract infection in children	2003	10	652	x	
Modes of administration of antibiotics for symptomatic severe urinary tract infections	2007	15	1743		x
One dose per day compared to multiple doses per day of gentamicin for treatment of suspected or proven sepsis in neonates	2011	11	574	x	
Interventions for primary vesicoureteric reflux	2011	20	2324	x	
Corticosteroid therapy for nephrotic syndrome in children	2015	34	3033	x	
Interventions for idiopathic steroid-resistant nephrotic syndrome in children	2010	14	449	x	
Lipid-lowering agents for nephrotic syndrome	2013	5	203		x
Interventions for preventing and treating kidney disease in Henoch-Schönlein Purpura (HSP)	2009	11	1230	x	
Treatment for lupus nephritis	2012	50	2846		x
Non-immunosuppressive treatment for IgA nephropathy	2011	56	2838		x
Protein restriction for children with chronic kidney disease	2007	2	250	x	
Oral protein calorie supplementation for children with chronic disease	1999	3	135	x	
Parenteral versus oral iron therapy for adults and children with chronic kidney disease	2012	28	2098		x
Interventions for bone disease in children with chronic kidney disease	2010	15	369	x	
Vitamin D compounds for people with chronic kidney disease requiring dialysis	2009	60	2773		x
Growth hormone for children with chronic kidney disease	2012	16	809	x	
Treatment for peritoneal dialysis-associated peritonitis	2014	42	2433		x
Biocompatible dialysis fluids for peritoneal dialysis	2014	36	2719		x
Steroid avoidance or withdrawal for kidney transplant recipients	2009	30	5949		x
Pharmacological interventions for hypertension in children	2014	21	3454	x	

tion. *Phase IV* trials, so-called *postmarketing surveillance trials*, are long-term studies aimed to rule out or detect rare side effects, evaluate effects on morbidity and mortality, and assess the interaction with other factors.

This classification can also be related to other treatments than drugs, like surgical interventions, physiotherapy, or psychological treatments.

Study Protocol

Besides aspects of preparation and organization of a study, the objectives, design, methods, and statistical considerations (e.g., sample size, analysis) should be described in advance in this document. The SPIRIT 2013 statement (Standard Protocol Items: Recommendations for Interventional Trials) provides a summary of the content of a good study protocol which can be used as guidance [11, 12].

Patient Population

The patient population included into a study should be as representative as possible of the population which the treatment is intended for. This is essential for the external validity of the study results and should be considered carefully when defining the inclusion and exclusion criteria.

Control Group

Investigators are often biased towards treating all future patients with a new therapy and may avoid randomization out of the belief that the new treatment is better or in order to collect more information on the new therapy from a given population size. However, in single-arm trials patient selection can be influenced intentionally in a way to increase the chance of showing preferable outcomes under the new therapy, e.g., by selecting less ill patients. Hence, including a control group is essential to prove efficacy and safety of a new treatment and to account for placebo effects or spontaneous improvements [13]. Hence, the prospective randomized control group design is considered as gold standard. Subjects in the control group will receive either standard treatment or, in case no standard therapy exists, placebo or no treatment. Alternatively, patients treated in the

past or recruited for other studies can serve as "historical" or "external" controls. However, inclusion of such controls retains the risk of introducing bias through patient selection, differences in patient care and variation of observation quality [8].

Methods to Prevent Bias

There are various sources of systematic bias(es) when estimating treatment effects in clinical trials, which can be reduced or eliminated by trial design and other methods. In the following we describe some of these approaches and provide illustrations by clinical trial examples.

Screening

The selection of subjects for a study is a major potential source of bias ("selection bias"). Systematic collection of basic data of all screened patients is helpful to ensure transparency of the recruitment process since the representativity of the study participants can be assessed. Pseudonymized documentation of the criteria resulting in trial ineligibility and recording of the number of patients not willing to participate is an essential component of the screening procedure.

Randomization

If the primary objective of a study is the comparison of different treatments, the groups must be as similar as possible aside from the study treatments given. This includes known influencing factors (confounders) but also unknown factors which cannot be accounted for in the statistical analysis. Prospective random assignment of subjects to study arms is the most important design method for reduction of biases [14]. Centralized randomization is recommended in multicentre trials to rule out any local influence on treatment allocation. Central randomization is usually conducted via fax, telephone or Web-based systems.

In trials with small population sizes – as is usually the case in pediatric nephrology – important prognostic factors impacting on treatment success can be unequally distributed in the study population despite proper randomization. In some situations even small differences in the composition of the comparator groups can lead to false-negative or false-positive trial results. To avoid such imbalances, stratified randomization can be performed by separating the study population according to important prognostic factors and randomizing the subgroups separately.

Blinding

Expectations from physicians, patients and study nurses regarding the allocated treatment can influence outcomes, consciously or unconsciously, resulting in bias concerning the observed treatment effects [15]. Equality of care and reporting of unbiased outcome data can be guaranteed through blinding of as many involved parties as possible. In medication studies placebo tablets or saline solution can be administered to the control and/or experimental group to enable blinding. In trials with a double-blind design neither the physician nor the patient knows which treatment the patient is assigned to. Double-blind study designs are desirable but not always possible, e.g., when comparing a surgical with a pharmacological therapy. A single-blind design involves blinding of only the patient or the physician. If neither the patient nor the physician is blinded the study is called open. Beyond that, a study can be conducted observer-blind, which means that an external observer is not aware of the treatment group when assessing the study endpoints.

Concealment of Allocation

When conducting an open or single-blind randomized trial, patients and/or physicians could be tempted to wait until the group the patient is randomized to has been determined, and then decide whether the patient participates in the study. To avoid such selection bias, randomization should be performed after informed consent has been given and the allocation result has to be documented unchangeably.

A recent meta-analysis of 34 trials on corticosteroid therapy for nephrotic syndrome in children illustrates the spectrum of methodological issues of clinical research in pediatric nephrology [16]. Only half of the studies were rated as at low risk for selection bias; in four studies group allocation was performed by alternation, which

allows for manipulation and therefore high risk of selection bias. Twenty-seven of the 34 studies were categorized as at high risk for performance bias since they were conducted in an open fashion or blinding was not mentioned. Twenty-six studies were additionally graded as at high risk for detection bias, i.e., bias in assessing outcome data, only in six studies blinding was maintained throughout the trial.

Choice of Outcomes of Interest

In a clinical trial, efficacy is evaluated based on a pre-defined primary endpoint which reflects the therapeutic effect. The variable serving as primary endpoint should be reliable, validated and, especially in Phase III trials, clinically relevant [17]. When an outcome of primary interest occurs only after an extended observation period, as is commonly the case for outcomes like death or cardiovascular events, or when the outcome is difficult or expensive to measure, a surrogate endpoint can be chosen. The use of an outcome as surrogate is only acceptable after validation and showing high correlation between the surrogate and the outcome of primary interest [18]. For example, in pharmacological nephroprotection trials there is an ongoing discussion whether short-term changes in proteinuria can be used as a surrogate for long-term kidney survival [19]. Likewise, it is controversial whether the rate of change in glomerular filtration rate can serve as a surrogate for time to end-stage renal disease [20]. Often several outcomes are combined to a composite endpoint to increase the likelihood of observing an event [21]. As an example, a composite endpoint could be time to renal failure as defined by 50 % eGFR loss or progression to end-stage renal disease, as used in the ESCAPE study [9]. This approach is applicable in a meaningful way only when accepting the assumption that the individual endpoints are of similar clinical importance and the effects on the single components are in the same direction.

Other endpoints of interest for analysis of further objectives of the study are defined as secondary endpoints and analysed for descriptive purposes.

Definition of Analysis Populations

Generally, in a clinical trial different analysis sets are defined. Depending on the type of primary hypotheses tested the primary analysis should be based either on the intention-to-treat population (ITT) or the per-protocol population (PP). The ITT population comprises all patients allocated to the study regardless of the kind and amount of treatment they actually received. In this way the comparability regarding known and unknown confounders as achieved by randomization will be maintained. When evaluating a superiority hypothesis, the ITT population should be the primary analysis set as recommended by the International Conference on Harmonisation Guideline [17]. Deviations to the protocol can result in more similar effects in the different groups and make it more difficult to show existing treatment effects. Additionally this approach better reflects "real world usage". In contrast, the PP population consists of all patients treated as defined in the study protocol without major protocol violations. In superiority trials the PP population is used for sensitivity analysis. In non-inferiority trials both analysis sets have equal importance [22]. The results of the study are most persuasive if both analyses lead to the same conclusion.

In addition, for analysis of safety aspects a "safety population" is defined, which usually contains all patients who received at least one dose of study medication. These patients are analysed in the group they were treated with.

Statistical Analysis

Statistical Analysis Plan

In confirmatory phase III trials the statistical analysis is usually described in detail in a Statistical Analysis Plan (SAP) after finalization of study protocol. This ensures that data-driven hypothesis testing is avoided and type I error is controlled. A pre-defined Statistical Analysis Plan is also recommended for observational studies as it increases the stringency of data analysis [23].

Type I and Type II Error

For statistical proof of treatment effects significance tests are often applied. In the planning phase a so called null hypothesis and an alternative hypothesis have to be defined. The null hypothesis (denoted H_0) states the event space which should be rejected, e.g., the treatment effects are equal and no difference between the groups exists. The alternative (denoted H_A) contains the contrary event space, e.g., the treatment effects are unequal and there is a difference between the groups. Even if the aim is to show that an experimental treatment is superior to a standard treatment the hypotheses should be formulated two-sided, leaving statistical analysis open for differences in both directions. Only in special situations one-sided testing is indicated [24].

Decisions based on statistical tests are associated with uncertainty. There is the risk to falsely reject the null hypothesis when in fact there is no difference between the groups (Type I error), and the risk that the null hypothesis has to be maintained when in fact the alternative is true (Type II error). The probability of making a Type I error is controlled through the predefined significance level α, commonly set to 5 %. The result of a statistical test, the p-value, is compared with this significance level to decide whether the observed treatment difference is consistent with the null hypothesis or not.

Particularly type II error issues are frequently encountered in studies of pediatric kidney diseases, where enrolment is notoriously difficult and endpoints often take long time to occur. An illustrative example of design-related enrolment issues impacting on trial power is the PLUTO trial in fetuses with lower urinary tract obstruction [25]. The trial aimed to compare the postnatal outcome of fetuses undergoing prenatal vesicoamniotic stenting vs no treatment and was powered to yield a clinically relevant result with enrolment of 75 subjects per arm. Unfortunately, many investigators and parents, when forced to make a rapid decision in an emotionally stressful situation, tended to opt for either interruption of pregnancy (n = 68) or entering a registry rather undergoing randomized treatment (n = 45). As a result, within 4 years only 31 cases were randomized in 7 of 21 participating centers. Of these, two cases randomized for conservative treatment still received a stent later on and three decided for termination of pregnancy after enrolment. The ITT analysis yielded a non-significant difference between the trial arms but was grossly underpowered to find a difference, which is even more unfortunate as the per-protocol analysis actually suggested a benefit of the intervention at borderline significance. Hence, the clinical benefit of a potentially useful intervention could not be ascertained despite a large multi-center effort due unsurmountable enrolment difficulties.

A successful example for a solution to a type II error problem is the ESCAPE trial. A trend towards improved preservation of kidney function by intensified blood pressure control was apparent at the end of the 3-year observation period which, however, did not reach significance. The investigators decided to extend the study period and indeed were able to demonstrate a significant benefit of the intervention (35 % risk reduction) after 5 years [9].

Statistical significance does not necessarily imply clinical relevance. Increasing sample size may result in small *p*-values even when the effect is relatively small and clinically irrelevant. Clinical relevance cannot be derived from statistical significance, whereas an existing difference can be overlooked by evaluating only a small study population. To avoid missing a true effect the probability of making a type II error, called β, has to be controlled for. Through sample size calculation it can be assured that the study has a predefined power 1- β to detect a truly existing effect given the assumptions hold true. The probability of not showing a difference when in fact it exists is often set to 20 or 10 %, which corresponds to a power of 80 and 90 % respectively.

Types of Statistical Hypotheses

In *superiority trials* the aim is to demonstrate a difference in treatment effects between two or more groups. A non-significant result cannot be interpreted as equality in treatment efficacy. In some instances one assumes a priori that an experimental treatment has a similar or clinically irrelevant smaller effect than standard treatment but provides advantages regarding other aspects such as fewer side effects. In these cases the objective is to show *non-inferiority*. The corresponding alternative hypothesis is formulated as the effect in the experimental group not being smaller than the effect in the control group minus a predefined non-inferiority margin defining the maximal acceptable amount of inferiority rated as clinically irrelevant. In non-inferiority trials the aim and the corresponding hypotheses require testing in a pre-specified direction, therefore one-sided testing is performed. For proof of *equivalence* two one-sided tests are necessary to demonstrate that treatment effects are, to some amount, equal. The interested reader is referred to [26, 27].

Endpoints

Mainly there are three different types of variables focused on in clinical studies. *Qualitative* outcomes classify each patient into one of several predefined categories. The simplest case is two categories, leading to a binary outcome, e.g., events like switch to dialysis. CKD stage is an example of a categorical variable. When a *quantitative* measure comes into consideration, like eGFR, it is usually preferable to use it as a continuous outcome rather than to dichotomize it into a qualitative outcome (e.g., eGFR <30 vs. ≥30) due to the higher statistical power of using information from continuous variables. In this way, smaller sample sizes are needed to reach the same statistical power [28].

Descriptive Analysis

Data analysis starts with a statistical description of the study population(s). Qualitative measures should be described by absolute and relative frequencies, and continuous measures by mean and standard deviation or, in case of non-normal data distribution, by median and inter quartile range, i.e., the difference from the 25th to the 75th distribution percentile. Time-to-event outcomes are often not normally distributed. In this case it is meaningful to state median survival times and x-year survival rates.

Statistical Testing

To adequately control the type I error, i.e., erroneous rejection of the null hypothesis, only one primary endpoint should preferentially be defined and analysed statistically [17]. Testing more than one endpoint has to be handled adequately to avoid inflating the type I error and must be considered in sample size calculation. Secondary outcomes are described and interpreted only in an exploratory way.

A wide range of statistical tests exists with different areas of application. On the one hand the choice depends on the level of measurement of the endpoint. For example, some tests require that the data are normally distributed. When this assumption is not reasonable, non-parametric tests can be applied which do not assume a specific underlying distribution of the data. However, the Student's t-test for comparison of two independent groups, applicable to continuous data, has been shown to be robust against deviations from the normal distribution for sample sizes <30 [29].

Often treatments are compared between independent groups of patients. Repeated measurements in the same patient typically obtained before and after an intervention, are dependent or "paired." This is also the case in groups with pairs regarding certain attributes as encountered in matched case-control studies. Such paired data require application of specific statistical tests. A list of common statistical tests is provided in Table 7.2. A more comprehensive overview can be found in [31].

Confidence Intervals

Significance tests do not provide information on how much better a treatment is in comparison to another. Confidence intervals are a useful method to quantitate treatment differences and therefore are more informative than significance tests and p-values alone. The confidence interval is reported commonly at the 90 or 95 % confidence level; this interval covers the true but unknown treatment difference which is just a point estimator with the respective probability.

Time-to-Event Analysis

When considering time-to-event endpoints, such as time to renal failure or time to recurrence of nephrotic syndrome, methods of survival analysis are useful. The individual time interval from the start of observation to a certain event is the basis of event time analysis, most commonly visualized using Kaplan-Meier (KM) graphs [32, 33]. Subjects who have been lost to follow up without

Table 7.2 Commonly used statistical tests

Statistical test	Description
Chi-square test	Comparison of binary data in two or more independent groups. Also applicable for categorical endpoints with more than two categories
McNemar test	Comparison of binary data but for two paired samples
Student's t-test	Comparison of means of two samples with the assumption of normally distributed data. Variants for unpaired and paired data
Analysis of variance (ANOVA)	Overall comparison of means for more than two groups
Wilcoxon's rank sum test	Non-parametric alternative to Student's t-test. Also known as the Mann-Whitney U test
Kruskal-Wallis test	Extension of the Wilcoxon's rank sum test for overall comparison of more than two unpaired groups
Friedman test	Non-parametric test for comparing more than two paired samples
Log rank test	Non-parametric test for comparing survival distributions of two or more independent groups

Used with permission from du Prel et al. [30]

reaching the study endpoint are still informative in KM survival analysis as their last observation is included as "censored." Since it is not known what will happen to such patients after the last contact this procedure is called right-censoring. Other forms of censoring, not further discussed here, are left-censoring or interval-censoring. An example of a Kaplan Meier survival analysis is shown in Fig. 7.1 [34]. Survival curves of individual treatment groups can be compared statistically using the log rank test [35, 36], which compares the number of patients per group who experienced an event at each event time, taking into account the patients at risk. Stratified analysis can be performed to account for the presence of known prognostic factors. Multivariable methods such as Cox regression are available if the effect of several prognostic factors on the event time are to be checked simultaneously. Using the Cox model, the treatment effect on survival time is estimated, adjusted for the prognostic factors.

From the regression coefficients hazard ratios are estimated, which indicate the relative increase or decrease of risk of an event with respect to a prognostic factor compared to its reference expression [37].

Dealing with Missing Values

Missing data are a common problem in clinical research and not completely avoidable also in very well-planned and well-conducted studies. In the past, missing values were often handled inadequately [38]. Missing values can be categorized according to the reason why they were not recorded. If observed values and missing values do not differ systematically one speaks from *missing completely at random* (MCAR). For example this arises if a laboratory measurement is missing since it could not be determined because an instrument was temporarily defective or not available; or when a patient moves to another center for reasons independent of treatment resulting in a drop-

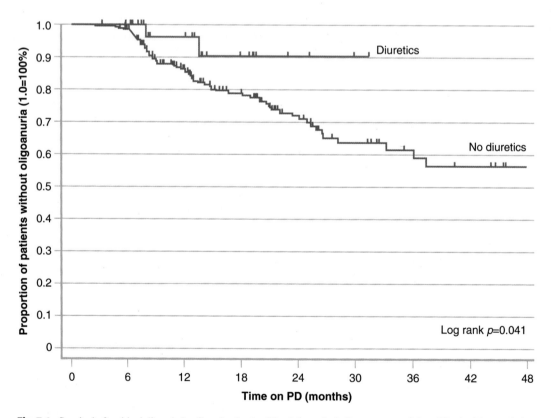

Fig. 7.1 Survival of residual diuresis by diuretics intake. The tick marks indicate censored data (Used with permission of Nature Publishing Group from Ha et al. [34])

out with missing values for subsequent follow-ups. *Missing at random* (MAR) is present if observed variables serve as an explanation for occurrence of missing values and any systematic difference between observed and missing values can be ascribed to other observed variables. For example, this would be the case if a laboratory parameter is higher in adolescents than in younger children and at the same time missing observations are more frequent in the adolescent population. If missing values depend on unobserved variables this means the values are *missing not at random* (MNAR) [39]. Since it is not possible to distinguish between MAR and MNAR based on the observed data, methods for handling missing values must be chosen carefully and sensitivity analyses carried out to examine the influence of different methods of handling missing data on the study results [40].

Intuitively the most straightforward way of dealing with missing data in the outcomes of interest or covariates required for the analysis appears to exclude observations and/or patients in case of missing values and to perform the analysis only with complete cases. However, this may result in information loss and at worst in bias if the MCAR assumption does not hold true. To ensure validity of study results the intention-to-treat analysis should contain as many study patients as possible [17]. Therefore, *imputation of missing values* is a meaningful way to deal with this problem [41]. A complete-case analysis omitting observations or patients with missing values in variables considered in analysis can be performed in addition as a sensitivity analysis.

A common but not recommended imputation method is the "*last observation carried forward* (LOCF)" approach [42]. As the name implies the last observed value is used as substitute for a missing value. Another approach are *best- and worst-case scenarios*, which are often used as sensitivity analysis. Here worst possible values are assumed for the control group and best possible values for the experimental group and vice versa. Higgins [43] provided a framework for *imputing binary missing values* based on the individual reasons for withdrawal instead of applying the same method to all patients.

The *multiple imputation* method randomly inserts ("imputes") estimates of the missing values based on a specified (regression) model incorporating information on other observed variables associated with the variable to be imputed. The procedure is repeated several times resulting in multiple imputed data sets. After analysing each data set separately the results are combined in an appropriate way.

In studies investigating repeated measures over time the analysis can be performed based on *mixed effect models* (MMRM) which do not formally impute missing values but consider all available observations per patient without missing values.

The interested reader is referred to the pertinent literature for further information [39, 44].

Multiple Testing

Multiple statistical testing within an experiment or clinical trial increases the risk of type I error, i.e., false-positive findings. The most appropriate handling of multiple testing depends on the respective research setting. Assume a study on organ transplantation where a significant treatment effect on two endpoints must be demonstrated to achieve a positive study result [45]. In such a case no adjustment for multiple testing is necessary. However, if showing a treatment effect on at least one of several co-primary endpoints is sufficient to prove efficacy, the chance of making a false-positive decision accumulates. Multiplicity problems also arise when comparing more than two treatment groups or subgroups or more than one time point of interest. In such cases appropriate methods must be applied to control the type I error rate to the intended overall significance level (e.g., 5 %). This has also consequences on power and sample size and must be taken into consideration at the planning stage.

Different approaches exist to avoid inflation of the type I error. Adjusting the nominal significance levels of the single tests is one way. The Bonferroni method divides the overall significance level α by the number of tests k carried out. A single test result can then be interpreted as statistically significant if the p-value is smaller than α/k. There are less conservative strategies, e.g., the Holms procedure.

Another approach is a priori ordering of the individual hypotheses (e.g., according to clinical relevance) with hierarchical testing. At this, a hypothesis is tested only if the above hypotheses have shown significance. A further option is testing according to the closed testing principle. At the beginning, a global hypotheses (e.g., overall comparison of three groups) is tested, e.g., by ANOVA or Kruskal-Wallis test. If this yields a significant result, individual specified hypotheses (e.g., two-group comparisons) are examined. A comprehensive overview is given in [46] and [47], and the regulatory point of view in [48].

Sample Size Calculation

The sample size, i.e., the number of patients to be included in a study, is a key aspect in planning studies of adequate statistical power. In clinical phase III studies, the aim is to include on the one hand as many patients as necessary to assure detection of a clinically relevant treatment difference with a high probability, and on the other hand as few as possible to avoid unnecessary exposure to an inferior therapy and to conserve resources.

The study design and kind of primary endpoint determine the test method used for analysis and consequently affect also the necessary sample size. The sample size is amongst others determined by:

- α: the maximally tolerable type I error (in case of two-sided testing commonly set to 5 %)
- β: the maximally tolerable type II error (commonly 20 %, frequently 10 %) or the complementary probability 1- β, i.e., the power to discover an existing difference (usually 80–90 %).
- Effect size: the pre-specified size of the clinically relevant difference between the treatments. When using an event time as primary endpoint the effect can be expressed as hazard ratio (HR), i.e., the ratio of the median survival times in the experimental and the control group.

In summary, the smaller α and β and the smaller the expected effect, the greater the number of patients that must be included into the study to ensure that a treatment difference can be demonstrated. On the other hand, if the assumed effect size is too optimistic, the power to detect a clinically meaningful difference may not be sufficient, and the probability is high that an existing effect cannot be demonstrated.

If the expected variability of a treatment effect is uncertain, it is difficult to calculate sample size appropriately. In such a situation, an internal pilot study can be designed to obtain information on the effect size variability from an initial number of patients and subsequently adjust the sample size for the final trial [49].

In studies of survival time, the required sample size is also influenced by two other factors: the duration of patient recruitment and the duration of follow-up. Both aspects also play an important role from an ethical perspective. When calculating the required sample size, it is therefore advisable to discuss these issues in the context of available resources. Also, the pure observation period should always be chosen so that at least an estimate of the median survival times in the two groups is possible. When applying a group-sequential or adaptive design, the number and nature of planned interim analyses should be considered in sample size calculation. To achieve the necessary number of patients for the confirmatory analysis, the percentage of assumed drop-outs has to be considered.

Interim Analyses

In the framework of adaptive study designs, pre-specified interim analyses provide the possibility to adapt the initial study plan regarding different aspects (e.g., endpoints, sample size, treatment arms, study population). Adequate statistical methods must be applied to control the type I error [50]. The study protocol must contain a description on how to handle the results of an interim analysis, whether and who will be informed and under which circumstances the study will be terminated (due to futility or early proof of efficacy). Interim analyses can have different purposes. If efficacy is demonstrated at an early stage of the trial, the number of study participants receiving the inferior treatment can be minimized and the superior treatment made available earlier. Early discontinuation of a study due to proof of efficacy or insufficient likelihood of showing efficacy at the end of the study reduces duration and costs.

The conduct of unplanned interim analyses with the intention to have a look on the primary endpoint during the conduct of a clinical trial without applying suitable statistical methods can introduce bias and inflation of type I error and is therefore not justified.

Data and Safety Monitoring Board (DSMB)

An independent Data and Safety Monitoring Board (DSMB) periodically reviews the progress of the study, safety data and data quality to ensure ethical conduct and protection of the rights and welfare of the patients. Based on the provided data the DSMB also gives recommendations whether the study should be terminated or continued based on the evaluation of serious adverse events, early positive results (in case of interim analysis) or the impossibility to finalize the study as planned [14, 17].

Publications

Clinical trials must be carried out in accordance with mandatory standards. These include the ICH guidelines authored by the International Conference on Harmonisation, which are available on the internet at http://www.ich.org/. Publication of the results should follow the CONSORT statement (Consolidated Standards of Reporting Trials), which designates standards for the publication of controlled clinical trials and their compliance and facilitates the adherence and readability by means of a checklist and a flowchart [51].

Clinical Research in Pediatric and Rare Disease Populations

Researchers in the field of pediatric nephrology are often confronted with the problem of small sample sizes and the low incidence of disease entities and treatment outcomes since most childhood kidney diseases are rare. The wide spectrum of manifestation ages, underlying genetic abnormalities and associated comorbidi-

ties add to the heterogeneity of the populations. These circumstances represent major challenges to clinical trials regarding enrolment, duration and costs. Consequently, many studies performed in this field are underpowered and prone to type II errors, i.e., not proofing a treatment difference when in fact one is present [52].

In the following, we outline several strategies to tackle the challenges of clinical trials in the context of rare diseases and small populations. From the statistical point of view, the power of a study can be maximized by the choice of appropriate study designs and statistical methods. In addition, efforts can be made to increase the available number of patients by clinical research collaborations and to increase families' willingness to participate in a clinical trial. Further information on ways to conduct clinical research in small populations can be found in the literature [4, 53–57].

Statistical Approaches

In a *crossover study* patients receive the experimental and control treatments one after the other with a wash-out phase in-between. Since each patient serves as his own control, total sample size can be reduced as compared to the classic parallel group design. However, the crossover study design is only appropriate when investigating diseases which quickly return into a stable condition after the end of treatment and when evaluating short-term endpoints available at the end of the first treatment period [58]. An example of such a crossover trial is the study published by Pieper et al. comparing sevelamer with calcium acetate in children with CKD [59]. Sometimes an alternative study design can be preferable to the classic randomized controlled trial. Such alternatives include *early-escape, randomized placebo-phase, risk-based allocation and n-of-1* trial designs [57, 60]. In an early-escape design, the time exposed to ineffective treatments is reduced through withdrawal of patients from the study if a pre-specified response is not observed. In a randomized placebo-phase trial all patients receive the experimental treatment but at different start times. The focus is on survival times with the hypothesis that patients starting treatment sooner respond sooner compared to those with longer waiting time. In contrast, the risk-based allocation design is a non-randomized design. Patients at high risk receive the potentially superior treatment, whereas patients at lower risk are allocated to the control group. N-of-1 trials have the aim to find the best treatment for an individual patient applying methods like randomization, blinding and wash-out phases.

When outcomes are measured at different time points one can analyze and compare the time points each by each. A more powerful approach is to include all obtained information in a single model, which increases the power and therefore allows reducing the sample size when considered at the planning stage.

Multivariable methods, e.g., analysis of variance, analysis of covariance, linear and logistic regression or proportional hazards models, are applied to adjust for potential prognostic factors or imbalances between groups. Thereby treatment effects can be estimated more precisely and the power of the study increases. Such methods are also meaningful in cases of heterogeneous study populations.

Besides the opportunity of defining *surrogate* or *composite endpoints* as primary endpoint to improve the feasibility of a study, *continuous outcomes* provide more information than *categorical* ones [28]. This should be considered when choosing the primary endpoint and calculating the required sample size.

Bayesian approaches are a further option for planning and analyzing clinical trials. Hereby, prior knowledge on treatment effects is incorporated via suitable *a priori* distributions which might lead to a slightly reduced sample size compared to "classical" approaches. These are not yet frequently used in phase III trials but more commonly in phase I and II trials. An introduction to Bayesian methods together with a discussion on advantages and disadvantages is given in [61].

Clinical Research Infrastructures

Careful choice of study design and statistical methods allows decreasing sample size to a certain extent. However, there are limits and the need to think about ways to increase the number of patients available for a clinical trial remains. In most instances, *multicenter efforts* will be required to assemble sufficiently large patient populations for adequately powered studies. There are numerous examples of successful collaborative research initiatives in pediatric nephrology. Historically, most trial activities have been initiated and promoted by national professional societies. In recent years, international collaborations have started to emerge that are empowered to gather sufficiently large populations even of patients with rare disorders. Unfortunately, such investigator-driven collaborations are often hampered by the high regulatory demands given by Good Clinical Practice standards and the heterogeneity of national clinical research regulations. As a result, the majority of clinical trial activities in pediatric nephrology are currently industry-driven. Despite a recent surge of industry interest in studying kidney disease populations in response to legislative measures enforcing pediatric trial programs for new drugs, many clinically relevant research questions remain unaddressed since they are outside the scope of trial programs focused on pediatric drug approval. Nonetheless, a few industry-independent investigator-driven clinical trial consortia have been established such as the European Study Consortium on Kidney Diseases Affecting Pediatric Patients (ESCAPE Network).

Furthermore, alternative types of studies can be considered for clinical research when objectives other than proof of treatment efficacy are of interest. In *patient registries* information on patients with certain diseases or indications are collected. A broad range of clinical data accumulating in daily routine is systematically collected in an external database. Gliklich et al. define patient registries as „an organized system that uses observational study methods to collect uniform data (clinical and other) to evaluate specified outcomes for a population defined by a particular disease, condition, or exposure, and that serves one or more predetermined scientific, clinical, or policy purposes" [62]. No procedures additional to clinical practice are carried out for the registry. Such registries can become an important data source to researchers since they may comprise a very large number of children who are often followed over extensive time periods. Clinical registries can be focused on specific diseases or disease groups (e.g., the PodoNet Registry for Steroid Resistant Nephrotic Syndrome, www.podonet. org) or on certain treatments (e.g., the International Pediatric Dialysis Network (IPDN) Registry, www.pedpd.org). Registries and observational studies in general reflect "real world usage" and complement findings from interventional studies. In addition, they can serve as a platform for multicenter clinical trials and as a source for external and historical controls to clinical trials [4]. However, registries also have limitations. Their usually voluntary nature commonly leads to a high rate of implausible and missing data and unsteady follow-up. Also, selection bias can be present resulting in non-representative population structures and biased analyses. The growing use of Web-based registry data entry greatly facilitates data collection and opens possibilities for automated plausibility checks and enforced completeness of data entries. Carefully planned, conducted, maintained and analyzed to ensure reliable results, state-of-the-art patient registries contribute to high-quality research.

In conclusion, thorough planning, conduct and analysis of clinical trials are essential on the way to evidence based medicine. In the field of pediatric nephrology researchers are faced with some challenges to deal with. Improvements regarding sample size can be made but with limitations. Efforts should be made in all directions to tap the full potential to provide high-quality research [30]. Counseling by a biostatistician can be helpful when planning a clinical trial.

Electronic Medical Records for Pediatric Patient Management and Research

The recent spread of electronic medical records (EMR) has opened a new window of opportunity for clinical research. While adoption has varied across practices, facilities, and healthcare delivery systems, utilization of EMR has become more widespread. In the United States, hospital EMR adoption tripled between 2009 and 2013,

and EMR adoption has been even more prevalent in other developed countries [63, 64]. As EMRs have become more ubiquitous, their functionality has become better understood, allowing innovative EMR applications, including clinical and translational research.

The EMR is, essentially, a comprehensive, electronic adaptation of paper patient charts. While this is a vast oversimplification, the concept of digitalized paper charting effectively illustrates EMR content; it contains all the data generated through the routine provision of patient care including demographics, daily progress notes, physician orders, medications, vital signs, test results, etc.. The analogy falls short, however, when trying to portray the volume of the content. To accurately describe the scale of the data available when the delivery of healthcare is codified electronically, one would need to envision a stack of all the charts of all the patients seen at a medical center since its inception. As an objective example, routine provision of care to hospitalized children at our institution generates, on average, 900 discrete data points per patient per day (care of a critically ill child generates between 2000 and 2500 data points per day). Across our inpatient population, this equates to 222,000 data points per day or 80,000,000 data points per year. In actuality, this understates the available volume of data since it excludes ambulatory care visits and the narrative data contained within clinical notes.

The extent of available data is one of the most striking advantages of EMR-enabled research. Pediatric research has long been plagued by small sample sizes, and the ability to generate massive cohorts is appealing. Furthermore, the actual generation and capture of data are without cost to the researcher. This is advantageous since data acquisition in prospective studies is labor and resource intensive. Additionally, EMR-enabled research offers near universal generalizability [65, 66]. The delivery of patient care occurs in an uncontrolled, real-world setting devoid of artificial study constructs; interventions and outcomes can be studied in a population not subjected to inclusion or exclusion criteria. Finally, beyond the repository of data, the EMR offers an interventional platform. It represents the intersection of data generation and care delivery; research findings can be integrated into the EMR itself to deliver outcome improvement at the point of care.

This is not to say that EMR-enabled research is without shortcomings; it will never replace the randomized controlled trial (RCT). A discussion of EMR-related limitations, including barriers to data extraction and manipulation as well as the potential for confounding and bias, will be presented subsequently. However, EMR-enabled research represents an emerging methodology [67, 68] and fundamental knowledge of the technique is important for all academic pediatric nephrologists. The purpose of this chapter is to describe EMR-enabled research, giving examples of techniques, methods, and study designs.

Retrospective, Observational Studies

The majority of EMR-enabled research to date could be best classified as retrospective and observational. Although the patient data itself is collected prospectively in real time as patients receive care, hypotheses are derived and analytics are applied retrospectively. Patients receive interventions; treatments and monitoring are performed in a non-experimental fashion according to locally derived standards of care. Retrospectively, data can be extracted, validated, merged, and analyzed (Fig. 7.2).

EMR data can be used to create *case series or cohorts of patients with rare diseases*. A single practitioner may have seen only one or two cases of an uncommon condition, whereas the number of cases across an institution may be five or ten times that. Additionally, EMR-enabled research relies upon institutional memory, rather than individual provider memory, to identify patients which increases case yield. Searching across the EMR for a particular diagnosis code or type of procedure is a relatively straightforward undertaking. Bioinformatic platforms such as the Stanford Translational Research Integrated Database Environment (STRIDE) or Informatics for Integrating Biology & the Bedside (i2b2) can further simplify the process [69, 70].

As an example, this methodology was used to study plastic bronchitis in children [71]. This uncommon and underreported disease in children was found to be present in 14 children amongst 205,100 pediatric patients at a single institution. Although they began with a single incident case, the authors were able to describe the epidemiology, including incident rates amongst several different subpopulations, pathologic findings, and treatment strategies. Similarly, this approach was used to investigate a potential link between two rare, previously unassociated diseases – eosinophilic gastrointestinal disorders (EGID) and the PTEN hamartoma tumor syndromes (PHTS) [72]. This hypothetical relationship was generated based upon clinical observation and provider recollection; however, by querying a cohort of 1,058,260 pediatric patients, the study found that there was indeed an association between the two diseases. Furthermore, the findings suggested that the tumor suppressor gene PTEN may play a role in the development of EGID.

EMR data can also be used *to create massive datasets for analysis*. These sets can be either immense cohorts of patients who each have relatively few data points, or more moderately sized patient cohorts that contain vast numbers of data points per patient. In either case, developing these datasets would be time and resource prohibitive if collected prospectively or in a randomized controlled fashion.

A terrific example of this approach examined ambulatory hypertension across a cohort of 14,187 children (ages 3–18) who had been seen at least three times for well child care [73]. The study found that while 507 (3.6%) children met criteria for hypertension, only 131 (26%) were ever diagnosed with hypertension; nearly three-quarters of pediatric hypertension was missed. Risk factors for under diagnosis included younger age and fewer elevated blood pressure readings. Patients who were obese or had more severely elevated blood pressures were more likely to be correctly diagnosed. A similar study examined obesity diagnosis trends across 60,711 children and found that overweight, obesity, and severe obesity were also under diagnosed [74]. Interestingly, they found a trend towards more accurate diagnosis over the 8 year study period; this trend corresponded to the perceived increase in attentiveness directed at weight related problems which occurred over the timeframe. A third example evaluated the association between administration of hypotonic maintenance fluid and the subsequent development of hyponatremia in hospitalized children [75]. This study created the largest such cohort to date and was able to confirm that hypotonic fluids are associated with an increased risk of hyponatremia. However, the study demonstrated clearly that additional patient and disease factors contribute to hyponatremic risk, some perhaps more so than fluid tonicity.

As EMR implementation becomes more universal, the amount of data increases and the impact of the findings become more substantial. For example, using deidentified data from the National Health Service (NHS) in England, a research group evaluated retinopathy of prematurity (ROP) screening practices in preterm infants weighing less than 1500 g [76]. Remarkably, the study included data from 94 % of all neonatal units in England, and by so doing, identified novel risk factors for non-adherence to ROP screening guidelines.

Although EMR data can be used to analyze disease processes and pathophysiology, studies have also been performed in order *to provide normative data*. Currently, good normative data exist for ambulatory pediatric patients (i.e., blood pressure ranges and growth charts); however, similar data are sparse for hospitalized children.

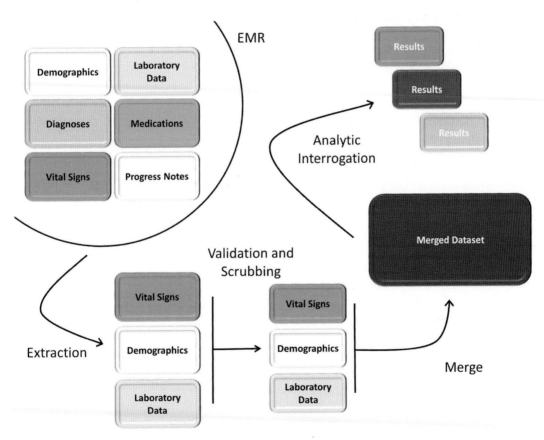

Fig. 7.2 EMR-enabled data extraction, validation, and analysis. Utilization of EMR data for research purposes requires several interconnected processes. Data is extracted from the EMR; careful attention must be paid to determine which elements are required in order to optimize analytic success and minimize personal health information (PHI) related risk. Once extracted, the data must be cleaned and validated. Validated data elements are merged into a unified database through various linking identifiers. This database can then be subjected to analytic interrogation

By extracting nurse documented vital signs for 14,014 pediatric hospitalizations, one study was able to devise heart and respiratory rate percentile curves for inpatients [77]. A similar study in adults identified 63,177 patients (drawn from a population of 1.7 million patients) with normal electrocardiograms (ECG) [78]. This allowed the researchers to devise patient-specific normal ECG parameter ranges and identify novel ECG associations with demographic characteristics and disease states.

An Interventional Platform to Improve Quality of Care

In addition to being a clinical data repository created through the routine delivery of patient care, the EMR offers an ideal platform to *implement research findings*. Data suggest that it can take practitioners over a decade to implement the findings of even the highest quality research on an everyday basis [79]. The EMR offers the capacity to deliver research findings, prediction algorithms, and best practice recommendations directly at the point of care; information can be distributed at the physician-EMR interface. This may allow more successful and widespread adoption of interventions which are known to improve patient outcomes.

One example of this approach integrated decision support with computerized physician order entry (CPOE). At the time of study initiation, the best available data suggested that a red blood cell transfusion threshold set at hemoglobin <7 g/dL was optimal in hemodynamically stable patients. The study found that providing this information to practitioners at the time of order entry resulted in an institution wide, statistically significant reduction in PRBC transfusions without a concomitant increase in mortality [80]. Another example used an automated reporting alert to address the harm associated with administration of nephrotoxic medications. The authors created an automated alert based upon medication administration data which identified patients who were receiving a predefined set of nephrotoxins [81]. Once these patients were identified, more robust serum creati-

nine monitoring was performed and medication substitution was suggested. Through the implementation of this automated alerting system, the authors were able to reduce the intensity of nephrotoxin associated acute kidney injury (AKI). Given that AKI has been associated with poorer short and long term outcomes, mitigation of AKI severity has the potential to reduce harm and improve care.

The fact that the majority of EMR data can be placed within a chronologic continuum makes it possible to use EMR data to *predict events*. The ability to prevent an adverse event or injury such as AKI is likely to have a far greater impact than the ability to mitigate it. We have used predictive analytics across a massive administrative database to identify AKI-associated clinical factors [82]. Although EMR data were not used, the study demonstrated the feasibility of applying high-content, high-throughput machine learning techniques to pediatric clinical data. The temporal nature of EMR data allows a researcher to anchor an event such as AKI, the development of hypertension, or even death, in time; this allows a clear delineation between pre-event data and post-event data. The pre-event data can then be used to derive a predictive algorithm.

Looking Ahead and Future Directions

The aforementioned studies and methodologies have really only begun to explore EMR related research possibilities. One of the most exciting areas of EMR research surrounds *use of narrative data* and the application of natural language processing (NLP) techniques. Although the EMR contains massive amounts of discrete data such as vital signs and laboratory results, potentially even more data are contained in the textual information found within narrative clinical notes.

A comprehensive discussion of NLP techniques is beyond the scope of this chapter; however, several examples may best explain how this technology can take advantage of even the non-discrete EMR data. One such study applied NLP to evaluate medication related adverse events, using cilostazol as an illustrative case [83]. This medication, which is used to treat claudication in adults, carries a black box warning since other medications in its drug class have been associated with increased mortality in the setting of congestive heart failure; the warning has been applied to this medication despite the fact that this risk has never been associated with cilstazol itself. Applying NLP to all textual documents in patients receiving cilostazol found no evidence of increased cardiovascular complications or mortality in high risk patients with CHF who were receiving the medication. The authors suggested that, "in the wild," cilostazol might be safe in this population; without text analytics, such a study would not have been feasible. In 2011, 26 research groups participated in the i2b2 Challenge which was designed to use NLP to detect emotions within suicide notes [84]. This concept may best illustrate the capacity of narrative text within the EMR. While some text may be rendered redundant by discrete data elements, there will always be data which is most efficiently captured textually – data for which there is no discrete proxy. For example, the discrete data contained within the EMR poorly captures environmental patient exposures and risks. We have hypothesized that the textual information contained within social work notes may be able to identify environmental exposures, risk factors which are otherwise not available. Although NLP has been less commonly applied within pediatrics, there are some research groups who are applying the technology to children. For example, one group analyzed the clinical notes of pediatric patients with chronic uveitis and juvenile idiopathic arthritis [85]. They were able to confirm four known disease associations as well as identify one novel association between allergic conditions and uveitis.

Some investigators have also begun to explore the interface between *EMR data and genomics*. The ability to link genetic and clinical information would allow correlation of genotypes and phenotypes, improve genome-wide association studies (GWAS), and create a platform for delivery of true pediatric systems medicine [86–89].

One such example of this evaluated genetic variants in obese children. The authors successfully linked EMR data with genotypic data for 2860 children and performed a GWAS with BMI z-scores [88]. They were able to demonstrate that genetic variants in the FTO gene, a known risk factor for obesity in adults, were associated with higher BMI in children as well. Although EMR-wide availability of genetic material has previously been a limitation, development of pediatric bio repositories may be able to overcome this difficultly. Researchers at Vanderbilt University have taken an opt-out approach to unused blood samples obtained through the routine provision of patient care. Essentially, unless patients opt-out, any leftover blood from drawn samples are retained within their local bio repository and linked with EMR data in a deidentified manner [87]. By so doing, the research team has available genetic material which can be analyzed along with EMR data. Efforts such as these may lead us toward a true systems medicine approach where the aim is to intervene early to prevent disease rather than reacting to a disease once it becomes manifest [89].

Limitations in EMR-Enabled Research

While EMR data offer a number of benefits, research using this data is subject to certain significant limitations. To begin, EMR-enabled research is almost always retrospective and observational. Thus, it can be challenging to prove causality and many of the findings are best described as associations. One of the most challenging aspects of this research is the *potential for bias and confounding*. When physicians provide clinical care, there are often patient factors which effect both treatment decisions and outcomes; retrospectively, it can be challenging to eliminate these biases. Additionally, it can be particularly difficult to determine disease severity retrospectively; many aspects of the patient's condition may confound the findings of these studies. Therefore, researchers need to be comprehensive and creative in their attempts to address bias and confounding.

An additional limitation is *missing or flawed data*. In many situations, EMR workflows poorly capture data elements. For example, we have found that heights are not obtained or recorded at every hospitalization; this is especially true in the ICU setting. While there are certain methods that can be used to impute missing data, nothing compares to having the actual data present. Flawed or incorrect data are harder to address. It's quite challenging to determine when a weight is entered in pounds instead of kilograms after the fact, or when a decimal place is mistakenly moved one digit to the right. However, EMR-enabled research can generate massive datasets, and unless the data are flawed systematically, many such errors end up having marginal impact.

Finally, the *scale of the data* can, at times, be a limitation. Manipulation of large data tables can be challenging and analysis of the myriad data elements often requires a high-content, high-throughput analytic technique such as those typically applied to genomic or proteomic analysis. Data elements are often stored in disparate locations within the EMR and manipulation can require linking identifiers. With the correct personnel in place, however, this is a limitation which can be overcome.

Summary

In summary, although subject to certain intrinsic limitations, EMR-enabled research offers near limitless possibilities. The ability to develop immense retrospective cohorts containing many data elements is one of the most striking features. Perhaps more important, however, is the potential for the EMR to become a platform for intervention and integration of EMR-enabled research findings. The EMR exists at the intersection of care delivery, clinical and translational research, and quality improvement. With time, it is possible that EMR-enabled research will allow us to "learn from every patient at every visit" and deliver high-quality clinical decision support in real time at the point of care [90].

Regulatory and Ethical Aspects in Pediatric Research

Fundamentally, children represent a particularly challenging research population from an ethics standpoint. Although regulations that pertain specifically to pediatric patients exist, investiga-tors must also properly apply ethical principles which were primarily developed for adult participants. Although research has been conducted on children for hundreds of years, the past half century has brought much focus to this particularly vulnerable population.

Historical Perspective

Historical examples demonstrating the need for pediatric-specific research guidelines abound; many of these examples are controversial from an ethical perspective. Both the cowpox and the rabies vaccines were tested initially in children [91–93]. Although now the potential benefit seems to greatly outweigh the potential harm, at the time, the absence of a pediatric-specific ethical construct likely made such determinations problematic. Other examples include the radioisotope experiments at Fernald and the hepatitis studies of Krugman [91, 94]. In these situations, even a rudimentary framework did not adequately safeguard pediatric patients due to inadequate risk disclosure, the absence of balancing benefit, the potential for coercion, and the exploitation of particularly vulnerable populations, even by pediatric standards [92, 95]. In many ways, the current pediatric ethics construct was born from these cases and those like them; however, this structure was clearly build upon a foundation of the biomedical ethical principles developed in adults.

The first international code of research ethics, the Nuremberg Code (1947), was developed in response to the experimentation performed by Nazi scientists in concentration camps during the second world war; interestingly, its provisions actually prohibited research in children [91, 96]. The provisions stated that any participants in medical research were required to provide informed consent. Children, without the legal and developmental capacity to give this consent, were excluded from participation, according to the code. Nearly two decades later, The Declaration of Helskinki (1964), which is often considered the underpinning of current ethical standards, was developed [91, 96, 97]. The Declaration allowed consent to be obtained by a legal guardian, thus allowing research to be conducted in children. A revision to the Declaration (1983) supplemented this proxy consent with an assenting procedure that was to be performed whenever possible in minors, underscoring the role of the child in the process [96]. In 1977, the National Commission for Protection of Human Subjects of Biomedical and Behavioral Research was commissioned by the United States Congress to addresses the specific issues surrounding the role of children in biomedical research; the Belmont Report (1979) outlines the findings of the Commission, highlighting the importance of three ethical principles: respect for persons, beneficence, and justice [96–98].

Principles of Biomedical Ethics and Their Relevance to Children

In addition to the three principles outlined in the Belmont Report, many biomedical ethicists have added the concept of nonmaleficence [99, 100]. These four principles will be discussed with a specific focus on pediatric research.

Respect for Persons
This concept centers on respect for individual autonomy [91, 98, 99]. The process of informed consent is probably the most tangible aspect of this provision. Any individual who participates in research, must do so of their own volition. Furthermore, they must be provided with a comprehensive explanation of the risks and benefits; withholding or inadequately providing information pertinent to the research is contrary to this principle. Perhaps most relevant to children is the idea that those who are incapable of autonomy, due to disability (mental incapacity), environment (prisoners), or maturity/development (children) deserve special consideration and protection. Children, by definition, are legally and often developmentally, unable to give fully informed consent. Thus, the consent/assent process is one aspect of research that is fundamentally different in children and adults. Although the parents may fully understand the risks and benefits, the child may not

completely comprehend them; this is more likely with younger children and more complex processes. Older children (usually above age 7) are asked to give assent; this process is similar, but less comprehensive than the consent process. Essentially the child is asked to confirm that they understand the research/benefits/harms and that they agree to participate in the study. In younger children, or those who are unable to provide assent developmentally, proxy consent from the parent or parents takes the place of individual consent.

Beneficence
The concept of beneficence centers on maximizing benefit and minimizing risk [91, 98, 99]. Clearly, to benefit from research, children must participate; thus, this concept underscores the need for medical research in pediatric patients. At the same time, however, pediatric participants must be protected from risk given their inability to completely provide informed consent and their inherently vulnerable nature [99]. One way to conceptualize the balance of benefit and risk is the risk stratification system set up by the Code of Federal Regulations (45 CFR 46) [91, 101, 102]. The first risk category specified is that of "no greater than minimal risk." In this situation, children can be included in research even if there is no potential benefit to the individual subject. The second category is that of "greater than minimal risk." In this situation, children may participate if there is likely to be a direct benefit to the individual child; the benefit to risk ratio, however, must be favorable. Children may also participate in the absence of a direct benefit if the study is likely to generate novel, relevant information about the child's disease or disorder; in such a situation, the risk must be no more than "a minor increase over minimal risk." Clearly, categorization of studies hinges on our ability to accurately assess the concepts of minimal risk and minor increase over minimal risk. Application of these concepts can prove challenging; one study by Shah and colleagues demonstrated significant variability in the application of both the minimal risk and direct benefit concepts amongst Internal Review Board (IRB) chairs [103].

Justice

The concept of justice in medical research emphasizes the importance of equal and fair distribution of research benefits and risks [91, 96–98]. According to this concept, it would be unethical to completely exclude research in pediatric patients since they would not be afforded the opportunity to benefit. However, it also clearly suggests that research should not be conducted in children for the sole purpose of benefiting other populations. The notion of justice within medical research highlights the need for prudent and insightful selection of participant populations within pediatric research.

Nonmaleficence

The concept of nonmaleficence can be summarized by the phrase, "primum non nocere," which is familiar to medical students far and wide [99, 100]. Any research which is conducted in humans must be governed by the principle of "doing no harm." While clearly harm can occur as a result of research procedures and interventions, the research must be designed upon a foundation of harm avoidance; regardless of the purported benefit or novelty of one's research, one cannot intentionally intend to harm participants. Although this standard seems self-evident, there are a number of historical examples where it was disregarded or erroneous applied. Given the particularly vulnerable nature of children, this concept gains additional traction when applied to pediatric research.

Conclusions

Medical research has been the key to our modern day understanding of disease pathophysiology and the basis for the majority of our treatment paradigms. Indeed, even our knowledge of normal organ and systemic function has been born from experimentation. The significance and magnitude of our collective research efforts are manifested in a myriad of ways every day that we participate in the provision of medical care to patients. However, we cannot ignore the instances where such knowledge was gained unethically and dishonorably; in these situations the benefit gained from the data can never overcome the harmful and inequitable nature of the research. It is our duty as academicians to continue to strive for high quality research performed in an ethical manner. The fact that children are legally and developmentally unable to agree to participate in experimental protocols should constantly remind us that this population, while deserving of consideration for inclusion, needs special protection and additional foresight.

References

1. Foster BJ, Warady BA. Clinical research in pediatric nephrology: challenges, and strategies to address them. J Nephrol. 2009;22(6):685–93.
2. Sackett DL, Rosenberg WM, Gray JA, Haynes RB, Richardson WS. Evidence based medicine: what it is and what it isn't. BMJ. 1996;312(7023):71–2.
3. CEBM Center for Evidence Based Medicine; http://www.cebm.net/index.aspx?o=1025.
4. CPMP. Guideline on clinical trials in small populations. 2006. CHMP/EWP/83561/2005.
5. Cochrane online library; http://www.cochranelibrary.com/app/content/browse/page/?context=editorial-group/Renal%20Group.
6. National Kidney Foundation Kidney Disease Outcomes Quality Initiative (NKF KDOQI); https://www.kidney.org/professionals/guidelines.
7. International Society of Nephrology. Kidney Disease – Improving global Outcomes (KDIGO); http://kdigo.org/home/guidelines/.
8. Pocock SJ. Clinical trials: a practical approach. Chichester: Wiley; 1983.
9. The ESCAPE Trial Group. Strict blood-pressure control and progression of renal failure in children. N Engl J Med. 2009;361(17):1639–50.
10. Keren R, Carpenter MA, Hoberman A, Shaikh N, Matoo TK, Chesney RW, et al. Rationale and design issues of the Randomized Intervention for Children with Vesicoureteral Reflux (RIVUR) study. Pediatrics. 2008;122 Suppl 5:S240–50.
11. Chan AW, Tetzlaff JM, Altman DG, Laupacis A, Gøtzsche PC, Krleža-Jerić K, et al. SPIRIT 2013 statement: defining standard protocol items for clinical trials. Ann Intern Med. 2013;158(3):200–7.
12. Chan AW, Tetzlaff JM, Gøtzsche PC, Altman DG, Mann H, Berlin JA, et al. SPIRIT 2013 explanation and elaboration: guidance for protocols of clinical trials. BMJ. 2013;346:e7586.
13. ICH E10. Choice of control group and related issues in clinical trials. 2000. http://www.ich.org/fileadmin/Public_Web_Site/ICH_Products/Guidelines/Efficacy/E10/Step4/E10_Guideline.pdf.

14. ICH E6. Guideline for good clinical practice. 1996. http://www.ich.org/fileadmin/Public_Web_Site/ ICH_Products/Guidelines/Efficacy/E6_R1/Step4/ E6_R1__Guideline.

15. Schulz KF, Grimes DA. Blinding in randomised trials: hiding who got what. Lancet. 2002;359(9307): 696–700.

16. Hahn D, Hodson EM, Willis NS, Craig JC. Corticosteroid therapy for nephrotic syndrome in children. Cochrane Database Syst Rev. 2015;(3):CD001533.

17. ICH E9. Statistical principles for clinical trials. 1998. http://www.ich.org/fileadmin/Public_Web_ Site/ICH_Products/Guidelines/Efficacy/E9/Step4/ E9_Guideline.pdf.

18. Molenberghs G, Burzykowski T, Alonso A, Buyse M. A perspective on surrogate endpoints in controlled clinical trials. Stat Methods Med Res. 2004;13(3):177–206.

19. Lambers Heerspink HJ, Kröpelin TF, Hoekman J, de Zeeuw D, the Reducing Albuminuria as Surrogate Endpoint (REASSURE) Consortium. Drug-induced reduction in albuminuria is associated with subsequent renoprotection: a meta-analysis. J Am Soc Nephrol. 2015;26(8):2055–64.

20. Weldegiorgis M, de Zeeuw D, Heerspink HJ. Renal end points in clinical trials of kidney disease. Curr Opin Nephrol Hypertens. 2015;24(3):284–9.

21. Chi GYH. Some issues with composite endpoints in clinical trials. Fundam Clin Pharmacol. 2005;19(6): 609–19.

22. Lesaffre E. Superiority, equivalence, and noninferiority trials. Bull NYU Hosp Jt Dis. 2008;66(2):150–4.

23. Thomas L, Peterson ED. The value of statistical analysis plans in observational research: defining high-quality research from the start. JAMA. 2012;308(8):773–4.

24. Bland JM, Altman DG. One and two sided tests of significance. BMJ. 1994;309(6949):248.

25. Morris RK, Malin GL, Quinlan-Jones E, Middleton LJ, Hemming K, Burke D, et al. Percutaneous vesicoamniotic shunting versus conservative management for fetal lower urinary tract obstruction (PLUTO): a randomised trial. Lancet. 2013; 382(9903):1496–506.

26. Rothmann MD, Wiens BL, Chan ISF. Design and analysis of non-inferiority trials. London: Chapman and Hall; 2012.

27. FDA. Guidance for industry: non-inferiority clinical trials. 2010. http://www.fda.gov.

28. Altman DG, Royston P. The cost of dichotomising continuous variables. BMJ. 2006;332(7549):1080.

29. Rasch D, Guiard V. The robustness of parametric statistical methods. Psychol Sci. 2004;46:175–208.

30. du Prel JB, Röhrig B, Hommel G, Blettner M. Choosing statistical tests: part 12 of a series on evaluation of scientific publications. Dtsch Arztebl Int. 2010;107(19):343–8.

31. Altman D. Practical statistics for medical research. London: Chapman and Hall; 1991.

32. Kaplan EL, Meier P. Nonparametric estimation from incomplete observations. J Am Stat Assoc. 1958;53(282):457–81.

33. Bland JM, Altman DG. Survival probabilities (the Kaplan-Meier method). BMJ. 1998;317(7172):1572.

34. Ha IS, Yap HK, Munarriz RL, Zambrano PH, Flynn JT, Bilge I, et al. Risk factors for loss of residual renal function in children treated with chronic peritoneal dialysis. Kidney Int. 2015;88(3):605–13.

35. Peto R, Peto J. Asymptotically efficient rank invariant test procedures. J R Stat Soc Ser A (General). 1972;135(2):185–207.

36. Bland JM, Altman DG. The logrank test. BMJ. 2004;328(7447):1073.

37. Cox RD. Regression models and life-tables. J R Stat Soc Ser B (Methodological). 1972;34(4): 187–220.

38. Wood AM, White IR, Thompson SG. Are missing outcome data adequately handled? A review of published randomized controlled trials in major medical journals. Clin Trials. 2004;1(4):368–76.

39. Sterne JAC, White IR, Carlin JB, Spratt M, Royston P, Kenward MG, et al. Multiple imputation for missing data in epidemiological and clinical research: potential and pitfalls. BMJ. 2009;338:b2393.

40. Little RJ, Rubin DB. Statistical analysis with missing data. 2nd ed. New York: Wiley; 2002.

41. CPMP. Guideline on missing data in confirmatory clinical trials. 2009. CPMP/EWP/1776/99.

42. Lane P. Handling drop-out in longitudinal clinical trials: a comparison of the LOCF and MMRM approaches. Pharm Stat. 2008;7(2):93–106.

43. Higgins JPT, White IR, Wood AM. Imputation methods for missing outcome data in meta-analysis of clinical trials. Clin Trials. 2008;5(3):225–39.

44. van Buuren S. Flexible imputation of missing data. London: Chapman and Hall; 2012.

45. Offen W, Chuang-Stein C, Dmitrienko A, Littman G, Maca J, Meyerson L, et al. Multiple co-primary endpoints: medical and statistical solutions: a report from the multiple endpoints expert team of the pharmaceutical research and manufacturers of America. Drug Inf J. 2007;41(1):31–46.

46. Moyé LA. Multiple analyses in clinical trials: fundamentals for investigators. New York: Springer; 2003.

47. Dmitrienko A, Tamhane AC, Bretz F, editors. Multiple testing problems in pharmaceutical statistics. Boca Raton: Chapman & Hall/CRC Biostatistics Series; 2009.

48. CPMP. Points to consider on multiplicity issues in clinical trials. 2002. CPMP/EWP/908/99.

49. Friede T, Kieser M. Sample size recalculation in internal pilot study designs: a review. Biom J. 2006;48(4):537–55.

50. Friede T, Kieser M. A comparison of methods for adaptive sample size adjustment. Stat Med. 2001;20(24):3861–73.

51. Moher D, Schulz KF, Altman DG. The CONSORT statement: revised recommendations for improving the quality of reports of parallel-group randomized trials. Ann Intern Med. 2001;134(8):657–62.
52. Lilford R, Stevens AJ. Underpowered studies. Br J Surg. 2002;89(2):129–31.
53. van der Lee JH, Wesseling J, Tanck MWT, Offringa M. Efficient ways exist to obtain the optimal sample size in clinical trials in rare diseases. J Clin Epidemiol. 2008;61(4):324–30.
54. Behera M, Kumar A, Soares HP, Sokol L, Djulbegovic B. Evidence-based medicine for rare diseases: implications for data interpretation and clinical trial design. Cancer Control. 2007;14(2):160–6.
55. Griggs RC, Batshaw M, Dunkle M, Gopal-Srivastava R, Kaye E, Krischer J, et al. Clinical research for rare disease: opportunities, challenges, and solutions. Mol Genet Metab. 2009;96(1):20–6.
56. Augustine EF, Adams HR, Mink JW. Clinical trials in rare disease: challenges and opportunities. J Child Neurol. 2013;28(9):1142–50.
57. National Research Council. Small clinical trials: issues and challenges. Washington, DC: The National Academies Press; 2001.
58. Senn S. Practical statistics for medical research. Cross-over trials in clinical research. New York: Wiley; 1993.
59. Pieper AK, Haffner D, Hoppe B, Dittrich K, Offner G, Bonzel KE, et al. A randomized crossover trial comparing sevelamer with calcium acetate in children with CKD. Am J Kidney Dis. 2006;47(4): 625–35.
60. Feldman B, Wang E, Willan A, Szalai JP. The randomized placebo-phase design for clinical trials. J Clin Epidemiol. 2001;54(6):550–7.
61. FDA. Guidance for the use of Bayesian statistics in medical device clinical trials. 2010. http://www.fda.gov/RegulatoryInformation/Guidances/ucm071072.htm.
62. Gliklich RE, Dreyer NA. Registries for evaluating patient outcomes: a user's guide. 2nd ed. Rockville: Agency for Healthcare Research and Quality (US); 2010.
63. Charles D, King J, Patel V, MF F. Adoption of electronic health record systems among U.S. non-federal acute care hospitals: 2008–2012. Office of the National coordinator for health information technology. Mar 2013;ONC Data Brief, no 9.
64. Schoen C, Osborn R, Squires D, Doty M, Rasmussen P, Pierson R, Applebaum S. A survey of primary care doctors in ten countries shows progress in use of health information technology, less in other areas. Health Aff. 2012;31(12):2805–16.
65. Stewart WF, Shah NR, Selna MJ, Paulus RA, Walker JM. Bridging the inferential gap: the electronic health record and clinical evidence. Health Aff (Millwood). 2007;26(2):w181–91.
66. Wasserman RC. Electronic Medical Records (EMRs), epidemiology, and epistemology: reflec-

tions on emrs and future pediatric clinical research. Acad Pediatr. 2011;11(4):280–7.
67. Dean BB, Lam J, Natoli JL, Butler Q, Aguilar D, Nordyke RJ. Review: use of electronic medical records for health outcomes research: a literature review. Med Care Res Rev MCRR. 2009;66(6):611–38.
68. Lin J, Jiao T, Biskupiak JE, McAdam-Marx C. Application of electronic medical record data for health outcomes research: a review of recent literature. Expert Rev Pharmacoecon Outcomes Res. 2013;13(2):191–200.
69. Lowe H, Ferris T, Hernandez P, Weber S. STRIDE – an integrated standards-based translational research informatics platform. AMIA Annu Symp Proc. 2009;2009:391–5.
70. Kohane IS, Churchill SE, Murphy SN. A translational engine at the national scale: informatics for integrating biology and the bedside. J Am Med Inform Assoc JAMIA. 2012;19(2):181–5.
71. Kunder R, Kunder C, Sun HY, Berry G, Messner A, Frankovich J, Roth S, Mark J. Pediatric plastic bronchitis: case report and retrospective comparative analysis of epidemiology and pathology. Case Rep Pulmonol. 2013;2013:8.
72. Henderson CJ, Ngeow J, Collins MH, Martin LJ, Putnam PE, Abonia JP, Marsolo K, Eng C, Rothenberg ME. Increased prevalence of eosinophilic gastrointestinal disorders (EGID) in pediatric PTEN hamartoma tumor syndromes (PHTS). J Pediatr Gastroenterol Nutr. 2014;58(5):553–60.
73. Hansen ML, Gunn PW, Kaelber DC. Underdiagnosis of hypertension in children and adolescents. JAMA. 2007;298(8):874–9.
74. Benson L, Baer HJ, Kaelber DC. Trends in the diagnosis of overweight and obesity in children and adolescents: 1999–2007. Pediatrics. 2009;123(1):e153–8. doi:10.1542/peds.2008-1408.
75. Carandang F, Anglemyer A, Longhurst CA, Krishnan G, Alexander SR, Kahana M, Sutherland SM. Association between maintenance fluid tonicity and hospital-acquired hyponatremia. J Pediatr Us. 2013;163(6):1646–51.
76. Wong HS, Santhakumaran S, Statnikov Y, Gray D, Watkinson M, Modi N, Collaborative tUN. Retinopathy of prematurity in English neonatal units: a national population-based analysis using NHS operational data. Arch Dis Child Fetal Neonatal Ed. 2014;99:F196–202.
77. Bonafide CP, Brady PW, Keren R, Conway PH, Marsolo K, Daymont C. Development of heart and respiratory rate percentile curves for hospitalized children. Pediatrics. 2013;131(4):e1150–7.
78. Ramirez AH, Schildcrout JS, Blakemore DL, Masys DR, Pulley JM, Basford MA, Roden DM, Denny JC. Modulators of normal electrocardiographic intervals identified in a large electronic medical record. Heart Rhythm. 2011;8(2):271–7.
79. Westfall JM, Mold J, Fagnan L. PRactice-based research—"blue highways" on the nih roadmap. JAMA. 2007;297(4):403–6.

80. Adams ES, Longhurst CA, Pageler N, Widen E, Franzon D, Cornfield DN. Computerized physician order entry with decision support decreases blood transfusions in children. Pediatrics. 2011;127(5):e1112–9.

81. Goldstein SL, Kirkendall E, Nguyen H, Schaffzin JK, Bucuvalas J, Bracke T, Seid M, Ashby M, Foertmeyer N, Brunner L, Lesko A, Barclay C, Lannon C, Muething S. Electronic health record identification of nephrotoxin exposure and associated acute kidney injury. Pediatrics. 2013;132(3):e756–67.

82. Sutherland SM, Ji J, Sheikhi FH, Widen E, Tian L, Alexander SR, Ling XB. AKI in hospitalized children: epidemiology and clinical associations in a national cohort. Clin J Am Soc Nephrol. 2013;8(10):1661–9.

83. Leeper NJ, Bauer-Mehren A, Iyer SV, Lependu P, Olson C, Shah NH. Practice-based evidence: profiling the safety of cilostazol by text-mining of clinical notes. PLoS One. 2013;8(5):e63499.

84. Pak A, Bernhard D, Paroubek P, Grouin C. A combined approach to emotion detection in suicide notes. Biomed Inform Insights. 2012;5 Suppl 1:105–14.

85. Cole TS, Frankovich J, Iyer S, Lependu P, Bauer-Mehren A, Shah NH. Profiling risk factors for chronic uveitis in juvenile idiopathic arthritis: a new model for EHR-based research. Pediatr Rheumatol Online J. 2013;11(1):45. doi:10.1186/1546-0096-11-45.

86. Gottesman O, Kuivaniemi H, Tromp G, Faucett WA, Li R, Manolio TA, Sanderson SC, Kannry J, Zinberg R, Basford MA, Brilliant M, Carey DJ, Chisholm RL, Chute CG, Connolly JJ, Crosslin D, Denny JC, Gallego CJ, Haines JL, Hakonarson H, Harley J, Jarvik GP, Kohane I, Kullo IJ, Larson EB, McCarty C, Ritchie MD, Roden DM, Smith ME, Bottinger EP, Williams MS, e MN. The Electronic Medical Records and Genomics (eMERGE) network: past, present, and future. Genet Med Off J Am Coll Med Genet. 2013;15(10):761–71.

87. McGregor TL, Van Driest SL, Brothers KB, Bowton EA, Muglia LJ, Roden DM. Inclusion of pediatric samples in an opt-out biorepository linking DNA to de-identified medical records: pediatric BioVU. Clin Pharmacol Ther. 2013;93(2):204–11.

88. Namjou B, Keddache M, Marsolo K, Wagner M, Lingren T, Cobb B, Perry C, Kennebeck S, Holm IA, Li R, Crimmins NA, Martin L, Solti I, Kohane I,

Harley JB. EMR-linked GWAS study: investigation of variation landscape of loci for body mass index in children. Front Genet. 2013;4:268.

89. Tegner J, Abugessaisa I. Pediatric systems medicine: evaluating needs and opportunities using congenital heart block as a case study. Pediatr Res. 2013;73(4–2):508–13.

90. Frankovich J, Longhurst CA, Sutherland SM. Evidence-based medicine in the EMR era. N Engl J Med. 2011;365(19):1758–9.

91. Diekema DS. Conducting ethical research in pediatrics: a brief historical overview and review of pediatric regulations. J Pediatr. 2006;149(1 Suppl):S3–11.

92. Burns JP. Research in children. Crit Care Med. 2003;31(3 Suppl):S131–6.

93. Geison GL. Pasteur's work on rabies: reexamining the ethical issues. Hastings Cent Rep. 1978;8(2):26–33.

94. Krugman S. The Willowbrook hepatitis studies revisited: ethical aspects. Rev Infect Dis. 1986;8(1):157–62.

95. Goldby S. Experiments at the Willowbrook State School. Lancet. 1971;1(7702):749.

96. Boss RD. Ethics for the pediatrician: pediatric research ethics: evolving principles and practices. Pediatr Rev Am Acad Pediatr. 2010;31(4):163–5.

97. Diekema DS. Ethical issues in research involving infants. Semin Perinatol. 2009;33(6):364–71.

98. The Belmont report: ethical principles and guidelines for the protection of human subjects of research. 18 Apr 1979; http://www.hhs.gov/ohrp/humansubjects/guidance/belmont.html.

99. Pinxten W, Dierickx K, Nys H. Ethical principles and legal requirements for pediatric research in the EU: an analysis of the European normative and legal framework surrounding pediatric clinical trials. Eur J Pediatr. 2009;168(10):1225–34.

100. Beauchamp TL. Methods and principles in biomedical ethics. J Med Ethics. 2003;29(5):269–74.

101. Laventhal N, Tarini BA, Lantos J. Ethical issues in neonatal and pediatric clinical trials. Pediatr Clin North Am. 2012;59(5):1205–20.

102. Code of federal regulations: public welfare, protection of human subjects. 1/15/09; http://www.hhs.gov/ohrp/humansubjects/guidance/45cfr46.html.

103. Shah S, Whittle A, Wilfond B, Gensler G, Wendler D. How do institutional review boards apply the federal risk and benefit standards for pediatric research? JAMA. 2004;4(291):476–82.

Part II

Disorders of Renal Development

Structural Development of the Kidney

8

Jacqueline Ho

The kidney presents in the highest degree the phenomenon of sensibility; the power of reacting to various stimuli in a direction which is appropriate for the survival of the organism; a power of adaptation which almost gives one the idea that its component parts must be endowed with intelligence (E. Starling 1909)

Introduction

As recognized by Starling, the mammalian kidney has evolved to provide critical adaptive regulatory mechanisms, such as the excretion of waste, and the maintenance of water, electrolyte and acid-base homeostasis. These regulatory functions require the coordinate development of specific cell types within a precise pattern so that body fluid composition can be closely monitored and regulated. The developmental program that controls this pattern is a highly dynamic process involving the interplay between multiple factors. Defects in kidney development result in a spectrum of structural and functional disorders that are the topics of other chapters in this book. To provide a framework for understanding the

J. Ho
Department of Pediatrics, Rangos Research Building,
Children's Hospital of Pittsburgh of UPMC,
4401 Penn Avenue, Pittsburgh, PA 15224, USA
e-mail: jacqueline.ho2@chp.edu

developmental origins of these disorders, the structural of the kidney will be outlined in this chapter.

Overview of Human Kidney Development

Human kidney development begins in the fifth week of gestation, with the first functioning nephrons making urine by the ninth week [1]. The formation of new nephrons continues until approximately 32–34 weeks gestation [2, 3]. Further renal growth is the result of growth and maturation of already formed nephrons, rather than the generation of new nephrons. Remarkably, there exists wide variability in the number of nephrons that occur naturally in humans, from 200,000 to 1.8 million per person [4]. In humans that suffer fetal or perinatal renal injury, the developing kidney is incapable of compensating for irreversible nephron loss by either accelerating the rate of nephron formation ex utero in infants born prematurely, or by de novo generation of nephrons once nephrogenesis is completed [2, 5]. Thus, the number of nephrons formed at birth is thought to be an important determinant of renal function later in life.

This concept is supported by the association of renal failure in humans with oligomeganephronia [6, 7], and by the demonstration of reduced

© Springer-Verlag Berlin Heidelberg 2016
D.F. Geary, F. Schaefer (eds.), *Pediatric Kidney Disease*, DOI 10.1007/978-3-662-52972-0_8

glomerular number in humans with primary hypertension and chronic kidney disease [8, 9]. Quantitative analyses in humans and rodents using stereological methods of glomerular counting in renal autopsy specimens have revealed a relationship between birth weight and glomerular number [4, 10]. The latter data are consistent with the "Barker Hypothesis," which proposes that adult disease has fetal origins and is based on epidemiological studies showing a correlation between birth weight and the incidence of cardiovascular disease [11, 12]. Equally important is the normal structural development of each nephron (or nephron pattern), which is critical for nephron function. Abnormal nephron pattern results in renal dysplasia. Consequently, mechanisms that control congenital nephron endowment and nephron pattern are likely to be crucial for programming long-term as well as short-term renal survival.

Our understanding of human kidney development historically began with histological descriptions of microdissected human fetal kidney autopsy specimens performed by Edith Potter and Vitoon Osathanondh [1, 13, 14]. Their seminal work was complemented by analyses of mouse kidney development performed by Lauri Saxen [15]. The mammalian kidney derives from two parts of the metanephros, its embryonic precursor. The first part is the ureteric bud, which gives rise to the collecting duct system, including the cortical and medullary collecting ducts, the renal calyces, the renal pelvis, the ureter, and trigone of the bladder [2, 15]. The second part is the metanephric mesenchyme, which differentiates into all the epithelial cell types comprising the mature nephron, including the visceral and parietal epithelium of the glomerulus, the proximal convoluted tubule, the ascending and descending limbs of the Loops of Henle, and the distal convoluted tubule [2, 15]. Reciprocal signals between these two tissues are critical for normal kidney development.

The molecular and genetic control of kidney morphogenesis is the subject of several recent comprehensive reviews [16–22]. Mutational analyses in mice have yielded much insight into the molecular pathways that regulate key events during the formation of nephrons, including the specification and differentiation of the metanephric mesenchyme, ureteric bud induction, renal branching morphogenesis, nephron segmentation and glomerulogenesis. The phenotypes resulting from murine gene mutations also serve as paradigms for renal malformations (viz. renal agenesis, duplex kidney) that predict roles for corresponding human gene mutations in the pathogenesis of these conditions (Table 8.1). Thus, advances in human genomics and mammalian developmental genetics have accelerated the tempo of discovery in the field of developmental nephrology, providing novel insights into the genetic, epigenetic and environmental factors that impact nephron number and pattern. In the following sections, the morphologic events and molecular underpinnings of these developmental processes will be described.

Origin of the Mammalian Kidney

The mammalian kidney is derived from the intermediate mesoderm of the urogenital ridge, which develops along the posterior abdominal wall of the developing fetus between the dorsal somites and the lateral plate mesoderm. The Wolffian Duct (also known as the mesonephric or nephric duct) is a paired embryonic epithelial tubule extending in an anterior-posterior orientation on either side of the midline, which arises from the intermediate mesoderm. The Wolffian Duct is divided into three segments – the pronephros, mesonephros, and metanephros (Fig. 8.1). At its anterior end, the pronephros forms the renal anlage in fish [24] and frogs [25], but degenerates in mammals. The mid-portion of the Wolffian Duct, the mesonephros, gives rise to male reproductive organs including the rete testis, efferent ducts, epididymis, vas deferens, seminal vesicle, and prostate [26]. In females, the mesonephric portion of the Wolffian Duct degenerates. The caudal portion of the Wolffian Duct, the metanephros, becomes the mature mammalian kidney. The posterior segment of the Wolffian Duct ultimately communicates with the cloaca to form the trigone of the bladder [26].

Table 8.1 Mouse mutations exhibiting defects in kidney morphogenesis and predominant accompanying renal phenotypes

Mutant gene	Predominant mutant renal malformation phenotype
Failed ureteric bud outgrowth	
Metanephric mesenchyme-derived	Renal aplasia
Eya1	
Fgf9/20	
Fgfr1/2	
Gdnf	
Lhx1	
Osr1	
Pax2	
Sall1	
Six1	
Wt1	
Ureteric Bud-derived	
Emx2	
Gata3	
Gfrα1	
Hoxa11/Hoxd11/Hoxc11	
Hs2st	
Itgα8	
Lhx1	
Pax2/8	
Ret	
Ectopic ureteric bud outgrowth	
Bmp4	Duplex collecting system
Foxc1	
Robo2	
Slit2	
Spry1	
Decreased ureteric bud branching	
Fgfr2	Renal hypoplasia,
Foxd1	Renal dysplasia
Pod1	
Raldh2	
Rarα/Rarβ2	
Spry2	
Wnt11	
Defective renal medulla formation	
Fgf7	Medullary dysplasia
Fgf10	
Gpc3	
p57^{KIP2}	

(continued)

Table 8.1 (continued)

Mutant gene	Predominant mutant renal malformation phenotype
Agt	Hydronephrosis
Agtr1	
Agtr2	
Bmp4	
Bmp5	
Defective tubulogenesis	
Bmp7	Renal hypoplasia,
Brn1	Renal dysplasia
Fgf8	
Pod1	
Lhx1	
Notch1	
Notch2	
Psen1/ Psen2	
Rbpsuh	
Six2	
Wnt4	
Wnt9b	
Defective glomerulogenesis	
Jag1	Glomerular malformation
Notch2	
Pdgfβ	
Pdgfrβ	
Pod1	
Vegf	
Col4α3/Col4α4/Col4α5	Loss of glomerular filtration selectivity
Lamb	
Lmx1β	
Mafβ	
Wt1	

Several molecules have been identified as necessary in establishing the immediate precursors to the ureteric bud and metanephric mesenchyme of the developing metanephros in the intermediate mesoderm. The regional specification of metanephric mesenchyme at the posterior intermediate mesoderm next to the Wolffian Duct requires function of the transcription factor, *Odd-skipped related 1 (Osr1)* [27]. The establishment and development of the Wolffian Duct requires the function of the transcription factors, *Paired box gene 2 (Pax2)* [28], *Pax8* [29], *Lim homeobox 1 (Lhx1)* [30], *Gata binding protein 3 (Gata3)* [31] and the tyrosine kinase receptor, *Ret* [32], as well as *Osr1*, prior to onset of ureteric bud induction.

Cell-fate tracing studies using the transcription factor, *Osr1*, have identified *Osr1*-expressing cells of the intermediate mesoderm as the origin of the principle cellular components of the metanephric kidney: the main body of the nephron, vascular and interstitial cell types, and the Wolffian Duct [33]. Interactions amongst the different cellular derivatives of *Osr1*-expressing cells are critical for kidney development. The ureteric bud forms as an outgrowth of the Wolffian Duct in response to external cues provided by the surrounding metanephric mesenchyme. Signals

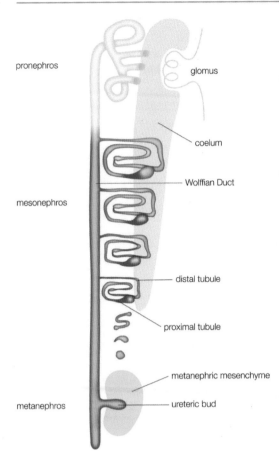

pronephros

glomus

coelum

Wolffian Duct

mesonephros

distal tubule

proximal tubule

metanephric mesenchyme

metanephros

ureteric bud

Fig. 8.1 Schematic overview of kidney development. Mammalian kidney development begins with the formation of the Wolffian duct, which is divided into three segments: pronephros, mesonephros and metanephros. The pronephros degenerates in mammals, whereas the mesonephros forms the male reproductive organs (rete testis, efferent ducts, epididymis, vas deferens, seminal vesicles and prostate). The metanephros becomes the mature mammalian kidney, and forms via inductive interactions between the metanephric mesenchyme and the ureteric bud (Used with permission of Springer Science + Business Media from Moritz [23])

that promote and direct ureteric bud branching morphogenesis originate from all derivative cell types of the metanephric mesenchyme, including induced and uninduced mesenchyme [34–36], stromal cells [37–41], and angioblasts [42, 43], as well as the ureteric bud itself [44]. The metanephric mesenchyme, in turn, originates from undifferentiated cells in the intermediate mesoderm adjacent to the Wolffian Duct, to form nephrons and the renal stroma [33]. Similarly, the

metanephric mesenchyme responds to inductive cues supplied by the ureteric bud and renal stroma to initiate nephron formation [16, 19, 45–47]. Subsequent patterning and differentiation of the cell types of the nephron is highly dependent on factors supplied by developing epithelial and stromal cells [40, 48, 49].

Induction of Nephrons from the Metanephric Mesenchyme

Once induced by the ureteric bud, the metanephric mesenchyme condenses around the ureteric bud tip, resulting in formation of the cap mesenchyme (Fig. 8.2a, b). The cap mesenchyme is thought to represent a population of nephron progenitors, as these cells have the capacity to self-renew to generate an appropriate number of nephrons at the end of kidney development, and to differentiate into the multiple cell types required to form a mature nephron [51, 52]. The molecules that regulate the specification, proliferation, survival and differentiation of nephron progenitors are of great interest to researchers, because an improved understanding of these processes may guide the development of novel cell-based therapies for chronic kidney disease.

The differentiation of the cap mesenchyme involves a process termed *mesenchymal-epithelial transformation* (MET). A localized cluster of cells separates from the cap mesenchyme under the ureteric bud tip, and acquires epithelial characteristics, becoming a "pre-tubular aggregate" (Fig. 8.2a, b) [53]. Simultaneous with epithelialization, an internal cavity forms within the pre-tubular aggregate, at which point the structure is termed a renal vesicle. The renal vesicle subsequently forms a connection with its neighbouring ureteric bud ampulla, permitting the ureteric bud lumen to communicate with the internal cavity of the renal vesicle. Further differentiation of the renal vesicle in a spatially organized proximal-distal pattern results in formation of the glomerular and tubular segments of the mature nephron.

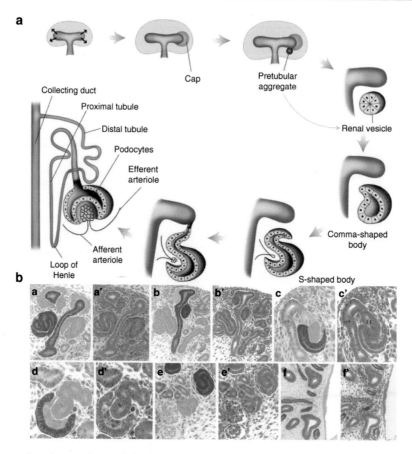

Fig. 8.2 Stages of nephrogenesis. (**a**) Induction of the metanephric mesenchyme by the ureteric bud promotes aggregation of the cap mesenchyme around the tip of the ureteric bud. The cap mesenchyme subsequently undergoes a mesenchymal to epithelial transition to form the pretubular aggregate, followed by a polarized renal vesicle. A cleft forms in the renal vesicle giving rise to the comma- shaped body. The development of the S-shaped body involves the formation of a proximal cleft which is subsequently invaded by angioblasts and starts the process of glomerulogenesis. Fusion of S-shaped body occurs with the collecting ducts. (Used with permission of Springer Science + Business Media from Moritz [23]). (**b**) Series of matched-pair histological images from a developing metanephric kidney with colouring for specific developmental stages. (*a, a′*) The ureteric tip and renal cortical collecting duct are in red, with the cap mesenchyme in green. Derivatives of the cap mesenchyme include the comma-shaped body in light blue and S-shaped body in dark blue. (*b, b′*) Next to the ureteric bud and renal cortical collecting duct (*red*) is a pretubular aggregate (*yellow*), a renal vesicle (*dark blue*), capillary loop stage developing glomerulus (*green*) and renal tubules (*light blue*). (*c, c′*) Segments of the S-shaped body include the visceral epithelium (*red*), parietal epithelium (*dark blue*), medial segment (*green*), distal segment (*yellow*) and renal junctional tubule (*light blue*). (*d, d′*) Segments of the capillary loop stage developing glomerulus include the visceral epithelium (*red*), parietal epithelium (*dark blue*), presumptive mesangium (*green*) and renal tubule (*light blue*). (*e, e′*) Image of the cortex of the metanephros showing different stages of glomerular development: an S-shaped body (*dark blue*), capillary loop stage (*green*) and maturing glomeruli (*yellow*). (*f, f′*) Image of the renal medulla and pelvis of the metanephros showing the renal medullary interstitium (*yellow*), medullary collecting ducts (*red*), immature loop of Henle (*dark blue*), renal medullary vasculature (*green*) and renal pelvic urothelial lining (*blue*) (Used with permission of Elsevier from Little et al. [50])

Specification of the Metanephric Mesenchyme

The formation of the metanephric mesenchyme is genetically marked by up-regulated expression of the transcription factors *Wilms tumour 1 (Wt1)* [54], *Sal-like 1 (Sall1)* [55], *Pax2* [28], *Cbp/p300- interacting transactivator, with Glu/Asp-rich carboxy-terminal domain, 1 (Cited1)* [56] and *sine oculis homeobox homolog 2 (Six2)* [57], and by expression of transmembrane molecules *cadherin-11* [58] and *α8 integrin* (Fig. 8.3a, b) [62]. *Sall1* [55], *Six1* [63], *Eyes absent homolog 1 (Eya1)* [64, 65] and the secreted peptide growth factor, *Glial-derived neurotrophic factor (Gdnf)* [66], are expressed in intermediate mesoderm in the presumptive metanephric mesenchyme. *Wt1*, *Cited1* and *Six2* expression is induced in the cap mesenchyme at the onset of ureteric bud outgrowth [54, 56, 57]. *Pax2* [67] and *Lhx1* [68] are also expressed in cap mesenchyme and its early epithelial derivatives.

Phenotypic analyses of mice with targeted gene deletions or tissue-specific inactivation of conditional alleles for these transcription factors have been informative regarding their role in specification of the cap mesenchyme, and subsequent induction of ureteric bud outgrowth. Homozygous deletion in many of these genes (including: *Eya1* [65], *Six1* [63], *Pax2* [69, 70], *Wt1* [54], *Sall1* [55], *Six2* [57] and *Lhx1* [68, 71]) causes ureteric bud outgrowth failure, and results in bilateral renal agenesis or severe renal dysgenesis with variable penetrance depending on the gene involved (Fig. 8.3e, f). Shared features of these mutant phenotypes include arrest of ureteric bud induction, loss of cap mesenchyme and/ or arrest of mesenchymal-epithelial induction. Of note, the arrest of ureteric bud induction is commonly the result of loss of *Gdnf* expression in the metanephric mesenchyme, which is critical for ureteric bud induction (discussed below in Sect. Ureteric Bud Induction and Branching).

The mechanism responsible for renal agenesis/ severe dysgenesis in each of these mutants is variable, however. For example, *Pax2* mutants fail to form the posterior Wolffian Duct from which derives the ureteric bud [70]. In contrast, *Lhx1* [68, 72] and *Sall1* [55] mutants initiate, but do not complete, ureteric bud induction. *Wt1* mutants also exhibit failed ureteric bud induction and show apoptosis of the metanephric mesenchyme [54] (Fig. 8.3e, f). Tissue recombination experiments show that isolated metanephric mesenchyme explants from *Wt1* knock-out mice are neither competent to respond to signals from wild-type ureteric buds, nor able to induce growth and branching of isolated wild-type ureteric bud explants [54, 73]. In contrast, *Sall1*-deficient mesenchyme, which express *Wt1*, responds to a heterologous inducer in ex vivo tissue recombination experiments [55], suggesting that *Sall1* functions downstream of *Wt1* in a genetic regulatory cascade. Taken together, these data present an emerging image of intricate interplay between transcription factors that are required for the establishment of the nephric duct, subsequent specification of the cap mesenchyme, induction of *Gdnf* expression, and regulation of the differentiation capacity of the cap mesenchyme in response to inductive cues from surrounding ureteric and stromal cells.

There is a growing body of work defining the signals required to induce and regulate nephron progenitors, resulting in the expression of the above-mentioned transcription factors that signify a nephron progenitor cell fate. These signals are responsible for maintaining a delicate balance between the ability of nephron progenitors to self-renew (or, proliferate) and differentiate into multiple cell-types during nephrogenesis. Of these, the growth factor, *Wingless-type MMTV integration site family 9b (Wnt9b)*, is required in the ureteric bud for induction of the cap mesenchyme (Fig. 8.3b). The loss of *Wnt9b* activity results in failure of the cap mesenchyme to undergo MET [74]. Moreover, recent data suggest that *Wnt9b* plays an important role in regulating the balance between nephron progenitor differentiation and self-renewal, in cooperation with signals mediated by stromal cells [47, 75].

Fibroblast growth factor (FGF) signaling has also been shown to be critical in regulating nephron progenitors. The FGF ligands belong to a large family of secreted peptides that signal through their cognate receptor tyrosine kinases, FGFRs. Several FGFs are expressed in the developing kidney, including FGF2, FGF7, FGF8, and FGF10 [41, 76, 77] (Fig. 8.3a–h′). Two FGF ligands, *Fgf9* and *Fgf20*, have been shown to be critical in regulating nephron progenitor survival, proliferation and competence to respond to inductive signals in mice and humans, with loss of these signals regulating in renal agenesis [78]. These in vivo findings were supported by in vitro studies showing that the addition of FGF1, 2, 9 and 20 protein results in the ability to maintain early nephron progenitor cells in culture [79]. In addition, in vivo

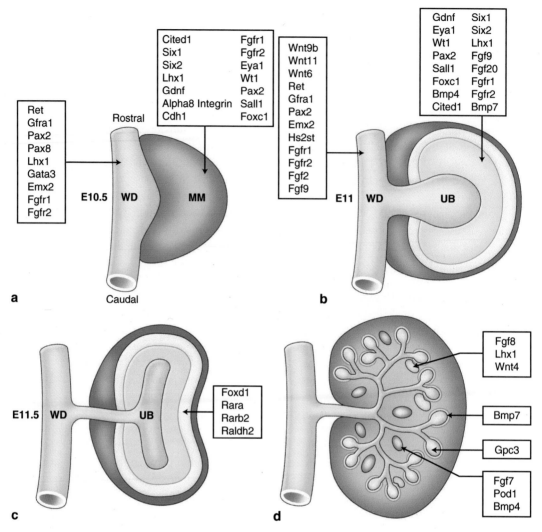

Fig. 8.3 Molecules involved in specification of the metanephric mesenchyme and nephron induction. (**a**) The mammalian kidney starts to develop when the ureteric bud forms at the caudal end of the Wolffian Duct (*WD*) at about embryonic day (**e**) 10.5 in mice. The ureteric bud grows into the metanephric mesenchyme (*MM*) and (**b**) induces the mesenchyme that is adjacent to the tips of the ureteric bud (*UB*) to condense to form the cap mesenchyme, as well as the stromal cells that are peripheral to the cap. (**c**) The cap mesenchyme induces the ureteric bud to branch from E11.5 onwards. (**d**) In association with ureteric branching morphogenesis, mesenchymal cells are induced at each ureteric bud tip to undergo a mesenchymal-to-epithelial transformation to form the nephron. *Bmp7* bone morphogenetic protein 7, *Emx2* empty spiracles 2, *Eya1* eyes absent 1, *Fgf7* fibroblast growth factor 7, *Foxc1* forkhead box C1, *Foxd1* forkhead box D1, *Gdnf1* glial cell-line-derived neurotrophic factor 1, *Gfra1* glial cell-line derived neurotrophic factor receptor-α1, *Gpc3* glypican-3, *Hs2st* heparan sulfate 2-O-sulphotransferase 1, *Pax1* paired-box gene 1, *Rara* retinoic acid receptor-α, *Ret* Ret proto-oncogene, *Sall1* sal-like 1.; *Wnt* wingless-related, *Wt1* wilms tumour 1 (Used with permission from Nature Publishing Group from Vainio and Lin [59]); Representative kidney phenotypes of mice with targeted deletions affecting nephron progenitors and nephron induction. (**e**, **f**) Histological transverse sections from E11.5 embryos showing a wild-type (**e**) and *Wt1* mutant embryo (**f**) with the ureteric bud (*U*), Wolffian duct (*W*) and metanephric mesenchyme (*M*) labeled. (**e′**, **f′**) At higher magnification, a cluster of apoptotic cells with dark nuclear fragments is visualized in the Wt1 mutant kidney, resulting in loss of nephron progenitors (*arrow*) (Used with permission of Elsevier from Kreidberg et al. [60]); (**g**, **h′**) Loss of *Wnt4* results in renal hypoplasia and failure of nephron induction, with no epithelial to mesenchymal transition when comparing control (**g**, **g′**) to control kidneys (**h**, **h′**) (Used with permission of Nature Publishing Group from Stark et al. [61])

Fig. 8.3   (continued)

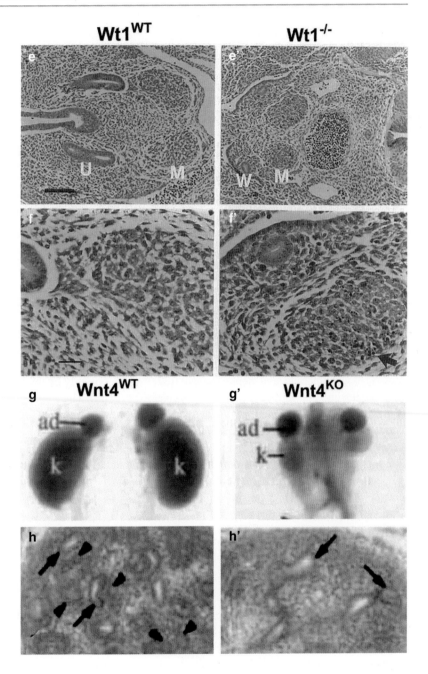

data are consistent with a functionally important role for *Fgfr1* and *Fgfr2* in the metanephric mesenchyme during kidney development, with loss of *Fgr1* and *Fgfr2* function in the metanephric mesenchyme resulting in renal agenesis [80–82].

In vitro studies demonstrate an interaction between FGF and Bone Morphogenetic Protein (BMP) signaling. *Bmp7* inhibits mesenchymal apoptosis and, in conjunction with FGF2, maintains the competence of mesenchyme to respond to inductive signals (Fig. 8.3a–h'). However, the combined effects of BMP7 and FGF2 in kidney organ culture block tubulogenesis [83]. This in vitro observation has led to the speculation that *Bmp7* functions with FGF2 to balance mesenchymal differentiation and renewal [17].

Consistent with this hypothesis is the demonstration in mice deficient for *Bmp7* of developmental arrest and rudimentary kidneys without inhibiting the differentiation of already induced cells, which is likely to due failure to expand and renew the epithelial precursor population [84, 85].

The regulation of nephron progenitor survival is likely to be important as well. Archetypal organ culture experiments have demonstrated that isolated metanephric mesenchyme undergoes apoptosis unless induced by co-culture with ureteric buds or a heterologous inducer (e.g., spinal cord) [15, 35]. These data suggest that the default program for the mesenchyme is death, unless induction otherwise occurs [53]. Several soluble factors have been described to be essential to prevent apoptosis, e.g., Epidermal growth factor (EGF), FGF2, and BMP7 [45, 83, 86]. However, inhibition of apoptosis by pharmacologic or genetic manipulation causes defects in ureteric bud branching and nephrogenesis [87, 88], suggesting that alterations in cell survival disrupt important functional interactions between mesenchymal and epithelial cells. Possible roles for apoptosis in the metanephric mesenchyme include regulation of nephron number or establishment of tissue boundaries between cells destined to become epithelial or stromal [89, 90].

Nephron Induction

Seminal experiments involving isolated kidney rudiments cultured ex vivo established the role of ureteric bud-derived secreted factors in providing inductive cues for cap mesenchyme to undergo epithelial differentiation to initiate tubulogenesis [35]. The isolation of ureteric bud cell lines has subsequently facilitated the identification of several secreted factors that function individually or in combination to cause mesenchymal-epithelial conversion and tubulogenesis in vitro, including FGF2 [91], leukemia inhibitory factor (LIF) [46, 92, 93], transforming growth factor-β2 (TGFβ2) [93, 94], and growth/differentiation factor-11 (GDF-11) [93, 95].

Wnt genes also play a key role in epithelial conversion, as suggested by the observation that cells expressing WNT proteins are potent inducers of tubulogenesis in isolated metanephric mesenchyme [96, 97]. A genetic requirement for *Wnt4* in MET is revealed by the demonstration of the arrest of the cap mesenchyme, and the inability to form pretubular aggregates, in *Wnt4* mutant mice [74] (Fig. 8.3d, g, h). The effects of Wnt signals are modulated by mesenchymal-derived secreted Wnt binding proteins including secreted Frizzled-related protein (sFrp). sFrp antagonizes the actions of Wnt4 and Wnt9b by binding secreted Wnt proteins in vitro and preventing them from activating membrane-bound Wnt receptors [98]. Similar to the induction of nephron progenitors, FGF signaling is also critical for MET. Mice with deletions in *Fgf8* fail to undergo tubulogenesis, and the data suggest that *Wnt4* and *Fgf8* cooperate in the conversion of mesenchymal to epithelial cells, possibly by up-regulating *Lhx1* expression [99, 100]. The transcription factor, *Lhx1*, is uniformly expressed in renal vesicles [68], and conditional knockout of *Lhx1* in metanephric mesenchyme causes developmental arrest at the renal vesicle stage [68].

Ureteric Bud Induction and Branching

Ureteric bud formation is initiated at week 5 of human fetal gestation and at embryonic day 10.5 (E10.5) in mice. Signals from the metanephric mesenchyme induce the ureteric bud to form, elongate, and invade the mesenchyme (Fig. 8.4a). Further development of the collecting duct system involves a process termed *branching morphogenesis*, defined as the formation of branched tubules [104]. Renal branching morphogenesis may be considered as a sequence of related events, which include: (i) outgrowth of the ureteric bud; (ii) iterative branching of the ureteric bud and derivation of its daughter collecting ducts; (iii) patterning of the cortical and medullary collecting duct system; and (iv) formation of the pelvicalyceal system.

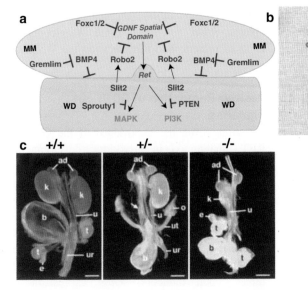

Fig. 8.4 Schematic demonstrating the molecular control of ureteric bud branching. (**a**) Glial cell-line derived neurotrophic factor (*GDNF*) is secreted from the mesenchyme (*grey*) and binds to the Ret receptor to induce a thickening of the WD (*pink*); the WD will then elongate to form the UB. Binding of GDNF to RET leads to activation of the MAPK and PI3K signal transduction pathways. These pathways are negatively regulated by SPROUTY1 and PTEN, respectively. SLIT2/ROBO2 and FOXC1 and FOXC2 inhibit the spatial GDNF expression domain and limit UB outpouching to a single site. BMP4 inhibits branching, in a manner that is opposed by Gremlin. RED Inhibitory, Green stimulatory, Grey MM and GDNF spatial domain, Pink WD (Used with permission of Springer Science + Business Media from Bridgewater and Rosenblum [101]); Representative kidney phenotypes of mice having targeted mutations affecting branching morphogenesis. (**b**) Severe bilateral renal hypoplasia in *Ret* null mutants. *A* adrenal, *K* kidney, *U* ureter, *B* bladder (Used with permission of Nature Publishing Group from Schuchardt et al. [102]); (**c**) Bilateral renal agenesis in *GDNF* mutant mice (Used with permission of Nature Publishing Group from Pichel et al. [103])

Ureteric Bud Induction and Outgrowth

Genes encoding *Gdnf* [105], its tyrosine kinase receptor *Ret* [106], and its co-receptor *Gfrα-1* [107], are recognized as crucial regulators of ureteric bud outgrowth. Targeted mutagenesis of *Gdnf* in mice causes bilateral renal aplasia due to ureteric bud outgrowth failure [108, 109] (Fig. 8.4b). Similarly, homozygous deletion of *Ret* or *Gfrα1* causes the same defect [106, 110–113] (Fig. 8.4c). However, in 20–40 % of *Gdnf−/−* or *Ret−/−* mutant offspring, the aplastic renal phenotype is not fully penetrant and initial ureteric bud outgrowth is evident [106, 108], indicating that ureteric bud outgrowth is not under the exclusive control of GDNF-RET signaling. Other molecular pathways likely to play important roles include signaling through integrins, as revealed by the demonstration that approximately 50 % of mouse embryos deficient in the *α8* integrin gene show termination of ureteric bud outgrowth at the point of contact with the metanephric mesenchyme [62]. Likewise, 100 % of mice with a homozygous null mutation in the gene *heparan sulfate 2-sulfotransferase (Hs2st)* [114], which is involved in proteoglycan synthesis, show a similar phenotype.

The downstream effect of GDNF-RET signalling is ureteric bud proliferation, cell survival and branching of the epithelium, and recent data are shedding light on the molecules involved in these processes. The ETS transcription factors, *Etv4* and *Etv5*, are up-regulated in response to RET signaling, and loss of both transcription factors results in bilateral renal agenesis [115]. *Etv4* and *Etv5* function is necessary for the expression of several key genes in the ureteric bud tip, such as *Wnt11, Chemokine (C-X-C motif) receptor 4*

(*Cxcr4*), *Matrix metallopeptidase 14* (*Mmp14*), *Myb proto-oncogene* (*Myb*) and *Met proto-oncogene* (*Met*) [115]. *Wnt11* is expressed in ureteric bud tips [116, 117]. Loss of *Wnt11* in mice results in reduced levels of GDNF in the metanephric mesenchyme and reduced ureteric bud branching morphogenesis, suggesting that Wnt11 functions to maintain *Gdnf* expression in the metanephric mesenchyme [118]. In vitro, GDNF stimulates cell proliferation in cultured primary ureteric bud cells [119], as well as in collecting ducts of whole kidney explants [116, 120]. GDNF does not, however, stimulate cell proliferation in isolated ureteric bud explants, although it does promote ureteric bud cell survival by inhibiting apoptosis [105]. Thus, while GDNF may exert direct inhibitory effects on apoptosis, it may require the presence of other factors for its proliferative effects in the ureteric bud lineage.

Failure to induce ureteric bud outgrowth results in renal agenesis, which occurs unilaterally or bilaterally if the ureteric bud fails to form on one or both Wolffian Ducts, respectively [121]. Additional signals are required to restrict the number of ureteric buds induced to form from the Wolffian Duct, as revealed by the demonstration of renal and urogenital malformations in humans and mice when ectopic outgrowth of multiple ureteric buds from a single Wolffian Duct is observed (e.g., duplex kidney) [122]. Moreover, the relative position of ureteric bud outgrowth from the Wolffian Duct appears to be crucial to formation of a single ureter and competent vesico-ureteral junction. A relationship between ectopic positioning of ureteric bud outgrowth and vesico-ureteral reflux is largely supported by evidence from Mackie and Stephens who described defects in vesico-ureteral junction formation in patients with ureteral duplications [123]. Based on their observations, they postulated that when outgrowth of the ureteric bud occurs at an ectopic site, the final site of the ureteral orifice in the bladder will be ectopic [123]. These data are supported by phenotypic analyses of mice with mutations in *Bmp4* [124], *Roundabout, axon guidance receptor, homolog 2* (*Robo2*) [125], components of the renin-angiotensin cascade [88, 126] and *Fgfr2* [127, 128] which show ureteral duplications or vesico-ureteral reflux and demonstrate ectopic placement of ureteric bud formation on the Wolffian Duct.

Positive Regulation of GDNF-ret Signaling

Stemming from the importance of the GDNF-RET signaling axis in early kidney development, considerable attention has been given to identifying the genes that regulate the function of *Gdnf* and *Ret*. Prior to kidney development, *Gdnf* is expressed along the entire length of the intermediate mesoderm parallel to the Wolffian Duct [105]. Likewise, *Ret* is expressed throughout the Wolffian Duct at this stage [32]. At the time of ureteric bud induction, *Gdnf* expression is restricted to the posterior intermediate mesoderm, marking the location of the presumptive metanephric mesenchyme in close proximity to the site of ureteric bud outgrowth. When the ureteric bud begins to invade the metanephric mesenchyme, *Ret* expression becomes spatially restricted to the tips of ureteric bud branches [32]. In vitro studies involving the application of GDNF-soaked agarose beads demonstrate that the entire length of the Wolffian Duct is competent to respond to ectopic GDNF and initiate the morphogenetic program for ureteric bud branching [105, 116]. These data suggest that the spatial activity of GDNF-RET signaling must be tightly regulated for a single ureteric bud to form. The demonstration of renal malformations including duplex kidney and hydronephrosis in transgenic mice that ectopically express *Gdnf* or *Ret* throughout the length of the Wolffian Duct further underscores the importance of posterior restriction of GDNF-RET signaling activity to establishing normal renal number and form [129, 130].

Functional and genetic evidence support the role of three transcription factor genes expressed in intermediate mesoderm – *Eya1*, *Six1*, and *Pax2* – in a molecular cascade which promotes *Gdnf* expression during kidney development (Fig. 8.3a). *Eya1* and *Six1* are placed at the top of this cascade based on the loss of *Gdnf* expression in mice mutant for either *Eya1* or *Six1* [131]. *Eya1* is expressed in an overlapping domain with

Gdnf in the presumptive metanephric mesenchyme at the time of ureteric bud outgrowth [65]. *Eya1* knock-out mice exhibit renal agenesis resulting from failed ureteric bud outgrowth due to loss of *Gdnf* expression [65]. *Six1* null mice also show failed ureteric bud induction, normal *Eya1* expression, and subsequent apoptosis of the mesenchyme [63]. *Pax2* is expressed in the intermediate mesoderm and directly activates *Gdnf* transcription [67].

In addition to *Eya1*, *Six1*, and *Pax2*, other activators of *Gdnf* expression have been identified, including the paralogous genes *Homeobox A11 (Hoxa11)*, *Hoxc11*, and *Hoxd11*. Compound inactivation of at least two of these genes causes renal aplasia and loss of *Gdnf* and *Six2* expression [132]. Since *Eya1* and *Pax2* expression are normal in hox compound mutant mice, it has been suggested that hox genes maintain *Gdnf* expression by cooperating with *Eya1* to induce *Six1 and Six2* expression [131]. An additional regulatory mechanism for the maintenance of *Gdnf* expression involves *Empty spiracles homolog 2 (Emx2)*, a transcription factor expressed in the Wolffian Duct [133]. *Emx2* null mice exhibit bilateral renal agenesis due to failure of the ureteric bud to form its first branch following induction [133]. Morphogenetic arrest in these mutants is associated with down-regulation of ureteric bud markers *Ret*, *Pax2*, *Lhx1* as well as *Gdnf* in the metanephric mesenchyme. Tissue recombination experiments between isolated wild-type and mutant *Emx2* kidney rudiments reveal that the mutant ureteric bud is incompetent to induce metanephric mesenchyme [133]. These data suggest *Emx2* may be important in the nascent ureteric bud for providing cues to maintain *Gdnf* expression in the mesenchyme and sustain ureteric bud branching morphogenesis.

Negative Regulation of GDNF-ret Signaling

Negative regulation of *Gdnf* expression is equally important in controlling both the location, and number, of ureteric buds induced. At least three genes – *Foxc1*, *Slit2*, and *Robo2* – are involved in restricting *Gdnf* expression to the posterior intermediate mesoderm (Fig. 8.4a). In support of this conclusion is the demonstration of ectopic ureteric bud formation, multiple ureters, hydroureter and anterior expansion of *Gdnf* expression in *Forkhead box C1 (Foxc1)*, *Slit homolog 2 (Slit2)*, or *Robo2* homozygous null mutant mice [125, 134]. *Foxc1* encodes a transcription factor expressed in an overlapping domain with *Gdnf* in the intermediate mesoderm [134]. The mechanism of defective ureteric bud induction in *Foxc1*[-/-] mutant mice is thought to result from an anterior expansion of *Eya1* and *Gdnf* expression in the intermediate mesoderm, leading to ectopic GDNF stimulation of Wolffian Duct budding [134]. The secreted protein SLIT2 and its receptor ROBO2 are encoded by genes best known for their roles in axon guidance functioning as chemorepellents that cause axons or migrating cells to move away from the source of SLIT2 [135, 136]. In the developing kidney, *Slit2* is primarily expressed in the Wolffian Duct, whereas *Robo2* is detected in a complementary pattern in the metanephric mesenchyme [137]. In *Slit2* and *Robo2* mutant mice, *Gdnf* expression is also expanded anteriorly in the posterior intermediate mesoderm; however, this expansion of *Gdnf* expression occurs independent of alterations in the expression of *Foxc1*, *Eya1*, and *Pax2* [125]. Consequently, SLIT2 and ROBO2 are likely to function in a parallel pathway to restrict GDNF-RET activity during ureteric bud outgrowth.

The gene *Sprouty1 (Spry1)* is implicated in a negative feedback loop involving GDNF-RET signaling and their downstream effector, *Wnt11*. *Spry1* is expressed along the length of the Wolffian Duct with highest levels of expression in the posterior duct [136] (Fig. 8.4a). Loss of *Spry1* function in mice results in renal malformations including multiple ureters, multiplex kidneys, and hydroureter [138, 139]. *Spry1*[-/-] mutants exhibit ectopic ureteric bud induction, and show increased expression of *Gdnf* in the metanephric mesenchyme, expanded expression of GDNF-RET target genes such as *Wnt11*, and increased sensitivity to GDNF in metanephric culture. The role of *Spry1* as a negative regulator of renal branching morphogenesis is further supported by the demonstration of decreased ureteric bud branching in transgenic mice that ectopically express human *SPRY2*, a related homologue, throughout the Wolffian Duct [140].

A second example of negative feedback in renal branching morphogenesis involves secreted growth factors belonging to the Bone Morphogenetic Protein (BMP) family. Several BMPs including *Bmp -2, -4, -5, -6,* and *-7* and their receptors are expressed in the developing kidney in distinct but partially overlapping domains [141–144]. Kidney organ culture studies have revealed inhibitory roles for BMP -2, -4, and -7 in ureteric bud branching morphogenesis [145–148]. However, convincing evidence that BMPs modulate ureteric bud outgrowth in vivo is provided only for *Bmp4* [124] (Fig. 8.4a). Mice heterozygous for *Bmp4* exhibit ectopic or duplicated ureteric buds, associated with a spectrum of renal malformations including hypodysplastic kidneys, hydroureteronephrosis and ureteral duplications [149, 150]. *Bmp4* is expressed in stromal cells immediately adjacent to the Wolffian Duct and the early ureteric bud [124, 141]. The abnormal sites of ureteric bud outgrowth in *Bmp4+/-* mice led to the proposal that BMP4 may act by antagonizing the local effect of GDNF-RET signaling at the preferential site of ureteric induction on the Wolffian Duct [124]. Support for this hypothesis is provided by the demonstration that BMP4 can block the ability of GDNF to induce ureteric bud outgrowth from Wolffian Duct in vitro [67, 151]. Exogenous BMP4 also inhibits further ureteric bud branching in vitro in an asymmetric manner [145, 146], suggesting that BMP4 may have additional roles in three-dimensional growth of the ureteric bud/collecting system.

Renal Branching Morphogenesis

Renal branching morphogenesis commences between the fifth and sixth week of gestation in humans [2], and at E11.5 in mice [15] when the ureteric bud invades the metanephric mesenchyme and forms a T-shaped, branched structure (Fig. 8.3c). This T-shaped structure subsequently undergoes further iterative branching events to generate approximately 15 generations of branches. In human kidney development, the first 9 generations of branching are completed by approximately 15 weeks gestation [2]. During this time, new nephrons are induced through reciprocal inductive interactions between the newly formed tips of the ureteric bud and surrounding metanephric mesenchyme. By the 20th–22nd week of gestation, ureteric bud branching is completed, and the remainder of collecting duct development occurs by extension of peripheral (or cortical) segments and remodeling of central (or medullary) segments [2]. During these final stages, new nephrons form predominantly through the induction of approximately four to seven nephrons around the tips of terminal collecting duct branches which have completed their branching program, while retaining the capacity to induce new nephron formation [2, 15].

Analysis of renal branching morphogenesis in organ culture systems employing kidneys of transgenic mice expressing the fluorescent reporter, enhanced green fluorescent protein (EGFP), in the ureteric bud lineage have been informative regarding the sequence and pattern of branching events that occur following the formation of the initial T structure [152, 153]. Throughout renal branching morphogenesis, the branching ureteric bud recapitulates a patterned, morphogenetic sequence. This sequence includes: (1) expansion of the advancing ureteric bud branch at its leading tip (called the ampulla); (2) division of the ampulla causing the formation of new ureteric bud branches; and (3) elongation of the newly formed branch segment.

Proliferation and Apoptosis in Branching Morphogenesis

During branching morphogenesis, cell proliferation is highly conspicuous at the tips of the ureteric bud/collecting duct branches where inductive and branching events occur [89]. In contrast, cell proliferation is detected at lower levels in the medulla and renal papilla [89]. Localized cell proliferation appears to contribute to evagination of the ureteric bud from the Wolffian Duct and formation of ampullae. During ureteric bud induction, proliferation rates are highest on the side of the Wolffian Duct where the ureteric bud forms [120]. As the ureteric bud generates new branches, proliferation rates are higher in branch tips than in trunks [44, 120, 154].

In contrast to metanephric mesenchyme which undergoes apoptosis in the absence of an inducer, isolated ureteric bud cells do not demonstrate apoptosis when cultured ex vivo [155]. The mechanism underlying cellular preservation in this context is unclear, and may reflect an intrinsic survival tendency imparted to ureteric bud-derived cells. Evidence that cell survival is regulated during renal branching morphogenesis is provided by several studies in which dysregulated apoptosis and cell proliferation are associated with defective collecting duct development. For example, increased branched ureteric bud cell proliferation and subsequent medullary collecting duct cell apoptosis were observed in *Glypican 3*[−/−] (*Gpc3*) mice which exhibit profound cystic degeneration of the medullary collecting duct system [156, 157] (Fig. 8.3d). Also, increased apoptosis was associated with collecting duct cyst formation in mice mutated for genes associated with cell survival, including *B-cell lymphoma 2* (*bcl2*) [158] and *transcription factor AP2* (*AP-2*) [159]. Moreover, apoptosis was a prominent feature of dilated collecting ducts in experimental models of fetal and neonatal urinary tract obstruction [160, 161]. These data suggest a relationship between collecting duct apoptosis and two frequent features of renal dysplasia – cystogenesis and urinary tract dilatation.

Signaling Molecules in Branching Morphogenesis

In addition to its role as a potent stimulus for ureteric bud induction, GDNF has been shown in vivo and in vitro to be a stimulus for subsequent ureteric bud branching [116, 130]. The ability of GDNF to induce ureteric bud branching in vivo is revealed by the demonstration of multiple branched ureteric buds in transgenic mice which express *Gdnf* ectopically in the Wolffian Duct lineage [130]. However, in vitro studies show that recombinant GDNF is not sufficient to induce robust branching in isolated ureteric bud culture [105, 162]. These latter data suggest that

other factors cooperate with GDNF-RET to control ureteric bud branching.

One of these factors is WNT signaling. For example, *Wnt11* is expressed at the tips of the ureteric bud, and in mice that are deficient for *Wnt11*, there are defects in branching morphogenesis and consequent renal hypoplasia [117, 118] (Fig. 8.3b). The data suggest that *Wnt11* functions, at least in part, by maintaining normal GDNF expression of GDNF, and conversely, *Wnt11* expression is reduced in the absence of GDNF-RET signaling. Beta-catenin is a critical effector regulating downstream transcriptional targets of the canonical WNT pathway. The loss of b-catenin in the ureteric epithelium results in abnormal branching, loss of expression of key genes in the ureteric bud tip, and premature expression of differentiated collecting duct epithelia genes [163, 164]. Together, this suggests parallel signaling pathways that act in concert to regulate branching morphogenesis.

In addition to Wnts, in vitro studies testing the effects of recombinant FGFs on isolated ureteric bud cultures indicate that all members of the FGF family support growth and cell proliferation of the ureteric bud [76]. These observations are consistent with the demonstration of decreased ureteric bud branching, decreased cell proliferation, and increased ureteric bud apoptosis in mice following conditional mutational inactivation of the FGF receptor gene, *Fgfr2*, in the ureteric bud lineage [81, 165, 166] (Fig. 8.3b). Interestingly, FGF family members exert unique spatial effects on ureteric bud cell proliferation in vitro. For example, FGF10 preferentially stimulates cell proliferation at the ureteric bud tips, whereas FGF7 induces cell proliferation in a non-selective manner throughout the developing collecting duct system [76]. These data suggest that multiple FGF family members may function coordinately to control three-dimensional growth of the developing collecting duct system. FGF7 has also been shown to induce the expression of the Sprouty gene, *Spry2*, in developing collecting ducts in vitro [140]. Consequently, FGF7 may also participate with *Spry2* in a feedback loop that controls ureteric bud branching by regulating *Gdnf* and *Wnt11* expression.

Several other secreted peptides, including hepatocyte growth factor (HGF), transforming growth factor alpha (TGFα), EGF, and FGF1 stimulate branching morphogenesis in vitro [76, 167–169]. However, in vivo evidence does not support essential roles for these factors since kidney development is normal when genes encoding these proteins are mutated in mice [170–172]. Thus, other mechanisms may compensate for their loss of function during kidney development.

GDNF, FGF7, and TGF-β have also been shown to promote the expression of tissue inhibitors of metalloproteinases (TIMPs) from cultured ureteric bud cells [173, 174]. TIMPS regulate the local activity of extracellular matrix metalloproteases (MMPs), which are implicated in altering the composition of the extracellular matrix to facilitate branch initiation. This concept is supported by the demonstration that TIMPs block ureteric bud branching in vitro [173, 175]. Consequently, growth factors may play an important role in regulating the local activity of matrix-degrading proteases by controlling TIMP expression.

Formation of Nephrons

Proximal-distal patterning of nephron epithelial cell fate, as reflected by the formation of tubular and glomerular cell fate domains, is a crucial step in nephron segmentation. Nephron segmentation begins with the sequential formation of two clefts in the renal vesicle, the earliest epithelial derivative of nephron progenitors [2] (Fig. 8.2a, b). Creation of a lower cleft, termed the vascular cleft, heralds formation of the comma-shaped body. The comma-shaped body is a transient structure that rapidly undergoes morphogenetic conversion into an S-shaped structure (termed S-shaped body) upon generation of an upper cleft. The S-shaped body is characterized by three segments or limbs. The middle and upper limbs give rise to the tubular segments of the mature nephron. While the middle limb of the S-shaped body gives rise to the proximal convoluted tubule [2], the descending and ascending limbs of the loops of Henle and the distal convoluted tubule originate from the upper limb of the S-shaped body [2, 15] (Fig. 8.5a). As the vascular cleft broadens and deepens, the lower limb of the S-shaped body forms a cup-shaped unit (Fig. 8.5b). Epithelial cells lining the inner wall of this cup will comprise the visceral glomerular epithelium, or podocytes. Cells lining the outer wall of the cup will form parietal glomerular epithelium, or Bowman's capsule.

All parts of the developing nephron increase in size as they become mature. However, the most striking changes consist of increased tortuosity of the proximal convoluted tubule, and elongation of the loop of Henle [2]. Cellular maturation of the proximal tubule involves transition from columnar to cuboidal epithelium, elaboration of apical and basal microvilli, and gradual increase in tubular diameter and length [179]. The human kidney at birth shows marked heterogeneity in proximal tubule length as one progresses from the outer cortex to the inner cortex [180]. Uniformity in proximal tubule length is achieved by 1 month of life, which subsequently lengthens at a uniform rate. Prospective cells of the loop of Henle are thought to be first positioned at the junctional region of the middle and upper limbs of the S-shaped body near the vascular pole of the glomerulus, where it will form the macula densa [181]. The descending and ascending limbs of the presumptive loop of Henle are first recognizable as a U-shaped structure in the periphery of the developing renal cortex, termed the nephrogenic zone [181, 182]. Maturation of the primitive loop involves elongation of both ascending and descending limbs through the cortico-medullary boundary. Continued maturation involves differentiation of descending and ascending limb epithelia [183]. Development of the presumptive distal tubule involves elongation of the connecting segment, which joins with the ureteric bud/collecting duct.

Longitudinal growth of the medulla contributes to lengthening of the loops of Henle such that all but a small percentage of the loops of Henle extend below the corticomedullary junction in full term newborn infants [2]. As the kidney increases in size post-natally, the loops of

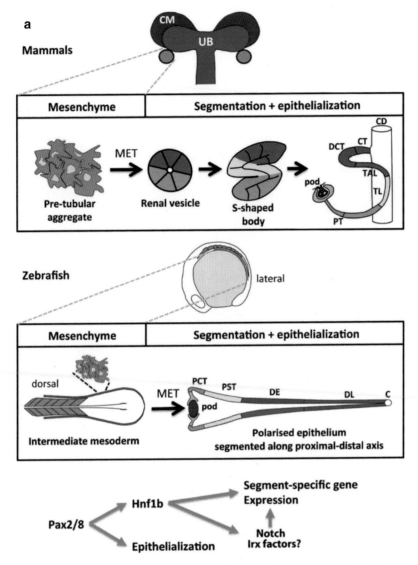

Fig. 8.5 Schematic of nephron segmentation. (**a**) The stages of mammalian metanephric nephron developed are shown, with colors denoting the segmentation of the renal vesicle, S-shaped body and mature nephron (Used with permission of Springer Science + Business Media from Naylor and Davidson [176]); (**b**) Dual section in situ hybridization and immunohistochemistry for Wt1 (*brown*) and Wnt4 (*purple*) in the mouse kidney at embryonic day 15.5. (1) Wt1 and Wnt4 expression in a pretubular aggregate. (2) Wt1 in a pretubular aggregate (*arrowhead*) and the proximal portion of the renal vesicle (*arrow*). (3) Wt1 expression in the lower limb of the comma-shaped body. (4) Wt1 in the podocytes and parietal epithelium of the proximal segment of an early S-shape body. (5) Wt1 in podocyte and parietal epithelium of the proximal segment of an S-shape body (Used with permission of Springer Science + Business Media from Georgas et al. [177]); (**c**) Representative kidney phenotype of mice with a conditional mutation affecting nephron segmentation. Loss of Notch2 in the metanephric mesenchyme results in loss of proximal nephron elements (glomeruli, proximal tubules and S-shaped bodies). *Red arrows* glomeruli, *green* proximal tubule, *yellow* S-shaped bodies; turquoise, collecting duct (Used with permission from Cheng et al. [178])

b

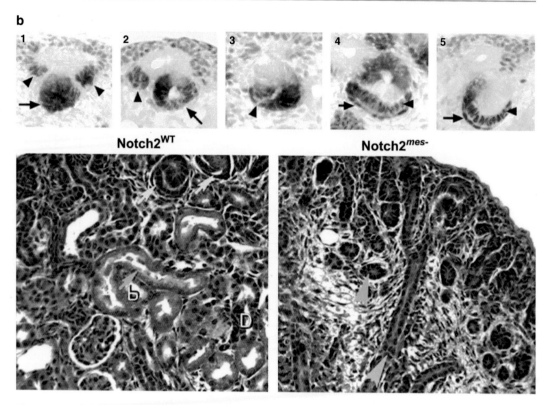

Fig. 8.5 (continued)

Henle further elongate and reach the inner two-thirds of the renal medulla in the mature kidney. Functional development of the kidney's urine concentrating mechanism is dependent on elongation of the loops of Henle during nephrogenesis since longer loops favour urine concentrating capacity. In the extremely premature fetus, the loops of Henle are short owing to the relative distance between the renal capsule and the renal papilla. Consequently, the urine concentrating capacity of the premature kidney is limited by generation of a shallow medullary tonicity gradient.

Nephron Segmentation

Proximal-distal patterning of nephron epithelial cell fate, as reflected by the formation of glomerular and tubular cell fate domains, is a crucial step in nephron segmentation. One mechanism for patterning glomerular and tubu-

lar cell fates in the S-shaped body appears to be dependent on negative feedback between *Wt1* and *Pax2* [184–186] (Fig. 8.5b). During early kidney development, the expression patterns of *Pax2* and *Wt1* become restricted in S-shaped bodies such that the expression domain of *Pax2* is complementary to the corresponding domain for *Wt1*. *Wt1* expression is restricted to glomerular epithelial precursors, which give rise to podocytes later in the glomerular development [187]. In contrast, *Pax2* expression is restricted to that portion which gives rise to tubular epithelial precursors of the proximal and distal nephron segments, and is later repressed in differentiated tubular epithelium [99, 188]. The precise roles for *Wt1* or *Pax2* in nephron differentiation is not evident from the analyses of renal phenotypes in mice with targeted *Wt1* or *Pax2* mutations since these mutants fail to form kidneys [54, 70]. However, evidence from transgenic mice that over-express PAX2 in all nephrogenic cell types illustrates the importance of spatially restricting *Pax2* expression during early nephrogenesis since these mice exhibit dysplastic kidneys with defective differentiation of both tubular and glomerular epithelia [189].

Two other transcription factors expressed at the renal vesicle stage, *Lhx1* and *Brn1*, also appear to be involved in initiating proximal-distal nephron epithelial cell fate patterning. While *Lhx1* is uniformly expressed in renal vesicles [68], *Brain specific homeobox 1 (Brn1)* expression occurs in a more spatially restricted pattern in renal vesicles [182]. Conditional knockout of *Lhx1* in the metanephric mesenchyme causes developmental arrest at the renal vesicle stage, and results in loss of *Brn1* expression [68]. In contrast, targeted deletion of *Brn1* in the metanephric mesenchyme does not prevent the early stages of nephron morphogenesis, but blocks formation of the loop of Henle, and suppresses terminal differentiation of distal nephron epithelia [182]. Taken together, these data suggest that *Brn1* functions downstream of *Lhx1* in a genetic hierarchy which establishes proximal and distal cell fates. An additional role for *Lhx1* in specifying podocyte cell fate is revealed by the analysis of *Lhx1* chimeric mutant mice [68].

Genetic evidence in mice suggests that the process for selecting which nephrogenic progenitors will comprise the proximal portion of the developing nephron (i.e., the podocytes and proximal convoluted tubule) is dependent on Notch signaling [190–192]. Conditional knock-out of *Notch2* and *Recombining binding protein suppressor of hairless (Rbpsuh)*, but not *Notch1*, in metanephric mesenchyme prior to nephron segmentation results in complete lack of both proximal tubule and glomerular epithelia [191] (Fig. 8.5c). Similar effects were observed in mutant mice when presenilin-mediated Notch activation was abrogated by mutagenesis of *Psen1* and *Psen2* [192], and in cultured metanephroi when Notch signaling is blocked following treatment with the γ-secretase inhibitor, DAPT [190]. Moreover, ectopic Notch activation in nephron progenitors results in premature differentiation and MET, with a preference towards proximal tubule cell fate [193].

Glomerulogenesis

During embryonic development, formation of the lower limb of the S-shaped body heralds the onset of glomerulogenesis [2, 194] (Fig. 8.6a). The vascular cleft provides an entry point to which progenitor endothelial and mesangial cells are recruited [197]. Cells residing along the inner surface of the lower S-shaped body limb represent nascent podocytes. At this stage, immature podocytes are proliferative and exhibit a columnar shape, apical cell attachments and a single-layer basement membrane [194]. Development of the glomerular capillary tuft is a dynamic process involving recruitment and proliferation of endothelial and mesangial cell precursors, formation of a capillary plexus, and concomitant assembly of podocytes and mesangial cells distributed around the newly formed capillary loops [194].

The origin of endothelial cell precursors is the subject of ongoing research. Experimental evidence involving autologous transplantation of embryonic kidney rudiments into adult renal cortex suggests that glomerular endothelial precursors, or angioblasts, originate from a unique subpopulation of induced metanephric mesenchyme that do not differentiate along epithelial lineages [197–199]. In contrast, an alternate theory is provided by evidence that glomerular capillaries originate from ingrowth of primitive sprouts from external vessels through experiments involving engraftment of rodent fetal kidneys onto avian chorioallantoic membrane [200]. These latter experiments support the potential role of angiogenesis in glomerular capillary tuft development.

Although clear cause and effect relationships are not known, recruitment of angioblasts and mesangial precursors into the vascular cleft results in deformation of the lower S-shaped body limb into a cup-like structure [2] (Fig. 8.6a). Formation of a primitive vascular plexus occurs at this so-called capillary loop stage. Podocytes of capillary loop stage glomeruli lose mitotic capacity [201] and begin to demonstrate complex cellular architecture, including the formation of actin-based cytoplasmic extensions, or foot

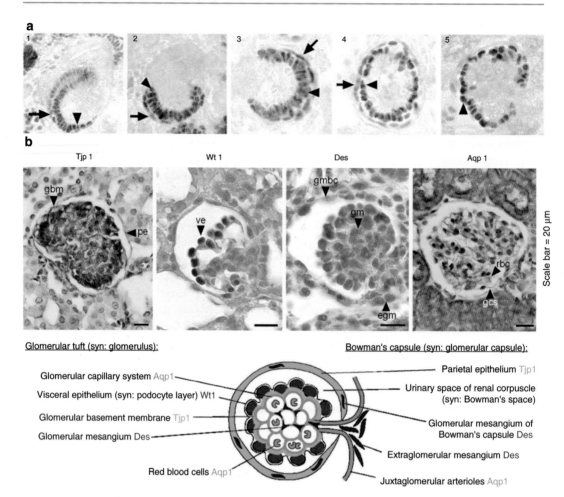

Fig. 8.6 Development of the glomerulus. (**a**) Immunohistochemical staining for Wt1 (*brown*) in the developing glomerulus. (1) Wt1 in podocytes and parietal epithelium in a late S-shaped body. Endothelial cells are recruited into the cup-shaped glomerular precursor region of the S-shaped body forming a primitive vascular tuft. (2, 3) Wt1 in podocytes and parietal epithelium in a capillary loop stage glomerulus. Podocyte precursors contact invading endothelial cells and begin to differentiate. In turn, endothelial cells form a primitive capillary plexus (capillary loop stage). (4, 5) Wt1 is strongly expressed in podocytes in maturing glomeruli. Parietal epithelial cells encapsulate the developing glomerulus. (**b**) Immunohistochemistry of maturing glomeruli using antibodies to Tjp1, Wt1, Des and Aqp1. Tjp1 expression in the glomerular basement membrane (*gbm*) and parietal epithelium (*pe*); Wt1 in podocytes or visceral epithelium (*ve*); Desmin in the extraglomerular mesangium (*egm*), glomerular mesangium of the Bowman's capsule (*gmbc*) and the glomerular mesangium (*gm*); and Aqp1 in endothelial cells of the glomerular capillary system (*gcs*) and red blood cells (*rbc*). Schematic of a developing glomerulus showing the structures present in both the adult and embryonic kidney. The developing glomerulus is composed of a central glomerular tuft, which contains a capillary loop network arising from the afferent arteriole termed the glomerular capillary system. Forming a

tight association with the endothelial cells of the capillaries is the visceral epithelium (or podocytes), a layer of highly specialised epithelial cells specific to the nephron. The fused basal lamina of the endothelial and visceral epithelial cells forms the glomerular basement membrane, an extracellular component of the renal corpuscle. In the interstitial spaces between the capillaries is the glomerular mesangium, a complex of mesangial cells and extracellular matrix. The glomerular tuft is surrounded by the Bowman's capsule, which is composed of the parietal epithelium, mesangium and the urinary space of the renal corpuscle. Extraglomerular mesangium located outside the renal corpuscle is a component of the juxtaglomerular complex and is associated with the afferent arteriole. The antibodies used to identify each of the structures are shown; Aqp1 (*orange*), Wt1 (*red*), Tjp1 (*green*) and Des (*blue*). (**a**, **b**: Used with permission of Springer Science + Business Media from Georgas [195]); (**c**) Representative kidney phenotype of mice with a conditional deletion affecting glomerulogenesis. Loss of VEGFA in the podocyte results in a failure of the glomerular endothelial cells to undergo fenestration and progressive loss of endothelial cells. +/+, wild-type glomerulus; −/−, VEGF-null glomerulus; green, Wt1 staining; red PECAM staining (Used with permission of the American Society for Clinical Investigation from Eremina et al. [196])

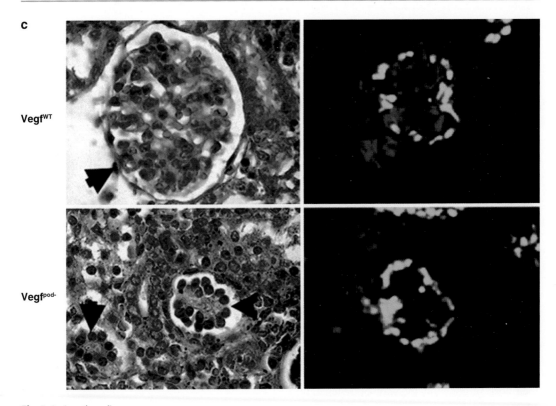

Fig. 8.6 (continued)

processes, and the formation of specialized intercellular junctions, termed slit diaphragms [202, 203] (Fig. 8.6b). Subsequent development of the glomerular capillary tuft involves extensive branching of capillaries and formation of endothelial fenestrae [2]. Mesangial cells, in turn, populate the core of the tuft and provide structural support to capillary loops through the deposition of extracellular matrix [204, 205]. The full complement of glomeruli in the fetal human kidney is attained by 32–34 weeks when nephrogenesis ceases [2]. At birth, superficial glomeruli, which are chronologically the last to be formed, are significantly smaller than juxtamedullary glomeruli, which are the earliest formed glomeruli [180]. Subsequent glomerular development involves hypertrophy, and glomeruli reach adult size by 3.5 years of age [180].

Podocyte Terminal Differentiation

Functional and genetic evidence support the role of Notch signaling in the determination of podocyte cell fate early in nephron development [190, 192]. Additional roles for the Notch receptor gene, *Notch2*, and its ligand, *Jagged1*, at later stages of glomerular capillary tuft assembly are revealed by the analysis of compound mutant mice which show avascular glomeruli or aneurysmal defects and absent mesangial cells in glomerular capillary tuft formation [206].

Following podocyte cell fate determination, the transcription factors *Wt1*, *podocyte expressed 1* (*Pod1*), *Lim homeobox 1b* (*Lmx1b*), and *Mafb* have been shown to have important roles in podocyte terminal differentiation. Loss of function mutations in *Pod1*, *Lmx1b*, and *Mafb* cause podocyte defects in mice which become evident at the capillary loop stage (in the case of *Pod1*) or later (in the case of *Lmx1b* and *Mafb*) [207–209]. Analysis of chimeric mice reveal that normal glomerular epithelial differentiation requires the function of *Pod1* in neighbouring stromal cells, suggesting that *Pod1* regulates stromal factors that act to promote podocyte cell fate [49]. In humans, *LMX1b* mutations are identified in patients with Nail-Patella Syndrome, which is associated with focal segmental glomerulosclerosis [210]. A role for *Wt1* in podocyte differentiation is suggested by the identification of *WT1* mutations in humans with Denys-Drash and Frasier Syndromes [211–213], which are inherited disorders associated with mesangial sclerosis, a form of glomerular disease characterized by defects in podocyte differentiation [214]. The demonstration of an identical glomerular phenotype in mice with targeted *Wt1* mutations genetically similar to the *WT1* mutation in humans with Denys-Drash and Frasier syndromes [215–218] serves as additional support that *Wt1* has important roles in podocyte differentiation.

Podocyte maturation coincides with a loss of mitotic activity and cell cycle blockade [201]. The limited capacity of mature podocytes to undergo cell proliferation has important implications on the glomerular response to injury since damaged podocytes are not capable of compensating for their loss of function by way of regeneration. Moreover, escape from cell cycle blockade in mature podocytes has been associated with severe changes in glomerular cytoarchitecture and a rapidly progressive decline in renal function, as demonstrated by the deleterious course of idiopathic collapsing and human immunodeficiency virus (HIV) nephropathies [219].

Glomerular Capillary Tuft Development

Several signaling systems are involved in the recruitment of endothelial and mesangial precursors during the formation and assembly of the glomerular capillary tuft. Vascular endothelial growth factor (VEGF) is secreted by podocyte precursors of early S-shaped bodies [220]. VEGF promotes recruitment of angioblasts into the vascular cleft [221]. This process is under tight regulatory control, as suggested by the demonstration of severe glomerular defects in mice when the gene dosage of *Vegf* is genetically manipulated [222, 223] (Fig. 8.6c). The local effects of VEGF are likely modulated by angiopoietin-1 and -2, which are expressed by podocytes and mesangial cells, respectively [224]. Recruitment of mesangial cells

is under the guidance of platelet-derived growth factor (PDGF)–B, expressed by endothelial cells, which binds to its receptor, PDGF receptor-β (PDGFRβ) [225]. The function of this axis is required for proliferation and assembly of glomerular capillaries and mesangium as revealed by the absence of glomerular capillary tufts in mice deficient for either *Pdgfβ* or *Pdgfrβ* [226, 227].

During the S-shaped stage, podocyte progenitors express a primitive glomerular basement membrane which is composed predominantly of laminin-1 and α-1 and α-2 subchains of type IV collagen [228]. During glomerular development, composition of the glomerular basement membrane undergoes transition as laminin-1 is replaced by laminin-11, and α-1 and α-2 type IV collagen chains are replaced by α-3, α-4, and α-5 subchains [228]. As demonstrated in several mouse models, failure of these changes results in severe structural and functional defects [229–231].

Formation of the Collecting System

Between the 22nd and 34th week of human fetal gestation [2], or E15.5-birth in mice [15], morphologic changes result in the establishment of peripheral (i.e., cortical) and central (i.e., medullary) domains in the developing kidney. The renal cortex, which represents 70 % of total kidney volume at birth [232], becomes organized as a relatively compact, circumferential rim of tissue surrounding the periphery of the kidney. The renal medulla, which represents 30 % of total kidney volume at birth [232], has a modified cone shape with a broad base contiguous with cortical tissue. The apex of the cone is formed by convergence of collecting ducts in the inner medulla, and is termed the papilla.

Distinct morphologic differences emerge between collecting ducts located in the medulla compared to those located in the renal cortex during this stage of kidney development. Medullary collecting ducts are organized into elongated, relatively unbranched linear arrays which converge centrally in a region devoid of glomeruli. In contrast, collecting ducts located in the renal cortex continue to induce metanephric mesenchyme. The specification of cortical and medullary domains is essential to the eventual function of the mature collecting duct system. The most central segments of the collecting duct system formed from the first five generations of ureteric bud branching undergo remodeling by increased growth and dilatation of these tubules to form the pelvis and calyces (reviewed in [233]).

The developing renal cortex and medulla exhibit distinct axes of growth. The renal cortex grows along a circumferential axis, resulting in a tenfold increase in volume while preserving compact organization of cortical tissue around the developing kidney [232]. In this manner, differentiating glomeruli and tubules maintain their relative position in the renal cortex with respect to the external surface of the kidney, or renal capsule. In contrast to the circumferential pattern of growth exhibited by the developing renal cortex, the developing renal medulla expands 4.5-fold in thickness along a longitudinal axis perpendicular to the axis of cortical growth [232]. This pattern of renal medulla growth is largely due to elongation of outer medullary collecting ducts [232]. The development of a medullary zone coincides with the appearance of stromal cells between the seventh and eighth generations of ureteric bud branches [232]. It has been suggested that stromal cells provide stimulatory cues to promote the growth of medullary collecting ducts [232]. Additional support for this hypothesis is provided by analyses of mutant mice lacking functional expression of the stromal transcription factors *Pod1* and *Forkhead box d1* (*Foxd1*) [37, 49, 234], which demonstrate defects in medullary collecting duct patterning.

In the developing collecting system, apoptosis is infrequently detected in the tips and trunks of the branching ureteric bud [89]. At later stages of embryonic and post-natal kidney development, apoptosis is prominent in the medullary regions of the rat collecting duct system that give rise to the calyces, renal pelvis and renal papilla [89]. The prominence of apoptosis in these regions suggests a potential role for apoptosis in remodeling the first three to five generations of the branched ureteric bud/developing collecting duct

system. The extent to which apoptosis contributes to this morphogenetic process is, however, unknown. Other suggested roles for medullary apoptosis include elimination of medullary interstitial cells as a mechanism for making room for new blood vessel ingrowth [235].

Medullary Patterning and Formation of the Pelvicalyceal System

Regional specification of cortical and medullary domains of the renal collecting duct system is a relatively late event in kidney development. At least five soluble growth factor genes (*Fgf7*, *Fgf10*, *Bmp4*, *Bmp5 and Wnt7b*), one proteoglycan gene (*Gpc3*), one cell cycle regulatory gene (*p57^{KIP2}*), and molecular components of the renin-angiotensin axis (*Angiotensinogen* (*Agt*), *Angiotensinogen receptor* 1 (*Agtr1*, *Agtr2*) are implicated in medullary collecting duct morphogenesis as revealed by the demonstration of defects in renal medulla development in mutant mice.

The kidneys of *Fgf7* null mice are characterized by marked underdevelopment of the papilla [41]. Similarly, *Fgf10* null kidneys exhibit modest medullary dysplasia with reduced numbers of loops of Henle and medullary collecting ducts, increased medullary stromal cells, and enlargement of the renal calyx [236]. Cellular responses to FGFs are modulated through interactions with cell surface proteoglycans [237]. Syndecans and glypicans are heparan sulfate proteoglycans expressed in developing collecting ducts [157, 238], and their expression is required for normal collecting duct growth and branching [114, 239]. Moreover, treatment of embryonic kidney explants with pharmacologic inhibitors of sulfated proteoglycan synthesis leads to loss of *Wnt11* expression at the ureteric bud branch tips [138], suggesting that sulfated proteoglycans interact with multiple mechanisms that control ureteric bud branching.

Functional and genetic evidence in humans and mice demonstrate that GPC3, a glycosylphosphotidylinositol (GPI) -linked cell surface heparan sulfate proteoglycan, is required for normal patterning of the medulla [156, 157]. Medullary dysplasia in the *Gpc3* deficient mouse arises from overgrowth of the ureteric bud and collecting ducts due to increased cell proliferation in the ureteric bud lineage [156], with subsequent destruction of these elements due to apoptosis [157]. The defect is thought to be caused by an altered cellular response of GPC3-deficient collecting duct cells to growth factors such as FGFs [157, 240, 241]. The defective renal medulla formation in *Gpc3* null mutant mice illustrates the importance of tightly regulated cell proliferation and apoptosis in this process.

Additional support for this concept is provided by the phenotypic analysis of mice carrying a null mutation for *p57^{KIP2}*, a cell cycle regulatory gene. *p57^{KIP2}* knock-out mice show medullary dysplasia characterized by a decreased number of inner medullary collecting ducts, in addition to abdominal, skeletal, and adrenal defects [242]. Genetic studies in humans and mice suggest a potential functional interaction between *p57^{KIP2}* and the insulin-like growth factor-2 (*IGF2*) gene in the formation of the renal medulla. For example, phenotypic features of mice with *p57^{KIP2}* null mutations are exhibited by approximately 15 % of individuals with Beckwith-Wiedemann Syndrome, a heterogeneous disorder characterized by somatic overgrowth and renal dysplasia [243]. Genetic linkage studies in humans with this syndrome have mapped the disease to chromosome 11p15.5, which harbours loci for *p57^{KIP2}* as well as for *IGF2* and *H19*. Murine *H19* mutations result in enhanced *Igf2* expression, but do not cause renal dysplasia [244]. However, *H19^{-/-}*; *p57^{KIP2 -/-}* double knock-out mice exhibit elevated serum levels of IGF2, and more severe renal dysplasia than that observed in *p57^{KIP2}* single knock-out mice [245]. These findings support an additional mechanism for the cause of renal medullary dysplasia resulting from dysregulated stimulation of cell proliferation through the inactivation of p57^{KIP2} and over-expression of IGF2.

Elaboration of the medullary collecting duct network is thought to require oriented cell divisions that permit elongation of the medullary collecting ducts through proliferation during development. One means by which this occurs is through the activity of the secreted factor, WNT7b, in up-regulating canonical Wnt signaling in medullary collecting ducts to promote oriented cell division and cell survival [246, 247]. Alpha3beta1 integrin and the receptor tyrosine kinase c-Met (receptor for hepatocyte growth factor) appear to coordinately regulate *Wnt7b* expression in the medullary collecting duct [247].

Development of the Ureteral Smooth Muscle

Urinary filtrate removal also requires coordinated ureteric contractions, which in turn is the result of development of a "pacemaker" at the base of the renal papilla and smooth muscle around the ureter. *Bmp4* heterozygous mutant mice develop both hydronephrosis and hydroureter [124], suggesting that *Bmp4* may play additional roles that involve formation of the ureter and renal pelvis. Support for this concept is provided by the finding in kidney explants that recombinant BMP4 induces smooth muscle actin, an early marker for smooth muscle differentiation, in peri-ureteric mesenchymal cells [145]. Moreover, mice mutant for *Bmp5* show similar defects in renal pelvis and ureter development [248]. Both *Bmp4* and *Bmp5* are expressed in mesenchymal cells lining the ureter and the developing renal pelvis [124, 141, 143], and BMP receptors *Bone morphogenetic protein receptor, type 1A* (*Alk3*) and *Bone morphogenetic protein receptor, type 1B* (*Alk6*) in neighbouring collecting ducts [124].

In addition to BMP signaling, the Sonic hedgehog (Shh) pathway plays a critical role in regulating ureteral mesenchymal development. SHH is secreted from the medullary collecting duct and ureteric stalk, and signals to the surrounding interstitium through its receptor, Patched1 (Ptch1) [249]. BMP4, together with SHH, induces the expression of the transcription factor, *Teashirt zinc finger homeobox 3* (Tshz3), which regulates the development of smooth muscle [250]. Interestingly, loss of the *Gli family zinc finger 3* (*Gli3*) repressor (resulting in inappropriate Hedgehog pathway activation) results in hydronephrosis due to ureteric dyskinesis and reduced numbers of pacemaker cells [251]. Mutations in *GLI3* are associated with Pallister-Hall syndrome in humans [252].

Mutations in genes encoding components of the renin-angiotensin axis also cause abnormalities in the development of the renal calyces, pelvis and ureter. Mice homozygous for a null mutation in *Agt* gene demonstrate progressive widening of the calyx and atrophy of the papillae and underlying medulla [253]. Identical defects occur in homozygous mutants for the *Agtr1* gene [254]. The underlying defect in these mutants appears to be decreased cell proliferation of the smooth muscle cell layer lining the renal pelvis, resulting in decreased thickness of this layer in the proximal ureter. Mutational inactivation of *Agtr2* results in a range of anomalies including vesico-ureteral reflux, duplex kidney, renal ectopia, uretero-pelvic or uretero-vesical junction stenoses, renal dysplasia or hypoplasia, multicystic dysplastic kidney, or renal agenesis [88]. Null mice demonstrate a decreased rate of apoptosis of the cells around the ureter, suggesting that *Agtr2* also plays a role in morphogenetic remodeling of the ureter.

Renal Stroma

Stromal cells are comprised of interstitial cells that secrete extracellular matrix and growth factors, to provide a supportive framework and developmental patterning signals around the developing nephrons and collecting system. In keeping with this idea, stromal cells are found in close proximity to developing nephrons and ureteric bud branches (Fig. 8.3c). Developmentally, stromal cells are derived from a population of *Foxd1*-expressing stromal progenitors [255]. As the renal cortex and medulla become morphologically distinct regions, stromal cells become defined geographically and molecularly into two separate populations – cortical stroma, which form interstitium between induced nephrons and express *Foxd1*, *Aldehyde dehydrogenase 1 family, member A2 (Raldh2)*, *Retinoic acid receptor α (Rarα)*, and *Rarβ2*; and medullary stroma,

which form interstitium between medullary collecting ducts and express *Fgf7*, *Pod1*, and *Bmp4*. Key roles for stromal cells in kidney development are suggested by the demonstration of defects in renal branching morphogenesis and nephronogenesis in mutant mice lacking stromal-expressed genes [37, 38, 40, 41, 124, 209]. By birth, many medullary stromal cells have undergone apoptosis and the space they once occupied is filled by developing loops of Henle [256]. Once nephrogenesis is complete, stromal cells differentiate into a diverse population which includes fibroblasts, lymphocyte-like cells, glomerular mesangial cells, renin-expressing cells and pericytes [255–257].

One important role for the renal stroma is regulation of *Ret* expression, and hence branching morphogenesis. Several factors expressed by stromal cells have been implicated in regulating *Ret* expression– *Raldh2*, *Foxd1*, and *Pod1*. RARα and RARβ2, members of the retinoic acid receptor (RAR) and retinoid X receptor (RXR) families of transcription factors, are both expressed in stromal cells and *Ret*-expressing ureteric bud branch tips [38]. *Rara* $^{-/-}$;*Rarβ2* $^{-/-}$ double mutant mice have small kidneys characterized by a decreased number of ureteric bud branches and loss of normal cortical stromal patterning between induced nephrons [38]. In the collecting ducts of *Rara* $^{-/-}$;*Rarβ2* $^{-/-}$ double mutant mice, *Ret* expression is down-regulated whereas *Gdnf* expression in the metanephric mesenchyme is maintained. The renal defect in these mice can be rescued by over-expressing a *Ret* transgene in the ureteric bud lineage [39]. Recent data suggest that retinoic acid derived from the renal stroma via the enzyme Raldh2 signals to the ureteric bud to up-regulate expression of *Rara* and *Rarβ2* to induce *Ret* expression in the ureteric bud [258].

Foxd1, and the basic helix loop helix transcription factor, *Pod1*, have roles in regulating the spatially restricted pattern of *Ret* expression during collecting duct development. *Foxd1* is most strongly expressed in the developing kidney in the cortical, or subcapsular, stroma [37, 40] (Fig. 8.3c). In contrast, *Pod1* is most abundant in medullary stromal cells [209, 259]. Homozygous deletion of either *Foxd1* or *Pod1* results in decreased renal branching morphogenesis and misexpression of *Ret* throughout the developing collecting system [37, 209]. These data suggest that stromal cues expressed under the control of *Foxd1* and *Pod1* are involved in inhibiting *Ret* expression in the truncal segments of the developing ureteric bud. It is not clear from the analyses of these mutants whether secreted stromal factors directly block *Ret* expression in collecting ducts. Since *Foxd1* and *Pod1* mutants show additional defects in nephron morphogenesis [37, 209], these stromal genes may indirectly control *Ret* expression through the production of nephron-derived factors that secondarily act on collecting duct cells to inhibit *Ret* expression.

Acknowledgements The author would like to express their gratitude to Tino Piscione for his contributions to the second edition of this chapter.

Glossary

Agt	Angiotensinogen
Agtr1	Angiotensinogen receptor 1
Agtr2	Angiotensinogen receptor 2
Alk3	Bone morphogenetic protein receptor, type 1A
Alk6	Bone morphogenetic protein receptor, type 1B
Ap-2	Transcription factor AP-2
Bcl2	B-cell lymphoma 2
Bmp4	Bone morphogenetic protein 4
Bmp5	Bone morphogenetic protein 5
Bmp7	Bone morphogenetic protein 7
Brn1	Brain specific homeobox 1
Cited1	Cbp/p300-interacting transactivator, with Glu/Asp-rich carboxy-terminal domain, 1
Cxcr4	Chemokine (C-X-C motif) receptor 4
Egf	Epidermal growth factor
Emx2	Empty spiracles homolog 2
Eya1	Eyes absent homolog 1
Etv4	ETS transcription factor 4
Etv5	ETS transcription factor 5
Fgf8	Fibroblast growth factor 8
Fgf9	Fibroblast growth factor 9
Fgf20	Fibroblast growth factor 20
Fgfr1	Fibroblast growth factor receptor 1
Fgfr2	Fibroblast growth factor receptor 2
Foxc1	Forkhead box C1
Foxd1	Forkhead box D1
Gata3	Gata binding protein 3
Gdnf	Glial-derived neurotrophic factor
Gdf11	Growth/differentiation factor-11
Gfrα-1	Glial-derived neurotrophic factor receptor alpha-1
Gpc3	Glypican 3
Gli3	Gli family zinc finger 3
Hgf	Hepatocyte growth factor
Hoxa11	Homeobox A11
Hoxc11	Homeobox C11
Hoxd11	Homeobox D11
Hs2st	Heparan sulfate 2-sulfotransferase
Igf2	Insulin-like growth factor 2
Lhx1	Lim homeobox 1
Lmx1b	Lim homeobox 1b
Met	Met proto-oncogene
Mmp14	Matrix metallopeptidase 14
Myb	Myb proto-oncogene
Osr1	Odd-skipped related1
Pax2	Paired box gene 2
Pax8	Paired box gene 8
Pdgfβ	Platelet derived growth factor beta
Pod1	Podocyte expressed 1
Psen1	Presenilin 1
Psen2	Presenilin 2
Ptch1	Patched1
Raldh2	Aldehyde dehydrogenase 1 family, member A2
Rarα	Retinoic acid receptor α
Rarβ2	Retinoic acid receptor β2
Rbpsuh	Recombining binding protein suppressor of hairless
Ret	Ret proto-oncogene
Robo2	Roundabout, axon guidance receptor, homolog 2
Sall1	Sal-like 1
sFrp	Secreted Frizzled-related protein
Shh	Sonic hedgehog
Six1	Sine oculis homeobox homolog 1
Six2	Sine oculis homeobox homolog 2
Slit2	Slit homolog 2
Spry1	Sprouty1
Timp	Tissue inhibitors of metalloproteinases
TGFα	Transforming growth factor alpha
TGFβ2	Transforming growth factor beta2
Tshz3	Teashirt zinc finger homeobox 3
Vegf	Vascular endothelial growth factor

Wnt4	Wingless-type MMTV integration site family 4
Wnt7b	Wingless-type MMTV integration site family 7b
Wnt9b	Wingless-type MMTV integration site family 9b
Wnt11	Wingless-type MMTV integration site family 11
Wt1	Wilms tumour 1

References

1. Osathanondh V, Potter EL. Development of human kidney as shown by microdissection. Arch Pathol. 1966;82:391–402.
2. Potter EL. Normal and abnormal development of the kidney. Chicago: Year Book Medical Publishers; 1972.
3. Hinchliffe SA, Sargent PH, Howard CV, Chan YF, van Velzen D. Human intrauterine renal growth expressed in absolute number of glomeruli assessed by the disector method and Cavalieri principle. Lab Invest. 1991;64(6):777–84.
4. Hughson M, Farris 3rd AB, Douglas-Denton R, Hoy WE, Bertram JF. Glomerular number and size in autopsy kidneys: the relationship to birth weight. Kidney Int. 2003;63(6):2113–22.
5. Rodriguez MM, Gomez AH, Abitbol CL, Chandar JJ, Duara S, Zilleruelo GE. Histomorphometric analysis of postnatal glomerulogenesis in extremely preterm infants. Pediatr Dev Pathol. 2004;7(1):17–25.
6. Brenner BM, Chertow GM. Congenital oligonephropathy and the etiology of adult hypertension and progressive renal injury. Am J Kidney Dis. 1994;23(2):171–5.
7. Brenner BM, Mackenzie HS. Nephron mass as a risk factor for progression of renal disease. Kidney Int. 1997;63:S124–7.
8. Keller G, Zimmer G, Mall G, Ritz E, Amann K. Nephron number in patients with primary hypertension. N Engl J Med. 2003;348(2):101–8.
9. Hoy WE, Hughson MD, Singh GR, Douglas-Denton R, Bertram JF. Reduced nephron number and glomerulomegaly in Australian Aborigines: a group at high risk for renal disease and hypertension. Kidney Int. 2006;70(1):104–10.
10. Manalich R, Reyes L, Herrera M, Melendi C, Fundora I. Relationship between weight at birth and the number and size of renal glomeruli in humans: a histomorphometric study. Kidney Int. 2000;58(2):770–3.
11. Barker DJ, Osmond C, Golding J, Kuh D, Wadsworth ME. Growth in utero, blood pressure in childhood and adult life, and mortality from cardiovascular disease. BMJ. 1989;298(6673):564–7. Clinical research ed.
12. Barker DJ, Eriksson JG, Forsen T, Osmond C. Fetal origins of adult disease: strength of effects and biological basis. Int J Epidemiol. 2002;31(6):1235–9.
13. Osathanondh V, Potter EL. Development of human kidney as shown by microdissection. II. Renal pelvis, calyces, and papillae. Arch Pathol. 1963;76:277–89.
14. Osathanondh V, Potter EL. Development of human kidney as shown by microdissection. III. Formation and interrelationship of collecting tubules and nephrons. Arch Pathol. 1963;76:66–78.
15. Saxen L. Organogenesis of the kidney. Cambridge: Cambridge University Press; 1987.
16. Piscione TD, Rosenblum ND. The molecular control of renal branching morphogenesis: current knowledge and emerging insights. Differentiation. 2002;70(6):227–46.
17. Dressler GR. The cellular basis of kidney development. Annu Rev Cell Dev Biol. 2006;22:509–29.
18. Costantini F. Renal branching morphogenesis: concepts, questions, and recent advances. Differentiation. 2006;74(7):402–21.
19. Shah MM, Sampogna RV, Sakurai H, Bush KT, Nigam SK. Branching morphogenesis and kidney disease. Development. 2004;131(7):1449–62.
20. Yu J, McMahon AP, Valerius MT. Recent genetic studies of mouse kidney development. Curr Opin Genet Dev. 2004;14(5):550–7.
21. Little MH, McMahon AP. Mammalian kidney development: principles, progress, and projections. Cold Spring Harb Perspect Biol. 2012;4:5. Research Support, N.I.H., Extramural Review.
22. Costantini F, Kopan R. Patterning a complex organ: branching morphogenesis and nephron segmentation in kidney development. Dev Cell. 2010;18(5):698–712. Research Support, N.I.H., Extramural Review.
23. Moritz K. Factors influencing mammalian kidney development: implications for health in adult life, morphological development of the kidney. Adv Anat Cell Biol. 2008;196:9–16.
24. Drummond IA, Majumdar A, Hentschel H, Elger M, Solnica-Krezel L, Schier AF, et al. Early development of the zebrafish pronephros and analysis of mutations affecting pronephric function. Development. 1998;125:4655–67.
25. Vize PD, Seufert DW, Carroll TJ, Wallingford JB. Model systems for the study of kidney development: use of the pronephros in the analysis of organ induction and patterning. Dev Biol. 1997;188:189–204.
26. Staack A, Donjacour AA, Brody J, Cunha GR, Carroll P. Mouse urogenital development: a practical approach. Differentiation. 2003;71(7):402–13.
27. James RG, Kamei CN, Wang Q, Jiang R, Schultheiss TM. Odd-skipped related 1 is required for development of the metanephric kidney and regulates formation and differentiation of kidney precursor cells. Development. 2006;133(15):2995–3004.
28. Dressler GR, Deutsch U, Chowdhury K, Nornes HO, Gruss P. Pax-2, a new murine paired-box-containing

gene and its expression in the developing excretory system. Development. 1990;109:787–95.

29. Bouchard M, Souabni A, Mandler M, Neubuser A, Busslinger M. Nephric lineage specification by Pax2 and Pax8. Genes Dev. 2002;16(22):2958–70. Research Support, Non-U.S. Gov't.

30. Fujii T, Pichel JG, Taira M, Toyama R, Dawid IB, Westphal H. Expression patterns of the murine LIM class homeobox gene lim1 in the developing brain and excretory system. Dev Dyn. 1994;1:73–83.

31. Grote D, Souabni A, Busslinger M, Bouchard M. Pax 2/8-regulated Gata 3 expression is necessary for morphogenesis and guidance of the nephric duct in the developing kidney. Development. 2006;133(1):53–61.

32. Pachnis V, Mankoo B, Costantini F. Expression of the c-ret proto-oncogene during mouse embryogenesis. Development. 1993;119:1005–17.

33. Mugford JW, Sipila P, McMahon JA, McMahon AP. Osr1 expression demarcates a multi-potent population of intermediate mesoderm that undergoes progressive restriction to an Osr1-dependent nephron progenitor compartment within the mammalian kidney. Dev Biol. 2008;324(1):88–98. Research Support, N.I.H., Extramural Research Support, Non-U.S. Gov't.

34. Erickson RA. Inductive interactions in the development of the mouse metanephros. J Exp Zool. 1968;169(1):33–42.

35. Grobstein C. Morphogenetic interaction between embryonic mouse tissues separated by a membrane filter. Nature. 1953;172:869–71.

36. Grobstein C. Inductive interaction in the development of the mouse metanephros. J Exp Zool. 1955;130:319–40.

37. Hatini V, Huh SO, Herzlinger D, Soares VC, Lai E. Essential role of stromal mesenchyme in kidney morphogenesis revealed by targeted disruption of Winged Helix transcription factor BF-2. Genes Dev. 1996;10:1467–78.

38. Mendelsohn C, Batourina E, Fung S, Gilbert T, Dodd J. Stromal cells mediate retinoid-dependent functions essential for renal development. Development. 1999;126:1139–48.

39. Batourina E, Gim S, Bello N, Shy M, Clagett-Dame M, Srinivas S, et al. Vitamin A controls epithelial/mesenchymal interactions through Ret expression. Nat Genet. 2001;27:74–8.

40. Levinson RS, Batourina E, Choi C, Vorontchikhina M, Kitajewski J, Mendelsohn CL. Foxd1-dependent signals control cellularity in the renal capsule, a structure required for normal renal development. Development. 2005;132(3):529–39.

41. Qiao J, Uzzo R, Obara-Ishihara T, Degenstein L, Fuchs E, Herzlinger D. FGF-7 modulates ureteric bud growth and nephron number in the developing kidney. Development. 1999;126:547–54.

42. Gao X, Chen X, Taglienti M, Rumballe B, Little MH, Kreidberg JA. Angioblast-mesenchyme induc-

tion of early kidney development is mediated by Wt1 and Vegfa. Development. 2005;132(24):5437–49.

43. Tufro-McReddie A, Norwood VF, Aylor KW, Botkin SJ, Carey RM, Gomez RA. Oxygen regulates vascular endothelial growth factor-mediated vasculogenesis and tubulogenesis. Dev Biol. 1997;183(2):139–49.

44. Meyer TN, Schwesinger C, Bush KT, Stuart RO, Rose DW, Shah MM, et al. Spatiotemporal regulation of morphogenetic molecules during in vitro branching of the isolated ureteric bud: toward a model of branching through budding in the developing kidney. Dev Biol. 2004;275(1):44–67.

45. Barasch J, Qiao J, McWilliams G, Chen D, Oliver JA, Herzlinger D. Ureteric bud cells secrete multiple factors, including bFGF, which rescue renal progenitors from apoptosis. Am J Physiol. 1997;273:F757–67.

46. Barasch J, Yang J, Ware CB, Taga T, Yoshida K, Erdjument-Bromage H, et al. Mesenchymal to epithelial conversion in rat metanephros is induced by LIF. Cell. 1999;99(4):377–86.

47. Das A, Tanigawa S, Karner CM, Xin M, Lum L, Chen C, et al. Stromal-epithelial crosstalk regulates kidney progenitor cell differentiation. Nat Cell Biol. 2013;15(9):1035–44.

48. Yang J, Blum A, Novak T, Levinson R, Lai E, Barasch J. An epithelial precursor is regulated by the ureteric bud and by the renal stroma. Dev Biol. 2002;246(2):296–310.

49. Cui S, Schwartz L, Quaggin SE. Pod1 is required in stromal cells for glomerulogenesis. Dev Dyn. 2003;226(3):512–22.

50. Little MH, et al. A high-resolution anatomical ontology of the developing murine genitourinary tract. Gene Expr Patterns. 2007;7(6):688.

51. Boyle S, Misfeldt A, Chandler KJ, Deal KK, Southard-Smith EM, Mortlock DP, et al. Fate mapping using Cited1-CreERT2 mice demonstrates that the cap mesenchyme contains self-renewing progenitor cells and gives rise exclusively to nephronic epithelia. Dev Biol. 2008;313(1):234–45.

52. Kobayashi A, Valerius MT, Mugford JW, Carroll TJ, Self M, Oliver G, et al. Six2 defines and regulates a multipotent self-renewing nephron progenitor population throughout mammalian kidney development. Cell Stem Cell. 2008;3(2):169–81.

53. Bard JB. Growth and death in the developing mammalian kidney: signals, receptors and conversations. Bioessays. 2002;24(1):72–82.

54. Kreidberg JA, Sariola H, Loring JM, Maeda M, Pelletier J, Housman D, et al. WT-1 is required for early kidney development. Cell. 1993;74:679–91.

55. Nishinakamura R, Matsumoto Y, Nakao K, Nakamura K, Sato A, Copeland NG, et al. Murine homolog of SALL1 is essential for ureteric bud invasion in kidney development. Development. 2001;128:3105–15.

56. Boyle S, Shioda T, Perantoni AO, de Caestecker M. Cited1 and Cited2 are differentially expressed in

the developing kidney but are not required for nephrogenesis. Dev Dyn Off Publ Am Assoc Anatomists. 2007;236(8):2321–30. Research Support, N.I.H., Extramural.

57. Self M, Lagutin OV, Bowling B, Hendrix J, Cai Y, Dressler GR, et al. Six2 is required for suppression of nephrogenesis and progenitor renewal in the developing kidney. Embo J. 2006;25(21):5214–28.

58. Cho EA, Patterson LT, Brookhiser WT, Mah S, Kintner C, Dressler GR. Differential expression and function of cadherin-6 during renal epithelium development. Development. 1998;125(5):803–12.

59. Vainio S, Lin Y. Coordinating early kidney development: lessons from gene targeting. Nat Rev Genet. 2002;4(7):535.

60. Kreidberg JA, et al. WT-1 is required for early kidney development. Cell. 1993;74(4):682.

61. Stark K, et al. Epithelial transformation of metanephric mesenchyme in the developing kidney regulated by Wnt-4. Nature. 1994;372(6507):682.

62. Müller U, Wang D, Denda S, Meneses JJ, Pedersen RA, Reichardt LF. Integrin a8b1 is critically important for epithelial-mesenchymal interactions during kidney morphogenesis. Cell. 1997;88:603–13.

63. Xu PX, Zheng W, Huang L, Maire P, Laclef C, Silvius D. Six1 is required for the early organogenesis of mammalian kidney. Development. 2003;130(14):3085–94.

64. Kalatzis V, Sahly I, El-Amraoui A, Petit C. Eya1 expression in the developing ear and kidney: towards the understanding of the pathogenesis of Branchio-Oto-Renal (BOR) syndrome. Dev Dyn. 1998;213:486–99.

65. Xu P-X, Adams J, Peters H, Brown MC, Heaney S, Maas R. Eya1-deficient mice lack ears and kidneys and show abnormal apoptosis of organ primordia. Nat Genet. 1999;23:113–7.

66. Hellmich HL, Kos L, Cho ES, Mahon KA, Zimmer A. Embryonic expression of glial cell-line derived neurotrophic factor (GDNF) suggests multiple developmental roles in neural differentiation and epithelial-mesenchymal interactions. Mech Dev. 1996;54:95–105.

67. Brophy PD, Ostrom L, Lang KM, Dressler GR. Regulation of ureteric bud outgrowth by Pax2-dependent activation of the glial derived neurotrophic factor gene. Development. 2001;128:4747–56.

68. Kobayashi A, Kwan KM, Carroll TJ, McMahon AP, Mendelsohn CL, Behringer RR. Distinct and sequential tissue-specific activities of the LIM-class homeobox gene Lim1 for tubular morphogenesis during kidney development. Development. 2005;132(12):2809–23. Research Support, N.I.H., Extramural Research Support, U.S. Gov't, P.H.S.

69. Rothenpieler UW, Dressler GR. Pax-2 is required for mesenchyme-to-epithelium conversion during kidney development. Development. 1993;119:711–20.

70. Torres M, Gomez-Pardo E, Dressler GR, Gruss P. Pax-2 controls multiple steps of urogenital development. Development. 1995;121:4057–65.

71. Tsang TE, Shawlot W, Kinder SJ, Kobayashi A, Kwan KM, Schughart K, et al. Lim1 activity is required for intermediate mesoderm differentiation in the mouse embryo. Dev Biol. 2000;223(1):77–90.

72. Shawlot W, Behringer RR. Requirement for Lim1 in head-organizer function. Nature. 1995;374:425–30.

73. Donovan MJ, Natoli TA, Sainio K, Amstutz A, Jaenisch R, Sariola H, et al. Initial differentiation of the metanephric mesenchyme is independent of WT1 and the ureteric bud. Dev Genet. 1999;24:252–62.

74. Carroll TJ, Park JS, Hayashi S, Majumdar A, McMahon AP. Wnt9b plays a central role in the regulation of mesenchymal to epithelial transitions underlying organogenesis of the mammalian urogenital system. Dev Cell. 2005;9(2):283–92.

75. Karner CM, Das A, Ma Z, Self M, Chen C, Lum L, et al. Canonical Wnt9b signaling balances progenitor cell expansion and differentiation during kidney development. Development. 2011;138(7):1247–57. Research Support, N.I.H., Extramural Research Support, Non-U.S. Gov't.

76. Qiao J, Bush KT, Steer DL, Stuart RO, Sakurai H, Wachsman W, et al. Multiple fibroblast growth factors support growth of the ureteric bud but have different effects on branching morphogenesis. Mech Dev. 2001;109(2):123–35.

77. Cancilla B, Davies A, Cauchi JA, Risbridger GP, Bertram JF. Fibroblast growth factor receptors and their ligands in the adult rat kidney. Kidney Int. 2001;60(1):147–55.

78. Barak H, Huh SH, Chen S, Jeanpierre C, Martinovic J, Parisot M, et al. FGF9 and FGF20 maintain the stemness of nephron progenitors in mice and man. Dev Cell. 2012;22(6):1191–207.

79. Brown AC, Adams D, de Caestecker M, Yang X, Friesel R, Oxburgh L. FGF/EGF signaling regulates the renewal of early nephron progenitors during embryonic development. Development. 2011;138(23):5099–112. Research Support, American Recovery and Reinvestment Act Research Support, N.I.H., Extramural Research Support, Non-U.S. Gov't.

80. Hains D, Sims-Lucas S, Kish K, Saha M, McHugh K, Bates CM. Role of fibroblast growth factor receptor 2 in kidney mesenchyme. Pediatr Res. 2008;64(6):592–8. Research Support, N.I.H., Extramural.

81. Poladia DP, Kish K, Kutay B, Hains D, Kegg H, Zhao H, et al. Role of fibroblast growth factor receptors 1 and 2 in the metanephric mesenchyme. Dev Biol. 2006;291(2):325–39. Research Support, N.I.H., Extramural.

82. Sims-Lucas S, Cusack B, Baust J, Eswarakumar VP, Masatoshi H, Takeuchi A, et al. Fgfr1 and the IIIc isoform of Fgfr2 play critical roles in the metanephric mesenchyme mediating early inductive events in kidney development. Dev Dyn Off Publ Am Assoc

Anatomists. 2011;240(1):240–9. Research Support, N.I.H., Extramural.

83. Dudley AT, Godin RE, Robertson EJ. Interaction between FGF and BMP signaling pathways regulates development of metanephric mesenchyme. Genes Dev. 1999;13:1601–13.

84. Dudley AT, Lyons KM, Robertson EJ. A requirement for bone morphogenetic protein-7 during development of the mammalian kidney and eye. Genes Dev. 1995;9:2795–807.

85. Luo G, Hofmann C, Bronckers ALJJ, Sohocki M, Bradley A, Karsenty G. BMP-7 is an inducer of nephrogenesis, and is also required for eye development and skeletal patterning. Genes Dev. 1995;9:2808–20.

86. Koseki C, Herzlinger D, Al-Awqati Q. Apoptosis in metanephric development. J Cell Biol. 1992;119(5):1327–33.

87. Araki T, Saruta T, Okano H, Miura M. Caspase activity is required for nephrogenesis in the developing mouse metanephros. Exp Cell Res. 1999;248(2):423–9.

88. Nishimura H, Yerkes E, Hohenfellner K, Miyazaki Y, Ma J, Hunley TE, et al. Role of the angiotensin type 2 receptor gene in congenital anomalies of the kidney and urinary tract, CAKUT, of mice and men. Mol Cell. 1999;3:1–10.

89. Coles HSR, Burne JF, Raff MC. Large-scale normal cell death in the developing rat kidney and its reduction by epidermal growth factor. Development. 1993;117:777–84.

90. Winyard PJD, Nauta J, Lirenman DS, Hardman P, Sams VR, Risdon RA, et al. Deregulation of cell survival in cystic and dysplastic renal development. Kidney Int. 1996;49:135–46.

91. Karavanov AA, Karavanova I, Perantoni A, Dawid IB. Expression pattern of the rat Lim-1 homeobox gene suggests a dual role during kidney development. Int J Dev Biol. 1998;42:61–6.

92. Stewart CL, Kaspar P, Brunet LJ, Bhatt H, Gadi I, Kontgen F, et al. Blastocyst implantation depends on maternal expression of leukaemia inhibitory factor. Nature. 1992;359(6390):76–9.

93. Plisov SY, Yoshino K, Dove LF, Higinbotham KG, Rubin JS, Perantoni AO. TGF beta 2, LIF and FGF2 cooperate to induce nephrogenesis. Development. 2001;128(7):1045–57.

94. Sanford LP, Ormsby I, Gittenberger-de Groot AC, Sariola H, Friedman R, Boivin GP, et al. TGFb2 knockout mice have multiple developmental defects that are non-overlapping with other TGFb knockout phenotypes. Development. 1997;124:2659–70.

95. McPherron AC, Lawler AM, Lee SJ. Regulation of anterior/posterior patterning of the axial skeleton by growth/differentiation factor 11. Nat Genet. 1999;22(3):260–4.

96. Herzlinger D, Qiao J, Cohen D, Ramakrishna N, Brown AMC. Induction of kidney epithelial morphogenesis by cells expressing wnt-1. Dev Biol. 1994;166:815–8.

97. Kispert A, Vainio S, McMahon AP. Wnt-4 is a mesenchymal signal for epithelial transformation of metanephric mesenchyme in the developing kidney. Development. 1998;125:4225–34.

98. Yoshino K, Rubin JS, Higinbotham KG, Uren A, Anest V, Plisov SY, et al. Secreted Frizzled-related proteins can regulate metanephric development. Mech Dev. 2001;102(1–2):45–55.

99. Grieshammer U, Cebrian C, Ilagan R, Meyers E, Herzlinger D, Martin GR. FGF8 is required for cell survival at distinct stages of nephrogenesis and for regulation of gene expression in nascent nephrons. Development. 2005;132(17):3847–57. Research Support, N.I.H., Extramural Research Support, Non-U.S. Gov't Research Support, U.S. Gov't, P.H.S.

100. Perantoni AO, Timofeeva O, Naillat F, Richman C, Pajni-Underwood S, Wilson C, et al. Inactivation of FGF8 in early mesoderm reveals an essential role in kidney development. Development. 2005;132(17):3859–71.

101. Bridgewater D, Rosenblum ND. Stimulatory and inhibitory signaling molecules that regulate renal branching morphogenesis. Pediatr Nephrol. 2009;24(9):1616.

102. Schuchardt A, et al. Defects in the kidney and enteric nervous system of mice lacking the tyrosine kinase receptor Ret. Nature. 1994;367(6461):382.

103. Pichel JG, et al. Defects in enteric innervation and kidney development in mice lacking GDNF. Nature. 1996;382(6586):74.

104. Hu MC, Rosenblum ND. Genetic regulation of branching morphogenesis: lessons learned from loss-of-function phenotypes. Pediatr Res. 2003;54(4):433–8.

105. Sainio K, Suvanto P, Davies J, Wartiovaara J, Wartiovaara K, Saarma M, et al. Glial-cell-line-derived neurotrophic factor is required for bud initiation from ureteric epithelium. Development. 1997;124:4077–87.

106. Schuchardt A, D'Agati V, Larsson-Blomberg L, Costantini F, Pachnis V. Defects in the kidney and enteric nervous system of mice lacking the tyrosine kinase receptor Ret. Nature. 1994;367:380–3.

107. Enomoto H, Araki T, Jackman A, Heuckeroth RO, Snider WD, Johnson EMJ, et al. GFRa 1-deficient mice have deficits in the enteric nervous system and kidneys. Neuron. 1998;21:317–24.

108. Pichel JG, Shen L, Sheng HZ, Granholm A-C, Drago J, Grinberg A, et al. Defects in enteric innervation and kidney development in mice lacking GDNF. Nature. 1996;382:73–6.

109. Sanchez MP, Silos-Santiago I, Frisen J, He B, Lira SA, Barbacid M. Renal agenesis and the absence of enteric neurons in mice lacking GDNF. Nature. 1996;382:70–3.

110. Schuchardt A, D'Agati V, Pachnis V, Costantini F. Renal agenesis and hypodysplasia in ret-k⁻ mutant mice result from defects in ureteric bud development. Development. 1996;122:1919–29.

111. Cacalano G, Farinas I, Wang LC, Hagler K, Forgie A, Moore M, et al. GFRalpha1 is an essential receptor component for GDNF in the developing nervous system and kidney. Neuron. 1998;21:53–62.

112. Jain S, Encinas M, Johnson Jr EM, Milbrandt J. Critical and distinct roles for key RET tyrosine docking sites in renal development. Genes Dev. 2006;20(3):321–33. Research Support, N.I.H., Extramural Research Support, Non-U.S. Gov't.

113. Jain S, Knoten A, Hoshi M, Wang H, Vohra B, Heuckeroth RO, et al. Organotypic specificity of key RET adaptor-docking sites in the pathogenesis of neurocristopathies and renal malformations in mice. J Clin Invest. 2010;120(3):778–90. Research Support, N.I.H., Extramural Research Support, Non-U.S. Gov't.

114. Bullock SL, Fletcher JM, Beddington RSP, Wilson VA. Renal agenesis in mice homozygous for a gene trap mutation in the gene encoding heparan sulfate 2-sulfotransferase. Genes Dev. 1998;12:1894–906.

115. Lu BC, Cebrian C, Chi X, Kuure S, Kuo R, Bates CM, et al. Etv4 and Etv5 are required downstream of GDNF and Ret for kidney branching morphogenesis. Nat Genet. 2009;41(12):1295–302. Research Support, N.I.H., Extramural Research Support, Non-U.S. Gov't.

116. Pepicelli CV, Kispert A, Rowitch D, McMahon AP. GDNF induces branching and increased cell proliferation in the ureter of the mouse. Dev Biol. 1997;192:193–8.

117. Kispert A, Vainio S, Shen L, Rowitch DH, McMahon AP. Proteoglycans are required for maintenance of *Wnt-11* expression in the ureter tips. Development. 1996;122:3627–37.

118. Majumdar A, Vainio S, Kispert A, McMahon J, McMahon AP. Wnt11 and Ret/Gdnf pathways cooperate in regulating ureteric branching during metanephric kidney development. Development. 2003;130(14):3175–85.

119. Towers PR, Woolf AS, Hardman P. Glial cell line-derived neurotrophic factor stimulates ureteric bud outgrowth and enhances survival of ureteric bud cells in vitro. Exp Nephrol. 1998;6:337–51.

120. Michael L, Davies JA. Pattern and regulation of cell proliferation during murine ureteric bud development. J Anat. 2004;204(4):241–55.

121. Piscione TD, Rosenblum ND. The malformed kidney: disruption of glomerular and tubular development. Clin Genet. 1999;56(5):343–58.

122. Woolf AS, Winyard PJ. Molecular mechanisms of human embryogenesis: developmental pathogenesis of renal tract malformations. Pediatr Dev Pathol. 2002;5(2):108–29.

123. Mackie GG, Stephens FD. Duplex kidneys: a correlation of renal dysplasia with position of the ureteral orifice. J Urol. 1975;114:274–80.

124. Miyazaki Y, Oshima Y, Fogo A, Hogan BLM, Ichikawa I. Bone morphogenetic protein 4 regulates the budding site and elongation of the mouse ureter. J Clin Invest. 2000;105:863–73.

125. Grieshammer U, Le M, Plump AS, Wang F, Tessier-Lavigne M, Martin GR. SLIT2-mediated ROBO2 signaling restricts kidney induction to a single site. Dev Cell. 2004;6(5):709–17.

126. Tsuchida S, Matsusaka T, Chen X, Okubo S, Niimura F, Nishimura H, et al. Murine double nullizygotes of the angiotensin type 1A and 1B receptor genes duplicate severe abnormal phenotypes of angiotensinogen nullizygotes. J Clin Invest. 1998;101:755–60.

127. Hains DS, Sims-Lucas S, Carpenter A, Saha M, Murawski I, Kish K, et al. High incidence of vesicoureteral reflux in mice with Fgfr2 deletion in kidney mesenchyma. J Urol. 2010;183(5):2077–84. Research Support, N.I.H., Extramural.

128. Walker KA, Sims-Lucas S, Di Giovanni VE, Schaefer C, Sunseri WM, Novitskaya T, et al. Deletion of fibroblast growth factor receptor 2 from the peri-wolffian duct stroma leads to ureteric induction abnormalities and vesicoureteral reflux. PLoS One. 2013;8(2):e56062. Research Support, N.I.H., Extramural.

129. Srinivas S, Wu Z, Chen C-M, D'Agati V, Costantini F. Dominant effects of RET receptor misexpression and ligand-independent RET signaling on ureteric bud development. Development. 1999;126:1375–86.

130. Shakya R, Jho EH, Kotka P, Wu Z, Kholodilov N, Burke R, et al. The role of GDNF in patterning the excretory system. Dev Biol. 2005;283(1):70–84.

131. Brodbeck S, Englert C. Genetic determination of nephrogenesis: the Pax/Eya/Six gene network. Pediatr Nephrol. 2004;19(3):249–55.

132. Wellik DM, Hawkes PJ, Capecchi MR. Hox11 paralogous genes are essential for metanephric kidney induction. Genes Dev. 2002;16(11):1423–32.

133. Miyamoto N, Yoshida M, Kuratani S, Matuso I, Aizawa S. Defects of urogenital development in mice lacking *Emx2*. Development. 1997;124:1653–64.

134. Kume T, Deng K, Hogan BL. Murine forkhead/winged helix genes Foxc1 (Mf1) and Foxc2 (Mfh1) are required for the early organogenesis of the kidney and urinary tract. Development. 2000;127:1387–95.

135. Tessier-Lavigne M, Goodman CS. The molecular biology of axon guidance. Science. 1996;274:1123–33.

136. Brose K, Bland KS, Wang KH, Arnott D, Henzel W, Goodman CS, et al. Slit proteins bind Robo receptors and have an evolutionarily conserved role in repulsive axon guidance. Cell. 1999;96:795–806.

137. Piper M, Georgas K, Yamada T, Little M. Expression of the vertebrate Slit gene family and their putative receptors, the Robo genes, in the developing murine kidney. Mech Dev. 2000;94:213–7.

138. Basson MA, Akbulut S, Watson-Johnson J, Simon R, Carroll TJ, Shakya R, et al. Sprouty1 is a critical regulator of GDNF/RET-mediated kidney induction. Dev Cell. 2005;8(2):229–39.

139. Basson MA, Watson-Johnson J, Shakya R, Akbulut S, Hyink D, Costantini FD, et al. Branching morphogenesis of the ureteric epithelium during kidney development is coordinated by the opposing functions of GDNF and Sprouty1. Dev Biol. 2006;299(2):466–77.

140. Chi L, Zhang S, Lin Y, Prunskaite-Hyyrylainen R, Vuolteenaho R, Itaranta P, et al. Sprouty proteins regulate ureteric branching by coordinating reciprocal epithelial Wnt11, mesenchymal Gdnf and stromal Fgf7 signalling during kidney development. Development. 2004;131(14):3345–56.

141. Dudley AT, Robertson EJ. Overlapping expression domains of bone morphogenetic protein family members potentially account for limited tissue defects in BMP7 deficient embryos. Dev Dyn. 1997;208:349–62.

142. Godin RE, Robertson EJ, Dudley AT. Role of BMP family members during kidney development. Int J Dev Biol. 1999;43:405–11.

143. Dewulf N, Verschueren K, Lonnoy O, Morén A, Grimsby S, Vande Spiegle K, et al. Distinct spatial and temporal expression patterns of two type 1 receptors for bone morphogenetic proteins during mouse embryogenesis. Endocrinology. 1995;136:2652–63.

144. Verschueren K, Dewulf N, Goumans MJ, Lonnoy O, Feijen A, Grimsby S, et al. Expression of type I and type IB receptors for activin in midgestation mouse embryos suggests distinct functions in organogenesis. Mech Dev. 1995;52:109–23.

145. Raatikainen-Ahokas A, Hytonen M, Tenhunen A, Sainio K, Sariola H. Bmp-4 affects the differentiation of metanephric mesenchyme and reveals an early anterior-posterior axis of the embryonic kidney. Dev Dyn. 2000;217:146–58.

146. Cain JE, Nion T, Jeulin D, Bertram JF. Exogenous BMP-4 amplifies asymmetric ureteric branching in the developing mouse kidney in vitro. Kidney Int. 2005;67(2):420–31.

147. Piscione TD, Yager TD, Gupta IR, Grinfeld B, Pei Y, Attisano L, et al. BMP-2 and OP-1 exert direct and opposite effects on renal branching morphogenesis. Am J Physiol. 1997;273:F961–75.

148. Piscione TD, Phan T, Rosenblum ND. BMP7 controls collecting tubule cell proliferation and apoptosis via Smad1-dependent and -independent pathways. Am J Physiol. 2001;280:F19–33.

149. Pope IV JC, Brock III JW, Adams MC, Stephens FD, Ichikawa I. How they begin and how they end: classis and new theories for the development and deterioration of congenital anomalies of the kidney and urinary tract, CAKUT. J Am Soc Nephrol. 1999;10:2018–28.

150. Ichikawa I, Kuwayama F, Pope JC, Stephens FD, Miyazaki Y. Paradigm shift from classic anatomic theories to contemporary cell biological views of CAKUT. Kidney Int. 2002;61(3):889–98.

151. Bush KT, Sakurai H, Steer DL, Leonard MO, Sampogna RV, Meyer TN, et al. TGF-beta superfam-

ily members modulate growth, branching, shaping, and patterning of the ureteric bud. Dev Biol. 2004;266(2):285–98.

152. Watanabe T, Costantini F. Real-time analysis of ureteric bud branching morphogenesis in vitro. Dev Biol. 2004;271(1):98–108.

153. Lin Y, Zhang S, Tuukkanen J, Peltoketo H, Pihlajaniemi T, Vainio S. Patterning parameters associated with the branching of the ureteric bud regulated by epithelial-mesenchymal interactions. Int J Dev Biol. 2003;47(1):3–13.

154. Fisher CE, Michael L, Barnett MW, Davies JA. Erk MAP kinase regulates branching morphogenesis in the developing mouse kidney. Development. 2001;128(21):4329–38.

155. Perantoni AO, Williams CL, Lewellyn AL. Growth and branching morphogenesis of rat collecting duct anlagen in the absence of metanephrogenic mesenchyme. Differentiation. 1991;48:107–13.

156. Cano-Gauci DF, Song H, Yang H, McKerlie C, Choo B, Shi W, et al. Glypican-3-deficient mice exhibit developmental overgrowth and some of the renal abnormalities typical of Simpson-Golabi-Behmel syndrome. J Cell Biol. 1999;146:255–64.

157. Grisaru S, Cano-Gauci D, Tee J, Filmus J, Rosenblum ND. Glypican-3 modulates BMP- and FGF-mediated effects during renal branching morphogenesis. Dev Biol. 2001;231:31–46.

158. Sorenson CM, Rogers SA, Korsmeyer SJ, Hammerman MR. Fulminant metanephric apoptosis and abnormal kidney development in bcl-2-deficient mice. Am J Physiol. 1995;268:F73–81.

159. Moser M, Pscherer A, Roth C, Becker J, Mücher G, Zerres K, et al. Enhanced apoptotic cell death of renal epithelial cells in mice lacking transcription factor AP-2ß. Genes Dev. 1997;11:1938–48.

160. Chevalier RL. Growth factors and apoptosis in neonatal ureteral obstruction. J Am Soc Nephrol. 1996;7:1098–105.

161. Tarantal AF, Han VK, Cochrum KC, Mok A, daSilva M, Matsell DG. Fetal rhesus monkey model of obstructive renal dysplasia. Kidney Int. 2001;59:446–56.

162. Qiao J, Sakurai H, Nigam SK. Branching morphogenesis independent of mesenchymal-epithelial contact in the developing kidney. Proc Natl Acad Sci U S A. 1999;96:7330–5.

163. Bridgewater D, Cox B, Cain J, Lau A, Athaide V, Gill PS, et al. Canonical WNT/beta-catenin signaling is required for ureteric branching. Dev Biol. 2008;317(1):83–94.

164. Marose TD, Merkel CE, McMahon AP, Carroll TJ. Beta-catenin is necessary to keep cells of ureteric bud/Wolffian duct epithelium in a precursor state. Dev Biol. 2008;314(1):112–26.

165. Sims-Lucas S, Cusack B, Eswarakumar VP, Zhang J, Wang F, Bates CM. Independent roles of Fgfr2 and Frs2alpha in ureteric epithelium. Development. 2011;138(7):1275–80. Research Support, N.I.H., Extramural.

166. Zhao H, Kegg H, Grady S, Truong HT, Robinson ML, Baum M, et al. Role of fibroblast growth factor receptors 1 and 2 in the ureteric bud. Dev Biol. 2004;276(2):403–15.

167. Barros EJG, Santos OFP, Matsumoto K, Nakamura T, Nigam SK. Differential tubulogenic and branching morphogenetic activities of growth factors: implications for epithelial tissue development. Proc Natl Acad Sci U S A. 1995;92:4412–6.

168. Cantley LG, Barros EJG, Gandhi M, Rauchman M, Nigam SK. Regulation of mitogenesis, motogenesis, and tubulogenesis by hepatocyte growth factor in renal collecting duct cells. Am J Physiol. 1994;267:F271–80.

169. Montesano R, Soriano JV, Pepper MS, Orci L. Induction of epithelial branching tubulogenesis in vitro. J Cell Physiol. 1997;173:152–61.

170. Bladt F, Riethmacher D, Isenmann S, Aguzzi A, Birchmeier C. Essential role for the c-*met* receptor in the migration of myogenic precursor cells into the limb bud. Nature. 1995;376:768–71.

171. Threadgill DW, Dlugosz AA, Hansen LA, Tennenbaum T, Lichti U, Yee D, et al. Targeted disruption of mouse EGF receptor: effect of genetic background on mutant phenotype. Science. 1995;269:230–4.

172. Uehara Y, Minowa O, Mori C, Shiota K, Kuno J, Noda T, et al. Placental defect and embryonic lethality in mice lacking hepatocyte growth factor/scatter factor. Nature. 1995;373(6516):702–5.

173. Barasch J, Yang J, Qiao JY, Tempst P, Erdjument-Bromage H, Leung W, et al. Tissue inhibitor of metalloproteinase-2 stimulates mesenchymal growth and regulates epithelial branching during morphogenesis of the rat metanephros. J Clin Invest. 1999;103:1299–307.

174. Sakurai H, Nigam SK. In vitro branching tubulogenesis: implications for developmental and cystic disorders, nephron number, renal repair, and nephron engineering. Kidney Int. 1998;54:14–26.

175. Pohl M, Sakurai H, Bush KT, Nigam SK. Matrix metalloproteinases and their inhibitors regulate in vitro ureteric bud branching morphogenesis. Am J Physiol. 2000;279:F891–900.

176. Naylor RW, Davidson AJ. Hnf1beta and nephron segmentation. Pediatr Nephrol. 2014;29(4):659–64.

177. Georgas K, et al. Use of dual section mRNA in situ hybridisation/ immunohistochemistry to clarify gene expression patterns during the early stages of nephron development in the embryo and in the mature nephron of the adult mouse kidney. Histochem Cell Biol. 2008;130:937.

178. Cheng HT, et al. Notch2, but not Notch1, is required for proximal cell fate acquisition in the mammalian nephron. Development. 2007;134(4):803.

179. Evan AP, Gattone 2nd VH, Schwartz GJ. Development of solute transport in rabbit proximal tubule. II. Morphologic segmentation. Am J Physiol. 1983;245(3):F391–407.

180. Fetterman GH, Shuplock NA, Philipp FJ, Gregg HS. The growth and maturation of human glomeruli and proximal convolutions from term to adulthood: studies by microdissection. Pediatrics. 1965;35:601–19.

181. Neiss WF. Histogenesis of the loop of Henle in the rat kidney. Anat Embryol. 1982;164(3):315–30.

182. Nakai S, Sugitani Y, Sato H, Ito S, Miura Y, Ogawa M, et al. Crucial roles of Brn1 in distal tubule formation and function in mouse kidney. Development. 2003;130(19):4751–9.

183. Neiss WF, Klehn KL. The postnatal development of the rat kidney, with special reference to the chemo-differentiation of the proximal tubule. Histochemistry. 1981;73(2):251–68.

184. Majumdar A, Lun K, Brand M, Drummond IA. Zebrafish no isthmus reveals a role for pax2.1 in tubule differentiation and patterning events in the pronephric primordia. Development. 2000;127(10):2089–98.

185. Wallingford JB, Carroll TJ, Vize PD. Precocious expression of the Wilms' tumor gene xWT1 inhibits embryonic kidney development in Xenopus laevis. Dev Biol. 1998;202(1):103–12.

186. Ryan G, Steele-Perkins V, Morris JF, Rauscher 3rd FJ, Dressler GR. Repression of Pax-2 by WT1 during normal kidney development. Development. 1995;121(3):867–75.

187. Pelletier J, Schalling M, Buckler AJ, Rogers A, Haber DA, Housman D. Expression of the Wilms' tumor gene WT1 in the murine urogenital system. Genes Dev. 1991;5:1345–56.

188. Dressler GR, Douglass EC. Pax-2 is a DNA-binding protein expressed in embryonic kidney and Wilms tumor. Proc Natl Acad Sci U S A. 1992;89:1179–83.

189. Dressler GR, Wilkinson JE, Rothenpieler UW, Patterson LT, Silliams-Simons L, Westphal H. Deregulation of Pax-2 expression in transgenic mice generates severe kidney abnormalities. Nature. 1993;362:65–7.

190. Cheng HT, Miner JH, Lin M, Tansey MG, Roth K, Kopan R. Gamma-secretase activity is dispensable for mesenchyme-to-epithelium transition but required for podocyte and proximal tubule formation in developing mouse kidney. Development. 2003;130(20):5031–42.

191. Cheng HT, Kim M, Valerius MT, Surendran K, Schuster-Gossler K, Gossler A, et al. Notch2, but not Notch1, is required for proximal fate acquisition in the mammalian nephron. Development. 2007;134(4):801–11.

192. Wang P, Pereira FA, Beasley D, Zheng H. Presenilins are required for the formation of comma- and S-shaped bodies during nephrogenesis. Development. 2003;130(20):5019–29.

193. Boyle SC, Kim M, Valerius MT, McMahon AP, Kopan R. Notch pathway activation can replace the requirement for Wnt4 and Wnt9b in mesenchymal-to-epithelial transition of nephron stem cells. Development. 2011;138(19):4245–54. Research Support, N.I.H., Extramural.

194. Kreidberg JA. Podocyte differentiation and glomerulogenesis. J Am Soc Nephrol. 2003;14(3):806–14.

195. Georgas K. Use of dual section mRNA in situ hybridisation/ immunohistochemistry to clarify gene expression patterns during the early stages of nephron development in the embryo and in the mature nephron of the adult mouse kidney. Histochem Cell Biol. 2008;130:932–7.

196. Eremina V, et al. Glomerular-specific alterations of VEGF-A lead to distinct congenital and acquired renal diseases. J Clin Invest. 2003;111(5):712.

197. Robert B, St John PL, Hyink DP, Abrahamson DR. Evidence that embryonic kidney cells expressing flk-1 are intrinsic, vasculogenic angioblasts. Am J Physiol. 1996;271(3 Pt 2):F744–53.

198. Hyink DP, Tucker DC, St John PL, Leardkamolkarn V, Accavitti MA, Abrass CK, et al. Endogenous origin of glomerular endothelial and mesangial cells in grafts of embryonic kidneys. Am J Physiol. 1996;270(5 Pt 2):F886–99.

199. Ricono JM, Xu YC, Arar M, Jin DC, Barnes JL, Abboud HE. Morphological insights into the origin of glomerular endothelial and mesangial cells and their precursors. J Histochem Cytochem. 2003;51(2):141–50.

200. Sariola H, Ekblom P, Lehtonen E, Saxen L. Differentiation and vascularization of the metanephric kidney grafted on the chorioallantoic membrane. Dev Biol. 1983;96(2):427–35.

201. Nagata M, Nakayama K, Terada Y, Hoshi S, Watanabe T. Cell cycle regulation and differentiation in the human podocyte lineage. Am J Pathol. 1998;153(5):1511–20.

202. Garrod DR, Fleming S. Early expression of desmosomal components during kidney tubule morphogenesis in human and murine embryos. Development. 1990;108(2):313–21.

203. Pavenstadt H, Kriz W, Kretzler M. Cell biology of the glomerular podocyte. Physiol Rev. 2003;83(1):253–307.

204. Ekblom P. Formation of basement membranes in embryonic kidney: an immunohistological study. J Cell Biol. 1981;91:1–10.

205. Sariola H, Timpl R, von der Mark K, Mayne R, Fitch JM, Linsenmayer TF, et al. Dual origin of glomerular basement membrane. Dev Biol. 1984;101:86–96.

206. McCright B, Gao X, Shen L, Lozier J, Lan Y, Maguire M, et al. Defects in development of the kidney, heart and eye vasculature in mice homozygous for a hypomorphic Notch2 mutation. Development. 2001;128:491–502.

207. Sadl V, Jin F, Yu J, Cui S, Holmyard D, Quaggin S, et al. The mouse Kreisler (Krml1/MafB) segmentation gene is required for differentiation of glomerular visceral epithelial cells. Dev Biol. 2002;249(1):16–29.

208. Miner JH, Morello R, Andrews KL, Li C, Antignac C, Shaw AS, et al. Transcriptional induction of slit diaphragm genes by Lmx1b is required in podocyte differentiation. J Clin Invest. 2002;109(8):1065–72.

209. Quaggin SE, Schwartz L, Cui S, Igarashi P, Deimling J, Post M, et al. The basic-helix-loop-helix protein pod1 is critically important for kidney and lung organogenesis. Development. 1999;126:5771–83.

210. Dreyer SD, Zhou G, Baldini A, Winterpacht A, Zabel B, Cole W, et al. Mutations in LMX1B cause abnormal skeletal patterning and renal dysplasia in nail patella syndrome. Nat Genet. 1998;19:47–50.

211. Barbaux S, Niaudet P, Gubler M-C, Grünfeld J-P, Jaubert F, Kuttenn F, et al. Donor splice-site mutations in WT1 are responsible for Frasier syndrome. Nat Genet. 1997;17:467–70.

212. Klamt B, Koziell A, Poulat F, Wieacker P, Scambler P, Berta P, et al. Frasier syndrome is caused by defective alternative splicing of WT1 leading to an altered ratio of WT1+/−KTS splice isoforms. Hum Mol Genet. 1998;7:709–14.

213. Coppes MJ, Liefers GJ, Higuchi M, Zinn AB, Balfe JW, Williams BR. Inherited WT1 mutation in Denys-Drash syndrome. Cancer Res. 1992;52(21):6125–8.

214. Yang Y, Jeanpierre C, Dressler GR, Lacoste M, Niaudet P, Gubler MC. WT1 and PAX-2 podocyte expression in Denys-Drash syndrome and isolated diffuse mesangial sclerosis. Am J Pathol. 1999;154(1):181–92.

215. Gao F, Maiti S, Sun G, Ordonez NG, Udtha M, Deng JM, et al. The Wt1+/R394W mouse displays glomerulosclerosis and early-onset renal failure characteristic of human Denys-Drash syndrome. Mol Cell Biol. 2004;24(22):9899–910.

216. Patek CE, Little MH, Fleming S, Miles C, Charlieu JP, Clarke AR, et al. A zinc finger truncation of murine WT1 results in the characteristic urogenital abnormalities of Denys-Drash syndrome. Proc Natl Acad Sci U S A. 1999;96(6):2931–6.

217. Hammes A, Guo JK, Lutsch G, Leheste JR, Landrock D, Ziegler U, et al. Two splice variants of the Wilms' tumor 1 gene have distinct functions during sex determination and nephron formation. Cell. 2001;106(3):319–29.

218. Guo JK, Menke AL, Gubler MC, Clarke AR, Harrison D, Hammes A, et al. WT1 is a key regulator of podocyte function: reduced expression levels cause crescentic glomerulonephritis and mesangial sclerosis. Hum Mol Genet. 2002;11(6):651–9.

219. Barisoni L, Kriz W, Mundel P, D'Agati V. The dysregulated podocyte phenotype: a novel concept in the pathogenesis of collapsing idiopathic focal segmental glomerulosclerosis and HIV-associated nephropathy. J Am Soc Nephrol. 1999;10(1):51–61.

220. Kitamoto Y, Tokunaga H, Tomita K. Vascular endothelial growth factor is an essential molecule for mouse kidney development: glomerulogenesis and nephrogenesis. J Clin Invest. 1997; 99(10):2351–7.

221. Tufro A, Norwood VF, Carey RM, Gomez RA. Vascular endothelial growth factor induces

nephrogenesis and vasculogenesis. J Am Soc Nephrol. 1999;10(10):2125–34.

222. Eremina V, Cui S, Gerber H, Ferrara N, Haigh J, Nagy A, et al. Vascular endothelial growth factor a signaling in the podocyte-endothelial compartment is required for mesangial cell migration and survival. J Am Soc Nephrol. 2006;17(3):724–35.

223. Eremina V, Sood M, Haigh J, Nagy A, Lajoie G, Ferrara N, et al. Glomerular-specific alterations of VEGF-A expression lead to distinct congenital and acquired renal diseases. J Clin Invest. 2003;111(5):707–16.

224. Woolf AS, Yuan HT. Angiopoietin growth factors and Tie receptor tyrosine kinases in renal vascular development. Pediatr Nephrol. 2001; 16(2):177–84.

225. Lindahl P, Hellström M, Kalén M, Karlsson L, Pekny M, Pekna M, et al. Paracrine PDGF-B/PDGF-Rß signaling controls mesangial cell development in kidney glomeruli. Development. 1998;125:3313–22.

226. Leveen P, Pekny M, Gebre-Medhin S, Swolin B, Larsson E, Betsholtz C. Mice deficient for PDGF B show renal, cardiovascular, and hematological abnormalities. Genes Dev. 1994;8:1875–87.

227. Soriano P. Abnormal kidney development and hematological disorders in PDGF ß-receptor mutant mice. Genes Dev. 1994;8:1888–96.

228. Miner JH, Sanes JR. Collagen IV alpha 3, alpha 4, and alpha 5 chains in rodent basal laminae: sequence, distribution, association with laminins, and developmental switches. J Cell Biol. 1994;127(3):879–91.

229. Miner JH, Li C. Defective glomerulogenesis in the absence of laminin alpha5 demonstrates a developmental role for the kidney glomerular basement membrane. Dev Biol. 2000;217(2):278–89.

230. Miner JH, Sanes JR. Molecular and functional defects in kidneys of mice lacking collagen alpha 3(IV): implications for Alport syndrome. J Cell Biol. 1996;135(5):1403–13.

231. Noakes PG, Miner JH, Gautam M, Cunningham JM, Sanes JR, Merlie JP. The renal glomerulus of mice lacking s-laminin/laminin ß2: nephrosis despite molecular compensation by laminin ß1. Nat Genet. 1995;10:400–6.

232. Cebrian C, Borodo K, Charles N, Herzlinger DA. Morphometric index of the developing murine kidney. Dev Dyn. 2004;231(3):601–8.

233. Al-Awqati Q, Goldberg MR. Architectural patterns in branching morphogenesis in the kidney. Kidney Int. 1998;54:1832–42.

234. Bard J. A new role for the stromal cells in kidney development. Bioessays. 1996;18(9):705–7.

235. Loughna S, Landels E, Woolf AS. Growth factor control of developing kidney endothelial cells. Exp Nephrol. 1996;4(2):112–8.

236. Ohuchi H, Hori Y, Yamasaki M, Harada H, Sekine K, Kato S, et al. FGF10 acts as a major ligand for FGF receptor 2 IIIb in mouse multi-organ

development. Biochem Biophys Res Commun. 2000;277:643–9.

237. Bonneh-Barkay D, Shlissel M, Berman B, Shaoul E, Admon A, Vlodavsky I, et al. Identification of glypican as a dual modulator of the biological activity of fibroblast growth factors. J Biol Chem. 1997;272:12415–21.

238. Bernfield M, Hinkes MT, Gallo RL. Developmental expression of the syndecans: possible function and regulation. Development. 1993;Suppl.:205–12.

239. Davies J, Lyon M, Gallagher J, Garrod D. Sulphated proteoglycan is required for collecting duct growth and branching but not nephron formation during kidney development. Development. 1995;121:1507–17.

240. Jackson SM, Nakato H, Sugiura M, Jannuzi A, Oakes R, Kaluza V, et al. dally, a drosophila glypican, controls cellular responses to the TGF-ß-related morphogen, Dpp. Development. 1997;124:4113–20.

241. Tsuda M, Kamimura K, Nakato H, Archer M, Staatz W, Fox B, et al. The cell-surface proteoglycan *dally* regulates *wingless* signalling in Drosophila. Nature. 1999;400:276–80.

242. Zhang P, Liégeois NJ, Wong C, Finegold M, Thompson JC, Silverman A, et al. Altered cell differentiation and proliferation in mice lacking p57^{KIP2} indicates a role in Beckwith-Wiedemann syndrome. Nature. 1997;387:151–8.

243. Hatada I, Ohashi H, Fukushima Y, Kaneko Y, Inoue M, Komoto Y, et al. An imprinted gene p57^{KIP2} is mutated in Beckwith-Wiedemann syndrome. Nat Genet. 1996;14:171–3.

244. Leighton PA, Ingram RS, Eggenschwiler J, Efstratiadis A, Tilghman SM. Disruption of imprinting caused by deletion of the H19 gene region in mice. Nature. 1995;375:34–9.

245. Caspary T, Cleary MA, Perlman EJ, Zhang P, Elledge SJ, Tilghman SM. Oppositely imprinted genes p57(Kip2) and Igf2 interact in a mouse model for Beckwith-Wiedemann syndrome. Genes Dev. 1999;13(23):3115–24.

246. Yu J, Carroll TJ, Rajagopal J, Kobayashi A, Ren Q, McMahon AP. A Wnt7b-dependent pathway regulates the orientation of epithelial cell division and establishes the cortico-medullary axis of the mammalian kidney. Development. 2009;136(1):161–71. Research Support, N.I.H., Extramural Research Support, Non-U.S. Gov't.

247. Liu Y, Chattopadhyay N, Qin S, Szekeres C, Vasylyeva T, Mahoney ZX, et al. Coordinate integrin and c-Met signaling regulate Wnt gene expression during epithelial morphogenesis. Development. 2009;136(5):843–53.

248. Green MC. Mechanism of the pleiotropic effects of the short-ear mutant gene in the mouse. J Exp Zool. 1968;176:129–50.

249. Yu J, Carroll TJ, McMahon AP. Sonic hedgehog regulates proliferation and differentiation of

mesenchymal cells in the mouse metanephric kidney. Development. 2002;129(22):5301–12. Research Support, Non-U.S. Gov't Research Support, U.S. Gov't, P.H.S.

250. Caubit X, Lye CM, Martin E, Core N, Long DA, Vola C, et al. Teashirt 3 is necessary for ureteral smooth muscle differentiation downstream of SHH and BMP4. Development. 2008;135(19):3301–10. Research Support, Non-U.S. Gov't.

251. Cain JE, Islam E, Haxho F, Blake J, Rosenblum ND. GLI3 repressor controls functional development of the mouse ureter. J Clin Invest. 2011;121(3):1199–206. Research Support, Non-U.S. Gov't.

252. Bose J, Grotewold L, Ruther U. Pallister-Hall syndrome phenotype in mice mutant for Gli3. Hum Mol Genet. 2002;11(9):1129–35. Research Support, Non-U.S. Gov't.

253. Niimura F, Labostky PA, Kakuchi J, Okubo S, Yoshida H, Oikawa T, et al. Gene targeting in mice reveals a requirement for angiotensin in the development and maintenance of kidney morphology and growth factor regulation. J Clin Invest. 1995;96:2947–54.

254. Miyazaki Y, Tsuchida S, Nishimura H, Pope IV JC, Harris RC, McKanna JM, et al. Angiotensin induces the urinary peristaltic machinery during the perinatal period. J Clin Invest. 1998;102:1489–97.

255. Humphreys BD, Lin SL, Kobayashi A, Hudson TE, Nowlin BT, Bonventre JV, et al. Fate tracing reveals the pericyte and not epithelial origin of myofibroblasts in kidney fibrosis. Am J Pathol. 2010;176(1):85–97. Research Support, N.I.H., Extramural Research Support, U.S. Gov't, Non-P.H.S.

256. Cullen-McEwen LA, Caruana G, Bertram JF. The where, what and why of the developing renal stroma. Nephron Exp Nephrol. 2005;99(1):e1–8.

257. Lemley KV, Kriz W. Anatomy of the renal interstitium. Kidney Int. 1991;39(3):370–81.

258. Rosselot C, Spraggon L, Chia I, Batourina E, Riccio P, Lu B, et al. Non-cell-autonomous retinoid signaling is crucial for renal development. Development. 2010;137(2):283–92. Research Support, N.I.H., Extramural Research Support, Non-U.S. Gov't.

259. Quaggin SE, Vanden Heuvel GB, Igarashi P. Pod-1, a mesoderm-specific basic-helix-loop-helix protein expressed in mesenchymal and glomerular epithelial cells in the developing kidney. Mech Dev. 1998;71:37–48.

Functional Development of the Nephron

9

Aoife Waters

Abbreviations

ACE	Angiotensin converting enzyme
ACEI	Angiotensin converting enzyme inhibitors
ADH	Antidiuretic hormone
ANP	Atrial natriuretic peptide
AQ2	Aquaporin-2
AT1	Angiotensin type 1 receptors
BK	Bradykinin
CA	Carbonic anhydrase
cAMP	Cyclic adenosine monophosphate
CCD	Cortical collecting duct
CD	Collecting duct
cGMP	Cyclic guanosine monophosphate
COX-2	Cyclooxygenase type-2
DDAVP	Desmopressin
ELBW	Extremely low birth weight
ENaC	Epithelial sodium channel
ET	Endothelin
FGF-23	Fibroblast growth factor 23
GA	Gestational age
GFB	Glomerular filtration barrier
GFR	Glomerular filtration rate
GH	Growth hormone
IGF-1	Insulin growth factor-1
KK	Kallikrein
NaCl	Sodium chloride
NAG	N-acetyl-β-D-glucosaminidase
NaPII	Sodium-phosphate type 2 co-transporter
NCC	Sodium chloride co-transporter
NHE3	Sodium-hydrogen antiporter 3
NKCC2	Sodium-potassium-chloride cotransporter
NO	Nitric oxide
PGs	Prostaglandins
PTH	Parathyroid hormone
RAS	Renin – angiotensin – aldosterone system
ROMK	Renal outer medullary potassium channel
RVR	Renal vascular resistance
TALH	Thick ascending limb of loop of Henle
TRPV5	Transient receptor potential cation channel subfamily V member 5
TTKG	Transtubular potassium gradient
VMNP	Vasomotor nephropathy

General Overview of Antenatal, Perinatal, and Postnatal Fluid and Electrolyte Homeostasis

Fluid and electrolyte homeostasis in the fetus is controlled by the placenta. As a result, the placenta receives a significant proportion of the fetal cardiac output (33 %), whereas the fetal kidneys

A. Waters
Department of Nephrology, Great Ormond Street Hospital NHS Foundation Trust,
Great Ormond Street, London WC1N 3JH, UK
e-mail: aoife.waters@ucl.ac.uk

© Springer-Verlag Berlin Heidelberg 2016
D.F. Geary, F. Schaefer (eds.), *Pediatric Kidney Disease*, DOI 10.1007/978-3-662-52972-0_9

receive only 2.5 % even in late gestation [1]. The low fetal renal blood flow results in a low creatinine clearance which correlates well with gestational age (Fig. 9.1a, b). Urine production begins at approximately 10 weeks of gestation in the human kidney. This coincides with the acquisition of the first capillary loops by the inner medullary metanephric nephrons. Subsequently, hourly fetal urine production increases from 5 ml at 20 weeks to approximately 50 ml at 40 weeks [4]. After 20 weeks, the kidneys provide over 90 % of the amniotic fluid volume [5]. Severe oligohydramnios due to abnormal fetal renal function in the second trimester can result in pulmonary hypoplasia and in severe cases, Potter's syndrome [6].

At birth, the newborn consists largely of water, with total body water comprising 75 % of body weight at full term and about 80–85 % in preterm infants [7]. Adaptation to the extrauterine environment involves an increase in glomerular filtration with an immediate postnatal natriuresis. High circulating levels of atrial natriuretic peptide in the newborn are responsible for the postnatal physiological natriuresis [8]. In addition, maturation of tubular function occurs postnatally [9]. Changes include an increase in resorptive surface area, transporter number and function, together with further modification of paracrine regulatory mechanisms [9]. In the following section, we will discuss the developmental changes in the neonatal kidney that are necessary for extrauterine

a

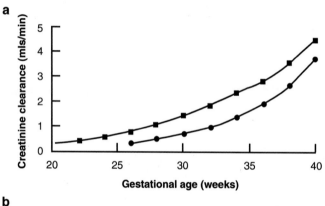

b

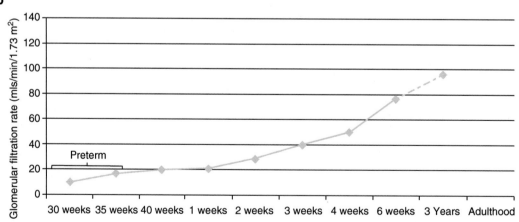

Fig. 9.1 (a, b) (a) Creatinine clearance for human fetuses from 20 weeks. (■) and corresponding preterm neonates (●). Creatinine clearance increases with increasing gestational age (Used with permission of John Wiley and Sons from Haycock [2]) (b) GFR doubles over the first 2 weeks of life in term infants and reaches almost 50 mls/min/1.73 m² between 2 and 4 weeks after birth and adult values by 2 years of age (Used with permission of Vieux R et al. [3])

adaptation. Regulatory mechanisms of the mature kidney will be discussed elsewhere.

Glomerular Function in the Fetal, Perinatal, and Postnatal Period

Glomerular filtration is the transudation of plasma across the glomerular filtration barrier (GFB) and is the first step in the formation of urine (Fig. 9.2). Filtration depends both on Starling's forces and an adequate renal blood flow [10]. The total glomerular filtration rate (GFR) is the sum of the GFR of each single functioning nephron, SNGFR [where SNGFR=(k × S) × (Δ P–Δ π)]. Δ P, is the hydrostatic pressure difference between the glomerular capillary pressure (P_{GC}) and the hydrostatic pressure in Bowman's space (P_{BS}). Δπ is the oncotic pressure difference between the glomerular capillary

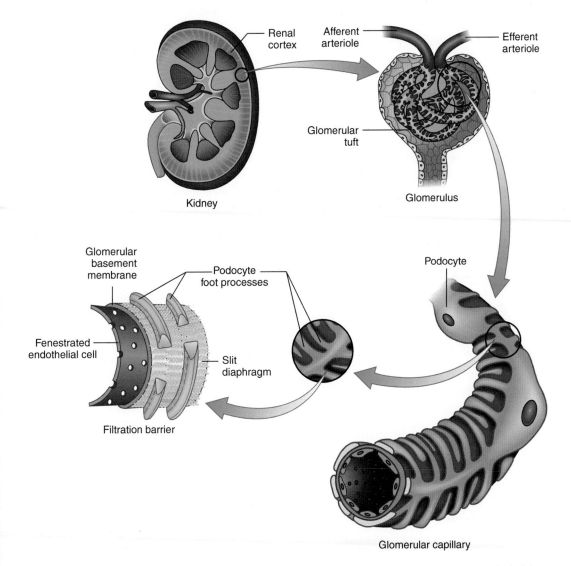

Fig. 9.2 Schematic of the structure and function of the glomerular filtration barrier. It consists of layers that block the passage of plasma macromolecules and also maintain plasma oncotic pressure. A fenestrated capillary endothelium lines each capillary loop. A porous glomerular basement membrane attached to highly dynamic epithelial cells (podocytes) is on the other side of this lining. The slit diaphragm is the prime barrier to filtration of plasma macromolecules. This slit diaphragm consists of podocytes that have interdigitating foot processes with neighbor podocytes and are connected to each other by a platform of signaling molecules

pressure (π_{GC}) and the oncotic pressure in Bowman's space (π_{BS}). K_f is the product of the hydraulic permeability of glomerular capillary walls (k) and the surface area available for filtration, (S), ($K_f = k \times S$). In an adult, the rate of glomerular filtration is about 100–120 ml/min/1.73 m². Even though the term neonate has the full number of glomeruli, its GFR is about 30 ml/min/1.73 m². In this section, we will discuss the functional development of glomerular filtration in the perinatal period.

Fetal GFR

During nephrogenesis, the increase in renal mass parallels an increase in fetal GFR [11]. Indeed, fetal GFR correlates well with both gestational age and body weight [11]. Preterm infants of 30 week gestational age have a creatinine clearance of less than 10 ml/min/1.73 m² within the first 24–40 h of birth [12], whereas creatinine clearance in term infants is higher and ranges between 10 and 40 ml/min/1.73 m² [13]. A study involving 275 neonates aged between 27 and 31 weeks gestation reported GFR reference values as 3rd, 10th, 50th, 90th, and 97th percentiles and provide useful reference ranges of the various gestational ages (Table 9.1) [3].

All four determinants of SNGFR contribute to the maturational increase in GFR to varying degrees [14]. Mean arterial pressure increases during fetal development and an increase in P_{GC} occurs as a result [15]. An increase in renal plasma flow leads to a further increase in SNGFR

[16]. In addition, the oncotic pressure also rises with advancing gestational age [17]. However, the increase in P_{GC} is greater than that observed for π_{GC}, favoring ultrafiltration.

Fetal renal blood flow can be measured by Doppler ultrasound techniques and increases from 20 ml/min at 25 weeks of gestation to more than 60 ml/min at 40 weeks [12]. Fetal renal blood flow is low due to the high renal vascular resistance (RVR) [1, 18]. RVR depends on arteriolar tone and on the number of resistance vessels. As nephrogenesis proceeds, there is an increase in the number of glomerular vessels and in preterm infants born before 36 weeks gestation, the postnatal fall in RVR can, in part be attributable to new nephron formation [18]. Concomitantly, a re-distribution of RBF occurs from the inner medullary nephrons to the more superficial cortical nephrons. The superficial cortex is the site of more recent glomerulogenesis and the increase in SNGFR of the superficial nephrons significantly contributes to the increase in total GFR [14, 19].

Assessment of fetal glomerular function is possible by measurement of fetal serum cystatin C, α1-microglobulin and β2-microglobulin [20]. Cystatin C is a proteinase inhibitor involved in intracellular catabolism of proteins, produced by all nucleated cells, freely filtered across glomeruli and completely catabolized and reabsorbed in the proximal tubule. Fetal serum cystatin C is independent of gestational age and has been shown to have a high specificity (92 %) for the prediction of postnatal kidney dysfunction. Reference intervals were calculated in a study of 129 cordocenteses

Table 9.1 Glomerular filtration rate reference values in premature infants

	Glomerular filtration rate, ml/min/1.73 m²								
	Day 7			Day 14			Day 21		
Gestational age at birth	10th	Median	90th	10th	Median	90th	10th	Median	90th
27 weeks	8.7	13.4	18.1	11.5	16.2	20.9	13.3	18	22.7
28 weeks	11.5	16.2	20.9	14.4	19.1	23.8	16.1	20.8	25.5
29 weeks	14.4	19.1	23.8	17.2	21.9	26.6	19	23.7	28.4
30 weeks	17.2	21.9	26.6	20.1	24.8	29.4	21.8	26.5	31.2
31 weeks	20.1	24.8	29.5	22.9	27.6	32.3	24.7	29.4	34.1

Used with permission from Vieux et al. [3]

involving 54 fetuses without renal disease [21]. Mean serum cystatin C levels were 1.6 mg/l with 2.0 mg/l being the upper limit of normal. In the same study, the authors showed that fetal serum β2-microglobulin decreased significantly with gestational age and the upper limit could be calculated from 7.19 to 0.052 × gestational age in weeks. In the same study, serum β2-microglobulin was demonstrated to have a higher sensitivity (87 %) than cystatin C in predicting postnatal renal dysfunction. Both tests therefore, may be used to assess fetal glomerular function in antenatally diagnosed renal malformations.

Neonatal GFR

A rapid rise in GFR occurs in term infants over the first 4 days of life. Preterm infants also experience a rise in GFR but the rise occurs more slowly than that in term neonates [22]. Overall, a doubling of GFR is seen over the first 2 weeks of life in term infants and reaches almost 50 ml/min/1.73 m2 between 2 and 4 weeks after birth and adult values by 2 years of age (Fig. 9.1b) [23, 24]. Postnatally, the mean arterial pressure increases and consequently, an increase in glomerular hydraulic pressure occurs resulting in an increase in GFR. A dramatic postnatal fall in RVR with redistribution of intrarenal blood flow from the juxtamedullary nephrons to the superficial cortical nephrons also contributes to the increased GFR. The fraction of cardiac output supplying the neonatal kidneys increases to 15–18 % over the first 6 weeks of life [25]. In addition, an increase in the area available for glomerular filtration also contributes to the increase in GFR seen postnatally [14]. Glomerular size, glomerular basement membrane surface area and capillary permeability to macromolecules all contribute to the increase in GFR seen from the neonatal period to adulthood [26]. Maturation of glomerular filtration also occurs, as result of changes in both afferent and efferent arteriolar tone. A decrease in renal vasoconstrictors and activation of renal vasodilators occurs over the first 2 weeks of life and will be discussed in the following section.

Neonatal renal function is often assessed by measurement of serum creatinine which is derived from creatinine and phosphocreatine of muscles and therefore reflects muscle mass. The serum creatinine concentration in the neonate is determined by maturation of the renal tubules, the total muscle mass of the body, glomerular filtration rate and tubular secretion. Several studies have now shown that the plasma creatinine in most infants actually increases after birth (Table 9.2) [27–30]. This is consistent with the idea that the tubules in the neonate are reabsorbing creatinine and not secreting it. Clearly, this has important implications for misinterpreting a rising creatinine in many neonatal ICU (NICU) patients as renal impairment.

Emerging evidence suggests that Cystatin C is a more reliable marker of GFR in the neonatal period. A recent report involving 60 preterm (<37 weeks' GA) and 40 term infants studied from birth demonstrated that Creatinine-based equations consistently underestimated GFR, whereas Cystatin C and combined equations were more consistent with referenced inulin clearance studies [31].

Vasoregulatory Mechanisms of the Neonatal Kidney

Renal Vasoconstrictors in the Developing Nephron

The Renin-Angiotensin System (RAS)
The renin – angiotensin system plays an important role in the regulation of renal blood flow and glomerular filtration. Angiotensin II is a potent

Table 9.2 Reference values for serum creatinine levels in term neonates

Age	Serum creatinine, mg/dL		
	10th	Median	90th
Day 1	0.49	0.62	0.79
Day 3	0.37	0.48	0.61
Week 1	0.31	0.38	0.50
Week 2	0.27	0.35	0.45
Week 4	0.23	0.28	0.36

Used with permission of Springer Science + Business Media from Boer et al. [27]

vasoconstrictor of the efferent arteriole causing a resultant increase in P_{GC} and therefore, GFR. Both plasma renin activity and angiotensin II levels are high in the neonate. Renal angiotensin converting enzyme (ACE) levels are higher than adult levels during first 2 weeks of life and expression is localized to the proximal tubules and capillaries in the developing human kidney [32, 33]. Expression of angiotensinogen and ACE increases during late gestation and peaks after birth [34, 35]. In addition, the number of angiotensin type 1 receptors (AT1) are also twice that of adult levels at 2 weeks of age [35, 36]. AT2 receptors, on the other hand, are more abundant in the fetal kidney with progressive downregulation during fetal maturation. In contrast, AT1 receptors undergo upregulation as the fetal kidney matures [36, 37].

Animal studies have shown that angiotensin II constricts the fetal renal arteries via the AT1 receptor and during fetal life plays an important role in controlling the resistance of the umbilical arteries and therefore, the total fetal peripheral vascular resistance [38]. Maintenance of arterial pressure and baroreceptor control of heart rate and renal sympathetic nerve activity is controlled by circulating and endogenous angiotensin II in newborn lambs [39]. Therefore, the RAS plays a significant role in maintaining blood pressure as well as vascular resistance in the developing fetus.

Indeed, the importance of the fetal RAS is highlighted by studies reporting cases of ACE fetopathy with the use of angiotensin converting enzyme inhibitors (ACEI) in pregnancy. Maternal ACEI can result in decreased placental perfusion, fetal hypotension, oligohydramnios and neonatal renal failure [40]. Recently, mutations in genes coding for renin, angiotensinogen, ACE and AT1 have been described in association with autosomal recessive renal tubular dysgenesis with fetal hypotension [41]. Both inherited and acquired defects of the RAS, therefore, can alter fetal renal haemodynamics with deleterious effects on renal development.

Renal Nerves and Catecholamines

The high RVR in the perinatal period can in part be due to increased renal sympathetic nerve activity (through α1 receptor stimulation) and ris-

ing circulating catecholamine levels [42]. The renal sympathetic nerves cause renal vasoconstriction, primarily of the afferent arteriole which results in a decrease in P_{GC} and glomerular filtration rate (Fig. 9.3) [44]. Renal sympathetic nerve activity increases immediately after birth in sheep and plasma epinephrine and norepinephrine increase several fold immediately following birth [45, 46]. A fall in catecholamine levels subsequently occurs over the first few days of life [47]. Renal denervation in maturing piglets has been shown to increase RBF demonstrating the role of renal nerves in maintaining high RVR. The sympathetic nervous system also has an important secondary role by stimulating the release of

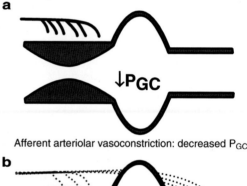

Afferent arteriolar vasoconstriction: decreased P_{GC}

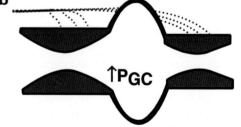

Efferent arteriolar vasoconstriction: increased P_{GC}

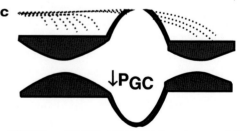

Afferent>>>efferent vasoconstriction: decreased P_{GC}

Fig. 9.3 (a–c) The renal nerves constrict the renal vasculature, causing decreases in renal blood flow and glomerular filtration (Used with permission of John Wiley and Sons from Denton et al. [43])

renin. Rodent studies have shown that renin – containing cells and nerve fibers are detected at 17 days of gestation, in close spatial relationship along the main branches of the renal artery [48]. Innervation of renin – containing cells follows the centrifugal pattern of renin distribution and nephrovascular development. The density and organization of nerve fibers increases with age along the arterial vascular tree [48]. Therefore, an interplay between increased sympathetic nerve activity and high plasma renin is likely for the high RVR during the perinatal period.

Endothelin

Endothelin (ET) is a potent vasoconstrictor secreted by the endothelial cells of renal vessels, mesangial cells, and distal tubular cells in response to angiotensin II, bradykinin, epinephrine and shear stress [48]. Renal vasomotor tone is exquisitely sensitive to endothelin. An increase in RVR occurs following ET- induced contraction of glomerular arterioles (afferent > efferent) with a subsequent reduction in GFR [49]. In the first days of life, ET is elevated both in term and preterm neonates. A subsequent reduction in ET levels occur after the first week of life [50]. Newborn rat kidneys have a higher number of ET receptors than adult rat kidneys. A comparable binding affinity for ET has also been shown [51]. In addition, ET can also cause vasodilatation. Activation of ET_B receptors on the vascular endothelium evokes the release of vasodilators. The renal vasculature of fetal renal lambs reacts with vasodilatation to low doses of ET which may be due to the secondary release of nitric oxide (NO) which blunts the vasoconstrictor effects of ET [52, 53]. Endothelin, therefore, may have both vasoconstrictor effects and vasodilatory effects on the neonatal kidney.

Renal Vasodilators in the Developing Nephron

Prostaglandins

The major prostaglandins (PGs), PGE_2, PGD_2, and PGI_2, increase RBF by stimulating afferent arteriolar vasodilatation, free water clearance, urine flow, and natriuresis. PGs are synthesized by the fetal and neonatal kidney [54]. Alterations in the synthetic and catabolic activity of renal prostaglandins occur with advancing gestational and postnatal age. Concomitant alterations in RBF, GFR, water and electrolyte excretion occur, suggesting an important role for PGs in renal functional development.

Newborns have high circulating levels of PGs that counteract the highly activated vasoconstrictor state of the neonatal microcirculation [55]. The deleterious renal vasoconstrictor effect of PG synthesis inhibitors illustrates the protective role of PGs in the immature kidney. Long – term maternal indomethacin treatment may decrease fetal urine output enough to alter amniotic fluid volume [56]. Severe renal impairment leading to fetal or neonatal death has been reported with the use of PG synthesis inhibitors which include indomethacin [57]. Neonatal indomethacin therapy may cause transient dose-related renal dysfunction characterized by a decrease in urine output. Renal dysfunction depends in part, on dosage, timing of therapy, and the cardiovascular and renal status of the infant prior to treatment [58]. In addition, recent data from studies in rodents with targeted gene disruption have shown that cyclooxygenase type-2 (COX-2) are necessary for late stages of kidney development and lack of COX-2 activity leads to pathological change in cortical architecture and eventually to renal failure [59]. Therefore, both the RAS and PGs are not only important for renal hemodynamics but are also necessary for kidney development.

Nitric Oxide

Nitric oxide (NO) plays a major role in maintaining basal renal vascular tone in the mature kidney. Through activation of its second messenger, cGMP, NO results in vasodilatation, modification of renin release and change in glomerular filtration rate [60]. Nitric oxide plays an important role in the maintenance of glomerular filtration in the developing kidney. Animal studies have shown that inhibition of NO synthesis by infusion with L-arginine analogues significantly decreases GFR in the developing kidney but not in the adult [61–63]. Treatment with angiotensin receptor blockers abolishes the decrease in GFR observed in the developing kidneys treated with L-arginine analogues [63]. Therefore, NO plays a critical role in the developing kidney by counteregulating the vasoconstricting effects of angiotensin II and protecting the immature kidney.

The Kallikrein-Kinin System

Bradykinin (BK) is a vasodilator and diuretic peptide, produced by the action of kallikrein (KK), an enzyme produced by the collecting duct epithelial cells. Activation of the BK-2 receptor by BK stimulates NO and PG production resulting in vasodilation and natriuresis. An endogenous kallikrein-kinin system is expressed in the developing kidney with higher neonatal expression than that found in adult kidneys [64, 65]. Renal expression and urinary excretion of KK rapidly rises in the postnatal period with excretion of KK correlating well with the rise in RBF [66, 67]. Blockade of the BK-2 receptor results in renal vasoconstriction in newborn rabbits, demonstrating the renal vasodilatory action of BK in the neonatal kidney [68].

Disordered Vasoregulatory Mechanisms

Vasomotor Nephropathy (VMNP)

Vasomotor nephropathy (VMNP) is defined as renal dysfunction due to reduced renal perfusion, and the preterm infant is particularly vulnerable to VMNP [69]. The main causes of neonatal acute renal failure are prerenal mechanisms and include hypotension, hypovolemia, hypoxemia and neonatal septicemia. Hypotension itself can stimulate vasoconstrictive mediators such as angiotensin II, cause renal vasoconstriction and hypoperfusion and further reduce the GFR in the newborn. The treatment of neonatal hypotension can involve inotropic support and dopamine is usually considered as the first line agent. Dopamine itself has a direct effect on renal function via renal dopaminergic receptors located in the renal arteries, glomeruli, proximal and distal tubules [70]. At low doses (0.5–2 µg/kg/min), dopamine causes renal vasodilatation and increases GFR and electrolyte excretion. In neonatal intensive care units, higher doses of dopamine (6–10 µg/kg/min) are needed to achieve systemic cardiovascular effects. Such doses have an opposite effect on renal function, causing renal vasoconstriction and reduction in sodium and water excretion [71]. Hypoxemia itself reduces renal blood flow and GFR. In a study of severely asphyxiated neonates 61 % developed acute renal failure [72]. Hypoxemia stimulates ET, ANP and PG release. In addition, mechanical ventilation can reduce venous return and cardiac output and can thus cause renal hypoperfusion and impair renal function [69]. Therefore, in the neonate, VMNP can result from disturbances of glomerular hemodynamics, through complex interplay of the renal vasoregulatory mechanisms.

Water Transport in the Developing Kidney

Term neonates can dilute their urine to an osmolality as low 50 mOsm/l which is similar to adults [73]. However, the ability to excrete a water load is limited by the neonate's low GFR. As a result, the newborn infant is largely water, with total body water comprising 75 % of body weight at full term and about 80–85 % in babies between 26 and 31 weeks gestation [7]. Under normal physiological conditions, the kidneys have to excrete this water load during the first week of life [74]. Therefore, maximal concentrating abilities are not necessary at birth and in fact, are low in the neonatal period. A progressive increase in concentrating capacity occurs postnatally and in term infants reaches adult levels by the first month of life (Fig. 9.4) [75]. In the premature neonate, concentrating capacity is maximal at about 500 mOsm/l for a more prolonged period [76] which places the sick premature infant at greater risk for serious disturbances in water and electrolyte homeostasis [77]. The reasons for the limited concentrating capacity include diminished responsiveness of the collecting ducts to antidiuretic hormone (ADH), anatomical immaturity of the renal medulla and decreased medullary concentration of sodium chloride (NaCl) and

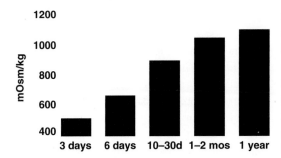

Fig. 9.4 Renal concentrating capacity increases in the postnatal period in the term infant, reaching adult values by the first month of life (Used with permission of BMJ Publishing Group from Polacek et al. [75])

urea [78, 79] In the following section, we will discuss each of these components in detail.

Antidiuretic Hormone in the Development of Water Transport

Normal ADH Physiology

ADH exerts its antidiuretic effect in the collecting duct (CD) via the V_2 receptor on the basolateral membrane of the principal and inner medullary CD cells [80, 81]. Binding of ADH to the V_2 receptor results in activation of adenyl cyclase, increased cAMP and activation of protein kinase A. Subsequent phosphorylation of the cytoplasmic COOH terminus at serine 256 of the aquaporin-2 water channel (AQ2) occurs and results in the insertion of AQ2 into the apical membrane of the CD cells [82–84]. Water enters the cells via AQ2 and exits the cell via the AQ3 and AQ4 water channels located on the basolateral membrane of the CD cells [85]. Water reabsorption depends on a hypertonic medullary interstitium, which drives water from the luminal fluid across the tubular epithelium [86].

Development of Water Transport in the Collecting Duct

Neonatal low urine concentrating capacity is not attributable to low ADH levels. During labour, ADH levels are elevated which is consistent with the raised intracranial pressure and hypoxemia acting as stimuli for ADH release [87]. Despite

adequate ability to secrete ADH, no correlation exists between ADH levels and urine osmolality in the first 3 weeks of life [88]. ADH stimulation of the neonatal cortical collecting duct results in a lower permeability response to water than that seen in the adult [89, 90]. The response to ADH does, however, improve with age [91]. Similarly, studies have shown that the concentrating capacity is even lower in infants who have sustained neonatal asphyxia [92]. V_2 receptor mRNA expression is observed in rodents as early as day 16 of gestation in cells of the developing medullary and cortical CD [93]. During the first 2 weeks of life in rats, the number of receptors does not change. By the fifth week of life, the number of receptors reaches adult levels [94]. However, the low response of the immature kidney to ADH is more likely to be due to immaturity of the intracellular second messenger systems rather than inadequate receptor number. ADH binding sites precede the onset of adenyl cyclase responsiveness [95]. In addition, ADH stimulation of adenyl cyclase generation is markedly lower in the neonatal period and is only about one-third that of the cAMP response seen in the adult CCD [96]. However, even when cAMP generation is rescued using cAMP analogs, the hydraulic permeability of isolated, microperfused rabbit CCD remains low [97]. Intracellular phosphodiesterases degrade cAMP. Indeed, an increase in phosphodiesterase IV and inhibition of the production of cAMP by PGE2 acting through EP3 receptors has been shown to inhibit adenyl cyclase generation on ADH stimulation. Therefore, cAMP inhibition likely accounts for the immature kidney's reduced response to ADH [98, 99].

AQ-2 levels (mRNA and protein) are lower in early postnatal life and reach maximal expression at 10 weeks of age (Fig. 9.5) [100]. AQ2 trafficking can be appropriately stimulated by dehydration and DDAVP in the immature kidney but the urine osmolality remains low [100]. Glucocorticoids regulate the AQ2 expression which increase expression of both AQ2 protein and mRNA in the infant and not in the adult [101]. The expression of AQ3 and AQ4 does not change significantly after birth and they do not

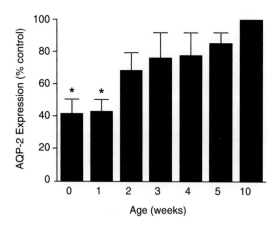

Fig. 9.5 Aquaporin-2 (AQ2) expression between 0 and 10 weeks of age. An increase in protein expression occurs in the postnatal period (Used with permission from Bonilla-Felix [78])

seem to play a role in the maturation of water transport in the CD [102].

Tonicity of the Developing Medullary Interstitium

In addition to low CD responsiveness to ADH, two other factors are responsible for the low concentrating capacity of the neonatal nephron. The medullary interstitium of the neonate has a low tonicity due to a low concentration of NaCl and urea [103]. Factors such as low protein intake, low sodium transport by the thick ascending loop of Henle [104], immaturity of the medullary architecture with shorter loops of Henle [105, 106] and alterations in urea transport [107] all contribute to the lower tonicity of the medullary interstitium. The activity of the Na-K-ATPase in the thick ascending limb of Henle's loop increases after birth, with the most pronounced increase in activity between the second and third week of life, correlating well with the increase in urine concentrating capacity [108]. The loops of Henle elongate and penetrate the medulla, forming tubulovascular units that are completed by the fourth postnatal week in rodents [109].

The medulla/cortex urea ratio increases over the first 3 weeks of life in newborn rabbits [103]. Rodent studies have shown that there is a striking increase in the number of urea transporters during the first 2 weeks of life [107]. The urea transporters prevent the loss of urea from the medulla into the circulation thereby ensuring a high concentration of urea in the medullary interstitium. Renal concentrating capacity is dependent on dietary protein intake [103] and infants fed on high protein diets show a significant improvement in urinary concentrating capacity [92, 110].

In summary, the neonatal kidney's ability to concentrate urine is dependent on a number of steps involving the ADH – signal transduction pathway (Fig. 9.6), the maturation of Henle's loop and tonicity of the medullary interstitium.

Postnatal Urine Flow

Oliguria is the most helpful sign of renal impairment in the neonate and a delay in the first void in a newborn may signal a renal disorder. Pre-term neonates void earlier than term or post-term neonates [111] and the majority of normal newborns void within the first 24 h of life regardless of gestational age. Therefore, any neonate who remains anuric beyond the first day of life should be evaluated for renal insufficiency. The factors determining urine output include water balance, solute load and renal concentrating ability.

Minimum urine volume (L) = Urine solutes to be excreted/ urine osmolality (max). As a result, a neonate receiving the usual renal solute load (7–15 mOsm/kg daily) with a maximal renal concentrating capacity of 500 mOsm/kg would require a minimal urine output of approximately 1 ml/kg per hour to remain in solute balance. Since acute renal failure results in progressively positive solute balance, a urine flow rate less than 1 ml/kg per hour has become an accepted criterion for the definition of oliguria in the neonate.

Sodium Transport in the Developing Kidney

Adaptation to the extrauterine environment involves a physiological natriuresis in the immediate postnatal period with preterm infants losing up to 16 % of their birth weight in the first 3 days of life and term infants losing slightly less [112].

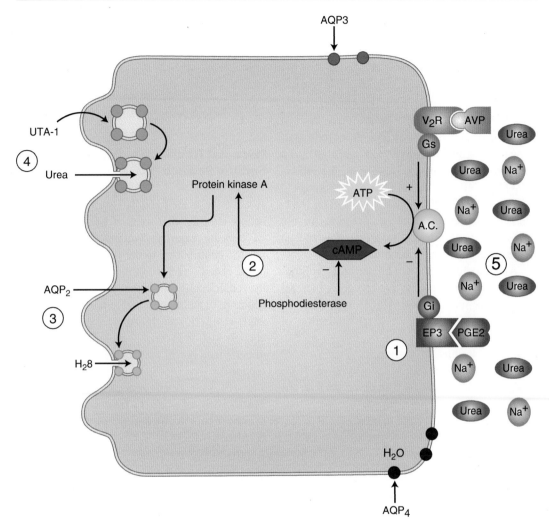

Fig. 9.6 The immature kidney's response to ADH: Responsible mechanisms are illustrated as follows: *1* Inhibition of cAMP generation by PGE₂ through EP3 receptor, *2* rapid degradation of formed cAMP resulting from increased phosphodiesterase activity, *3* low expres-sion of AQP2 during early postnatal life, *4* low expression of UTA-1 during early postnatal life, *5* low concentration of urea and sodium in the medullary interstitium resulting from low rates of sodium transport, low dietary protein intake, and low expression of urea transporters

Human neonates remain in negative sodium balance for the first 4 days of life and then shift to a positive sodium balance by the second and third weeks of life (Fig. 9.7) [113]. Sodium conservation occurs because sodium is essential for growth in the neonate. In contrast to term neonates, preterm infants less than 35 weeks of gestation do not tolerate sodium deprivation, and hyponatremia may develop due to tubular immaturity and sodium wasting [114]. For this reason sodium supplementation is important. Thus, the sodium requirements for a term newborn range from 1 to 1.5 mEq/kg. daily, whereas the requirements for a pre-term neonate range from 3 to 5 mEq/kg daily. Sodium supplementation in the preterm infant enhances the cumulative weight gain following the initial postnatal diuresis [113]. In the following section, we will discuss the mechanisms involved in the postnatal natriuresis and then the factors involved in the neonatal transition from negative to positive sodium balance.

Early Postnatal Natriuresis

High perinatal circulating levels of atrial natriuretic peptide (ANP) have been implicated in the
immediate postnatal natriuresis seen in both term
and preterm infants [8]. ANP is a natriuretic hormone produced within the cardiac myocytes and
released by stretch of the atrial wall. At birth, pulmonary vascular resistance falls and left atrial
venous return increases, stimulating the release
of ANP. ANP exerts a number of physiological
effects including an increase in glomerular filtration rate, natriuresis, diuresis, inhibition of renin
and aldosterone release, vasorelaxation and an
increase in vascular permeability [115].

ANP modulates sodium homeostasis by binding to physiologically active receptors increasing intracellular cGMP [116]. Inhibition of
sodium transport occurs through inhibition of
apical sodium channels in renal tubular epithelial cells, leading to natriuresis. Plasma ANP
concentration decreases with maturation [117,
118]. A fall in right atrial volume occurs over the
first 4 days of fetal life with parallel reductions
in ANP concentration and urinary cGMP excretion [119]. In addition, a decrease in cGMP

production per ANP binding site has been shown
to occur rapidly in the suckling period in neonatal rats [120]. Therefore, sodium excretion is
reduced after the first few postnatal days and the
neonatal kidney subsequently aims to conserve
sodium.

Neonatal Transition to Positive Sodium Balance

A reduction in the fractional excretion of sodium
occurs after the first week of life with fractions
<1 % in the majority of infants (Fig. 9.8) [122].
Factors contributing to the decrease in the fractional excretion of sodium include maturation of
the sodium transport mechanisms in the postnatal
nephron, in addition to high circulating levels of
angiotensin II, catecholamines, glucocorticoids
and a reduction in atrial natriuretic peptide. Each
of these factors will be discussed in the following
section.

Maturation of Sodium Transport Mechanisms in the Developing Nephron

A progressive maturation of each tubular segment occurs in the postnatal kidney [123]. Each
tubular segment will be discussed separately in
the following section.

Proximal Tubule

Solute transport in the neonatal proximal tubule
is similar to that in the adult and follows both
chloride and bicarbonate reabsorption. Several
animal studies have shown an increase in the
activity of the Na^+/H^+ exchanger as the neonate
matures [124, 125]. In addition, an increase in
activity of the chloride/formate exchanger has
also been shown to occur [126]. The Na-K-
ATPase transporter plays a key role in sodium
reabsorption in the proximal tubule and slower
transport has been shown in neonates compared
to adults, with a progressive maturation occurring from birth (Fig. 9.9) [127, 128]. In guinea
pigs, posttranslational increase in the α1 and β1
subunits of the Na-K-ATPase transporter occurs
immediately after birth [129].

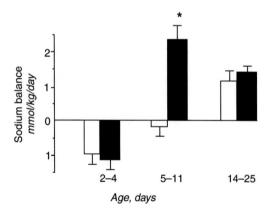

Fig. 9.7 Net external sodium balance for preterm infants
in the first 3 weeks of life. Symbols are: (□) control
infants; (■) sodium-supplemented infants, 4–5 mEq/kg/
day; *$P<0.0005$ vs. controls. In the first 2–4 days after
birth, infants undergo natriuresis regardless of sodium
intake, whereas by 1 week, supplemented infants achieve
positive sodium balance sooner than controls (Used with
permission of BMJ Publishing Group from Al-Dahhan
et al. [113])

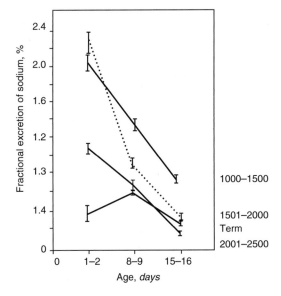

Fig. 9.8 Fractional excretion of sodium during the first 2 weeks of life in preterm and term infants. Sodium is conserved despite an increase in GFR (Used with permission of Elsevier from Chevalier [121])

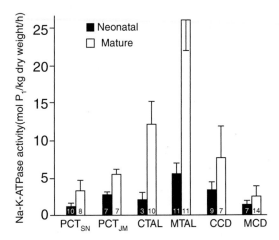

Fig. 9.9 Na+/K+ ATPase activity in the neonatal and adult nephron. The Na+/K+/ATPase activity is lower in the neonate compared to the adult (Used with permission of Schmidt and Horster [127])

Loop of Henle

NaCl transport in the thick ascending limb occurs by paracellular and transcellular pathways via the apical NKCC2 and NHE3 exchangers. The basolateral cell membrane utilizes the Na-K-ATPase to extrude sodium. Transcription of NKCC2 is observed early in development, prior to the onset of filtration in the descending loop of Henle. Physiological studies show, however, that the NKCC2 is unlikely to be functional until postnatally, as a low reabsorptive capacity has been shown for this segment in early postnatal life [109]. Compared to the adult, the expression of all of these transporters is lower in the neonate [130–133]. A postnatal five to tenfold increase in activity of the Na-K-ATPase co-transporter occurs and is greater than that seen in other tubular segments (Fig. 9.9) [127, 134]. Na-K-ATPase consists of a catalytic (α subunit) and a regulatory (β subunit). Both the $\alpha 1$ and $\beta 1$ isoforms are present in the mature kidney. On the other hand, the $\alpha 1$ subunit is detected early in fetal life whereas the $\beta 1$ subunit is detected only after birth. Interestingly, the $\beta 2$ isoform is expressed in the fetal kidney and in contrast to the adult, Na-K-ATPase is expressed on both the apical and basolateral cell membranes. After birth, the $\beta 2$ isoform is downregulated and the $\alpha 1$ and $\beta 1$ isoforms are upregulated [135]. Heterodimerization of the $\alpha 1$ and $\beta 1$ isoforms is essential for the function of the Na-K-ATPase. Of note, treatment with glucocorticoid hormones increases the synthesis of mRNA for both the catalytic and regulatory subunits of the Na-K-ATPase. During postnatal life there is a 20% increase in the amount of sodium reabsorbed along this segment, which reflects functional maturation of transporters, an increase in the resorptive surface area and maturation mechanisms of hormonal control.

Distal Tubule

The Na+-Cl⁻ (NCC) co-transporter is the major sodium influx co-transporter in the distal tubule. In the mature nephron, NCC is expressed along the entire distal tubule, starting beyond the NKCC-expressing post-macular segment and ending at the transition into the collecting tubules [136]. During development, NCC mRNA is detected in distal tubule segments before the expression of NKCC2 mRNA and sodium-phosphate type 2 co-transporter (NaPII) mRNA. Later in development, the NCC expression proceeds gradually into the post-macula segment of the thick ascending limb of the loop of Henle [132].

Cortical Collecting Duct

Fine-tuning of sodium reabsorption occurs in the CCD where the amiloride-sensitive epithelial sodium channel (ENaC) plays an important role. ENaC is located on the apical membrane distal tubular, cortical and outer medullary collecting duct cells [137]. ENaC is comprised of three subunits, α,β and γ. Rodent studies show that the amount of total renal embryonic rat ENaC subunit mRNA is low but increases from murine gestational day 16–19 [138]. A sharp rise to almost adult levels occurs in the first three postnatal days [139]. After birth, the mRNA for α ENaC increases, whereas that for β- and γ-decreases. In the immature kidney, the greatest expression is seen in the terminal collecting duct for all three subunits. As the kidney matures, the expression in the cortical distal nephron increases and in rodents is complete by the ninth postnatal day [140]. Endogenous glucocorticoids do not appear to have any effect on the pre-natal maturation of ENaC in the kidney [141]. Although this response has long been assumed to be solely the result of liganded nuclear hormone receptors trans-activating αENaC, epigenetic controls of basal and aldosterone-induced transcription of αENaC in the collecting duct were recently described [142].

The Na-K-ATPase is also present in the CCD on the basolateral cell membrane.

Tracer uptake assays of individual CCDs have shown that the activity of the Na-K-ATPase increases within the same time interval as it takes for maturation of the net transepithelial reabsorption of sodium and potassium [143]. The capacity of the CCD to reabsorb sodium increases immediately after birth [144] and reflects the increase in expression of the aforementioned sodium channels.

Developmental Paracrine Regulation of Renal Sodium Excretion

Renin: Angiotensin: Aldosterone System (RAS)

Studies have shown that the RAS is involved in renal tubular sodium reabsorption in the neonate. Acute volume expansion in neonatal rat pups results in natriuresis and AT1 blockade attenuates the natriuretic response, demonstrating that angiotensin II mediates sodium reabsorption via the ATI receptor [145]. The proximal tubule is the likely site of sodium reabsorption because angiotensin II augments sodium reabsorption in the proximal tubule in adult rats during volume contraction [146]. In addition, angiotensin II stimulates aldosterone which stimulates sodium reabsorption in the thick ascending limb of the loop of Henle as well as the distal tubule and the collecting duct. Preterm neonates without sodium supplementation demonstrate markedly increased plasma renin and aldosterone activity compared to their sodium supplemented counterparts, indicating that the neonatal RAS is involved in sodium homeostatic mechanisms [147].

Catecholamines

Catecholamines stimulate NaCl and water reabsorption by the proximal tubule, ascending limb of Henle's loop, distal tubule and collecting duct. Circulating plasma catecholamines are high in the neonatal period and then fall over the first few days of life as discussed earlier (see Section on "Development of Glomerular Filtration"). Catecholamines stimulate an increase in renin release which promotes sodium reabsorption. In addition, dopamine acting via the D2 receptor in preterm neonates, enhances sodium reabsorption in the proximal tubule [148].

Glucocorticoids and Thyroid Hormone

Plasma cortisol levels increase markedly after birth [149]. Maturation of the Na+/H+ exchanger occurs under the influence of glucocorticoids as demonstrated by the attenuated postnatal increase of Na^+/H^+ exchanger activity, protein and mRNA abundance in the brush border of proximal tubular cells of adrenalectomized newborn rodents [150]. Glucocorticoids also play a role in the maturation of transporters along the entire nephron [151, 152].

Thyroid hormone plays a role in the maturation of the paracellular pathways of sodium reabsorption [153]. Hypothyroid animals have paracellular tubular chloride permeability to that seen in the mature nephron. In addition, thyroid hormone, which increases sharply after birth, plays a role in the regulation of the Na⁺/K⁺ ATPase activity [154].

Fractional Excretion of Sodium

In the oliguric term neonate (urine flow less than 1 ml/kg per hour) fractional excretion of sodium of less than 2.5 % suggests a pre-renal cause, such as volume depletion, hypoalbuminemia or reduced cardiac output [155]. The criterion of 2.5 % is valid after the first 10 days of life in the low birth weight newborn after the period of postnatal natriuresis [122]. In addition, very low birth weight infants have greater fractional sodium excretion due to immaturity of the sodium reabsorptive capacity [156].

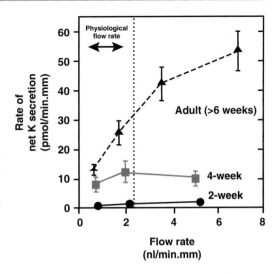

Fig. 9.10 Net potassium secretion in maturing rabbits (Used with permission of Elsevier from Zhou and Satlin [163])

Potassium Transport in the Developing Kidney

Like sodium, potassium is critical for somatic growth and an increase in total body potassium content is associated with growth [157]. In contrast to the adult, neonates greater than 30 weeks gestational age (GA) must maintain a positive potassium balance [157, 158]. Premature newborns, as a result, tend to have higher plasma potassium concentrations than children [158]. In utero, the placenta transports potassium from the mother to the fetus [159]. Interestingly, potassium levels >6.5 mmol/l are observed in 30–50 % of very low birth weight infants in the first 48 h in the absence of potassium intake and not after 72 h [160]. A shift from the intracellular to the extracellular fluid compartment, as a result of either Na/K pump failure and/or a limited renal potassium excretory capacity have been postulated to account for this increase [161, 162].

Renal potassium excretion is determined by the rate of potassium excretion by the principal cells of the distal tubule and collecting duct. Net potassium secretion cannot be detected in microperfused CCD of newborn rabbits until after the third week of life (Fig. 9.10) [164] and flow – stimulated transport is not detected until after the first postnatal month [165].

Maturation of Potassium Transport Mechanisms in the Developing Nephron

Maturation of tubular transport mechanisms will be discussed for each tubular segment in this section.

Proximal Tubule and Loop of Henle

In the mature nephron, 65 % of the filtered potassium load is reabsorbed passively in the proximal tubule [166] and only 10 % reaches the early distal tubule. In contrast, 35 % of the filtered potassium load reaches the distal tubule of the newborn rat [167]. Therefore, postnatal maturation of the TALH is required for further potassium reabsorption. Indeed, both the diluting capacity and Na-K-ATPase activity increase after birth [108, 127]. As discussed earlier, transcription of NKCC2 is observed early in development, prior to the onset of filtration in the descending loop of Henle but is unlikely to be functional until postnatally in view of the low reabsorptive capacity shown for this segment in early postnatal life [104]. Apical ROMK has been detected in the TALH at an earlier developmental stage compared to the CCD. Functional analyses on ROMK in the developing TALH have not been performed.

Cortical Collecting Duct

In the fully differentiated CCD, two types of potassium channels are involved in potassium secretion – (i) the ROMK channel mediates potassium secretion under baseline conditions [168, 169] and (ii) the maxi -K^+ channel which mediates flow-stimulated potassium secretion [170]. ROMK has only been shown in principal cells of the CCD. Maxi- K^+ exists in both the principal and intercalated cells of the CCD [170]. In isolated CCDs of neonatal rabbits, apical ROMK channels are not detected in the first 7 days of life and subsequently, a three-fold increase in the number of ROMK channels is seen in the principal cells of CCD between the third and fifth week of life [171]. The initial increase in expression follows 1 week after an increase in ENaC activity is detected [172]. Also, expression of the ROMK protein on apical cell membranes of the thick ascending limb of the loop of Henle and occasional CCD in the inner cortex and outer medulla is detected in 1-week old animals [173] by indirect immuno-fluorescence studies. By 3 weeks of age expression has increased to involve the mid-and outer CCDs [173]. Maxi-K+ channels mediate flow stimulated K+ secretion and do not appear to be functional in 4-week old rabbits subjected to a sixfold increase in tubular flow rate [165]. However, a small but significant increase in net potassium secretion after 5 weeks of age is observed. An associated increase in the mRNA and protein expression of the α subunit of the maxi-K^+ channel is seen on the apical surface of the intercalated cells of the CCD [165]. In addition, to potassium excretion, potassium reabsorption also occurs in the distal nephron via the apical H^+/K^+ ATPase. Fluorescent functional assays identify significant H^+/K^+ ATPase activity on the apical cell membranes of neonatal intercalated cells [174] which suggests that neonatal collecting ducts have a capacity to retain potassium. Indeed, a longitudinal prospective study of fractional potassium excretion in 23–31 week GA infants demonstrated that despite a threefold increase of filtered potassium, the renal excretion fell by half between 26 and 30 weeks [157]. This study supports the idea that the developing kidney has the capacity for potassium reabsorption.

Regulation of Potassium Balance in the Neonate

Table 9.3 illustrates the factors which acutely regulate plasma potassium in the neonate. The immature kidney displays an insensitivity to aldosterone despite high circulating levels of aldosterone [158]. The number of mineralocorticoid receptors, the receptor affinity and degree of nuclear binding of hormone-receptor is similar in adult and neonatal rats [175]. Aldosterone insensitivity may result from immature intracellular signal transduction mechanisms. Aldosterone insensitivity in the immature kidney is supported by the low trans-tubular potassium gradients (TTKG) reported in 27 week GA infants compared to 30-week infants followed over the first 5 days of postnatal life [176]. However, the low TTKG may also reflect a low secretory ability. Glucocorticoids have a significant effect on potassium balance in extremely LBW infants during the first week of life. Infants whose mothers received a full course of prenatal steroids had no hyperkalemia

Table 9.3 Neonatal potassium regulation

	Effect on cell uptake of K+
Physiologic	
Plasma K concentration	
↑	↑
↓	↓
Insulin	↑
Catecholamines	
α-agonists	↓
β-agonists	↑
Pathologic	
Acid-base balance	
Acidosis	↓
Alkalosis	↑
Hyperosmolality	↑ cell efflux
Cell breakdown	↑ cell efflux

Used with permission of Elsevier from Zhou and Satlin [163]

(>6.5 mmol/L) and a less negative potassium balance at the end of the first week of life [177]. Several studies have shown that glucocorticoids upregulate the expression of the Na^+/K^+ ATPase [178] resulting in a decrease of the intracellular to extracellular potassium shift.

Acid-Base Regulation in the Developing Kidney

The term neonate has a lower bicarbonate concentration than the adult (Fig. 9.11) [179, 180]. In the low birth weight newborn, total bicarbonate may be as low as 15 mmol/l during the early postnatal period and is within normal limits [179]. Bicarbonate gradually increases with increasing glomerular filtration rate. Misdiagnosis of renal tubular acidosis may occur if one does not take into account, the physiologically low plasma bicarbonate in neonates. In addition, neonates need to excrete 2–3 mEq/Kg/day of acid due to their high protein intake and formation of new

bone. The neonate has a reduced ability to respond to an acid load while ammoniagenesis and titratable acidity mature after 4–6 weeks in the low birth weight newborn [181]. Renal regulation of acid – base balance undergoes complex changes during development and will be discussed in detail.

Proximal Tubule Handling of Bicarbonate in the Neonate

Neonatal bicarbonate reabsorption in the proximal tubule is one third that of the adult [182] and is due to lower activity of the similar transporters present in the adult [183]. The number of apical NHE3 antiporters is lower than that in the mature nephron and has about one-third the activity [124]. The H^+/ATPase does not appear to be active in the neonate while the basolateral Na-K-ATPase has about one-half of activity compared to the adult [184]. The carbonic anhydrase type IV isoform which is expressed

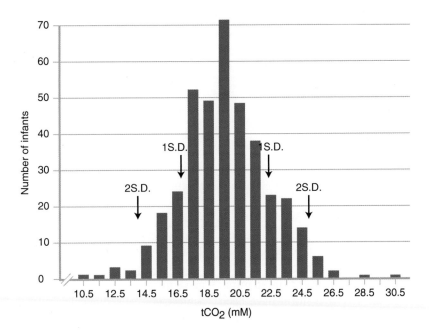

Fig. 9.11 Frequency distribution of serum total bicarbonate (tCO_2) in low birth weight neonates during first month of life. Mean is approximately 20 mM with normal range plus/minus 2 standard deviations (S.D.) is 14.5–24.5 mM (Used with permission of Elsevier from Schwartz et al. [179])

on the brush border of proximal tubular epithelial cells has a lower activity in the developing nephron of rabbits but activity does increase during maturation and parallels the increase in bicarbonate reabsorption occurring in the proximal tubule [185]. Ammoniagenesis does occur in the neonatal kidney but at a much lower rate compared to the adult [186, 187]. Glutamine and activity of the deaminating enzyme, glutaminase is lower in the neonatal kidney while glutaminate, an inhibitor of glutaminase is higher. Neonates, as a result, cannot generate the same amount of ammonia during an acid load and take a longer time to recover their acid – base balance.

Thick Ascending Limb of Henle's Loop

While transcription of NKCC2 is observed early in development, NKCC2 is unlikely to be functional until postnatally as a low reabsorptive capacity has been shown for this segment in early postnatal life [104]. As discussed earlier, the expression of all of the TALH transporters is lower in the neonate [130–133]. As a result, bicarbonate and ammonium reabsorption occur at a lower rate compared to the adult. A postnatal five to tenfold increase in activity of the Na-K-ATPase co-transporter has been shown and is greater than that seen in other tubular segments (Fig. 9.9) [127, 134].

Cortical Collecting Duct

Microperfusion studies of neonatal rabbit kidneys demonstrate a lower capacity to secrete acid compared to their adult controls [188]. The neonatal number of intercalated cells is half that of the adult [189–191]. In addition, lower levels of the CA II isoform have been shown in neonatal rat kidneys [191, 192]. The CA II isoform is important for the function of the α intercalated cell and may be indicative of the increase in acid secreting capability of the developing CCD.

Regulation of Maturational Acid-Base Homeostatic Mechanisms

Glucocorticoids

Glucocorticoids can stimulate bicarbonate reabsorption and a developmental increase in circulating cortisol levels precedes the increase in bicarbonate reabsorption [193]. Pregnant rabbits injected with glucocorticoids give birth to neonatal rabbits with proximal tubular bicarbonate reabsorption rates similar to that of adults [193]. An increase in NHE3 antiporters occurs with prenatal glucocorticoids [194]. Adrenalectomy prevents this maturational increase in NHE3 antiporter expression at both the level of protein and mRNA. Therefore, the maturational increase in glucocorticoids is responsible for the postnatal increase seen in proximal tubule acidification.

Renal Calcium Handling in the Developing Kidney

Higher calcium and phosphorus levels are required for the growing skeleton in the fetus [195, 196]. The placenta actively transports calcium by a calcium pump in the basal membrane to maintain a high fetal:maternal calcium ratio [197]. The elevated fetal calcium suppresses PTH release [198]. PTH is the main regulator of calcium metabolism after birth. Circulating fetal calcium levels increase with advancing gestational age and at term the fetus is hypercalcemic relative to the maternal levels [199]. The serum calcium levels fall over the first 24 h in the absence of the placenta. As a result, PTH secretion is stimulated [200] but the response to the falling calcium is not sufficient such that a physiological nadir of serum calcium occurs in the first 2 days of life. This nadir is still within the adult range but represents a significant decrease compared to fetal levels [198]. Term infants typically achieve normal serum calcium levels by the second week of life with typical circulating concentrations of ionized calcium in neonates being in the range of 1–1.5 mmol/l (2–3 mEq/L) [201]. After birth, the kidney plays an important role in calcium and phosphorus homeostasis. The amount of calcium excreted increases over the first 2 weeks of life [202], and normal Ca/creatinine values are accordingly higher in infants. The most common cause of hypercalciuria in the neonate is iatrogenic. The risk of nephrocalcinosis is increased when calciuric drugs such as frusemide and glucocorticoids are administered. As a result, neonates with bronchopulmonary dysplasia are at increased risk for the development of nephrocalcinosis. Substitution of frusemide with thiazide diuretics will reduce this risk.

In the mature nephron, calcium reabsorption in the proximal tubule occurs by the paracellular (80%) and transcellular (20%) pathways. Calcium diffuses across an apical cell membrane into the cell down its electrochemical gradient, via Ca^{2+} channels. Calcium is extruded across the basolateral cell membrane via the $3Na^+/Ca^{2+}$ antiporter and a Ca^{2+}ATPase. Little is known about the ontogeny of such transporters in the developing nephron. In the distal nephron, active calcium reabsorption occurs through the highly Ca^{2+} – selective TRPV5 channel and binds to calbindin/D28K. The calbindin/D28K ferries Ca^{2+} to the basolateral $3Na^+/Ca^{2+}$ exchanger (NCX1) and the plasma membrane ATPase (PMCA1b) extruding calcium into the blood compartment. Animal studies have shown that the expression of TRPV6, calbindin/D9K, TRPV5 and calbindin/D28K are expressed in the kidneys of fetal mice at gestational age 18 days [203]. TRPV6 reaches a maximum level at 1 week of age and then decreases to <10% of TRPV5 expression, suggesting a possible role for TRPV6 during developmental regulation of calcium homeostasis. The expression of TRPV5 calbindin/D28K peaks at the third postnatal week and then falls [203]. Further functional studies are required to ascertain the response and ontogeny of the calcium transport proteins in the developing kidney.

Renal Phosphate Handling in the Developing Kidney

Phosphate is of critical importance to body functions particularly during periods of growth. Neonates excrete only 60% of intestinally absorbed phosphate and have a higher phosphate concentration than that of adults [204]. In neonates, the transtubular reabsorption of phosphate is high. Neonates reabsorb 99% of the filtered load of phosphate on the first day of life and 90% by the end of the first week [205]. Micropuncture studies performed on guinea pig neonatal proximal tubules demonstrated a higher phosphate reabsorption rate than adult guinea pigs [206]. Reabsorption does not occur through the 2Na+/Pi IIa antiporter but rather through its developmental isoform, the 2Na+/Pi IIc antiporter, the expression of which is higher in weaning animals and has a reduced function in adults [207].

Regulation of Renal Phosphate Handling in the Developing Kidney

The increased phosphate reabsorption in the early postnatal period is thought to be multifactorial. Parathyroidectomy in immature rats results in a greater increase in the maximal tubular phosphate reabsorption than in mature rats suggesting a role for PTH in neonatal phosphaturia [208]. However, a decline in resorptive capacity is also observed with age in the presence of parathyroid glands suggesting that there is an enhanced capacity of the immature tubule to reabsorb phosphate. In addition, responsiveness to PTH increases threefold during the first few weeks of life suggesting a maturation of second messenger systems [209]. In the mature nephron Klotho and PTH both increase the expression and activity of the 2Na+/Pi symporter [210] resulting in phosphaturia. Future research will provide an interesting insight into the ontogeny of Klotho and FGF-23, a phosphaturic hormone, during maturation of the renal phosphate transport systems.

Growth hormone (GH) has also been shown to upregulate 2Na+/Pi symporter in micropuncture studies performed on 4 week old rat proximal tubules, an effect that is independent of PTH [211, 212]. The mechanism enhancing the GH effect is unknown as developmental differences in the expression of GH receptors have not been shown. Both GH and IGF-1 mRNA have been localized to the apical membrane of proximal tubular epithelial cells suggesting a role of the GH/IGF-1 axis in Pi reabsorption [213].

Magnesium Handling in the Developing Kidney

In the adult kidney, 80% of total serum magnesium is filtered and >95% is reabsorbed along the nephron [214]. The proximal tubule reabsorbs 15–20% in the adult kidney but interestingly 70% in the developing proximal tubule [214]. A maturational decrease in the paracellular permeability at the level of the tight junction has been suggested as a reason for the decline in proximal magnesium reabsorption. From early childhood on, the majority of magnesium transport (70% of the filtered load) occurs in the loop of Henle. The DCT reabsorbs 5–10%. Transport in the TALH is passive and paracellular driven by the lumen positive transepithelial voltage and involves paracellin-1, a member of the claudin family involved in tight junction formation [215]. Active and transcellular reabsorption of magnesium occurs in the DCT and probably through the apical TRPM6 channel [216]. Ontogeny of the TRPM6 channel and its family members and paracellin-1 requires further research.

Renal Glucose Handling in the Developing Kidney

In the mature nephron, more than 99% of the filtered glucose is reabsorbed [217]. Glucosuria is more common among neonates, with the highest levels in preterm infants [218]. The maximum tubular reabsorption of glucose is lower in preterm and term infants than in adults [219]. Age-related differences in glucose transport activity correlate with differences in sodium conductance. Changes in membrane permeability to sodium affect membrane potential, a factor which modifies glucose reabsorption. Therefore, factors such as an increase in cell membrane surface area, in basolateral Na+/K+-ATPase, increased density of transporter proteins and the development of

new nephrons are implicated in the increase in glucose resorptive capacity observed as the fetus matures [220–222].

Renal Amino Acid Handling in the Developing Kidney

Amino acids are reabsorbed in the proximal one third of the proximal tubule in an active, sodium – dependent process [223]. Specific amino acid transport systems on the luminal cell membrane reabsorb the amino acids by secondary active transport against an uphill concentration gradient along with sodium. Aminoaciduria is frequently observed in the neonate. Factors include decreased activity of the amino acid-sodium cotransporter, increased Na+/H+ exchange at the luminal membrane and decreased activity of the Na+/K+/ATPase at the basolateral membrane [224]. Of note, not all of the amino acids are wasted to the same degree [224]. Developmental differences have been shown for the amino acid system and the glycine transporter systems [225, 226].

Assessment of Renal Functional Maturation

Renal functional maturation can be measured by either glomerular or tubular indicators. Glomerular function is assessed by serum creatinine levels, Cystatin C, urinary microalbumin, immunoglobulin G and GFR. Tubular function can be assessed by the fractional excretion of sodium or urinary alpha 1-microglobulin and urinary levels of other tubular proteins normally reabsorbed by the proximal tubule such as N-acetyl-β-D-glucosaminidase (NAG), beta-2-microglobulin [227, 228]. All markers have been closely associated with gestational age. A decrease in urinary tubular proteins occurs with increasing gestational age [229].

Acknowledgments The author would like to express her gratitude to Tino Piscione for his contributions to the second edition of this chapter.

References

1. Rudolph AM. Distribution and regulation of blood flow in the fetal and neonatal lamb. Circ Res. 1985;57:811–21.

2. Haycock GB. Development of glomerular filtration and tubular sodium reabsorption in the human fetus and newborn. Br J Urol. 1998;81 suppl 2:33–8.

3. Vieux R, Hascoet JM, Merdariu D, et al. Glomerular filtration rate reference values in very preterm infants. Pediatrics. 2010;125:e1186–92.

4. Rabinowitz R, Peters MT, Vyas S, Campbell S, Nicolaides KH. Measurement of fetal urine production in normal pregnancy by real-time ultrasonography. Am J Obstet Gynecol. 1989;161:1264–6.

5. Vanderheyden T, Kumar S, Fisk NM. Fetal renal impairment. Semin Neonatol. 2003;8:279–89.

6. Potter EL. Bilateral renal agenesis. J Pediatr. 1946;29:68–76.

7. Friis-Hansen B. Water distribution in the foetus and newborn infant. Acta Paediatr Scand Suppl. 1983;305:7–11.

8. Tulassay T, Seri I, Rascher W. Atrial natriuretic peptide and extracellular volume contraction after birth. Acta Paediatr Scand. 1987;76:444–6.

9. Baum M, Quigley R, Satlin L. Maturational changes in renal tubular transport. Curr Opin Nephrol Hypertens. 2003;12:521–6.

10. Pappenheimer JR. Permeability of glomerulomembranes in the kidney. Klin Wochenschr. 1955; 33:362–5.

11. Kleinman LI, Lubbe RJ. Factors affecting the maturation of renal PAH extraction in the new-born dog. J Physiol. 1972;223:411–8.

12. Veille JC, Hanson RA, Tatum K, Kelley K. Quantitative assessment of human fetal renal blood flow. Am J Obstet Gynecol. 1993;169: 1399–402.

13. Chevalier RL. Developmental renal physiology of the low birth weight pre-term newborn. J Urol. 1996;156:714–9.

14. Spitzer A, Edelmann Jr CM. Maturational changes in pressure gradients for glomerular filtration. Am J Physiol. 1971;221:1431–5.

15. Ichikawa I, Maddox DA, Brenner BM. Maturational development of glomerular ultrafiltration in the rat. Am J Physiol. 1979;236:F465–71.

16. Aperia A, Herin P. Development of glomerular perfusion rate and nephron filtration rate in rats 17–60 days old. Am J Physiol. 1975;228:1319–25.

17. Allison ME, Lipham EM, Gottschalk CW. Hydrostatic pressure in the rat kidney. Am J Physiol. 1972;223:975–83.

18. Gruskin AB, Edelmann Jr CM, Yuan S. Maturational changes in renal blood flow in piglets. Pediatr Res. 1970;4:7–13.

19. Aperia A, Broberger O, Herin P, Joelsson I. Renal hemodynamics in the perinatal period. A study in lambs. Acta Physiol Scand. 1977;99:261–9.

20. Nguyen C, Dreux S, Heidet L, Czerkiewicz I, Salomon LJ, Guimiot F, Schmitz T, Tsatsaris V, Boulot P, Rousseau T, Muller F. Fetal serum α-1 microglobulin for renal function assessment: comparison with β2-microglobulin and cystatin C. Prenat Diagn. 2013;33(8):775–81.

21. Bokenkamp A, Dieterich C, Dressler F, Muhlhaus K, Gembruch U, Bald R, Kirschstein M. Fetal serum concentrations of cystatin C and beta2-microglobulin as predictors of postnatal kidney function. Am J Obstet Gynecol. 2001;185:468–75.

22. Aperia A, Broberger O, Elinder G, Herin P, Zetterstrom R. Postnatal development of renal function in pre-term and full-term infants. Acta Paediatr Scand. 1981;70:183–7.

23. Bueva A, Guignard JP. Renal function in preterm neonates. Pediatr Res. 1994;36:572–7.

24. Guignard JP, Torrado A, Da Cunha O, Gautier E. Glomerular filtration rate in the first three weeks of life. J Pediatr. 1975;87:268–72.

25. Paton JB, Fisher DE, DeLannoy CW, Behrman RE. Umbilical blood flow, cardiac output, and organ blood flow in the immature baboon fetus. Am J Obstet Gynecol. 1973;117:560–6.

26. Fetterman GH, Shuplock NA, Philipp FJ, Gregg HS. The growth and maturation of human glomeruli and proximal convolutions from term to adulthood: studies by microdissection. Pediatrics. 1965;35: 601–19.

27. Boer DP, de Rijke YB, Hop WC, Cransberg K, Dorresteijn EM. Reference values for serum creatinine in children younger than 1 year of age. Pediatr Nephrol. 2010;25:2107–13.

28. Miall LS, Henderson MJ, Turner AJ, et al. Plasma creatinine rises dramatically in the first 48 h of life in preterm infants. Pediatrics. 1999;104, e76.

29. Auron A, Mhanna MJ. Serum creatinine in very low birth weight infants during their first days of life. J Perinatol. 2006;26:755–60.

30. Jacobelli S, Bonsante F, Ferdinus C, et al. Factors affecting postnatal changes in serum creatinine in preterm infants with gestational age <32 weeks. J Perinatol. 2009;29:232–6.

31. Abitbol CL, Seeherunvong W, Galarza MG, Katsoufis C, Francoeur D, Defreitas M, Edwards-Richards A, Master Sankar Raj V, Chandar J, Duara S, Yasin S, Zilleruelo G. Neonatal kidney size and function in preterm infants: what is a true estimate of glomerular filtration rate? J Pediatr. 2014;164: 1026–31.

32. Kotchen TA, Strickland AL, Rice TW, Walters DR. A study of the renin-angiotensin system in newborn infants. J Pediatr. 1972;80:938–46.

33. Wolf G. Angiotensin II and tubular development. Nephrol Dial Transplant. 2002;17 Suppl 9:48–51.

34. Niimura F, Okubo S, Fogo A, Ichikawa I. Temporal and spatial expression pattern of the angiotensinogen gene in mice and rats. Am J Physiol. 1997;272: R142–7.

35. Yosipiv IV, El-Dahr SS. Developmental biology of angiotensin-converting enzyme. Pediatr Nephrol. 1998;12:72–9.

36. Tufro-McReddie A, Harrison JK, Everett AD, Gomez RA. Ontogeny of type 1 angiotensin II receptor gene expression in the rat. J Clin Invest. 1993;91:530–7.

37. Kakuchi J, Ichiki T, Kiyama S, Hogan BL, Fogo A, Inagami T, Ichikawa I. Developmental expression of renal angiotensin II receptor genes in the mouse. Kidney Int. 1995;47:140–7.

38. Segar JL, Barna TJ, Acarregui MJ, Lamb FS. Responses of fetal ovine systemic and umbilical arteries to angiotensin II. Pediatr Res. 2001;49:826–33.

39. Segar JL, Minnick A, Nuyt AM, Robillard JE. Role of endogenous ANG II and AT1 receptors in regulating arterial baroreflex responses in newborn lambs. Am J Physiol. 1997;272:R1862–73.

40. Robillard JE, Weismann DN, Gomez RA, Ayres NA, Lawton WJ, VanOrden DE. Renal and adrenal responses to converting-enzyme inhibition in fetal and newborn life. Am J Physiol. 1983;244:R249–56.

41. Lacoste M, Cai Y, Guicharnaud L, Mounier F, Dumez Y, Bouvier R, Dijoud F, Gonzales M, Chatten J, Delezoide AL, et al. Renal tubular dysgenesis, a not uncommon autosomal recessive disorder leading to oligohydramnios: role of the renin-angiotensin system. J Am Soc Nephrol. 2006;17:2253–63.

42. Nakamura KT, Matherne GP, McWeeny OJ, Smith BA, Robillard JE. Renal hemodynamics and functional changes during the transition from fetal to newborn life in sheep. Pediatr Res. 1987;21:229–34.

43. Denton KM, Luff SE, Shweta A, Anderson WP. Differential neural control of glomerular ultrafiltration. Clin Exp Pharmacol Physiol. 2004;31:380–6.

44. DiBona GF, Kopp UC. Neural control of renal function. Physiol Rev. 1997;77:75–197.

45. Buckley NM, Brazeau P, Gootman PM, Frasier ID. Renal circulatory effects of adrenergic stimuli in anesthetized piglets and mature swine. Am J Physiol. 1979;237:H690–5.

46. Smith FG, Smith BA, Guillery EN, Robillard JE. Role of renal sympathetic nerves in lambs during the transition from fetal to newborn life. J Clin Invest. 1991;88:1988–94.

47. Segar JL, Mazursky JE, Robillard JE. Changes in ovine renal sympathetic nerve activity and baroreflex function at birth. Am J Physiol. 1994;267:H1824–32.

48. Pupilli C, Gomez RA, Tuttle JB, Peach MJ, Carey RM. Spatial association of renin-containing cells and nerve fibers in developing rat kidney. Pediatr Nephrol. 1991;5:690–5.

49. Naicker S, Bhoola KD. Endothelins: vasoactive modulators of renal function in health and disease. Pharmacol Ther. 2001;90:61–88.

50. Mattyus I, Zimmerhackl LB, Schwarz A, Brandis M, Miltenyi M, Tulassay T. Renal excretion of endothelin in children. Pediatr Nephrol. 1997;11:513–21.

51. Abadie L, Blazy I, Roubert P, Plas P, Charbit M, Chabrier PE, Dechaux M. Decrease in endothelin-1 renal receptors during the 1st month of life in the rat. Pediatr Nephrol. 1996;10:185–9.

52. Bogaert GA, Kogan BA, Mevorach RA, Wong J, Gluckman GR, Fineman JR, Heymann MA. Exogenous endothelin-1 causes renal vasodilation in the fetal lamb. J Urol. 1996;156:847–53.

53. Semama DS, Thonney M, Guignard JP. Role of endogenous endothelin in renal haemodynamics of newborn rabbits. Pediatr Nephrol. 1993;7:886–90.

54. Gleason CA. Prostaglandins and the developing kidney. Semin Perinatol. 1987;11:12–21.

55. Guignard JP, Gouyon JB, John EG. Vasoactive factors in the immature kidney. Pediatr Nephrol. 1991;5:443–6.

56. Cantor B, Tyler T, Nelson RM, Stein GH. Oligohydramnios and transient neonatal anuria: a possible association with the maternal use of prostaglandin synthetase inhibitors. J Reprod Med. 1980;24:220–3.

57. Simeoni U, Messer J, Weisburd P, Haddad J, Willard D. Neonatal renal dysfunction and intrauterine exposure to prostaglandin synthesis inhibitors. Eur J Pediatr. 1989;148:371–3.

58. Marpeau L, Bouillie J, Barrat J, Milliez J. Obstetrical advantages and perinatal risks of indomethacin: a report of 818 cases. Fetal Diagn Ther. 1994;9:110–5.

59. Jensen BL, Stubbe J, Madsen K, Nielsen FT, Skott O. The renin-angiotensin system in kidney development: role of COX-2 and adrenal steroids. Acta Physiol Scand. 2004;181:549–59.

60. Bachmann S, Mundel P. Nitric oxide in the kidney: synthesis, localization, and function. Am J Kidney Dis. 1994;24:112–29.

61. Ballevre L, Solhaug MJ, Guignard JP. Nitric oxide and the immature kidney. Biol Neonate. 1996;70:1–14.

62. Bogaert GA, Kogan BA, Mevorach RA. Effects of endothelium-derived nitric oxide on renal hemodynamics and function in the sheep fetus. Pediatr Res. 1993;34:755–61.

63. Solhaug MJ, Wallace MR, Granger JP. Nitric oxide and angiotensin II regulation of renal hemodynamics in the developing piglet. Pediatr Res. 1996;39:527–33.

64. El-Dahr SS, Figueroa CD, Gonzalez CB, Muller-Esterl W. Ontogeny of bradykinin B2 receptors in the rat kidney: implications for segmental nephron maturation. Kidney Int. 1997;51:739–49.

65. El-Dahr SS. Spatial expression of the kallikrein-kinin system during nephrogenesis. Histol Histopathol. 2004;19:1301–10.

66. El-Dahr SS, Chao J. Spatial and temporal expression of kallikrein and its mRNA during nephron maturation. Am J Physiol. 1992;262:F705–11.

67. Robillard JE, Lawton WJ, Weismann DN, Sessions C. Developmental aspects of the renal kallikrein-like activity in fetal and newborn lambs. Kidney Int. 1982;22:594–601.

68. Toth-Heyn P, Guignard JP. Endogenous bradykinin regulates renal function in the newborn rabbit. Biol Neonate. 1998;73:330–6.
69. Toth-Heyn P, Drukker A, Guignard JP. The stressed neonatal kidney: from pathophysiology to clinical management of neonatal vasomotor nephropathy. Pediatr Nephrol. 2000;14:227–39.
70. Felder RA, Felder CC, Eisner GM, Jose PA. The dopamine receptor in adult and maturing kidney. Am J Physiol. 1989;257:F315–27.
71. Seri I. Cardiovascular, renal, and endocrine actions of dopamine in neonates and children. J Pediatr. 1995;126:333–44.
72. Karlowicz MG, Adelman RD. Nonoliguric and oliguric acute renal failure in asphyxiated term neonates. Pediatr Nephrol. 1995;9:718–22.
73. Rodriguez-Soriano J, Vallo A, Castillo G, Oliveros R. Renal handling of water and sodium in infancy and childhood: a study using clearance methods during hypotonic saline diuresis. Kidney Int. 1981;20:700–4.
74. Rodriguez G, Ventura P, Samper MP, Moreno L, Sarria A, Perez-Gonzalez JM. Changes in body composition during the initial hours of life in breast-fed healthy term newborns. Biol Neonate. 2000;77:12–6.
75. Polacek E, Vocel J, Neugebauerova L, Sebkova M, Vechetova E. The osmotic concentrating ability in healthy infants and children. Arch Dis Child. 1965;40:291–5.
76. Sujov P, Kellerman L, Zeltzer M, Hochberg Z. Plasma and urine osmolality in full-term and preterm infants. Acta Paediatr Scand. 1984;73:722–6.
77. Day GM, Radde IC, Balfe JW, Chance GW. Electrolyte abnormalities in very low birthweight infants. Pediatr Res. 1976;10:522–6.
78. Bonilla-Felix M. Development of water transport in the collecting duct. Am J Physiol Renal Physiol. 2004;287:F1093–101.
79. Edelmann CM, Barnett HL, Troupkou V. Renal concentrating mechanisms in newborn infants. Effect of dietary protein and water content, role of urea, and responsiveness to antidiuretic hormone. J Clin Invest. 1960;39:1062–9.
80. Grantham JJ, Burg MB. Effect of vasopressin and cyclic AMP on permeability of isolated collecting tubules. Am J Physiol. 1996;211:255–9.
81. Sands JM, Nonoguchi H, Knepper MA. Vasopressin effects on urea and H2O transport in inner medullary collecting duct subsegments. Am J Physiol. 1987;253:F823–32.
82. Fushimi K, Sasaki S, Marumo F. Phosphorylation of serine 256 is required for cAMP-dependent regulatory exocytosis of the aquaporin-2 water channel. J Biol Chem. 1997;272:14800–4.
83. Fushimi K, Uchida S, Hara Y, Hirata Y, Marumo F, Sasaki S. Cloning and expression of apical membrane water channel of rat kidney collecting tubule. Nature. 1993;361:549–52.
84. Nielsen S, Chou CL, Marples D, Christensen EI, Kishore BK, Knepper MA. Vasopressin increases water permeability of kidney collecting duct by inducing translocation of aquaporin-CD water channels to plasma membrane. Proc Natl Acad Sci U S A. 1995;92:1013–7.
85. Liu H, Wintour EM. Aquaporins in development – a review. Reprod Biol Endocrinol. 2005;3:18.
86. Knepper MA, Nielsen S, Chou CL, DiGiovanni SR. Mechanism of vasopressin action in the renal collecting duct. Semin Nephrol. 1994;14:302–21.
87. Hadeed AJ, Leake RD, Weitzman RE, Fisher DA. Possible mechanisms of high blood levels of vasopressin during the neonatal period. J Pediatr. 1979;94:805–8.
88. Rees L, Forsling ML, Brook CG. Vasopressin concentrations in the neonatal period. Clin Endocrinol (Oxf). 1980;12:357–62.
89. Horster MF, Zink H. Functional differentiation of the medullary collecting tubule: influence of vasopressin. Kidney Int. 1982;22:360–5.
90. Siga E, Horster MF. Regulation of osmotic water permeability during differentiation of inner medullary collecting duct. Am J Physiol. 1991;260:F710–6.
91. Ivanova LN, Zelenina MN, Melidi NN, Solenov EI, Khegaĭ II. Vasopressin: the ontogeny of antidiuretic action at the cellular level. Fiziol Zh SSSR Im I M Sechenova. 1989;7:970–9.
92. Svenningsen NW, Aronson AS. Postnatal development of renal concentration capacity as estimated by DDAVP-test in normal and asphyxiated neonates. Biol Neonate. 1974;25:230–41.
93. Ostrowski NL, Young 3rd WS, Knepper MA, Lolait SJ. Expression of vasopressin V1a and V2 receptor messenger ribonucleic acid in the liver and kidney of embryonic, developing, and adult rats. Endocrinology. 1993;133:1849–59.
94. Ammar A, Roseau S, Butlen D. Postnatal ontogenesis of vasopressin receptors in the rat collecting duct. Mol Cell Endocrinol. 1992;86:193–203.
95. Rajerison RM, Butlen D, Jard S. Ontogenic development of antidiuretic hormone receptors in rat kidney: comparison of hormonal binding and adenylate cyclase activation. Mol Cell Endocrinol. 1976; 4:271–85.
96. Bonilla-Felix M, John-Phillip C. Prostaglandins mediate the defect in AVP-stimulated cAMP generation in immature collecting duct. Am J Physiol. 1994;267:F44–8.
97. Bonilla-Felix M, Vehaskari VM, Hamm LL. Water transport in the immature rabbit collecting duct. Pediatr Nephrol. 1999;13:103–7.
98. Quigley R, Chakravarty S, Baum M. Antidiuretic hormone resistance in the neonatal cortical collecting tubule is mediated in part by elevated phosphodiesterase activity. Am J Physiol Renal Physiol. 2004;286:F317–22.
99. Negishi M, Sugimoto Y, Hayashi Y, Namba T, Honda A, Watabe A, Narumiya S, Ichikawa A. Functional interaction of prostaglandin E receptor EP3 subtype with guanine nucleotide-binding proteins, showing

low-affinity ligand binding. Biochim Biophys Acta. 1993;1175:343–50.

100. Bonilla-Felix M, Jiang W. Aquaporin-2 in the immature rat: expression, regulation, and trafficking. J Am Soc Nephrol. 1997;8:1502–9.

101. Yasui M, Marples D, Belusa R, Eklof AC, Celsi G, Nielsen S, Aperia A. Development of urinary concentrating capacity: role of aquaporin-2. Am J Physiol. 1996;271:F461–8.

102. Yamamoto T, Sasaki S, Fushimi K, Ishibashi K, Yaoita E, Kawasaki K, Fujinaka H, Marumo F, Kihara I. Expression of AQP family in rat kidneys during development and maturation. Am J Physiol. 1997;272:F198–204.

103. Forrest Jr JN, Stanier MW. Kidney composition and renal concentration ability in young rabbits. J Physiol. 1996;187:1–4.

104. Horster M. Loop of Henle functional differentiation: in vitro perfusion of the isolated thick ascending segment. Pflugers Arch. 1978;78:15–24.

105. Cha JH, Kim YH, Jung JY, Han KH, Madsen KM, Kim J. Cell proliferation in the loop of henle in the developing rat kidney. J Am Soc Nephrol. 2001;12:1410–21.

106. Liu W, Morimoto T, Kondo Y, Iinuma K, Uchida S, Imai M. "Avian-type" renal medullary tubule organization causes immaturity of urine-concentrating ability in neonates. Kidney Int. 2001;60:680–93.

107. Kim YH, Kim DU, Han KH, Jung JY, Sands JM, Knepper MA, Madsen KM, Kim J. Expression of urea transporters in the developing rat kidney. Am J Physiol Renal Physiol. 2002;282:F530–40.

108. Zink H, Horster M. Maturation of diluting capacity in loop of Henle of rat superficial nephrons. Am J Physiol. 1977;233:F519–24.

109. Speller AM, Moffat DB. Tubulo-vascular relationships in the developing kidney. J Anat. 1977;123:487–500.

110. Edelmann Jr CM, Barnett HL, Stark H. Effect of urea on concentration of urinary nonurea solute in premature infants. J Appl Physiol. 1966;21:1021–5.

111. Clark DA. Times of first void and first stool in 500 newborns. Pediatrics. 1977;60:457–9.

112. Hansen JD, Smith CA. Effects of withholding fluid in the immediate postnatal period. Pediatrics. 1953;12:99–113.

113. Al-Dahhan J, Haycock GB, Nichol B, Chantler C, Stimmler L. Sodium homeostasis in term and preterm neonates. III. Effect of salt supplementation. Arch Dis Child. 1984;59:945–50.

114. Engelke SC, Shah BL, Vasan U, Raye JR. Sodium balance in very low-birth-weight infants. J Pediatr. 1978;93:837–41.

115. Goetz KL. Physiology and pathophysiology of atrial peptides. Am J Physiol. 1988;254:E1–15.

116. Chevalier RL. Atrial natriuretic peptide in renal development. Pediatr Nephrol. 1993;7:652–6.

117. Kikuchi K, Shiomi M, Horie K, Ohie T, Nakao K, Imura H, Mikawa H. Plasma atrial natriuretic polypeptide concentration in healthy children from birth to adolescence. Acta Paediatr Scand. 1988;77:380–4.

118. Weil J, Bidlingmaier F, Dohlemann C, Kuhnle U, Strom T, Lang RE. Comparison of plasma atrial natriuretic peptide levels in healthy children from birth to adolescence and in children with cardiac diseases. Pediatr Res. 1986;20:1328–31.

119. Bierd TM, Kattwinkel J, Chevalier RL, Rheuban KS, Smith DJ, Teague WG, Carey RM, Linden J. Interrelationship of atrial natriuretic peptide, atrial volume, and renal function in premature infants. J Pediatr. 1990;116:753–9.

120. Semmekrot B, Chabardes D, Roseau S, Siaume-Perez S, Butlen D. Developmental pattern of cyclic guanosine monophosphate production stimulated by atrial natriuretic peptide in glomeruli microdissected from kidneys of young rats. Pflugers Arch. 1990;416:519–25.

121. Chevalier RL. The moth and the aspen tree: sodium in early postnatal development. Kidney Int. 2001;59(5):1617–25.

122. Ross B, Cowett RM, Oh W. Renal functions of low birth weight infants during the first two months of life. Pediatr Res. 1977;11:1162–4.

123. Spitzer A. The role of the kidney in sodium homeostasis during maturation. Kidney Int. 1982;21:539–45.

124. Baum M. Neonatal rabbit juxtamedullary proximal convoluted tubule acidification. J Clin Invest. 1990;85:499–506.

125. Guillery EN, Karniski LP, Mathews MS, Robillard JE. Maturation of proximal tubule Na+/H+ antiporter activity in sheep during transition from fetus to newborn. Am J Physiol. 1994;267:F537–45.

126. Guillery EN, Huss DJ. Developmental regulation of chloride/formate exchange in guinea pig proximal tubules. Am J Physiol. 1995;269:F686–95.

127. Schmidt U, Horster M. Na-K-activated ATPase: activity maturation in rabbit nephron segments dissected in vitro. Am J Physiol. 1977;233:F55–60.

128. Fukuda Y, Bertorello A, Aperia A. Ontogeny of the regulation of Na+, K(+)-ATPase activity in the renal proximal tubule cell. Pediatr Res. 1991;30:131–4.

129. Guillery EN, Huss DJ, McDonough AA, Klein LC. Posttranscriptional upregulation of Na(+)-K(+)-ATPase activity in newborn guinea pig renal cortex. Am J Physiol. 1997;273:F254–63.

130. Biemesderfer D, Rutherford PA, Nagy T, Pizzonia JH, Abu-Alfa AK, Aronson PS. Monoclonal antibodies for high-resolution localization of NHE3 in adult and neonatal rat kidney. Am J Physiol. 1997;273:F289–99.

131. Igarashi P, Vanden Heuvel GB, Payne JA, Forbush 3rd B. Cloning, embryonic expression, and alternative splicing of a murine kidney-specific Na-K-Cl cotransporter. Am J Physiol. 1995;269:F405–18.

132. Schmitt R, Ellison DH, Farman N, Rossier BC, Reilly RF, Reeves WB, Oberbaumer I, Tapp R, Bachmann S. Developmental expression of sodium

entry pathways in rat nephron. Am J Physiol. 1999;276:F367–81.

133. Bachmann S, Bostanjoglo M, Schmitt R, Ellison DH. Sodium transport-related proteins in the mammalian distal nephron – distribution, ontogeny and functional aspects. Anat Embryol (Berl). 1999; 200:447–68.

134. Rane S, Aperia A. Ontogeny of Na-K-ATPase activity in thick ascending limb and of concentrating capacity. Am J Physiol. 1985;249:F723–8.

135. Burrow CR, Devuyst O, Li X, Gatti L, Wilson PD. Expression of the beta2-subunit and apical localization of Na+-K+-ATPase in metanephric kidney. Am J Physiol. 1999;277:F391–403.

136. Obermuller N, Bernstein P, Velazquez H, Reilly R, Moser D, Ellison DH, Bachmann S. Expression of the thiazide-sensitive Na-Cl cotransporter in rat and human kidney. Am J Physiol. 1995;269: F900–10.

137. Duc C, Farman N, Canessa CM, Bonvalet JP, Rossier BC. Cell-specific expression of epithelial sodium channel alpha, beta, and gamma subunits in aldosterone-responsive epithelia from the rat: localization by in situ hybridization and immuno cytochemistry. J Cell Biol. 1994;127:1907–21.

138. Vehaskari VM, Hempe JM, Manning J, Aviles DH, Carmichael MC. Developmental regulation of ENaC subunit mRNA levels in rat kidney. Am J Physiol. 1998;274:C1661–6.

139. Horster M. Embryonic epithelial membrane transporters. Am J Physiol Renal Physiol. 2000;279: F982–96.

140. Watanabe S, Matsushita K, McCray Jr PB, Stokes JB. Developmental expression of the epithelial Na+ channel in kidney and uroepithelia. Am J Physiol. 1999;276:F304–14.

141. Nakamura K, Stokes JB, McCray Jr PB. Endogenous and exogenous glucocorticoid regulation of ENaC mRNA expression in developing kidney and lung. Am J Physiol Cell Physiol. 2002;283:C762–72.

142. Kone BC. Epigenetics and the control of the collecting duct epithelial sodium channel. Semin Nephrol. 2013;33(4):383–91.

143. Constantinescu AR, Lane JC, Mak J, Zavilowitz B, Satlin LM. Na(+)-K(+)-ATPase-mediated basolateral rubidium uptake in the maturing rabbit cortical collecting duct. Am J Physiol Renal Physiol. 2000;279:F1161–8.

144. Vehaskari VM. Ontogeny of cortical collecting duct sodium transport. Am J Physiol. 1994;267: F49–54.

145. Chevalier RL, Thornhill BA, Belmonte DC, Baertschi AJ. Endogenous angiotensin II inhibits natriuresis after acute volume expansion in the neonatal rat. Am J Physiol. 1996;270:R393–7.

146. Quan A, Baum M. Endogenous angiotensin II modulates rat proximal tubule transport with acute changes in extracellular volume. Am J Physiol. 1998;275:F74–8.

147. Sulyok E. In: Spitzer A, editor. The kidney during development: morphogenesis and function. New York: Masson; 1982. p. 273.

148. Sulyok E. Dopaminergic control of neonatal salt and water metabolism. Pediatr Nephrol. 1988;2:163–5.

149. Magyar DM, Fridshal D, Elsner CW, Glatz T, Eliot J, Klein AH, Lowe KC, Buster JE, Nathanielsz PW. Time-trend analysis of plasma cortisol concentrations in the fetal sheep in relation to parturition. Endocrinology. 1980;107:155–9.

150. Gupta N, Tarif SR, Seikaly M, Baum M. Role of glucocorticoids in the maturation of the rat renal Na+/H+ antiporter (NHE3). Kidney Int. 2001;60: 173–81.

151. Guillery EN, Karniski LP, Mathews MS, Page WV, Orlowski J, Jose PA, Robillard JE. Role of glucocorticoids in the maturation of renal cortical Na+/H+ exchanger activity during fetal life in sheep. Am J Physiol. 1995;268:F710–7.

152. Celsi G, Nishi A, Akusjarvi G, Aperia A. Abundance of Na(+)-K(+)-ATPase mRNA is regulated by glucocorticoid hormones in infant rat kidneys. Am J Physiol. 1991;260:F192–7.

153. Shah M, Quigley R, Baum M. Maturation of proximal straight tubule NaCl transport: role of thyroid hormone. Am J Physiol Renal Physiol. 2000;278:F596–602.

154. McDonough AA, Brown TA, Horowitz B, Chiu R, Schlotterbeck J, Bowen J, Schmitt CA. Thyroid hormone coordinately regulates Na+-K+-ATPase alpha- and beta-subunit mRNA levels in kidney. Am J Physiol. 1988;254:C323–9.

155. Mathew OP, Jones AS, James E, Bland H, Groshong T. Neonatal renal failure: usefulness of diagnostic indices. Pediatrics. 1980;65:57–60.

156. Siegel SR, Oh W. Renal function as a marker of human fetal maturation. Acta Paediatr Scand. 1976;65:481–5.

157. Delgado MM, Rohatgi R, Khan S, Holzman IR, Satlin LM. Sodium and potassium clearances by the maturing kidney: clinical-molecular correlates. Pediatr Nephrol. 2003;18:759–67.

158. Sulyok E, Nemeth M, Tenyi I, Csaba IF, Varga F, Gyory E, Thurzo V. Relationship between maturity, electrolyte balance and the function of the renin-angiotensin-aldosterone system in newborn infants. Biol Neonate. 1979;35:60–5.

159. Serrano CV, Talbert LM, Welt LG. Potassium deficiency in the pregnant dog. J Clin Invest. 1964;43:27–31.

160. Lorenz JM, Kleinman LI, Markarian K. Potassium metabolism in extremely low birth weight infants in the first week of life. J Pediatr. 1997;131:81–6.

161. Sato K, Kondo T, Iwao H, Honda S, Ueda K. Internal potassium shift in premature infants: cause of nonoliguric hyperkalemia. J Pediatr. 1995;126:109–13.

162. Stefano JL, Norman ME, Morales MC, Goplerud JM, Mishra OP, Delivoria-Papadopoulos M. Decreased erythrocyte Na+, K(+)-ATPase activity associated

with cellular potassium loss in extremely low birth weight infants with non oliguric hyperkalemia. J Pediatr. 1993;122:276–84.

163. Zhou H, Satlin LM. Renal potassium handling in healthy and sick newborns. Semin Perinatol. 2004;28(2):103–11.

164. Satlin LM. Postnatal maturation of potassium transport in rabbit cortical collecting duct. Am J Physiol. 1994;266:F57–65.

165. Woda CB, Miyawaki N, Ramalakshmi S, Ramkumar M, Rojas R, Zavilowitz B, Kleyman TR, Satlin LM. Ontogeny of flow-stimulated potassium secretion in rabbit cortical collecting duct: functional and molecular aspects. Am J Physiol Renal Physiol. 2003;285:F629–39.

166. Giebisch G. Renal potassium transport: mechanisms and regulation. Am J Physiol. 1998;274:F817–33.

167. Lelievre-Pegorier M, Merlet-Benichou C, Roinel N, de Rouffignac C. Developmental pattern of water and electrolyte transport in rat superficial nephrons. Am J Physiol. 1983;245:F15–21.

168. Frindt G, Palmer LG. Low-conductance K channels in apical membrane of rat cortical collecting tubule. Am J Physiol. 1989;256:F143–51.

169. Wang WH, Schwab A, Giebisch G. Regulation of small-conductance K+ channel in apical membrane of rat cortical collecting tubule. Am J Physiol. 1990;259:F494–502.

170. Pacha J, Frindt G, Sackin H, Palmer LG. Apical maxi K channels in intercalated cells of CCT. Am J Physiol. 1991;261:F696–705.

171. Satlin LM, Palmer LG. Apical K+ conductance in maturing rabbit principal cell. Am J Physiol. 1997;272:F397–404.

172. Satlin LM, Palmer LG. Apical Na+ conductance in maturing rabbit principal cell. Am J Physiol. 1996;270:F391–7.

173. Zolotnitskaya A, Satlin LM. Developmental expression of ROMK in rat kidney. Am J Physiol. 1999;276:F825–36.

174. Hunter M, Lopes AG, Boulpaep EL, Giebisch GH. Single channel recordings of calcium-activated potassium channels in the apical membrane of rabbit cortical collecting tubules. Proc Natl Acad Sci U S A. 1984;81:4237–9.

175. Stephenson G, Hammet M, Hadaway G, Funder JW. Ontogeny of renal mineralocorticoid receptors and urinary electrolyte responses in the rat. Am J Physiol. 1984;247:F665–71.

176. Rodriguez-Soriano J, Ubetagoyena M, Vallo A. Transtubular potassium concentration gradient: a useful test to estimate renal aldosterone bio-activity in infants and children. Pediatr Nephrol. 1990;4:105–10.

177. Omar SA, DeCristofaro JD, Agarwal BI, LaGamma EF. Effect of prenatal steroids on potassium balance in extremely low birth weight neonates. Pediatrics. 2000;106:561–7.

178. Celsi G, Wang ZM, Akusjarvi G, Aperia A. Sensitive periods for glucocorticoids' regulation of Na+, K(+)-ATPase mRNA in the developing lung and kidney. Pediatr Res. 1993;33:5–9.

179. Schwartz GJ, Haycock GB, Edelmann Jr CM, Spitzer A. Late metabolic acidosis: a reassessment of the definition. J Pediatr. 1979;95:102–7.

180. Edelmann CM, Soriano JR, Boichis H, Gruskin AB, Acosta MI. Renal bicarbonate reabsorption and hydrogen ion excretion in normal infants. J Clin Invest. 1967;46:1309–17.

181. Kerpel-Fronius E, Heim T, Sulyok E. The development of the renal acidifying processes and their relation to acidosis in low-birth-weight infants. Biol Neonate. 1970;15:156–68.

182. Schwartz GJ, Evan AP. Development of solute transport in rabbit proximal tubule. I. HCO-3 and glucose absorption. Am J Physiol. 1983;245:F382–90.

183. Baum M, Quigley R. Ontogeny of proximal tubule acidification. Kidney Int. 1995;48:1697–704.

184. Schwartz GJ, Brown D, Mankus R, Alexander EA, Schwartz JH. Low pH enhances expression of carbonic anhydrase II by cultured rat inner medullary collecting duct cells. Am J Physiol. 1994;266: C508–14.

185. Winkler CA, Kittelberger AM, Watkins RH, Maniscalco WM, Schwartz GJ. Maturation of carbonic anhydrase IV expression in rabbit kidney. Am J Physiol Renal Physiol. 2001;280:F895–903.

186. Goldstein L. Renal ammonia and acid excretion in infant rats. Am J Physiol. 1970;218:1394–8.

187. Goldstein L. Ammonia metabolism in kidneys of suckling rats. Am J Physiol. 1971;220:213–7.

188. Mehrgut FM, Satlin LM, Schwartz GJ. Maturation of HCO3- transport in rabbit collecting duct. Am J Physiol. 1990;259:F801–8.

189. Kim J, Tisher CC, Madsen KM. Differentiation of intercalated cells in developing rat kidney: an immunohistochemical study. Am J Physiol. 1994;266:F977–90.

190. Satlin LM, Matsumoto T, Schwartz GJ. Postnatal maturation of rabbit renal collecting duct. III. Peanut lectin-binding intercalated cells. Am J Physiol. 1992;262:F199–208.

191. Satlin LM, Schwartz GJ. Postnatal maturation of rabbit renal collecting duct: intercalated cell function. Am J Physiol. 1987;253:F622–35.

192. Karashima S, Hattori S, Ushijima T, Furuse A, Nakazato H, Matsuda I. Developmental changes in carbonic anhydrase II in the rat kidney. Pediatr Nephrol. 1998;12:263–8.

193. Baum M, Quigley R. Prenatal glucocorticoids stimulate neonatal juxtamedullary proximal convoluted tubule acidification. Am J Physiol. 1991;261: F746–52.

194. Baum M, Moe OW, Gentry DL, Alpern RJ. Effect of glucocorticoids on renal cortical NHE-3 and NHE-1 mRNA. Am J Physiol. 1994;267:F437–42.

195. David L, Anast CS. Calcium metabolism in newborn infants. The interrelationship of parathyroid function and calcium, magnesium, and phosphorus

metabolism in normal, "sick," and hypocalcemic newborns. J Clin Invest. 1974;54:287–96.

196. Moniz CF, Nicolaides KH, Tzannatos C, Rodeck CH. Calcium homeostasis in second trimester fetuses. J Clin Pathol. 1986;39:838–41.

197. Care AD. The placental transfer of calcium. J Dev Physiol. 1991;15:253–7.

198. Kovacs CS, Kronenberg HM. Maternal-fetal calcium and bone metabolism during pregnancy, puerperium, and lactation. Endocr Rev. 1997;18:832–72.

199. Hsu SC, Levine MA. Perinatal calcium metabolism: physiology and pathophysiology. Semin Neonatol. 2004;9:23–36.

200. Saggese G, Baroncelli GI, Bertelloni S, Cipolloni C. Intact parathyroid hormone levels during pregnancy, in healthy term neonates and in hypocalcemic preterm infants. Acta Paediatr Scand. 1991;80: 36–41.

201. Wandrup J, Kroner J, Pryds O, Kastrup KW. Age-related reference values for ionized calcium in the first week of life in premature and full-term neonates. Scand J Clin Lab Invest. 1988;48:255–60.

202. Karlen J, Aperia A, Zetterstrom R. Renal excretion of calcium and phosphate in preterm and term infants. J Pediatr. 1985;106:814–9.

203. Song Y, Peng X, Porta A, Takanaga H, Peng JB, Hediger MA, Fleet JC, Christakos S. Calcium transporter 1 and epithelial calcium channel messenger ribonucleic acid are differentially regulated by 1,25 dihydroxyvitamin D3 in the intestine and kidney of mice. Endocrinology. 2003;144:3885–94.

204. Brodehl J, Gellissen K, Weber HP. Postnatal development of tubular phosphate reabsorption. Clin Nephrol. 1982;17:163–71.

205. Hohenauer L, Rosenberg TF, Oh W. Calcium and phosphorus homeostasis on the first day of life. Biol Neonate. 1970;15:49–56.

206. Kaskel FJ, Kumar AM, Feld LG, Spitzer A. Renal reabsorption of phosphate during development: tubular events. Pediatr Nephrol. 1988;2:129–34.

207. Segawa H, Kaneko I, Takahashi A, Kuwahata M, Ito M, Ohkido I, Tatsumi S, Miyamoto K. Growth-related renal type II Na/Pi cotransporter. J Biol Chem. 2002;277:19665–72.

208. Haramati A, Mulroney SE, Webster SK. Developmental changes in the tubular capacity for phosphate reabsorption in the rat. Am J Physiol. 1988;255:F287–91.

209. Imbert-Teboul M, Chabardes D, Clique A, Montegut M, Morel F. Ontogenesis of hormone-dependent adenylate cyclase in isolated rat nephron segments. Am J Physiol. 1984;247:F316–25.

210. Hu MC, Shi M, Zhang J, Pastor J, Nakatani T, Lanske B, Razzaque MS, Rosenblatt KP, Baum MG, Kuro-o M, Moe OW. Klotho: a novel phosphaturic substance acting as an autocrine enzyme in the renal proximal tubule. FASEB J. 2010;24:3438–50.

211. Mulroney SE, Lumpkin MD, Haramati A. Antagonist to GH-releasing factor inhibits growth and renal Pi reabsorption in immature rats. Am J Physiol. 1989;257:F29–34.

212. Woda CB, Halaihel N, Wilson PV, Haramati A, Levi M, Mulroney SE. Regulation of renal NaPi-2 expression and tubular phosphate reabsorption by growth hormone in the juvenile rat. Am J Physiol Renal Physiol. 2004;287:F117–23.

213. Hammerman MR, Karl IE, Hruska KA. Regulation of canine renal vesicle Pi transport by growth hormone and parathyroid hormone. Biochim Biophys Acta. 1980;603:322–35.

214. de Rouffignac C, Quamme G. Renal magnesium handling and its hormonal control. Physiol Rev. 1994;74:305–22.

215. Simon DB, Lu Y, Choate KA, Velazquez H, Al-Sabban E, Praga M, Casari G, Bettinelli A, Colussi G, Rodriguez-Soriano J, et al. Paracellin-1, a renal tight junction protein required for paracellular Mg2+ resorption. Science. 1999;285:103–6.

216. Voets T, Nilius B, Hoefs S, van der Kemp AW, Droogmans G, Bindels RJ, Hoenderop JG. TRPM6 forms the Mg2+ influx channel involved in intestinal and renal Mg2+ absorption. J Biol Chem. 2004;279:19–25.

217. Rossi R, Danzebrink S, Linnenburger K, Hillebrand D, Gruneberg M, Sablitzky V, Deufel T, Ullrich K, Harms E. Assessment of tubular reabsorption of sodium, glucose, phosphate and amino acids based on spot urine samples. Acta Paediatr. 1994;83: 1282–6.

218. Arant Jr BS. Developmental patterns of renal functional maturation compared in the human neonate. J Pediatr. 1978;92:705–12.

219. Brodehl J, Franken A, Gellissen K. Maximal tubular reabsorption of glucose in infants and children. Acta Paediatr Scand. 1972;61:413–20.

220. Beck JC, Lipkowitz MS, Abramson RG. Characterization of the fetal glucose transporter in rabbit kidney. Comparison with the adult brush border electrogenic Na+-glucose symporter. J Clin Invest. 1988;82:379–87.

221. LeLievre-Pegorier M, Geloso JP. Otogeny of sugar transport in fetal rat kidney. Biol Neonate. 1980;38:16–24.

222. Robillard JE, Sessions C, Kennedy RL, Smith Jr FG. Maturation of the glucose transport process by the fetal kidney. Pediatr Res. 1978;12:680–4.

223. Silbernagl S. The renal handling of amino acids and oligopeptides. Physiol Rev. 1988;68:911–1007.

224. Zelikovic I, Chesney RW. Development of renal amino acid transport systems. Semin Nephrol. 1989;9:49–55.

225. Baerlocher KE, Scriver CR, Mohyuddin F. The ontogeny of amino acid transport in rat kidney. I. Effect on distribution ratios and intracellular metabolism of proline and glycine. Biochim Biophys Acta. 1971;249:353–63.

226. Baerlocher KE, Scriver CR, Mohyuddin F. The ontogeny of amino acid transport in rat kidney.

II. Kinetics of uptake and effect of anoxia. Biochim Biophys Acta. 1971;249:364–72.

227. Muller F, Dommergues M, Bussieres L, Lortat-Jacob S, Loirat C, Oury JF, Aigrain Y, Niaudet P, Aegerter P, Dumez Y. Development of human renal function: reference intervals for 10 biochemical markers in fetal urine. Clin Chem. 1996;42:1855–60.

228. Ojala R, Ala-Houhala M, Harmoinen AP, Luukkaala T, Uotila J, Tammela O. Tubular proteinuria in pre-term and full-term infants. Pediatr Nephrol. 2006;21:68–73.

229. Awad H, el-Safty I, el-Barbary M, Imam S. Evaluation of renal glomerular and tubular functional and structural integrity in neonates. Am J Med Sci. 2002;324:261–6.

Disorders of Kidney Formation

10

Norman D. Rosenblum and Indra R. Gupta

Introduction

Congenital anomalies of the kidneys and urinary tract, otherwise known as CAKUT, are classical disorders of development that are the most common cause of renal failure in children [1, 2]. These disorders encompass a spectrum of entities including renal agenesis, renal hypodysplasia, multicystic kidney dysplasia, duplex renal collecting systems, ureteropelvic junction obstruction, ureterovesical junction obstruction, megaureter, posterior urethral valves and vesicoureteral reflux. While congenital disorders like autosomal recessive and autosomal dominant polycystic kidney disease, nephronophthisis, and heritable nephrotic syndrome could also be considered as disorders of kidney formation, these generally occur later in kidney development as part of terminal cell differentiation events. However, some of the genes that cause nephronophthisis are also reported in children with

CAKUT. In this chapter, we discuss disorders that arise during the early inductive events that lead to the formation of the kidneys and the urinary tracts. Both tissues arise from a common primordial tissue known as the mesonephric duct and thus, congenital kidney and urinary tract malformations commonly co-occur. In this chapter, we will focus on renal disorders encompassed within CAKUT and discuss their etiology, clinical manifestations and management. Other disorders within CAKUT with significant urinary tract pathology like ureteropelvic junction obstruction, ureterovesical junction obstruction, megaureter, posterior urethral valves and vesicoureteral reflux are discussed in other chapters.

Classification and Definition of Renal Malformations

Congenital malformations of the kidney can be defined at the macroscopic level by changes in size, shape, location or number or microscopically by changes within specific lineages like the ureteric bud, the metanephric mesenchyme, or combinations of both [3]. In clinical practice, most congenital renal malformations are defined grossly using imaging methods like ultrasound and nuclear medicine scans. Sometimes renal tissue is obtained from biopsies or from nephrectomies, and in these cases, histological definitions of renal hypoplasia, renal dysplasia, and multicystic renal dysplasia can be utilized for

N.D. Rosenblum (✉)
Division of Nephrology, Department of Pediatrics,
Hospital for Sick Children, University of Toronto,
686 Bay St, Rm 16-9-706, Toronto, ON M5G 0A4,
Canada
e-mail: norman.rosenblum@sickkids.ca

I.R. Gupta
Division of Nephrology, Department of Pediatrics,
Montreal Children's Hospital, McGill University,
2300 Tupper Street, Montreal, Quebec
H3H 1P3, Canada
e-mail: indra.gupta@muhc.mcgill.ca

© Springer-Verlag Berlin Heidelberg 2016
D.F. Geary, F. Schaefer (eds.), *Pediatric Kidney Disease*, DOI 10.1007/978-3-662-52972-0_10

classification. One can group congenital malformations of the kidney as follows:

- Changes in size
  - Renal Hypoplasia
  - Renal Dysplasia
- Changes in shape
  - Multicystic Renal Dysplasia
  - Renal Fusion
- Changes in location
  - Renal Ectopia
  - Renal Fusion
- Changes in number
  - Renal Duplication
  - Renal Agenesis

When induction events do not occur at the right time or location during embryogenesis, the kidneys may fail to form (agenesis, hypoplasia, dysplasia), the kidneys may form, but in the wrong location (ectopia +/− hypoplasia/dysplasia), the kidneys may fail to migrate to the correct location (fusion +/− hypoplasia/dysplasia) or there may be multiple induction events that arise (duplication). Malformations can be either unilateral or bilateral. Importantly from animal models and from human studies, disorders of renal formation are frequently observed with concurrent lower urinary tract malformations. In these cases, it is not clear if the impairment in induction of the kidney is primary or secondary to urinary tract obstruction. Renal agenesis refers to congenital absence of the kidney and ureter. Typically, renal malformations defined as renal hypoplasia or dysplasia are grossly small in size, defined as less than two SD below the mean for kidney length or weight [3–5]. Simple renal hypoplasia is defined as a small kidney with a reduced number of nephrons and normal architecture. Renal dysplasia is defined by the presence of malformed kidney tissue elements. Characteristic microscopic abnormalities include abnormal differentiation of mesenchymal and epithelial elements, a decreased number of nephrons, loss of corticomedullary differentiation and the presence of dysplastic elements including cartilage and bone (Fig. 10.1a–d). As stated, dysplastic or hypoplastic kidneys are typically small,

but can range in size and appear normal or even large due to the presence of multiple cysts or coincident urinary tract obstruction with hydronephrosis. The multicystic dysplastic kidney (MCDK) is an extreme form of renal dysplasia and is defined grossly as a non-reniform collection of cysts.

Epidemiology and Longterm Outcomes of Renal Malformations

The prevalence of renal and urinary tract malformations is 0.3–17 per 1000 liveborn and stillborn infants [6, 7]. Due to their common embryonic origin from the mesonephric duct, lower urinary tract abnormalities are found in about 50 % of patients with renal malformations and include vesicoureteral reflux (25 %), ureteropelvic junction obstruction (11 %), and ureterovesical junction obstruction (11 %) [8]. Renal malformations are commonly detected in the antenatal period and account for 20–30 % of all anomalies detected [9]: upper urinary tract dilatation is the most frequent abnormality that is observed. All major organs are formed between the fourth and eighth week of gestation: the aortic arches undergo transformation, the cloacal membrane ruptures, and the kidneys begin to form. Renal malformations are therefore observed in association with non-renal malformations in about 30 % of cases [6]. Indeed, there are over 100 multi-organ syndromes associated with renal and urinary tract malformations [10] (Table 10.1).

Bilateral renal agenesis occurs in 1:3000–10,000 births and males are affected more often than females. Unilateral renal agenesis has been reported with a prevalence of 1:1000 autopsies. The incidence of unilateral hypoplasia/dysplasia is 1 in 3000–5000 births (1:3640 for the MCDK) compared to 1 in 10,000 for bilateral dysplasia [11]. The male to female ratio for bilateral and unilateral renal hypo/dysplasia is 1.32:1 and 1.92:1, respectively [12]. Nine percent of first degree relatives of patients with bilateral renal agenesis or bilateral renal hypoplasia/dysplasia have some type of renal malformation [13]. The incidence of renal ectopia is 1 in 1000 from

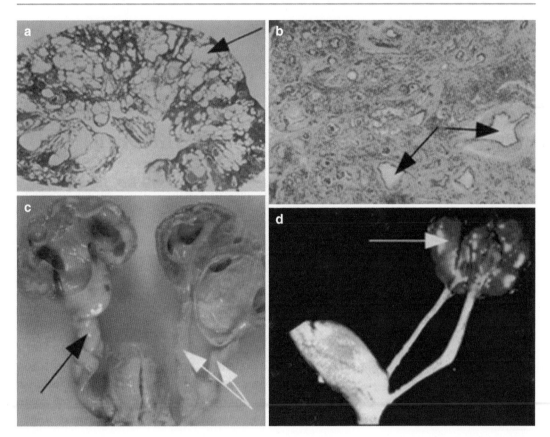

Fig. 10.1 Anatomical features of human renal and lower urinary tract malformations. (**a**) Multicystic dysplastic kidney characterized by numerous cysts (*arrow*) distorting the renal architecture. (**b**) Dysplastic renal tissue demonstrating lack of recognizable nephron elements, dilated tubules, large amounts of stromal tissue and primitive ducts (*arrows*) characterized by epithelial tubules with fibromuscular collars. (**c**) Ureteral duplication (*right, white arrows*) and dilated ureter (*left, black arrow*) associated with a ureterocoele. All ureters are obstructed at the level of the bladder and are associated with hydronephrosis. (**d**) Crossed fused ectopia with fused orthotopic and heterotopic kidneys (*arrow*)

autopsies, while from clinical studies, it is estimated to be less frequent at 1 in 10,000 patients [14]. Males and females are equally affected. Renal ectopia is bilateral in 10 % of cases; when unilateral, there is a slight predilection for the left side. The incidence of fusion anomalies is estimated to be about 1 in 600 infants [15].

While congenital renal malformations are relatively frequent birth defects, there is a wide spectrum of outcomes from no symptoms at all to chronic kidney disease with a spectrum of severity to mortality in the newborn period or later in life. The range in phenotypic severity makes it extremely difficult to counsel patients with certainty. Melo et al. reported a prevalence of CAKUT of 1.77 per 100 live births (524 cases of CAKUT in 29,653 newborns) in a tertiary care unit and a mortality rate of 24 % in those affected (126/524) [7]. Amongst the 524 cases, risk factors for early mortality were the co-existence of non-renal and non-urinary tract organ disease, prematurity, low birth weight, oligohydramnios, and renal involvement (renal agenesis, renal hypodysplasia, multicystic renal dysplasia). Quirino et al. reported on the clinical course of 822 children with prenatally detected CAKUT that were followed for a median time of 43 months [16]. Their results demonstrate that most affected children do well: 29 % of the children had urinary tract infection, 2.7 % had hypertension, 6 % had chronic

Table 10.1 Most frequent syndromes, chromosomal abnormalities and metabolic disorders with renal or urinary tract malformation

Syndromes
Beckwith-Wiedemann
Cerebro-oculo-renal
CHARGE
DiGeorge
Ectrodactyly, ectodermal dysplasia and cleft/lip palates
Ehlers Danlos
Fanconi pancytopenia syndrome
Fraser
Fryns
Meckel
Marfan
MURCS Association
Oculo-auriculo-vertebral (Goldenhar)
Oculo-facial-digital (OFD)
Pallister-Hall
Renal cyst and diabetes
Simpson-Golabi-Behmel (SGBS)
Tuberous sclerosis
Townes Brock
VATER
WAGR
Williams Beuren
Zelweger (cerebrohepatorenal)
Chromosomal abnormalities
Trisomy 21
Klinefelter
DiGeorge, 22q11
45, X0 (Turner)
(XXY) Kleinfelter
Tri 9 mosaic, Tri 13, Tri 18, del 4q, del 18q, dup3q, dup 10q
Triploidy
Metabolic disorders
Peroxysomal
Glycosylation defect
Mitochondriopathy
Glutaric aciduria type II
Carnitine palmitoyl transferase II deficiency

kidney disease, and 1.5 % died during followup. Celedon et al. studied 176 children with chronic renal failure secondary to renal dysplasia, reflux nephropathy or urinary tract obstruction with a minimum of 5 years of followup [17]. They noted

that patients with a urine albumin to creatinine ratio greater than 200 mg/mmol deteriorated faster compared to those with less than 50 mg/mmol (-6.5 ml/min/1.73 m^2 year vs. -1.5 ml/min/1.73 m^2 year). They also observed that those children with more than two febrile urinary tract infections deteriorated faster than those with less than two infections (median -3.5 ml/min/1.73 m^2 vs. -2 ml/min/1.73 m^2 year). Similar differences were noted for children with hypertension when compared to those without. Finally they noted that the rate of decline in eGFR was greater during puberty (-4 ml/min/1.73 m^2/year vs. -1.9 ml/min/1.73 m^2/year). They noted no differences in deterioration of eGFR when comparing children with one or two functioning kidneys. In contrast, Sanna-Cherchi et al. examined the risk of progression to ESRD in patients with CAKUT. They found that by the age of 30 years, 58 out of 312 patients had initiated dialysis. They also noted that the risk for dialysis was significantly higher for patients with a solitary kidney [18]. The same group reported that patients with bilateral hypodysplasia, solitary kidney, or posterior urethral valves with renal hypodysplasia had a higher risk of dialysis requirement at 30 years when compared to patients with unilateral renal hypodysplasia or horseshoe kidney, and the risk was even higher if there was coexistence of vesicoureteric reflux. Most recently, Wuhl et al. compared patients with CAKUT to age-matched patients with other causes of renal failure who were receiving some form of renal replacement therapy and registered within the European Dialysis and Transplant Association Registry [19]. Of 212,930 patients ranging in age from 0 to 75 years who commenced renal replacement therapy (RRT), very few, 2.2 % (4765) had renal failure secondary to CAKUT. Importantly, the median age for requirement of renal replacement therapy was 31 years in the CAKUT cohort versus 61 years in the non-CAKUT cohort, suggesting that most children are likely to require dialysis and/or transplantation as adults. CAKUT was the most frequent cause of need for RRT in all pediatric age groups and peaked in incidence in the 15–19 year old group. Taken together, many questions remain in understanding the long-term outcome of CAKUT, but clearly most children are surviving into adulthood, and thus there is a need for adult nephrologists to understand these disorders as well.

Abnormal Molecular Signaling in the Malformed Kidney

Human renal development is complete by 34 weeks gestation [3]. Thus, by definition, renal malformation is a problem of disordered renal embryogenesis. The morphologic, cellular, and genetic events that underlie normal renal development are reviewed in Chaps. 8 and 9. During human kidney development, two primordial tissues, the ureteric bud and the metanephric mesenchyme, undergo epithelial morphogenesis to form the final metanephric kidney [20]. The kidneys and the ureters arise from two epithelial tubes that extend along the length of the embryo, the mesonephric ducts. An epithelial swelling emerges from the mesonephric duct and is known as the ureteric bud. The ureteric bud invades the adjacent undifferentiated mesenchyme and induces the formation of the metanephric mesenchyme. Reciprocal signaling between the ureteric bud and the metanephric mesenchyme induces the ureteric bud to elongate and bifurcate in a process known as branching morphogenesis that ultimately gives rise to the collecting duct system of the adult kidney. The process of ureteric bud branching morphogenesis is critical for kidney development: each ureteric bud tip induces the adjacent ventrally located metanephric mesenchyme to undergo mesenchymal-to-epithelial transition and this determines the final number of nephrons formed in utero. Perturbations in ureteric bud outgrowth, branching morphogenesis and mesenchymal-to-epithelial transition are thought to underlie the majority of the malformations described in humans.

Failure of ureteric bud outgrowth and invasion of the metanephric blastema are events antecedent to renal agenesis or severe renal dysplasia. Studies in the mouse embryo, a model of human renal development, have identified genes that control ureteric bud outgrowth, ureteric bud

branching morphogenesis, and mesenchymal-to-epithelial transition. Some of these genes are mutated in human renal malformations also characterized by agenesis or severe dysplasia [reviewed by [21]]. If the ureteric bud fails to emerge, the ureter and the kidney do not develop, while if the ureteric bud emerges from an abnormal location, the ureter that forms will not connect to the bladder properly and potentially result in obstruction and/or vesico-ureteric reflux with a malformed kidney. Indeed, a pathogenic role for abnormal ureteric bud outgrowth from the mesonephric duct was first hypothesized based on the clinical-pathological observation that abnormal insertion of the ureter into the lower urinary tract is frequently associated with a duplex kidney. Moreover, the renal parenchyma associated with the ureter with ectopic insertion into the bladder is frequently dysplastic [22]. The local environment of transcription factors and signalling pathways is therefore critical to the successful formation of an intact kidney-urinary tract. While a large number of transcription factors and ligand-receptor signalling pathways have been identified that regulate kidney development [21, 23], we will focus on the function of a few selected molecules that have been implicated in human congenital renal malformations: *Gdnf-Ret, EYA1, Six1, Sall1, Pax2, HNF1b, Shh*, and components of the renin-angiotensin-system.

The central ligand-receptor signalling pathway that leads to the outgrowth of the ureteric bud from the mesonephric duct is the GDNF-GFRA1-RET signalling pathway. Glial cell derived neurotrophic factor (GDNF) is a ligand expressed by the metanephric blastema that interacts with the tyrosine kinase receptor, RET, and its co-receptor GFRα1, both expressed on the surface of the mesonephric duct to initiate outgrowth of the ureteric bud. Mutational inactivation of *Gdnf, Gfra1, or Ret* in mice causes bilateral renal agenesis due to failure of ureteric bud outgrowth demonstrating the importance of this pathway [24–27]. Similarly, when GDNF-soaked beads are positioned adjacent to cultured murine mesonephric ducts, multiple ectopic ureteric buds emerge, demonstrating the potency of this signalling pathway [28]. The expression domain of GDNF is therefore tightly regulated in the nephrogenic mesenchyme and the metanephric mesenchyme.

A network of transcription factors promotes *Gdnf* expression: *Eya1*, *Six1*, *Sall1*, and *Pax2*, while *Foxc1* restricts *Gdnf* expression [29]. Another ligand-receptor complex that limits the domain of *Gdnf* expression is the secreted factor SLIT2 and its receptor ROBO2 [30]. *Slit2* is expressed in the mesonephric duct, while *Robo2* is expressed in the nephrogenic mesenchyme Bone morphogenetic protein 4 also negatively regulates the expression domain of *Gdnf* such that the ureteric bud emerges in the correct location [31].

EYA1 is expressed in metanephric mesenchymal cells in the same spatial and temporal pattern as GDNF. Mice with EYA1 deficiency demonstrate renal agenesis and failure of GDNF expression [32]. EYA1 functions in a molecular complex that includes SIX1 and together they translocate to the nucleus to regulate *Gdnf* expression. Therefore, mutational inactivation of *Six1* in mice also results in renal agenesis or severe dysgenesis [33]. Like GDNF, SIX1 and EYA1, SALL1 is expressed in the metanephric mesenchyme prior to and during ureteric bud invasion. Mutational inactivation of *Sall1* in mice causes renal agenesis or severe dysgenesis and a marked decrease in GDNF expression [34]. Thus, EYA1, SIX1 and SALL1 function upstream of GDNF to positively regulate its expression, thereby controlling ureteric bud outgrowth.

PAX2 is another transcription factor that is expressed in the mesonephric duct, the ureteric bud and in metanephric blastema cells induced by ureteric bud branch tips [35]. Mice with a *Pax2* mutation identical in type to that found in humans with Renal Coloboma syndrome (RCS) exhibit decreased ureteric bud branching and renal hypoplasia. Investigation of the mechanisms controlling abnormal ureteric bud branching in a murine model of RCS (*Pax2^{1Neu}*) revealed that increased ureteric bud cell apoptosis decreases the number of ureteric bud branches and glomeruli formed. Remarkably, rescue of ureteric bud cell apoptosis normalizes the mutant phenotype [36]. *Pax2* appears to function upstream of *Gdnf* since in *Pax2* null mice, no

Gdnf expression is detected and the PAX2 protein can activate the Gdnf promoter [37].

PAX2 and HNF1β, another transcription factor, are co-expressed in the mesonephric duct and the ureteric bud lineage. Constitutive inactivation of HNF1β is embryonic-lethal in the mouse at gastrulation prior to the formation of the kidneys, but by using tetraploid and diploid embryo complementation, homozygous mutant embryos were able to proceed past gastrulation. The latter study demonstrated that HNF1β is critical for mesonephric duct integrity, ureteric bud branching morphogenesis, and early nephron formation [38]. Another group conditionally inactivated HNF1β in the proximal tubule, loop of Henle and collecting ducts and noted that null mice had cystic kidneys with cysts arising predominantly from collecting duct and loop of Henle segments [39]. The renal phenotype was severe, leading to death from renal failure in the newborn period. Importantly cystic kidneys from null animals demonstrated downregulation of Uromodulin, Pkd2, and Pkhd1, suggesting that HNF1β may regulate genes associated with cyst formation [39]. Compound heterozygous mice bearing null alleles for *Pax2* and *Hnf1β* show severe CAKUT phenotypes including hypoplasia of the kidneys, caudal ectopic aborted ureteric buds, duplex kidneys, megaureters and hydronephrosis [40]. These phenotypes were much more severe than *Pax2* heterozygous null or *Hnf1β* heterozygous null mice, strongly suggesting that *Pax2* and *Hnf1β* genetically interact in a common kidney developmental pathway.

Sonic Hedgehog (SHH) is a secreted protein that controls a variety of critical processes during embryogenesis. In mammals, SHH acts to control gene transcription via three members of the GLI family of transcription factors, GLI1, GLI2 and GLI3. A pathogenic role for truncated GLI3 was demonstrated in mice engineered such that the normal *GLI3* allele was replaced with the truncated isoform. These mice are characterized by renal agenesis or dysplasia similar to humans with Pallister Hall Syndrome (PHS) [41]. Subsequent analysis of renal embryogenesis in mice deficient in SHH and GLI3 suggests that the truncated form of GLI3 represses genes like PAX2 and SALL1 that are required for the initiation of renal development [42]. Loss of Hedgehog signalling and increased formation of GLI3 repressor have also been implicated in non-obstructive hydronephrosis and urinary pacemaker dysfunction in mice [43]. Interestingly, some patients with Pallister Hall Syndrome do manifest hydronephrosis, although the underlying mechanisms are unclear.

In postnatal renal physiology, the renin-angiotensin system (RAS) plays a critical role in fluid and electrolyte homeostasis and in the control of blood pressure. Renin cleaves angiotensinogen (AGT) to generate angiotensin (Ang) I which is cleaved by angiotensin-converting enzyme (ACE) to yield Ang II. Ang II is the main effector peptide growth factor of the RAS and acts on two major receptors: AT1R and AT2R. The role of the RAS during kidney development appears to differ somewhat in humans versus rodents, but the metanephric kidney expresses all components of the pathway in both species. Angiotensin is expressed in the ureteric bud lineage and the stromal mesenchyme, while renin is expressed by mesenchymal cells destined to form vascular precursors in the kidney. ACE is expressed slightly later during kidney development in differentiated mesenchymal structures including glomeruli, proximal tubules and collecting ducts. The receptors AT1R and AT2R are expressed in the ureteric bud lineage and in metanephric mesenchymal cells [44]. Mutations of AGT, renin, ACE, or AT1R all result in CAKUT phenotypes in the mouse that are characterized by renal malformations with hypoplasia of the medulla and the papillae and hydronephrosis [45]. Mice with mutations in AT2R also exhibit CAKUT, but a wider range of phenotypes is observed that includes renal hypo/dysplasia, duplicated collecting systems, vesico-ureteric reflux, and hydronephrosis [46]. Importantly, genetic inactivation of the RAS pathway in mice does not result in renal tubular dysgenesis as observed in humans with similar mutations. It is postulated this may be due to differences between the species: in humans, RAS activity (renin and ANG II levels) reaches its peak during fetal life while nephrogenesis is occurring, while in rodents, RAS activity peaks postnatally from weeks 2–6, when nephrogenesis has ceased.

These temporal differences likely explain the lack of concordance between genetic mouse models and affected humans [47].

Ureteric bud branching and modelling of the lower urinary tract with its insertion into the bladder is also controlled by Vitamin A and its signaling effectors [48, 49]. Expression of RET, the receptor for GDNF, is controlled by members of the retinoic acid receptor family of transcription factors that function in the Vitamin A signaling pathway. These members, including RAR alpha and RAR beta2, are expressed in stromal cells surrounding *Ret*-expressing ureteric bud branch tips [49, 50]. Mice deficient in these receptors exhibit a decreased number of ureteric bud branches and diminished expression of *Ret*. These observations are consistent with the finding that Vitamin A deficiency during pregnancy causes renal hypoplasia in the rat fetus [51]. A similar observation has been noted in a human study where maternal Vitamin A deficiency was associated with congenital renal malformation [52].

In summary, genetic and nutritional factors like Vitamin A and folic acid [52–54] interact to control ureteric bud outgrowth, ureteric bud branching, nephrogenesis, and ureter formation. The number of nephrons is likely determined by a complex combination of factors including genetic variants, environmental events and stochastic factors. This could explain the variable number of nephrons in humans, ranging from approximately 230,000–1,800,000 [55]. Loss-of-function mutations in developmental genes can impair nephron formation in utero and depending on the magnitude of this effect, renal insufficiency may present at birth, childhood, adolescence or adulthood. Despite evidence in animals that depletion of protein, total calories or micronutrients causes renal hypoplasia, their contribution to human CAKUT remains unclear and an important area of future investigation.

Human Renal Malformations with a Defined Genetic Etiology

In humans, congenital renal malformations are more frequently sporadic than familial in occurrence. This may be due to the fact that infants with severe renal malformations have only recently survived: prior to the late 1970s, chronic dialysis was not offered as a therapy for children and this continues to be the case in much of the developing world because of a lack of resources [56]. Therefore, it is only in the past 30 years that children with congenital renal malformations have survived and been able to reproduce and potentially transmit deleterious gene mutations. Therefore, congenital renal malformations appear as sporadic events over time. Genetic haploinsufficiency for many of the aforementioned transcription factors (*Eya1*, *Six1* etc.) can result in a severe renal developmental phenotype; therefore, de novo heterozygous mutations continue to arise. However, as reported by others, incomplete penetrance with variable expressivity is frequently observed in genetic studies of CAKUT, especially in regards to many of the transcription factors described previously [57]. Congenital renal malformations can occur in isolation, as part of CAKUT, or as part of a syndrome with organ malformations. Importantly, familial cases and extra-renal symptoms are sometimes unrecognized if carefully phenotyping is not performed. A careful evaluation of family history reveals a clustering of isolated or syndromic urinary tract and renal malformations in more than 10 % of the cases [58]. Knowledge of the most frequent syndromes, a careful clinical examination and appropriately selected investigations are critical to the clinical approach to these disorders.

Mutations in more than 30 genes have been identified in children with renal development anomalies, generally as part of a multi-organ syndrome (Table 10.2). Some of these syndromes and their associated genes are described here. The most frequent syndromes in which renal malformations are encountered are listed in Tables 10.1 and 10.2. For a complete list of syndromes featuring renal malformations; the reader is referred to McKusick's Online Mendelian Inheritance in Man.[1]

----

[1] http://www.ncbi.nlm.nih.gov/

Genetic Causes of CAKUT

The GDNF/RET Signaling Pathway

The proto-oncogene *RET*, a tyrosine kinase receptor, and its ligand, GDNF, play a pivotal role during early nephrogenesis and enteric nervous system development. Activating *RET* mutations cause multiple endocrine neoplasia, whereas inactivating mutations lead to Hirschsprung disease. A number of human studies have demonstrated that patients with CAKUT have mutations in the RET/GDNF signaling pathway [89–92]. A study of 122 patients with CAKUT identified heterozygous deleterious sequence variants in GDNF or RET in 6/122 patients, 5 %, while another group screened 749 families from all over the world and identified three families with heterozygous mutations in RET [89, 93]. Similar findings have been reported in studies of fetuses with bilateral or unilateral renal agenesis [90, 92].

Branchio-oto-Renal Syndrome

The association of branchial (B), otic (O) and renal (R) anomalies was first described by Fraser and Melnick [94, 95]. Major diagnostic criteria consist of hearing loss (95 %), branchial defects (49–69 %), ear pits (83 %) and renal anomalies (38–67 %) [96, 97]. The association of these three major features defines the classical BOR syndrome (OMIM # 113650). Yet, many patients have only one or two of these major features in association with other minor features such as external ear anomalies, preauricular tags or other facial abnormalities (Table 10.3). Hearing loss can be conductive, sensorineural, or mixed.

The frequency of BOR syndrome has been estimated to be 1 in 40,000 births [98]. The transmission is autosomal dominant with incomplete penetrance and variable expressivity. Renal malformations include unilateral or bilateral renal agenesis, hypodysplasia as well as malformation of the lower urinary tract including vesicoureteral reflux, pyeloureteral obstruction, and ureteral duplication. Different renal malformations can be observed in the same family; moreover, some individuals have normal kidneys (BO syndrome, OMIM 120502). Other infrequent abnormalities

Table 10.2 Human gene mutations exhibiting defects in renal morphogenesis

Primary disease	Gene (s)	Kidney phenotype	References
Alagille syndrome	*JAGGED1, NOTCH2*	Cystic dysplasia	[59–61]
Apert syndrome (overlaps with Pfeiffer syndrome and Crouzon syndrome)	*FGFR2, FGFR1*	Hydronephrosis, VUR	[62, 63]
Beckwith-Wiedemann syndrome	*CDKN1C(p57^{KIP)2}), H19, LIT1, NSD1*	Medullary dysplasia, nephromegaly, collecting duct abnormalties, cysts, VUR, hydronephrosis, Wilm's tumor	[64, 65]
Branchio-oto-renal (BOR) syndrome	*EYA1, SIX1, SIX5*	Unilateral or bilateral agenesis/dysplasia, hypoplasia, collecting system anomalies	[66–68]
Campomelic dysplasia	*SOX9*	Dysplasia, hydronephrosis	[69, 70]
Duane radial ray (Okihiro) syndrome	*SALL4*	UNL agenesis, VUR, malrotation, cross-fused ectopia, pelviectasis	[71]
Fraser syndrome	*FRAS1, GRIP1, FREM2, FREM1*	Agenesis, dysplasia, CAKUT	[72–75]
Hyoparathyroidism, sensorineural deafness and renal anomalies (HDR) syndrome	*GATA3*	Dysplasia, VUR, CAKUT,mesangioproliferative glomerulonephritis	[76, 77]
Kallmann syndrome	*KAL1, FGFR1,FGF8 PROK2, PROK2R, CHD7, NELF, HS6ST1*	Agenesis	[78, 79]
Mammary-Ulnar syndrome	*TBX3*	Dysplasia	[80]
Pallister-Hall syndrome	*GLI3*	Dysplasia	[42, 81]
Renal-coloboma syndrome	*PAX2*	Hypoplasia, vesico-ureteral reflux	[82]
Renal tubular dysgenesis	RAS components, *REN, AGT, AGTR1, ACE*	Tubular dysplasia	[83]
Renal cysts and diabetes syndrome	*HNF1β*	Dysplasia, hypoplasia	[84]
Simpson-Golabi Behmel syndrome	*GPC3*	medullary dysplasia	[85]
Smith Lemli Opitz syndrome	*DHCR7*	Agenesis, dysplasia	[86]
Townes-Brock syndrome	*SALL1*	Hypoplasia, dysplasia, VUR	[87]
Zellweger syndrome	*PEX1*	VUR, cystic dysplasia	[88]

Table 10.3 Major and minor criteria for the diagnosis of BOR syndrome

Major features	Minor features
Deafness	External ear anomalies
Branchial anomalies	Preauricular tags
Preauricular pits	Other facial anomalies
Renal malformations	Cataracts
	Lacrimal duct stenosis

have been described in patients with the BOR syndrome. These include aplasia of the lacrimal ducts, congenital cataracts and anterior segment anomalies [94, 95]. Characteristic temporal bone findings include cochlear hypoplasia (four out of five of normal size with only two turns), dilation of the vestibular aqueduct, bulbous internal auditory canals, deep posterior fossae, and acutely-angled promontories [97].

Approximately 40 % of patients with BOR syndrome have a mutation in the EYA1 gene [96], while it is estimated that 5 % may have a mutation in SIX1 [66]. Mutations in another SIX family member, SIX5 have also been reported [67], although its role in BOR has also been questioned [99]. Both EYA1 and SIX1 are co-expressed in the developing otic, branchial and renal tissue [32, 100], where they function in a transcriptional complex that regulates cell proliferation and cell survival [101–103]. EYA1 and SIX1 control the expression of PAX2 and GDNF in the metanephric mesenchyme [104]. The EYA1 protein contains a highly conserved region called the *eyes absent* homologous region encoded within exons 9–16 which is the site of most mutations identified to date. A list of *EYA1* mutations can be found on the website of Iowa University http://www.healthcare.uiowa.edu/labs/pendredandbor/slcMutations.htm.[2]

The wide spectrum of phenotypic features associated with *EYA1* mutations complicates the approach to making a diagnosis of BOR syndrome [96]. A reasonable approach is to limit analysis of *EYA1* to families in which at least one member fulfils the criteria for classical BOR syndrome (Table 10.3). Investigations should include a family history, and examination of relatives to look for preauricular pits, lacrimal duct stenosis, and branchial fistulae and/or cysts. Hearing studies and renal ultrasound should be done in all first degree relatives.

Molecular testing can confirm the diagnosis and provide genetic recurrence risk information to families. However, variability of the phenotype even with the same mutation does not permit accurate prediction of the disease severity. Within the same family, a given mutation may be associated with renal malformation in some individuals, but not in others. This discrepancy might be explained by stochastic factors that impact the formation of the kidneys or by other unlinked genetic events that may act in synergy with the EYA1 protein during nephrogenesis.

Townes-Brocks Syndrome and VATER/VACTERL Associations

Townes-Brocks syndrome (TBS) is an autosomal dominant malformation syndrome usually defined by a triad of anomalies including imperforate anus, dysplastic ears, and thumb malformations [105]. A wide spectrum of additional features includes renal malformations, congenital heart defects, hand and foot malformations, hearing loss, and eye anomalies [106, 107]. Intelligence is usually normal. REAR Syndrome (renal-ear-anal-

radial) has also been used to describe this condition [108]. Its incidence is reported to be 1:250,000 live births [109]. The presentation of TBS is highly variable within and between affected families. Importantly, SALL1, is the only gene implicated in TBS and it encodes a C_2H_2 zinc finger transcription factor that is required for the normal development of the limbs, nervous system, ears, anus, heart and kidneys [87, 110].

The detection rate of SALL1 mutations in patients with TBS appears to be higher when malformations of the hands, the ears, and the anus are present [111]. However, genetic testing is further complicated by the fact that the phenotypic features of TBS can resemble other disorders like VACTERL association, Goldenhar syndrome, Oculo-Auriculo-Vertebral spectrum, Pallister-Hall syndrome and even BOR syndrome. TBS features overlap those seen in the VACTERL association (anal, radial and renal malformations). In contrast to VACTERL association, TBS is associated with ear anomalies and deafness and it is not characterized by tracheo-oesophageal fistula or vertebral anomalies.

VACTERL association is defined by the presence of at least three of the following congenital malformations: vertebral anomalies, anal atresia, cardiac defects, tracheo-esophageal defects, renal malformations, and limb anomalies [112]. It is reported to occur in 1:10,000–40,000 of all live births. Renal anomalies are reported in 50–80 % of patients and include unilateral or bilateral renal agenesis, horseshoe kidney, cystic kidneys, dysplastic kidneys, and they can be accompanied by urinary tract and genital defects [113, 114]. Ninety percent of VACTERL cases appear to be sporadic with little evidence of heritability [114]. In a subset of patients there is evidence of heritability [114–116], and genes that interact with the Sonic Hedgehog pathway have been implicated [117, 118]. The presence of a single umbilical artery on ultrasound has been associated with a variety of congenital birth defects, including VACTERL syndrome [119]. It has been hypothesized that the single umbilical artery is a risk factor for a placental defect that may affect nutrient supply for multiple organs simultaneously during development [120].

---

[2]http://www.medicine.uiowa.edu/pendredandbor/

An important diagnosis to consider in patients suspected to have VACTERL syndrome is Fanconi's anemia. Patients with Fanconi's anemia can phenocopy VACTERL syndrome, but also exhibit bone marrow failure manifest as pancytopenia. They can also develop malignancies like acute myelogenous leukemia secondary to their propensity for chromosomal instability manifest as spontaneous cytogenetic aberrations. Patients with Fanconi's anemia also frequently demonstrate skin pigmentation (café au lait spots), microcephaly, growth retardation and microphtalmia. There are at least nine different gene mutations implicated in Fanconi's anemia and they are inherited as X-linked or recessive disorders. It has been reported that approximately 5 % of patients with confirmed Fanconi's anemia have features consistent with VACTERL syndrome [121]. Therefore the diagnosis of Fanconi's anemia needs to be carefully considered in all patients with VACTERL syndrome and confirmed if needed by performing chromosomal breakage studies [112, 121].

Renal-Coloboma Syndrome

Renal Coloboma Syndrome (RCS) (also named papillo-renal syndrome) is an autosomal dominant disorder characterized by the association of renal hypoplasia, vesicoureteric reflux and optic nerve coloboma from a mutation in *Pax2* [122]. The prevalence of the syndrome is unknown, but approximately 100 families have been reported [123]. A wide range of renal malformations are observed in RCS. Oligomeganephronic hypoplasia, renal dysplasia and vesicoureteric reflux are the most frequent malformations but multicystic dysplasia [124] and ureteropelvic junction obstruction have also been described [57, 124, 125]. Similarly, the ocular phenotype is extremely variable. The most common finding is an optic disc pit associated with vascular abnormalities and cilio-retinal arteries, with mild visual impairment limited to blind spot enlargement, the "morning glory" anomaly [126]. In other cases, the only ocular anomaly is optic nerve dysplasia with an abnormal vessel pattern and no functional consequence (Fig. 10.2a, b). In contrast, a large coloboma of the optic nerve or of the chorioretina and the morning glory anomaly can be responsible for a severe visual impairment [127]. Coloboma and the related anomalies are probably the consequence of an incomplete closure of the embryonic fissure of the optic cup. Other extrarenal manifestations can include sensorineural hearing loss, joint laxity, Arnold Chiari malformation and seizures of unknown cause [128, 129]. In addition to its expression in the developing kidney and in the optic fissure, *PAX2* is also

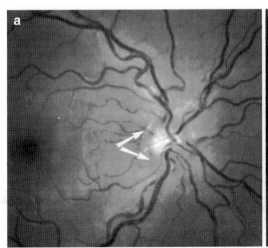
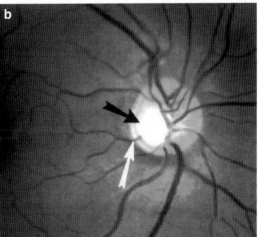

Fig. 10.2 Optic disc appearance in two patients with Renal Coloboma Syndrome and PAX2 mutations: (**a**) Characteristic features of optic disk coloboma with a deep temporal excavation (*arrowheads*). (**b**) The optic disk is dysplastic with thickening (black *arrow*) and emergence of abnormal vessels ("morning glory anomaly *white arrow*")

expressed in the hindbrain during its development. However, neurological symptoms are not usually present in RCS.

PAX2 is a transcription factor of the paired-box family of homeotic genes that is expressed in the mesonephros and in the metanephros during renal development. In 1995, Sanyanusin et al. reported heterozygous mutations in two RCS families [82]. Since then, more than 30 mutations have been reported, most of them lying in exons 2–4 that encode the paired domain that binds to DNA or in exons 7–9 that encode the transactivation domain [123, 130]. Other gene(s) are probably also responsible for this syndrome since *PAX2* mutations are not found in approximately 50 % of RCS patients. Importantly the RCS phenotype is highly variable even in patients harboring the same *PAX2* mutation suggesting that modifier genes might be implicated.

Optic nerve coloboma occurs frequently as an isolated anomaly or as a feature of many other multiorgan syndromes such as the CHARGE association, the COACH syndrome and the acro-renal-ocular syndrome. As optic nerve coloboma and the related disorders can be easily misdiagnosed, it is likely that the prevalence of RCS is underestimated. It is wise to examine the fundus in every patient with renal hypo-dysplasia, and conversely to perform renal ultrasound and serum creatinine in every patient with optic nerve coloboma.

Renal Cyst and Diabetes Syndrome

Mutations in the *TCF2* gene encoding the transcription factor HNF1β were initially found in patients with diabetes type MODY5, Maturity Onset Diabetes of the Young [131, 132]. Diabetes mellitus is present in approximately 60 % of all the cases reported, usually occurs before 25 years of age, and is often associated with pancreatic atrophy [133–135]. In some patients, a subclinical deficiency of pancreatic exocrine functions has been demonstrated [133]. Additional features have been described including a wide spectrum of renal phenotypes (Table 10.4). The presence of cysts is the most consistent feature of the renal phenotype, leading to the name, "Renal Cysts and Diabetes (RCAD) Syndrome." The cysts are

Table 10.4 Renal cyst and diabetes syndrome

Main features[a]
Fetal large hyperechoic kidneys
Renal hypodysplasia with cortical microcysts
Diabetes mellitus (MODY type 5)
Occasional features
Genital malformations
Female: vaginal aplasia, rudimentary or bicornuate uterus
Male: epididymal cysts, atresia of the vas deferens, asthenospermia, hypospadias
Hyperuricemia, rarely gout (reduced uric acid fraction excretion)
Hypomagnesemia
Moderate elevation of liver enzymes
Subclinical defect of exocrine pancreatic functions

[a]Age at onset and severity of these symptoms are highly variable

usually cortical, bilateral and small [136]. Mutations in the *TCF2* gene have also been found in association with a variety of renal development disorders such as renal hypo/dysplasia, multicystic dysplastic kidneys, renal agenesis, horseshoe kidneys, ureteropelvic junction obstruction as well as clubbing and tiny diverticulae of the calyces [137–139]. The most specific finding when histology is available is the presence of cortical glomerular cysts with dilatation of the Bowman spaces (glomerulocystic dysplasia) [140]. Other nonspecific lesions such as cystic renal dysplasia, interstitial fibrosis or oligomeganephronia have also been reported. Antenatal presentations with enlarged hyperechoic kidneys or macroscopic cysts can occur [141, 142].

Various genital tract malformations have been reported mostly in females. These include vaginal aplasia, rudimentary uterus, bicornuate uterus, uterus didelphys and double vagina. In males, hypospadias, epididymal cysts, and agenesis of the vas deferens have been reported [133]. These genital anomalies have been described in approximately 10–15 % of patients with *TCF2* mutations, but these malformations might be underestimated especially in paediatric reports. Reduced fractional excretion of uric acid (<15 %) and moderate hyperuricemia is observed in some cases and is usually asymptomatic. The hyperuricemia is thought to reflect altered urate transport by the kidney and impaired glomerular filtration [143]. Serum hypomagnesemia has also been reported and this may be due to the fact that HNF1β regulates FXYD2 that is needed for distal tubule reabsorption of magnesium [144]. A similar mechanism may be at work to explain the altered urate transport observed in these patients since HNF1β can activate the promoter of URAT1 that regulates urate transport in the proximal tubule [145]. Moderate elevation of liver enzymes is a common finding, but severe hepatopathy has not been reported.

HNF1β is a homeotic transcription factor, which is involved in the development of the pancreas, the kidneys, the liver and intestine. More than 50 mutations have been reported, most of which are located in the first four exons that encode the DNA-binding domain. In more than one-third of the cases, the gene is entirely deleted [134, 136, 145]. Such alterations are not detected by conventional amplification and screening methods. Importantly, deletions are infrequently transmitted by the parents but appear de novo in the proband. Analysis of *TCF2* can thus be recommended not only in patients with a family history of RCAD syndrome but also in cases with renal cysts when polycystic disease or nephronophthisis are unlikely. The presence of cortical bilateral cysts is probably the most typical finding. Reduced uric acid fractional excretion, elevation of liver enzymes, hypomagnesemia, glucose intolerance and abnormalities of the genital tract should be systemically sought and *TCF2* analyzed if one of these symptoms is present. As observed in other syndromes, phenotypic variability can be observed between families and also in family members with the same mutation, suggesting a role for environmental and genetic factors.

Kallmann Syndrome

Kallmann syndrome (KS) is defined by the presence of hypogonadotropic hypogonadism and deficiency of the sense of smell (anosmia or hyposmia) [146]. Some affected individuals exhibit unilateral renal agenesis, cleft lip and/or palate, selective tooth agenesis, bimanual syn-

kinesis and hearing impairment [147]. Other CAKUT phenotypes including duplex systems, hydronephrosis, and vesicoureteric reflux have been rarely reported. Anosmia/hyposmia is related to the absence or hypoplasia of the olfactory bulbs and tracts. Hypogonadism is due to a deficiency in gonadotropin-releasing hormone (GnRH). The GnRH-synthesizing neurons migrate during development from the olfactory epithelium to the forebrain along the olfactory nerve pathway [148, 149]. KS is genetically heterogeneous with eight genes reported including *KAL1*, an X-chromosome encoded gene that gives rise to the extracellular matrix protein anosmin-1 [150], *FGF8* (Fibroblast growth factor 8) [151] and *FGFR1* (Fibroblast Growth Factor Receptor 1), mutated in autosomal dominant forms of KS [152], *PROK2* (*prokinectin-2*) and *PROKR2* (*prokinectin-2 receptor*) [153], *CHD7, NELF, and HS6ST1* [78]. Chromodomain helicase DNA-binding protein 7 (CHD7) is a transcriptional regulator that binds to enhancer elements in the nucleus. It is implicated in CHARGE syndrome that is characterized by choanal atresia, malformations of the heart, the inner ear, and the retina, and in Kallman syndrome. In the largest study to date of 219 patients with Kallman syndrome, mutations were most commonly observed in the FGF pathway (either FGF8 or FGFR1), in KAL1, in the PROK2/PROKR2 pathway and in CHD7 [78]. Importantly in this study, unilateral renal agenesis was only observed in patients with KAL1 mutations (reported in 18 %,3/17), or in patients with no mutation in the above-mentioned eight genes where the frequency was noted to be 17 % (4/23). Patients with *KAL1* mutations are typically male since the disorder is X-linked and they demonstrate a much more severe reproductive phenotype compared to patients with other mutations with small testes, absent puberty, and micropenis. Females with KAL1 mutations typically present with partial pubertal development manifesting as spontaneous breast development in the absence of hormonal treatment. KAL1 is expressed in the developing human metanephric kidney at 11 weeks of gestation [154].

Renal Tubular Dysgenesis and Mutations of RAS System Elements

The differential diagnosis of oligohydramnios with neonatal renal failure includes a spectrum of diagnoses including bilateral renal dysplasia, posterior urethral valves, and polycystic kidney disease. All of these diagnoses are typically detectable and distinguishable on antenatal ultrasound imaging of the kidneys and the urinary tracts. The presence of normal kidneys on antenatal ultrasound in combination with oligo- or anhydramnios should strongly suggest the diagnosis of renal tubular dysgenesis [155]. Renal tubular dysgenesis (RTD) is a severe perinatal disorder characterized by absence or paucity of differentiated proximal tubules, early severe oligohydramnios, and perinatal death. The latter is usually due to pulmonary hypoplasia and skull ossification defects [156]. This condition has also been described in clinical conditions associated with renal ischemia including the twin–twin transfusion syndrome, major cardiac malformations, severe liver diseases, fetal or infantile renal artery stenosis [157] and in fetuses that are exposed in utero to angiotensin-converting enzyme (ACE) inhibitors, angiotensin II (AngII) receptor antagonists [158] or non-steroidal anti-inflammatory medications [155]. All of these environmental insults are postulated to lead to chronic hypoperfusion of the fetal kidneys with upregulation of the renin-angiotensin system. The absence or paucity of proximal tubules is believed to be secondary to chronic renal hypoperfusion [47]. Mutations in the genes which encode components of the renin-angiotensin system have been identified in some families [83]. Mutations in the Angioconverting enzyme (ACE) gene are seen in 65.5% of cases, while mutations in the Renin (REN) are observed in 20% of cases. Mutations in angiotensinogen (AGT) and in the angiotensinogen type I receptor (ATR1) occur much less frequently [159]. It has been suggested that if there is no expression of the renin protein on immunohistochemistry of the kidneys, then the Renin gene should first be assessed. Similarly, the plasma renin activity should be measured in the newborn with suspected genetic renal tubular dysgenesis and if elevated, this should prompt an analysis of genes downstream of the REN gene [160].

CHD1L, CHD7 and CHARGE Syndrome

Chromodomain helicase DNA binding protein 1-like protein, CHD1L, belongs to the Snf2 family of helicase-related ATP-hydrolyzing proteins and contains a helicase-like region that is similar to other family members, such as CHD7 which is implicated in CHARGE syndrome. Indeed, CHARGE syndrome is associated with CAKUT phenotypes including horseshoe kidneys, renal agenesis, VUR and renal cysts, in ~20% of patients carrying CHD7 Mutations [161].

Chromatin-remodelling and -modifying enzymes like CHD1L and CHD7 are predicted to play key roles in differentiation, development and tumour pathogenesis via effects on chromatin structure and accessibility. Brockeschmidt et al. screened 85 patients with CAKUT and identified three patients with heterozygous missense variants in CHD1L [162]. The same paper reported that CHD1L was expressed in early ureteric bud and comma- and S-shaped structures during human kidney development. In the postnatal human kidney, CHD1L was expressed in the cytoplasm of tubular cells in all nephron segments. Similarly, Hwang et al. reported that 5 out of 650 families had heterozygous mutations in CHD1L: the affected individuals had a spectrum of CAKUT phenotypes including renal dysplasia, posterior urethral valves, UVJ obstruction and horseshoe kidneys [93]. It is not yet known if these patients will also be at greater risk for malignancies given that CHD1L is known to be an oncogene in hepatocellular carcinoma [163].

DSTYK and CAKUT

DSTYK is a dual serine-threonine and tyrosine protein kinase that is co-expressed with fibroblast growth factor receptors in the developing mouse and human kidney in both metanephric mesenchyme and ureteric bud cells. Sanna Cherchi et al. discovered that 7/311 patients with CAKUT had heterozygous mutations in this gene and suggested that this is a relatively common gene variant in CAKUT [164].

Copy Number Variants, CAKUT and Neuropsychiatric Disorders

Copy number variants are stretches of DNA that are larger than 1 kb in length with the potential to contribute to functional variation and disease. Rare CNVs have been implicated in neuropsychiatric and craniofacial syndromes, and in syndromes with CAKUT [165, 166]. Sanna-Cherchi et al., examined the burden of rare CNVs in individuals with congenital renal malformations and observed that 10% (55/522) had these variants compared to 0.2% of population control [166]. Interestingly, deletions at the HNF1β locus (chromosome 17q12) and the locus for DiGeorge syndrome (chromosome 22q11) were most frequently noted, suggesting these are "hotspots" for copy number variation. In addition, 90% of the CNVs associated with congenital renal malformations were previously reported to predispose to developmental delay or neuropsychiatric disease, suggesting that there are shared pathways implicated in renal and central nervous system development. Similarly, Handrigan et al. demonstrated that copy number variants at chromosome 16q24.2 are associated with autism spectrum disorder, intellectual disability, and congenital renal malformations [165].

Genetic Causes of Isolated (Non Syndromic) Renal Malformation

In the majority of children with renal malformation, neither a syndrome nor a Mendelian pattern of inheritance is obvious. It appears that in a substantial proportion of such cases, genes that control nephrogenesis are mutated. A recent study on a cohort of 100 patients with renal hypodysplasia and renal insufficiency demonstrated that 16% of them had mutations in one gene encoding for a transcription factor [57]. The majority of mutations were identified in *TCF2* (HNF1β) (especially in the subset with kidney cysts) and *PAX2*. *EYA1* and *SALL1* mutations were found in single cases. Some of the mutations that were identified in these genes were de novo mutations explaining the sporadic appearance of RHD. Careful analysis of patients with *TCF2* and *PAX2* mutations

Table 10.5 Clinical indications to search for a renal anomaly

Exposure to teratogens
ACE inhibitors and angiotensin receptor blockers
Alcohol
Alkylating agents
Cocaine
Folic acid antagonists
Vitamin A congeners
Maternal diabetes
Findings on physical examination
High imperforate or anteriorly positioned anus
Abnormal external genitalia
Supernumerary nipples
Preauricular pits and ear tags, cervical cysts or fistula
Hearing loss
Aniridia
Coloboma or optic disc dysplasia
Hemihypertrophy
Single umbilical artery
Other
Hyperglycemia

revealed the presence of extrarenal symptoms in only half, supporting previous reports that *TCF2* and *PAX2* mutations can be responsible for isolated renal tract anomalies or at least CAKUT malformations with minimal extrarenal features [125, 136]. This study demonstrates that subtle extrarenal symptoms in syndromal RHD can easily be missed. Genetic testing in children with RHD should be preceded by a thorough clinical evaluation for extrarenal symptoms, including eye, ear, and metabolic anomalies. The presence of nonrenal anomalies increases the likelihood of detecting a specific genetic abnormality (Table 10.5). In addition, mutations in genes that are usually associated with syndromes can occur in patients with isolated RHD.

Clinical Approach to Renal Malformation

The majority of renal malformations are now diagnosed antenatally, largely because of the widespread use and sensitivity of fetal ultrasound. The sensitivity of prenatal ultrasound screening for renal malformations is about 82 % and the mean time at which these malformations are detected is 23 weeks gestation [6]. In general, urinary tract malformations detected antenatally are isolated and present as mild hydronephrosis with no therapeutic consequences. Parents should be reassured (see Chaps. 4 and 38). In contrast, bilateral forms of renal agenesis, severe dysgenesis, bilateral ureteric obstruction, or obstruction of the bladder outlet or the urethra can cause severe oligohydramnios as early as 18 weeks. Because amniotic fluid is critical to lung development, oligohydramnios as early as the second trimester can result in lung hypoplasia, a potentially fatal disorder. The oligohydramnios sequence, termed Potter's syndrome, in its most severe form consists of a typical facial appearance characterized by pseudoepicanthus, recessed chin, posteriorly rotated, flattened ears and flattened nose, as well as decreased fetal movement, musculoskeletal features including clubfoot and clubhand, hip dislocation, joint contractures and pulmonary hypoplasia. The renal prognosis can be evaluated antenatally. Poor outcome can be predicted when there is severe oligohydramnios, and small and hyperechogenic kidneys. Normative data on kidney dimensions including kidney length from antenatal ultrasound imaging are available from the 15th week of gestation and can be used to determine if a kidney is small, suggesting some type of renal dysplasia, or increased in size, as observed in autosomal recessive polycystic kidney disease [167]. Amniotic fluid analysis may be of help in some cases if the fetus is suspected to have a trisomy. Trisomy 21, 18, and 13 are all associated with CAKUT [168–170]. Antenatal diagnosis and assessment of the renal prognosis are important for consideration of early termination in cases of fatal (or eventually severe renal disease) and to prepare parents and medical staff for the likelihood of neonatal renal insufficiency. Other organ malformations should be sought carefully and, if detected, a karyotype should be done. Some authors have suggested that fetal urine analysis may be helpful to determine fetal renal prognosis and to decide on in utero therapy if congenital lower urinary tract obstruction is noted. Morris et al. performed a systematic review of the literature on fetal urine analysis and concluded that none of the analytes examined had sufficient accuracy to predict poor postnatal renal function [171].

The clinical presentation of renal malformation in the postnatal period is dependent on the amount of functioning renal mass, the presence of bilateral urinary tract obstruction and the occurrence of urinary tract infection. Bilateral renal agenesis or severe dysplasia is likely to present soon after birth with decreased renal function. This may be accompanied by oliguria. Alternatively, patients may present with a flank mass or an asymptomatic abnormality detected by renal imaging.

A detailed history and careful physical examination should be carried out on all infants with an antenatally detected renal malformation. An early (within 24 h of life) renal ultrasound is recommended for newborns with a history of oligohydramnios, progressive antenatal hydronephrosis, distended bladder on antenatal sonograms, and bilateral severe hydroureteronephrosis. In male infants, a distended bladder and bilateral hydroureteronephrosis may be secondary to posterior urethral valves, a condition which requires immediate renal imaging and clinical intervention. In general, unilateral anomalies do not require urgent investigation after birth. Renal ultrasound for unilateral hydronephrosis is not recommended within the first 72 h of life because urine output gradually increases over the first 24–48 h of life as renal plasma flow and glomerular filtration rate increase [172]. Thus, the degree of urinary tract dilatation can be underestimated during this period of transition.

A careful examination of the genitalia and the position of the anus are part of the initial assessment since CAKUT can occur in the context of cloacal malformations and with genital tract defects in females and males. The mesonephric duct gives rise to the developing kidneys, urinary tracts and the male genital tracts, therefore a careful examination of the testes, the epididymis, and the ductus deferens is important. Congenital epididymal cysts are the most frequent anomaly noted in association with mesonephric duct anomalies and are usually asymptomatic. Other male genital duct anomalies that may occur in the context of CAKUT include an absent, ectopic or duplicated ductus deferens. Seminal vesicle cysts may also arise and typically present after puberty as pelvic pain or with urinary symptoms like dysuria, polyuria, or urinary retention [173]. Adjacent to the mesonephric ducts are the paired Mullerian or paramesonephric ducts that give rise to the Fallopian tubes, the uterus, the cervix, and the upper two thirds of the vagina. Because Mullerian duct development is tightly linked to the growth and elongation of the mesonephric ducts, CAKUT is also observed with concurrent female Mullerian duct anomalies. Indeed the syndrome Mayer-Rokitansky-Kuster-Hauser syndrome describes women with normal female external genitalia, but Mullerian duct anomalies that include aplasia of the uterus, the cervix, and the upper vagina. In a large cohort of 284 women with this syndrome, roughly 30% of them had associated CAKUT anomalies including renal agenesis, horseshoe kidney, ectopic kidney, and urinary tract defects including duplications [174]. Females with Mullerian ducts anomalies are typically discovered because of primary amenorrhea, dyspareunia, infertility, and/or obstetric complications [175]. In females with CAKUT and a suspected Mullerian duct anomaly, MRI imaging may be indicated to define the anatomical defect with better precision.

Clinical Approach to Specific Malformations

Unilateral Renal Agenesis
A diagnosis of unilateral renal agenesis depends on the certainty that a second kidney does not exist in the pelvis or some other ectopic location. Since absence of one kidney induces compensatory hypertrophy in the existing kidney, the presence of a large kidney on one side suggests the possibility of unilateral renal agenesis. Interestingly, compensatory hypertrophy has been observed to begin as early as 20 weeks of gestation: van Vuuren et al. examined 67 fetuses with a diagnosis of multicystic dysplastic kidney or unilateral renal agenesis and noted that 87% of

the cases of multicystic dysplastic kidney and 100% of the cases of unilateral renal agenesis exhibited compensatory hypertrophy of the contralateral kidney with kidney length greater than the 95th % for gestational age [176]. Since unilateral agenesis is associated with contralateral urinary tract abnormalities including ureteropelvic junction obstruction and vesicoureteral reflux in 20–40% of the cases [177–179], imaging of the contralateral side is suggested. Management of affected patients involves determining the functional status of the contralateral kidney. If the contralateral kidney is normal, the longterm renal functional outcome is usually excellent, although a recent study suggests that some patients may in fact have a poor long-term outcome and require dialysis [18]. It is therefore reasonable to propose that individuals with a single functioning kidney should have their blood pressure measured, urine tested for protein, and renal function measured periodically throughout life. While some have suggested that children with single kidneys should avoid contact/collision sports, at least one study suggests that kidney injuries occur much less frequently than other organ injuries, and thus sports restriction may not be indicated solely on the basis of having a single kidney [180].

Renal Hypoplasia
Unless associated with other malformations, renal hypoplasia can be asymptomatic. Unilateral hypoplasia is often discovered as an incidental finding during an abdominal sonogram or other imaging study. In contrast, patients with bilateral renal hypoplasia are at risk for decreased renal function and chronic kidney disease.

Renal Dysplasia
The dysplastic kidney is generally smaller than normal. However, cystic elements can contribute to large kidney size, the most extreme example being the multicystic dysplastic kidney (see below). During the antenatal period, unilateral disease is likely to be discovered as an incidental finding. This may also be the case for bilateral renal dysplasia unless it is associated with oligohydramnios. After birth, bilateral renal dysplasia

may limit glomerular filtration causing renal failure that is usually progressive. Postnatal ultrasonagraphy of the dysplastic kidney is characterized by small size, increased echogenicity, loss of corticomedullary differentiation and cortical cysts. Renal dysplasia is strongly associated with dilatation of the upper and lower urinary tract from vesicoureteric reflux, posterior urethral valves, and/or other urinary tract obstruction [181]. Accordingly, imaging of the lower urinary tract should be performed to determine whether these abnormalities are present.

Multicystic Dysplastic Kidney

The MCDK presents by ultrasonagraphy as a large cystic non-reniform mass in the renal fossa and by palpation as a flank mass. The MCDK is nonfunctional, a condition that can be demonstrated by imaging with MAG3 or DTPA radionuclide scanning. The MCDK is usually unilateral. If bilateral, it is fatal. Complications of MCDK include hypertension (0.01–0.1 %). Wilm's tumour and renal cell carcinoma have also been described in MCDK but the incidence of malignant complications is not significantly different from the general population [182]. In 25 % of cases the contralateral urinary tract is abnormal. Contralateral abnormalities can include rotational or positional anomalies, renal hypoplasia, vesicoureteric reflux and ureteropelvic junction obstruction [11]. Contralateral UPJ obstruction occurs in 5–10 % of cases.

Gradual reduction in renal size and eventual resolution of the mass of the MCDK is common. At 2 years, an involution in size by ultrasound has been noted in up to 60 % of the affected kidneys. Complete disappearance of the MCDK can occur in a minority of patients (3–4 %) by the time of birth, and in 20–25 % by 2 years. Increase in the size of MCDK can be seen in some cases. Several reports suggest that if the kidney length of the MCDK is less than 6.2 cm on the initial postnatal US, then complete resolution is likely to occur [183, 184]. The contralateral kidney shows compensatory hypertrophy by ultrasound evaluation.

Management of patients with MCDK has shifted from routine nephrectomy in the past, to observation and medical therapy. Because of the risk of associated anomalies in the contralateral kidney, the possibility of VUR should be evaluated and blood pressure should be measured. Renal ultrasound is generally recommended at an interval of 3 months for the first year of life and then every 6 months up to involution of the mass, or at least up to 5 years. Compensatory hypertrophy of the contralateral kidney is expected and should be monitored by renal ultrasound. Medical therapy is usually effective in treating hypertension in the small number of affected patients, but nephrectomy may be curative in resistant cases. One study estimated the mean probability of a child with unilateral MCKD to develop hypertension as 5.4 out of 1000 children with MCKD [182].

Renal Ectopia

Normally, the kidneys lie on either side of the spine in the lumbar region and are located in the retroperitoneal renal fossae. Rapid caudal growth during embryogenesis results in migration of the developing kidney from the pelvis to the retroperitoneal renal fossa. With ascension, comes a 90° rotation from a horizontal to a vertical position with the renal hilum finally directed medially. Migration and rotation are complete by 8 weeks of gestation.

Simple congenital ectopy refers to a low lying kidney that failed to ascend normally. It most commonly lies over the pelvic brim or in the pelvis and is termed a pelvic kidney. Less commonly, the kidney may lie on the contralateral side of the body, a state that is termed crossed ectopy without fusion. Clinical presentation can be asymptomatic or symptomatic. Asymptomatic presentation is when the ectopic kidney has been diagnosed coincidentally such as might occur during routine antenatal sonography. Symptomatic presentation occurs with urinary tract infections. Symptoms such as abdominal pain or fever may occur. On examination, an abdominal mass may be palpable. Other presenting features include hematuria, incontinence, renal insufficiency and hypertension [14]. A high incidence of urological abnormalities has been associated with renal ectopia. Vesicoureteral reflux is the most common, occurring in 20 % of crossed renal ectopia and 30 % of simple renal ectopia. In bilateral simple renal ectopia, there is a higher incidence of VUR, occurring in 70 % of cases. Other associated urological abnormalities include contralateral renal dysplasia (4 %), cryptorchidism (5 %) and hypospadias (5 %) [14]. Reduced renal function is commonly observed by radionuclide scan in the ectopic kidney. Female genital anomalies such as agenesis of the uterus and vagina [185] or unicornuate uterus [186] have also been associated with ectopic kidneys. Other anomalies described include adrenal, cardiac and skeletal anomalies. Clinical assessment should therefore include a careful physical examination for other anomalies. Renal ultrasonography will help with diagnosis and defining the underlying anatomy. A VCUG should be undertaken, particularly if there is hydronephrosis, given the risk of VUR and obstruction. A DMSA scan is also recommended to assess for differential renal function.

Renal Fusion

Renal fusion is defined as the fusion of two kidneys. The most common fusion anomaly is the horseshoe kidney, in which fusion occurs at one pole of each kidney, usually the lower pole. The fused kidney may lie in the midline (symmetric horseshoe kidney) or the fused part may lie lateral to the midline (asymmetric horseshoe kidney). In a crossed fused ectopic kidney, the kidney from one side has crossed the midline to fuse with the kidney on the other side. Fusion is thought to occur before the kidneys ascend from the pelvis to their normal dorsolumbar position. This is usually between the fourth to ninth weeks of gestation. As a result, fusion anomalies seldom assume the high position of normal kidneys. The blood supply may therefore come from vessels such as the iliac arteries. Abnormal rotation is also associated with early fusion of the developing kidneys. The pelvis of each kidney lies anteriorly and the ureter, therefore, traverses over the isthmus of a horseshoe kidney or the anterior surface of the fused kidney. Ureteric compression may occur due to external compression by a traversing aberrant artery. The majority of patients

may be asymptomatic. Some, however, develop obstruction which presents with loin pain, hematuria and may be associated with urinary tract infections due to urinary stasis or vesicoureteric reflux. Renal calculi may occur in up to 20 % of cases [187]. Other associated urological anomalies include ureteral duplication, ectopic ureter and retrocaval ureter. Genital anomalies such as bicornuate and/or septate uterus, hypospadias, and undescended testis have also been described. Associated nonrenal anomalies involve the gastrointestinal tract (anorectal malformations such as imperforate anus, malrotation, and Meckel diverticulum) the central nervous system (neural tube defects), and the skeleton (rib defects, clubfoot, or congenital hip dislocation). Investigations should include static imaging (renal ultrasound) and functional imaging (DMSA scan) and a VCUG.

Acknowledgement The authors would like to thank Dr. Remi Salomon for his contributions to the previous version of this chapter in the first edition of this volume.

References

1. Ardissino G, Dacco V, Testa S, Bonaudo R, Claris-Appiani A, Taioli E, et al. Epidemiology of chronic renal failure in children: data from the ItalKid project. Pediatrics. 2003;111(4 Pt 1):e382–7.
2. Studies NAPRTaC. Annual dialysis report 2011.
3. Potter EL. Normal and abnormal development of the kidney. Chicago: Year Book Medical Publishers; 1972.
4. Han BK, Babcock DS. Sonographic measurements and appearance of normal kidneys in children. AJR Am J Roentgenol. 1985;145(3):611–6.
5. Dinkel EEM, Dittrich M, Peters H, Berres M, Schulte-Wissermann H. Kidney size in childhood. Sonographical growth charts for kidney length and volume. Pediatr Radiol. 1985;15:38–43.
6. Wiesel A, Queisser-Luft A, Clementi M, Bianca S, Stoll C. Prenatal detection of congenital renal malformations by fetal ultrasonographic examination: an analysis of 709,030 births in 12 European countries. Eur J Med Genet. 2005;48(2):131–44.
7. Melo BF, Aguiar MB, Bouzada MC, Aguiar RL, Pereira AK, Paixao GM, et al. Early risk factors for neonatal mortality in CAKUT: analysis of 524 affected newborns. Pediatr Nephrol. 2012;27(6): 965–72.
8. Piscione TD, Rosenblum ND. The malformed kidney: disruption of glomerular and tubular development. Clin Genet. 1999;56(5):341–56.

9. Queisser-Luft A, Stolz G, Wiesel A, Schlaefer K, Spranger J. Malformations in newborn: results based on 30,940 infants and fetuses from the Mainz congenital birth defect monitoring system (1990–1998). Arch Gynecol Obstet. 2002;266(3):163–7.

10. Limwongse CCS, Cassidy SB. Syndromes and malformations of the urinary tract. In: Barratt TMAE, Harmon WE, editors. Pediatric nephrology. 4th ed. Baltimore: Williams & Wilkins; 1999. p. 427–49.

11. Winyard P, Chitty L. Dysplastic and polycystic kidneys: diagnosis, associations and management. Prenat Diagn. 2001;21(11):924–35.

12. Harris J, Robert E, Kallen B. Epidemiologic characteristics of kidney malformations. Eur J Epidemiol. 2000;16(11):985–92.

13. Roodhooft AM, Birnholz JC, Holmes LB. Familial nature of congenital absence and severe dysgenesis of both kidneys. N Engl J Med. 1984;310(21):1341–5.

14. Guarino N, Tadini B, Camardi P, Silvestro L, Lace R, Bianchi M. The incidence of associated urological abnormalities in children with renal ectopia. J Urol. 2004;172(4 Pt 2):1757–9; discussion 9.

15. Weizer AZ, Silverstein AD, Auge BK, Delvecchio FC, Raj G, Albala DM, et al. Determining the incidence of horseshoe kidney from radiographic data at a single institution. J Urol. 2003;170(5):1722–6.

16. Quirino IG, Diniz JS, Bouzada MC, Pereira AK, Lopes TJ, Paixao GM, et al. Clinical course of 822 children with prenatally detected nephrouropathies. Clin J Am Soc Nephrol. 2012;7(3):444–51.

17. Gonzalez Celedon C, Bitsori M, Tullus K. Progression of chronic renal failure in children with dysplastic kidneys. Pediatr Nephrol. 2007;22(7): 1014–20.

18. Sanna-Cherchi S, Ravani P, Corbani V, Parodi S, Haupt R, Piaggio G, et al. Renal outcome in patients with congenital anomalies of the kidney and urinary tract. Kidney Int. 2009;76(5):528–33.

19. Wuhl E, van Stralen KJ, Verrina E, Bjerre A, Wanner C, Heaf JG, et al. Timing and outcome of renal replacement therapy in patients with congenital malformations of the kidney and urinary tract. Clin J Am Soc Nephrol. 2013;8(1):67–74.

20. Costantini F. Genetic controls and cellular behaviors in branching morphogenesis of the renal collecting system. Wiley Interdiscip Rev Dev Biol. 2012;1(5):693–713.

21. Chai OH, Song CH, Park SK, Kim W, Cho ES. Molecular regulation of kidney development. Anat Cell Biol. 2013;46(1):19–31.

22. Schwarz R, Stephens F, Cussen L. The pathogenesis of renal dysplasia[1] II. The significance of lateral and medial ectopy of the ureteric orifice. Investig Urol. 1981;19(September):97–100.

23. Hu MC, Rosenblum ND. Genetic regulation of branching morphogenesis: lessons learned from loss-of-function phenotypes. Pediatr Res. 2003; 54(4):433–8.

24. Schuchardt A, D'Agati V, Larsson-Blomberg L, Costantini F, Pachnis V. Defects in the kidney and enteric nervous system of mice lacking the tyrosine kinase receptor Ret. Nature. 1994;367:380–3.

25. Schuchardt A, D'Agati V, Pachnis V, Costantini F. Renal agenesis and hypodysplasia in ret-k⁻ mutant mice result from defects in ureteric bud development. Development. 1996;122:1919–29.

26. Enomoto H, Araki T, Jackman A, Heuckeroth R, Snider W, Johnson E, et al. GFRa1-deficient mice have deficits in the enteric nervous system and kidneys. Neuron. 1998;21:317–24.

27. Pichel J, Shen L, Sheng H, Granholm A-C, Drago J, Grinberg A, et al. Defects in enteric innervation and kidney development in mice lacking GDNF. Nature. 1996;382:73–6.

28. Maeshima A, Sakurai H, Choi Y, Kitamura S, Vaughn DA, Tee JB, et al. Glial cell-derived neurotrophic factor independent ureteric bud outgrowth from the Wolffian duct. J Am Soc Nephrol. 2007;18(12):3147–55.

29. Reidy KJ, Rosenblum ND. Cell and molecular biology of kidney development. Semin Nephrol. 2009;29(4):321–37.

30. Grieshammer U, Ma L, Plump A, Wang F, Tessier-Lavigne M, Martin G. SLIT2-mediated ROBO2 signaling restricts kidney induction to a single site. Dev Cell. 2004;6(May):709–17.

31. Miyazaki Y, Oshima K, Fogo A, Hogan B, Ichikawa I. Bone morphogenetic protein 4 regulates the budding site and elongation of the mouse ureter. J Clin Investig. 2000;105(7):863–73.

32. Xu PX, Adams J, Peters H, Brown MC, Heaney S, Maas R. Eya1-deficient mice lack ears and kidneys and show abnormal apoptosis of organ primordia. Nat Genet. 1999;23(1):113–7.

33. Xu PX, Zheng W, Huang L, Maire P, Laclef C, Silvius D. Six1 is required for the early organogenesis of mammalian kidney. Development. 2003; 130(14):3085–94.

34. Nishinakamura R, Matsumoto Y, Nakao K, Nakamura K, Sato A, Copeland NG, et al. Murine homolog of SALL1 is essential for ureteric bud invasion in kidney development. Development. 2001;128(16):3105–15.

35. Dressler G, Deutsch U, Chowdhury K, Nornes H, Gruss P. Pax2, a new murine paired-box-containing gene and its expression in the developing excretory system. Development. 1990;109:787–95.

36. Dziarmaga A, Eccles M, Goodyer P. Suppression of ureteric bud apoptosis rescues nephron endowment and adult renal function in Pax2 mutant mice. J Am Soc Nephrol. 2006;17(6):1568–75.

37. Brophy PD, Ostrom L, Lang KM, Dressler GR. Regulation of ureteric bud outgrowth by Pax2-dependent activation of the glial derived neurotrophic factor gene. Development. 2001;128(23): 4747–56.

38. Lokmane L, Heliot C, Garcia-Villalba P, Fabre M, Cereghini S. vHNF1 functions in distinct regulatory circuits to control ureteric bud branching and early nephrogenesis. Development. 2010;137(2):347–57.

39. Gresh L, Fischer E, Reimann A, Tanguy M, Garbay S, Shao X, et al. A transcriptional network in polycystic kidney disease. EMBO J. 2004;23(7): 1657–68.

40. Paces-Fessy M, Fabre M, Lesaulnier C, Cereghini S. Hnf1b and Pax2 cooperate to control different pathways in kidney and ureter morphogenesis. Hum Mol Genet. 2012;21(14):3143–55.

41. Bose J, Grotewold L, Ruther U. Pallister-hall syndrome phenotype in mice mutant for Gli3. Hum Mol Genet. 2002;11(9):1129–35.

42. Hu MC, Mo R, Bhella S, Wilson CW, Chuang PT, Hui CC, et al. GLI3-dependent transcriptional repression of Gli1, Gli2 and kidney patterning genes disrupts renal morphogenesis. Development. 2006; 133(3):569–78.

43. Cain JE, Islam E, Haxho F, Blake J, Rosenblum ND. GLI3 repressor controls functional development of the mouse ureter. J Clin Invest. 2011;121(3): 1199–206.

44. Yosypiv IV. Renin-angiotensin system in ureteric bud branching morphogenesis: implications for kidney disease. Pediatr Nephrol. 2014;29(4): 609–20.

45. Yosypiv IV. Renin-angiotensin system in ureteric bud branching morphogenesis: insights into the mechanisms. Pediatr Nephrol. 2011;26(9):1499–512.

46. Nishimura H, Yerkes E, Hohenfellner K, Miyazaki Y, Ma J, Hunley T, et al. Role of the angiotensin type 2 receptor gene in congenital anomalies of the kidney and urinary tract, CAKUT, of mice and men. Mol Cell. 1999;3(January):1–10.

47. Gubler MC, Antignac C. Renin-angiotensin system in kidney development: renal tubular dysgenesis. Kidney Int. 2010;77(5):400–6.

48. Batourina E, Choi C, Paragas N, Bello N, Hensle T, Costantini F, et al. Distal ureter morphogenesis depends on epithelial cell remodeling mediated by vitamin A and Ret. Nat Genet. 2002;32:109–15.

49. Batourina E, Gim S, Bello N, Shy M, Clagett-Dame M, Srinivas S, et al. Vitamin A controls epithelial/mesenchymal interactions through Ret expression. Nat Genet. 2001;27(January):74–8.

50. Mendelsohn C, Batourina E, Fung S, Gilbert T, Dodd J. Stromal cells mediate retinoid-dependent functions essential for renal development. Development. 1999;126:1139–48.

51. Lelievre-Pegorier M, Vilar J, Ferrier ML, Moreau E, Freund N, Gilbert T, et al. Mild vitamin A deficiency leads to inborn nephron deficit in the rat. Kidney Int. 1998;54(5):1455–62.

52. Goodyer P, Kurpad A, Rekha S, Muthayya S, Dwarkanath P, Iyengar A, et al. Effects of maternal vitamin A status on kidney development: a pilot study. Pediatr Nephrol. 2007;22(2):209–14.

53. Czeizel AE, Dobo M, Vargha P. Hungarian cohort-controlled trial of periconceptional multivitamin supplementation shows a reduction in certain congenital abnormalities. Birth Defects Res A Clin Mol Teratol. 2004;70(11):853–61.

54. Hernandez-Diaz S, Werler MM, Walker AM, Mitchell AA. Folic acid antagonists during pregnancy and the risk of birth defects. N Engl J Med. 2000;343(22):1608–14.

55. Nyengaard JR, Bendtsen TF. Glomerular number and size in relation to age, kidney weight, and body surface in normal man. Anat Rec. 1992;232(2):194–201.

56. Warady BA, Schaefer F, Alexander SR, editors. Pediatric dialysis. 2nd ed. New York: Springer; 2012.

57. Weber S, Moriniere V, Knuppel T, Charbit M, Dusek J, Ghiggeri GM, et al. Prevalence of mutations in renal developmental genes in children with renal hypodysplasia: results of the ESCAPE study. J Am Soc Nephrol. 2006;17(10):2864–70.

58. Schwaderer AL, Bates CM, McHugh KM, McBride KL. Renal anomalies in family members of infants with bilateral renal agenesis/adysplasia. Pediatr Nephrol. 2007;22(1):52–6.

59. Oda T, Elkahloun AG, Pike BL, Okajima K, Krantz ID, Genin A, et al. Mutations in the human Jagged1 gene are responsible for Alagille syndrome. Nat Genet. 1997;16(3):235–42.

60. Kamath BM, Podkameni G, Hutchinson AL, Leonard LD, Gerfen J, Krantz ID, et al. Renal anomalies in Alagille syndrome: a disease-defining feature. Am J Med Genet A. 2012;158A(1):85–9.

61. McDaniell R, Warthen DM, Sanchez-Lara PA, Pai A, Krantz ID, Piccoli DA, et al. NOTCH2 mutations cause Alagille syndrome, a heterogeneous disorder of the notch signaling pathway. Am J Hum Genet. 2006;79(1):169–73.

62. Wilkie AO, Slaney SF, Oldridge M, Poole MD, Ashworth GJ, Hockley AD, et al. Apert syndrome results from localized mutations of FGFR2 and is allelic with Crouzon syndrome. Nat Genet. 1995;9(2):165–72.

63. Seyedzadeh A, Kompani F, Esmailie E, Samadzadeh S, Farshchi B. High-grade vesicoureteral reflux in Pfeiffer syndrome. Urol J. 2008;5(3):200–2.

64. Hatada I, Ohashi H, Fukushima Y, Kaneko Y, Inoue M, Komoto Y, et al. An imprinted gene p57KIP2 is mutated in Beckwith-Wiedemann syndrome. Nat Genet. 1996;14(2):171–3.

65. Goldman M, Smith A, Shuman C, Caluseriu O, Wei C, Steele L, et al. Renal abnormalities in beckwith-wiedemann syndrome are associated with 11p15.5 uniparental disomy. J Am Soc Nephrol. 2002;13(8): 2077–84.

66. Kochhar A, Orten DJ, Sorensen JL, Fischer SM, Cremers CW, Kimberling WJ, et al. SIX1 mutation screening in 247 branchio-oto-renal syndrome families: a recurrent missense mutation associated with BOR. Hum Mutat. 2008;29(4):565.

67. Hoskins BE, Cramer CH, Silvius D, Zou D, Raymond RM, Orten DJ, et al. Transcription factor SIX5 is mutated in patients with branchio-oto-renal syndrome. Am J Hum Genet. 2007;80(4):800–4.

68. Abdelhak S, Kalatzis V, Heilig R, Compain S, Samson D, Vincent C, et al. A human homologue of

the Drosophila eyes absent gene underlies Branchio-Oto -Renal(BOR) syndrome and identifies a novel gene family. Nat Genet. 1997;15:157–64.

69. Houston CS, Opitz JM, Spranger JW, Macpherson RI, Reed MH, Gilbert EF, et al. The campomelic syndrome: review, report of 17 cases, and follow-up on the currently 17-year-old boy first reported by Maroteaux et al in 1971. Am J Med Genet. 1983;15(1):3–28.

70. Wagner T, Wirth J, Meyer J, Zabel B, Held M, Zimmer J, et al. Autosomal sex reversal and campomelic dysplasia are caused by mutations in and around the SRY-related gene SOX9. Cell. 1994;79(6):1111–20.

71. Sakaki-Yumoto M, Kobayashi C, Sato A, Fujimura S, Matsumoto Y, Takasato M, et al. The murine homolog of SALL4, a causative gene in Okihiro syndrome, is essential for embryonic stem cell proliferation, and cooperates with Sall1 in anorectal, heart, brain and kidney development. Development. 2006;133(15):3005–13.

72. McGregor L, Makela V, Darling SM, Vrontou S, Chalepakis G, Roberts C, et al. Fraser syndrome and mouse blebbed phenotype caused by mutations in FRAS1/Fras1 encoding a putative extracellular matrix protein. Nat Genet. 2003;34(2):203–8.

73. Alazami AM, Shaheen R, Alzahrani F, Snape K, Saggar A, Brinkmann B, et al. FREM1 mutations cause bifid nose, renal agenesis, and anorectal malformations syndrome. Am J Hum Genet. 2009;85(3):414–8.

74. Jadeja S, Smyth I, Pitera JE, Taylor MS, van Haelst M, Bentley E, et al. Identification of a new gene mutated in Fraser syndrome and mouse myelencephalic blebs. Nat Genet. 2005;37(5):520–5.

75. Vogel MJ, van Zon P, Brueton L, Gijzen M, van Tuil MC, Cox P, et al. Mutations in GRIP1 cause Fraser syndrome. J Med Genet. 2012;49(5):303–6.

76. Van Esch H, Groenen P, Nesbit MA, Schuffenhauer S, Lichtner P, Vanderlinden G, et al. GATA3 haploinsufficiency causes human HDR syndrome. Nature. 2000;406(6794):419–22.

77. Chenouard A, Isidor B, Allain-Launay E, Moreau A, Le Bideau M, Roussey G. Renal phenotypic variability in HDR syndrome: glomerular nephropathy as a novel finding. Eur J Pediatr. 2013;172(1):107–10.

78. Costa-Barbosa FA, Balasubramanian R, Keefe KW, Shaw ND, Al-Tassan N, Plummer L, et al. Prioritizing genetic testing in patients with Kallmann syndrome using clinical phenotypes. J Clin Endocrinol Metab. 2013;98(5):E943–53.

79. Franco B, Guioli S, Pragliola A, Incerti B, Bardoni B, Tonlorenzi R, et al. A gene deleted in Kallmann's syndrome shares homology with neural cell adhesion and axonal path-finding molecules. Nature. 1991;353(6344):529–36.

80. Bamshad M, Lin RC, Law DJ, Watkins WC, Krakowiak PA, Moore ME, et al. Mutations in human TBX3 alter limb, apocrine and genital development in ulnar-mammary syndrome. Nat Genet. 1997;16(3):311–5.

81. Kang S, Graham Jr JM, Olney AH, Biesecker LG. GLI3 frameshift mutations cause autosomal dominant Pallister-Hall syndrome. Nat Genet. 1997;15(3):266–8.

82. Sanyanusin P, Schimmenti L, McNoe L, Ward T, Pierpont M, Sullivan M, et al. Mutation of the PAX2 gene in a family with optic nerve colobomas, renal anomalies and vesicoureteric reflux. Nat Genet. 1995;9:358–64.

83. Gribouval O, Gonzales M, Neuhaus T, Aziza J, Bieth E, Laurent N, et al. Mutations in genes in the renin-angiotensin system are associated with autosomal recessive renal tubular dysgenesis. Nat Genet. 2005;37(9):964–8.

84. Bohn S, Thomas H, Turan G, Ellard S, Bingham C, Hattersley AT, et al. Distinct molecular and morphogenetic properties of mutations in the human HNF1beta gene that lead to defective kidney development. J Am Soc Nephrol. 2003;14(8):2033–41.

85. Pilia G, Hughes-Benzie RM, MacKenzie A, Baybayan P, Chen EY, Huber R, et al. Mutations in GPC3, a glypican gene, cause the Simpson-Golabi-Behmel overgrowth syndrome. Nat Genet. 1996;12(3):241–7.

86. Tint GS, Irons M, Elias ER, Batta AK, Frieden R, Chen TS, et al. Defective cholesterol biosynthesis associated with the Smith-Lemli-Opitz syndrome. N Engl J Med. 1994;330(2):107–13.

87. Kohlhase J, Wischermann A, Reichenbach H, Froster U, Engel W. Mutations in the SALL1 putative transcription factor gene cause Townes-Brocks syndrome. Nat Genet. 1998;18(1):81–3.

88. Preuss N, Brosius U, Biermanns M, Muntau AC, Conzelmann E, Gartner J. PEX1 mutations in complementation group 1 of Zellweger spectrum patients correlate with severity of disease. Pediatr Res. 2002;51(6):706–14.

89. Chatterjee R, Ramos E, Hoffman M, VanWinkle J, Martin DR, Davis TK, et al. Traditional and targeted exome sequencing reveals common, rare and novel functional deleterious variants in RET-signaling complex in a cohort of living US patients with urinary tract malformations. Hum Genet. 2012; 131(11):1725–38.

90. Skinner MA, Safford SD, Reeves JG, Jackson ME, Freemerman AJ. Renal aplasia in humans is associated with RET mutations. Am J Hum Genet. 2008;82(2):344–51.

91. Yang Y, Houle AM, Letendre J, Richter A. RET Gly691Ser mutation is associated with primary vesicoureteral reflux in the French-Canadian population from Quebec. Hum Mutat. 2008;29(5):695–702.

92. Jeanpierre C, Mace G, Parisot M, Moriniere V, Pawtowsky A, Benabou M, et al. RET and GDNF mutations are rare in fetuses with renal agenesis or other severe kidney development defects. J Med Genet. 2011;48(7):497–504.

93. Hwang DY, Dworschak GC, Kohl S, Saisawat P, Vivante A, Hilger AC, et al. Mutations in 12 known dominant disease-causing genes clarify many congenital anomalies of the kidney and urinary tract. Kidney Int. 2014;85(6):1429–33.

94. Fraser FC, Ling D, Clogg D, Nogrady B. Genetic aspects of the BOR syndrome – branchial fistulas, ear pits, hearing loss, and renal anomalies. Am J Med Genet. 1978;2(3):241–52.

95. Melnick M, Bixler D, Silk K, Yune H, Nance WE. Autosomal dominant branchiootorenal dysplasia. Birth Defects Orig Artic Ser. 1975;11(5): 121–8.

96. Chang EH, Menezes M, Meyer NC, Cucci RA, Vervoort VS, Schwartz CE, et al. Branchio-oto-renal syndrome: the mutation spectrum in EYA1 and its phenotypic consequences. Hum Mutat. 2004;23(6): 582–9.

97. Chen A, Francis M, Ni L, Cremers CW, Kimberling WJ, Sato Y, et al. Phenotypic manifestations of branchio-oto-renal syndrome. Am J Med Genet. 1995;58(4):365–70.

98. Fraser FC, Sproule JR, Halal F. Frequency of the branchio-oto-renal (BOR) syndrome in children with profound hearing loss. Am J Med Genet. 1980;7(3):341–9.

99. Krug P, Moriniere V, Marlin S, Koubi V, Gabriel HD, Colin E, et al. Mutation screening of the EYA1, SIX1, and SIX5 genes in a large cohort of patients harboring branchio-oto-renal syndrome calls into question the pathogenic role of SIX5 mutations. Hum Mutat. 2011;32(2):183–90.

100. Ozaki H, Watanabe Y, Ikeda K, Kawakami K. Impaired interactions between mouse Eya1 harboring mutations found in patients with branchio-oto-renal syndrome and Six, Dach, and G proteins. J Hum Genet. 2002;47(3):107–16.

101. Available from: www.cscc.unc.edu/rivur/.

102. Li X, Oghi KA, Zhang J, Krones A, Bush KT, Glass CK, et al. Eya protein phosphatase activity regulates Six1-Dach-Eya transcriptional effects in mammalian organogenesis. Nature. 2003;426(6964):247–54.

103. Ruf RG, Xu PX, Silvius D, Otto EA, Beekmann F, Muerb UT, et al. SIX1 mutations cause branchio-oto-renal syndrome by disruption of EYA1-SIX1-DNA complexes. Proc Natl Acad Sci U S A. 2004;101(21):8090–5.

104. Sajithlal G, Zou D, Silvius D, Xu PX. Eya 1 acts as a critical regulator for specifying the metanephric mesenchyme. Dev Biol. 2005;284(2):323–36.

105. Miller EM, Hopkin R, Bao L, Ware SM. Implications for genotype-phenotype predictions in Townes-Brocks syndrome: case report of a novel SALL1 deletion and review of the literature. Am J Med Genet A. 2012;158A(3):533–40.

106. Townes PL, Brocks ER. Hereditary syndrome of imperforate anus with hand, foot, and ear anomalies. J Pediatr. 1972;81(2):321–6.

107. O'Callaghan M, Young ID. The Townes-Brocks syndrome. J Med Genet. 1990;27(7):457–61.

108. Kurnit DM, Steele MW, Pinsky L, Dibbins A. Autosomal dominant transmission of a syndrome of anal, ear, renal, and radial congenital malformations. J Pediatr. 1978;93(2):270–3.

109. Martinez-Frias ML, Bermejo Sanchez E, Arroyo Carrera I, Perez Fernandez JL, Pardo Romero M, Buron Martinez E, et al. The Townes-Brocks syndrome in Spain: the epidemiological aspects in a consecutive series of cases. An Esp Pediatr. 1999;50(1):57–60.

110. Kohlhase J. SALL1 mutations in Townes-Brocks syndrome and related disorders. Hum Mutat. 2000;16(6):460–6.

111. Marlin S, Blanchard S, Slim R, Lacombe D, Denoyelle F, Alessandri JL, et al. Townes-Brocks syndrome: detection of a SALL1 mutation hot spot and evidence for a position effect in one patient. Hum Mutat. 1999;14(5):377–86.

112. Solomon BD. VACTERL/VATER association. Orphanet J Rare Dis. 2011;6:56.

113. Rittler M, Paz JE, Castilla EE. VACTERL association, epidemiologic definition and delineation. Am J Med Genet. 1996;63(4):529–36.

114. Solomon BD, Pineda-Alvarez DE, Raam MS, Bous SM, Keaton AA, Velez JI, et al. Analysis of component findings in 79 patients diagnosed with VACTERL association. Am J Med Genet A. 2010;152A(9):2236–44.

115. Brown AK, Roddam AW, Spitz L, Ward SJ. Oesophageal atresia, related malformations, and medical problems: a family study. Am J Med Genet. 1999;85(1):31–7.

116. van Rooij IA, Wijers CH, Rieu PN, Hendriks HS, Brouwers MM, Knoers NV, et al. Maternal and paternal risk factors for anorectal malformations: a Dutch case-control study. Birth Defects Res A Clin Mol Teratol. 2010;88(3):152–8.

117. Stankiewicz P, Sen P, Bhatt SS, Storer M, Xia Z, Bejjani BA, et al. Genomic and genic deletions of the FOX gene cluster on 16q24.1 and inactivating mutations of FOXF1 cause alveolar capillary dysplasia and other malformations. Am J Hum Genet. 2009;84(6):780–91.

118. Garcia-Barcelo MM, Wong KK, Lui VC, Yuan ZW, So MT, Ngan ES, et al. Identification of a HOXD13 mutation in a VACTERL patient. Am J Med Genet A. 2008;146A(24):3181–5.

119. Tongsong T, Wanapirak C, Piyamongkol W, Sudasana J. Prenatal sonographic diagnosis of VATER association. J Clin Ultrasound. 1999;27(7): 378–84.

120. Murphy-Kaulbeck L, Dodds L, Joseph KS, Van den Hof M. Single umbilical artery risk factors and pregnancy outcomes. Obstet Gynecol. 2010;116(4): 843–50.

121. Faivre L, Portnoi MF, Pals G, Stoppa-Lyonnet D, Le Merrer M, Thauvin-Robinet C, et al. Should chromosome breakage studies be performed in patients with VACTERL association? Am J Med Genet A. 2005;137(1):55–8.

122. Weaver RG, Cashwell LF, Lorentz W, Whiteman D, Geisinger KR, Ball M. Optic nerve coloboma associated with renal disease. Am J Med Genet. 1988;29(3):597–605.

123. Bower M, Salomon R, Allanson J, Antignac C, Benedicenti F, Benetti E, et al. Update of PAX2 mutations in renal coloboma syndrome and establishment of a locus-specific database. Hum Mutat. 2012;33(3):457–66.

124. Fletcher J, Hu M, Berman Y, Collins F, Grigg J, McIver M, et al. Multicystic dysplastic kidney and variable phenotype in a family with a novel deletion mutation of PAX2. J Am Soc Nephrol. 2005; 16(9):2754–61.

125. Salomon R, Tellier AL, Attie-Bitach T, Amiel J, Vekemans M, Lyonnet S, et al. PAX2 mutations in oligomeganephronia. Kidney Int. 2001;59(2): 457–62.

126. Dureau P, Attie-Bitach T, Salomon R, Bettembourg O, Amiel J, Uteza Y, et al. Renal coloboma syndrome. Ophthalmology. 2001;108(10):1912–6.

127. Parsa CF, Silva ED, Sundin OH, Goldberg MF, De Jong MR, Sunness JS, et al. Redefining papillorenal syndrome: an underdiagnosed cause of ocular and renal morbidity. Ophthalmology. 2001;108(4): 738–49.

128. Eccles MR, Schimmenti LA. Renal-coloboma syndrome: a multi-system developmental disorder caused by PAX2 mutations. Clin Genet. 1999;56(1): 1–9.

129. Schimmenti LA, Cunliffe HE, McNoe LA, Ward TA, French MC, Shim HH, et al. Further delineation of renal-coloboma syndrome in patients with extreme variability of phenotype and identical PAX2 mutations. Am J Hum Genet. 1997;60(4):869–78.

130. Bower M, Eccles M, Heidet L, Schimmenti LA. Clinical utility gene card for: renal coloboma (Papillorenal) syndrome. Eur J Hum Genet. 2011;19(9).

131. Coffinier C, Thepot D, Babinet C, Yaniv M, Barra J. Essential role for the homeoprotein vHNF1/HNF1beta in visceral endoderm differentiation. Development. 1999;126(21):4785–94.

132. Kolatsi-Joannou M, Bingham C, Ellard S, Bulman MP, Allen LI, Hattersley AT, et al. Hepatocyte nuclear factor-1beta: a new kindred with renal cysts and diabetes and gene expression in normal human development. J Am Soc Nephrol. 2001;12(10): 2175–80.

133. Bellanne-Chantelot C, Chauveau D, Gautier JF, Dubois-Laforgue D, Clauin S, Beaufils S, et al. Clinical spectrum associated with hepatocyte nuclear factor-1beta mutations. Ann Intern Med. 2004;140(7):510–7.

134. Bellanne-Chantelot C, Clauin S, Chauveau D, Collin P, Daumont M, Douillard C, et al. Large genomic rearrangements in the hepatocyte nuclear factor-1beta (TCF2) gene are the most frequent cause of maturity-onset diabetes of the young type 5. Diabetes. 2005;54(11):3126–32.

135. Edghill EL, Bingham C, Ellard S, Hattersley AT. Mutations in hepatocyte nuclear factor-1beta and their related phenotypes. J Med Genet. 2006;43(1):84–90.

136. Ulinski T, Lescure S, Beaufils S, Guigonis V, Decramer S, Morin D, et al. Renal phenotypes related to hepatocyte nuclear factor-1beta (TCF2) mutations in a pediatric cohort. J Am Soc Nephrol. 2006;17(2):497–503.

137. Bingham C, Bulman MP, Ellard S, Allen LI, Lipkin GW, Hoff WG, et al. Mutations in the hepatocyte nuclear factor-1beta gene are associated with familial hypoplastic glomerulocystic kidney disease. Am J Hum Genet. 2001;68(1):219–24.

138. Bingham C, Ellard S, Cole TR, Jones KE, Allen LI, Goodship JA, et al. Solitary functioning kidney and diverse genital tract malformations associated with hepatocyte nuclear factor-1beta mutations. Kidney Int. 2002;61(4):1243–51.

139. Lindner TH, Njolstad PR, Horikawa Y, Bostad L, Bell GI, Sovik O. A novel syndrome of diabetes mellitus, renal dysfunction and genital malformation associated with a partial deletion of the pseudo-POU domain of hepatocyte nuclear factor-1beta. Hum Mol Genet. 1999;8(11):2001–8.

140. Rizzoni G, Loirat C, Levy M, Milanesi C, Zachello G, Mathieu H. Familial hypoplastic glomerulocystic kidney. A new entity? Clin Nephrol. 1982;18(5):263–8.

141. Bingham C, Ellard S, Allen L, Bulman M, Shepherd M, Frayling T, et al. Abnormal nephron development associated with a frameshift mutation in the transcription factor hepatocyte nuclear factor-1 beta. Kidney Int. 2000;57(3):898–907.

142. Decramer S, Parant O, Beaufils S, Clauin S, Guillou C, Kessler S, et al. Anomalies of the TCF2 gene are the main cause of fetal bilateral hyperechogenic kidneys. J Am Soc Nephrol. 2007;18(3):923–33.

143. Bingham C, Hattersley AT. Renal cysts and diabetes syndrome resulting from mutations in hepatocyte nuclear factor-1beta. Nephrol Dial Transplant. 2004;19(11):2703–8.

144. Adalat S, Woolf AS, Johnstone KA, Wirsing A, Harries LW, Long DA, et al. HNF1B mutations associate with hypomagnesemia and renal magnesium wasting. J Am Soc Nephrol. 2009;20(5):1123–31.

145. Kikuchi R, Kusuhara H, Hattori N, Kim I, Shiota K, Gonzalez FJ, et al. Regulation of tissue-specific expression of the human and mouse urate transporter 1 gene by hepatocyte nuclear factor 1 alpha/beta and DNA methylation. Mol Pharmacol. 2007;72(6):1619–25.

146. Karstensen HG, Tommerup N. Isolated and syndromic forms of congenital anosmia. Clin Genet. 2012;81(3):210–5.

147. Tsai PS, Gill JC. Mechanisms of disease: insights into X-linked and autosomal-dominant Kallmann syndrome. Nat Clin Pract Endocrinol Metab. 2006;2(3):160–71.

148. Naftolin F, Harris GW, Bobrow M. Effect of purified luteinizing hormone releasing factor on normal and

hypogonadotrophic anosmic men. Nature. 1971;232(5311):496–7.

149. Schwanzel-Fukuda M, Bick D, Pfaff DW. Luteinizing hormone-releasing hormone (LHRH)-expressing cells do not migrate normally in an inherited hypogonadal (Kallmann) syndrome. Brain Res Mol Brain Res. 1989;6(4):311–26.

150. Cariboni A, Pimpinelli F, Colamarino S, Zaninetti R, Piccolella M, Rumio C, et al. The product of X-linked Kallmann's syndrome gene (KAL1) affects the migratory activity of gonadotropin-releasing hormone (GnRH)-producing neurons. Hum Mol Genet. 2004;13(22):2781–91.

151. Falardeau J, Chung WC, Beenken A, Raivio T, Plummer L, Sidis Y, et al. Decreased FGF8 signaling causes deficiency of gonadotropin-releasing hormone in humans and mice. J Clin Invest. 2008;118(8):2822–31.

152. Dode C, Levilliers J, Dupont JM, De Paepe A, Le Du N, Soussi-Yanicostas N, et al. Loss-of-function mutations in FGFR1 cause autosomal dominant Kallmann syndrome. Nat Genet. 2003;33(4):463–5.

153. Dode C, Teixeira L, Levilliers J, Fouveaut C, Bouchard P, Kottler ML, et al. Kallmann syndrome: mutations in the genes encoding prokineticin-2 and prokineticin receptor-2. PLoS Genet. 2006; 2(10):e175.

154. Duke VM, Winyard PJ, Thorogood P, Soothill P, Bouloux PM, Woolf AS. KAL, a gene mutated in Kallmann's syndrome, is expressed in the first trimester of human development. Mol Cell Endocrinol. 1995;110(1–2):73–9.

155. John U, Benz K, Hubler A, Patzer L, Zenker M, Amann K. Oligohydramnios associated with sonographically normal kidneys. Urology. 2012;79(5): 1155–7.

156. Kumar D, Moss G, Primhak R, Coombs R. Congenital renal tubular dysplasia and skull ossification defects similar to teratogenic effects of angiotensin converting enzyme (ACE) inhibitors. J Med Genet. 1997;34(7):541–5.

157. Mahieu-Caputo D, Dommergues M, Delezoide AL, Lacoste M, Cai Y, Narcy F, et al. Twin-to-twin transfusion syndrome. Role of the fetal renin-angiotensin system. Am J Pathol. 2000;156(2):629–36.

158. Barr Jr M, Cohen Jr MM. ACE inhibitor fetopathy and hypocalvaria: the kidney-skull connection. Teratology. 1991;44(5):485–95.

159. Gubler MC. Renal tubular dysgenesis. Pediatr Nephrol. 2014;29(1):51–9.

160. Uematsu M, Sakamoto O, Ohura T, Shimizu N, Satomura K, Tsuchiya S. A further case of renal tubular dysgenesis surviving the neonatal period. Eur J Pediatr. 2009;168(2):207–9.

161. Jongmans MC, Admiraal RJ, van der Donk KP, Vissers LE, Baas AF, Kapusta L, et al. CHARGE syndrome: the phenotypic spectrum of mutations in the CHD7 gene. J Med Genet. 2006;43(4):306–14.

162. Brockschmidt A, Chung B, Weber S, Fischer DC, Kolatsi-Joannou M, Christ L, et al. CHD1L: a new candidate gene for congenital anomalies of the kidneys and urinary tract (CAKUT). Nephrol Dial Transplant. 2012;27(6):2355–64.

163. Ma NF, Hu L, Fung JM, Xie D, Zheng BJ, Chen L, et al. Isolation and characterization of a novel oncogene, amplified in liver cancer 1, within a commonly amplified region at 1q21 in hepatocellular carcinoma. Hepatology. 2008;47(2):503–10.

164. Sanna-Cherchi S, Sampogna RV, Papeta N, Burgess KE, Nees SN, Perry BJ, et al. Mutations in DSTYK and dominant urinary tract malformations. N Engl J Med. 2013;369(7):621–9.

165. Handrigan GR, Chitayat D, Lionel AC, Pinsk M, Vaags AK, Marshall CR, et al. Deletions in 16q24.2 are associated with autism spectrum disorder, intellectual disability and congenital renal malformation. J Med Genet. 2013;50(3):163–73.

166. Sanna-Cherchi S, Kiryluk K, Burgess KE, Bodria M, Sampson MG, Hadley D, et al. Copy-number disorders are a common cause of congenital kidney malformations. Am J Hum Genet. 2012;91(6): 987–97.

167. van Vuuren SH, Damen-Elias HA, Stigter RH, van der Doef R, Goldschmeding R, de Jong TP, et al. Size and volume charts of fetal kidney, renal pelvis and adrenal gland. Ultrasound Obstet Gynecol. 2012;40(6):659–64.

168. Kupferman JC, Druschel CM, Kupchik GS. Increased prevalence of renal and urinary tract anomalies in children with Down syndrome. Pediatrics. 2009;124(4):e615–21.

169. Cereda A, Carey JC. The trisomy 18 syndrome. Orphanet J Rare Dis. 2012;7:81.

170. Iliopoulos D, Sekerli E, Vassiliou G, Sidiropoulou V, Topalidis A, Dimopoulou D, et al. Patau syndrome with a long survival (146 months): a clinical report and review of literature. Am J Med Genet A. 2006;140(1):92–3.

171. Morris RK, Quinlan-Jones E, Kilby MD, Khan KS. Systematic review of accuracy of fetal urine analysis to predict poor postnatal renal function in cases of congenital urinary tract obstruction. Prenat Diagn. 2007;27(10):900–11.

172. Bueva A, Guignard JP. Renal function in preterm neonates. Pediatr Res. 1994;36(5):572–7.

173. Mure PY, Sabatier-Laval E, Dodat H. Malformations of male internal genitalia originating from the Wolffian duct. Arch Pediatr. 1997;4(2):163–9.

174. Oppelt PG, Lermann J, Strick R, Dittrich R, Strissel P, Rettig I, et al. Malformations in a cohort of 284 women with Mayer-Rokitansky-Kuster-Hauser syndrome (MRKH). Reprod Biol Endocrinol. 2012;10:57.

175. Behr SC, Courtier JL, Qayyum A. Imaging of mullerian duct anomalies. Radiographics. 2012;32(6): E233–50.

176. van Vuuren SH, van der Doef R, Cohen-Overbeek TE, Goldschmeding R, Pistorius LR, de Jong TP. Compensatory enlargement of a solitary functioning kidney during fetal development. Ultrasound Obstet Gynecol. 2012;40(6):665–8.

177. Cascio S, Paran S, Puri P. Associated urological anomalies in children with unilateral renal agenesis. J Urol. 1999;162(3 Pt 2):1081–3.

178. Kaneyama K, Yamataka A, Satake S, Yanai T, Lane GJ, Kaneko K, et al. Associated urologic anomalies in children with solitary kidney. J Pediatr Surg. 2004;39(1):85–7.

179. Krzemien G, Roszkowska-Blaim M, Kostro I, Wojnar J, Karpinska M, Sekowska R. Urological anomalies in children with renal agenesis or multicystic dysplastic kidney. J Appl Genet. 2006;47(2):171–6.

180. Grinsell MM, Butz K, Gurka MJ, Gurka KK, Norwood V. Sport-related kidney injury among high school athletes. Pediatrics. 2012;130(1):e40–5.

181. Shibata S, Nagata M. Pathogenesis of human renal dysplasia: an alternative scenario to the major theories. Pediatr Int. 2003;45(5):605–9.

182. Narchi H. Risk of hypertension with multicystic kidney disease: a systematic review. Arch Dis Child. 2005;90(9):921–4.

183. Rabelo EA, Oliveira EA, Silva GS, Pezzuti IL, Tatsuo ES. Predictive factors of ultrasonographic involution of prenatally detected multicystic dysplastic kidney. BJU Int. 2005;95(6):868–71.

184. Hains DS, Bates CM, Ingraham S, Schwaderer AL. Management and etiology of the unilateral multicystic dysplastic kidney: a review. Pediatr Nephrol. 2009;24(2):233–41.

185. D'Alberton A, Reschini E, Ferrari N, Candiani P. Prevalence of urinary tract abnormalities in a large series of patients with uterovaginal atresia. J Urol. 1981;126(5):623–4.

186. Fedele L, Bianchi S, Agnoli B, Tozzi L, Vignali M. Urinary tract anomalies associated with unicornuate uterus. J Urol. 1996;155(3):847–8.

187. Raj GV, Auge BK, Assimos D, Preminger GM. Metabolic abnormalities associated with renal calculi in patients with horseshoe kidneys. J Endourol. 2004;18(2):157–61.

Miriam Schmidts and Philip L. Beales

Cilia in the Historic Context

Cilia are evolutionarily well conserved, hair-like structures projecting from the surface of most cells in vertebrates and are broadly divided into motile and non-motile cilia. While non-motile cilia can be found as single organelles on most cells in mammals, the occurrence of motile cilia in bundles of multiple (hundreds) is restricted to certain tissues in vertebrates such as the respiratory tract, the reproductive system (epididymidis and oviduct), the ependyma lining the brain ventricles and the embryonic node where they are involved in fluid movement and mucociliary clearance. Also, the flagellum of mammalian sperm has a very similar structure to motile cilia.

M. Schmidts (✉)
Department of Pediatrics, Genetics Division, Center for Pediatrics and Adolescent Medicine, University Hospital Freiburg, Mathildenstrasse 1,79100, Freiburg, Germany

Department of Human Genetics, Genome Research, Radboud University Hospital Nijmegen, Geert Grooteplain Zuid 10, Nijmegen, 6525 GA, The Netherlands
e-mail: miriam.schmidts@radboudumc.nl

P.L. Beales
Department of Genetics and Genomics Medicine, Institute of Child Health, University College London, 30 Guilford Street, London WC1N 1EH, UK
e-mail: p.beales@ucl.ac.uk

In vertebrate photoreceptor cells within the retina, a modified ciliary structure called "connecting cilium" links inner and outer segment of those cells. See Figs. 11.1a–c and 11.2a–k for examples of cilia visualisation.

Although the existence of cilia has been described as early as the 1800s by Purkinje and Valentin [3, 4], their significance for mammalian development, organ maintenance and clinical disease has only been fully appreciated in the last two decades. Cilia were regarded as functionless cellular extensions for many years as no link between this organelle and human disease was made despite the fact that dextrocardia had already been visualised by Leonardo da Vinci in the fifteenth century and in 1793, the Scottish pathologist Matthew Baillie mentioned situs inversus in his book *The Morbid Anatomy of Some of the Most Important Parts of the Human Body*. As published by Afzelius in 1979 [5], we realise today that situs abnormalities result from (mainly motile) ciliary dysfunction in the embryonic node. The function of non-motile, so called primary cilia remained elusive for even longer; however, when "rediscovered," their role in (cystic) kidney disease was one of the initial ciliary functions acknowledged [6, 7], Since then, a large number of (inherited) human diseases have been identified to result from ciliary malfunction [8–10]. See Table 11.1 for a summary of ciliary diseases with renal involvement and their underlying genetic cause.

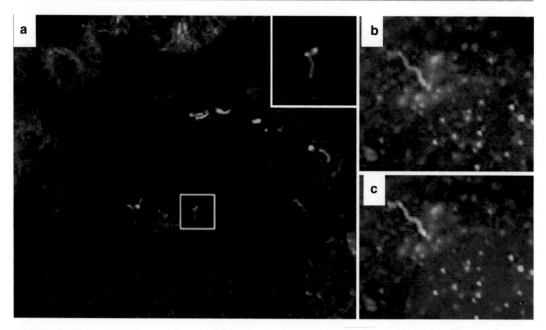

Fig. 11.1 (**a–c**) Mammalian cilia visualised by Immunofluorescence. (**a, b**) Antibody staining of WT IFT172 in human control fibroblasts showing axonemal and pericentriolar localization in comparison to acetylated tubulin (anti-acetylated alpha tubulin, mouse monoclonal antibody) marking the ciliary axoneme shown in (**c**). Images reprinted with permission from "Defects in the IFT-B component IFT172 cause Jeune and Mainzer-Saldino syndromes in humans", Halbritter et al. [1])

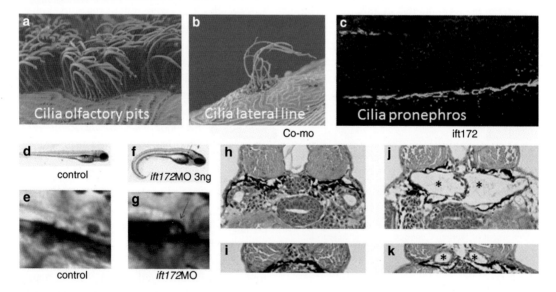

Fig. 11.2 (**a–k**) Zebrafish cilia and *ift172* knockdown mimicking the human renal phenotype: (**a, b**) Motile Cilia in the olfactory pits and Cilia in the lateral line organ (scanning electron microscopy). (**c**) *green*: Cilia in the zebrafish pronephric duct visualised by immunofluorescence (mouse anti-acetylated tubulin antibody followed by anti-mouse monoclonal antibody). Nuclei are shown in *blue* and visualised using DAPI. (**d**) Wildtype zebrafish embryo 4 days post fertilisation, shown from the side compared to a 4 days old embryo after *ift172* knockdown using antisense morpholino (**f**). *Ift172* knockdown results in formation of a glomerular cyst (**g**) not present in the wildtype embryo (**e**). (**j, k**) HE staining of zebrafish embryo sections showing glomerular cysts after *ift172* knockdown not present in the wildtype embryo (**h, i**) (**d–g** Used with permission from Halbritter et al. [1]; **h–k** Used with permission from Westhoff et al. [2])

Table 11.1 Summary of ciliary diseases with renal involvement and their underlying genetic causes

Disease	Renal phenotype	Retinopathy	Skeletal phenotype	Obesity	Developmental delay	Situs inversus	Other	Gene
Autosomal-dominant Polycystic Kidney Disease (ADPKD)	Always; polycystic	–	–	–	–	–	Increased risk for cerebral blood vessel aneurysma, liver involvement possible	*PKD1* *PKD2*
Autosomal-recessive polycystic Kidney Disease (ARPKD)	Always; polycystic	–	–	–	–	–	Frequent liver disease, possible pancreatic cysts	Fibrocystin (*PKHD1*)
Medullary cystic kidney disease (MCKD1/2)	Always; cysts at the cortico-medullary junction		–	–	–	–	Extensive salt wasting	*MUC1, Uromodulin*
Nephronophthisis (NPHP)	Always; NPHP	–	No	–	–	Rarely, especially *NPHP2/INVS* mutation carriers		*NPHP1, NPHP2 (Inversin), NPHP3, NPHP4, NPHP5 (IQCB-1) NPHP6 (CEP290), NPHP7 (GLIS2), NPHP8 (RPGRIP1L), NPHP9 (NEK8), NPHP10 (SDCCAG8), NPHP11 (TMEM67, Meckelin), NPHP12 (TTC21B), NPHP13 (WDR19), NPHP14 (ZNF423), NPHP15 (CEP164), NPHP16 (ANKS6)*
Joubert Syndrome (JS) and JS related disorders, including Senior-Loken syndrome, Cogan syndrome	Often; mainly NPHP-like, rarely cystic	Frequent in JSRD	Sometimes polydactyly	–	Very often	Rarely	Pathognomic "molar tooth sign" on brain MRI images; ataxia, ocular motor apraxia, hypoventilation	*TMEM216, AHI1, NPHP1, CEP290, TMEM67, RPGRIP1L, ARL13B CC2D2A, CXORF5, TTC21B, KIF7 TCTN1, TMEM237, CEP41, TMEM138, C5ORF42, TCTN3, ZNF423, TMEM231, CSPP1, PDE6D*

(continued)

Table 11.1 (continued)

Disease	Renal phenotype	Retinopathy	Skeletal phenotype	Obesity	Developmental delay	Situs inversus	Other	Gene
BBS	~30 %, mainly NPHP-like, rarely cystic,	+	Often polydactyly	Always	Very often	Rarely	Hypogonoadism	BBS1, BBS2, BBS3 (ARL6), BBS4, BBS5, BBS6 (MKKS), BBS7, BBS8 (TTC8), BBS9, BBS10, BBS11 (TRIM32), BBS13 (MKS1), BBS14 (CEP290), BBS15 (C2ORF86), BBS17 (LZTFL1), BBS18 (BBIP1), BBS19 (IFT27)
Alstrom syndrome	Often	+	–	Always	–	–	Frequent cardiomyopathy, sensorineural hearing loss, hepatic disease	Alms1
Meckel-Gruber syndrome	Often; NPHP like or cystic	na	Often orofacial clefting		na (early lethality)	Sometimes	Occipital encephalocele	MKS1, MKS2 (TMEM216), MKS3 (TMEM67), MKS4 (CEP290), MKS5 (RPGRIP1L), MKS6 (CC2D2A), MKS7 (NPHP3), MKS8 (TCTN2), MKS9 (B9D1), MKS10 (B9D2), MKS11 (TMEM231)
Orofacial digital syndrome (OFD)	Renal malformations	Usually not	Often polysyndactyly, orofacial clefting	–		Rarely	Lobulated tongue, heart defects, agenesis of the corpus callosum, conductive hearing loss, cerebellar atrophy described	OFD1 (CXORF5), TCTN3, C5orf42, DDX59

Short Rib-Polydactyly Syndrome (SRPS)	Often; NPHP-like or cystic	Usually not evident	Often polydactyly, short ribs, shortened long bones, brachydactyly, abnormal pelvis configuration, sometimes orofacial clefting	–	na (early lethality)	Rarely	Always lethal perinatally due to cardiorespiratory insufficiency	DYNC2H1, NEK1, WDR60, WDR34, WDR35
Jeune Asphyxiating Thoracic Dystrophy (JATD)	<30%, mainly NPHP-like, rarely cystic	Rarely	Short ribs, short long bones, rarely polydactyly, abnormal pelvis configuration, scoliosis, cone shaped epiphyses	Single cases	–	–	Sometimes retinal degeneration, mainly in cases with renal disease;	DYNC2H1, WDR34, WDR60, IFT80, IFT172, IFT140, WDR19 (IFT144), TTC21B (IFT139), CSPP1
Mainzer-Saldino-Syndrome (MSS)	Always; mainly NPHP-like, rarely cystic	Always	(Mildly) shortened ribs, cone shaped epiphyses	–	Single cases	Not described	Always retinal degenration	IFT140, IFT172
Sensenbrenner syndrome (CED)	Very often; mainly NPHP-like	Often	(Mildly) shortened ribs, brachydactyly, craniosynostosis	–	Sometimes	Usually not	Thin and sparse growing hair, nail dysplasia (ectodermal defects), heart defects	IFT122, WDR19 (IFT144) IFT43, WDR35

Ciliary Ultrastructure

The ciliary research field originates from the protozoan flagellar research undertaken since the 1950s and was therefore initially more focussed on motile cilia, possibly also because those were easier to detect due to their moving features. Electron microscopy is an essential imaging technique for visualisation these cilia also lack the central pair (9+0 structure). In motile cilia, so-called inner and outer dynein arms extend from the outer microtubule pairs and those outer pairs are connected to the central pair via radial spokes. This complex construction enables sliding of the microtubules generating ciliary movement. Dynein arms and radial spokes are absent from non-motile primary ciliary.

This ciliary *axoneme* is anchored to and extends from the *basal body* which itself lies within the cytosol and is derived from the mother centriole after cell division. Along its vertical axis, the primary cilium can be structurally divided into different sub-compartments: *the ciliary tip, the ciliary body, the ciliary necklace* [11], *the transition zone* [12], *the so-called inversin compartment* [13] *and the basal body* [14, 15]. The specialise cellular plasma membrane at the ciliary insertion site is referred to as the *ciliary pocket* (Fig. 11.3 for a schematic of ciliary structures). As cilia lack organelles such as endoplasmatic reticulum and Golgi and therefore no protein synthesis occurs within the cilium, all ciliary proteins are produced within the cellular cytosol, and transported to the cilium. Within the cilium, so called **Intraflagellar Transport** (**IFT**) enables protein trafficking from the ciliary base to the tip and vice versa (Fig. 11.3 for a schematic of ciliary ultrastructure and Fig. 11.4 for a schematic of IFT). Figure 11.5a–c shows a schematic

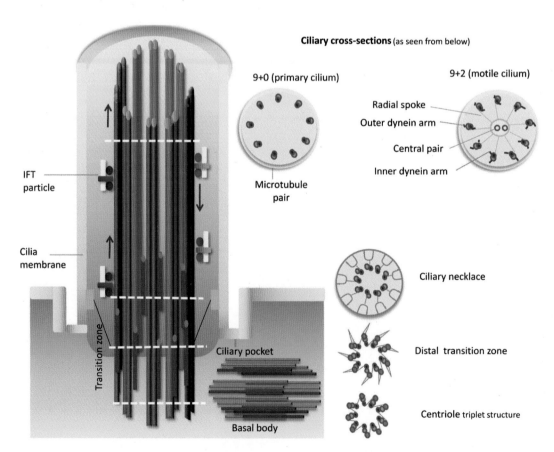

Fig. 11.3 Simplified schematic of the ciliary ultrastructure

of ciliary protein complex localisation and IFT defects are visualised in Fig. 11.6a, b.

Although cilia extend from the cell body and are surrounded by specialised plasma membrane forming the "*ciliary membrane*," cilia represent a distinct cellular compartment with the so called "*transition zone*" which acting as a barrier between the cilium and the rest of the cell [22, 23]. At the transition zone, the microtubule triplets of the basal body transform into the axonemal microtubule doublets. As the protein and lipid composition of the ciliary axoneme and ciliary membrane is distinct from the cell body, selective recruitment of components and transport of those components into the cilium is required. How this is precisely undertaken is still unclear, but some progress in understanding has been made in recent years. Interestingly, the connecting cilium of retinal photoreceptors is very similar in its structure to the ciliary transition zone and many proteins encoded by genes found to carry mutations leading to nephronophthisis

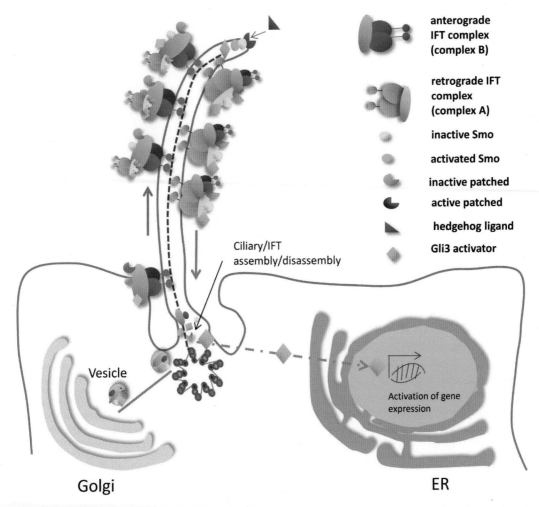

Fig. 11.4 Simplified schematic of Intraflagellar Transport (IFT) and it's relation to hedgehog signalling. Hedgehog signalling pathway components such as smoothened (smo) and patched localise to the cilium and require anterograde IFT to localise to the ciliary tip where binding of the hedgehog ligand (*blue triangle*) activates the smoothened inhibitor patched (*orange*) which in turn releases smoothened (*yellow*). Activated smoothened (*green ball*) releases GLI3 activator from its inhibitor SUFU (not shown). Gli3 activator (*green rectangle*) requires retrograde IFT to translocate to the nucleus where it activates genes involved in chondrogenic and osteogenic differentiation [16–19]

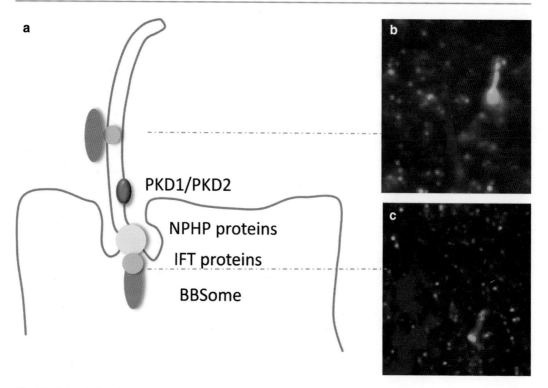

Fig. 11.5 (a–c) Localisation of major ciliary protein complexes. (**a**) Schematic of protein-complex localisation: While Bardet-Biedl-Syndrome (BBS) proteins and intraflagellar transport (IFT) proteins are detected both at the ciliary base and along the ciliary axoneme, many proteins encoded by genes mutated in nephronophthisis localise to the ciliary transition zone. (**b**) Immunofluorescence image of axonemal IFT140 localisation (*green*). (**c**) Immunofluorescence image of IFT140 localisation at the base of the cilium (*green*). The ciliary axoneme is marked in *red* using anti-acetylated tubulin antibody (**b**, **c**) used with permission of John Wiley and Sons from Schmidts et al. [20]

(often with retinal degeneration) localise to the ciliary transition zone as well as the photoreceptor connecting cilium. This implicates a function of these proteins in "gate keeping" (between cytosol and ciliary axoneme as well as between inner and outer photoreceptor segment) [12, 23]. Two highly specialised areas occur within the ciliary membrane: the *ciliary necklace*, initially described by Gilula and Satir 1972 [11] where the microtubules of the basal body are connected to the plasma membrane and the base of a plasma membrane invagination around the proximal ciliary axoneme, the ciliary pocket [24]. The "*inversin compartment*" is found in the proximal ciliary region the ciliary necklace, the transitional zone and the basal body [13]. Mutations in *INVS* encoding Inversin cause nephronophthisis type 2. Please also refer to the nephronophthisis chapter of this book (Chap. 13) for details.

Ciliary Assembly

As described above, proteins necessary to build a cilium cannot be synthesized within the cilium but have to be transported to the building site. How exactly ciliary components get to the cilium and the precise process of the transformation of the mother centriole (the older of the two centrioles) into a basal body from where the cilium is assembled has not been understood in all its depth to date. Ciliogenesis is tightly linked to the cell cycle: dividing cells do not exhibit a cilium, cilia are only observed during the G1 cell cycle phase or when cells are quiescent. At least some ciliary proteins seem to reach the ciliary building site by vesicular transport: ciliary vesicles (post-Golgi vesicles) traffic close to the ciliary building site and merge there with the plasma membrane [25]. In this process of sorting membrane proteins

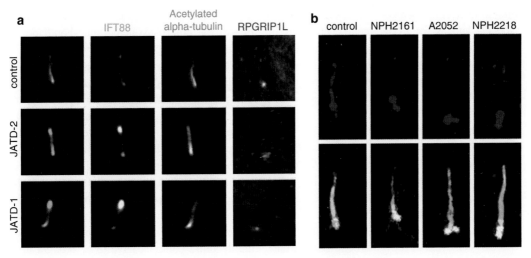

Fig. 11.6 (**a, b**) Visualisation of disturbed intraflagellar transport by Immunofluorescence. (**a**) Compared with controls, IFT88 accumulates in distal ends of cilia in fibroblasts from Jeune Syndrome patients (JATD-1 and -2) carrying mutations in the dynein-2 complex protein dync2h1 leading to impaired retrograde intraflagellar transport (IFT). Cells were stained with anti-IFT88 (*green*); anti-acetylated α tubulin (marker for the ciliary axoneme, *cyan*); and anti-RPGRIP1L (marker for the ciliary base, *red*) (Reprinted with permission from [21]) (**b**) Fibroblasts of patients with biallelic mutations in the anterograde IFT component IFT172 show decreased axonemal and increased basal body staining of IFT140 (*red*) compared to controls. The ciliary axoneme is marked with anti-acetylated-tubulin antibody (*green*), basal bodies are marked in *blue* using anti-g-tubulin antibody (Reprinted with permission from Exome sequencing identifies DYNC2H1 mutations as a common cause of asphyxiating thoracic dystrophy (Jeune syndrome) without major polydactyly, renal or retinal involvement. **a** Used with permission of BMJ Publishing Group from Schmidts et al. [21]; **b** Halbritter et al. [1])

to cilia, Bardet-Biedl syndrome proteins have been shown to be essential in assembling a coat that traffics membrane proteins to the cilium [26, 27]. Ciliogenesis is thought to start with the basal body docking to ciliary vesicles which then fuse with the plasma membrane, probably at the site of the ciliary pocket [28–32]. One of the proteins promoting this process has been identified as CEP164 and mutations in the *CEP164* gene cause nephronopthisis in humans [33, 34]. The fact that primary cilia and flagella only ever extend from the mother centriole could be due to the lack of subdistal appendages at the daughter centriole which seem to play a crucial role in anchoring the basal body to the plasma membrane [35]. Cilia stability seems to also depend on posttranslational modification of tubulin, including acetylation [36, 37], glutamylation [38, 39] and farnesylation. The latter seems of particular importance as Thomas et al. identified a homozygous *PDE6D* mutation Joubert syndrome which impaired the targeting of another known joubert protein, INPP5E to the cilium [40].

Cilia and Cell Cycle

As indicated above, ciliogenesis is interlinked with the cell cycle: dividing cells do not normally exhibit cilia, those only become visible after the cell's exit from cell cycle. When cells divide, one centrosome stays within the mother cell while the other can be found in the daughter cell. After cell division, the centrioles duplicate and the original centrioles from which duplication occurs are referred to as "mother centrioles." Once a cell has left cell cycle again, the cilium is built from this mother centriole [41]. When cells re-enter the cell cycle, cilia need to be disassembled which seems to be initiated by Percentrin-1 (PCM1) mediated recruitment of Polo-like kinase 1 (Plk1) to the pericentriolar material [42, 43]. While it has been accepted for many decades that ciliogenesis is linked to mitotic exit of the cell, the possibility that cilia themselves might influence cell cycle progression has only been recently taken into account. For example, the IFT protein Ift88 seems required for spindle orientation during mitosis [44]. Lack of

Ift88 in mice leads to a polycystic kidney pheno-type [7] and as for cystic renal phenotypes in humans, it remains controversial to which extent and at what time point cellular hyperproliferation contributes to the initiation and/or progression of disease [45]. The INPP5E protein (genetic muta-tions can cause a Joubert phenotype with renal dis-ease) and the tumor suppressor protein VHL (mutations in the VHL gene cause Von-Hippel-Lindau syndrome which is associated with cystic renal disease) are both involved in stabilising cilia by inhibiting AURKA triggered ciliary disassem-bly for cell-cycle re-entry [46–48]. The question how cilia influence cell cycle, how they are influ-enced by cell cycle and how this contributes to cili-opathy, especially polycystic phenotypes, is difficult to resolve as proteins encoded by genes mutated in ciliopathy subjects often have multiple extra-ciliary functions which might influence cell-cycle progression independently of the cilium. For example, several genes mutated in subjects with nephronophthisis such as *ZNF423*, *CEP164* and *NEK8* have been linked to DNA damage repair and therefore directly to cell cycle progression [34, 49]. It is, however, of note that, except for VHL, no increased rate of malignancies has been demon-strated for humans affected by ciliopathies to date.

Intraflagellar Transport (IFT)

Transport of ciliary proteins along the axoneme is undertaken via IFT, an energy dependent pro-cess. Kosminski et al. were the first to notice this process in 1993 [50]. IFT is a highly conserved transport mechanism along cilia and flagellae from the green algae *Chlamydomonas* to verte-brates and mammals including humans. Building a cilium from the base to the tip is largely depen-dent on anterograde IFT [51]. Counter-intuitively, the anterograde IFT complex transporting pro-teins from the ciliary base to the tip is named "complex B" while the complex enabling retro-grade transport from the ciliary tip back to the base is called "complex A." Motor for the antero-grade complex is kinesin-2 while the cytoplasmic dynein-2 complex enables transport from the cili-ary tip back to the base. Although named

"cytoplasmic dynein," the latter complex local-ises to the ciliary axoneme and should not be confused with the cytoplasmic dynein-1 complex which enables transport along microtubules within the cell body and along neuronal axons. The precise composition of the dynein-2 com-plex has still not been completely elucidated; however, it is assumed that it ressembles dynein-1 complex, a homodimer consisting of two heavy chains, two light-intermediate chains, two inter-mediate chains and two light chains. IFT-complex A and B are multiprotein assemblies functioning as an adaptor system between the motor com-plexes and cargo. As IFT-A complex proteins and the dynein-2 complex have to be brought up to the ciliary tip before they can fullfill their func-tion in retrograde transport back from the tip to the base and vice versa, kinesin-2 and IFT com-plex B must be transported back to the base after they have reached the ciliary tip, it is evident that both complexes must be transported as cargo by each other [25, 52, 53]. Knockout mice for the kinesin-2 component *Kif3a*, the dynein-2 motor heavy chain *Dync2h1* or IFT components often exhibit fewer or shorter cilia and are lethal around midgestation, indicating the fundamental role of these highly conserved proteins during develop-ment [43]. Kidney specific gene disruption or hypomorphic mutations often cause renal cysts in mice [7, 54, 55]. Human mutations in genes encoding dynein-2 complex components and IFT particles mainly cause ciliary chondrodysplasias with variable extraskeletal involvement [1, 20, 21,56–69] and mutations in the IFT-A compo-nent *TTC21B/IFT139* and in the IFT-B compo-nent *IFT27* were recently identified in Bardet-Biedl-Syndrome [68, 70]. For more details also see the human disease section below and Fig. 11.4 for a schematic of IFT and its rela-tion to hedgehog signalling.

Ciliary Signalling Pathways

Single non-motile (primary) cilia are considered sensory organelles involved in multiple signal-ling pathways transducing both signals from the cellular surroundings to the cells as well as modifying cell signalling pathways within the cell [71, 72]. As mentioned above, cilia and ciliary proteins have been highly conserved throughout evolution and mutations in genes encoding ciliary components often result in complex developmental defects in vertebrates. This can be attributed to disturbances of fundamental signalling pathways essential for embryogenesis, organogenesis and proper tissue maintenance.

Hedgehog Signalling

The best explored cilia-regulated cellular pathway is hedgehog signalling [16, 17, 73]. Hedgehog signalling crucially influences chondrogenic (and subsequently osteogenic) proliferation and differentiation [74]. Mouse models of ciliary chondrodysplasias, e.g., knockout mice for *Evc* (mutations in the EVC1 and EVC2 gene cause Ellis-van Creveld-Syndrome in humans), *Dync2h1* and *Ift80* (associated with Jeune Syndrome and Short-Rib-Polydactyly Syndrome type III in humans) indicate that IFT defects lead to imbalances in the hedgehog signalling pathway [18, 75, 76]. Lack of hedgehog signal transduction leads to decreased chondrogenic proliferation and imbalanced chondrogenic differentiation at the growth plates which impairs bone growth. As a result' mice, as well as human subjects with mutations in these genes as well as in *IFT144/WDR19*, exhibit shortened ribs and long bones. Lack of Ift80 or Ift144 also induces polydactyly in mice, a hallmark of dysregulated hedgehog signalling [18, 75–77].

The hedgehog signaling pathway operates via ciliary trafficking: the pathway components smoothened (smo) and patched move via anterograde IFT to the ciliary tip, where smo becomes activated and releases GLI3 activator. The latter is subsequently transported back to the base of the cilium via retrograde IFT and enters the cell body and nucleus where it activates genes regulating chondrogenic and osteogenic differentiation and proliferation (simplified schematic in Fig. 11.4).

Apart from altered bone growth, impaired hedgehog signalling leads to complex developmental defects in mammals including polydactyly, heart defects, midline defects such as clefting and holoprosencephaly. Renal abnormalities, especially ectopic kidneys but also cystic-dysplastic changes, can also be observed in mice [78] and human subjects affected by Smith-Lemli-Opitz syndrome, a condition thought to result from altered hedgehog signalling due to a cholesterol biosynthesis defect [79]. However, neither human subjects with *IFT80-* nor *EVC1/EVC2* mutation nor the corresponding mouse models exhibit a renal phenotype. On the other hand, human subjects with mutations in other IFT genes such as *WDR19/IFT144*, *TTC21B/IFT139*, *IFT140*, *IFT43*, *WDR35* or *IFT172* genes are affected by childhood-onset cystic or nehronopthisis-like renal disease [1, 20, 64, 65, 67–69], and in knockout mouse models for *IFT140* or *IFT172*, early onset cystic (dysplastic) kidney disease is observed [55, 80]. While it seems likely that the skeletal phenotype observed in those subjects is due to imbalances in the hedgehog pathway secondary to IFT defects, this does not necessarily apply to the renal phenotype as no changes in the hedgehog pathway were noted in kidneys from *Ift140* knockout mice prior to the onset of cystogenesis [55].

Wnt Signalling and Planar Cell Polarity (PCP)

The role of cilia and ciliary proteins in regulating wnt signalling is subject of an ongoing discussion recently reviewed by Wallingford and Mitchell [81]. Wnt signalling can be roughly divided into a so-called "canonical" pathway branch involving wnt/beta-catenin and a so called "non-canonical" or planar cell polarity (PCP) branch. Canonical Wnt/beta-catenin dependent signalling occurs after extracellular wnt ligand binds to transmembrane Frizzled receptors which stabilize beta-catenin. Beta-catenin subsequently localises to the nucleus to activate further target genes [82]. The non-canonical or PCP pathway is mediated via Frizzled and the large transmembrane proteins Vangl2 and Celsr and involves cytoplasmic regulatory proteins such as

Dishevelled (Dvl). PCP describes the process of orientation of cells and their structures along an axis in an epithelial plane in a coordinated manner [83]. Classical PCP readouts exist for all species from *drosophila* flies over *xenopus* frogs to mammals, including orientation of hair on the fly wing, convergent extension (axis elongation by cell intercalation) of the anterior-posterior body axis of frog embryos and orientation of hair cells in the inner ear of mice.

The first indication that proteins encoded by genes defective in human ciliopathies play a role in PCP came from Bardet-Biedl-Syndrome mouse models displaying typical PCP-related defects in the cochlea [84]. Further initial experiments suggested that the ciliary protein encoded by *NPHP2*, *Inversin* (*Invs*), inhibits Dvl-mediated transduction of the canonical wnt pathway while promoting a shift towards PCP signalling [85], proposing that Inversin might act as a switch between canonical and non-canonical/PCP Wnt signalling [85]. This would imply that in an inversin-deficient state such as in nephronophthisis patients with Inversin mutations, non-canonical wnt signalling might be expanded and PCP signalling reduced. In line with the assumption that cilia might act as a negative regulator of canonical wnt signalling, increased canonical wnt signalling was found in cells deficient for Bardet-Biedl-Syndrome proteins BBS1, BBS4 and MKKS and the anterograde IFT motor protein KIF3A [86], in mice mutant for *Kif3a*, *Ift88* and *Ofd1* [87] as well as in kidney-specific *Ift20* knockout mice exhibiting a cystic renal phenotype [88]. However, no abnormalities in wnt signalling were found by Ocbina et al. in the absence of cilia in mice mutant for *Kif3a*, *Ift88*, *Ift72* [89] and in *ift88* zebrafish mutants [90]. The relationship between cilia and wnt signalling therefore remains unclear.

Loss of ciliary proteins such as Ift88 and *Kif3a* in mice results in developmental defects resembling those expected for loss of PCP including mis-orientated inner ear kinocilia [91]. Also, renal tubules elongate during development using a process strongly resembling convergent extension, depending on the non-canonical wnt ligand *Wnt9b*, where loss of Wnt9b leads to renal cyst formation [92]. Furthermore, *Ift20* disruption in mice causes cystic renal disease and in those kidneys, mitotic spindle mis-orientation has been described [88]. As mis-orientated mitotic spindles could affect orientated cell division (OCD), and OCD is the basis for planar cell polarity and necessary for postnatal tubule elongation, loss of OCD might contribute to cystic phenotypes [93]. This is supported by observations in Kif3a, Pkd1, Tsc1/2 and Hnf1b-deficient mice [94–96]. Last, the wnt-regulator Dvl might also control apical docking and planar polarisation of basal bodies from which cilia extend in epithelial cells [97]. Ciliary polarity, which in turn could potentially define cellular polarity, is influenced by the anaphase promoting complex APC/C [98]. These findings, together with the suggestion that the nephronophthisis protein Inversin might act as a switch from canonical wnt towards PCP signalling [85], has led to the hypothesis that cystic and NPHP-phenotypes observed in ciliopathies might result from disturbed PCP. However, loss of OCD and/or PCP might not be the cyst-initiating event as mice mutant for the murine homologue of PKHD1, the Fibrocystin gene causing ARPKD in humans, do not develop cysts despite disrupted OCD [99]. Moreover, cysts can be present despite normal OCD as shown in mice lacking IFT140 in the kidneys [55]. Recent work in the Xenopus model suggests nevertheless that tubular morphogenesis requires planar cell polarity (PCP) and non-canonical Wnt signalling [100].

Flow Hypothesis, Ca- Signalling/ Mechanosensation and mTOR

In 2001, Praetorius and Spring observed increased intracellular calcium levels after flow induced bending of primary cilia on canine kidney cells [101] and subsequently demonstrated that loss of cilia abolishes the flow-induced calcium influx [102]. This was subsequently confirmed in mice with ciliary defects due to *Ift88* deficiency [103]. The *Polycystin-1* and *Polycystin-2* (*PKD1* and *PKD2*) genes, mutated in subjects with ADPKD, are thought to play a role in this mechanosensation and calcium influx process [104, 105]. However, loss of mechanosensation and/or flow induced calcium influx alone is probably not sufficient to cause cystic kidney disease and Polycystin-1, although required for maintenance of tubular morphology in the long run, does not appear essential in the short or intermediate term. Possibly a second exogenous harmful event such as kidney injury is required for cyst formation in the long term [93]. How lack of flow and subsequently reduced calcium influx might lead to cystogenesis has not been clearly established. Delayed or reduced clearance of intracellular cAMP may be involved as accumulation of cAMP was noticed in cystic renal tissue [106]. This in turn might lead to increased MAP kinase signalling stimulating both cell proliferation and fluid secretion into the cyst lumen. Interestingly, fluid flow also induces phosphorylation of a key regulator of cardiac hypertrophy, histone deacetylase 5 (HDAC5) via polycystin-mediated mechanosensation. This leads to myocyte enhancer factor 2C (MEF2C)-dependent transcriptional events in the nucleus and kidney-specific knockout of *Mef2c* results in extensive renal tubule dilatation and cysts whereas *Hdac5* heterozygosity or treatment with an HDAC inhibitor reduces cyst formation in *Pkd2–/–* mouse embryos, indicating a potential treatment target [107].

Based on the observations that human subjects with tuberous sclerosis due to *TSC2* mutations develop cystic renal disease, TSC2 (Tuberin) is considered a negative regulator of mTor signalling [108], Polycystin-1 interacts with Tuberin and mTor activity is elevated in cystic tissues [109, 110], a hypothesis evolved that mTor signalling might be involved in the initiation and/or progression of cystic renal disease and that inhibition of such signalling could delay disease progression. However, while in a rodent model the mTORC1 inhibitor Rapamycin significantly delayed cyst progression [111], a clinical trial using everolimus in human PKD subjects ended with disappointing results: despite slowing down cyst expansion, renal function was not better preserved in everolimus treated subjects compared to controls. Possibly the administered dose was insufficient or more likely, the timepoint of treatment initiation was chosen too late with regards

to the disease course to achieve stabilisation of renal function [112]. Nevertheless, mTor signalling seems to play a role in progression of cystic kidney disease and is potentially connected to flow-induced cilia bending: when cells are grown in a flow chamber, flow leads to Lkb1 induced mTor inhibition resulting in smaller cell size [113]. Flow might further regulate cilia length, potentially also through mTor signalling as cilia length is reduced under flow and increased within cysts where flow is absent [95]. Likewise, mTor inhibitors seem to decrease cilia length reflecting the effects of flow [93, 114].

Yap-Hippo Signalling

The hippo-signalling pathway has emerged in recent years as an important pathway controlling cell and organ growth, stem cell function, regeneration functions and tumor suppression. Dysregulation of hippo signalling was initially noticed to lead to initiation and maintenance of cancerous growth [115]. More recently evidence for this pathway has emerged indicating its fundamental role for developmental processes, including kidney and eye development in mammals. Knockout mice for one of the main pathway components, *Yes-associated protein-1* (*Yap1*), die during early gestation with major developmental defects including yolk sack and axis elongation defects [116] while heterozygous *YAP1* loss of function mutations lead to optic fissure closure defects and possibly also cleft-lip palate, hearing loss, learning difficulties and hematuria with incomplete penetrance in humans [117]. More importantly, inactivation of another major pathway molecule, TAZ, in mice leads to polycystic kidneys (glomerulocystic disease), severe urinary concentrating defects and pulmonary emphysema [118, 119]. The renal phenotype partially resembles that of nephronophthisis patients. Further, NPHP3, NPHP4 and NPHP9/NEK8, products of genes mutated in subjects with nephronophthisis and Meckel-Gruber Syndrome, seem to be involved in Hippo-pathway regulation [120–122]. It is of note, however, that YAP1 is not only directly implicated in the hippo signalling pathway but also modulates WNT signalling via β-catenin-interaction [123], BMP signalling via interaction with Smad7 [124] as well as NOTCH signalling through up-regulation of *JAG1* [125] so that the observed developmental defects in patients with *YAP1* mutations are probably not solely effects of impaired hippo signalling. Moreover, *YAP1* itself is up-regulated by hedgehog signalling [126] raising the possibility that disturbed hedgehog signalling in ciliopathy/nephro-nophthisis subjects might contribute to the observed abnormalities in hippo signalling.

The substantial cross-talk between major developmental signalling pathways including wnt, hedgehog, hippo, notch and mTor [127] leaves the actual molecular basis of a developmental defect such as nephronophthisis uncertain. Nonetheless, in view of the clear renal phenotype observed in TAZ-deficient mice and well established protein-protein interactions between NPHP proteins and TAZ, dysregulated hippo signalling is one of the best candidates so far regarding the primary molecular pathomechanism leading to nephronophthisis like disorders.

Other Cilia Associated Cell Signalling Pathways

Excellent overviews of how the cilium orchestrates cellular signalling pathways during development and tissue repair have been provided by Christensen et al. [128] and Satir et al. [129]. Due to space constraints, not all pathways can be discussed here in detail so we will only scratch the surface of the relationship between cilia and TGF-beta signalling. Clathrin-dependent endocytosis governs TGF-beta signalling and interestingly, TGF-β receptors localise to endocytotic vesicles at the ciliary base and to the ciliary tip in vitro. Activation of SMAD2/3 at the ciliary base has been observed. TGF-β signalling seems to be reduced in the absence of cilia in fibroblasts lacking Ift88 suggesting that cilia might regulate TGF-β signalling and that the cilium could represent a compartment for clathrin-dependent

endocytotic regulation of signal transduction [130]. Increased TGF-beta signalling has been associated with increased interstitial fibrosis in progressive renal dysfunction in ADPKD and other renal conditions. Most interestingly, the PPAR-γ agonist rosiglitazone, reversing a downstream effect of TGFß, was nephro-protective and prolonged survival in an ADPKD rodent model via inhibition of TGF-ß induced renal fibrosis [131]. If this effect is also applicable to humans remains to be established.

Cilia in Renal Disease

The clinical aspects of human ciliopathies with renal involvement are discussed in more detail in the polycystic kidney disease and nephronophthisis chapters of this book (Chaps. 12 and 13, respectively). We will here give a short introduction and overview, mainly focusing on conditions resulting from mutations in IFT and BBS genes. Please also see Table 11.1 for a summary of ciliopathies with renal involvement.

Polycystic Kidney Disease (ADPKD and ARPKD)

The classic ciliary polycystic renal diseases are represented by autosomal dominant polycystic kidney disease (ADPKD) and autosomal recessive polycystic kidney disease (ARPKD). The hallmark of both diseases is extensive cystic enlargement of both kidneys. ADPKD is one of the most common monogenetic disorders with an incidence of 1 in 600–800 live births in the western world and clinical signs of ADPKD usually become manifest in adulthood [132]. In affected subjects, heterozygous mutations in either PKD1 or PKD2, encoding for Polycystin 1 and Polycystin 2, have been identified and it is common belief that a second acquired somatic mutation is necessary for the initiation of cystogenesis ("second hit hypothesis"). Gene dosage at least of PKD1 probably plays a role for the severity of the phenotype, which rarely can mimic ARPKD [133].

With a frequency of 1:20,000 live births, ARPKD is a lot less common than ADPKD and is inherited in an autosomal-recessive manner. Two mutated germline alleles are present from the very beginning causing a very early disease onset due to loss of Fibrocystin function, the protein encoded by the *PKHD1* gene. Increased renal echogeneity and cysts are usually present prenatally and biliary dysgenesis resulting in intrahepatic bile duct dilatation and congenital hepatic fibrosis (Caroli disease) occurs frequently. Fibrocystin co-localises with PKD2 at the ciliary axoneme and the ciliary base; however, its exact function has remained elusive [134].

As outlined above, flow mediated ciliary bending might activate calcium influx and it has been suggested that PKD1 and PKD2 proteins together function as a Ca^{2+}-permeable receptor channel complex [104, 135, 136]. Further, Polycystins interact with the tuberous sclerosis protein Tuberin which is known to influence mTor signalling and the mTor pathway was found to be overactivated in cystic epithelia from Polycystin-deficient kidneys. However, despite major efforts over the past two decades, the exact pathomechanism for cystogenesis in ADPKD and ARPKD remains to be defined and to date, efficient pharmacological treatment remains to be developed. For more details on ciliary signalling pathways please refer to the above sections and the polycystic kidney disease chapter of this book, Chap. 12.

Syndromal Nephronophthisis (NPHP)

For a detailed description of Nephronophthisis, including isolated Nephronophthisis, Joubert Syndrome, Senior-Loken Syndrome and Cogan Syndrome, please refer Chap. 13. Nephronophthisis can be translated as "vanishing nephrons" or "vanishing kidney" and in contrast to ADPKD and ARPKD, where increasing numbers of cysts and increasing cyst volumes lead to larger kidneys, in subjects affected by NPHP or NPHP-like renal disease kidneys appear normal or small in size, often with increased echogenicity in ultrasound images. Many genes

have been identified to date causing either isolated NPHP or NPHP combined with extrarenal symptoms which could be described as "syndromal" NPHP. These extrarenal symptoms include retinal degeneration, cerebellar malformations, skeletal dysplasia including polydactyly, situs inversus, obesity and learning difficulties. There is excessive genetic and phenotypic heterogeneity, meaning that not only the clinical symptoms overlap between different syndromes with NPHP- or NPHP-like renal phenotypes but also mutations in one and the same gene can cause different phenotypes. We will focus in this chapter on selected phenotypes of "syndromal NPHP" including Bardet-Biedl-Syndrome resulting from mutations in BBS genes and ciliary skeletal dysplasias such as Short-rib polydactyly syndrome (SRPS), Jeune Syndrome (JATD), Mainzer-Saldino Syndrome and Sensenbrenner Syndrome (CED), consequences of impaired intraflagellar transport (IFT).

Bardet-Biedl-Syndrome (LMBBS, BBS)

Among the first human ciliopathy diseases recognised as such was Bardet-Biedl-Syndrome (BBS, Laurence-Moon-Bardet-Biedl-Syndrome, LMBBS) and therefore this condition is often referred as an example of a classical complex developmental phenotype resulting from hereditary cilia malfunction. The main features of BBS are polydactyly, developmental delay, obesity, retinal degeneration, cystic or, more commonly, NPHP-like renal disease and hypogenitalism [137]. BBS is very rare with an estimated frequency varying between 1:160,000 in northern European populations to 1:13,500 and 1:17,500 in isolated consanguineous communities such as in Kuwait and Newfoundland. Like other ciliopathies, BBS is a genetically very heterogenous disease with mutations in 19 genes identified to date and there is considerable genetic and phenotypic overlap (especially regarding eyes and kidneys) with other ciliopathies such as Meckel-Gruber-Syndrome and Senior-Loken-syndrome. Perinatally, BBS can be difficult to distinguish from McKusick-Kaufman syndrome if polydactyly and hydrometrocolpos are present [138]. Although BBS represents an autosomal-recessive condition, in individual cases more than two mutated alleles at two different loci have been found to be necessary to cause the phenotype ("triallelic inheritance") [139, 140]. However, the vast majority of cases are inherited in the classical recessive manner [141]. Nevertheless, several "modifier" genes have been described which may influence the phenotype. While genotype-phenotype correlations have proven difficult to establish, mutations in certain genes seem to predispose for more severe kidney involvement. Mutations in *BBS6*, *BBS10* and *BBS12* are associated with renal disease at an overall frequency of 30–86 %; however, this includes minor anomalies and the majority of patients do not progress to renal failure [142].

While some of the proteins encoded by genes mutated in BBS localise to the ciliary transition zone (e.g., CEP290), others localise further proximal to the basal body area and axonemal localisation has been observed as well. BBS proteins seem to form two different major protein complexes: the so-called BBSome and the BBS chaperone complex where the formation of the BBSome requires the function of the BBS chaperone complex. Data from mouse and zebrafish models indicate a role for BBS genes

in intracellular and intraflagellar trafficking of ciliary components. Therefore, although the BBSome does not seem to be required for ciliary assembly itself, due to its trafficking function specific signalling receptors and transmembrane proteins no longer reach the cilium in subjects affected by BBS, leading to organ-specific signalling abnormalities and subsequently the characteristic developmental defects [26, 143, 144]. While the loss of function of BBS and IFT proteins conceivably leads to retinal degeneration due to impaired transport of molecules such as rhodopsin along the connecting cilium between the inner and outer segments of photoreceptor cells, the mechanism for (NPHP-like) renal disease in BBS and IFT-related diseases as largely remains elusive. As discussed above, imbalances in the hippo signalling pathway seem to play a role in classical nephronophthisis. To which extent this applies to BBS has not yet been investigated. While polydactyly in BBS as well as indirectly IFT-dependent disorders point towards a hedgehog-based mechanism at least for the skeletal phenotype, a contribution of misregulated hedgehog signalling to the renal phenotype has yet to be proven. Clinical hallmarks of BBS are shown in Fig. 11.7a–h.

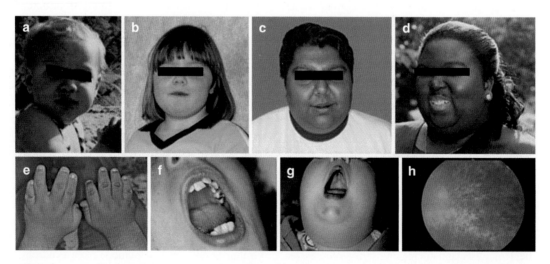

Fig. 11.7 (**a–h**) Clinical hallmarks of Bardet-Biedl-Syndrome (BBS). (**a–d**) Dysmorphic facial features including a flat nasal bridge, retrognathia, small mouth, malar hypoplasia, deep-set eyes, downward slanting palpebral fissures, hypertelorism (**e**) Brachydactyly and scars from removal of accessory digits. (**f**, **g**) High arched palate and dental crowding. (**h**) Rod-cone dystrophy in fundoscopy (All: used with permission of Nature Publishing Group from Forsythe and Beales [145])

Alström Syndrome

Alström syndrome is a very rare autosomal-recessive ciliopathy occurring with a frequency of 1:500,000–1:1,000,000 but can be more common amongst consanguineous populations. Over 100 mutations in a single large gene, *Alms1*, have been published to date. Clinical characteristics include obesity, retinal dysfunction, cardiomyopathy, hearing loss, hepatic involvement, renal disease and hypogonadism, resembling the BBS phenotype; however, with higher lethality due to cardiac complications [146]. In contrast to BBS, polydactyly and developmental delay are not common features. The Alms1 protein localises to the base of the cilium [147] and knockdown of *Alms1* in kidney epithelial cells in vitro causes shortened cilia and seems to abrogate calcium influx in response to mechanical stimuli. In a mouse model of Alström syndrome, loss of cilia from the kidney proximal tubules was observed [148]. *Alms1*-disrupted mice also recapitulate the neurosensory deficits observed in humans with Alström Syndrome and their cochleae display signs of disturbed planar cell polarity abnormal orientation of hair cell stereociliary bundles which seemed to be prematurely lost when the mice grow older [149]. Alms1 has further been implicated in cell cycle control, and intracellular transport as well as the recycling endosome pathway [150]. To which extent disturbance any of these processes contributes to the renal phenotype still requires further investigation.

Joubert-Syndrome Related Disorders (JSRD)

Joubert syndrome (JS) is a very rare neurodevelopmental, mostly autosomal recessive but rarely X-linked disorder characterised by the so-called molar tooth sign (MTS). MTS represents a complex midbrain-hindbrain malformation visible on brain imaging. Anatomical correlate is hypo-dysplasia of the cerebellar vermis, abnormally deep interpeduncular fossa at the level of the isthmus and upper pons, and horizontalized, thickened and elongated superior cerebellar peduncles [151]. The estimated incidence is 1/80,000–1/100,000 live births. Clinically, neurological features such hypotonia at birth, ataxia, developmental delay, abnormal eye movements and neonatal breathing dysregulation are predominant but multiple extra-neurological symptoms occur. JS and Joubert Syndrome related disorders (JSRD) can be classified in six phenotypic subgroups: isolated JS; JS with ocular defect; JS with renal defect; JS with oculo-renal defects; JS with hepatic defect and JS with orofaciodigital defects.

JS/JSRD are genetically heterogenous and there is marked phenotypical variability even within families. JS with renal defect (JS-R) is characterized by additional juvenile nephronophthisis but no retinal disease and mainly caused by mutations in *NPHP* and *RPGRIP1L*. JS with oculo-renal defects (JS-OR) occurs mainly due to mutations in *CEP290*, a transition zone protein encoding gene also found defective in BBS. Mutations in *TMEM67*, a gene also found to cause Meckel-Gruber Syndrome, have been identified in JS with hepatic defects, choreoretinal or optic nerve colobomas and NPH, indicating that Meckel-Gruber Syndrome (MKS) can be clinically regarded as the severe end of the JS spectrum. Genetically, MKS is allelic to JSRD in 7 loci. JS with oro-facio-digital defects (JS-OFD) displays a slightly different phenotype from all of the above with bifid or lobulated tongue (sometimes referred to as hamartomas in the literature), multiple oral frenulae and mesaxial polydactyly with Y-shaped metacarpals and occurs as a consequence of mutations in *TMEM216*. Mutations in this gene can also cause isolated JS as well as MKS and mutations in *C5orf42* have recently been identified in subjects with an OFDVI phenotype in addition to subjects with isolated JS [152–155].

Many of the genes involved in JS/JSRD have been found to localise to the transition zone in cilia where they might exhibit a special gatekeeping function for ciliary protein entry [156]. For more details on the renal phenotype please refer to Chap. 13.

Ciliary Chondrodysplasias

An excellent overview of skeletal chondrodysplasias is given in a recent review article by Huber and Cormier-Daire [157]. Ciliary chondrodysplasias represent a genetically and phenotypically heterogeous group of very rare (1:20,000- <1:1,000,000), mainly autosomal-recessively inherited conditions with the major hallmark of skeletal involvement, mainly short/hypoplastic ribs and polydactyly, but also a variable degree of extraskeletal involvement. While *Short-Rib Polydactyly Syndrome (SRPS)* is inevitably lethal perinatally, 20–60 % lethality has been reported for *Jeune Asphyxiating Thoracic Dystrophy Syndrome (JATD)*. Polydactyly, a ubiquitous feature in SRPS, is rarely observed in JATD. Radiologically, trident acetabulum with spurs is a pathognomic sign for JATD but can also be observed in some SRPS cases as well as Ellis-van Creveld syndrome (EVC). In SRPS, extraskeletal manifestations such as cardiac defects, orofacial clefting, cerebral, renal, liver or pancreatic abnormalities as well has situs inversus have been observed. In JATD, up to 30 % of the patients develop kidney disease, often accompanied by retinal degeneration. Elevated liver enzymes are common but only a handful cases of liver failure have been reported in the literature. Clinical hallmarks of JATD are shown in Fig. 11.8a–f.

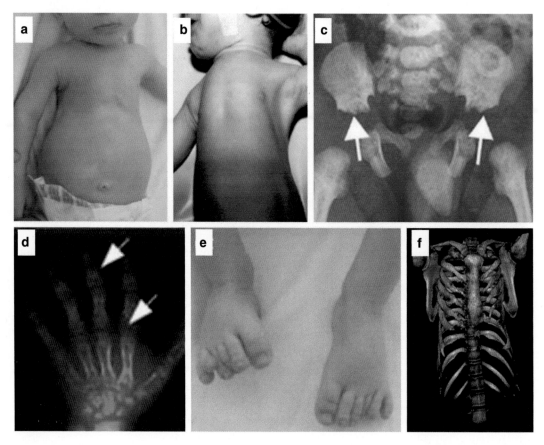

Fig. 11.8 (a–f) Clinical hallmarks of Jeune Syndrome. (a, b) Narrow thorax with short ribs. (c) Trident acetabulum with spurs. (d) Cone shaped epiphyses. (e) Polydactyly (f) 3D-Reconstruction from thoracic CT scan demonstrating long narrow thorax with short ribs (a, e Used with permission from Halbritter et al. [1]; b, c, f Used with permission of BMJ Publishing Group from Schmidts et al. [21]; d Used with permission of John Wiley and Sons from Schmidts et al. [20])

JATD also shares clinical features with *Mainzer-Saldino Syndrome*, which can be described as JATD with obligate renal and retinal disease; both conditions are summarised under "cono-renal syndromes" as cone shaped epiphyses of the phalanges are frequently observed on x-rays [157]. Clinical hallmarks of Mainzer-Saldino-Syndrome are shown in Fig. 11.9a–h.

Mutations in genes encoding several components of the retrograde IFT motor complex dynein-2 such as *DYNC2H1*, *WDR34* and *WDR60* as well as the IFT-B component *IFT80* have been identified in patients with *JATD and SRPS*, indicating that these conditions are allelic and JATD represents the milder end of the SRPS phenotypic spectrum [56, 58, 60–62, 158, 159], Mutations in genes encoding retrograde IFT (IFT-A) components such as *IFT43* [67], *IFT121/WDR35* [65], *IFT122* [63], *IFT139/TTC21B* [68], *IFT144/WDR19* [64] and *IFT140* [20, 69] have likewise been found to cause ciliary chondrodsyplasias with renal involvement such as Sensenbrenner Syndrome/Cranioectodermal Dysplasia (CED), JATD/Mainzer-Saldino Syndrome and SRPS, and isolated Nephronophthisis (*WDR19*). Interestingly,

in contrast to most JATD patients with mutations in genes encoding dynein-2 components who present with a severe thorax phenotype but usually preserved kidney funtion if they survive, the majority of patients described with mutations in IFT-A encoding genes as well as the IFT-B component IFT172 present with a milder thoracic phenotype but experience severe renal involvement with end-stage renal disease [1, 20, 21, 56–69]. In striking contrast to other ciliopathies such as BBS where up to two thirds of affected human subjects carry two null alleles (stop- or frameshift mutations), patients with ciliary chondrodysplasias usually harbour at least 1 missense allele. This is in line with findings from IFT-mutant mouse models where complete loss of IFT-protein function results in early embryonic death before midgestation (see also IFT section of this chapter) and one can assume that this also applies to humans, suggesting a more important role for IFT proteins compared to BBS proteins for ciliary function and embryonic development.

Likewise, human mutations have only been identified in two anterograde IFT (IFT-B) complex components to date: *IFT80* and

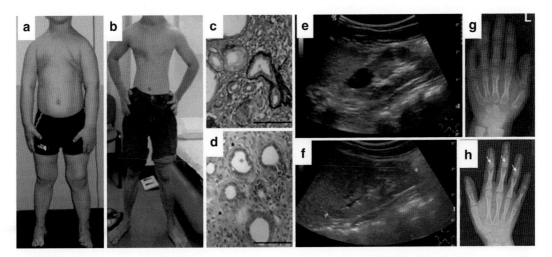

Fig. 11.9 (**a–h**) Clinical hallmarks of Mainzer-Saldino-Syndrome. (**a**, **b**) Mildly narrowed thorax. (**c**, **d**) Histological pictures of a renal biopsy. (**e**, **f**) Ultrasound images showing increased echogeneity and small renal cysts. (**g**, **h**) Cone shaped epiphyses (**b–h** Used with permission of Elsevier from Perrault et al. [69]; **a**, **e–g** Used with permission of John Wiley and Sons from Schmidts et al. [20])

IFT172. While *IFT80* mutations seem to cause a mild thoracic phenotype without extraskeletal involvement [57], *IFT172* mutations lead to a more complex phenotype with renal, liver and retinal involvement [1]. This might be due a more central role of IFT172 within complex-B or could also result from additional roles of IFT172 outside of IFT. The fact that in humans, mutations in more genes encoding IFT-A than IFT-B components have been identified to date again could point to a more essential role of IFT-B compared to IFT-A so that IFT-B mutations might be incompatible with embryonic development beyond very early stages. See also Fig. 11.6a, b for a visualisation of IFT defects observed in fibroblasts from ciliary chondrodysplasia patients.

SRPS can also be caused by mutations in the serine-threonine kinase *NEK1* [160] which acts within the DNA damage response pathway [161]. In humans affected by SRPS, kidney function cannot be followed due to neonatal death from respiratory failure, but mice carrying mutations in *Nek1* exhibit cystic renal disease [162]. Nek1 binds to the kinesin-2 component Kif3a [163], and kidney specific loss of Kif3a causes cystic disease [54]. Moreover, NEK1 and TAZ proteins interact physically to maintain normal levels of Polycystin 2 [164], so it seems possible that surviving patients would present with cystic or nephronophthisis-like renal involvement. Surprisingly, while impaired function of IFT proteins and Kif3a results in cystic kidney disease in mice, the combined knockout of *Kif3a* and *Pkd1* resulted in a milder rather than more severe phenotype, suggesting the existence of a cilia-dependent, as yet unidentified cyst growth promoting pathway [165]. No human mutations have been identified in *KIF3A* or other components of the kinesin-2 complex to date; presumably such mutations would lead to an early embryonic lethal phenotype.

Although mutations in some genes seem to be able to cause both JATD and *Sensenbrenner-Syndrome/CED* as mentioned above, the clinical phenotype is slightly different in CED where additional ectodermal defects such as dysplastic finger- and toe-nail, sparse and slow growing hair and teeth abnormalities are frequently observed. The thoracic phenotype is usually milder than in JATD and polydactyly not usually observed; however, craniosynostosis has been described and human subjects frequently present with renal involvement [166]. Clinical hallmarks of Sensenbrenner syndrome are shown in Fig. 11.10a–c.

While the skeletal features observed in skeletal chondrodysplasias, especially polydactyly, point towards imbalances in the hedgehog pathway as a molecular origin of disease, the molecular pathogenesis of renal disease in subjects with IFT and dynein-2 mutations has remained elusive as neither hedgehog- nor wnt signalling defects could be established as causative for the kidney phenotype in mouse models (see the IFT and hedgehog signalling sections of this chapter for more details). However, given the NPHP-like phenotype observed, hippo signalling might be a good candidate pathway leading to the renal phenotype in this group of ciliopathies.

Summary and Conclusion

Cilia are antenna-like structures projecting from most cells and hundreds of years after their first notion, we begin to acknowledge some of their essential function in human development, including the kidney. Extensive phenotypic and genetic heterogeneity has created a slightly chaotic picture of ciliopathies in the past and many aspects of these complex inherited conditions have remained unclear. Despite linking ciliopathies to imbalances in multiple fundamental cell signalling pathways, the molecular basis of disease, especially kidney mal-development, is still largely elusive to date.

Acknowledgment We apologize to all colleagues whose findings could not be cited due to space constraints. Miriam Schmidts and Philip L. Beales acknowledge funding from the Dutch Kidney Foundation, DKF (KOUNCII, CP11.18). Miriam Schmidts is funded by an Action Medical Research UK Clinical Training Fellowship (RTF-1411) and Philip L. Beales receives funding from the European Community's Seventh Framework Programme FP7/2009; 241955, SYSCILIA, the Wellcome Trust and is an NIHR Senior Investigator.

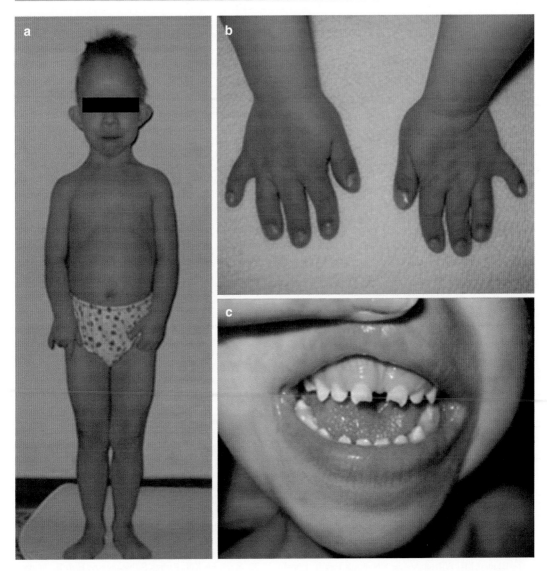

Fig. 11.10 (**a–c**) Clinical hallmarks of Sensenbrenner Syndrome (CED). Four-year-old girl displaying short extremities, mildly shortened and narrowed thorax, thin sparse hair, dolichocephaly, prominent forehead, full, hypertelorism, small flat nose, prominent auricles (**a**). (**b**) Brachydactyly. (**c**) Small abnormally shaped teeth (All: used with permission of Elsevier from Walczak-Sztulpa et al. [63])

References

1. Halbritter J, Bizet AA, Schmidts M, Porath JD, Braun DA, Gee HY, et al. Defects in the IFT-B component IFT172 cause Jeune and Mainzer-Saldino syndromes in humans. Am J Hum Genet. 2013; 93(5):915–25.
2. Westhoff JH, Giselbrecht S, Schmidts M, Schindler S, Beales PL, Tonshoff B, et al. Development of an automated imaging pipeline for the analysis of the zebrafish larval kidney. PLoS ONE. 2013;8(12): e82137.
3. Wheatley DN. Landmarks in the first hundred years of primary (9 + 0) cilium research. Cell Biol Int. 2005;29(5):333–9.
4. G PJaV. De phaenomeno generali et fundamentali motus vibratorii continui in membranis cum externis tum internis animalium plurimorum et superiorum et inferiorum ordinum obvii. In: A S, editor. Commentatio Physiologica. Wratislaviae1835.
5. Afzelius BA. The immotile-cilia syndrome and other ciliary diseases. Int Rev Exp Pathol. 1979;19:1–43.
6. Murcia NS, Richards WG, Yoder BK, Mucenski ML, Dunlap JR, Woychik RP. The Oak Ridge Polycystic Kidney (orpk) disease gene is required

for left-right axis determination. Development. 2000;127(11):2347–55.

7. Pazour GJ, Dickert BL, Vucica Y, Seeley ES, Rosenbaum JL, Witman GB, et al. Chlamydomonas IFT88 and its mouse homologue, polycystic kidney disease gene tg737, are required for assembly of cilia and flagella. J Cell Biol. 2000;151(3): 709–18.

8. Fliegauf M, Benzing T, Omran H. When cilia go bad: cilia defects and ciliopathies. Nat Rev Mol Cell Biol. 2007;8(11):880–93.

9. Baker K, Beales PL. Making sense of cilia in disease: the human ciliopathies. Am J Med Genet C: Semin Med Genet. 2009;151C(4):281–95.

10. Hildebrandt F, Benzing T, Katsanis N. Ciliopathies. N Engl J Med. 2011;364(16):1533–43.

11. Gilula NB, Satir P. The ciliary necklace. A ciliary membrane specialization. J Cell Biol. 1972;53(2): 494–509.

12. Fliegauf M, Horvath J, von Schnakenburg C, Olbrich H, Muller D, Thumfart J, et al. Nephrocystin specifically localizes to the transition zone of renal and respiratory cilia and photoreceptor connecting cilia. J Am Soc Nephrol. 2006;17(9):2424–33.

13. Shiba D, Yamaoka Y, Hagiwara H, Takamatsu T, Hamada H, Yokoyama T. Localization of Inv in a distinctive intraciliary compartment requires the C-terminal ninein-homolog-containing region. J Cell Sci. 2009;122(Pt 1):44–54.

14. Wheatley DN. Cilia and centrioles of the rat adrenal cortex. J Anat. 1967;101(Pt 2):223–37.

15. Wheatley DN. Primary cilia in normal and pathological tissues. Pathobiology. 1995;63(4):222–38.

16. Goetz SC, Ocbina PJ, Anderson KV. The primary cilium as a Hedgehog signal transduction machine. Methods Cell Biol. 2009;94:199–222.

17. Huangfu D, Liu A, Rakeman AS, Murcia NS, Niswander L, Anderson KV. Hedgehog signalling in the mouse requires intraflagellar transport proteins. Nature. 2003;426(6962):83–7.

18. Ruiz-Perez VL, Blair HJ, Rodriguez-Andres ME, Blanco MJ, Wilson A, Liu YN, et al. Evc is a positive mediator of Ihh-regulated bone growth that localises at the base of chondrocyte cilia. Development. 2007;134(16):2903–12.

19. Quinlan RJ, Tobin JL, Beales PL. Modeling ciliopathies: primary cilia in development and disease. Curr Top Dev Biol. 2008;84:249–310.

20. Schmidts M, Frank V, Eisenberger T, Al Turki S, Bizet AA, Antony D, et al. Combined NGS approaches identify mutations in the intraflagellar transport gene IFT140 in skeletal ciliopathies with early progressive kidney disease. Hum Mutat. 2013;34(5):714–24.

21. Schmidts M, Arts HH, Bongers EM, Yap Z, Oud MM, Antony D, et al. Exome sequencing identifies DYNC2H1 mutations as a common cause of asphyxiating thoracic dystrophy (Jeune syndrome) without major polydactyly, renal or retinal involvement. J Med Genet. 2013;50(5):309–23.

22. Williams CL, Li C, Kida K, Inglis PN, Mohan S, Semenec L, et al. MKS and NPHP modules cooperate to establish basal body/transition zone membrane associations and ciliary gate function during ciliogenesis. J Cell Biol. 2011;192(6):1023–41.

23. Reiter JF, Blacque OE, Leroux MR. The base of the cilium: roles for transition fibres and the transition zone in ciliary formation, maintenance and compartmentalization. EMBO Rep. 2012;13(7): 608–18.

24. Rohatgi R, Snell WJ. The ciliary membrane. Curr Opin Cell Biol. 2010;22(4):541–6.

25. Rosenbaum J. Intraflagellar transport. Curr Biol. 2002;12(4):R125.

26. Nachury MV, Loktev AV, Zhang Q, Westlake CJ, Peranen J, Merdes A, et al. A core complex of BBS proteins cooperates with the GTPase Rab8 to promote ciliary membrane biogenesis. Cell. 2007;129(6): 1201–13.

27. Jin H, White SR, Shida T, Schulz S, Aguiar M, Gygi SP, et al. The conserved Bardet-Biedl syndrome proteins assemble a coat that traffics membrane proteins to cilia. Cell. 2010;141(7):1208–19.

28. Poole CA, Flint MH, Beaumont BW. Analysis of the morphology and function of primary cilia in connective tissues: a cellular cybernetic probe? Cell Motil. 1985;5(3):175–93.

29. Sorokin S. Centrioles and the formation of rudimentary cilia by fibroblasts and smooth muscle cells. J Cell Biol. 1962;15:363–77.

30. Rattner JB, Sciore P, Ou Y, van der Hoorn FA, Lo IK. Primary cilia in fibroblast-like type B synoviocytes lie within a cilium pit: a site of endocytosis. Histol Histopathol. 2010;25(7):865–75.

31. Ghossoub R, Molla-Herman A, Bastin P, Benmerah A. The ciliary pocket: a once-forgotten membrane domain at the base of cilia. Biol Cell. 2011;103(3): 131–44.

32. Avasthi P, Marshall WF. Stages of ciliogenesis and regulation of ciliary length. Differentiation. 2012;83(2):S30–42.

33. Schmidt KN, Kuhns S, Neuner A, Hub B, Zentgraf H, Pereira G. Cep164 mediates vesicular docking to the mother centriole during early steps of ciliogenesis. J Cell Biol. 2012;199(7):1083–101.

34. Chaki M, Airik R, Ghosh AK, Giles RH, Chen R, Slaats GG, et al. Exome capture reveals ZNF423 and CEP164 mutations, linking renal ciliopathies to DNA damage response signaling. Cell. 2012;150(3):533–48.

35. Kim S, Dynlacht BD. Assembling a primary cilium. Curr Opin Cell Biol. 2013;25(4):506–11.

36. Shida T, Cueva JG, Xu Z, Goodman MB, Nachury MV. The major alpha-tubulin K40 acetyltransferase alphaTAT1 promotes rapid ciliogenesis and efficient mechanosensation. Proc Natl Acad Sci U S A. 2010;107(50):21517–22.

37. Kalebic N, Sorrentino S, Perlas E, Bolasco G, Martinez C, Heppenstall PA. alphaTAT1 is the major alpha-tubulin acetyltransferase in mice. Nat Commun. 2013;4:1962.

38. O'Hagan R, Barr MM. Regulation of tubulin glutamylation plays cell-specific roles in the function and stability of sensory cilia. Worm. 2012;1(3):155–9.

39. Pathak N, Obara T, Mangos S, Liu Y, Drummond IA. The zebrafish fleer gene encodes an essential regulator of cilia tubulin polyglutamylation. Mol Biol Cell. 2007;18(11):4353–64.

40. Thomas S, Wright KJ, Le Corre S, Micalizzi A, Romani M, Abhyankar A, et al. A homozygous PDE6D mutation in Joubert syndrome impairs targeting of farnesylated INPP5E protein to the primary cilium. Hum Mutat. 2014;35(1):137–46.

41. Paridaen JT, Wilsch-Brauninger M, Huttner WB. Asymmetric inheritance of centrosome-associated primary cilium membrane directs ciliogenesis after cell division. Cell. 2013;155(2):333–44.

42. Wang G, Chen Q, Zhang X, Zhang B, Zhuo X, Liu J, et al. PCM1 recruits Plk1 to the pericentriolar matrix to promote primary cilia disassembly before mitotic entry. J Cell Sci. 2013;126(Pt 6):1355–65.

43. Norris DP, Grimes DT. Mouse models of ciliopathies: the state of the art. Dis Model Mech. 2012; 5(3):299–312.

44. Delaval B, Bright A, Lawson ND, Doxsey S. The cilia protein IFT88 is required for spindle orientation in mitosis. Nat Cell Biol. 2011;13(4):461–8.

45. Pan J, Seeger-Nukpezah T, Golemis EA. The role of the cilium in normal and abnormal cell cycles: emphasis on renal cystic pathologies. Cell Mol Life Sci. 2013;70(11):1849–74.

46. Bielas SL, Silhavy JL, Brancati F, Kisseleva MV, Al-Gazali L, Sztriha L, et al. Mutations in INPP5E, encoding inositol polyphosphate-5-phosphatase E, link phosphatidyl inositol signaling to the ciliopathies. Nat Genet. 2009;41(9):1032–6.

47. Jacoby M, Cox JJ, Gayral S, Hampshire DJ, Ayub M, Blockmans M, et al. INPP5E mutations cause primary cilium signaling defects, ciliary instability and ciliopathies in human and mouse. Nat Genet. 2009;41(9):1027–31.

48. Xu J, Li H, Wang B, Xu Y, Yang J, Zhang X, et al. VHL inactivation induces HEF1 and Aurora kinase A. J Am Soc Nephrol. 2010;21(12):2041–6.

49. Choi HJ, Lin JR, Vannier JB, Slaats GG, Kile AC, Paulsen RD, et al. NEK8 links the ATR-regulated replication stress response and S phase CDK activity to renal ciliopathies. Mol Cell. 2013;51(4):423–39.

50. Kozminski KG, Johnson KA, Forscher P, Rosenbaum JL. A motility in the eukaryotic flagellum unrelated to flagellar beating. Proc Natl Acad Sci U S A. 1993;90(12):5519–23.

51. Cole DG, Diener DR, Himelblau AL, Beech PL, Fuster JC, Rosenbaum JL. Chlamydomonas kinesin-II-dependent intraflagellar transport (IFT): IFT particles contain proteins required for ciliary assembly in Caenorhabditis elegans sensory neurons. J Cell Biol. 1998;141(4):993–1008.

52. Pazour GJ, Rosenbaum JL. Intraflagellar transport and cilia-dependent diseases. Trends Cell Biol. 2002;12(12):551–5.

53. Cole DG, Snell WJ. SnapShot: intraflagellar transport. Cell. 2009;137(4):784–e1.

54. Lin F, Hiesberger T, Cordes K, Sinclair AM, Goldstein LS, Somlo S, et al. Kidney-specific inactivation of the KIF3A subunit of kinesin-II inhibits renal ciliogenesis and produces polycystic kidney disease. Proc Natl Acad Sci U S A. 2003;100(9): 5286–91.

55. Jonassen JA, SanAgustin J, Baker SP, Pazour GJ. Disruption of IFT complex A causes cystic kidneys without mitotic spindle misorientation. J Am Soc Nephrol. 2012;23(4):641–51.

56. Dagoneau N, Goulet M, Genevieve D, Sznajer Y, Martinovic J, Smithson S, et al. DYNC2H1 mutations cause asphyxiating thoracic dystrophy and short rib-polydactyly syndrome, type III. Am J Hum Genet. 2009;84(5):706–11.

57. Beales PL, Bland E, Tobin JL, Bacchelli C, Tuysuz B, Hill J, et al. IFT80, which encodes a conserved intraflagellar transport protein, is mutated in Jeune asphyxiating thoracic dystrophy. Nat Genet. 2007;39(6):727–9.

58. Merrill AE, Merriman B, Farrington-Rock C, Camacho N, Sebald ET, Funari VA, et al. Ciliary abnormalities due to defects in the retrograde transport protein DYNC2H1 in short-rib polydactyly syndrome. Am J Hum Genet. 2009;84(4):542–9.

59. Baujat G, Huber C, El Hokayem J, Caumes R, Do Ngoc Thanh C, David A, et al. Asphyxiating thoracic dysplasia: clinical and molecular review of 39 families. J Med Genet. 2013;50(2):91–8.

60. McInerney-Leo AM, Schmidts M, Cortes CR, Leo PJ, Gener B, Courtney AD, et al. Short-rib polydactyly and Jeune syndromes are caused by mutations in WDR60. Am J Hum Genet. 2013;93(3):515–23.

61. Schmidts M, Vodopiutz J, Christou-Savina S, Cortes CR, McInerney-Leo AM, Emes RD, et al. Mutations in the gene encoding IFT dynein complex component WDR34 cause Jeune asphyxiating thoracic dystrophy. Am J Hum Genet. 2013;93(5):932–44.

62. Huber C, Wu S, Kim AS, Sigaudy S, Sarukhanov A, Serre V, et al. WDR34 mutations that cause short-rib polydactyly syndrome type III/severe asphyxiating thoracic dysplasia reveal a role for the NF-kappaB pathway in cilia. Am J Hum Genet. 2013;93(5): 926–31.

63. Walczak-Sztulpa J, Eggenschwiler J, Osborn D, Brown DA, Emma F, Klingenberg C, et al. Cranioectodermal Dysplasia, Sensenbrenner syndrome, is a ciliopathy caused by mutations in the IFT122 gene. Am J Hum Genet. 2010;86(6):949–56.

64. Bredrup C, Saunier S, Oud MM, Fiskerstrand T, Hoischen A, Brackman D, et al. Ciliopathies with skeletal anomalies and renal insufficiency due to mutations in the IFT-A gene WDR19. Am J Hum Genet. 2011;89(5):634–43.

65. Gilissen C, Arts HH, Hoischen A, Spruijt L, Mans DA, Arts P, et al. Exome sequencing identifies WDR35 variants involved in Sensenbrenner syndrome. Am J Hum Genet. 2010;87(3):418–23.

66. Mill P, Lockhart PJ, Fitzpatrick E, Mountford HS, Hall EA, Reijns MA, et al. Human and mouse mutations in WDR35 cause short-rib polydactyly syndromes due to abnormal ciliogenesis. Am J Hum Genet. 2011;88(4):508–15.

67. Arts HH, Bongers EM, Mans DA, van Beersum SE, Oud MM, Bolat E, et al. C14ORF179 encoding IFT43 is mutated in Sensenbrenner syndrome. J Med Genet. 2011;48(6):390–5.

68. Davis EE, Zhang Q, Liu Q, Diplas BH, Davey LM, Hartley J, et al. TTC21B contributes both causal and modifying alleles across the ciliopathy spectrum. Nat Genet. 2011;43(3):189–96.

69. Perrault I, Saunier S, Hanein S, Filhol E, Bizet AA, Collins F, et al. Mainzer-Saldino syndrome is a ciliopathy caused by IFT140 mutations. Am J Hum Genet. 2012;90(5):864–70.

70. Aldahmesh MA, Li Y, Alhashem A, Anazi S, Alkuraya H, Hashem M, et al. IFT27, encoding a small GTPase component of IFT particles, is mutated in a consanguineous family with Bardet-Biedl syndrome. Hum Mol Genet. 2014;23(12):3307–15.

71. Eggenschwiler JT, Anderson KV. Cilia and developmental signaling. Annu Rev Cell Dev Biol. 2007;23: 345–73.

72. Goetz SC, Anderson KV. The primary cilium: a signalling centre during vertebrate development. Nat Rev Genet. 2010;11(5):331–44.

73. Huangfu D, Anderson KV. Cilia and Hedgehog responsiveness in the mouse. Proc Natl Acad Sci U S A. 2005;102(32):11325–30.

74. Kronenberg HM. Developmental regulation of the growth plate. Nature. 2003;423(6937):332–6.

75. Ocbina PJ, Eggenschwiler JT, Moskowitz I, Anderson KV. Complex interactions between genes controlling trafficking in primary cilia. Nat Genet. 2011;43(6):547–53.

76. Rix S, Calmont A, Scambler PJ, Beales PL. An Ift80 mouse model of short rib polydactyly syndromes shows defects in hedgehog signalling without loss or malformation of cilia. Hum Mol Genet. 2011;20(7): 1306–14.

77. Ashe A, Butterfield NC, Town L, Courtney AD, Cooper AN, Ferguson C, et al. Mutations in mouse Ift144 model the craniofacial, limb and rib defects in skeletal ciliopathies. Hum Mol Genet. 2012;21(8): 1808–23.

78. Hu MC, Mo R, Bhella S, Wilson CW, Chuang PT, Hui CC, et al. GLI3-dependent transcriptional repression of Gli1, Gli2 and kidney patterning genes disrupts renal morphogenesis. Development. 2006; 133(3):569–78.

79. Kelley RI, Hennekam RC. The Smith-Lemli-Opitz syndrome. J Med Genet. 2000;37(5):321–35 [Review].

80. Friedland-Little JM, Hoffmann AD, Ocbina PJ, Peterson MA, Bosman JD, Chen Y, et al. A novel murine allele of intraflagellar transport protein 172 causes a syndrome including VACTERL-like features with hydrocephalus. Hum Mol Genet. 2011;20(19):3725–37.

81. Wallingford JB, Mitchell B. Strange as it may seem: the many links between Wnt signaling, planar cell polarity, and cilia. Genes Dev. 2011;25(3):201–13.

82. van Amerongen R, Nusse R. Towards an integrated view of Wnt signaling in development. Development. 2009;136(19):3205–14.

83. Vladar EK, Antic D, Axelrod JD. Planar cell polarity signaling: the developing cell's compass. Cold Spring Harb Perspect Biol. 2009;1(3):a002964.

84. Ross AJ, May-Simera H, Eichers ER, Kai M, Hill J, Jagger DJ, et al. Disruption of Bardet-Biedl syndrome ciliary proteins perturbs planar cell polarity in vertebrates. Nat Genet. 2005;37(10):1135–40.

85. Simons M, Gloy J, Ganner A, Bullerkotte A, Bashkurov M, Kronig C, et al. Inversin, the gene product mutated in nephronophthisis type II, functions as a molecular switch between Wnt signaling pathways. Nat Genet. 2005;37(5):537–43.

86. Gerdes JM, Liu Y, Zaghloul NA, Leitch CC, Lawson SS, Kato M, et al. Disruption of the basal body compromises proteasomal function and perturbs intracellular Wnt response. Nat Genet. 2007;39(11): 1350–60.

87. Corbit KC, Shyer AE, Dowdle WE, Gaulden J, Singla V, Chen MH, et al. Kif3a constrains beta-catenin-dependent Wnt signalling through dual ciliary and non-ciliary mechanisms. Nat Cell Biol. 2008;10(1):70–6.

88. Jonassen JA, San Agustin J, Follit JA, Pazour GJ. Deletion of IFT20 in the mouse kidney causes misorientation of the mitotic spindle and cystic kidney disease. J Cell Biol. 2008;183(3):377–84.

89. Ocbina PJ, Tuson M, Anderson KV. Primary cilia are not required for normal canonical Wnt signaling in the mouse embryo. PLoS ONE. 2009;4(8):e6839.

90. Huang P, Schier AF. Dampened Hedgehog signaling but normal Wnt signaling in zebrafish without cilia. Development. 2009;136(18):3089–98.

91. Jones C, Roper VC, Foucher I, Qian D, Banizs B, Petit C, et al. Ciliary proteins link basal body polarization to planar cell polarity regulation. Nat Genet. 2008;40(1):69–77.

92. Karner CM, Chirumamilla R, Aoki S, Igarashi P, Wallingford JB, Carroll TJ. Wnt9b signaling regulates planar cell polarity and kidney tubule morphogenesis. Nat Genet. 2009;41(7):793–9.

93. Kotsis F, Boehlke C, Kuehn EW. The ciliary flow sensor and polycystic kidney disease. Nephrol Dial Transplant. 2013;28(3):518–26.

94. Patel V, Li L, Cobo-Stark P, Shao X, Somlo S, Lin F, et al. Acute kidney injury and aberrant planar cell polarity induce cyst formation in mice lacking renal cilia. Hum Mol Genet. 2008;17(11):1578–90.

95. Bonnet CS, Aldred M, von Ruhland C, Harris R, Sandford R, Cheadle JP. Defects in cell polarity underlie TSC and ADPKD-associated cystogenesis. Hum Mol Genet. 2009;18(12):2166–76.

96. Verdeguer F, Le Corre S, Fischer E, Callens C, Garbay S, Doyen A, et al. A mitotic transcriptional switch in polycystic kidney disease. Nat Med. 2010;16(1):106–10.

97. Park TJ, Mitchell BJ, Abitua PB, Kintner C, Wallingford JB. Dishevelled controls apical docking and planar polarization of basal bodies in ciliated epithelial cells. Nat Genet. 2008;40(7):871–9.

98. Ganner A, Lienkamp S, Schafer T, Romaker D, Wegierski T, Park TJ, et al. Regulation of ciliary polarity by the APC/C. Proc Natl Acad Sci U S A. 2009;106(42):17799–804.

99. Nishio S, Tian X, Gallagher AR, Yu Z, Patel V, Igarashi P, et al. Loss of oriented cell division does not initiate cyst formation. J Am Soc Nephrol. 2010;21(2):295–302.

100. PMID 23143599 Nat Genet 2012;44(12):1382–7. doi:10.1038/ng.2452

101. Praetorius HA, Spring KR. Bending the MDCK cell primary cilium increases intracellular calcium. J Membr Biol. 2001;184(1):71–9.

102. Praetorius HA, Spring KR. Removal of the MDCK cell primary cilium abolishes flow sensing. J Membr Biol. 2003;191(1):69–76.

103. Liu W, Murcia NS, Duan Y, Weinbaum S, Yoder BK, Schwiebert E, et al. Mechanoregulation of intracellular Ca2+ concentration is attenuated in collecting duct of monocilium-impaired orpk mice. Am J Physiol Renal Physiol. 2005;289(5):F978–88.

104. Nauli SM, Alenghat FJ, Luo Y, Williams E, Vassilev P, Li X, et al. Polycystins 1 and 2 mediate mechanosensation in the primary cilium of kidney cells. Nat Genet. 2003;33(2):129–37.

105. Xu C, Rossetti S, Jiang L, Harris PC, Brown-Glaberman U, Wandinger-Ness A, et al. Human ADPKD primary cyst epithelial cells with a novel, single codon deletion in the PKD1 gene exhibit defective ciliary polycystin localization and loss of flow-induced Ca2+ signaling. Am J Physiol Renal Physiol. 2007;292(3):F930–45.

106. Cowley Jr BD. Calcium, cyclic AMP, and MAP kinases: dysregulation in polycystic kidney disease. Kidney Int. 2008;73(3):251–3.

107. Xia S, Li X, Johnson T, Seidel C, Wallace DP, Li R. Polycystin-dependent fluid flow sensing targets histone deacetylase 5 to prevent the development of renal cysts. Development. 2010;137(7):1075–84.

108. Inoki K, Li Y, Zhu T, Wu J, Guan KL. TSC2 is phosphorylated and inhibited by Akt and suppresses mTOR signalling. Nat Cell Biol. 2002;4(9):648–57.

109. Shillingford JM, Murcia NS, Larson CH, Low SH, Hedgepeth R, Brown N, et al. The mTOR pathway is regulated by polycystin-1, and its inhibition reverses renal cystogenesis in polycystic kidney disease. Proc Natl Acad Sci U S A. 2006;103(14):5466–71.

110. Distefano G, Boca M, Rowe I, Wodarczyk C, Ma L, Piontek KB, et al. Polycystin-1 regulates extracellular signal-regulated kinase-dependent phosphorylation of tuberin to control cell size through mTOR

and its downstream effectors S6K and 4EBP1. Mol Cell Biol. 2009;29(9):2359–71.

111. Tao Y, Kim J, Schrier RW, Edelstein CL. Rapamycin markedly slows disease progression in a rat model of polycystic kidney disease. J Am Soc Nephrol. 2005;16(1):46–51.

112. Walz G, Budde K, Mannaa M, Nurnberger J, Wanner C, Sommerer C, et al. Everolimus in patients with autosomal dominant polycystic kidney disease. N Engl J Med. 2010;363(9):830–40.

113. Boehlke C, Kotsis F, Patel V, Braeg S, Voelker H, Bredt S, et al. Primary cilia regulate mTORC1 activity and cell size through Lkb1. Nat Cell Biol. 2010;12(11):1115–22.

114. Yuan S, Li J, Diener DR, Choma MA, Rosenbaum JL, Sun Z. Target-of-rapamycin complex 1 (Torc1) signaling modulates cilia size and function through protein synthesis regulation. Proc Natl Acad Sci U S A. 2012;109(6):2021–6.

115. Johnson R, Halder G. The two faces of Hippo: targeting the Hippo pathway for regenerative medicine and cancer treatment. Nat Rev Drug Discov. 2014;13(1):63–79.

116. Morin-Kensicki EM, Boone BN, Howell M, Stonebraker JR, Teed J, Alb JG, et al. Defects in yolk sac vasculogenesis, chorioallantoic fusion, and embryonic axis elongation in mice with targeted disruption of Yap65. Mol Cell Biol. 2006;26(1):77–87.

117. Williamson KA, Rainger J, Floyd JA, Ansari M, Meynert A, Aldridge KV, et al. Heterozygous loss-of-function mutations in YAP1 cause both isolated and syndromic optic fissure closure defects. Am J Hum Genet. 2014;94(2):295–302.

118. Hossain Z, Ali SM, Ko HL, Xu J, Ng CP, Guo K, et al. Glomerulocystic kidney disease in mice with a targeted inactivation of Wwtr1. Proc Natl Acad Sci U S A. 2007;104(5):1631–6.

119. Makita R, Uchijima Y, Nishiyama K, Amano T, Chen Q, Takeuchi T, et al. Multiple renal cysts, urinary concentration defects, and pulmonary emphysematous changes in mice lacking TAZ. Am J Physiol Renal Physiol. 2008;294(3):F542–53.

120. Habbig S, Bartram MP, Muller RU, Schwarz R, Andriopoulos N, Chen S, et al. NPHP4, a cilia-associated protein, negatively regulates the Hippo pathway. J Cell Biol. 2011;193(4):633–42.

121. Frank V, Habbig S, Bartram MP, Eisenberger T, Veenstra-Knol HE, Decker C, et al. Mutations in NEK8 link multiple organ dysplasia with altered Hippo signalling and increased c-MYC expression. Hum Mol Genet. 2013;22(11):2177–85.

122. Habbig S, Bartram MP, Sagmuller JG, Griessmann A, Franke M, Muller RU, et al. The ciliopathy disease protein NPHP9 promotes nuclear delivery and activation of the oncogenic transcriptional regulator TAZ. Hum Mol Genet. 2012;21(26):5528–38.

123. Rosenbluh J, Nijhawan D, Cox AG, Li X, Neal JT, Schafer EJ, et al. beta-Catenin-driven cancers require a YAP1 transcriptional complex for

survival and tumorigenesis. Cell. 2012;151(7): 1457–73.

124. Aragon E, Goerner N, Xi Q, Gomes T, Gao S, Massague J, et al. Structural basis for the versatile interactions of Smad7 with regulator WW domains in TGF-beta pathways. Structure. 2012;20(10):1726–36.

125. Tschaharganeh DF, Chen X, Latzko P, Malz M, Gaida MM, Felix K, et al. Yes-associated protein up-regulates jagged-1 and activates the notch pathway in human hepatocellular carcinoma. Gastroenterology. 2013;144(7):1530–42.e12.

126. Fernandez LA, Northcott PA, Dalton J, Fraga C, Ellison D, Angers S, et al. YAP1 is amplified and up-regulated in hedgehog-associated medulloblastomas and mediates sonic hedgehog-driven neural precursor proliferation. Genes Dev. 2009;23(23): 2729–41.

127. Shimobayashi M, Hall MN. Making new contacts: the mTOR network in metabolism and signalling crosstalk. Nat Rev Mol Cell Biol. 2014;15(3): 155–62.

128. Christensen ST, Pedersen SF, Satir P, Veland IR, Schneider L. The primary cilium coordinates signaling pathways in cell cycle control and migration during development and tissue repair. Curr Top Dev Biol. 2008;85:261–301.

129. Satir P, Pedersen LB, Christensen ST. The primary cilium at a glance. J Cell Sci. 2010;123(Pt 4): 499–503.

130. Clement CA, Ajbro KD, Koefoed K, Vestergaard ML, Veland IR, Henriques de Jesus MP, et al. TGF-beta signaling is associated with endocytosis at the pocket region of the primary cilium. Cell Rep. 2013;3(6):1806–14.

131. Liu Y, Dai B, Xu C, Fu L, Hua Z, Mei C. Rosiglitazone inhibits transforming growth factor-beta1 mediated fibrogenesis in ADPKD cyst-lining epithelial cells. PLoS ONE. 2011;6(12):e28915.

132. Guay-Woodford LM. Renal cystic diseases: diverse phenotypes converge on the cilium/centrosome complex. Pediatr Nephrol. 2006;21(10):1369–76.

133. Kleffmann J, Frank V, Ferbert A, Bergmann C. Dosage-sensitive network in polycystic kidney and liver disease: multiple mutations cause severe hepatic and neurological complications. J Hepatol. 2012;57(2):476–7.

134. Harris PC, Torres VE. Polycystic kidney disease. Annu Rev Med. 2009;60:321–37.

135. Mochizuki T, Wu G, Hayashi T, Xenophontos SL, Veldhuisen B, Saris JJ, et al. PKD2, a gene for polycystic kidney disease that encodes an integral membrane protein. Science. 1996;272(5266):1339–42.

136. Hughes J, Ward CJ, Peral B, Aspinwall R, Clark K, San Millan JL, et al. The polycystic kidney disease 1 (PKD1) gene encodes a novel protein with multiple cell recognition domains. Nat Genet. 1995;10(2): 151–60.

137. Beales PL, Elcioglu N, Woolf AS, Parker D, Flinter FA. New criteria for improved diagnosis of Bardet-

Biedl syndrome: results of a population survey. J Med Genet. 1999;36(6):437–46.

138. Forsythe E, Beales PL. Bardet-Biedl syndrome. Eur J Hum Genet. 2013;21(1):8–13.

139. Katsanis N, Ansley SJ, Badano JL, Eichers ER, Lewis RA, Hoskins BE, et al. Triallelic inheritance in Bardet-Biedl syndrome, a Mendelian recessive disorder. Science. 2001;293(5538):2256–9.

140. Eichers ER, Lewis RA, Katsanis N, Lupski JR. Triallelic inheritance: a bridge between Mendelian and multifactorial traits. Ann Med. 2004;36(4):262–72.

141. Redin C, Le Gras S, Mhamdi O, Geoffroy V, Stoetzel C, Vincent MC, et al. Targeted high-throughput sequencing for diagnosis of genetically heterogeneous diseases: efficient mutation detection in Bardet-Biedl and Alstrom syndromes. J Med Genet. 2012;49(8):502–12.

142. Imhoff O, Marion V, Stoetzel C, Durand M, Holder M, Sigaudy S, et al. Bardet-Biedl syndrome: a study of the renal and cardiovascular phenotypes in a French cohort. Clin J Am Soc Nephrol. 2011;6(1): 22–9.

143. Sheffield VC. The blind leading the obese: the molecular pathophysiology of a human obesity syndrome. Trans Am Clin Climatol Assoc. 2010;121: 172–81; discussion 81–2.

144. Nachury MV, Seeley ES, Jin H. Trafficking to the ciliary membrane: how to get across the periciliary diffusion barrier? Annu Rev Cell Dev Biol. 2010;26:59–87.

145. Forsythe E, Beales PL. Bardet Biedl syndrome. Eur J Hum Gen. 2012;21:8–13.

146. Marshall JD, Maffei P, Beck S, Barrett TG, Paisey R, Naggert JK. Clinical utility gene card for: Alstrom Syndrome – update 2013. Eur J Hum Genet. 2013;21(11).

147. Hearn T, Spalluto C, Phillips VJ, Renforth GL, Copin N, Hanley NA, et al. Subcellular localization of ALMS1 supports involvement of centrosome and basal body dysfunction in the pathogenesis of obesity, insulin resistance, and type 2 diabetes. Diabetes. 2005;54(5):1581–7.

148. Li G, Vega R, Nelms K, Gekakis N, Goodnow C, McNamara P, et al. A role for Alstrom syndrome protein, alms1, in kidney ciliogenesis and cellular quiescence. PLoS Genet. 2007;3(1):e8.

149. Jagger D, Collin G, Kelly J, Towers E, Nevill G, Longo-Guess C, et al. Alstrom syndrome protein ALMS1 localizes to basal bodies of cochlear hair cells and regulates cilium-dependent planar cell polarity. Hum Mol Genet. 2011;20(3):466–81.

150. Collin GB, Marshall JD, King BL, Milan G, Maffei P, Jagger DJ, et al. The Alstrom syndrome protein, ALMS1, interacts with alpha-actinin and components of the endosome recycling pathway. PLoS ONE. 2012;7(5):e37925.

151. Maria BL, Quisling RG, Rosainz LC, Yachnis AT, Gitten J, Dede D, et al. Molar tooth sign in Joubert

syndrome: clinical, radiologic, and pathologic significance. J Child Neurol. 1999;14(6):368–76.

152. Brancati F, Dallapiccola B, Valente EM. Joubert syndrome and related disorders. Orphanet J Rare Dis. 2010;5:20.

153. Iannicelli M, Brancati F, Mougou-Zerelli S, Mazzotta A, Thomas S, Elkhartoufi N, et al. Novel TMEM67 mutations and genotype-phenotype correlates in meckelin-related ciliopathies. Hum Mutat. 2010;31(5):E1319–31.

154. Valente EM, Dallapiccola B, Bertini E. Joubert syndrome and related disorders. Handb Clin Neurol. 2013;113:1879–88.

155. Lopez E, Thauvin-Robinet C, Reversade B, Khartoufi NE, Devisme L, Holder M, et al. C5orf42 is the major gene responsible for OFD syndrome type VI. Hum Genet. 2014;133(3):367–77.

156. Betleja E, Cole DG. Ciliary trafficking: CEP290 guards a gated community. Curr Biol. 2010;20(21):R928–31.

157. Huber C, Cormier-Daire V. Ciliary disorder of the skeleton. Am J Med Genet C: Semin Med Genet. 2012;160C(3):165–74.

158. El Hokayem J, Huber C, Couve A, Aziza J, Baujat G, Bouvier R, et al. NEK1 and DYNC2H1 are both involved in short rib polydactyly Majewski type but not in Beemer Langer cases. J Med Genet. 2012;49(4):227–33.

159. Cavalcanti DP, Huber C, Sang KH, Baujat G, Collins F, Delezoide AL, et al. Mutation in IFT80 in a fetus with the phenotype of Verma-Naumoff provides molecular evidence for Jeune-Verma-Naumoff dysplasia spectrum. J Med Genet. 2011;48(2):88–92.

160. Thiel C, Kessler K, Giessl A, Dimmler A, Shalev SA, von der Haar S, et al. NEK1 mutations cause short-rib polydactyly syndrome type majewski. Am J Hum Genet. 2011;88(1):106–14.

161. Chen Y, Chen CF, Riley DJ, Chen PL. Nek1 kinase functions in DNA damage response and checkpoint control through a pathway independent of ATM and ATR. Cell Cycle. 2011;10(4):655–63.

162. Upadhya P, Birkenmeier EH, Birkenmeier CS, Barker JE. Mutations in a NIMA-related kinase gene, Nek1, cause pleiotropic effects including a progressive polycystic kidney disease in mice. Proc Natl Acad Sci U S A. 2000;97(1):217–21.

163. Surpili MJ, Delben TM, Kobarg J. Identification of proteins that interact with the central coiled-coil region of the human protein kinase NEK1. Biochemistry. 2003;42(51):15369–76.

164. Yim H, Sung CK, You J, Tian Y, Benjamin T. Nek1 and TAZ interact to maintain normal levels of polycystin 2. J Am Soc Nephrol. 2011;22(5):832–7.

165. Ma M, Tian X, Igarashi P, Pazour GJ, Somlo S. Loss of cilia suppresses cyst growth in genetic models of autosomal dominant polycystic kidney disease. Nat Genet. 2013;45(9):1004–12.

166. Arts HH, Knoers NV. Current insights into renal ciliopathies: what can genetics teach us? Pediatr Nephrol. 2013;28(6):863–74.

Polycystic Kidney Disease: ADPKD and ARPKD

Max Christoph Liebau and Carsten Bergmann

Introduction

Polycystic kidney disease (PKD) is a clinically and genetically heterogeneous group of disorders with phenotypes ranging from manifestation in utero to clinically silent disease well into adulthood. Progressive fibrocystic renal changes are often accompanied by severe hepatobiliary changes or other extrarenal abnormalities [1–7]. While single renal cysts are a common and usually benign finding in adults, bilateral cystic kidneys require careful clinical workup to identify the underlying genetic disorder, especially in children. Even though there are still more questions than answers, substantial progress has been made in unravelling the etiology of cystic kidney disease. Despite numerous underlying genetic causes, recent findings suggest that cystogenic processes share common phenotypic abnormalities [1, 4]. It has been shown that PKD-associated proteins co-localize in multimeric complexes at distinct subcellular epithelial sites and compel-ling evidence suggests that primary cilia play a central pathogenic role [1–4, 8]. The insights gained within the last 15 years including ground-breaking basic science progress regarding the role of cilia in cystogenesis have led to the establishment of multiple clinical trials evaluating emerging therapeutic strategies [9]. Several promising trials have already further extended our understanding of the pathophysiology of PKD and may have the potential for rational personalized therapies in future years.

Classification and Differential Diagnosis of Cystic Kidney Diseases

In their seminal studies, Osathanondh and Potter systematically classified renal cystic diseases into four distinct types [10]. Potter syndrome type I is referred to as autosomal recessive polycystic kidney disease (ARPKD), type II as renal cystic dysplasia, type III as autosomal dominant polycystic kidney disease (ADPKD), and type IV occurs when longstanding obstruction of either the kidney or ureter leads to cystic kidneys or hydronephrosis. Particularly types II–IV can be part of many syndromes. While this historical classification still has a great impact for concise pathoanatomical description, it is hardly to be reconciled with clinical and genetic entities.

Accurate diagnosis is essential both in the management of patients with PKD and in counselling their families. Notably, cystic kidneys are an

M.C. Liebau (✉)
Department of Pediatrics, Division of Pediatric
Nephrology and Center for Molecular Medicine,
University Hospital of Cologne, Kerpener Strasse 62,
50937 Cologne, Germany
e-mail: max.liebau@uk-koeln.de

C. Bergmann (✉)
Renal Division, Department of Medicine,
University of Freiburg Medical Center,
Hugstetter Straße 55, 79106 Freiburg, Germany
e-mail: carsten.bergmann@uniklinik-freiburg.de

© Springer-Verlag Berlin Heidelberg 2016
D.F. Geary, F. Schaefer (eds.), *Pediatric Kidney Disease*, DOI 10.1007/978-3-662-52972-0_12

important feature of numerous genetic syndromes, such as the dominant disorders tuberous sclerosis, branchio-oto-renal syndrome and von Hippel-Lindau disease or the recessively inherited Joubert, Bardet-Biedl and Zellweger syndromes.

Six straightforward questions that can be answered by the patient and sonographic examination may be helpful to narrow down potential diagnosis [9].

In a first general consideration it is important to differentiate a kidney with a single or a few cyst(s) from a cystic kidney. Cysts within the kidneys are fairly common in elderly persons [11] and usually do not impose problems or require treatment. Especially in young children, however, even a single cyst should raise suspicion. Two useful investigations in the evaluation of a child with early onset of cystic renal disease of unknown underlying disease entity might be ultrasound of the parents and measurement of blood pressure [12]. If ADPKD is clinically suspected and the parents are younger than 30 years, the grandparents may also be considered for renal ultrasound [13]. Ultrasound-based diagnostic criteria in patients at risk for ADPKD have been established and are discussed in more detail below [14, 15]. A second important question addresses the age of the patient at the time of presentation. While cysts in the kidney may appear in childhood in ADPKD, clinical symptoms usually only present way into adulthood. ARPKD fetuses and a minor subset of ADPKD patients may be identified because of oligohydramnion during pregnancy. As discussed in detail in a separate chapter of this book, juvenile nephronophthisis (NPH) classically presents with polyuria and polydipsia in school children. Thirdly the localization of cysts may give a hint. Cysts in NPH are found at the cortico-medullary border, whereas in ADPKD cysts localize to all parts of the kidney. As mentioned above cystic kidney disorders may be accompanied by extrarenal symptoms. Thus, the fourth question aims to find out where else symptoms occur and what kind of clinical presentation can be found in addition to cystic kidneys. Classical hints may be retinitis pigmentosa presenting with initial night blindness later progressing to almost complete loss of vision in case of syndromes accompanied

by NPH, liver cysts in ADPKD and congenital hepatic fibrosis in ARPKD. Furthermore, kidney and cyst size can point to the correct diagnosis. Kidneys in NPH tend to be normal-sized or small, whereas ARPKD and ADPKD kidneys are large. Cysts are typically tiny in early stages of ARPKD, but may resemble ADPKD cysts during the course of the disease. Finally, family history is important. Ten percent of ADPKD patients do not show a positive family history [16]. ARPKD and NPH are usually inherited recessively with healthy parents. Naturally, recessive disorders can be found more frequently in offspring of consanguineous couples. With these six pieces of information at hand a potential diagnosis can be identified in many cases. Nonetheless, clinical diagnosis can be challenging due to overlapping syndromes and symptoms, and particularly in these cases establishing a genetic diagnosis is helpful.

The two major inherited PKDs are ADPKD and ARPKD [4, 6]. This chapter focuses on these two disorders; a thorough discussion of other cystic kidney disease entities is given in further sections of this book. We aim to summarize the current state of knowledge concerning the structure and function of genes and proteins underlying polycystic kidney disease, to explore the cellular pathophysiology and clinical consequences of changes in mutant genes, and to discuss emerging therapeutic approaches.

Autosomal Dominant Polycystic Kidney Disease (ADPKD)

Epidemiology and Morphology

ADPKD is the most common inherited renal disease and one of the commonest Mendelian human disorders overall with a frequency of 1/500–1000 [17, 18]. This approximates to about 12.5 million affected individuals worldwide. ADPKD is among the most common causes of end stage renal disease (ESRD); about 5–10 % of all patients requiring renal replacement therapy (kidney transplant or dialysis) are affected by ADPKD. Overall, the disease is a major health care issue of socio-economic interest.

ADPKD   ARPKD

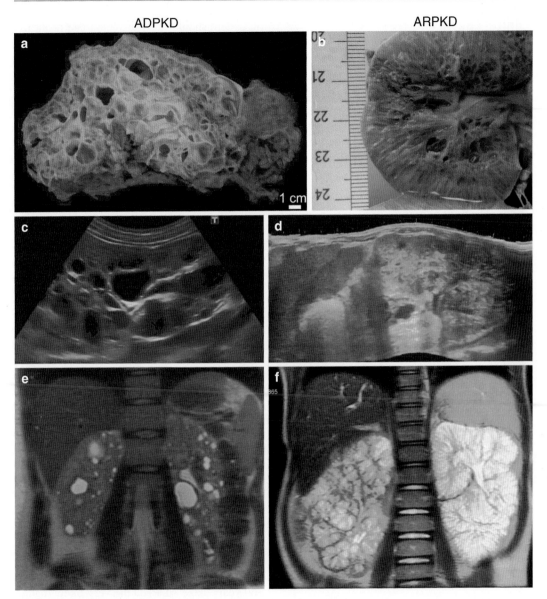

Fig. 12.1 (**a**) Macroscopic appearance of advanced-stage ADPKD (**a**) and ARPKD kidneys (**b**). On cut section, multiple cysts in the cortex and medulla can be seen that vary considerably in size and appearance, from a few millimetres to diameters of many centimeters in the ADPKD kidney, while ubiquitous small dilatations can be seen in the ARPKD kidney. These findings can also be recapitulated by ultrasound (**c**, **d**) and T2-weighted magnetic resonance imaging (MRI; **e**, **f**) (Used with permission of Springer Science + Business Media from Liebau and Serra [9]; with thanks to Andreas Serra (Zürich, Switzerland), Bernd Hoppe (Bonn, Germany), Lisa Guay-Woolford, Washington, USA)

Histopathologically, renal cysts are fluid-filled epithelia-lined cavities that generally arise from tubular segments. ADPKD is characterized by the formation and progressive enlargement of renal cysts in all segments of the nephron. In contrast to ARPKD in which the cysts usually remain connected with the tubular lumen, cysts in ADPKD become disconnected from the tubular space. Renal cysts in ADPKD vary considerably in size and appearance, from a few millimetres to many centimeters (Fig. 12.1a–f).

Clinical Course and Treatment

ADPKD is a systemic disorder with profound extrarenal cystic and non-cystic complications, which are summarized in Table 12.1. Among the most important extrarenal manifestations commonly seen in adults are cysts in other epithelial organs (especially in the liver and less commonly in the pancreas) and cardiovascular abnormalities. In pediatric patients, however, extrarenal disease features are only rarely observed.

Renal Involvement

Despite significant extrarenal disease burden in many ADPKD patients, the kidneys are usually in the center of interest. While there are currently no well-established disease-specific treatment options, it is crucial to prevent and effectively manage complications such as arterial hypertension and urinary tract infections to slow progression to ESRD. Renal insufficiency and ESRD in ADPKD is treated with standard medical management and renal replacement therapy as outlined in other chapters of this book.

ADPKD diagnosis is usually established by ultrasound. About 95 % of the disease carriers exhibit the characteristic ultrasonographic features of ADPKD at age 20, and almost all patients do so at age 30. It is less clear what proportion of carriers can already be identified by ultrasound in childhood. Even a single kidney cyst in a pediat-

ric patient should raise suspicion and result in a diagnostic work-up encompassing a careful record of family and medical history, physical examination and, where required, further abdominal imaging. These patients usually show an onset of clinical symptoms not until adulthood and should be distinguished from those with an early-manifesting clinical course. Still, as novel treatment approaches are emerging, it may become more important to identify ADPKD patients at an early stage of disease. Various early markers of renal disease have been suggested and are currently under investigation [20]. In a study by the Denver Polycystic Kidney Disease Research Group, approximately 60 % of children younger than 5 years of age, and 75–80 % of children 5–18 years of age with a *PKD1* mutation had renal cysts detectable by ultrasound [21]. In the early 1990s, Bear and colleagues proposed a rate of false negative ultrasonographic diagnosis of about 35 % below the age of 10 years [22]. Simple cysts are extremely rare in childhood [11]. Ravine et al. found nil prevalence of cysts in individuals aged 15–29 years [15].

Especially in children with a positive family history, ADPKD will be the most likely underlying condition for a child with renal cysts. In adults aged ≤39 years with a positive family history of ADPKD, the diagnosis of ADPKD can be established with high sensitivity and specificity by the presence of three kidney cysts uni- or bilaterally as detected by ultrasound [14]. Two cysts on each side for patients aged 40–59 years and four cysts on each side for patients aged >60 years make ADPKD the very likely diagnosis according to the modified Ravine criteria [14]. Fewer than two cysts in persons at risk aged >40 years practically exclude ADPKD. In 420 children with a positive family history of ADPKD, ultrasound screening detected renal cysts in 49 % of individuals at the age of 15 years [23].

Magnetic resonance imaging (MRI) and computed tomography (CT) have higher detection rates, especially for small cysts. Given this, MRI may be a helpful tool to discover small cysts, e.g., to detect affected persons prior to living kidney donation, but unmodified application of the

Table 12.1 Extrarenal manifestations of ADPKD

Manifestation	Prevalence
Hepatic cysts	>90 %
Arterial hypertension	Up to 70 %
Left ventricular hypertrophy	Up to 70 %
Valvular abnormalities	Up to 20 %
Intracranial aneurysm	6–16 %
Abdominal aorta aneurysm	5–10 %
Diverticula	Up to 40 %
Hernias	Up to 45 %
Bronchiectasis	Up to 37 %
Genitourinary cysts	39–60 %
Depression	Up to 60 %
Pain	Up to 60 %

Used with permission of Oxford University Press from Luciano and Dahl [19]

Ravine criteria to MRI and CT data would result in false-positive results [24, 25]. Novel high-resolution ultrasound equipment may also be more sensitive in detecting small cysts. New standard values have therefore been established for MRI-based cyst detection, revealing at least one cyst in about 60 % of healthy adults [25]. CT-based studies detected simple renal cysts in 24 % [26] and 27 % of patients over the age of 40 and 50 years, respectively [27]. Men had more cysts than women and cyst size as well as cyst number increased with age.

While there is consensus on the need for tight blood pressure control and early treatment of potential complications in children at risk for ADPKD [28–30], ethical concerns exist on the question whether or not an ADPKD diagnosis should be actively sought in asymptomatic children. As there is currently no established disease-controlling treatment that would need to be started during childhood, it has been argued that one should not take the right of self-determination from these children before these individuals are old enough to decide on their own what they consider best for them. Recently, KDIGO guidelines and recommendations have been framed for this and other issues around ADPKD [31].

The study by the CRISP (Consortium for Radiologic Imaging Studies of Polycystic Kidney Disease) consortium on ADPKD patients suggested that total kidney volume (TKV) as measured by MRI predicts renal function decline in ADPKD. TKV is therefore considered a good surrogate parameter for disease severity in ADPKD, even before renal function declines [9]. This is highly relevant as kidney function remains stable in ADPKD for a very long time even though kidneys may already be greatly cystic and fibrotic. ADPKD therefore constitutes a progressive kidney disorder that cannot be monitored based on serum creatinine measurements only. TKV could in this context be helpful to monitor the disease course and the response to interventions.

In detail, the CRISP consortium used annual MRI as well as GFR measurements by iothalamate clearance to monitor kidney and cyst volume in 232 young ADPKD patients with a GFR of >60 ml/min/1.72 m^2 over a period of 3 and 8 years [32]. Some 85 % of the patients had *PKD1* mutations and 15 % had *PKD2* mutations. TKV was calculated by a stereological approach from T1-weighted coronal images that were initially enhanced by gadolinium. Later studies were performed without contrast material, a protocol change that did not impair the accuracy of the TKV measurements [33]. As expected the CRISP study showed that the expected progression of cyst growth and kidney volume occurred prior to functional impairment with a mean rate of kidney growth of 5.3 % per year. Total cyst growth and total kidney growth were closely correlated. While PKD2 patients showed smaller kidney volumes and fewer cysts, the rate of cyst expansion was the same. These data suggested that the milder clinical course in PKD2 is rather due to a lower number of cysts, instead of a lower rate of cyst expansion. Rapid kidney growth was associated with a faster decline in kidney function and lower renal blood flow [32, 34]. Renal blood flow and age as well as gender, hypertension, and kidney volume predicted the loss of kidney function [35]. Kidney size was also associated with blood pressure: the larger the kidney, the more ADPKD patients suffered from hypertension [32].

The CRISP data have been supported and expanded by an ADPKD study in Switzerland [36] and most recently by the HALT-PKD trial [37]. The SUISSE ADPKD study showed that a semi-automated segmentation applied to measure cyst volume on T2-weighted pictures could reliably detect TKV changes in 100 patients within a 6-month period. Volume regressions were found in some of the patients and were attributed to the asymptomatic rupture of large cysts. Those researchers pointed out that kidney growth was solely due to an increase in cyst volume; however, kidney volume could be assessed more precisely than cyst volume [36].

Greater renal enlargement and fast renal growth were associated with a more rapid decrease in renal function. Even though the association of TKV with disease progression can be considered well-established by now, there are various aspects that need to be considered.

MRI-based TKV assessment is unsuitable as a routine clinical marker in pediatric practice, as TKV measurement is highly laborious and MRI would require sedation in young children. For the daily clinical work, ultrasound remains the method of choice [9], even more as the resolution of modern ultrasound equipment is excellent.

Chronic renal failure is present in about 50 % of ADPKD patients by the age of 60 years. On average, PKD2 is regarded to be significantly milder than PKD1 with a 20 years later median age of onset of end-stage renal disease (ESRD) (58.1 vs. 79.9 years) and a lower prevalence of arterial hypertension and urinary tract infections [17]. There is also evidence for a limited genotype-phenotype correlation in PKD1. In a recent large French cohort, patients with a proven truncating mutation were shown to have a more severe course than patients in whom a missense mutation was detected [38]. There is no evidence for any sex influence in PKD1; however, females affected by PKD2 were found to have a significantly longer median survival (71.0 vs. 67.3 years) than males. Another study corroborated these findings by a later mean age of onset of ESRD (76.0 vs. 68.1 years) in PKD2 females [39].

Early-Onset ADPKD and Clinical Spectrum of Renal Disease in Pediatric ADPKD

Clinical symptoms of ADPKD usually do not arise until the middle decades; however, there is striking phenotypic variability not only between but even within families, indicating that modifying genes, environmental factors and/or other mechanisms considerably influence the clinical course in ADPKD [40, 41]. In line with this, a small proportion of ADPKD patients presents with an early-manifesting clinical course [5]. Early manifestation in ADPKD has usually been defined as clinical symptoms (e.g., arterial hypertension, proteinuria, impaired renal function) occurring before the age of 15 years. Among these are cases with significant peri-/neonatal morbidity and mortality sometimes indistinguishable from those with severe ARPKD. Conflicting data exist on the precise incidence of early-manifesting ADPKD cases

that may result in reduced fitness and, thus, may equal the portion of spontaneous autosomal dominant *PKD* mutations. While most authors propose a figure of about 2 % [42], Sweeney and Avner even suggested a prevalence of up to 5 % [6, 43]. Given the prevalence rates for ADPKD (1/400–1000) and ARPKD (1/20,000), it is plausible that the total number of patients with early-onset ADPKD seen in paediatric nephrology clinics may be comparable to those of the children with ARPKD. Importantly, mutations in *TCF2/HNF1-beta*, which initially were mainly found in children with bilateral cystic dysplasia [44], can result in PKD-mimicking phenotypes [5, 45].

Longitudinal studies of children with ADPKD demonstrated that severe renal enlargement at a young age and/or hypertension are risk factors for accelerated renal growth [46–48]. Many clinical symptoms such as pain, hematuria, proteinuria, stones and hypertension are associated with large kidney size. Furthermore, a large cyst number in early childhood is a predictor for faster progression of structural abnormalities. A study evaluating annual MRI scans of 77 ADPKD individuals aged between 4 and 21 years over a period of 5 years revealed that patients with high blood pressure ($\geq$95th percentile) displayed larger TKVs and greater increases in fractional cyst volume than patients with normal blood pressure [49]. The fractional increase in cyst volume after correction for body surface area was 4.7 ± 1.2 %/year in children with high blood pressure compared to 1.7 ± 1.2 %/year in children with normal blood pressure. TKV was calculated from T1-weighted images, whereas T2-weighted images were used for cyst volume quantification. Children with high blood pressure were found to have more cysts and higher serum creatinine values [49]. Conclusively, larger kidneys are associated with increased morbidity and more rapid progression to ESRD.

Intriguingly, in children with ADPKD, renal involvement is commonly asymmetric (including asymmetric kidney enlargement) and even unilateral in a small minority at early stages of the disease [50]. As in ARPKD, the kidneys can present as large and hyperechoic bilateral masses with decreased corticomedullary differentiation. While the ultrasonographic kidney pattern in ADPKD and ARPKD often becomes quite similar and hard to distinguish with progressive disease, the radiographic features in early disease course are often easier to distinguish. Unlike ARPKD, in which the cysts are usually fusiform and tiny (<2 mm in diameter) often impressing as pepper-salt pattern on ultrasound, ADPKD kidneys are frequently characterized by greatly variable macrocysts (up to several centimeters in diameter) even in small children [9, 51].

While a significant proportion of adult ADPKD patients experience at least one episode of gross hematuria that is known to be a risk factor for the progression of renal disease [52–54], hematuria is not that common in children and occurs in only about 10 % of affected children at a mean age of 9 years [47].

Arterial Hypertension

Arterial hypertension in the first months of life is common in pediatric ADPKD patients even with normal renal function [42, 55, 56]. Hypertension should be identified as early as possible and aggressively treated, particularly in children under 12 years of age with more than ten renal cysts [57]. The precise pathogenesis of hypertension in PKD still remains to be elucidated; at least in part it appears to be mediated by activation of the intrarenal renin-angiotensin-aldosterone system (RAS), reduced renal blood flow, and increased sodium retention. Hence, RAS antagonists are the pharmacotherapy of first choice [58–61]. Hypertension in PKD is associated with increased cyst growth.

Intracerebral Aneurysms (ICA)

Intracerebral aneurysms (ICAs) are an important, specific cardiovascular comorbidity in ADPKD. However, the question of screening for ICAs in ADPKD patients has been a matter of ongoing debate [62–64]. A prevalence of about 8 % of asymptomatic ICAs has been estimated from large prospective series [65–67]. This number equals a rate four to five times above that found in the general population [63]. Pirson et al. concluded in their comprehensive review that the

prevalence of asymptomatic ICAs is about 6 % in ADPKD patients in the absence of a positive family history of ICA or SAH (subarachnoid hemorrhage) and approximately 16 % if family history is positive [64]. ICA prevalence in ADPKD patients increases with age and a study on 355 ADPKD patients only found one patient with an ICA, who was under 30 years of age [68].

MR angiography is the first-choice screening test; it does not require intravascular administration of contrast material and carries essentially no risk [64, 69]. The majority of ICAs detected by current MR and helical CT angiography techniques are small, measuring <6 mm in diameter and the majority also remains asymptomatic [63]. Screening may be applied to patients with a positive family history of aneurysms of SAH, previous aneurysm rupture, preparation for major elective surgery, high-risk occupations (e.g., airline pilots), and patient anxiety despite adequate information [63]. However, as interventions also carry risks, individualized decisions may be required for screening and potential treatment [70]. In addition to size, the location of the ICA has an impact of its probability to rupture. Furthermore, in ADPKD a family or personal history of ICA or SAH is clearly associated with ICA rupture, five times higher than in a control group [71, 72].

As the risk to develop novel aneurysms after a negative screening is small, repetitive imaging after 5–10 years has been recommended in patients with a positive family history in patients with unruptured intracranial aneurysms [63].

Liver Cysts

Simple, mostly solitary hepatic cysts are common with a prevalence of 2.5–10 % in the general population [73, 74]. These cysts must not be mixed up with the hepatic cysts observed in about 80–85 % of patients with ADPKD between 15 and 46 years of age. They usually gain in size and number as the renal cysts. Their incidence increases from 58 % in the age group of 15–24 years to 94 % in the group of 35–46 years [75]. Women may be more often and more severely affected, especially those who used estrogens, had multiple pregnancies or both [63, 76, 77]. There are some ADPKD families in whom hepatic cysts can be predominant with multiple cysts throughout the liver in the presence of very few renal cysts. These cases need to be distinguished, however, from autosomal dominant polycystic liver disease (PCLD) without renal involvement that is different from ADPKD at the phenotypic and genotypic level and is characterized by lack of renal cysts and progressive development of multiple (usually >20) liver cysts. Two separate genes, *PRKCSH* and *SEC63*, have been identified to cause familial PCLD [78, 79]. Recent work has linked signalling events affected in ADPKD and PCLD to common pathophysiological pathways [8, 80, 81].

Irrespective of the underlying entity, the pathogenesis, manifestations, and management of hepatic cysts are similar. Liver cysts usually arise from progressive dilatation of abnormal ducts in biliary hamartomas [82]. Hamartomas are the result of a ductal plate malformation (DPM) of small intrahepatic bile ducts. These small bile ducts have lost continuity with the remaining biliary tree explaining the non-communicating nature of the cysts [83]. The smooth transition between various different disease entities is illustrated by the fact that DPM is usually associated with congenital hepatic fibrosis and hyperplastic biliary ducts. While these histologic findings are mandatory in ARPKD [84], they have been anecdotally reported also in ADPKD patients [85–87].

Liver cysts only rarely result in clinical problems and complications appear much less common than complications of renal cysts. Usually, hepatic, pancreatic, or ovarian cysts are not observed before puberty; however, there are case reports of children affected in the first year of life [88, 89]. In case of cyst infection, surgical drainage has been recommended as the exclusive use of antibiotics may be ineffective [90]. To differentiate a complicated from an uncomplicated hepatic cyst, MRI imaging is the most sensitive technique although ultrasound may provide good results too [76]. Massive liver enlargement secondary to hepatic cysts may result in disabling discomfort. These individuals may benefit from percutaneous sclerotherapy when one or

a few large cysts are present [89]. Occasionally, more aggressive surgical intervention with fenestration, partial hepatectomy or even liver transplantation may be required [76, 77, 91]. Furthermore, as discussed below somatostatin analogues are currently under investigation in first clinical trials [92–99]. Further complications might result from hemorrhage into a cyst that may cause severe acute abdominal pain, fever, elevated liver enzymes and possibly mimic acute cholecystitis or hepatic abscess. Exceptionally rare is a ruptured cyst that gives rise to hemoperitoneum.

In addition, other abnormalities may occur including mitral valve prolapse (usually without clinical significance), left ventricular hypertrophy, aneurysms of the abdominal aorta, diverticular disease, hernia, chronic back pain, cystic lesions in the genitourinary tract, the pancreas and the lung, hematuria, urinary tract infection, kidney stones, deregulated phosphate homeostasis, and arachnoidal cysts as well as pain and depression [9, 63, 100] (Table 12.1).

Genetic

Marquardt is thought to be the first who postulated genetic heterogeneity of polycystic kidney diseases when stating in 1935: "In surviving individuals, cystic kidneys are inherited dominantly. In non-viable individuals, cystic kidneys are recessive" [101]. It took more than 35 years from that point of view before Blyth and Ockenden demonstrated in a systematic analysis that age at presentation alone is not a reliable criterion for defining genetic heterogeneity [102]. Parental renal ultrasound, however, is still the most important classification criterion in most cases to distinguish between ARPKD and ADPKD.

As the name implies, ADPKD is transmitted in an autosomal dominant fashion, i.e., virtually all individuals who inherit a mutated *PKD* germline allele will develop renal cysts by age 30–40. The majority of ADPKD patients (~85 %) carry a germline mutation in the *PKD1* gene on chromosome 16p13.3 [100, 103, 104], whereas about

15 % harbour a mutation in the *PKD2* gene on chromosome 4q21 [105].

PKD1 and PKD2 Genes and Their Encoded Polycystin-1 and -2 Proteins

PKD1 is a large gene with a longest open reading frame transcript of 46 exons predicted to encode a 4302 aa multidomain integral membrane glycoprotein (polycystin-1). *PKD2* has 15 exons encoding a 5.3 kb transcript that is translated into a 968 aa protein (polycystin-2). In keeping with the systemic nature of ADPKD, the two polycystins are widely expressed in tissues others than kidney. The systemic character is further emphasized by mouse models with homozygous *Pkd1* or *Pkd2* mutations [106–109]. Some of these mice are embryonically lethal and display severe cardiovascular anomalies along with renal and pancreatic cysts. The expression of polycystin-1 and -2 is developmentally regulated with highest levels during late fetal and early neonatal life. Renal expression is highest in distal tubule and collecting duct epithelial cells. Notably, the majority of cysts in ADPKD originate from collecting ducts.

Although the two-hit model of tumorigenesis supposed by Knudson is too simplistic, it may still provide a reasonable basis of our understanding of ADPKD. According to these data, second-hit mutation and resulting loss of heterozygosity (LOH) has been proposed as the mechanism underlying cyst formation in ADPKD. The considerable intrafamilial phenotypic variation, focal cyst formation with evidence of epithelial cell clonality within individual cysts, as well as the detection of somatic mutations in cells lining renal and hepatic cysts are all in keeping with this theory [110–114]. However, numerous findings rule out the two-hit model of a germline mutation on one allele and a somatic mutation on the other as the sole cause of cystogenesis. Patients and mice have been described that carry germline mutations in both *PKD1* and *PKD2* (double-heterozygotes) and, thus, are to be regarded as "homozygously" affected in every cell of the organism [115, 116]. In contradiction to a simple two-hit theory, not every renal tubular cell or nephron in these individuals may give

rise to a cyst. Therefore, the second-hit mutation to the other *PKD* gene may act as a modifying factor that boosts the risk of cyst development and/or drives cyst progression, rather than initiating cyst events [5]. As regards mechanisms underlying cystogenesis in ADPKD, it is worth noting that increased as well as decreased polycystin-1 expression may result in cyst formation [108, 117, 118]. Also, haploinsufficiency of *Pkd1* itself has been demonstrated to suffice to elicit a cystic phenotype [119]. Finally, the timepoint of *Pkd1* inactivation crucially determines the severity of the cystic phenotype in mice [120]. Furthermore ischemia [121–123], nephrotoxic injury [124] and immunological events [125, 126] may affect cystogenesis and it has been suggested that these events might represent a required third or even further additional hit [127, 128]. Taking all data together, the two-hit model of cyst formation initially proposed for ADPKD is no longer a tenable theory as an exclusive explanation for the complex process of cystogenesis.

The predicted structure of polycystin-1 and polycystin-2 indicates that they are glycosylated integral membrane proteins (Fig. 12.2). Polycystin-2 is predicted to have six transmembrane passes with cytoplasmic N- and C-termini. It is believed to function as a divalent cation channel, particularly involved in cellular Ca^{2+} signalling, a member of the transient receptor potential (TRP) protein superfamily [130].

Polycystin-1 is a huge integral membrane glycoprotein with an extensive amino-terminal extracellular region, 11 transmembrane passes, and a short 200 aa cytoplasmic carboxy-terminus. The intracellular C-terminus is predicted to contain several different potential phosphorylation sites and is supposed to mediate protein interactions, by, e.g., a heterotrimeric G-protein activation site and a coiled-coil domain that has been demonstrated to interact with the C-terminus of polycystin-2 [131–133]. The large extracellular portion of polycystin-1 contains numerous structural motifs including 16 copies of the immunoglobulin-like PKD domain, two cysteine-flanked leucine-rich repeats, the WSC homology domain (a cell-wall integrity and stress response

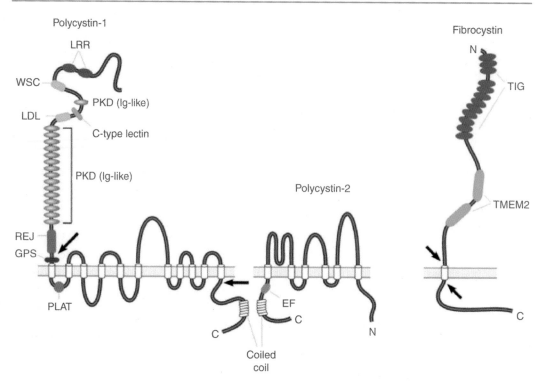

Fig. 12.2 Structures of polycystin-1, polycystin-2, and polyductin/fibrocystin. (*LRR* leucine-rich repeats, *WSC* cell wall integrity and stress response component 1, *PKD* (*Ig-like*) Ig-like domains, *LDL* low density lipoprotein domain, *REJ* receptor for egg jelly, *GPS* proteolytic G protein-coupled receptor proteolytic site, *PLAT* lipoxygenase domain, *EF* EF hand domain, *TIG* immunoglobulin-like domains, *TMEM2* homology with TMEM2 protein). Polycystin-1 and fibrocystin undergo cleavage at sites indicated by the *arrows* (Used with permission of Springer Science + Business Media from Ibraghimov-Beskrovnaya and Bukanov [129])

component) and a C-type lectin domain, which are putatively involved in protein-protein or protein-carbohydrate interactions. In this context it is noteworthy that Hogan et al. found urinary exosomes with abundant expression of polycystin-1, polycystin-2 and the ARPKD protein fibrocystin among others [134]. It has been proposed that polycystin-1 and polycystin-2 form a chemo- and mechanosensing protein complex which senses fluid flow in the renal tubule and controls cell growth and differentiation [1, 4, 104, 135]. Bending of the primary cilia leads to an increase in intracellular calcium potentially via a polycystin-1-dependent mechanism [136, 137] and the ratio of polycystin-1 to polycystin-2 has been shown to regulate pressure sensing [138]. As recently reviewed in more detail, polycystin-1 is involved in the regulation of multiple intracellular signalling pathways [139].

PKD1/PKD2 Mutation Spectrum and Routine Diagnostic Testing

Mutation analysis of the *PKD1* gene is complicated by genomic duplication of the first 33 exons at six other sites on chromosome 16p. Many of these pseudogenes are expressed as mRNA transcripts, but probably do not encode proteins. Both *PKD1* and *PKD2* mutations are scattered throughout the genes' coding regions exhibiting marked allelic heterogeneity with most mutations being unique to single families (private mutations) [140–142]. The majority of mutations presumably truncate the resulting protein and thus are assumed to be pathogenic; however, a considerable proportion of changes are novel amino acid substitutions that are difficult to evaluate with respect to their significance.

Whereas diagnostic genetic testing of ADPKD is a complex task, the clinical and sonographic diagnosis is usually straightforward. Thus, mutation analysis can usually be restricted to particular circumstances. These include (1) individuals with suspected ADPKD without a positive family history, (2) donor screening of a young relative willing to donate one of his healthy kidneys with ambiguous ultrasonographic or MRI findings, (3) a request for prenatal diagnosis in families with early-onset ADPKD. However, much more cost- and time-efficient approaches based on next-generation sequencing (NGS) may change the approach and spectrum of indications in the very near future.

Genotype-Phenotype Correlations

The wide range of age at attainment of ESRD observed within families clearly illustrates the limitations of simple genotype-phenotype correlation analysis. While no genotype-phenotype correlations have been identified for *PKD2* [16, 143], certain associations have been established in *PKD1* where mutations 5′ to the median are associated with a slightly earlier age at onset of ESRD (53 vs. 56 years) [144] Moreover, the median position of the *PKD1* mutation was found to be located further 5′ in families with a vascular phenotype of intracranial aneurysms and subarachnoid haemorrhage [145]. Most recently, *PKD1* mutations resulting in a truncated protein were shown to have a more severe phenotype than *PKD1* missense mutations [38]. *PKD1* missense mutations, however, were still more severe than *PKD2* mutations. In addition, the presence of mutations in multiple PKD genes can result in a more severe phenotype [146]. However, for genetic counselling and the prediction of the outcome of an individual patient, these genotype-phenotype correlations are only of limited value.

Data on families with early-manifesting offspring clearly corroborate a common familial modifying background for early and severe disease expression; conclusive data of underlying mechanisms are still lacking and a matter of ongoing research. Most seriously discussed mechanisms are anticipation, imprinting, and the segregation of modifying genes. However, data published on anticipation and imprinting are rather inconsistent. Segregation of modifying

alleles being inherited from the unaffected parent is an intriguing possibility [147]. The recurrence risk of about 25% for similarly early-onset ADPKD in siblings [148] fits to this hypothesis and it is further supported by the low incidence of in utero presentation of ADPKD in second degree relatives in these families. Anecdotal reports of second degree relatives also affected by early-onset ADPKD may thus be explained by chance segregation of a modifying gene in these families. Indeed, it was recently found that parallel mutations in multiple PKD genes may occur in ADPKD patients with early and severe manifestation. These patients carried mutations in PKD genes including *HNF1β* or a mutation *in trans* affecting the other *PKD1* allele in addition to the expected germline mutation [5, 146]. However, this mechanism is unlikely to explain all cases with early-onset ADPKD. For example, in a published case from Finland an affected mother had four offspring with in utero onset PKD with two different unrelated husbands [149]. In another pedigree, early-onset ADPKD was reported in mother and daughter [12]. To fit with the theory of complementary segregation of modifying variants, every unaffected parent in these families would have been expected to carry a rare modifying allele by chance. Conclusively, the mechanisms underlying early-onset ADPKD still require further examination.

Autosomal Recessive Polycystic Kidney Disease (ARPKD)

Epidemiology and Morphology

ARPKD is much rarer than its dominant counterpart with a proposed incidence among Caucasians of about 1 in 20,000 live births corresponding to a carrier frequency of approximately 1:70 in non-isolated populations [150–152]. The exact incidence is unknown since published studies vary in the cohorts of patients examined (e. g., autopsied patients vs. moderately affected patients followed by pediatricians), and some severely affected babies may die perinatally without a definitive diagnosis. Isolated populations may have higher prevalences, e.g., Kääriäinen reported an incidence of 1:8000 in Finland [149]. As mentioned before, among children with polycystic kidney diseases in departments of pediatric nephrology, there may be a significant number of individuals affected with early-onset ADPKD possibly resembling ARPKD.

Histologic changes can vary depending on the age of presentation and the extent of cystic involvement. However, usually ARPKD can be reliably diagnosed pathoanatomically [6]. Principally, the kidneys are symmetrically enlarged (up to ten times normal size) in affected neonates and retain their reniform contour (Fig. 12.1a–f and Table 12.2). Macroscopically, the cut surface demonstrates the cortical extension of fusiform or cylindrical spaces arranged radially throughout the renal parenchyma from medulla to cortex (Fig. 12.1a–f). Invariable histological manifestations are fusiform dilations of renal collecting ducts and distal tubuli lined by columnar or cuboidal epithelium that usually remain in contact with the urinary system (unlike ADPKD), whereas glomerular cysts (as in ADPKD) or dysplastic elements (e.g., cartilage;

Table 12.2 Clinical manifestations of ARPKD and ADPKD

	ARPKD	ADPKD
Incidence	1:20,000	1:500–1:1000
Macroscopic renal findings	Symmetrical, massively enlarged, reniform kidneys	Symmetrical, enlarged, reniform kidneys
Localization of renal cysts	Dilated collecting ducts an distal tubuli	Cysts derived from all parts of nephron
Ultrasound and diameter of renal cysts	Increased echogenicity of renal parenchyma. "Salt-and-pepper"-pattern. Small, sometimes invisible cysts (<2 mm). More ADPKD-like pattern with advancing age	Cysts of different sizes in cortex and medulla. Usually several large cysts
Hepatic pathology	Mandatory: ductal plate malformation/ congenital hepatic fibrosis with hyperplastic biliary ducts and portal fibrosis (may impress as Caroli syndrome)	"Liver cysts". Common in adults, rare in children. Occasionally ductal plate malformation/congenital hepatic fibrosis
Associated anomalies	Lung hypoplasia. Rarely pancreatic cysts. Single case reports of intracranial aneurysms	Pancreatic cysts and/or cysts in other epithelial organs. Familiarly clustered intracranial aneurysms, abdominal Aorta aneurysms. Diverticula. Hernia. Bronchiectasis
Main clinical manifestations	Neonatal respiratory distress/failure due to pulmonary hypoplasia. Renal insufficiency. Portal hypertension. Hyponatremia. Hypertension	Arterial hypertension. Proteinuria. Hematuria. Arterial hypertension. Renal insufficiency. Pain
Risk for siblings	25 %	50 % (except in rare cases of spontaneous mutation with virtually no risk)
Risk for own children	<1 % (unless unaffected parent is related to affected partner, or ARPKD is known in the unaffected partner's family)	50 % (also for patients with spontaneous mutations)
Manifestation in affected family members	About 20 % gross intrafamilial variability	Often similar within the same family
Parental kidneys	No alterations	Usually one affected parent (unless parents are <30 years or in case of spontaneous mutation)
Prognosis	Substantial mortality in patients with neonatal respiratory distress. Severe complications due to portal hypertension	Median age of end stage renal disease: 53 years (PKD1) vs. 69 years (PKD2)

as in Meckel-Gruber syndrome, etc.) are usually not evident in ARPKD kidneys (Fig. 12.3a, b). During early fetal development, a transient phase of proximal tubular cyst formation has been identified that is largely absent by birth, however [153]. As mentioned above, with advancing clinical course and development of larger renal cysts accompanied by interstitial fibrosis, ARPKD kidney structure may increasingly resemble the pattern observed in ADPKD [9]. However, ARPKD kidneys usually do not progress to grow unlimited but may at some point stop growing. Liver changes are obligatory for ARPKD and characterized by dysgenesis of the hepatic portal triad attributable to defective remodelling of the ductal plate with hyperplastic biliary ducts and congenital hepatic fibrosis (CHF) (Fig. 12.4a, b) [82]. These hepatobiliary changes subsumed as ductal plate malformation (DPM) are present from early embryonic development (first trimester) on and lead to progressive portal fibrosis. At later stages, fibrous septa may link different portal tracts by intersecting the hepatic parenchyma often leading to portal hypertension; however, the remaining liver parenchyma usually develops normally and hepatocellular function initially often remains stable [154–156]. Thus, liver enzymes, except for cholestasis parameters that are sometimes elevated, are characteristically not

increased. As extensively discussed for ADPKD, liver cysts usually arise from DPM and biliary ectasia and there obviously exist smooth transitions to extensive dilations of both intra- and extrahepatic bile ducts and forms like Caroli's disease/syndrome [82].

Clinical Course and Treatment

While ADPKD is usually a disease of adults with no more than 2–5 % of patients displaying an early manifesting clinical course, ARPKD is typically an infantile disease. However, the clinical spectrum is much more variable than generally presumed [157]. Despite dramatic advances in neonatal and intensive care over the past decades, the short-term and long-term morbidity and mortality of ARPKD remain substantial. Despite the establishment of consensus expert recommendations treatment is symptomatic and opinion-based [158]. Ages at diagnosis and initial clinical features are listed in Table 12.3, which summarizes results of various clinical studies on ARPKD. Notably, these studies differ widely by their selection criteria of patients and their mode of data analysis. Patients of German and North American studies [151, 162, 165] were mostly recruited at pediatric nephrology departments.

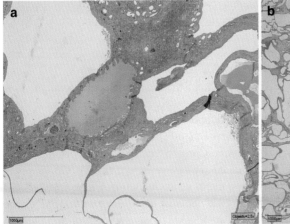
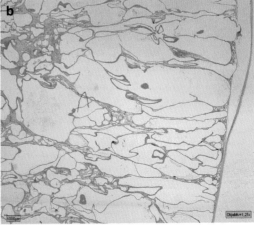
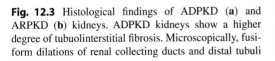

Fig. 12.3 Histological findings of ADPKD (**a**) and ARPKD (**b**) kidneys. ADPKD kidneys show a higher degree of tubulointerstitial fibrosis. Microscopically, fusiform dilations of renal collecting ducts and distal tubuli lined by columnar or cuboidal epithelium can be observed in ARPKD. These dilated collecting ducts run perpendicular to the renal capsule (Courtesy of Dr. Heike Göbel, Instite for Pathology, University Hospital of Cologne)

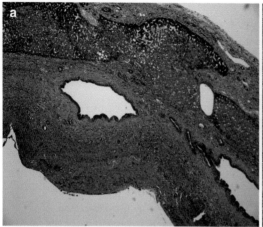
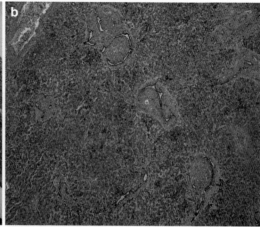

Fig. 12.4 Histological liver findings. Hepatic cysts (**a**) and the obligatory hepatobiliary changes in ARPKD subsumed as ductal plate malformation (DPM, **b**) characterized by dysgenesis of the hepatic portal triad with hyperplastic biliary ducts and congenital hepatic fibrosis (CHF) (Courtesy of Dr. Uta Drebber, Institute for Pathology, University Hospital of Cologne)

As a consequence, individuals with an early lethal form of ARPKD were underrepresented. Gagnadoux et al. [55] and Capisonda et al. [164] reported clinical outcomes of patients from specialized single centers. Most of the individuals in the study by Roy et al. [163] had previously been reported by Kaplan et al. who exclusively included patients with pathoanatomically proven CHF [161]. Kääriäinen et al. analysed mainly data obtained from Finnish death registers [160]. Inclusion criteria of the study by Cole et al. were diagnosis within the first year of life and survival of the neonatal period [159]. Gunay-Aygun et al. prospectively studied a cohort of 90 patients with the clinical diagnosis of ARPKD surviving beyond the first 6 months of age with admission to the NIH Clinical Center and follow-up visits every 1–2 years [152, 167].

Overall, the majority of cases are identified late in pregnancy or at birth. Severely affected fetuses display a "Potter" oligohydramnios phenotype with pulmonary hypoplasia (Fig. 12.5), a characteristic facies, and contracted limbs with club feet. Despite the advances of neonatal intensive care medicine with sophisticated methods of mechanical ventilation and/or surfactant application, mortality remains high in affected neonates and early detection of oligohydramnios seems to be associated with worse outcome [168]. As many as 30 % of affected neonates die shortly after birth from respiratory insufficiency. The respiratory distress in these severely affected children is mainly caused by a critical degree of pulmonary hypoplasia due to in utero renal dysfunction leading to oligo-/anhydramnios.

Hyponatremia related to a urine dilution defect is often present in the newborn period, but usually resolves over time [151, 161, 165]. Advances in mechanical ventilation, feeding and other supportive measures as well as further improvements in renal replacement therapies have increased the survival rates of ARPKD patients with some of them reaching adulthood. In the largest study published so far on almost 200 ARPKD patients with known *PKHD1* mutation status, survival rates of those patients who survived the first month of life were 94 % at 5 years and 92 % at 10 years of age [165].

Renal failure is rarely a cause of neonatal demise. Chronic renal failure was first detected at a mean age of 4 years in patients of the survey by Bergmann et al. including mainly patients followed in pediatric nephrology units [165]. Infants with ARPKD may have a transient improvement in their glomerular filtration rate (GFR) due renal maturation in the first 6 months of life [159]. However, subsequently, a progressive but highly variable decrease in renal function occurs. The

Table 12.3 Summary of clinical findings in ARPKD patients

	Patients (n)	Age at diagnosis	Renal function	Kidney length	Hypertension (% on drug treatment)	Growth retardation	Anemia	Evidence of portal hypertension	Survival rate	Death rate in the first year of life
Cole et al. [159]	17	100% 1–12 months (inclusion criterion)	35% GFR <40 29% ESRD	NA	100% (drug treatment or BP>95th percentile)	NA	NA	35%	1 year: 88%	12%
Kääriäinen et al. [160]	73 (18 neonatal survivors)	23% prenatal 31% <1 month 16% 1–12 months 30% >1 year	82% GFR <90	NA	61%	6% <2.5 SD	NA	50% (hepatomegaly)	1 year: 19%	81%
Gagnadoux et al. [55]	33	33% <1 month 55% 1–18 months 12% 6–11 year	42% GFR <80 21% ESRD	100% >2 SD	76%	18% <4 SD	NA	39%	1 year: 91%	9%
Kaplan et al. [161]	55	42% <1 month 42% 1–12 months 16% >1 year	58% serum creatinine >100 µmol/l	NA	65%	NA	NA	47%	1 year: 79% 10 years: 51% 15 years: 46%	24%
Zerres et al. [162]	115	10% prenatal 41% <1 month 23% 1–12 months 26% >1 year	72% GFR <3rd percentile for age 10% ESRD	68% >2 SD	70%	25% <2 SD	NA	46%	1 year: 89% 3 years: 88%	9%
Roy et al. [163]	52	85% <1 year 15% >1 year	33% ESRD (by 15 years)	NA	60% (by 15 years)	NA	NA	23% (8/35)	NA	26%

(continued)

Table 12.3 (continued)

	Patients (n)	Age at diagnosis	Renal function	Kidney length	Hypertension (% on drug treatment)	Growth retardation	Anemia	Evidence of portal hypertension	Survival rate	Death rate in the first year of life
Guay-Woodford and Desmond [151]	166	46 % prenatal 27 % <1 month 11 % 1–12 months 16 % >1 year	42 % GFR <3rd percentile for age. 13 % ESRD	NA	65 %	24 % <2 SD	NA	15 %	1 year: 79 % 5 years: 75 %	8 % death rate in patients surviving the first month of life
Capisonda et al. [164]	31	32 % prenatal 23 % <1 month 19 % 1–12 months 26 % >1 year	51 % GFR <80 16 % ESRD	NA	55 %	NA	NA	37 %	1 year: 87 % 9 years: 80 %	13 %
Bergmann et al. [165]	186 (164)	23 % prenatal 31 % <1 month 16 % 1–12 months 30 % >1 year	86 % GFR <3rd percentile. Median age for CRF 4 years 29 % ESRD 8 @ 10 years)	92 % >2 SD	76 % (80 % M, 72 % F)	16 % <2 SD (23 % M, 10 % F)	14 % (9 % M, 19 % F)	44 % (41 % M/47 % F), 38 % splenomegaly, 15 % esophageal varices 2 % ascites	1 year: 85 % 5 years: 84 % 10 years: 82 %	15 %
Gunay-Aygun et al. [156]	73	43 % <1 month (perinatal) 57 % >1 month (non-perinatal)	Mean GFR 61 vs. 89 ml/min/1.73 m² for perinatal and non perinatal patients	Mean SD: 6.3 for perinatal and 4.5 for non-perinatal patients	71 %	NA	NA	72 % splenomegaly 31 % varices	NA	NA (survival for >6 months inclusion criterion)

BP blood pressure, *ESRD* end stage renal disease, *NA* not available, *SD* standard deviation

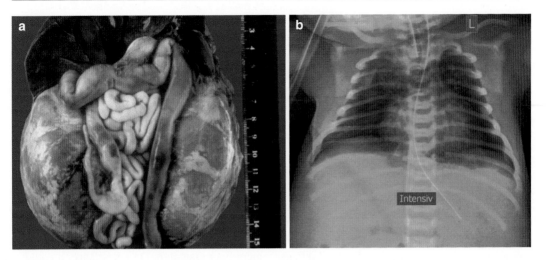

Fig. 12.5 Abdominal situs of an ARPKD patient with symmetrically enlarged kidneys that maintain their reniform configuration (**a**) and chest X-ray of a patient with pulmonary hypoplasia due to ARPKD (**b**)

management of children with declining renal function should follow the standard guidelines established for chronic renal insufficiency in other pediatric patients. Peritoneal dialysis (PD) and hemodialysis have both been successfully used in ARPKD neonates and infants. PD has been recommended as the chronic modality of choice for infants with stage 5 chronic kidney disease by the European Pediatric Dialysis Working Group [169] as nutrition can be optimized and vascular access can be preserved for later use. In the German study [165], ESRD occurred in 29 % of patients at 10 years and 58 % at 20 years which is much lower than the previously reported 50 % of ARPKD patients progressing to ESRD within the first decade of life [159, 163]. In the NIH cohort patients with perinatal presentation showed worse renal follow-up than those with non-perinatal presentation [170]. While 25 % of the perinatally symptomatic patients required renal replacement therapy by the age of 11 years, 25 % of the non-perinatal patients required kidney transplantation by age 32 years. Also corticomedullary involvement on high resolution ultrasound was associated with worse renal function in comparison with medullary involvement only. Kidney volume correlated inversely with function, although with wide variability [170]. Renal transplantation is the treatment of choice for individuals with ESRD. In case of massively enlarged kidneys, native nephrectomies may be warranted to allow allograft placement. Nephrectomy has also been proposed for pulmonary indications, to facilitate feeding and to improve blood pressure control [171–176]. However, supportive evidence for beneficial effects of nephrectomy is very limited and very careful consideration of the potential benefits against the risk of potentially accelerated loss of renal function and subsequent renal replacement therapy early in life are required.

Arterial hypertension usually develops in the first few months of life and affects up to 80 % of children with ARPKD (Table 12.2). Hypertension can be difficult to control in these children and may require multi-drug treatment. Hypertension needs early and aggressive treatment with careful blood pressure monitoring to prevent sequelae of hypertension (e.g., cardiac hypertrophy, congestive heart failure) and deterioration of renal function [155]. RAS antagonists (ACE inhibitors or AT1 receptor blockers) are regarded the treatment of choice. Further effective antihypertensive options are calcium channel blockers, beta blockers (particularly in patients with signs of CHF and portal hypertension), and diuretics (especially loop agents) [151, 177]. It has been proposed that the epithelial sodium channel blocker amiloride can be used to decrease intracellular cAMP concentrations that may result in Pseudo-Liddle syndrome [178]. As previously discussed for ADPKD, the pathophysiology of hypertension in ARPKD is not clearly understood. Although peripheral vein renin values are not usually elevated in hypertensive ARPKD patients and although the precise mechanism still remains unclear [155], the pathogenesis of hypertension may be mediated, at least in part, by dysregulation of renal sodium transport and activation of the RAS [179, 180] leading to increased intravascular volume [161].

By ultrasound, children with ARPKD typically have characteristic bilateral large echogenic kidneys with poor corticomedullary differentiation; macrocysts are uncommon in small infants, although they may be observed with advanced clinical course when ARPKD and ADPKD often become hard to differentiate by their sonographic appearance [181–183]. In a study by Bergmann et al. 92 % of ARPKD patients had a kidney length above or on the 97th centile for age [165]. In no case the kidney size was decreased and SD scores ranged from 0 to 17. In contrast to ADPKD, clear correlations were neither observed between kidney length and renal function nor between kidney length and duration of the disease.

In keeping with generally prolonged survival in ARPKD, for many patients the hepatobiliary complications come to dominate the clinical picture [155, 156]. While hepatocellular function is usually preserved, these individuals develop sequelae of portal hypertension and may present with hematemesis or melena due to bleeding oesophageal varices and/or hypersplenism with consequent pancytopenia. Primary management of variceal bleeding may include endoscopic approaches, such as sclerotherapy or variceal banding. In some patients, portosystemic shunting or liver-kidney transplantation (sequential or combined) can be considered as a viable therapeutic option but it needs to be pointed out that renal function contributes to disposal of ammonia. Therefore, impaired renal function in ARPKD patients makes portosystemic shunting less attractive [184]. A serious, potentially lethal complication in ARPKD especially after kidney transplantation is ascending suppurative cholangitis that may cause fulminant hepatic failure. It always requires diligent evaluation with aggressive antimicrobial treatment. Noteworthy, ARPKD patients may not display the typical clinical findings of cholangitis; thus, every patient with unexplained recurrent sepsis, particularly with gram-negative organisms, should be critically evaluated for this diagnosis [155, 156, 185].

Another aspect depicted in clinical studies on ARPKD was the renal-hepatobiliary morbidity pattern [151, 156, 165]. While most patients usually show uniform disease progression, individual ARPKD patients present with an organ-specific phenotype, i.e., either an (almost) exclusive renal phenotype or a predominant or mere liver phenotype. In accordance, it could be demonstrated that *PKHD1* mutations can cause isolated congenital hepatic fibrosis or Caroli's disease [142]. Noteworthy, in mouse models for *Pkhd1* the liver phenotype is stronger than renal involvement [186–189].

Somewhat surprisingly, several patients carrying two convincing *PKHD1* mutations were reported that were clinically asymptomatic until advanced adulthood and may have a normal life expectancy [157]. While these cases suggest some sort of alertness, overall, they may be exceptions to the rule.

ARPKD is one of the two major indications for combined liver and kidney transplantation during childhood, next to primary hyperoxaluria that is discussed in detail elsewhere in this book [190, 191]. The best timing and strategy for combined transplantation is still a matter of debate and usually requires individualized decision-making. Moreover, there is some preliminary evidence that adult ARPKD patients beyond the age of 40 years may have a slightly increased risk to develop hepatic tumors, especially cholangiocarcinoma [192, 193]. Thus, overall, ARPKD is an important cause of renal- and liver-related morbidity and mortality in children with a still severely diminished life expectancy.

Genetics

Given its autosomal recessive mode of inheritance, the recurrence risk for subsequent pregnancies of parents of an affected child is 25 %.

Males and females are equally affected. As indicated by formal genetics, unaffected siblings harbour a two-thirds risk of being a carrier for ARPKD. By definition, heterozygous carriers do not show any clinical disease manifestations. Healthy siblings, other relatives and patients themselves seeking genetic counselling for their own family planning can be reassured of a low risk for offspring with ARPKD when neither the partner is related with the index family nor a case of ARPKD is known in the partner's pedigree. At an assumed heterozygosity rate of 1:70, the estimated risk is 1:140 for offspring of patients, 1:420 for offspring of patients' healthy siblings and 1:560 for offspring of patients' healthy uncles/aunts.

Based on age at presentation and relative degrees of renal and hepatic involvement, Blyth and Ockenden originally stratified ARPKD patients into four phenotypic entities (perinatal, neonatal, infantile, juvenile) [102]. They hypothesized four distinct genes to be responsible for ARPKD. Doubts on the correctness of this hypothesis arose with the description of affected sibships with significant discordance in disease onset and manifestation [194–196]. These observations led to the proposal that the entire spectrum of ARPKD is caused by multiple allelism in a single gene [197]. This hypothesis was confirmed by mapping the gene underlying ARPKD to the short arm of chromosome 6 and demonstrating that all phenotypic variants are compatible with linkage to this single locus [198, 199].

PKHD1 Gene and Polyductin/ Fibrocystin Protein

In 2002, two groups independently identified the sequence of the *PKHD1* gene providing the basis for direct genotyping [200, 201]. *PKHD1* is amongst the largest disease genes in the human genome, extending over a genomic segment of at least 470 kb and including a minimum of 86 exons. Both *PKHD1* and its murine orthologue undergo a complex and extensive pattern of alternative splicing, generating transcripts highly variable in size. In accordance with the disease phenotype, the gene is highly expressed in fetal and adult kidney and at lower levels in liver [200,

202]. Weak expression is present in other tissues too, including pancreas and arterial wall. The longest *PKHD1* transcript contains 67 exons encoding a protein of 4074 amino acids.

The predicted full-length protein (termed fibrocystin or polyductin) represents a novel integral membrane protein with a signal peptide at the amino terminus of its extensive, highly glycosylated extracellular domain, a single transmembrane (TM)-spanning segment, and a short cytoplasmic C-terminal tail containing potential protein kinase A phosphorylation sites (Fig. 12.2). The ~3860 amino acid extracellular portion contains several IPT and IPT-like domains that can be found in cell surface receptors and transcription factors. Between the IPT domains and the TM segment, multiple PbH1 repeats are present, a motif also found in polysaccharidases that may bind to carbohydrate moieties such as glycoproteins on the cell surface and/or in the basement membrane. Based on the structural features of the deduced protein and on the human ARPKD phenotype, fibrocystin might be involved in cellular adhesion, repulsion and proliferation. In addition, the domain and structural analyses suggest that the potential *PKHD1* gene products may be involved in intercellular signalling and function as receptor, ligand and/or membrane-associated enzyme [200].

In common with most other cystoproteins, fibrocystin is localized to primary cilia with concentration in the basal body area [203–207]. As part of acquisition of epithelial polarity during kidney development, fibrocystin becomes localized to the apical zone of nephron precursor cells and subsequently to the basal bodies at the origin of primary cilia in fully differentiated epithelial cells [208]. Its peculiar subcellular localization and known interactions with polycystin-2 and CAML place fibrocystin suggest that it may be involved both in microtubule organization, a characteristic centrosomal function, and in mechano- or chemosensation, the key functions of the primary cilia [4].

In addition, there is preliminary evidence of fibrocystin isoproteins which may be secreted in exosomes and undergo posttranslational processing [203–207, 209, 210]. However, the number of alternative *PKHD1* transcripts that are actually translated into protein and exert biological function(s) is as yet unknown. It will be important to establish which isoforms are essential for renal and hepatobiliary integrity to better understand the role of fibrocystin in the etiology of ARPKD. The distribution of mutations over the entire *PKHD1* gene suggests that the longest transcript is necessary for proper fibrocystin function in kidney and liver. Thus, it might be proposed that a critical amount of the full-length protein is required for normal function. Alternatively, it might be hypothesized that mutations disrupt a critical functional stoichiometric or temporal balance between the different protein isoforms which is normally maintained by elaborate, tightly regulated splicing patterns.

PKHD1 Mutation Spectrum and Routine Diagnostic Testing

The large size of *PKHD1*, its presumably complex pattern of splicing and still very limited knowledge of the encoded protein's function(s) pose significant challenges to DNA-based diagnostic testing. Further requirements for investigation are set by the extensive allelic heterogeneity with a high number of missense mutations and private mutations in non-isolate populations [142, 165, 211–215]. Thus, it was crucial to set up a locus-specific database for *PKHD1* (www. humgen.rwth-aachen.de).

Homozygous or compound heterozygous mutations in *PKHD1* are found in approximately 80 % of ARPKD patients, ranging from individuals with perinatal demise to moderately affected adults [165, 167, 170, 214, 215]. At least one mutation is even found in more than 95 % of families screened. One reason for missing mutations may have been the limited sensitivity of the screening methods (e.g., SSCP, DHPLC) used in earlier studies. Moreover, silent exonic changes and intronic sequence variations may also have an effect on *PKHD1* splicing, e.g., by affecting splice enhancer or silencer sites [216]. Functional and mRNA studies are usually needed to prove a possible pathogenic effect of such changes [217]. "Missing" mutations may also reside in regulatory elements. In addition, genomic rearrangements occur in the *PKHD1* gene [166]. In patients without any detectable *PKHD1* mutation misdiagnosis of ARPKD should be considered. ARPKD can be mimicked by mutations in a number of other genes [154]. Finally, evidence for genetic heterogeneity has been found in a small subset of families.

The most common mutation c.107C>T (p.Thr36Met) in exon 3 accounts for approximately 15–20 % of mutated alleles [212]. It is unclear whether it represents an ancestral change or occurs due to a frequent mutational event. Ultimately, it cannot be excluded that some of the mutated c.107C>T alleles represent a founder effect in the Central European population where it is particularly frequent [218]. However, there is compelling evidence that c.107C>T constitutes a mutational "hotspot." c.107C>T was identified in a multitude of obviously unrelated families of different ethnic origins on various haplotypes [165]. Besides c.107C>T there are no mutational hotspots, but marked allelic heterogeneity at *PKHD1* with the majority of mutations unique to a single family in "non-isolate" populations. Given the size of the *PKHD1* gene with absence of mutational hotspots, conventional *PKHD1* molecular testing by Sanger sequencing can thus be a time-consuming, labour-intensive process. For this, diagnostic testing has been simplified by the characterization of an algorithm for *PKHD1* that allows for detection of most mutations by analysis of only a subset of fragments and facilitates robust *PKHD1* mutation analysis in a routine diagnostic setting [150, 219]. However, next-generation sequencing (NGS) further streamlines this process and makes molecular genetic diagnostics much more efficient [154].

Genotype-Phenotype Correlations

The task to set up genotype-phenotype correlations for *PKHD1* is hampered by multiple allelism and the high rate of different compound heterozygotes. Genotype-phenotype correlations can be drawn for the type of mutation rather than for the site of individual mutations [211]. Almost all patients carrying two truncating mutations display a severe phenotype with peri- or neonatal demise while patients surviving the neonatal period bear at least one missense mutation. Although the converse did not apply and some missense changes are as devastating as truncating mutations, missense changes are more frequently observed among patients with a moderate clinical course. No significant clinical differences could be observed between patients with two missense mutations and those patients harbouring a truncating mutation in trans; thus, the milder mutation obviously defines the phenotype [165].

Loss of function probably explains the uniformly early demise of patients carrying two truncating alleles. A critical amount of the full-length fibrocystin protein seems to be required for normal function that obviously cannot be compensated by alternative isoforms, which might be generated by reinitiation of translation at a downstream ATG codon. In contrast, missense mutations and small in-frame deletions may have more variable effects on protein function. Phenotypic diversity also reflects the variable extent to which different *PKHD1* missense mutations might compromise the function and/or abundance of the mutant protein. While some may result in hypomorphic alleles with reduced function allowing for a clinically milder course, others might represent loss-of-function variants. Recent evidence suggests that complex transcriptional profiles may further play a role in defining the patient's phenotype [220, 221].

As depicted by discordant siblings (see below) and patients with severe and early polycystic kidney disease, phenotypes cannot be simply explained on the basis of the *PKHD1* genotype, but likely depend on the background of other, potentially PKD-associated genes resulting in an increased mutational load for an individual patient [146, 222–225], epigenetic factors (e.g., alternative splicing) [226, 227], and environmental influences. Such modifiers will probably have their greatest impact on the phenotype in the setting of hypomorphic missense changes and may explain, at least in part, the highly variable clinical course resulting from missense mutations, whereas they are less likely to be relevant in null alleles.

Phenotypic Variability Among Affected Siblings

While the majority of ARPKD sibships display comparable clinical courses, about 20 % of pedigrees exhibit gross intrafamilial phenotypic variability with peri-/neonatal demise in one and survival into childhood or even adulthood in another affected sibling [195]. An even higher proportion of 20 out of 48 sibships (42 %) was observed among families with at least one neonatal survivor per family [165]. Adjusting for differing family sizes the risk for perinatal demise of a further affected child was 37 %. With regards to genetic counselling this rate is alarming given that the study cohort was representative for the spectrum of patients followed in pediatric nephrology units. Of course, phenotype categorization into "severe" and "moderate" is a simplified and artificial view given the considerably better prognosis for patients surviving the most critical neonatal period. Also, the survival chance of an affected neonate might depend on available intensive care facilities and parental awareness of ARPKD risk. Overall, caution should be warranted in predicting the clinical outcome of a further affected child. The phenomenon of discordant siblings illustrates that phenotypes cannot be simply explained on the basis of the *PKHD1* genotype alone. To characterize putative modifying factors will be one of the major tasks for future research.

Prenatal Diagnosis

In view of the recurrence risk of 25 %, the oftentimes devastating course of early manifestations of ARPKD and a usually similar clinical course among affected siblings, many parents of ARPKD children seek early and reliable prenatal diagnosis (PND) to guide future family planning. Frequently, ARPKD patients are identified by ultrasound only late in pregnancy or at birth. However, fetal sonography at the time when termination of pregnancy (TOP) is usually performed may fail to detect enlargement and increased echogenicity of kidneys or oligohydramnios secondary to poor fetal urine output [51]. Therefore, an early and reliable PND for ARPKD in "at risk" families is only feasible by molecular genetic analysis. This became feasible for families with ARPKD when *PKHD1* was mapped and finally cloned [212, 228]. The majority, albeit not all patients with typical ARPKD, is linked to this locus. In the past, indirect haplotype-based linkage analysis has often been performed for ARPKD in terms of prenatal diagnosis. However, due to the aforementioned reasons with phenocopies and evidence for further heterogeneity in ARPKD, haplotype-based prenatal diagnostics is not any longer state of the art and regarded as too risky without knowledge of *PKHD1* mutational status. It should only be performed in those families in which the diagnosis has been previously proven unequivocally. Conclusively, mutation analysis of the *PKHD1* gene should be performed as the basis for PND and genetic counselling [213, 228].

and demonstrated that *Tg737* and its homologue in the green algae *C. reinhardtii, Ift88*, are required for ciliogenesis [230].

As discussed in detail elsewhere in this book, cilia seem to act as cellular antennae, sensing the cellular environment and regulate multiple intracellular signalling pathways, including the mTOR pathway, sonic hedgehog signalling, and WNT signalling [1–4]. It has been suggested that cilia may act as mechano- or chemosensors which control proliferative and apoptotic mechanisms. For *Pkd1*, however, the massive renal phenotype of *Pkd1* knockout mice is more severe than the phenotype of "ciliary" knockout mice [231]. Notably, parallel loss of cilia even ameliorated the *Pkd1* knockout phenotype. Therefore, a cilia-dependent pathway can be postulated that triggers renal cyst growth and that is not explained by activation of known pathways such as MAPK/ERK, mTOR or cAMP [231]. See Fig. 12.6.

Pathomechanisms Underlying Cyst Formation: Primary Cilia

To unravel the still widely unknown molecular pathomechanisms of polycystic kidney disease (PKD), it will be crucial to first further characterize the involved proteins and signaling pathways. To understand genetic interaction, it needs to be modeled at the cellular level. As mentioned, it is noteworthy that most, if not all, cystoproteins, among them the polycystins and fibrocystin, appear to co-localize at the base and within primary cilia [1–4]. This puts the primary cilium at the centre of a putative common network of cystoproteins in which these proteins may interact with each other and converge into joint signaling cascades. The importance of primary renal cilia as critical organelles for architectural homeostasis of the kidney was first recognized when Barr and Sternberg found that the homologue of *PKD1* in *C. elegans* localizes to neuronal cilia and is involved in ciliary sensing [229]. In a landmark publication, Pazour identified the underlying mutation in *Tg737* in the *orpk* mouse, a model of autosomal recessive polycystic kidney disease,

Treatment Prospects

Currently, there is no curative treatment option for patients affected by PKDs to ameliorate or even regress the clinical course. However, given the insights into ciliary biology and dysregulated intracellular signaling pathways in different PKDs, novel treatment approaches in ADPKD have been suggested [17, 232].

Using different rodent models, various research groups have published promising data on treatment of PKD. Interestingly, the severity of cystic kidney disease in an inducible orthologous mouse model of *Pkd1* depends on the day of inactivation. Early inactivation in mice before postnatal day 13 results in severe polycystic kidney disease within 3 weeks, whereas inactivation at day 14 or later results in slow-onset PKD with cysts only after 5 months [120]. These insights may be highly relevant when testing potential therapeutic approaches in mouse models [233]. V2 receptor antagonists, mTOR inhibitors the somatostatin analog octreotide, the cyclin-dependent kinase (CDK) inhibitor (R-) roscovitine, Src

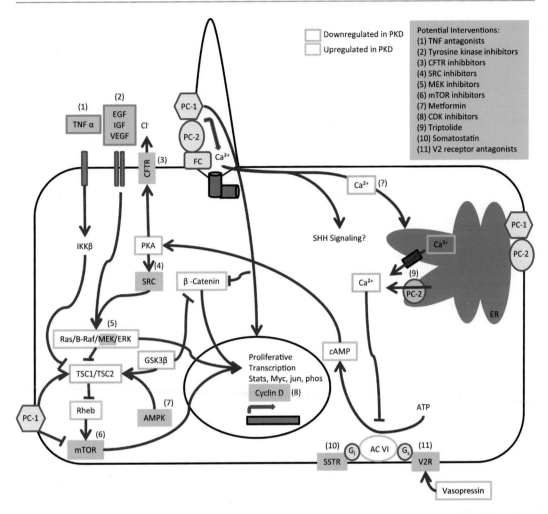

Fig. 12.6 Schematic presentation of polycystin-associated signalling pathways and potential pharmacological targets. Polycystin-1 (PC-1), polycystin-2 (PC-2), and fibrocystin/polyductin (FC) are located in primary cilia. PC2 is also located in the endoplasmic reticulum. The ciliary polycystin complex regulates ciliary calcium signals that may lead to calcium-induced calcium release from the endoplasmic reticulum. Reduction of calcium enhances cAMP accumulation, that is furthermore supported by activation of V2-receptors (V2R) but may be inhibited by activation of the somatostatin receptor (SSTR). cAMP stimulates chloride-driven fluid secretion. In PKD cAMP also stimulates cell proliferation in an src-, Ras-, and B-raf–dependent manner. Finally, Mammalian target of rapamycin (mTOR) is activated in cyst-lining PKD epithelia. *AC-VI* adenylyl cyclase type VI, *ATP* adenosine triphosphate, *CFTR* cystic fibrosis transmembrane conductance regulator, *ER* endoplasmic reticulum, *ERK* extracellular signal–regulated kinase, *MEK* mitogen-activated protein kinase kinase, *PKA* protein kinase A, *EGF* Epidermal Growth Factor, *IGF* Insulin-like growth factors, *VEGF* Vascular Endothelial Growth Factor, *CFTR* Cystic Fibrosis Transmembrane Conductance Regulator, *AMPK* AMP-activated protein kinase, *SHH* Sonic Hedgehog Signaling

inhibitors, pioglitazone, etanercept, and the traditional Chinese medicine-derived natural product triptolide have all been found to reduce kidney volume in murine models of PKD [17, 232]. Recently, inhibition of the HSP90 chaperone showed beneficial effects in a model of ADPKD [234].

Encouraged by these experimental results, various clinical trials for ADPKD have been inaugurated. Recent publications nicely summarize the pathophysiological considerations underlying those novel treatment approaches [17, 232, 235]. We will therefore only provide a brief overview here.

Vasopressin V₂ Receptor Antagonists

Briefly, the concept for the use of V2 receptor antagonists is based on the observation that tubular cells in ADPKD contain high levels of cAMP and that PKD patients show high levels of circulating vasopressin. Vasopressin induces intracellular increase of cAMP via the V2 receptor to increase fluid secretion into cysts via the CFTR channel. To inhibit the accumulation of renal cAMP as a known promoter of renal cystic enlargement, studies have been performed with V_2R antagonists in several orthologous animal models of human PKD [236–238]. The V2 receptor antagonist tolvaptan was investigated in the TEMPO 3/4 trial (Tolvaptan Efficacy and Safety in Management of PKD and Outcomes), a large phase 3, placebo-controlled, double-blind study in 18- to 50-year-old patients with a GFR of >60 ml/min but relatively large kidneys (>750 ml) as an indicator of progressive disease. After 3 years, Tolvaptan significantly reduced kidney growth rate (2.8 %; vs. 5.5 % in the control group) and lesser renal function decline or ADPKD-related adverse events (Fig. 12.7) [239]. There was, however, a higher discontinuation rate in the Tolvaptan group (23 % vs. 14 % in the control group) related to aquaresis and hepatic events [239]. While long-term follow-ups will need to confirm the beneficial effects of tolvaptan and although there are still many issues to reduce the disonctinuation rate, the TEMPO trial was the first convincing study to show effective treatment of ADPKD in humans.

Somatostatin Analogues

Another way to decrease intracellular cAMP is the use of a long-acting analog of somatostatin. Indeed, octreotide led to reduced renal and hepatic cyst growth in the PCK rat asa model of ARPKD, even though there was no improvement in renal function. These findings were also seen in various small clinical trials. A small randomized, crossover, placebo-controlled study found smaller kidney volume after treatment.

However, there were no differences in renal function [240]. Another randomized, double-blind, placebo-controlled trial on octreotide treatment for 1 year enrolled 42 patients with either ADPKD or autosomal dominant liver disease (ADPLD) with a baseline GFR of 70 ml/min or 71 ml/min, respectively [97]. MRI-assessed mean TKV in ADPKD patients after 1 year on octreotide did not increase (1,143 vs. 1129 ml) whereas it did in the placebo group (803 vs. 874 ml). There was no significant difference in GFR change between the octreotide and the placebo group and octreotide was tolerated well.

Subcutaneous lanreotide was used in another randomized, double-blind, placebo-controlled trial on patients with ADPLD or ADPKD [99]. Lanreotide was associated with a decrease in CT-assessed mean TKV (1000–983 ml), while TKV increased from 1115 to 1165 ml in the placebo group. There was a slight decrease in serum creatinine in the lanreotide group, while a slight increase was found in the placebo group. However, the difference was not statistically significant. Lanreotide was tolerated well.

The ALADIN trial (A Long-Acting somatostatin on Disease progression in Nephropathy due to autosomal dominant polycystic kidney disease) was the most recent trial on somatostatin analogues in ADPKD [241]. This multicenter, randomised, single-blind, placebo-controlled trial on 79 patients compared octreotide longacting release to placebo. A significant difference in MRI-measured TKV between control and intervention group was observed after 1 year, but mean TKV increase was only numerically and not significantly smaller in the octreotide group after 3 years. GFR decline seemed less pronounced in the intervention group, without reaching significance. Substantial differences in TKV and eGFR at baseline raised concerns (1557 ml in intervention group vs. 2161 ml in control group and 90 ml/min/1.73 m² in intervention group vs. 76 ml/min/1.73 m² in control group respectively). Serious adverse events were similarly found in both groups. The data lay the foundation for a larger and more powerful follow-up study.

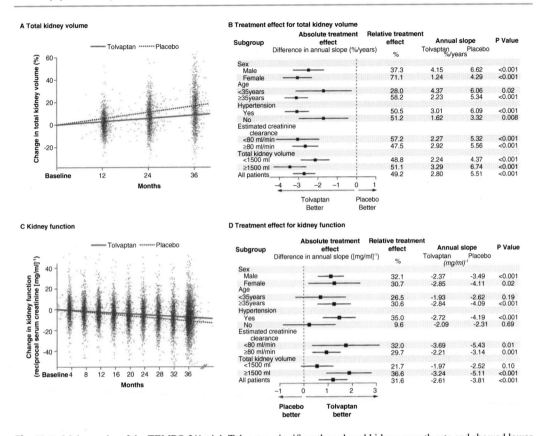

Fig. 12.7 Main results of the TEMPO 3/4 trial: Tolvaptan significantly reduced kidney growth rate and showed lower rates of renal function decline (Used with permission of Massachusetts Medical Society from Torres et al. [239])

Blood Pressure Control

As outlined above, blood pressure control is essential in PKD patients. The RAS may be activated in PKD patients [17], and hypertensive ADPKD patients have larger kidney volumes than age-matched normotensive control patients. A recent study evaluating the effects of ACE inhibition in children with ADPKD found no difference in the TKV growth rate assessed by ultrasonography [46]. The two HALT-PKD trials compared the combination of ACE inhibition (ACEI) with an angiotensin receptor blocker to ACEI alone in patients with an eGFR of either >60 (Study A) or 25–60 ml/min/1.73 m^2 (Study B) as well as standard blood pressure with low blood pressure targets in early-stage patients (Study A). Overall, more than 1000 ADPKD patients were enrolled [242, 243]. In these trials rigorous blood pressure control showed benefits over standard blood pres-

sure control in early ADPKD in terms of a reduced increase in total kidney volume, a greater decline in left ventricular mass index and less albuminuria. eGFR was not different among the groups. Side effects included more common dizziness and light-headedness in the low-blood pressure group [242].

mTOR Inhibition

Finally, mTOR activation has been observed in the cyst epithelium of ADPKD kidneys, and Polycystin-1 is a negative regulator of mTOR activation linking the mTOR pathway to ADPKD [244]. After promising results in animal models [244–251], four different trials studied mTOR inhibition in ADPKD. The two large trials on mTOR inhibition in ADPKD did not deliver a therapeutic breakthrough. The SUISSE ADPKD trial included 100 patients between 18 and 40 years of age at an early disease stage with an estimated creatinine clearance of at least 70 ml/min in an 18-month, open-label, randomized, controlled trial. Mean initial TKV was 907 cm^3 for the treatment group and 1003 cm^3 in the control group. Sirolimus was given at a target dose of 2 mg/day. The primary outcome was TKV after 18 months, which was blindly assessed on MRI scans. After 18 months there was no significant difference in TKV or GFR, but there was an increase in albuminuria in the sirolimus group [252]. This may be the result of impaired mTOR signalling, e.g., in glomerular cells. Recent insights into the significance of autophagy and mTOR signalling for podocyte function in health and disease may serve as a good explanation for this observation [253–257]. Walz et al. studied 433 patients with more advanced ADPKD in a 2-year, randomized, double-blind, placebo-controlled trial. Mean eGFR at baseline was 53 and 56 ml/min/1.73 m^2 in the treatment and control group respectively. A significant reduction of TKV was observed after 1 year of everolimus treatment, but this difference lost statistical significance after 2 years. Unfortunately, patients receiving everolimus had a significantly more rapid decline of eGFR after 2 years (8.9 vs. 7.7 ml/) [258]. Potential reasons for the discrepancy between the animal model findings and the results obtained in clinical trials are subject of ongoing discussion [233]. mTOR inhibitors might still be an option in selected patients with ADPKD or if administered in combination with other agents or in a tubule-specific way. However, they are not the magic bullets hoped for a couple of years ago [257].

Acknowledgements CB is an employee of Bioscientia/ Sonic Healthcare and holds a part-time faculty appointment at the University of Freiburg. His research lab received support from the Deutsche Forschungsgemeinschaft (DFG), Deutsche Nierenstiftung, and PKD Foundation. MCL was supported by the Köln Fortune and the GEROK program of the medical faculty of the University of Cologne, the Marga and Walter Boll-Stiftung and the PKD Familiäre Zystennieren e.V. (PKD Foundation) CB and MCL are supported by a grant from the German Ministry of Education and Research (Grant No. 01GM1515). We thank Klaus Zerres (Aachen, Germany) for his valuable contributions to the chapter originally published in the first edition of the book.

References

1. Fliegauf M, Benzing T, Omran H. When cilia go bad: cilia defects and ciliopathies. Nat Rev Mol Cell Biol. 2007;8(11):880–93.
2. Gerdes JM, Davis EE, Katsanis N. The vertebrate primary cilium in development, homeostasis, and disease. Cell. 2009;137(1):32–45.
3. Nigg EA, Raff JW. Centrioles, centrosomes, and cilia in health and disease. Cell. 2009;139(4):663–78.
4. Hildebrandt F, Benzing T, Katsanis N. Ciliopathies. N Engl J Med. 2011;364(16):1533–43.
5. Bergmann C. ARPKD and early manifestations of ADPKD: the original polycystic kidney disease and phenocopies. Pediatr Nephrol Berl Ger. 2015;30(1):15–30.
6. Sweeney Jr WE, Avner ED. Diagnosis and management of childhood polycystic kidney disease. Pediatr Nephrol Berl Ger. 2011;26(5):675–92.
7. Drenth JPH, Chrispijn M, Bergmann C. Congenital fibrocystic liver diseases. Best Pract Res Clin Gastroenterol. 2010;24(5):573–84.
8. Bergmann C, Weiskirchen R. It's not all in the cilium, but on the road to it: genetic interaction network in polycystic kidney and liver diseases and how trafficking and quality control matter. J Hepatol. 2012;56(5):1201–3.
9. Liebau MC, Serra AL. Looking at the (w)hole: magnet resonance imaging in polycystic kidney disease. Pediatr Nephrol Berl Ger. 2013;28(9):1771–83.
10. Osathanondh V, Potter EL. Pathogenesis of polycystic kidneys. Type 4 due to urethral obstruction. Arch Pathol. 1964;77:502–9.
11. McHugh K, Stringer DA, Hebert D, Babiak CA. Simple renal cysts in children: diagnosis and follow-up with US. Radiology. 1991;178(2):383–5.
12. Ogborn MR. Polycystic kidney disease – a truly pediatric problem. Pediatr Nephrol Berl Ger. 1994;8(6):762–7.
13. Bear JC, McManamon P, Morgan J, Payne RH, Lewis H, Gault MH, et al. Age at clinical onset and at ultrasonographic detection of adult polycystic kidney disease: data for genetic counselling. Am J Med Genet. 1984;18(1):45–53.
14. Pei Y, Obaji J, Dupuis A, Paterson AD, Magistroni R, Dicks E, et al. Unified criteria for ultrasonographic diagnosis of ADPKD. J Am Soc Nephrol JASN. 2009;20(1):205–12.
15. Ravine D, Gibson RN, Donlan J, Sheffield LJ. An ultrasound renal cyst prevalence survey: specificity data for inherited renal cystic diseases. Am J Kidney Dis Off J Natl Kidney Found. 1993;22(6):803–7.
16. Harris PC, Rossetti S. Determinants of renal disease variability in ADPKD. Adv Chronic Kidney Dis. 2010;17(2):131–9.
17. Torres VE, Harris PC. Autosomal dominant polycystic kidney disease: the last 3 years. Kidney Int. 2009;76(2):149–68.

18. Wilson PD. Polycystic kidney disease. N Engl J Med. 2004;350(2):151–64.
19. Luciano RL, Dahl NK. Extra-renal manifestations of autosomal dominant polycystic kidney disease (ADPKD): considerations for routine screening and management. Nephrol Dial Transplant Off Publ Eur Dial Transpl Assoc Eur Ren Assoc. 2014;29(2):247–54.
20. Helal I, Reed B, Schrier RW. Emergent early markers of renal progression in autosomal-dominant polycystic kidney disease patients: implications for prevention and treatment. Am J Nephrol. 2012;36(2):162–7.
21. Gabow PA, Kimberling WJ, Strain JD, Manco-Johnson ML, Johnson AM. Utility of ultrasonography in the diagnosis of autosomal dominant polycystic kidney disease in children. J Am Soc Nephrol JASN. 1997;8(1):105–10.
22. Bear JC, Parfrey PS, Morgan JM, Martin CJ, Cramer BC. Autosomal dominant polycystic kidney disease: new information for genetic counselling. Am J Med Genet. 1992;43(3):548–53.
23. Reed B, Nobakht E, Dadgar S, Bekheirnia MR, Masoumi A, Belibi F, et al. Renal ultrasonographic evaluation in children at risk of autosomal dominant polycystic kidney disease. Am J Kidney Dis Off J Natl Kidney Found. 2010;56(1):50–6.
24. Chapman AB, Wei W. Imaging approaches to patients with polycystic kidney disease. Semin Nephrol. 2011;31(3):237–44.
25. Nascimento AB, Mitchell DG, Zhang XM, Kamishima T, Parker L, Holland GA. Rapid MR imaging detection of renal cysts: age-based standards. Radiology. 2001;221(3):628–32.
26. Laucks Jr SP, McLachlan MS. Aging and simple cysts of the kidney. Br J Radiol. 1981;54(637):12–4.
27. Tada S, Yamagishi J, Kobayashi H, Hata Y, Kobari T. The incidence of simple renal cyst by computed tomography. Clin Radiol. 1983;34(4):437–9.
28. Boyer O, Gagnadoux M-F, Guest G, Biebuyck N, Charbit M, Salomon R, et al. Prognosis of autosomal dominant polycystic kidney disease diagnosed in utero or at birth. Pediatr Nephrol Berl Ger. 2007;22(3):380–8.
29. Pei Y. Diagnostic approach in autosomal dominant polycystic kidney disease. Clin J Am Soc Nephrol CJASN. 2006;1(5):1108–14.
30. Rizk D, Chapman A. Treatment of autosomal dominant polycystic kidney disease (ADPKD): the new horizon for children with ADPKD. Pediatr Nephrol Berl Ger. 2008;23(7):1029–36.
31. Chapman AB, et al. Autosomal Dominant Polycystic Kidney Disease (ADPKD): report from a Kidney Disease: Improving Global Outcomes (KDIGO) controversies conference. Kidney Int. 2015;88(1):17–27.
32. Grantham JJ, Torres VE, Chapman AB, Guay-Woodford LM, Bae KT, King Jr BF, et al. Volume progression in polycystic kidney disease. N Engl J Med. 2006;354(20):2122–30.
33. Bae KT, Tao C, Zhu F, Bost JE, Chapman AB, Grantham JJ, et al. MRI-based kidney volume measurements in ADPKD: reliability and effect of gadolinium enhancement. Clin J Am Soc Nephrol CJASN. 2009;4(4):719–25.
34. Torres VE, King BF, Chapman AB, Brummer ME, Bae KT, Glockner JF, et al. Magnetic resonance measurements of renal blood flow and disease progression in autosomal dominant polycystic kidney disease. Clin J Am Soc Nephrol CJASN. 2007;2(1):112–20.
35. Chapman AB. Approaches to testing new treatments in autosomal dominant polycystic kidney disease: insights from the CRISP and HALT-PKD studies. Clin J Am Soc Nephrol CJASN. 2008;3(4):1197–204.
36. Kistler AD, Poster D, Krauer F, Weishaupt D, Raina S, Senn O, et al. Increases in kidney volume in autosomal dominant polycystic kidney disease can be detected within 6 months. Kidney Int. 2009;75(2):235–41.
37. Torres VE, Chapman AB, Perrone RD, Bae KT, Abebe KZ, Bost JE, et al. Analysis of baseline parameters in the HALT polycystic kidney disease trials. Kidney Int. 2012;81(6):577–85.
38. Cornec-Le Gall E, Audrézet M-P, Chen J-M, Hourmant M, Morin M-P, Perrichot R, et al. Type of PKD1 mutation influences renal outcome in ADPKD. J Am Soc Nephrol JASN. 2013;24(6):1006–13.
39. Magistroni R, He N, Wang K, Andrew R, Johnson A, Gabow P, et al. Genotype-renal function correlation in type 2 autosomal dominant polycystic kidney disease. J Am Soc Nephrol JASN. 2003;14(5):1164–74.
40. Paterson AD, Magistroni R, He N, Wang K, Johnson A, Fain PR, et al. Progressive loss of renal function is an age-dependent heritable trait in type 1 autosomal dominant polycystic kidney disease. J Am Soc Nephrol JASN. 2005;16(3):755–62.
41. Persu A, Duyme M, Pirson Y, Lens XM, Messiaen T, Breuning MH, et al. Comparison between siblings and twins supports a role for modifier genes in ADPKD. Kidney Int. 2004;66(6):2132–6.
42. Sedman A, Bell P, Manco-Johnson M, Schrier R, Warady BA, Heard EO, et al. Autosomal dominant polycystic kidney disease in childhood: a longitudinal study. Kidney Int. 1987;31(4):1000–5.
43. Sweeney Jr WE, Avner ED. Molecular and cellular pathophysiology of autosomal recessive polycystic kidney disease (ARPKD). Cell Tissue Res. 2006;326(3):671–85.
44. Ulinski T, Lescure S, Beaufils S, Guigonis V, Decramer S, Morin D, et al. Renal phenotypes related to hepatocyte nuclear factor-1beta (TCF2) mutations in a pediatric cohort. J Am Soc Nephrol JASN. 2006;17(2):497–503.
45. Faguer S, Bouissou F, Dumazer P, Guitard J, Bellanné-Chantelot C, Chauveau D. Massively enlarged polycystic kidneys in monozygotic twins with TCF2/HNF-1beta (hepatocyte nuclear factor-1beta) heterozygous whole-gene deletion. Am

J Kidney Dis Off J Natl Kidney Found. 2007;50(6):1023–7.

46. Cadnapaphornchai MA, McFann K, Strain JD, Masoumi A, Schrier RW. Prospective change in renal volume and function in children with ADPKD. Clin J Am Soc Nephrol CJASN. 2009; 4(4):820–9.

47. Fick-Brosnahan GM, Tran ZV, Johnson AM, Strain JD, Gabow PA. Progression of autosomal-dominant polycystic kidney disease in children. Kidney Int. 2001;59(5):1654–62.

48. Shamshirsaz AA, Shamshirsaz A, Reza Bekheirnia M, Bekheirnia RM, Kamgar M, Johnson AM, et al. Autosomal-dominant polycystic kidney disease in infancy and childhood: progression and outcome. Kidney Int. 2005;68(5):2218–24.

49. Cadnapaphornchai MA, Masoumi A, Strain JD, McFann K, Schrier RW. Magnetic resonance imaging of kidney and cyst volume in children with ADPKD. Clin J Am Soc Nephrol CJASN. 2011; 6(2):369–76.

50. Fick-Brosnahan G, Johnson AM, Strain JD, Gabow PA. Renal asymmetry in children with autosomal dominant polycystic kidney disease. Am J Kidney Dis Off J Natl Kidney Found. 1999; 34(4):639–45.

51. Bergmann C, Zerres K. Autosomal dominant polycystic kidney disease (ADPKD) in children and young adults. In: Turner N, et al., editors. Oxford textbook of clinical nephrology. Oxford University Press; 2015.

52. Gabow PA, Duley I, Johnson AM. Clinical profiles of gross hematuria in autosomal dominant polycystic kidney disease. Am J Kidney Dis Off J Natl Kidney Found. 1992;20(2):140–3.

53. Gabow PA, Johnson AM, Kaehny WD, Kimberling WJ, Lezotte DC, Duley IT, et al. Factors affecting the progression of renal disease in autosomal-dominant polycystic kidney disease. Kidney Int. 1992;41(5):1311–9.

54. Johnson AM, Gabow PA. Identification of patients with autosomal dominant polycystic kidney disease at highest risk for end-stage renal disease. J Am Soc Nephrol JASN. 1997;8(10):1560–7.

55. Gagnadoux MF, Habib R, Levy M, Brunelle F, Broyer M. Cystic renal diseases in children. Adv Nephrol Necker Hosp. 1989;18:33–57.

56. MacDermot KD, Saggar-Malik AK, Economides DL, Jeffery S. Prenatal diagnosis of autosomal dominant polycystic kidney disease (PKD1) presenting in utero and prognosis for very early onset disease. J Med Genet. 1998;35(1):13–6.

57. Avner ED. Childhood ADPKD: answers and more questions. Kidney Int. 2001;59(5):1979–80.

58. Chapman AB, Schrier RW. Pathogenesis of hypertension in autosomal dominant polycystic kidney disease. Semin Nephrol. 1991;11(6):653–60.

59. Harrap SB, Davies DL, Macnicol AM, Dominiczak AF, Fraser R, Wright AF, et al. Renal, cardiovascular and hormonal characteristics of young adults with autosomal dominant polycystic kidney disease. Kidney Int. 1991;40(3):501–8.

60. Schrier RW. Renal volume, renin-angiotensin-aldosterone system, hypertension, and left ventricular hypertrophy in patients with autosomal dominant polycystic kidney disease. J Am Soc Nephrol JASN. 2009;20(9):1888–93.

61. Tkachenko O, Helal I, Shchekochikhin D, Schrier RW. Renin-Angiotensin-aldosterone system in autosomal dominant polycystic kidney disease. Curr Hypertens Rev. 2013;9(1):12–20.

62. Gibbs GF, Huston 3rd J, Qian Q, Kubly V, Harris PC, Brown Jr RD, et al. Follow-up of intracranial aneurysms in autosomal-dominant polycystic kidney disease. Kidney Int. 2004;65(5):1621–7.

63. Pirson Y. Extrarenal manifestations of autosomal dominant polycystic kidney disease. Adv Chronic Kidney Dis. 2010;17(2):173–80.

64. Pirson Y, Chauveau D, Torres V. Management of cerebral aneurysms in autosomal dominant polycystic kidney disease. J Am Soc Nephrol JASN. 2002;13(1):269–76.

65. Chapman AB, Rubinstein D, Hughes R, Stears JC, Earnest MP, Johnson AM, et al. Intracranial aneurysms in autosomal dominant polycystic kidney disease. N Engl J Med. 1992;327(13):916–20.

66. Huston 3rd J, Torres VE, Sulivan PP, Offord KP, Wiebers DO. Value of magnetic resonance angiography for the detection of intracranial aneurysms in autosomal dominant polycystic kidney disease. J Am Soc Nephrol JASN. 1993;3(12): 1871–7.

67. Ruggieri PM, Poulos N, Masaryk TJ, Ross JS, Obuchowski NA, Awad IA, et al. Occult intracranial aneurysms in polycystic kidney disease: screening with MR angiography. Radiology. 1994;191(1): 33–9.

68. Xu HW, Yu SQ, Mei CL, Li MH. Screening for intracranial aneurysm in 355 patients with autosomal-dominant polycystic kidney disease. Stroke J Cereb Circ. 2011;42(1):204–6.

69. Nicholas BA, Vricella GJ, Smith M, Passalacqua M, Gulani V, Ponsky LE. Contrast-induced nephropathy and nephrogenic systemic fibrosis: minimizing the risk. Can J Urol. 2012;19(1):6074–80.

70. Kaufmann TJ, Huston 3rd J, Mandrekar JN, Schleck CD, Thielen KR, Kallmes DF. Complications of diagnostic cerebral angiography: evaluation of 19,826 consecutive patients. Radiology. 2007; 243(3):812–9.

71. Belz MM, Hughes RL, Kaehny WD, Johnson AM, Fick-Brosnahan GM, Earnest MP, et al. Familial clustering of ruptured intracranial aneurysms in autosomal dominant polycystic kidney disease. Am J Kidney Dis Off J Natl Kidney Found. 2001;38(4): 770–6.

72. Chauveau D, Pirson Y, Le Moine A, Franco D, Belghiti J, Grünfeld JP. Extrarenal manifestations in autosomal dominant polycystic kidney disease. Adv Nephrol Necker Hosp. 1997;26:265–89.

73. Cheung J, Scudamore CH, Yoshida EM. Management of polycystic liver disease. Can J Gastroenterol J Can Gastroenterol. 2004;18(11):666–70.

74. Mathieu D, Vilgrain V, Mahfouz AE, Anglade MC, Vullierme MP, Denys A. Benign liver tumors. Magn Reson Imaging Clin N Am. 1997;5(2):255–88.

75. Bae KT, Zhu F, Chapman AB, Torres VE, Grantham JJ, Guay-Woodford LM, et al. Magnetic resonance imaging evaluation of hepatic cysts in early autosomal-dominant polycystic kidney disease: the Consortium for Radiologic Imaging Studies of Polycystic Kidney Disease cohort. Clin J Am Soc Nephrol CJASN. 2006;1(1):64–9.

76. Gevers TJG, Drenth JPH. Diagnosis and management of polycystic liver disease. Nat Rev Gastroenterol Hepatol. 2013;10(2):101–8.

77. Abu-Wasel B, Walsh C, Keough V, Molinari M. Pathophysiology, epidemiology, classification and treatment options for polycystic liver diseases. World J Gastroenterol WJG. 2013;19(35):5775–86.

78. Davila S, Furu L, Gharavi AG, Tian X, Onoe T, Qian Q, et al. Mutations in SEC63 cause autosomal dominant polycystic liver disease. Nat Genet. 2004;36(6):575–7.

79. Drenth JPH, te Morsche RHM, Smink R, Bonifacino JS, Jansen JBMJ. Germline mutations in PRKCSH are associated with autosomal dominant polycystic liver disease. Nat Genet. 2003;33(3):345–7.

80. Fedeles SV, Tian X, Gallagher A-R, Mitobe M, Nishio S, Lee SH, et al. A genetic interaction network of five genes for human polycystic kidney and liver diseases defines polycystin-1 as the central determinant of cyst formation. Nat Genet. 2011; 43(7):639–47.

81. Strazzabosco M, Somlo S. Polycystic liver diseases: congenital disorders of cholangiocyte signaling. Gastroenterology. 2011;140(7):1855–9, 1859.e1.

82. Desmet VJ. Ludwig symposium on biliary disorders – part I. Pathogenesis of ductal plate abnormalities. Mayo Clin Proc Mayo Clin. 1998;73(1):80–9.

83. Lazaridis KN, Strazzabosco M, Larusso NF. The cholangiopathies: disorders of biliary epithelia. Gastroenterology. 2004;127(5):1565–77.

84. Cobben JM, Breuning MH, Schoots C, ten Kate LP, Zerres K. Congenital hepatic fibrosis in autosomal-dominant polycystic kidney disease. Kidney Int. 1990;38(5):880–5.

85. Lipschitz B, Berdon WE, Defelice AR, Levy J. Association of congenital hepatic fibrosis with autosomal dominant polycystic kidney disease. Report of a family with review of literature. Pediatr Radiol. 1993;23(2):131–3.

86. Milutinovic J, Schabel SI, Ainsworth SK. Autosomal dominant polycystic kidney disease with liver and pancreatic involvement in early childhood. Am J Kidney Dis Off J Natl Kidney Found. 1989;13(4): 340–4.

87. Tamura H, Kato H, Hirose S, Itoyama S, Matsumura O, Nagasawa R, et al. An adult case of polycystic kidney disease associated with congenital hepatic fibrosis. Nihon Jinzo Gakkai Shi. 1994;36(8): 962–7.

88. Everson GT. Hepatic cysts in autosomal dominant polycystic kidney disease. Mayo Clin Proc Mayo Clin. 1990;65(7):1020–5.

89. Telenti A, Torres VE, Gross Jr JB, Van Scoy RE, Brown ML, Hattery RR. Hepatic cyst infection in autosomal dominant polycystic kidney disease. Mayo Clin Proc Mayo Clin. 1990;65(7):933–42.

90. Tan YM, Ooi LLPJ, Mack POP. Current status in the surgical management of adult polycystic liver disease. Ann Acad Med Singapore. 2002;31(2): 217–22.

91. Garcea G, Rajesh A, Dennison AR. Surgical management of cystic lesions in the liver. ANZ J Surg. 2013;83(7–8):E3–20.

92. Caroli A, Antiga L, Cafaro M, Fasolini G, Remuzzi A, Remuzzi G, et al. Reducing polycystic liver volume in ADPKD: effects of somatostatin analogue octreotide. Clin J Am Soc Nephrol CJASN. 2010; 5(5):783–9.

93. Chrispijn M, Nevens F, Gevers TJG, Vanslembrouck R, van Oijen MGH, Coudyzer W, et al. The long-term outcome of patients with polycystic liver disease treated with lanreotide. Aliment Pharmacol Ther. 2012;35(2):266–74.

94. Chrispijn M, Gevers TJG, Hol JC, Monshouwer R, Dekker HM, Drenth JPH. Everolimus does not further reduce polycystic liver volume when added to long acting octreotide: results from a randomized controlled trial. J Hepatol. 2013;59(1):153–9.

95. Gevers TJG, Chrispijn M, Wetzels JFM, Drenth JPH. Rationale and design of the RESOLVE trial: lanreotide as a volume reducing treatment for polycystic livers in patients with autosomal dominant polycystic kidney disease. BMC Nephrol. 2012; 13:17.

96. Gevers TJG, Inthout J, Caroli A, Ruggenenti P, Hogan MC, Torres VE, et al. Young women with polycystic liver disease respond best to somatostatin analogues: a pooled analysis of individual patient data. Gastroenterology. 2013;145(2):357–65.e1. –2.

97. Hogan MC, Masyuk TV, Page LJ, Kubly VJ, Bergstralh EJ, Li X, et al. Randomized clinical trial of long-acting somatostatin for autosomal dominant polycystic kidney and liver disease. J Am Soc Nephrol JASN. 2010;21(6):1052–61.

98. Hogan MC, Masyuk TV, Page L, Holmes 3rd DR, Li X, Bergstralh EJ, et al. Somatostatin analog therapy for severe polycystic liver disease: results after 2 years. Nephrol Dial Transplant Off Publ Eur Dial Transpl Assoc Eur Ren Assoc. 2012;27(9): 3532–9.

99. Van Keimpema L, Nevens F, Vanslembrouck R, van Oijen MGH, Hoffmann AL, Dekker HM, et al. Lanreotide reduces the volume of polycystic liver: a randomized, double-blind, placebo-controlled trial. Gastroenterology. 2009;137(5): 1661–8.e1. –2.

100. Torres VE, Harris PC, Pirson Y. Autosomal dominant polycystic kidney disease. Lancet. 2007;369(9569):1287–301.

101. Marquardt. Cystennieren, Cystenleber, und Cystenpancreas bei zwei Geschwistern. Universität Tübingen; 1935.

102. Blyth H, Ockenden BG. Polycystic disease of kidney and liver presenting in childhood. J Med Genet. 1971;8(3):257–84.

103. Hughes J, Ward CJ, Peral B, Aspinwall R, Clark K, San Millán JL, et al. The polycystic kidney disease 1 (PKD1) gene encodes a novel protein with multiple cell recognition domains. Nat Genet. 1995;10(2): 151–60.

104. Torres VE, Harris PC. Polycystic kidney disease: genes, proteins, animal models, disease mechanisms and therapeutic opportunities. J Intern Med. 2007; 261(1):17–31.

105. Mochizuki T, Wu G, Hayashi T, Xenophontos SL, Veldhuisen B, Saris JJ, et al. PKD2, a gene for polycystic kidney disease that encodes an integral membrane protein. Science. 1996;272(5266):1339–42.

106. Boulter C, Mulroy S, Webb S, Fleming S, Brindle K, Sandford R. Cardiovascular, skeletal, and renal defects in mice with a targeted disruption of the Pkd1 gene. Proc Natl Acad Sci U S A. 2001;98(21): 12174–9.

107. Kim K, Drummond I, Ibraghimov-Beskrovnaya O, Klinger K, Arnaout MA. Polycystin 1 is required for the structural integrity of blood vessels. Proc Natl Acad Sci U S A. 2000;97(4):1731–6.

108. Lu W, Peissel B, Babakhanlou H, Pavlova A, Geng L, Fan X, et al. Perinatal lethality with kidney and pancreas defects in mice with a targetted Pkd1 mutation. Nat Genet. 1997;17(2):179–81.

109. Lu W, Shen X, Pavlova A, Lakkis M, Ward CJ, Pritchard L, et al. Comparison of Pkd1-targeted mutants reveals that loss of polycystin-1 causes cystogenesis and bone defects. Hum Mol Genet. 2001;10(21):2385–96.

110. Brasier JL, Henske EP. Loss of the polycystic kidney disease (PKD1) region of chromosome 16p13 in renal cyst cells supports a loss-of-function model for cyst pathogenesis. J Clin Invest. 1997;99(2):194–9.

111. Koptides M, Mean R, Demetriou K, Pierides A, Deltas CC. Genetic evidence for a trans-heterozygous model for cystogenesis in autosomal dominant polycystic kidney disease. Hum Mol Genet. 2000;9(3): 447–52.

112. Qian F, Watnick TJ, Onuchic LF, Germino GG. The molecular basis of focal cyst formation in human autosomal dominant polycystic kidney disease type I. Cell. 1996;87(6):979–87.

113. Watnick T, He N, Wang K, Liang Y, Parfrey P, Hefferton D, et al. Mutations of PKD1 in ADPKD2 cysts suggest a pathogenic effect of trans-heterozygous mutations. Nat Genet. 2000;25(2): 143–4.

114. Watnick TJ, Torres VE, Gandolph MA, Qian F, Onuchic LF, Klinger KW, et al. Somatic mutation in individual liver cysts supports a two-hit model of cystogenesis in autosomal dominant polycystic kidney disease. Mol Cell. 1998;2(2):247–51.

115. Pei Y, Paterson AD, Wang KR, He N, Hefferton D, Watnick T, et al. Bilineal disease and trans-heterozygotes in autosomal dominant polycystic kidney disease. Am J Hum Genet. 2001;68(2):355–63.

116. Wu G, Tian X, Nishimura S, Markowitz GS, D'Agati V, Park JH, et al. Trans-heterozygous Pkd1 and Pkd2 mutations modify expression of polycystic kidney disease. Hum Mol Genet. 2002;11(16):1845–54.

117. Thivierge C, Kurbegovic A, Couillard M, Guillaume R, Coté O, Trudel M. Overexpression of PKD1 causes polycystic kidney disease. Mol Cell Biol. 2006;26(4):1538–48.

118. Happé H, Peters DJM. Translational research in ADPKD: lessons from animal models. Nat Rev Nephrol. 2014;10(10):587–601.

119. Lantinga-van Leeuwen IS, Dauwerse JG, Baelde HJ, Leonhard WN, van de Wal A, Ward CJ, et al. Lowering of Pkd1 expression is sufficient to cause polycystic kidney disease. Hum Mol Genet. 2004;13(24):3069–77.

120. Piontek K, Menezes LF, Garcia-Gonzalez MA, Huso DL, Germino GG. A critical developmental switch defines the kinetics of kidney cyst formation after loss of Pkd1. Nat Med. 2007;13(12):1490–5.

121. Bastos AP, Piontek K, Silva AM, Martini D, Menezes LF, Fonseca JM, et al. Pkd1 haploinsufficiency increases renal damage and induces microcyst formation following ischemia/reperfusion. J Am Soc Nephrol JASN. 2009;20(11):2389–402.

122. Patel V, Li LL, Cobo-Stark P, Shao X, Somlo S, Lin F, et al. Acute kidney injury and aberrant planar cell polarity induce cyst formation in mice lacking renal cilia. Hum Mol Genet. 2008;17(11):1578–90.

123. Takakura A, Contrino L, Zhou X, Bonventre JV, Sun Y, Humphreys BD, et al. Renal injury is a third hit promoting rapid development of adult polycystic kidney disease. Hum Mol Genet. 2009;18(14):2523–31.

124. Happé H, Leonhard WN, van der Wal A, van de Water B, Lantinga-van Leeuwen IS, Breuning MH, et al. Toxic tubular injury in kidneys from Pkd1-deletion mice accelerates cystogenesis accompanied by dysregulated planar cell polarity and canonical Wnt signaling pathways. Hum Mol Genet. 2009;18(14):2532–42.

125. Karihaloo A, Koraishy F, Huen SC, Lee Y, Merrick D, Caplan MJ, et al. Macrophages promote cyst growth in polycystic kidney disease. J Am Soc Nephrol JASN. 2011;22(10):1809–14.

126. Swenson-Fields KI, Vivian CJ, Salah SM, Peda JD, Davis BM, van Rooijen N, et al. Macrophages promote polycystic kidney disease progression. Kidney Int. 2013;83(5):855–64.

127. Weimbs T. Third-hit signaling in renal cyst formation. J Am Soc Nephrol JASN. 2011;22(5):793–5.

128. Zhou J. Polycystins and primary cilia: primers for cell cycle progression. Annu Rev Physiol. 2009;71: 83–113.

129. Ibraghimov-Beskrovnaya O, Bukanov N. Polycystic kidney diseases: from molecular discoveries to targeted therapeutic strategies. Cell Mol Life Sci CMLS. 2008;65(4):605–19.

130. Hofherr A, Köttgen M. TRPP channels and polycystins. Adv Exp Med Biol. 2011;704:287–313.

131. Hanaoka K, Qian F, Boletta A, Bhunia AK, Piontek K, Tsiokas L, et al. Co-assembly of polycystin-1 and -2 produces unique cation-permeable currents. Nature. 2000;408(6815):990–4.

132. Qian F, Germino FJ, Cai Y, Zhang X, Somlo S, Germino GG. PKD1 interacts with PKD2 through a probable coiled-coil domain. Nat Genet. 1997; 16(2):179–83.

133. Qian F, Boletta A, Bhunia AK, Xu H, Liu L, Ahrabi AK, et al. Cleavage of polycystin-1 requires the receptor for egg jelly domain and is disrupted by human autosomal-dominant polycystic kidney disease 1-associated mutations. Proc Natl Acad Sci U S A. 2002;99(26):16981–6.

134. Hogan MC, Manganelli L, Woollard JR, Masyuk AI, Masyuk TV, Tammachote R, et al. Characterization of PKD protein-positive exosome-like vesicles. J Am Soc Nephrol JASN. 2009;20(2):278–88.

135. Yoder BK. Role of primary cilia in the pathogenesis of polycystic kidney disease. J Am Soc Nephrol JASN. 2007;18(5):1381–8.

136. Nauli SM, Alenghat FJ, Luo Y, Williams E, Vassilev P, Li X, et al. Polycystins 1 and 2 mediate mechanosensation in the primary cilium of kidney cells. Nat Genet. 2003;33(2):129–37.

137. Praetorius HA, Spring KR. Bending the MDCK cell primary cilium increases intracellular calcium. J Membr Biol. 2001;184(1):71–9.

138. Sharif-Naeini R, Folgering JHA, Bichet D, Duprat F, Lauritzen I, Arhatte M, et al. Polycystin-1 and -2 dosage regulates pressure sensing. Cell. 2009; 139(3):587–96.

139. Gallagher AR, Germino GG, Somlo S. Molecular advances in autosomal dominant polycystic kidney disease. Adv Chronic Kidney Dis. 2010;17(2): 118–30.

140. Rossetti S, Harris PC. Genotype-phenotype correlations in autosomal dominant and autosomal recessive polycystic kidney disease. J Am Soc Nephrol JASN. 2007;18(5):1374–80.

141. Rossetti S, Strmecki L, Gamble V, Burton S, Sneddon V, Peral B, et al. Mutation analysis of the entire PKD1 gene: genetic and diagnostic implications. Am J Hum Genet. 2001;68(1):46–63.

142. Rossetti S, Torra R, Coto E, Consugar M, Kubly V, Málaga S, et al. A complete mutation screen of PKHD1 in autosomal-recessive polycystic kidney disease (ARPKD) pedigrees. Kidney Int. 2003;64(2):391–403.

143. Hateboer N, Veldhuisen B, Peters D, Breuning MH, San-Millán JL, Bogdanova N, et al. Location of mutations within the PKD2 gene influences clinical outcome. Kidney Int. 2000;57(4):1444–51.

144. Rossetti S, Burton S, Strmecki L, Pond GR, San Millán JL, Zerres K, et al. The position of the polycystic kidney disease 1 (PKD1) gene mutation correlates with the severity of renal disease. J Am Soc Nephrol JASN. 2002;13(5):1230–7.

145. Rossetti S, Chauveau D, Kubly V, Slezak JM, Saggar-Malik AK, Pei Y, et al. Association of mutation position in polycystic kidney disease 1 (PKD1) gene and development of a vascular phenotype. Lancet. 2003;361(9376):2196–201.

146. Bergmann C, von Bothmer J, Ortiz Brüchle N, Venghaus A, Frank V, Fehrenbach H, et al. Mutations in multiple PKD genes may explain early and severe polycystic kidney disease. J Am Soc Nephrol JASN. 2011;22(11):2047–56.

147. Fain PR, McFann KK, Taylor MRG, Tison M, Johnson AM, Reed B, et al. Modifier genes play a significant role in the phenotypic expression of PKD1. Kidney Int. 2005;67(4):1256–67.

148. Zerres K, Rudnik-Schöneborn S, Deget F. Childhood onset autosomal dominant polycystic kidney disease in sibs: clinical picture and recurrence risk. German Working Group on Paediatric Nephrology (Arbeitsgemeinschaft für Pädiatrische Nephrologie). J Med Genet. 1993;30(7):583–8.

149. Kääriäinen H. Polycystic kidney disease in children: a genetic and epidemiological study of 82 Finnish patients. J Med Genet. 1987;24(8):474–81.

150. Bergmann C, Küpper F, Dornia C, Schneider F, Senderek J, Zerres K. Algorithm for efficient PKHD1 mutation screening in autosomal recessive polycystic kidney disease (ARPKD). Hum Mutat. 2005;25(3):225–31.

151. Guay-Woodford LM, Desmond RA. Autosomal recessive polycystic kidney disease: the clinical experience in North America. Pediatrics. 2003;111(5 Pt 1):1072–80.

152. Gunay-Aygun M, Avner ED, Bacallao RL, Choyke PL, Flynn JT, Germino GG, et al. Autosomal recessive polycystic kidney disease and congenital hepatic fibrosis: summary statement of a first National Institutes of Health/Office of Rare Diseases conference. J Pediatr. 2006;149(2):159–64.

153. Nakanishi K, Sweeney Jr WE, Zerres K, Guay-Woodford LM, Avner ED. Proximal tubular cysts in fetal human autosomal recessive polycystic kidney disease. J Am Soc Nephrol JASN. 2000;11(4): 760–3.

154. Bergmann C. Autosomal recessive polycystic kidney disease. In: Kenny TD, Beales PL, Herausgeber, editors. Ciliopathies: a reference for clinicians. Oxford University Press; 2014.

155. Büscher R, Büscher AK, Weber S, Mohr J, Hegen B, Vester U, et al. Clinical manifestations of autosomal recessive polycystic kidney disease (ARPKD): kidney-related and non-kidney-related phenotypes. Pediatr Nephrol Berl Ger. 2014;29(10):1915–25.

156. Gunay-Aygun M, Font-Montgomery E, Lukose L, Tuchman Gerstein M, Piwnica-Worms K, Choyke P,

et al. Characteristics of congenital hepatic fibrosis in a large cohort of patients with autosomal recessive polycystic kidney disease. Gastroenterology. 2013; 144(1):112–21.e2.

157. Adeva M, El-Youssef M, Rossetti S, Kamath PS, Kubly V, Consugar MB, et al. Clinical and molecular characterization defines a broadened spectrum of autosomal recessive polycystic kidney disease (ARPKD). Medicine (Baltimore). 2006;85(1):1–21.

158. Guay-Woodford LM, Bissler JJ, Braun MC, Bockenhauer D, Cadnapaphornchai MA, Dell KM, et al. Consensus expert recommendations for the diagnosis and management of autosomal recessive polycystic kidney disease: report of an International Conference. J Pediatr. 2014;165(3):611–7.

159. Cole BR, Conley SB, Stapleton FB. Polycystic kidney disease in the first year of life. J Pediatr. 1987;111(5):693–9.

160. Kääriäinen H, Koskimies O, Norio R. Dominant and recessive polycystic kidney disease in children: evaluation of clinical features and laboratory data. Pediatr Nephrol Berl Ger. 1988;2(3):296–302.

161. Kaplan BS, Fay J, Shah V, Dillon MJ, Barratt TM. Autosomal recessive polycystic kidney disease. Pediatr Nephrol Berl Ger. 1989;3(1):43–9.

162. Zerres K, Rudnik-Schöneborn S, Deget F, Holtkamp U, Brodehl J, Geisert J, et al. Autosomal recessive polycystic kidney disease in 115 children: clinical presentation, course and influence of gender. Arbeitsgemeinschaft für Pädiatrische Nephrol Acta Paediatr Oslo Nor. 1996;85(4):437–45. 1992.

163. Roy S, Dillon MJ, Trompeter RS, Barratt TM. Autosomal recessive polycystic kidney disease: long-term outcome of neonatal survivors. Pediatr Nephrol Berl Ger. 1997;11(3):302–6.

164. Capisonda R, Phan V, Traubuci J, Daneman A, Balfe JW, Guay-Woodford LM. Autosomal recessive polycystic kidney disease: outcomes from a single-center experience. Pediatr Nephrol Berl Ger. 2003;18(2):119–26.

165. Bergmann C, Senderek J, Windelen E, Küpper F, Middeldorf I, Schneider F, et al. Clinical consequences of PKHD1 mutations in 164 patients with autosomal-recessive polycystic kidney disease (ARPKD). Kidney Int. 2005;67(3):829–48.

166. Bergmann C, Küpper F, Schmitt CP, Vester U, Neuhaus TJ, Senderek J, et al. Multi-exon deletions of the PKHD1 gene cause autosomal recessive polycystic kidney disease (ARPKD). J Med Genet. 2005;42(10):e63.

167. Gunay-Aygun M, Tuchman M, Font-Montgomery E, Lukose L, Edwards H, Garcia A, et al. PKHD1 sequence variations in 78 children and adults with autosomal recessive polycystic kidney disease and congenital hepatic fibrosis. Mol Genet Metab. 2010;99(2):160–73.

168. Mehler K, Beck BB, Kaul I, Rahimi G, Hoppe B, Kribs A. Respiratory and general outcome in neonates with renal oligohydramnios – a single-centre experience. Nephrol Dial Transplant Off Publ Eur Dial Transpl Assoc Eur Ren Assoc. 2011;26(11): 3514–22.

169. Zurowska AM, Fischbach M, Watson AR, Edefonti A, Stefanidis CJ, European Paediatric Dialysis Working Group. Clinical practice recommendations for the care of infants with stage 5 chronic kidney disease (CKD5). Pediatr Nephrol Berl Ger. 2013;28(9):1739–48.

170. Gunay-Aygun M, Font-Montgomery E, Lukose L, Tuchman M, Graf J, Bryant JC, et al. Correlation of kidney function, volume and imaging findings, and PKHD1 mutations in 73 patients with autosomal recessive polycystic kidney disease. Clin J Am Soc Nephrol CJASN. 2010;5(6):972–84.

171. Arbeiter A, Büscher R, Bonzel K-E, Wingen A-M, Vester U, Wohlschläger J, et al. Nephrectomy in an autosomal recessive polycystic kidney disease (ARPKD) patient with rapid kidney enlargement and increased expression of EGFR. Nephrol Dial Transplant. 2008;23(9):3026–9.

172. Bean SA, Bednarek FJ, Primack WA. Aggressive respiratory support and unilateral nephrectomy for infants with severe perinatal autosomal recessive polycystic kidney disease. J Pediatr. 1995;127(2): 311–3.

173. Beaunoyer M, Snehal M, Li L, Concepcion W, Salvatierra Jr O, Sarwal M. Optimizing outcomes for neonatal ARPKD. Pediatr Transplant. 2007;11(3): 267–71.

174. Shukla AR, Kiddoo DA, Canning DA. Unilateral nephrectomy as palliative therapy in an infant with autosomal recessive polycystic kidney disease. J Urol. 2004;172(5 Pt 1):2000–1.

175. Spechtenhauser B, Hochleitner BW, Ellemunter H, Simma B, Hörmann C, Königsrainer A, et al. Bilateral nephrectomy, peritoneal dialysis and subsequent cadaveric renal transplantation for treatment of renal failure due to polycystic kidney disease requiring continuous ventilation. Pediatr Transplant. 1999;3(3):246–8.

176. Sumfest JM, Burns MW, Mitchell ME. Aggressive surgical and medical management of autosomal recessive polycystic kidney disease. Urology. 1993;42(3):309–12.

177. Jafar TH, Stark PC, Schmid CH, Strandgaard S, Kamper A-L, Maschio G, et al. The effect of angiotensin-converting-enzyme inhibitors on progression of advanced polycystic kidney disease. Kidney Int. 2005;67(1):265–71.

178. Veizis EI, Carlin CR, Cotton CU. Decreased amiloride-sensitive Na+ absorption in collecting duct principal cells isolated from BPK ARPKD mice. Am J Physiol Renal Physiol. 2004;286(2):F244–54.

179. Goto M, Hoxha N, Osman R, Dell KM. The renin-angiotensin system and hypertension in autosomal recessive polycystic kidney disease. Pediatr Nephrol Berl Ger. 2010;25(12):2449–57.

180. Goto M, Hoxha N, Osman R, Wen J, Wells RG, Dell KM. Renin-angiotensin system activation in congenital hepatic fibrosis in the PCK rat model of autosomal recessive polycystic kidney disease. J Pediatr Gastroenterol Nutr. 2010;50(6):639–44.

181. Nahm A-M, Henriquez DE, Ritz E. Renal cystic disease (ADPKD and ARPKD). Nephrol Dial Transplant Off Publ Eur Dial Transpl Assoc Eur Ren Assoc. 2002;17(2):311–4.

182. Nicolau C, Torra R, Badenas C, Pérez L, Oliver JA, Darnell A, et al. Sonographic pattern of recessive polycystic kidney disease in young adults. Differences from the dominant form. Nephrol Dial Transplant Off Publ Eur Dial Transpl Assoc Eur Ren Assoc. 2000;15(9):1373–8.

183. Vester U, Kranz B, Hoyer PF. The diagnostic value of ultrasound in cystic kidney diseases. Pediatr Nephrol Berl Ger. 2010;25(2):231–40.

184. Srinath A, Shneider BL. Congenital hepatic fibrosis and autosomal recessive polycystic kidney disease. J Pediatr Gastroenterol Nutr. 2012;54(5):580–7.

185. Kashtan CE, Primack WA, Kainer G, Rosenberg AR, McDonald RA, Warady BA. Recurrent bacteremia with enteric pathogens in recessive polycystic kidney disease. Pediatr Nephrol Berl Ger. 1999;13(8):678–82.

186. Gallagher A-R, Esquivel EL, Briere TS, Tian X, Mitobe M, Menezes LF, et al. Biliary and pancreatic dysgenesis in mice harboring a mutation in Pkhd1. Am J Pathol. 2008;172(2):417–29.

187. Garcia-Gonzalez MA, Menezes LF, Piontek KB, Kaimori J, Huso DL, Watnick T, et al. Genetic interaction studies link autosomal dominant and recessive polycystic kidney disease in a common pathway. Hum Mol Genet. 2007;16(16):1940–50.

188. Moser M, Matthiesen S, Kirfel J, Schorle H, Bergmann C, Senderek J, et al. A mouse model for cystic biliary dysgenesis in autosomal recessive polycystic kidney disease (ARPKD). Hepatol Baltim Md. 2005;41(5):1113–21.

189. Woollard JR, Punyashtiti R, Richardson S, Masyuk TV, Whelan S, Huang BQ, et al. A mouse model of autosomal recessive polycystic kidney disease with biliary duct and proximal tubule dilatation. Kidney Int. 2007;72(3):328–36.

190. Brinkert F, Lehnhardt A, Montoya C, Helmke K, Schaefer H, Fischer L, et al. Combined liver-kidney transplantation for children with autosomal recessive polycystic kidney disease (ARPKD): indication and outcome. Transpl Int Off J Eur Soc Org Transplant. 2013;26(6):640–50.

191. Jalanko H, Pakarinen M. Combined liver and kidney transplantation in children. Pediatr Nephrol Berl Ger. 2014;29(5):805–14; quiz 812.

192. Telega G, Cronin D, Avner ED. New approaches to the autosomal recessive polycystic kidney disease patient with dual kidney-liver complications. Pediatr Transplant. 2013;17(4):328–35.

193. Turkbey B, Ocak I, Daryanani K, Font-Montgomery E, Lukose L, Bryant J, et al. Autosomal recessive polycystic kidney disease and congenital hepatic fibrosis (ARPKD/CHF). Pediatr Radiol. 2009;39(2):100–11.

194. Chilton SJ, Cremin BJ. The spectrum of polycystic disease in children. Pediatr Radiol. 1981;11(1):9–15.

195. Deget F, Rudnik-Schöneborn S, Zerres K. Course of autosomal recessive polycystic kidney disease (ARPKD) in siblings: a clinical comparison of 20 sibships. Clin Genet. 1995;47(5):248–53.

196. Kaplan BS, Kaplan P, de Chadarevian JP, Jequier S, O'Regan S, Russo P. Variable expression of autosomal recessive polycystic kidney disease and congenital hepatic fibrosis within a family. Am J Med Genet. 1988;29(3):639–47.

197. Zerres K, Völpel MC, Weiss H. Cystic kidneys. Genetics, pathologic anatomy, clinical picture, and prenatal diagnosis. Hum Genet. 1984;68(2):104–35.

198. Guay-Woodford LM, Muecher G, Hopkins SD, Avner ED, Germino GG, Guillot AP, et al. The severe perinatal form of autosomal recessive polycystic kidney disease maps to chromosome 6p21.1-p12: implications for genetic counseling. Am J Hum Genet. 1995;56(5):1101–7.

199. Zerres K, Mücher G, Bachner L, Deschennes G, Eggermann T, Kääriäinen H, et al. Mapping of the gene for autosomal recessive polycystic kidney disease (ARPKD) to chromosome 6p21-cen. Nat Genet. 1994;7(3):429–32.

200. Onuchic LF, Furu L, Nagasawa Y, Hou X, Eggermann T, Ren Z, et al. PKHD1, the polycystic kidney and hepatic disease 1 gene, encodes a novel large protein containing multiple immunoglobulin-like plexin-transcription-factor domains and parallel beta-helix 1 repeats. Am J Hum Genet. 2002;70(5):1305–17.

201. Ward CJ, Hogan MC, Rossetti S, Walker D, Sneddon T, Wang X, et al. The gene mutated in autosomal recessive polycystic kidney disease encodes a large, receptor-like protein. Nat Genet. 2002;30(3):259–69.

202. Nagasawa Y, Matthiesen S, Onuchic LF, Hou X, Bergmann C, Esquivel E, et al. Identification and characterization of Pkhd1, the mouse orthologue of the human ARPKD gene. J Am Soc Nephrol JASN. 2002;13(9):2246–58.

203. Masyuk TV, Huang BQ, Ward CJ, Masyuk AI, Yuan D, Splinter PL, et al. Defects in cholangiocyte fibrocystin expression and ciliary structure in the PCK rat. Gastroenterology. 2003;125(5):1303–10.

204. Menezes LFC, Cai Y, Nagasawa Y, Silva AMG, Watkins ML, Da Silva AM, et al. Polyductin, the PKHD1 gene product, comprises isoforms expressed in plasma membrane, primary cilium, and cytoplasm. Kidney Int. 2004;66(4):1345–55.

205. Wang S, Luo Y, Wilson PD, Witman GB, Zhou J. The autosomal recessive polycystic kidney disease protein is localized to primary cilia, with concentration in the basal body area. J Am Soc Nephrol JASN. 2004;15(3):592–602.

206. Ward CJ, Yuan D, Masyuk TV, Wang X, Punyashthiti R, Whelan S, et al. Cellular and subcellular localization of the ARPKD protein; fibrocystin is expressed on primary cilia. Hum Mol Genet. 2003;12(20): 2703–10.

207. Zhang M-Z, Mai W, Li C, Cho S, Hao C, Moeckel G, et al. PKHD1 protein encoded by the gene for autosomal recessive polycystic kidney disease associates with basal bodies and primary cilia in renal epithelial cells. Proc Natl Acad Sci U S A. 2004;101(8): 2311–6.

208. Follit JA, Li L, Vucica Y, Pazour GJ. The cytoplasmic tail of fibrocystin contains a ciliary targeting sequence. J Cell Biol. 2010;188(1):21–8.

209. Hiesberger T, Gourley E, Erickson A, Koulen P, Ward CJ, Masyuk TV, et al. Proteolytic cleavage and nuclear translocation of fibrocystin is regulated by intracellular Ca2+ and activation of protein kinase C. J Biol Chem. 2006;281(45):34357–64.

210. Kaimori J, Nagasawa Y, Menezes LF, Garcia-Gonzalez MA, Deng J, Imai E, et al. Polyductin undergoes notch-like processing and regulated release from primary cilia. Hum Mol Genet. 2007;16(8):942–56.

211. Bergmann C, Senderek J, Sedlacek B, Pegiazoglou I, Puglia P, Eggermann T, et al. Spectrum of mutations in the gene for autosomal recessive polycystic kidney disease (ARPKD/PKHD1). J Am Soc Nephrol JASN. 2003;14(1):76–89.

212. Bergmann C, Senderek J, Küpper F, Schneider F, Dornia C, Windelen E, et al. PKHD1 mutations in autosomal recessive polycystic kidney disease (ARPKD). Hum Mutat. 2004;23(5):453–63.

213. Bergmann C, Senderek J, Schneider F, Dornia C, Küpper F, Eggermann T, et al. PKHD1 mutations in families requesting prenatal diagnosis for autosomal recessive polycystic kidney disease (ARPKD). Hum Mutat. 2004;23(5):487–95.

214. Furu L, Onuchic LF, Gharavi A, Hou X, Esquivel EL, Nagasawa Y, et al. Milder presentation of recessive polycystic kidney disease requires presence of amino acid substitution mutations. J Am Soc Nephrol JASN. 2003;14(8):2004–14.

215. Losekoot M, Haarloo C, Ruivenkamp C, White SJ, Breuning MH, Peters DJM. Analysis of missense variants in the PKHD1-gene in patients with autosomal recessive polycystic kidney disease (ARPKD). Hum Genet. 2005;118(2):185–206.

216. Baralle D, Baralle M. Splicing in action: assessing disease causing sequence changes. J Med Genet. 2005;42(10):737–48.

217. Bergmann C, Frank V, Küpper F, Schmidt C, Senderek J, Zerres K. Functional analysis of PKHD1 splicing in autosomal recessive polycystic kidney disease. J Hum Genet. 2006;51(9):788–93.

218. Consugar MB, Anderson SA, Rossetti S, Pankratz VS, Ward CJ, Torra R, et al. Haplotype analysis improves molecular diagnostics of autosomal recessive polycystic kidney disease. Am J Kidney Dis Off J Natl Kidney Found. 2005;45(1):77–87.

219. Krall P, Pineda C, Ruiz P, Ejarque L, Vendrell T, Camacho JA, et al. Cost-effective PKHD1 genetic testing for autosomal recessive polycystic kidney disease. Pediatr Nephrol Berl Ger. 2014;29(2): 223–34.

220. Boddu R, Yang C, O'Connor AK, Hendrickson RC, Boone B, Cui X, et al. Intragenic motifs regulate the transcriptional complexity of Pkhd1/PKHD1. J Mol Med Berl Ger. 2014;92(10):1045–56.

221. Frank V, Zerres K, Bergmann C. Transcriptional complexity in autosomal recessive polycystic kidney disease. Clin J Am Soc Nephrol CJASN. 2014; 9(10):1729–36.

222. Guay-Woodford LM, Wright CJ, Walz G, Churchill GA. Quantitative trait loci modulate renal cystic disease severity in the mouse bpk model. J Am Soc Nephrol JASN. 2000;11(7):1253–60.

223. Liebau MC, Benzing T. Recent developments in genetic kidney diseases. Dtsch Med Wochenschr. 2011;136(19):1014–20. 1946.

224. Sommardahl C, Cottrell M, Wilkinson JE, Woychik RP, Johnson DK. Phenotypic variations of orpk mutation and chromosomal localization of modifiers influencing kidney phenotype. Physiol Genomics. 2001;7(2):127–34.

225. Zaghloul NA, Katsanis N. Functional modules, mutational load and human genetic disease. Trends Genet TIG. 2010;26(4):168–76.

226. Modrek B, Lee C. A genomic view of alternative splicing. Nat Genet. 2002;30(1):13–9.

227. Nissim-Rafinia M, Kerem B. Splicing regulation as a potential genetic modifier. Trends Genet TIG. 2002;18(3):123–7.

228. Zerres K, Senderek J, Rudnik-Schöneborn S, Eggermann T, Kunze J, Mononen T, et al. New options for prenatal diagnosis in autosomal recessive polycystic kidney disease by mutation analysis of the PKHD1 gene. Clin Genet. 2004;66(1):53–7.

229. Barr MM, Sternberg PW. A polycystic kidney-disease gene homologue required for male mating behaviour in C. elegans. Nature. 1999;401(6751):386–9.

230. Pazour GJ, Dickert BL, Vucica Y, Seeley ES, Rosenbaum JL, Witman GB, et al. Chlamydomonas IFT88 and its mouse homologue, polycystic kidney disease gene tg737, are required for assembly of cilia and flagella. J Cell Biol. 2000;151(3):709–18.

231. Ma M, Tian X, Igarashi P, Pazour GJ, Somlo S. Loss of cilia suppresses cyst growth in genetic models of autosomal dominant polycystic kidney disease. Nat Genet. 2013;45(9):1004–12.

232. Patel V, Chowdhury R, Igarashi P. Advances in the pathogenesis and treatment of polycystic kidney disease. Curr Opin Nephrol Hypertens. 2009;18(2): 99–106.

233. Watnick T, Germino GG. mTOR inhibitors in polycystic kidney disease. N Engl J Med. 2010;363(9): 879–81.

234. Seeger-Nukpezah T, Proia DA, Egleston BL, Nikonova AS, Kent T, Cai KQ, et al. Inhibiting the HSP90 chaperone slows cyst growth in a mouse

model of autosomal dominant polycystic kidney disease. Proc Natl Acad Sci U S A. 2013;110(31):12786–91.

235. Grantham JJ, Mulamalla S, Swenson-Fields KI. Why kidneys fail in autosomal dominant polycystic kidney disease. Nat Rev Nephrol. 2011;7(10):556–66.

236. Gattone 2nd VH, Wang X, Harris PC, Torres VE. Inhibition of renal cystic disease development and progression by a vasopressin V2 receptor antagonist. Nat Med. 2003;9(10):1323–6.

237. Torres VE, Wang X, Qian Q, Somlo S, Harris PC, Gattone 2nd VH. Effective treatment of an orthologous model of autosomal dominant polycystic kidney disease. Nat Med. 2004;10(4):363–4.

238. Wang X, Gattone 2nd V, Harris PC, Torres VE. Effectiveness of vasopressin V2 receptor antagonists OPC-31260 and OPC-41061 on polycystic kidney disease development in the PCK rat. J Am Soc Nephrol JASN. 2005;16(4):846–51.

239. Torres VE, Chapman AB, Devuyst O, Gansevoort RT, Grantham JJ, Higashihara E, et al. Tolvaptan in patients with autosomal dominant polycystic kidney disease. N Engl J Med. 2012;367(25):2407–18.

240. Ruggenenti P, Remuzzi A, Ondei P, Fasolini G, Antiga L, Ene-Iordache B, et al. Safety and efficacy of long-acting somatostatin treatment in autosomal-dominant polycystic kidney disease. Kidney Int. 2005;68(1):206–16.

241. Caroli A, Perico N, Perna A, Antiga L, Brambilla P, Pisani A, et al. Effect of longacting somatostatin analogue on kidney and cyst growth in autosomal dominant polycystic kidney disease (ALADIN): a randomised, placebo-controlled, multicentre trial. Lancet. 2013;382(9903):1485–95.

242. Schrier RW, Abebe KZ, Perrone RD, Torres VE, Braun WE, Steinman TI, et al. Blood pressure in early autosomal dominant polycystic kidney disease. N Engl J Med. 2015;372(10):976–7.

243. Torres VE, Abebe KZ, Chapman AB, Schrier RW, Braun WE, Steinman TI, et al. Angiotensin blockade in late autosomal dominant polycystic kidney disease. N Engl J Med. 2014;371:2267–76.

244. Shillingford JM, Murcia NS, Larson CH, Low SH, Hedgepeth R, Brown N, et al. The mTOR pathway is regulated by polycystin-1, and its inhibition reverses renal cystogenesis in polycystic kidney disease. Proc Natl Acad Sci U S A. 2006;103(14):5466–71.

245. Novalic Z, van der Wal AM, Leonhard WN, Koehl G, Breuning MH, Geissler EK, et al. Dose-dependent effects of sirolimus on mTOR signaling and polycystic kidney disease. J Am Soc Nephrol JASN. 2012;23(5):842–53.

246. Shillingford JM, Piontek KB, Germino GG, Weimbs T. Rapamycin ameliorates PKD resulting from conditional inactivation of Pkd1. J Am Soc Nephrol JASN. 2010;21(3):489–97.

247. Torres VE, Boletta A, Chapman A, Gattone V, Pei Y, Qian Q, et al. Prospects for mTOR inhibitor use in patients with polycystic kidney disease and hamartomatous diseases. Clin J Am Soc Nephrol CJASN. 2010;5(7):1312–29.

248. Wahl PR, Serra AL, Le Hir M, Molle KD, Hall MN, Wüthrich RP. Inhibition of mTOR with sirolimus slows disease progression in Han: SPRD rats with autosomal dominant polycystic kidney disease (ADPKD). Nephrol Dial Transplant Off Publ Eur Dial Transpl Assoc Eur Ren Assoc. 2006;21(3):598–604.

249. Wu M, Wahl PR, Le Hir M, Wackerle-Men Y, Wuthrich RP, Serra AL. Everolimus retards cyst growth and preserves kidney function in a rodent model for polycystic kidney disease. Kidney Blood Press Res. 2007;30(4):253–9.

250. Wu M, Arcaro A, Varga Z, Vogetseder A, Le Hir M, Wüthrich RP, et al. Pulse mTOR inhibitor treatment effectively controls cyst growth but leads to severe parenchymal and glomerular hypertrophy in rat polycystic kidney disease. Am J Physiol Renal Physiol. 2009;297(6):F1597–605.

251. Zafar I, Belibi FA, He Z, Edelstein CL. Long-term rapamycin therapy in the Han: SPRD rat model of polycystic kidney disease (PKD). Nephrol Dial Transplant Off Publ Eur Dial Transpl Assoc Eur Ren Assoc. 2009;24(8):2349–53.

252. Serra AL, Poster D, Kistler AD, Krauer F, Raina S, Young J, et al. Sirolimus and kidney growth in autosomal dominant polycystic kidney disease. N Engl J Med. 2010;363(9):820–9.

253. Cinà DP, Onay T, Paltoo A, Li C, Maezawa Y, De Arteaga J, et al. Inhibition of MTOR disrupts autophagic flux in podocytes. J Am Soc Nephrol JASN. 2012;23(3):412–20.

254. Gödel M, Hartleben B, Herbach N, Liu S, Zschiedrich S, Lu S, et al. Role of mTOR in podocyte function and diabetic nephropathy in humans and mice. J Clin Invest. 2011;121(6):2197–209.

255. Hartleben B, Gödel M, Meyer-Schwesinger C, Liu S, Ulrich T, Köbler S, et al. Autophagy influences glomerular disease susceptibility and maintains podocyte homeostasis in aging mice. J Clin Invest. 2010;120(4):1084–96.

256. Inoki K, Mori H, Wang J, Suzuki T, Hong S, Yoshida S, et al. mTORC1 activation in podocytes is a critical step in the development of diabetic nephropathy in mice. J Clin Invest. 2011;121(6):2181–96.

257. Liebau MC, Braun F, Höpker K, Weitbrecht C, Bartels V, Müller R-U, et al. Dysregulated autophagy contributes to podocyte damage in Fabry's disease. PLoS ONE. 2013;8(5):e63506.

258. Walz G, Budde K, Mannaa M, Nürnberger J, Wanner C, Sommerer C, et al. Everolimus in patients with autosomal dominant polycystic kidney disease. N Engl J Med. 2010;363(9):830–40.

Nephronophthisis and Autosomal Dominant Interstitial Kidney Disease (ADIKD)

13

Jens König, Beate Ermisch-Omran, and Heymut Omran

The Nephronophthisis Complex

The nephronophthisis complex comprises a clinically and genetically heterogeneous group of tubulointerstitial cystic disorders with an autosomal recessive inheritance pattern. It represents the most frequent genetic cause of end-stage renal disease in children and young adults. Nephronophthisis can be accompanied by anomalies in other organs, e.g., liver, pancreas, central nervous system, eyes and bones. There are several well described complex clinical syndromes which can feature the renal picture of nephronophthisis, including Senior-Løken syndrome, Joubert syndrome, COACH syndrome, Jeune syndrome, Meckel-Gruber syndrome and others. Because of extended clinical as well as genetic overlap, the term *nephronophthisis complex* was introduced. Due to this variability establishment of the correct diagnosis can become very challenging.

Nephronophthisis

Nephronophthisis literally means "vanishing of the nephrons." 1951 Fanconi et al. introduced the term *familial juvenile nephronophthisis* to describe a disease characterized by autosomal recessive inheritance, a defect in urinary concentrating capacity, severe anemia and progressive renal failure that leads to death before puberty [1, 2]. The incidence ranges around 1:50.000 in Europe and the USA. Thus, nephronophthisis belongs to the group of rare hereditary renal disorders. Renal histology is characterized by disintegrated tubular basement membranes, tubular atrophy and cyst formation, as well as a sclerosing tubulointerstitial nephropathy (Fig. 13.1) [3, 4]. Cortico-medullary cysts occur late in the disease process [5] and are only a facultative finding (Fig. 13.2a, b). Thus, although nephronophthisis has been referred to as cystic kidney disorder, cysts are not a hallmark of the disease.

Typical clinical signs comprise polyuria and polydipsia due to the reduced urinary concentrating capacity. Other clinical manifestations such as growth retardation and persisting primary or secondary enuresis might be a hint for the diagnosis but are only facultative findings. Urine analyses usually do not show any characteristic abnormalities. Proteinuria and arterial hypertension are not typically found before onset of renal failure. Because of the lack of disease-specific clinical features and the slow progress, many patients are only diagnosed when end-stage renal

J. König • H. Omran (✉) • B. Ermisch-Omran
Department of General Pediatrics, University
Children's Hospital Muenster, Albert-Schweitzer-
Campus 1, Muenster 48149, Germany
e-mail: jens.koenig@ukmuenster.de;
heymut.omran@ukmuenster.de; beate.ermisch-
omran@ukmuenster.de

© Springer-Verlag Berlin Heidelberg 2016
D.F. Geary, F. Schaefer (eds.), *Pediatric Kidney Disease*, DOI 10.1007/978-3-662-52972-0_13

disease has been reached. On ultrasound, nephronophthisis patients generally show normal or small-sized kidneys with increased echogenicity and a loss of cortico-medullary differentiation. Cysts, which are typically located at the cortico-medullary junction, often only occur late in the disease process [5] and are not an obligatory finding (Fig. 13.2a, b).

Depending on the onset of end-stage renal disease (ESRD) the terms infantile, juvenile, and adolescent nephronophthisis have been used. The

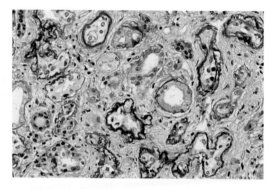

Fig. 13.1 PAS stained renal biopsy specimen depicting characteristic finding in "classical nephronophthisis" comprising tubular basement alterations with irregular thickening and thinning, tubular atrophy and cystic dilatation of tubules

juvenile form is the most common entity with a median age of 13 years at the onset of ESRD [6]. In infantile nephronophthisis end-stage renal disease is reached very early in life (median age 8 months) whereas in adolescent forms renal function is usually preserved until adulthood (median age 19 years). The above described renal phenotype and clinical course is very similar in most nephronophthisis variants. An exception to this rule is the infantile nephronophthisis, which is characterized by a distinct clinical course and pathology, and therefore will be addressed separately (see below). The typical clinical findings of the various nephronophthisis variants are summarized in Table 13.1.

Infantile Nephronophthisis

Infantile nephronophthisis differs from "classical nephronophthisis" variants in many respects. Infantile nephronophthisis (NPHP2; OMIM 602088) is characterized by an early disease onset which might start prior to birth or in early infancy. Infantile nephronophthisis leads to ESRD within the first 5 years of life [7–10]. While kidney size in "classical nephronophthisis variants" is normal or small, it is typically enlarged in infantile nephronophthisis. Patients often suffer from arterial hypertension and might

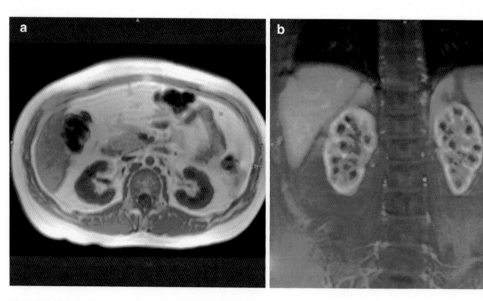

Fig. 13.2 Magnetic resonance tomography findings of the kidneys in a patient with nephronophthisis type 1. Please note the prominent cysts at the cortico-medullary junction on axial (**a**) and coronal (**b**) images

Table 13.1 Clinical and diagnostic findings in genetically characterized nephronophthisis variants

Nephronophthisis variants/types, allelic diseases	OMIM entry	Gene Mutation frequency	Age at ESRD [yrs] (median)	Isolated NPH	NPH associated with extrarenal manifestations (10–15%)						
					Joubert syndrome	Severe retinal degeneration	Tapetoretinal degeneration	OMA type Cogan II	Liver fibrosis	Situs inversus	Other symptoms
NPHP1/JBTS4/SLSN1	256100	NPHP1 20–25%	7–29 (13)	+	+ (2%, mild)	+ (10–15%)	+	+ (2%)	–	–	–
NPHP2	602088	Inversin 1–2%	0–5 (3)	+	–	+ (10%)	–	–	+	+	VSD, HT, OH
NPHP3/SLNS3/renal hepatic pancreatic syndrome1	604387	NPHP3 <1%	11–47 (19)	+	+	+ (10%)	+	–	+	+	MKS, CHD (AS, ASD, PDA, RVH)
NPHP4/SLSN4	606966	NPHP4 2–3%	6–35 (21)	+	+ (rare, mild)	+ (10–15%)	+	+ (rare)	+	–	LCA
NPHP5/SLSN5	609254	IQCB1 3–4%	6–32 (15)	–	–	+ (100%)	–	–	–	–	LCA
NPHP6/JBTS5/SLSN6/MKS4	610188	CEP290 1%	5–17 (12)	–	+	+ (100%)	+	+	+ (10%)	–	LCA, MKS, BBS, CHD, MO, ELE, BC, COACH syndrome
NPHP7	611498	GLIS2 0.1%	8	+	–	–	–	–	–	–	–
NPHP8/JBTS7/MKS5	611560	RPGRIP1L 0.5%	10, juvenile	+	+	+ (10%)	+	+	+		MKS, LCA, COACH syndrome, RHYNS-like (pituitary agenesis, partial GH deficiency)
NPHP9	613824	NEK8 <0.5%	3 (infantile, juvenile)	+	–	+ (30%)	?	–	–	–	MKS-like
NPHP10/SLSN7	613615	SDCCAG8 <0.5%	4–24	–	–	+ (rare)	+	–	–	–	BBS-like
NPHP11/JBTS6/MKS3	613550	TMEM67 (Meckelin) <0.5%	infantile	+	+	–	–	–	+	–	MKS, BBS, JADT, COACH syndrome

Table 13.1 (continued)

Nephronophthisis variants/types, allelic diseases	OMIM entry	Gene Mutation frequency	Age at ESRD [yrs] (median)	Isolated NPH	NPH associated with extrarenal manifestations (10–15%)						
					Joubert syndrome	Severe retinal degeneration	Tapetoretinal degeneration	OMA type Cogan II	Liver fibrosis	Situs inversus	Other symptoms
NPHP12/ JBTS11	613820	*TTC21B* <1%	+	+	+	–	–	–	–	–	JADT, MKS, BBS
NPHP13/ cranioectodermal dysplasia 4	614377	*WDRI9* ?	5–17 (12)	+	–	+	–	–	–	–	JADT, SS
NPHP14/JBTS19	614844	*ZNF423* ?	Infantile	?	+ (AD)	+		–	–	+	LCA, CVH
NPHP15	614845	*CEP164*	?	–	+	+	+	–	+		Obesity, BC, CVH, NYS, LCA, seizures
NPHP16	615382	*ANKS6* ?	Infantile, juvenile	+	–	–	–	–	+	+	CHD (AS, PS, PDA, CMP)
JBTS1	213300	*INPP5E*	?	(+)	+	+	+	+			
JBTS2	608091	*TMEM216*	Juvenile	(+)	+	(+)	(+)	+			
JBTS3	608629	*AHI1*	Juvenile, adult	(+)	+	(+)	(+)	(+)			
JBTS8		*ARL13B*	? (no)	no	+	–	–	(+)			MKS

AS aortic stenosis, *BBS* Bardet Biedl syndrome, *BC* bone changes, *CHD* congenital heart defect, *CMP* cardiomyopathy, *COACH* (cerebellar vermis hypoplasia, oligophrenia [cognitive dysfunction], ataxia, coloboma, hypotonia) syndrome, *COGAN* congenital oculomotor apraxia type Cogan II syndrome, *CVH* cerebellar vermis hypoplasia, *ELE* elevated liver enzymes, *HT* arterial hypertension, *JADT* Jeune asphyxiating thoracic dystrophy, *LCA* Leber congenital amaurosis, *MKS* Meckel Gruber syndrome (occipital encephalocele, polydactyly, microphthalmia, liver fibrosis), *MO* microphthalmus, *NYS* nystagmus, *OH* oligohydramnion, *OMA* okulomotor apraxia type Cogan II, *PDA* persistent ductus arteriosus, *PS* pulmonal stenosis, *RVH* right ventricular hypertrophy, *SS* Sensenbrenner syndrome, *VSD* ventricular septal defect

present with acute renal failure. In patients with *NPHP2* mutations end-stage renal disease was reached between the first and fifth year of life. Interestingly, in addition to the extrarenal symptoms mentioned below, associated *situs inversus* and ventricular septal defect of the heart have been reported. In one patient with a homozygous *NPHP2* mutation retinitis pigmentosa was already present at the age of 2 years [11]. Morphologically infantile nephronophtisis differs from juvenile forms by the presence of cortical microcysts and the absence of medullary cysts as well as typical tubular basement membrane changes [10].

Mutations of *NPHP2/INV* (9q22-q31) were the first gene defects identified in infantile nephronophthisis [7]. The gene product called *inversin* is located to renal monocilia and demonstrates interaction with multiple nephrocystins indicating that it is part of a large multi-protein complex and functioning as a switch between distinct Wnt signalling pathways [12]. Recently, mutations in several other genes have been reported in individuals with infantile nephronophthisis (Table 13.1): Loss-of function mutations in *NPHP3* typically result in early renal disease onset, whereas other types of mutations are associated with late renal disease. Mutations in *NPHP9/NEK8*, *TMEM67/MKS3/NPHP11*, *NPHP14/JBTS19*, and *ANKS6* have been also reported in early onset nephronophthisis. In a large proportion of individuals the renal phenotype is associated with extra-renal disease manifestations such as Meckel-Gruber or Joubert syndrome (Table 13.1).

Juvenile Nephronophhisis

In juvenile nephronophthisis the first and most important gene (*NPHP1*), localized on chromosome 2q12-q13 [13, 14], has been identified by positional cloning [15, 16]. Nephronophthisis type 1 (OMIM #256100) accounts for 27–62 % of nephronophthisis cases and is one of the most frequent genetic causes of end-stage renal disease in children and young adults [17, 18]. In the vast majority of *NPHP1* patients (94 %), large homozygous deletions of approximately 290 kb involving the *NPHP1* locus can be detected while only some patients carry point

mutations in combination with a heterozygous deletion [17, 19]. *NPHP1* encodes nephrocystin-1, a 733 amino-acid protein [15, 16]. A number of protein interaction partners, including p130^{CAS}, proline-rich tyrosine kinase 2 (Pyk2) and tensin have been identified which are supposed to function in focal adhesion complexes or at sites of cell-cell contact in polarized MDCK cells [20, 21]. In addition, the proteins involved in the nephronophthisis types −2, −3 and −4 associate with nephrocystin, suggesting assembly into a large multi-protein complex [7, 22–24]. Recent findings suggest that this protein complex is localized at the ciliary base (transition zone) playing a functional role in motile (respiratory cilia) and immotile cilia (renal monocilia, connecting cilia of the photoreceptor) [25, 26]. Interestingly, this expression can be used to demonstrate nephrocystin deficiency in patients with *NPHP1* deletions by analyzing ciliated nasal respiratory cells obtained by simple nasal brushings (Fig. 13.3a–c) [26].

In a renal survival analysis of patients with juvenile nephronophthisis end-stage renal failure was attained at a median age of 13.1 years, with an interquartile range of 11.3–17.3 years [6]. While the youngest child was 7 years, a single 29-year-old subject had not yet progressed to end-stage kidney disease. Hence, it is still conceivable that some individuals with homozygous *NPHP1* deletions may not progress to renal failure in later adulthood or even never at all. Bollee et al. (2002) confirmed that *NPHP1* mutations sometimes may not cause renal failure before adult age [27]. They reported four adults with chronic renal failure at the age of 19, 22, 22 and 25 years, respectively. It is important to note that renal imaging in these subjects revealed no (n = 2) or only one cortical cyst (n = 2). Thus, cysts at the cortico-medullary junction are not an obligatory finding in juvenile nephronophthisis. Other clinical manifestations such as polyuria and secondary enuresis might be a hint for the diagnosis but are only facultative findings in the disease. Proteinuria and hypertension are not typically found in nephronophthisis. However, these symptoms might develop especially when renal function deteriorates. In the four patients reported by

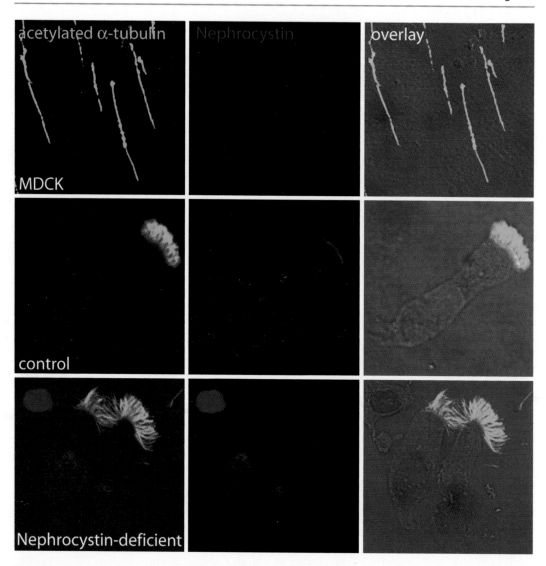

Fig. 13.3 High-resolution immunofluorescence micros-copy of Madin-Darby canine kidney (MDCK) cells and human respiratory cells. Nuclei are stained blue. (**a**) Renal monocilia of MDCK cells are stained with α-tubulin (*green*). Nephrocystin-1 (*red*) specifically localizes to the ciliary transition zone at the ciliary base. (**b**) Motile respi-ratory cilia of control cells are stained with α-tubulin (*green*). Nephrocystin-1 (*red*) also specifically localizes to the ciliary transition zone at the ciliary base. (**c**) In respira-tory cells of nephronophthisis patients with homozygous *NPHP1* deletions, nephrocystin is absent from the entire cell

Bollee et al. [27] proteinuria ranged from 0.2 to 1.6 g per day.

The most common extrarenal disease mani-festation in patients with juvenile nephronophthi-sis is tapeto-retinal degeneration. It is usually a milder type of retinitis pigmentosa. Some patients might even not complain of any symptoms, although specific retinal changes can be detected by a funduscopic ophthalmologic examination.

Other extra-renal manifestations such as cerebel-lar ataxia with vermis aplasia and mental retarda-tion (Joubert syndrome) and ocular motor apraxia type Cogan II (Cogan syndrome) have only been reported anecdotally [28, 29].

While *NPHP1* mutations represent the most frequent underlying genetic abnormality, several other gene defects can also account for juvenile nephronophthisis (Table 13.1) [22, 30].

Adolescent Nephronophthisis

Adolescent nephronophthisis was first identified as a new distinct disease variant based on clinical symptoms, renal pathology, and genetic findings in a large consanguineous 340-member Venezuelan kindred [31]. Genome-wide linkage analysis localized a region of homozygosity by descent on chromosome 3q within a critical genetic interval of 2.4 cM [31]. Fluorescence in situ hybridization refined the chromosomal assignment of *NPHP3* to chromosome 3q21-q22 [32].

Synteny between the human *NPHP3* locus on chromosome 3q and the *pcy* locus on mouse chromosome 9 has been demonstrated, providing the first evidence of synteny between a human and a spontaneous murine renal cystic disease [32]. The renal pathology observed in the recessive *pcy* mouse model of late-onset polycystic kidney disease comprised tubular basement membranes changes, tubular atrophy and dilatation, sclerosing tubulointerstitial nephropathy, and renal cyst development at the corticomedullary junction, resembling human adolescent nephronophthisis [32]. Demonstration of synteny suggested that both diseases are caused by recessive mutations of homologous genes.

Additional linkage analyses showed that some families with Senior-Løken syndrome also inherited the disease through a mutated gene residing in the same chromosomal region [33]. Subsequently, recessive mutations in the *NPHP3* gene were identified in patients with adolescent nephronophthisis [23]. *NPHP3* encodes a 1330-amino acid protein, which interacts with nephrocystin-1. In the adult kidney *NPHP3* expression was observed in distal tubules located at the cortico-medullary border, which corresponds to the site of cyst formation in adolescent nephronophthisis. Expression in retina and liver is in agreement with associated tapeto-retinal degeneration or hepatic fibrosis in patients carrying *NPHP3* mutations. In addition, a homozygous missense mutation in *NPHP3* was found to be most likely responsible for the polycystic kidney disease (*pcy*) mouse phenotype [23].

While *NPHP3* was the first gene found to cause adolescent nephronophthisis, other genetic defects such as *NPHP1* mutations can also cause adolescent or adult disease manifestations (Table 13.1)

Onset of end-stage renal failure in adolescent nephronophthisis occurs significantly later (median 19 years, interquartile range 16–25 years) than in juvenile nephronophthisis [31]. Clinical signs of adolescent nephronophthisis consist of renal symptoms such as polyuria, polydipsia, secondary enuresis, severe anemia and progressive renal failure [31]. Renal morphology is characterized by cysts at the corticomedullary junction. Renal histology shows the characteristic triad of irregularly thickened tubular basement membranes, atrophy and dilatation of tubules, and sclerosing tubulo-interstitial nephropathy [31].

In some patients with adolescent nephronophthisis carrying *NPHP3* mutations, extrarenal disease manifestations such as tapeto-retinal degeneration or hepatic fibrosis have been reported [23].

Extra-Renal Disease Manifestations

Nephronophthisis can be associated with extrarenal disease manifestations including ocular motor apraxia, retinitis pigmentosa, Leber congenital amaurosis, coloboma of the optic nerve, cerebellar vermis aplasia, liver fibrosis, cranioectodermal dysplasia, cone-shaped epiphyses, asphyxiating thoracic dysplasia (Jeune's syndrome), Ellis-van-Creveld syndrome, and rarely *situs inversus* (Table 13.1) [10, 34].

Senior-Løken Syndrome

The term Senior-Løken syndrome denotes the association of nephronophthisis and retinal degeneration [35, 36]. Two variants of retinal disorders have been described.

Leber congenital amaurosis (*LCA*), the most severe variant, is a clinically and genetically heterogeneous retinal disorder that occurs in infancy and is accompanied by profound visual loss, nystagmus, poor pupillary reflexes, and either a normal retina or varying degrees of atrophy and pigmentary changes [37–39]. Affected children exhibit the so-called oculodigital sign characterized by poking, rubbing and pressing of the eyes in order to mechanically stimulate the retina. The electroretinogram is extinguished or severely reduced [40]. All but one form of LCA is inherited as an autosomal recessive trait. LCA is a disorder of photoreceptors, caused by failed transport of rhodopsin and a loss of outer segments of the photoreceptor resulting in its ultimate cell death. Although LCA being a clinical diagnosis, molecular testing is currently available for many different genes, including several genes that can be associated with nephronophthisis such as *NPHP5* and *NPHP6/CEP290* [41] (Table 13.1). So far all reported Senior-Løken patients with *NPHP5* mutations presented with early severe LCA [42]. Thus nephronophthisis patients without any early retinal disease do not need to be screened for *NPHP5* mutations. In 21 patients with *NPHP5* mutations end-stage renal disease ranged between 6 and 32 years (median 15 years).

A milder retinopathy which can also be associated with nephronophthisis is referred to as *tapeto-retinal degeneration*. Usually patients suffer from severe tube-like restriction of visual fields and night blindness. Funduscopy reveals various degrees of atrophic and pigmentary retinal alterations. Mutations in several genes can result in tapeto-retinal degeneration (Table 13.1).

Joubert Syndrome

Joubert syndrome is an autosomal recessive disorder with a predicted incidence of 1:100,000. It is clinically characterized by muscular hypotonia, cerebellar ataxia, unusual eye movements, hyperpnea/apnea in infancy and variable degrees of cognitive impairment. The abnormal eye movements often comprise oculomotor apraxia with jerking head thrusting and a rotating nystagmus [29]. Retinopathy may be present depending on the underlying mutation (e.g., *NPHP6/CEP290*). Certain dysmorphic features have been described such as hypertelorism, broad forehead and unilateral or bilateral ptosis. There is high phenotopic variability even among family members. The unifying pathognomonic radiographic finding of Joubert syndrome is the so called "molar tooth sign," which is visible on the axial brain magnetic resonance imaging (MRI). It reflects a complex malformation of the midbrain and hindbrain, consisting of cerebellar vermis hypoplasia, increased interpeduncular distance at the pontomesencephalic junction and elongated superior cerebellar peduncles (Fig. 13.4a, b) [43]. We recommend regular laboratory screening for evidence of chronic renal failure, because depending on the underlying genetic defect a high proportion of

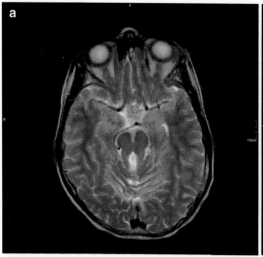
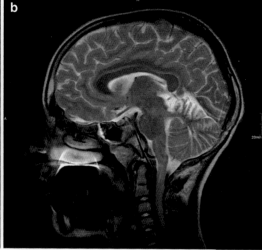

Fig. 13.4 Cranial magnetic resonance tomography findings in a patient with Joubert syndrome. (**a**) Axial T2-weighted image at the pontine level showing thickened superior cerebellar peduncles and umbrella-shaped fourth ventricle, giving the appearance of a molar tooth. (**b**) Sagittal T2-weighted image demonstrating prominent superior cerebellar peduncles running horizontally toward the brain stem, and cerebellar atrophy

individuals with Joubert syndrome can develop renal failure.

So far mutations in many different genes have been identified of which *AHI1*, *RPGRIP1L* and *CC2DA2* are the most frequently affected ones, each explaining about 10 % of cases (Table 13.1). Notably, mutations in some genes, such as *AHI1/JBTS3*, were initially not associated with nephronophthisis until recessive mutations were also found in subjects with Joubert syndrome and renal failure [44, 45]. One patient reached end-stage renal disease at the age of 16 years, and two others beyond 20 years of age. It is important to note that most patients diagnosed with *AHI1* mutations are still too young to tell whether they might develop renal failure at a later age.

The phenotype associated with NPHP6/*CEP290* mutations is mainly characterized by the neurological and neuroradiological features of Joubert syndrome associated with severe retinal and renal involvement [46, 47]. Other rare clinical findings included microphthalmus and elevated liver enzymes [47]. In a larger patient series (n = 12) end-stage renal disease was reached at a median age of 12 years but occurred as early as 5 years of age [46].

Clinical as well as genetic overlap makes it sometimes hard to differentiate Joubert syndrome from other ciliopathies such as Meckel-Gruber syndrome and to predict the clinical outcome. For individual genes, such as *NPHP6/JBTS5/SLSN6/MKS4/CEP290*, a correlation between the type of the two recessive mutations and the severity of disease has been demonstrated: two truncating mutations cause a severe early-onset disorder (as in Meckel-Gruber syndrome), whereas the presence of at least one missense mutation leads to a milder, late-onset phenotype with limited organ involvement (as in nephronophthisis) [48]. Because mutations of the *NPHP1* gene are also a rare cause of Joubert syndrome (see above), the *NPHP1* gene has also been referred to as *JBTS4*. Screening of 117 Joubert syndrome patients revealed mutations in *NPHP1* only in 2 % of cases, indicating that *NPHP1* is only a minor contributor in the pathogenesis of this disorder [45].

COACH Syndrome

The acronym COACH stands for the clinical key features cerebellar vermis hypoplasia, oligophrenia [cognitive dysfunction], congenital ataxia, coloboma and congenital hepatic fibrosis. COACH syndrome is a rare autosomal recessive disorder that shows substantial overlap with Joubert syndrome. In contrast to Joubert syndrome, the pathognomonic feature of this syndrome is the obligatory liver involvement caused by the malformation of the embryonic ductal plate resulting in fibrosis of the liver. Elevated liver enzymes, reduced blood flow in the portal vein and splenomegaly secondary to portal hypertension regularly develop during progression of the disease.

In up to 83 % of patients with COACH syndrome mutations in *MKS3/TMEM67* were identified, which makes this gene a genetic hotspot for ciliopathy patients with liver envolement [49].

Meckel Gruber Syndrome

Meckel-Gruber syndrome (MKS) is a neonatal lethal dysmorphic disorder affecting multiple organ systems (Fig. 13.5a–e). It follows an autosomal recessive inheritance and incidences from 1/13.500 to 1/40.000 live births have been reported. Typical clinical features comprise occipital encephalocele, bilateral cystic kidney dysplasia, hepatobiliary ductal plate malformation and postaxial polydactyly. Associated features might include severe cardiac anomalies, lung hypoplasia, *situs inversus*, severe malformations of the central nervous system, hydrocephalus, cleft palate, microphthalmia, developmental disorders of genitalia and skeletal deformities. Survival beyond the neonatal period is unusual, most affected individuals die in utero [50]. Prenatal ultrasonography documenting the combination of occipital encephalocele and polydactyly as well as elevated levels of alpha-fetoprotein in amnial fluid may lead to early diagnosis. Prenatal MRI can confirm typical additional malformations.

Mutations in several genes responsible for MKS or MKS-like phenotypes have been reported: *MKS1*, *MKS2/TMEM216*, *MKS3/TMEM67*, *NPHP6/JBTS5/MKS4/CEP290*, *NPHP8/JBTS7/*

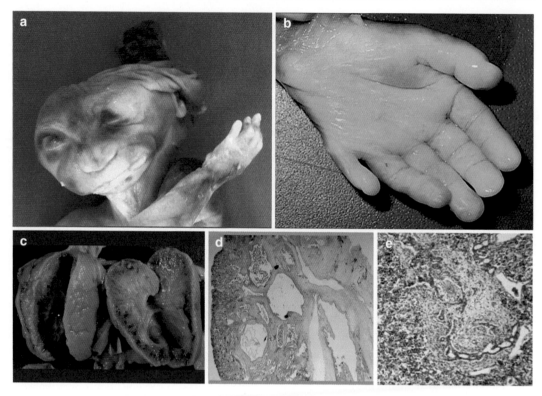

Fig. 13.5 Fetus with Meckel syndrome. (**a**) Phenotype with occipital meningoencephalocele and a massively malformed brain resembling anencephaly. (**b**) Postaxial hexadactyly. (**c**) Bilateral considerably enlarged kidneys interspersed with small, pinhead-sized cysts. (**d**) Cystic kidney with considerable interstitial fibrosis. (**e**) Ductal plate malformation characterized by dysgenesis of the hepatic portal triad with hyperplastic biliary ducts and congenital hepatic fibrosis (Used with permission of Springer Science + Business Media from Bergmann [48])

MKS5/RPGRIP1L, MKS6/CC2D2A, NPHP9/ NEK8, NPHP3/SLSN3, MKS8/TCTN2, NPHP11/ JBTS6, and *B9D1* [48]. Besides genetic heterogeneity there is significant clinical overlap with nephronophthisis and Joubert syndrome (Table 13.1). Current data suggest that severe truncating mutations cause MKS whereas milder, non-truncating mutations rather lead to Joubert or isolated nephronophthisis syndromes. In fact there are even some families in which one child is diagnosed with Joubert syndrome and another with MKS, indicating the presence of genetic modifiers influencing the clinical phenotype [41].

Congenital Oculomotor Apraxia Type Cogan II

Congenital oculomotor apraxia (COMA) type Cogan II is characterized by impairment of horizontal voluntary eye movements, ocular attraction movements, and optokinetic nystagmus [51]. Compensation for the defective horizontal eye movements is accomplished by jerky movements of the head. The disease is not progressive, and older patients may be able to compensate by an over-shooting thrust of the eyeballs rather than by head jerks. The condition can improve with age. Because individuals with COMA type Cogan II have an increased risk to develop chronic renal failure due to nephronophthisis, renal function should be analysed in regular intervals.

Some individuals also show cerebellar vermis hypoplasia with evidence of the molar tooth sign. Associations with other extra-renal disease manifestations such as retinal degeneration might also occur. Deletions in *NPHP1* have been described in few individuals with congenital COMA type Cogan II in combination with nephronophthisis [28]. So far mutations in several genes including

NPHP4/SLSN4, NPHP6/JBTS5/SLSN6/MKS4, and *NPHP8/JBTS7/MKS5* have been reported (Table 13.1).

RHYNS Syndrome

In 2001, Hedera and Gorski [52] reported two brothers with retinitis pigmentosa, growth hormone deficiency, and acromelic skeletal dysplasia. They proposed for this clinical picture the acronyme RHYNS syndrome (retinitis pigmentosa, hypopituitarism, nephronophthisis, and skeletal dysplasia). Recently mutations in *NPHP8/JBTS7/MKS5* have been reported. Some individuals had associated pituitary agenesis and partial growth hormone deficiency.

Mainzer-Saldino Syndrome

The association of cone-shaped phalangeal epiphyses and nephronophthisis has been referred to as Mainzer-Saldino syndrome [53, 54]. An additional association with retinitis pigmentosa, ataxia and hepatic fibrosis has been described [55, 56]. Recently mutations in the genes encoding components of the intraflagellar transport (IFT) components IFT140 and IFT172 have been reported in Mainzer Saldino syndrome as well as Jeune syndrome. For a detailed description of IFT and ciliary chondrodysplasias please refer to Chap. 11 of this book.

Boichis Disease

The association of nephronophthisis and hepatic fibrosis has been referred to as Boichis disease. Other associated findings are retinal degeneration [57–59].

Glomerulocystic Kidney Disease

Glomerulocystic disease is a descriptive term for a histopathological picture that is defined by a two- to threefold dilatation of the glomerulous Bowman's space [60]. It can be seen in very different cystic disease syndromes such as autosomal dominant and recessive polycystic kidney disease (ADPKD, ARPKD), renal cyst and diabetes syndrome (MODY V), Bardet-Biedl syndrome, tuberous sclerosis complex, orofaciodigital syndrome and several more. Glomerulocystic kidney disease can also be seen as a component of renal dysplasia caused by maternal drug intake during pregnancy, following haemolytic uremic syndrome or as a consequence of tubular obstruction [61].

Although in nephronophthisis the typical histological picture shows cysts at the corticomedullary junction reflecting a dilatation of the tubules rather than Bowman's space, in some rare cases also glomerulocystic transformations could be identified. Genetically, of the numerous *NPHP* genes only *NPHP3* is currently associated with glomerulocystic kidney disease. Families with *NPHP3* mutations presented a broad clinical spectrum including a variety of congenital anomalies of the kidney and urinary tract as well as early embryonic pattering defects resulting in *situs inversus*, polydactyly, structural heart defects, central nervous system malformations and preauricular fistulas [62].

Most of the syndromic renal cystic diseases mentioned above are associated with mutations in genes of which the proteins are expressed at the primary cilia or centrosome. Cilia are crucial for embryonic development and are involved in a variety of signalling pathways such as the Wnt, Hedgehog, Glis3 or Wwtr1 pathway [63]. The reason why mutations in these genes and the disruption of affected pathways sometimes affect the glomerular region and sometimes other parts of the kidney is currently seen in the developmental timing as well as the extent of the individual mutations on organogenesis [64].

Genetics

Up to date 16 different genes (*NPHP1-16*) have been described. Given that these genes only account for about 50 % of all nephronophthisis patients, further heterogeneity can be expected. *NPHP1* on chromosome 2q13 is the most commonly mutated gene and homozygous deletions of this gene account for about 20–60 % of the clinical cases [17, 18]. Heterozygous deletions were found in another 6 % of patients. The other *NPHP* genes described so far only contribute to a minor part. Noteworthy, mutations in *TMEM67/ NPHP11* have recently been identified in patients with a hepatic phenotype. Mutations in *NPHP2/ INVS* and *NPHP3* cause infantile and adolescent nephronophthisis but often do not manifest with typical nephronophthisis-like renal phenotype and may even mimic polycystic kidney disease (Table 13.1).

Cilia Hypothesis

The gene products of *NPHP1-18* are called nephrocystins. All nephrocystin proteins analyzed so far localize either to primary cilia or the ciliary base indicating that cilia function is essential to preserve renal architecture and integrity (Fig. 13.5a–e) [65, 66]. Primary cilia are evolutionarily conserved, membrane-bound, microtubular projections protruding from the cell surface. They are found on virtually all cell types in the human body and play an essential role in transducing signaling information from the extracellular milieu into the cell [67, 68]. Multiple intracellular pathways are involved such as Wnt, Notch, Hedgehog, and mammalian target of rapamycin (mTOR) signaling [69, 70]. Cystic kidney diseases including nephronophthisis have played a major role in discovering the physiological function of non-motile cilia within the last 15–20 years. Meanwhile, a large variety of renal and extrarenal inherited diseases have been linked to ciliary malfunction and being referred to as ciliopathies. For a detailed description of the cell biological background as well as the clinical variety of ciliopathies, please refer to Chap. 11 of this book.

Therapy

So far, there is no specific therapy correcting the genetic or functional defects in nephronophthisis or nephronophthisis associated ciliopathies. Thus, in the early stage of disease without renal impairment, the main goal is the correction of water and electrolyte imbalances by replacing the ongoing loss of water and salt due to the reduced urinary concentrating capacity. Consequent fluid supplementation is probably helpful in maintaining renal function by preventing intermittent renal hypoperfusion. Besides, so far no

medical interventions have been demonstrated to slow down the decline of renal function. Nevertheless the recent molecular insights into the pathogenesis of nephronophthisis are hoped to translate into novel therapeutic strategies in the foreseeable future.

Once disease progress reaches end-stage renal disease, renal transplantation is the therapy of choice. Patients with nephronophthisis are not at risk for recurrence of the primary disease and outcomes are excellent [71].

Autosomal Dominant Interstitial Kidney Disease (ADIKD)

Autosomal dominant interstitial kidney disease (ADIKD) is a rare and heterogeneous genetic disorder. It is characterized by autosomal dominant inheritance and a slowly progressive tubulointerstitial nephropathy leading to end-stage renal disease in late adulthood [72]. Although the clinical and histological presentation may show significant overlap with nephronophthisis [73, 74], there are two major differences: Nephronophthisis refers to autosomal recessive conditions that typically present in childhood and lead to ESRD in the teenage years while ADIKD is inherited in an autosomal dominant fashion and typically presents later in life, although manifestation in the first decade of life is occasionally observed. So far three genes were identified in which mutations lead to ADIKD: *UMOD* (16p12); *REN*; and *MUC1(1q21)*.

Terminology and Classification

The terminology for this heterogeneous disease complex is confusing. The term "medullary cystic kidney disease (MCKD)" has historically been used to describe the same condition. The term MCKD was abandoned since medullary cysts are not an obligatory feature; in fact most patients with ADIKD show no cysts at all. Another term commonly used by pediatric nephrologists is "familial juvenile hyperuricaemic nephropathy (FJHN)," describing a condition that is synonymous to what adult nephrologists used to call MCKD.

Nowadays the classification of the ADIKD is based upon the underlying genetic mutation, resulting in at least four subtypes:

1. Mutations in the *MUC1* gene encoding Mucin. This form in the past has been referred to as medullary cystic kidney disease type 1 (MCKD1) [75].
2. Mutations in the *UMOD* gene encoding uromodulin (Tamm-Horsfall-protein). This group represents the majority of cases and includes what in the past was referred to as MCKD2 or FJHN [76, 77].
3. Mutations in the *REN* gene encoding Renin.
4. ADIKD patients with no mutations in the genes listed above.

Pathophysiology

Mutations in the *MUC1* gene have recently been identified to cause the condition previously referred to as medullary cystic kidney disease type 1 (MCKD1). All affected individuals show a single cytosine insertion into one variable-number tandem repeat sequence within the *MUC1* coding region. Mucin 1 is expressed intracellularly in the loop of Henle, distal tubule and collecting duct as well as in the apical membrane of the collecting duct. Mutations of the *MUC1* gene result in an abnormal mucin 1 protein. The functional impact of these mutations is not yet understood. Knockout studies in mice indicate that mucin 1 is not an essential protein; hence, a dominant negative or gain-of function effect of *MUC1* mutations is discussed [78].

UMOD encodes the Tamm-Horsfall protein (THP), which is expressed exclusively at the luminal side of renal epithelial cells of the thick ascending loop of Henle. While THP is the most abundant protein in human urine [79], its function is not fully understood. THP seems to play an important role in maintaining the water-tight integrity of the thick ascending limb. At the same time it appears to facilitate the transport of the NaK2Cl-Cotransporter [80] as well as the ROMK potassium channel to the surface of epithelial cells in the thick ascending limb [81]. Exon 4 is a hot spot for *UMOD* mutations affecting EGF-like protein domains [79]. Mutant uromodulin proteins are unable to exit the endoplasmic reticulum, leading to intracellular accumulation of abnormal uromodulin followed by tubular cell atrophy and death. This might explain the progressive chronic kidney failure of *UMOD* patients. Yet the pathophysiological role of *UMOD* mutations in the development of hyperuricemia is not clearly understood.

Mutations in the *REN* gene leading to ADIKD are extremely rare and have been identified in less than 10 families to date. It appears that these mutations result in a disrupted translocation of preprorenin into the endoplasmic reticulum of renin expressing cells. As a consequence the cleavage of preprorenin into prorenin and further into renin is blocked. Low serum levels of renin and angiotensin result in arterial hypotension and presumably hypoxic damage to renal tubular cells. At the same time the accumulation of preprorenin in renal tubular cells leads to apoptosis of these cells as well [82]. As renin is essential for nephrogenesis, homozygous *REN* mutations are mostly incompatible with life.

Clinical Presentation

Clinical symptoms are very similar in all disease variants. They typically include early-onset hyperuricaemia, gout and slowly progressive chronic renal failure. Urine sediment is usually normal; in case of significant proteinuria or hematuria alternative causes should be ruled out. On ultrasound small cortico-medullary cysts might develop during the course of the disease but these are not an obligatory prerequisite for the diagnosis. Kidney size is normal or slightly reduced. Renal histological findings comprise tubular basement membrane disintegration, tubular atrophy with cyst development, and interstitial round cell infiltration associated with fibrosis resembling the findings observed in "classical nephronophthisis" (Fig. 13.1). Thus, imaging and histological findings cannot confirm the diagnosis. Instead, careful analysis of clinical and pedigree information should lead to genetic testing, which will establish the diagnosis. Clinical and diagnostic findings are summarized in Table 13.2.

Table 13.2 Genetical, clinical and diagnostic findings in autosomal dominant interstitial kidney disease (ADIKD) variants

ADIKD type, allelic disorders	OMIM entry	Gene	Renal imaging	Renal histology	Age at ESRD	Arterial hypertension	Hyperuricemia, gout	Other symptoms
ADIKD1 –	174000	MUC1	Normal (50%) or small kidneys, corticomedullary cysts (40%)	TIN, TIF, TBM, TA, TCD (NPHP-like)	50–76 years (median 62)	+ (50%)	+ (40%) + Adult onset (34–66 years)	Anemia Late: arterial hypotension (salt wasting)
ADIKD2 FJHN1 Glomerulocystic kidney disease (GCKD)	603860	UMOD	Normal (50%) or small kidneys, corticomedullary cysts (40%), echogenicity ↑ (10%)	TIN, TIF, TBM, TA, TCD (NPHP-like), glomerular cysts (GCKD)	16–70 year (median 42)	+ (50%)	+ (75%) Juvenile onset (6–20 year) + (65%) Teenage onset (♀ 17–62 years, ♂ 18–33 years)	Uromodulin excretion ↓↓, UAEF <6%
FJHN2 –	613092	REN	Normal or small echogenic kidneys, no cysts	TIN, TA, IF (nonspecific)	43–68 years (median 57)	+ Late onset (secondary to CKD)	+/– +/– Early onset (10–30 year)	Hypoproliferative anemia, arterial Hypotension (plasma renin ↓, salt wasting), uromodulin excretion ↓↓

Clinical Manifestation of MUC1 Mutations

In contrast to patients with *UMOD* or *REN* gene mutations, slowly progressive chronic renal failure is the first and main symptom in patients with *MUC1* mutations. Hyperuricemia and gout, if at all present, develop late in the course of the disease. Other clinical manifestations are uncommon. This was illustrated by the examination of six large Cypriot families including 72 affected individuals which enabled the localization of the *MUC1 gene* [75]. The disease led to end-stage renal disease at a mean age of 54 years, ranging from 36 to 80 years. Arterial hypertension was found in 51 % of affected individuals, but strictly related to renal function. In the course of disease the prevelance of hyperuricemia increased at approximately the same rate as in chronic renal failure from other causes. Cysts were detected sonographically in 40 % of tested gene carriers. Mainly corticomedullary or medullary but also cortical cysts were reported. Approximately half of the gene carriers had normal sized kidneys without cysts, and 11 % had small kidneys with increased echogenicity but without cysts. The lack of cysts in 60 % of affected subjects precludes any diagnostic value of renal cysts at least in the early stages of this disease.

In another 23 kindreds with a total of 128 affected individuals, ESRD was reached at a median age of 32 years [83], with a range from 5 to 76 years. Renal biopsy was performed in affected patients from 15 families, revealing histological findings identical to those found in "classical nephronophthisis." Hyperuricemia was only reported in 8 families, whereas hypertension was present in affected individuals from 13 of the 23 families.

Clinical Manifestation of UMOD Mutations

Patients affected by *UMOD* gene mutations are typically characterized by juvenile onset of hyperuricemia, gout, and progressive renal failure. Clinical features of both conditions vary in presence and severity. In the past familial juvenile hyperuricemic nephropathy has been discriminated from medullary cystic kidney disease mainly by the absence of renal cysts. However, as mentioned before, cysts are not obligatory in "medullary cystic kidney disease." Moreover, Hart and coworkers demonstrated that both disorders are allelic, explaining why not all affected individuals even within a pedigree will exhibit renal cysts [84].

In 2004, Scolari et al. presented a series of 205 patients from 31 families with *UMOD* mutations in which 75 % showed hyperuricemia and 65 % gout, although in subset of families neither symptom was present. In 70 % of the patients chronic kidney disease developed, leading to ESRD in 80 % of the subjects between the age of 20 and 70 years [85]. Comparable findings were reported in a series of 109 patients from 45 families and in another Italian kindred with ten affected individuals. The median age of end-stage renal disease was 54 (25–70) years [86] and 31 (16–54) years [76], respectively. The clinical course in homozygotes from consanguineous families seems to be more severe. In a large Spanish kindred with *UMOD* mutations one individual with recessive (bi-allelic) *UMOD* mutations was identified. The homozygous individual survived to adulthood, and presented with an earlier onset of hyperuricemia and faster progression to ESRD than heterozygous individuals [87].

Mild urinary concentrating defects are common and may present as persistent enuresis [85]. Wolf et al. [79] reported renal imaging of 12 individuals with *UMOD* mutations by either magnetic resonance imaging or ultrasound. This revealed in all families suspicious results with small kidneys, decreased parenchyma, or cysts. Renal histology of these cases showed microcysts in 4 out of 12 cases and in the others dilated or atrophic tubules, global sclerosis, extensive tubulo-interstitial atrophy with fibrosis, and signs of chronic diffuse inflammation.

Clinical Manifestation of REN Mutations

Patients with *REN* gene mutations present very similar to *UMOD* patients with early onset gout and development of chronic kidney disease. However, *REN* patients are somewhat older when presenting with gout for the first time

(20–30 years) and progression of renal failure is slower. End-stage renal failure usually occurs after the age of 40. Unlike in *UMOD* patients, *REN* mutations result in additional clinical symptoms caused by hyporeninism such as arterial hypotension, mild hyperkalemia and an increased risk of acute renal injury in a setting of volume depletion or application of non-steroidal inflammatory drugs. Moreover, hypoproliferative anemia can be seen in early childhood which may resolve during adolescence [82].

Therapy

As in nephronophthisis, no specific therapy is available to correct the genetic or functional defects in ADIKD. The symptomatic treatment strategies include the management of hyperuricemia, gout and progressive renal failure. Hyperuricemia should be treated with a xanthin oxidase inhibitor, usually allopurinol. It is still controversial whether allopurinol can slow down the decline of renal function since in most patients with ADIKD underexcretion rather than overproduction of uric acid is the main problem.

In ESRD, renal transplantation is a good option for ADIKD patients since the disease does not recur in transplanted kidneys. Family members of patients with *UMOD*, *REN* or *MUC1* mutations must undergo genetic testing before living donation.

Acknowledgements We are grateful to Heike Olbrich for preparation of tables and figures and her continuous support.

References

1. Fanconi G, Hanhart E, von Albertini A, Uhlinger E, Dolivo G, Prader A. Die familiäre juvenile nephronophthise. Helv Paediatr Acta. 1951;6:1–49.
2. Smith C, Graham J. Congenital medullary cysts of kidneys with severe refractory anemia. Am J Dis Child. 1945;69:369–77.
3. Waldherr R, Lennert T, Weber HP, Fodisch HJ, Scharer K. The nephronophthisis complex. A clinico-pathologic study in children. Virchows Arch [Pathol Anat]. 1982;394:235–54.
4. Zollinger HU, Mihatsch MJ, Edefonti A, Gaboardi F, Imbasciati E, Lennert T. Nephronophthisis (medullary cystic disease of the kidney). A study using electron microscopy, immunofluorescence, and a review of the morphological findings. Helv Paediatr Acta. 1980;35:509–30.
5. Blowey DL, Querfeld U, Geary D, Warady BA, Alon U. Ultrasound findings in juvenile nephronophthisis. Pediatr Nephrol. 1996;10:22–4.
6. Hildebrandt F, Strahm B, Nothwang HG, Gretz N, Schnieders B, Singh-Sawhney I, Kutt R, Vollmer M, Brandis M. Molecular genetic identification of families with juvenile nephronophthisis type 1: rate of progression to renal failure. APN Study Group. Arbeitsgemeinschaft fuer Paedatrische Nephrologie. Kidney Int. 1997;51:261–9.
7. Otto EA, Schermer B, Obara T, O'Toole JF, Hiller KS, Mueller AM, Ruf RG, Hoefele J, Beekmann F, Landau D, Foreman JW, Goodship JA, Strachan T, Kispert A, Wolf MT, Gagnadoux MF, Nivet H, Antignac C, Walz G, Drummond IA, Benzing T, Hildebrandt F. Mutations in INVS encoding inversin cause nephronophthisis type 2, linking renal cystic disease to the function of primary cilia and left-right axis determination. Nat Genet. 2003;34:413–20.
8. Haider NB, Carmi R, Shalev H, Sheffield VC, Landau D. A Bedouin kindred with infantile nephronophthisis demonstrates linkage to chromosome 9 by homozygosity mapping. Am J Hum Genet. 1998;63:1404–10.
9. Bodaghi E, Honarmand MT, Ahmadi M. Infantile nephronophthisis. Int J Pediatr Nephrol. 1987;8:207–10.
10. Gagnadoux MF, Bacri JL, Broyer M, Habib R. Infantile chronic tubulo-interstitial nephritis with cortical microcysts: variant of nephronophthisis or new disease entity ? Pediatr Nephrol. 1989;3:50–5.
11. O'Toole JF, Otto EA, Frishberg Y, Hildebrandt F. Retinitis pigmentosa and renal failure in a patient with mutations in INVS. Nephrol Dial Transplant. 2006;21:1989–91.
12. Simons M, Gloy J, Ganner A, Bullerkotte A, Bashkurov M, Kronig C, Schermer B, Benzing T, Cabello OA, Jenny A, Mlodzik M, Polok B, Driever W, Obara T, Walz G. Inversin, the gene product mutated in nephronophthisis type II, functions as a molecular switch between Wnt signaling pathways. Nat Genet. 2005;37:537–43.
13. Antignac C, Arduy CH, Beckmann JS, Benessy F, Gros F, Medhioub M, Hildebrandt F, Dufier JL, Kleinknecht C, Broyer M, Weissenbach J, Habib R, Cohen D. A gene for familial juvenile nephronophthisis (recessive medullary cystic kidney disease) maps to chromosome 2p. Nat Genet. 1993;3:342–5.
14. Hildebrandt F, Singh-Sawhney I, Schnieders B, Centofante L, Omran H, Pohlmann A, Schmaltz C, Wedekind H, Schubotz C, Antignac C. Mapping of a gene for familial juvenile nephronophthisis: refining the map and defining flanking markers on chromosome

2. APN Study Group. Am J Hum Genet. 1993;53:1256–61.

15. Hildebrandt F, Otto E, Rensing C, Nothwang HG, Vollmer M, Adolphs J, Hanusch H, Brandis M. A novel gene encoding an SH3 domain protein is mutated in nephronophthisis type 1. Nat Genet. 1997;17:149–53.

16. Saunier S, Calado J, Heilig R, Silbermann F, Benessy F, Morin G, Konrad M, Broyer M, Gubler MC, Weissenbach J, Antignac C. A novel gene that encodes a protein with a putative src homology 3 domain is a candidate gene for familial juvenile nephronophthisis. Hum Mol Genet. 1997;6:2317–23.

17. Hildebrandt F, Rensing C, Betz R, Sommer U, Birnbaum S, Imm A, Omran H, Leipoldt M, Otto E. Arbeitsgemeinschaft fuer Paediatrische Nephrologie (APN) Study Group: establishing an algorithm for molecular genetic diagnostics in 127 families with juvenile nephronophthisis. Kidney Int. 2001;59(2):434–45.

18. Hoefele J, Sudbrak R, Reinhardt R, Lehrack S, Hennig S, Imm A, Muerb U, Utsch B, Attanasio M, O'Toole JF, Otto E, Hildebrandt F. Mutational analysis of the NPHP4 gene in 250 patients with nephronophthisis. Hum Mutat. 2005;25(4):411.

19. Konrad M, Saunier S, Heidet L, Silbermann F, Benessy F, Calado J, Le Paslier D, Broyer M, Gubler MC, Antignac C. Large homozygous deletions of the 2q13 region are a major cause of juvenile nephronophthisis. Hum Mol Genet. 1996;5:367–71.

20. Donaldson JC, Dempsey PJ, Reddy S, Bouton AH, Coffey RJ, Hanks SK. Crk-associated substrate p130(Cas) interacts with nephrocystin and both proteins localize to cell-cell contacts of polarized epithelial cells. Exp Cell Res. 2000;256:168–78.

21. Benzing T, Gerke P, Hopker K, Hildebrandt F, Kim E, Walz G. Nephrocystin interacts with Pyk2, p130(Cas), and tensin and triggers phosphorylation of Pyk2. Proc Natl Acad Sci U S A. 2001;98(17):9784–9.

22. Mollet G, Salomon R, Gribouval O, Silbermann F, Bacq D, Landthaler G, Milford D, Nayir A, Rizzoni G, Antignac C, Saunier S. The gene mutated in juvenile nephronophthisis type 4 encodes a novel protein that interacts with nephrocystin. Nat Genet. 2002;32:300–5.

23. Olbrich H, Fliegauf M, Hoefele J, Kispert A, Otto E, Volz A, Wolf MT, Sasmaz G, Trauer U, Reinhardt R, Sudbrak R, Antignac C, Gretz N, Walz G, Schermer B, Benzing T, Hildebrandt F, Omran H. Mutations in a novel gene, NPHP3, cause adolescent nephronophthisis, tapeto-retinal degeneration and hepatic fibrosis. Nat Genet. 2003;34:455–9.

24. Mollet G, Silbermann F, Delous M, Salomon R, Antignac C, Saunier S. Characterization of the nephrocystin/nephrocystin-4 complex and subcellular localization of nephrocystin-4 to primary cilia and centrosomes. Hum Mol Genet. 2005;14:645–56.

25. Schermer B, Hopker K, Omran H, Ghenoiu C, Fliegauf M, Fekete A, Horvath J, Kottgen M, Hackl M, Zschiedrich S, Huber TB, Kramer-Zucker A, Zentgraf H, Blaukat A, Walz G, Benzing T. Phosphorylation by casein kinase 2 induces PACS-1 binding of nephrocystin and targeting to cilia. EMBO J. 2005;24:4415–24.

26. Fliegauf M, Horvath J, von Schnakenburg C, Müller D, Thumfart J, Schermer B, Pazour GJ, Neumann HPH, Zentgraf H, Benzing T, Omran H. Nephrocystin specifically localizes to the transition zone of renal and respiratory cilia and is absent in nephronophthisis patients with NPHP1 deletions. J Am Soc Nephrol. 2006;17:2424–33.

27. Bollee G, Fakhouri F, Karras A, Noel LH, Salomon R, Servais A, Lesavre P, Moriniere V, Antignac C, Hummel A. Nephronophthisis related to homozygous NPHP1 gene deletion as a cause of chronic renal failure in adults. Nephrol Dial Transplant. 2006;21(9):2660–3.

28. Betz R, Rensing C, Otto E, Mincheva A, Zehnder D, Lichter P, Hildebrandt F. Children with ocular motor apraxia type Cogan carry deletions in the gene (NPHP1) for juvenile nephronophthisis. J Pediatr. 2000;136:828–31.

29. Parisi MA, Bennett CL, Eckert ML, Dobyns WB, Gleeson JG, Shaw DWW, McDonald R, Eddy A, Chance PF, Glass IA. The NPHP1 gene deletion associated with juvenile nephronophthisis is present in a subset of individuals with Joubert syndrome. Am J Hum Genet. 2004;75:82–91.

30. Otto E, Hoefele J, Ruf R, Mueller AM, Hiller KS, Wolf MT, Schuermann MJ, Becker A, Birkenhager R, Sudbrak R, Hennies HC, Nurnberg P, Hildebrandt F. A gene mutated in nephronophthisis and retinitis pigmentosa encodes a novel protein, nephroretinin, conserved in evolution. Am J Hum Genet. 2002;71:1161–7.

31. Omran H, Fernandez C, Jung M, Häffner K, Fargier B, Waldherr R, Gretz N, Brandis M, Rüschendorf F, Reis A, Hildebrandt F. Identification of a new gene locus for adolescent nephronophthisis, on chromosome 3q22 in a large Venzuelan pedigree. Am J Hum Genet. 2000;66:118–27.

32. Omran H, Häffner K, Burth S, Fernandez C, Fargier B, Villaquiran A, Nothwang HG, Schnittger S, Lehrach H, Woo D, Brandis M, Sudbrak R, Hildebrandt F. Human adolescent nephronophthisis: gene locus synteny with polycystic kidney disease in pcy mice. J Am Soc Nephrol. 2001;12:107–13.

33. Omran H, Sasmaz G, Häffner K, Volz A, Olbrich H, Otto E, Wienker TF, Korinthenberg R, Brandis M, Antignac C, Hildebrandt F. Identification of a gene locus for Senior-Løken syndrome in the region of the nephronophthisis type 3 gene. J Am Soc Nephrol. 2002;13:75–9.

34. Hildebrandt F, Omran H. New insights: nephronophthisis-medullary cystic kidney disease. Pediatr Nephrol. 2001;16:168–76.

35. Løken AC, Hanssen O, Halvorsen S, Jølster NJ. Hereditary renal dysplasia and blindness. Acta Paediatr. 1961;50:177–84.

36. Senior B, Friedmann AI, Braudo JL. Juvenile familial nephropathy with tapetoretinal degeneration: a new oculo-renal dystrophy. Am J Opthalmol. 1961;52: 625–33.

37. Leber T. Über Retinitis pigmentosa und angeborene Amaurose. Albrecht von Graefe's Arch Klin Exp Ophthalmol. 1869;15:1–25.

38. Leber T. Über anormale Formen der Retinitis pigmentosa. Arch Ophthalmol. 1871;17:314–41.

39. François J. Leber's congenital tapeto-retinal degeneration. Int Ophthalmol Clin. 1968;8:929–47.

40. Franceschetti A, Dieterle P. L'importance diagnostique de l'éléctrorétinogramme dans le dégénérescences tapéto-rétinennes avec rétrécissement du champ visuel et héméralopie. Conf Neurol. 1954;14: 184–6.

41. Sattar S, Gleeson JG. The ciliopathies in neuronal development: a clinical approach to investigation of Joubert syndrome and Joubert syndrome-related disorders. Dev Med Child Neurol. 2011;53(9):793–8.

42. Otto EA, Loeys B, Khanna H, Hellemans J, Sudbrak R, Fan S, Muerb U, O'Toole JF, Helou J, Attanasio M, Utsch B, Sayer JA, Lillo C, Jimeno D, Coucke P, De Paepe A, Reinhardt R, Klages S, Tsuda M, Kawakami I, Kusakabe T, Omran H, Imm A, Tippens M, Raymond PA, Hill J, Beales P, He S, Kispert A, Margolis B, Williams DS, Swaroop A, Hildebrandt F. Nephrocystin-5, a ciliary IQ domain protein, is mutated in Senior-Løken syndrome and interacts with RPGR and calmodulin. Nat Genet. 2005;37:282–8.

43. Maria BL, Quisling RG, Rosainz LC, Yachnis AT, Gitten JC, Dede DE, Fennell E. Molar tooth sign in Joubert syndrome: clinical, radiologic, and pathologic significance. J Child Neurol. 1999;14:368–76.

44. Utsch B, Sayer JA, Attanasio M, Pereira RR, Eccles M, Hennies HC, Otto EA, Hildebrandt F. Identification of the first AHI1 gene mutations in nephronophthisis-associated Joubert syndrome. Pediatr Nephrol. 2006;21:32–5.

45. Parisi MA, Doherty D, Eckert ML, Shaw DW, Ozyurek H, Aysun S, Giray O, Al Swaid A, Al Shahwan S, Dohayan N, Bakhsh E, Indridason OS, Dobyns WB, Bennett CL, Chance PF, Glass IA. AHI1 mutations cause both retinal dystrophy and renal cystic disease in Joubert syndrome. J Med Genet. 2006;43:334–9.

46. Sayer JA, Otto EA, O'Toole JF, Nurnberg G, Kennedy MA, Becker C, Hennies HC, Helou J, Attanasio M, Fausett BV, Utsch B, Khanna H, Liu Y, Drummond I, Kawakami I, Kusakabe T, Tsuda M, Ma L, Lee H, Larson RG, Allen SJ, Wilkinson CJ, Nigg EA, Shou C, Lillo C, Williams DS, Hoppe B, Kemper MJ, Neuhaus T, Parisi MA, Glass IA, Petry M, Kispert A, Gloy J, Ganner A, Walz G, Zhu X, Goldman D, Nurnberg P, Swaroop A, Leroux MR, Hildebrandt F. The centrosomal protein nephrocystin-6 is mutated in Joubert syndrome and activates transcription factor ATF4. Nat Genet. 2006;38:674–81.

47. Valente EM, Silhavy JL, Brancati F, Barrano G, Krishnaswami SR, Castori M, Lancaster MA,

Boltshauser E, Boccone L, Al-Gazali L, Fazzi E, Signorini S, Louie CM, Bellacchio E, International Joubert Syndrome Related Disorders Study Group, Bertini E, Dallapiccola B, Gleeson JG. Mutations in CEP290, which encodes a centrosomal protein, cause pleiotropic forms of Joubert syndrome. Nat Genet. 2006;38:623–5.

48. Bergmann C. Educational paper: ciliopathies. Eur J Pediatr. 2012;171(9):1285–300.

49. Doherty D, Parisi MA, Finn LS, Gunay-Aygun M, Al-Mateen M, Bates D, Clericuzio C, Demir H, Dorschner M, van Essen AJ, Gahl WA, Gentile M, Gorden NT, Hikida A, Knutzen D, Ozyurek H, Phelps I, Rosenthal P, Verloes A, Weigand H, Chance PF, Dobyns WB, Glass IA. Mutations in 3 genes (MKS3, CC2D2A and RPGRIP1L) cause COACH syndrome (Joubert syndrome with congenital hepatic fibrosis). J Med Genet. 2010;47(1):8–21.

50. Alexiev BA, Lin X, Sun CC, Brenner DS. Meckel-Gruber syndrome: pathologic manifestations, minimal diagnostic criteria, and differential diagnosis. Arch Pathol Lab Med. 2006;130(8):1236–8.

51. Cogan DG. Heredity of congenital ocular motor apraxia. Trans Am Acad Ophthal Otolaryngol. 1972;76:60–3.

52. Hedera P, Gorski JL. Retinitis pigmentosa, growth hormone deficiency, and acromelic skeletal dysplasia in two brothers: possible familial RHYNS syndrome. Am J Med Genet. 2001;101:142–5.

53. Mainzer F, Saldino RM, Ozonoff MB, Minagi H. Familial nephropathy associated with retinitis pigmentosa, cerebellar ataxia and skeletal abnormalities. Am J Med. 1970;49:556–62.

54. Giedion A. Phalangeal cone shaped epiphysis of the hands (PhCSEH) and chronic renal disease: the conorenal syndromes. Pediatr Radiol. 1979;8:32–8.

55. Popovic-Rolovic M, Calic-Perisic N, Bunjevacki G, Negovanovic D. Juvenile nephronophthisis associated with retinal pigmentary dystrophy, cerebellar ataxia, and skeletal abnormalities. Arch Dis Child. 1976;51:801–3.

56. Robins DG, French TA, Chakera TM. Juvenile nephronophthisis associated with skeletal abnormalities and hepatic fibrosis. Arch Dis Child. 1976;51:799–801.

57. Boichis H, Passwell J, David R, Miller H. Congenital hepatic fibrosis and nephronophthisis: a family study. Q J Med. 1973;42:221–33.

58. Proesmans W, Van Damme B, Macken J. Nephronophthisis and tapetoretinal degeneration associated with liver fibrosis. Clin Nephrol. 1975;3: 160–4.

59. Delaney V, Mullaney J, Bourke E. Juvenile nephronophthisis, congenital hepatic fibrosis and retinal hypoplasia in twins. Q J Med. 1978;186:281–96. 66: 558–63.

60. Bernstein J. Glomerulocystic kidney disease – nosological considerations. Pediatr Nephrol. 1993;7: 464–70.

61. Bissler J, Siroky BJ, Yin H. Glomerulocystic kidney disease. Pediatr Nephrol. 2010;25:2049–59.

62. Bergmann C, Fliegauf M, Brüchle NO, Frank V, Olbrich H, Kirschner J, Schermer B, Schmedding I, Kispert A, Kränzlin B, Nürnberg G, Becker C, Grimm T, Girschick G, Lynch SA, Kelehan P, Senderek J, Neuhaus TJ, Stallmach T, Zentgraf H, Nürnberg P, Gretz N, Lo C, Lienkamp S, Schäfer T, Walz G, Benzing T, Zerres K, Omran H. Loss of nephrocystin-3 function can cause embryonic lethality, Meckel-Gruber-like-syndrome, situs inversus and renal-hepatic-pancreatic dysplasia. Am J Hum Genet. 2008;82:959–70.

63. Kang HS, Beak JY, Kim YS, Herbert R, Jetten AM. Glis 3 is associated with primary cilia and Wwtr1/TAZ and implicated in polycystic kidney disease. Mol Cell Biol. 2009;29:2556–69.

64. Piontek K, Menezes LF, Garcia-Gonzalez MA, Huso DL, Germino GG. A critical developmental switch defines the kinetics of kidney cyst formation after loss of pkd1. Nat Med. 2007;13:1490–5.

65. Badano JL, Teslovich TM, Katsanis N. The centrosome in human genetic disease. Nat Rev Genet. 2005;6:194–205.

66. Hildebrandt F, Otto E. Cilia and centrosomes: a unifying pathogenic concept for cystic kidney disease ? Nat Rev Genet. 2005;6:928–4.

67. Nauli SM, Alenghat FJ, Luo Y, Williams E, Vassilev P, Li X, Elia AE, Lu W, Brown EM, Quinn SJ, Ingber DE, Zhou J. Polycystins 1 and 2 mediate mechanosensation in the primary cilium of kidney cells. Nat Genet. 2003;33:129–37.

68. Watnick T, Germino G. From cilia to cyst. Nat Genet. 2003;34:355–6.

69. Kim S, Dynlacht BD. Assembling a primary cilium. Curr Opin Cell Biol. 2013;25(4):506–11.

70. Omran H. NPHP proteins: gatekeepers of the ciliary compartment. J Cell Biol. 2010;190(5):715–7.

71. Hamiwka LA, Midgley JP, Wade AW, Martz KL, Grisaru S. Outcomes of kidney transplantation in children with nephronophthisis: an analysis of the North American Pediatric Renal Trials and Collaborative Studies (NAPRTCS) Registry. Pediatr Transplant. 2008;12:878–82.

72. Gardner KD. Cystic diseases of the kidney: a perspective on medullary cystic disease. Birth Defects Orig Artic Ser. 1974;10:29–31.

73. Goldman SH, Walker SR, Merigan TCJ, Gardner KDJ, Bull JM. Hereditary occurrence of cystic disease of the renal medulla. N Engl J Med. 1966;274:984–92.

74. Strauss MB, Sommers SC. Medullary cystic disease and familial juvenile nephronophthisis. N Engl J Med. 1967;277:863–4.

75. Stavrou C, Koptides M, Tombazos C, Psara E, Patsias C, Zouvani I, Kyriacou K, Hildebrandt F, Christofides T, Pierides A, Deltas CC. Autosomal-dominant medullary cystic kidney disease type 1: clinical and molecular findings in six large Cypriot families. Kidney Int. 2002;62:1385–94.

76. Scolari F, Puzzer D, Amoroso A, Caridi G, Ghiggeri GM, Maiorca R, Aridon P, De Fusco M, Ballabio A, Casari G. Identification of a new locus for medullary cystic disease, on chromosome 16p12. Am J Hum Genet. 1999;64:1655–60.

77. Kamatani N, Moritani M, Yamanaka H, Takeuchi F, Hosoya T, Itakura M. Localization of a gene for familial juvenile hyperuricemic nephropathy causing underexcretion-type gout to 16p12 by genome-wide linkage analysis of a large family. Arthritis Rheum. 2000;43:925–9.

78. Kirby A, Gnirke A, Jaffe DB, Barešová V, Pochet N, Blumenstiel B, Ye C, Aird D, Stevens C, Robinson JT, Cabili MN, Gat-Viks I, Kelliher E, Daza R, DeFelice M, Hůlková H, Sovová J, Vylet'al P, Antignac C, Guttman M, Handsaker RE, Perrin D, Steelman S, Sigurdsson S, Scheinman SJ, Sougnez C, Cibulskis K, Parkin M, Green T, Rossin E, Zody MC, Xavier RJ, Pollak MR, Alper SL, Lindblad-Toh K, Gabriel S, Hart PS, Regev A, Nusbaum C, Kmoch S, Bleyer AJ, Lander ES, Daly MJ. Mutations causing medullary cystic kidney disease type 1 lie in a large VNTR in MUC1 missed by massively parallel sequencing. Nat Genet. 2013;45:299–303.

79. Wolf MT, Mucha BE, Attanasio M, Zalewski I, Karle SM, Neumann HP, Rahman N, Bader B, Baldamus CA, Otto E, Witzgall R, Fuchshuber A, Hildebrandt F. Mutations of the Uromodulin gene in MCKD type 2 patients cluster in exon 4, which encodes three EGF-like domains. Kidney Int. 2003;64:1580–7.

80. Mutig K, Kahl T, Saritas T, Godes M,Persson P, Bates J, Raffi H, Rampoldi L, Uchida S, Hille S, Dosche C, Kumar S, Castaneda-Bueno M, Gamba G, Bachmann S. Na + K + 2Cl-Cotransporter (NKCC2) is regulated by Tamm-Horsfall-Protein (THP). American Society of Nephrology Annual Meeting, 2008; abstract 134.

81. Renigunta A, Renigunta V, Saritas T, Decher N, Mutig K, Waldegger S. Tamm-Horsfall glycoprotein interacts with renal outer medullary potassium channel ROMK2 and regulates its function. J Biol Chem. 2011;286:2224–35.

82. Zivná M, Hůlková H, Matignon M, Hodanová K, Vylet'al P, Kalbácová M, Baresová V, Sikora J, Blazková H, Zivný J, Ivánek R, Stránecký V, Sovová J, Claes K, Lerut E, Fryns JP, Hart PS, Hart TC, Adams JN, Pawtowski A, Clemessy M, Gasc JM, Gubler MC, Antignac C, Elleder M, Kapp K, Grimbert P, Bleyer AJ, Kmoch S. Dominant renin gene mutations associated with early onset hyperuricemia, anemia and chronic kidney failure. Am J Hum Genet. 2009;85:204–13.

83. Wolf MT, Mucha BE, Hennies HC, Attanasio M, Panther F, Zalewski I, Karle SM, Otto EA, Deltas CC, Fuchshuber A, Hildebrandt F. Medullary cystic kidney disease type 1: mutational analysis in 37 genes based on haplotype sharing. Hum Genet. 2006;119:649–5.

84. Hart TC, Gorry MC, Hart PS, Woodard AS, Shihabi Z, Sandhu J, Shirts B, Xu L, Zhu H, Barmada MM, Bleyer AJ. Mutations of the UMOD gene are responsible for medullary cystic kidney disease 2 and familial juvenile hyperuricaemic nephropathy. J Med Genet. 2002;39(12):882–92.

85. Scolari F, Caridi G, Rampoldi L, Tardanico R, Izzi C, Pirulli D, Amoroso A, Casari G, Ghiggeri GM. Uromodulin storage disease: clinical aspects and mechanisms. Am J Kidney Dis. 2004;44:987–99.

86. Bollée G, Dahan K, Flamant M, Morinière V, Pawtowski A, Heidet L, Lacombe D, Devuyst O, Pirson Y, Antignac C, Knebelmann B. Phenotype and outcome in hereditary tubulointerstitial nephritis secondary to UMOD mutations. Clin J Am Soc Nephrol. 2011;6:2429–38.

87. Rezende-Lima W, Parreira KS, Garcia-Gonzalez M, Riveira E, Banet JF, Lens XM. Homozygosity for uromodulin disorders: FJHN and MCKD-type 2. Kidney Int. 2004;66:558–63.

Part IV

Glomerular Disorders

Hematuria and Proteinuria

14

Hui-Kim Yap and Perry Yew-Weng Lau

Introduction

The presence of blood or protein in the urine may be just a normal transient finding in children, usually accompanying a non-specific viral infection. More importantly, these findings may be an indicator of a kidney or urinary tract disorder. Macroscopic hematuria or the incidental finding of hematuria or proteinuria on urine dipstick examination is often an alarming occurrence to parents, bringing the child to medical attention. The etiology of hematuria and proteinuria includes a long list of conditions. Workup can be extensive, expensive and unnecessary as most children with isolated hematuria or isolated proteinuria have a benign etiology. On the other hand, persistent proteinuria can be an indicator of significant glomerular disease, as well as chronic kidney disease.

Hematuria

In a normal person, very few red blood cells are excreted into the urine. The red blood cells are believed to pass into the urine via the glomerulus. The pliability of the red blood cells allows them to squeeze through the capillary basement membrane. The normal red blood cell excretion rate can be greater after exercise. Glomerular inflammation results in damage to the capillary endothelium and glomerular basement membrane, resulting in increased passage of red blood cells into the urinary space. Macroscopic hematuria is visible to the naked eye while microscopic hematuria is usually detected by a urine dipstick test during a routine examination or by microscopic examination of the urine sediment.

A very small quantity of blood can discolor the urine. If fresh blood is present in the urine, the urine will be pink or red in color. If left standing even in the bladder, the urine will develop a hazy smoky or brown color. The brown color comes from the metheme derivative of the oxidized heme pigment. Some pigments and crystals, when present at a significant concentration, will cause color changes in the urine that can be misinterpreted as hematuria. Discoloration of urine can be due to intravascular hemolysis, rhabdomyolysis, metabolic disorders and a number of foods and drugs (Table 14.1).

H.-K. Yap (✉)
Department of Pediatrics, National University of Singapore, 1E Kent Ridge Road, NUHS Tower Block Level 12, Singapore 119228, Singapore
e-mail: hui_kim_yap@nuhs.edu.sg

P.Y.-W. Lau
Khoo Teck Puat-National University Children's Medical Institute, National University Hospital, 1E Kent Ridge Road, NUHS Tower Block Level 12, Singapore 119228, Singapore
e-mail: perry_lau@nuhs.edu.sg

© Springer-Verlag Berlin Heidelberg 2016
D.F. Geary, F. Schaefer (eds.), *Pediatric Kidney Disease*, DOI 10.1007/978-3-662-52972-0_14

Table 14.1 Causes of discoloration of urine

Dark yellow or orange urine	Normal concentrated urine
	Rifampicin
	Carotene
	Pyridium
	Warfarin
Dark brown or black urine	Bile pigments
	Methemoglobinemia
	Alanine, resorcinol
	Laxatives containing cascara or senna
	Alkaptonuria, homogentesic acid, melanin, tyrosinosis
	Thymol
	Methyldopa metabolite
	Copper
	Phenol poisoning
Red or pink urine	Red blood cells (hematuria)
	Free hemoglobin (hemoglobinuria)
	Myoglobin (myoglobinuria)
	Porphyrins
	Urates in high concentration (may produce a pinkish tinge)
	Foods (e.g., beetroot, rhubarb, blackberries, red dyes)
	Drugs (e.g., benzene, chloroquine, desferoxamine, phenazopyridine, phenolphthalein)

Definition

The definition of hematuria is based on urine microscopic examination findings of red blood cells of more than 5/µL in a fresh uncentrifuged midstream urine specimen [1] or more than three red blood cells/high-power field in the centrifuged sediment from 10 ml of freshly voided midstream urine. However, there is some controversy as to the amount of red blood cells required for the diagnosis of microscopic hematuria. Some investigators have used a definition of greater than two red blood cells/high-power field in 12 ml of a midstream urine specimen spun at 1,500 RPM for 5 min [2]. Other investigators have used a definition of ten red blood cells/high power field in a midstream urine collection [3]. A study using more stringent criteria has greater positive predictive value with regard to presence of disease but loses some negative predictive value. Regardless of the criterion used, important

cofactors to consider when a child has hematuria include the presence of proteinuria, urinary casts, hypertension, a family history of renal disease and other clinical or laboratory findings suggestive of renal or urinary tract disease.

Urine Dipstick

The urine dipstick utilizes the peroxidase-like activity of hemoglobin present in the urine. The hemoglobin peroxidase activity converts the chromogen tetramethyl benzidine incorporated in the dipstick into an oxidized form resulting in a green-blue color. It is important to follow the manufacturer's instructions of the dipstick closely. Delayed reading may produce false positive results. The test depends on free hemoglobin, which comes from hemolysis of the red blood cells in the urine. It is assumed that when there is significant hematuria, some of the red blood cells will always lyse and there will be sufficient free hemoglobin released to cause a positive test. The test is very sensitive, capable of detecting as little as 150 µg/L of free hemoglobin.

False positive results can occur in hemoglobinuria following intravascular hemolysis or in myoglobinuria after rhabdomyolysis. False positive results can also be due to the presence of oxidizing agents in the urine such as hypochlorite and microbial peroxidases associated with microbial contamination including urinary tract infection. Conversely, false negative results can be due to the presence of large amounts of reducing agents such as ascorbic acid or urine with high specific gravity in which the dipstick test is less sensitive.

Due to the very sensitive nature of the urine dipstick test, it is unwise to investigate based on a "trace" reading on the dipstick. Similarly, a child with dipstick reading of "1+" on one occasion and negative readings on subsequent dipstick testing is unlikely to benefit from further investigations. Only if the urine dipstick reading for blood is persistently greater than "trace" is further evaluation warranted. In clinical practice, it is important to confirm hematuria with urine microscopic examination. An absence of red blood cells in the urine with a positive dipstick reaction may suggest hemoglobinuria or myoglobinuria.

Urine Microscopy

Microscopic examination of the urine sediment is important in diagnosing and evaluating hematuria. When abundant, red blood cells are easy to identify by their characteristic biconcave disc appearance under microscopy. When scanty, red blood cells become distorted in the urine and it is difficult to differentiate them from other unidentified small objects.

Urine centrifugation is one way to solve this problem. After centrifugation and removal of supernatant, the deposit is resuspended in the remaining urine and examined under the microscope. Urine microscopic examination can have false negative results when the urine is of low specific gravity or has an alkaline pH. These conditions result in red blood cells hemolysing rapidly in standing urine, resulting in a positive urine dipstick test due to the free hemoglobin, but without the characteristic red blood cells seen by microscopy.

The morphology of the red blood cells may help identify the origin of the bleeding [4, 5]. Red blood cells from the lower urinary tract maintain their morphology whereas red blood cells from the glomeruli show great variation in shape, size and hemoglobin content due to sheering stresses on their surface in their passage from the capillary lumen through gaps in the glomerular basement membrane into the urinary space [6]. Phase-contrast microscopy on freshly voided urine allows this differentiation. Red blood cells that are more than 90–95 % isomorphic (i.e., of normal size and shape) are most commonly from the lower urinary tract. If more than 30 % of dysmorphic red blood cells (blebs, budding and segmental loss of membrane with reduction in red cell volume) are present, the hematuria is more likely to be of glomerular origin [7].

The presence of casts or crystals in the urine can be helpful. Red blood cell casts are always pathological and usually suggest glomerulonephritis. Identification of red blood cell casts should be done on fresh urine or acidic urine stored at 4 °C, as red blood cell casts disintegrate readily in alkaline urine, taking on a granular appearance. Hence the finding of granular casts in association with hematuria may indicate that the blood has originated from the kidneys. The low rate of red blood cell cast identification in conventional microscopy is probably related to the low speed centrifugation of the urine specimen at 400 g. Recently, a study using high speed centrifugation at 2,000 g for microscopy was able to increase the sensitivity of the red blood cell cast yield in the urine [8]. When white blood cells are also present in the urine, the presence of infection and interstitial or glomerular inflammatory disorders should be considered. Interstitial nephritis is even more likely if Wright stain of the urine shows the presence of eosinophils. Infections and poststreptococcal nephritis often have neutrophils on urinalysis. Hyaline casts are associated with proteinuria, and a few such casts may be found in concentrated early morning samples from healthy people. If the child has other findings suggestive of nephrolithiasis, the shape of the crystals may help to identify the chemical nature of the calculi. Calcium oxalate crystals may point to hypercalciuria.

Etiology

Hematuria may originate from the glomeruli, renal tubules and interstitium, or urinary tract (including collecting systems, ureters, bladder and urethra). A practical approach is to determine whether the hematuria is of glomerular or non-glomerular origin. The various causes of hematuria in children are listed in Table 14.2. In children, the source of bleeding is more often from the glomeruli than from the urinary tract.

There are four different clinical presentations of hematuria:

1. Child with red or dark-colored urine
2. Child with lower urinary tract symptoms
3. Child with clinical features of acute glomerulonephritis
4. Asymptomatic child with incidental finding of microscopic hematuria on urine dipstick

These four clinical presentations will be considered separately as the approach is different in each of these scenarios though there is an overlap in the causes.

Table 14.2 Causes of hematuria in children

Glomerular		Nonglomerular
Familial hematuria syndromes	Glomerulonephritis (GN)	Urinary tract infection
	Primary GN	Hypercalciuria
	Post-infectious acute GN	Renal calculi
	Membranoproliferative GN	Trauma
	Membranous nephropathy	Exercise-induced
	Rapidly progressive GN	Chemical cystitis such as cyclophosphamide
	IgA nephropathy	
	Secondary GN	Coagulopathy
	Systemic lupus erythematosus	Vascular malformations
	Henoch Schönlein purpura	Nutcracker syndrome
	Polyarteritis nodosa	Urinary schistosomiasis
	ANCA positive systemic vasculitis	Malignancy
		Renal: nephroblastoma
	Hemolytic uremic syndrome	Bladder:
	Renal vein thrombosis	rhabdomyosarcoma
	Interstitial nephritis	Menarche
	Cystic renal disease	Factitious

Child with Red or Dark-Colored Urine

The first step in the evaluation is to exclude red discoloration of urine due to certain foods or drugs, hemoglobinuria and myoglobinuria (Table 14.1). A urine microscopic examination is essential to confirm that the discoloration is due to red blood cells. Macroscopic hematuria of glomerular origin is usually described as brown, tea-colored or cola-colored, while that of lower urinary tract origin (bladder and urethra) is usually pink or red.

The causes of gross hematuria in children include:

1. Acute glomerulonephritis, especially if edema and hypertension are also present
2. Urinary tract infection, hemorrhagic cystitis, urethritis, perineal irritation, urolithiasis, hypercalciuria. These conditions are usually accompanied by voiding symptoms such as dysuria, frequency and urgency
3. Exercise-induced hematuria
4. Trauma
5. Coagulopathy
6. Malignancy
7. Recurrent gross hematuria suggestive of IgA nephropathy, nutcracker syndrome, Alport syndrome, CFHR5 nephropathy or *MYH9* disorders.

Exercise-induced hematuria is a transient hematuria that appears immediately after severe exercise such as long-distance running and usually disappears within 48 h. This is due to excessive increase in red cell excretion associated with severe exercise and is benign.

Trauma sufficient to cause hematuria is usually associated with an obvious history such as traumatic urethral catheterization or abdominal injury. Cases of radiological evaluation of hematuria after abdominal trauma with finding of previously unsuspected obstructed urinary tract such as pelvi-ureteric junction stenosis have been reported.

Children with bleeding disorders such as hemophilia or thrombocytopenia commonly have microscopic hematuria and may also develop gross hematuria. Sickle cell hemoglobinopathy can cause hematuria by causing infarction of the renal collecting systems [9].

Urinary tract tumors are rare. Children with nephroblastoma can have microscopic hematuria (rarely macroscopic hematuria). More commonly, nephroblastomas are discovered following evaluation of abdominal distension or abdominal masses rather than hematuria. Rhabdomyosarcoma of the bladder is extremely rare, and usually presents with voiding symptoms in addition to macroscopic hematuria.

The nutcracker phenomenon refers to compression of the left renal vein between the aorta and superior mesenteric artery before the left renal vein joins the inferior vena cava. This leads to left renal vein hypertension which may result in rupture of the thin walled vein into the renal calyceal fornix with the clinical presentation of intermittent gross or microscopic hematuria. In addition, the increased venous pressure within the renal circulation can promote the development of varices of the renal pelvis and ureter. This phenomenon with its associated symptoms of unilateral hematuria and left flank pain is defined as the nutcracker syndrome. It occasionally presents as a varicocele in boys or abnormal menstruation in pubertal girls, as a result of the development of venous varicosities of the gonadal vein [10]. Orthostatic proteinuria has also been reported in nutcracker syndrome although the exact mechanism is unknown [11]. Possible mechanisms include subtle glomerular lesions associated with hemodynamic abnormality, and an increased release in norepinephrine and angiotensin II on standing up [11]. Nutcracker syndrome occurs in relatively young and previously healthy patients with an asthenic habitus, and may be one of the important causes of gross or microscopic hematuria [12]. Diagnosis of this condition can be made by renal ultrasound imaging demonstrating compression of a pre-aortic left renal vein in the fork between the abdominal aorta and the proximal superior mesenteric artery, and Doppler flow scanning measuring the peak flow velocity ratio between the aorto-mesenteric portion and the hilar portion of the renal vein. The most accurate method for diagnosing the nutcracker syndrome is left renal venography with measurement of the pressure gradient between the left renal vein and the inferior vena cava. Such invasive examination is difficult to perform in children. Magnetic resonance angiography can be used to demonstrate the dilated left renal vein after passing between the aorta and superior mesenteric artery. An alternative is multidetector computed tomography which can detect the decrease in velocity of contrast enhancement to the parenchyma of the left kidney due to compression of left renal vein;

however, the radiation risk in childhood is not negligible [13]. Controversy exists as to the treatment of nutcracker syndrome. Spontaneous resolution of hematuria in 75 % of children with nutcracker syndrome followed up for 2 or more years has been reported following increase in the body mass index. [12, 14, 15] Surgical or radiological intervention are indicated for severe pain, significant hematuria and renal impairment, with percutaneous endovascular stent insertion being the preferred mode of therapy [16].

Children with IgA nephropathy and some of the familial hematuria syndromes (Table 14.2) can have macroscopic hematuria at the time of, or 1 or 2 days following, an upper respiratory tract infection, a phenomenon known as synpharyngitic hematuria. Their urine can be normal in between the bouts of hematuria but a considerable proportion has persistent microscopic hematuria between the attacks of gross hematuria. A family history of relatives with known hematuria, renal failure or deafness may suggest Alport syndrome but it must be remembered that a negative family history does not exclude Alport syndrome. CFHR5 nephropathy is a recently recognized condition that is endemic in the Greek Cypriot population and is extremely rare in the non-Cypriot population. It is caused by a mutation of the Complement Factor H-Related 5 (*CFHR5*) gene. Kidney biopsy invariably shows mesangial C3 deposition and molecular testing is required for the diagnosis [17].

Another group of rare disorders associated with macroscopic hematuria are the autosomal dominant thrombocytopathies (*MYH9* syndromes), namely the spectrum of May-Hegglin anomaly, Sebastian, Fechtner and Epstein syndromes [18–20]. Hematological features include giant platelets and cytoplasmic leukocyte inclusions (Döhle-like bodies) in the Fechtner syndrome. These syndromes are associated with basement membrane thickening and lamellation, sensorineural deafness and cataracts.

Recently, a syndrome in which hereditary angiopathy, nephropathy, aneurysms and muscle cramps (HANAC) linked to heterozygous mutations of COL4A1 gene has been described [21]. HANAC syndrome is extremely rare. The renal disease presents with microscopic or macroscopic hematuria and should be considered if there is family history of hematuria and intracerebral aneurysm and bleed in the adult patient.

Child with Associated Lower Urinary Tract Symptoms

Hematuria with accompanying dysuria, frequency, urgency, flank or abdominal pain may suggest a diagnosis of urinary tract infection, hypercalciuria or nephrolithiasis.

One third of urinary tract infections have associated hematuria, though this is usually microscopic in nature. Urinary tract infections are usually caused by bacteria but viruses, fungi and parasites are potential etiological agents. Acute hemorrhagic cystitis is characterized by gross hematuria and symptoms of bladder inflammation. It is associated with adenovirus type 11 and type 21. The macroscopic hematuria usually lasts 5 days and microscopic hematuria may persist for 2 or 3 days more [22]. Schistosomiasis is an important cause of hematuria to be considered in tropical Africa, Middle Eastern countries, Turkey, India, and also in immigrants from these areas [23]. It is caused by swimming in lakes and ponds infested with snails infected by the flatworm *Schistosoma haematobium*. The trapped eggs of the flatworm in the bladder and lower urinary tract cause an intense granulomatous inflammatory reaction resulting in hematuria. In developing countries, tuberculosis of the urinary tract is another cause of hematuria, both microscopic and macroscopic, especially in the context of a child with prolonged ill health [24].

Nephrolithiasis is rare in children. The incidence of stone disease in children has been reported to account for between 0.13 and 0.94 cases per 1,000 hospital admissions [25]. It can present with hematuria alone or hematuria with colic. The pain can be due to the presence of the renal stone or clots of blood passing down the ureter. An association between hematuria and hypercalciuria has been reported in children with asymptomatic macroscopic or microscopic hematuria without signs of renal stones [26]. Children with hypercalciuria can also have accompanying irritative urinary symptoms such

as dysuria, frequency and urgency. These children have increased urinary excretion of calcium despite normal serum calcium levels. The urinary calcium over creatinine ratio in a single urine specimen is a useful index of calcium excretion for screening and monitoring purposes. In a large study, the 97th percentile level of urinary calcium over creatinine ratio in children eating an unrestricted diet was 0.69 mmol/mmol, whereas in infancy, it can reach as high as 2.2 mmol/mmol [27].

Child with Clinical Features of Acute Glomerulonephritis

Acute nephritic syndrome is characterized by sudden onset of macroscopic hematuria, accompanied by hypertension, oliguria, edema and varying degree of renal insufficiency. This is due to acute glomerular injury. In children, the majority of cases of acute nephritic syndrome have a post-infectious etiology, most commonly following infection with group A β-hemolytic streptococcal infection of throat or skin. It is important to identify acute nephritic syndrome in a child with hematuria because urgent appropriate management can prevent morbidity and mortality due to uncontrolled hypertension, fluid overload and renal insufficiency.

Asymptomatic Child with Incidental Finding of Microscopic Hematuria on Urine Dipstick

Increased use of urine dipstick testing to screen for urinary tract infection in a febrile child or during routine school health examination in many countries has resulted in the detection of asymptomatic microscopic hematuria in children. Mass urine screening programs in school children have reported a prevalence of isolated microscopic hematuria in 0.21–0.94 % [28–30]. Of those children who were subsequently referred for evaluation of persistent microscopic hematuria, a glomerular pathology was the most likely cause in between 22.2 and 52.3 % of children based on either phase-contrast microscopy or renal biopsy findings [28, 30–32].

Isolated hematuria (without accompanying hypertension, significant proteinuria or renal impairment) in children is traditionally regarded as benign. However, recent publications describing the long-term follow-up of patients who presented initially with microscopic hematuria has challenged this view. An adjusted hazard ratio of 18.5 for the development of end-stage renal disease was observed in Israeli adolescents and young adults with persistent asymptomatic isolated microscopic hematuria over a period of 22 years in a population-based retrospective cohort study [33]. While the clinical outcome for many children presenting with isolated hematuria is good, the lifetime risk of renal disease is not insignificant and is dependent on the underlying pathology.

As microscopic hematuria and mild proteinuria may appear transiently during fever, illness or extreme exertion, it is therefore not cost-effective to subject every child to extensive investigations to find the cause of microscopic hematuria. One practical approach is to repeat the urine dipstick and microscopic urinalysis twice within 2 weeks after the initial result. If the hematuria resolves, no further tests are required. If microscopic hematuria persists on at least two of the three consecutive samples, then further evaluation is required [34].

The common diagnoses in children with persistent microscopic hematuria without proteinuria are familial benign hematuria, idiopathic hypercalciuria, and IgA nephropathy. It is increasingly recognized that there is a group of genetically heterogenous monogenic conditions causing microscopic hematuria that may or may not progress to end stage kidney disease over the second and seventh decade of life. This group of familial hematuric diseases is caused by mutations in one of several genes (Table 14.3). Familial benign hematuria, also known as thin basement membrane nephropathy (TBMN), is the most common cause of persistent microscopic hematuria in children occurring in at least 1 % of children worldwide [18]. It is inherited in an autosomal dominant fashion, and is frequently associated with heterozygous mutations of the *COL4A3* or *COL4A4* genes. Absence of a family history does not exclude the diagnosis of TBMN due to these mutations because there may be a de

novo mutation, the penetrance may not be complete, or family members may not be aware that they have microscopic hematuria [35]. The red blood cells in the urine are mainly dysmorphic and there may be red blood cell casts. Hearing deficits or eye abnormalities almost never occur in patients with TBMN or their family members. Universal thinning of glomerular basement membrane is seen on electron microscopy. A renal biopsy is usually not indicated if TBMN is suspected unless there are atypical features to suggest IgA nephropathy or Alport syndrome. The prognosis of TBMN is traditionally regarded as benign. However, it is now recognized that TBMN can be associated with an increased risk of renal failure in adulthood, with up to 50 % of patients developing various degrees of chronic kidney disease after the age of 50 years [36]. Hence, lifelong follow-up is recommended for children with persistent isolated microscopic hematuria due to suspected TBMN.

Glomerulopathy with fibronectin deposition (GFND) is another rare glomerulopathy inherited in an autosomal dominant manner and associated with massive deposition of fibronectin in the mesangium and subendothelial space. It is characterized by microscopic hematuria with proteinuria, hypertension and progression to end-stage kidney disease between the second and sixth decade of life [37, 38].

Clinical Approach

In approaching a child with hematuria, we should ensure that serious conditions are not missed, avoid unnecessary and expensive laboratory tests, reassure the family and provide guidelines for further studies if there is a change in the child's course. Obtaining a careful history and physical examination is the crucial first step in the evaluation.

History

It is helpful to find out both the timing of the urinary changes in terms of days or hours and the associated symptoms. Patients should be asked regarding history of recent trauma, exercise,

Table 14.3 Familial hematuric disorders

Etiology	Gene	Protein	Risk of end-stage disease
Autosomal dominant thin basement membrane nephropathy (TBMN)	COL4A3/A4 heterozygous	α3(IV) α4(IV)	14 % at median age of 60 years
X-linked Alport syndrome (males)	COL4A5 hemizygous	α5(IV)	>90 % at median age of 25 years
X-linked Alport syndrome (females)	COL4A5 heterozygous	α5(IV)	15 % at median age of 49 years
Autosomal recessive Alport syndrome	COL4A3/A4 heterozygous	α3(IV) α4(IV)	>90 % at median age of 15 years
Autosomal dominant HANAC syndrome	COL4A1 heterozygous	α1(IV)	Unknown
Autosomal dominant macrothrombocytopathies	MYH9 heterozygous	Nonmuscle myosin heavy chain IIA	30 % at a median age of 15 years
CFHR5 nephropathy (males)	CFHR5 heterozygous	Complement factor H-related protein 5	80 % at a median age of 49 years
CFHR5 nephropathy (female)	CFHR5 heterozygous	Complement factor H-related protein 5	20 % at a median age of 56 years
Glomerulopathy associated with fibronectin deposition	FN1	Fibronectin 1	Progression between second to sixth decade

passage of urinary stones, recent respiratory or skin infections and intake of medications (including over-the-counter medications, calcium or vitamin D supplementation) or herbal compounds. Associated symptoms may include fever, dysuria, urinary frequency and urgency, back pain, skin rashes, joint symptoms and face and leg swelling. Predisposing illnesses such as sickle cell disease or trait should be noted. The family history should search for documented hematuria, hypertension, intracerebral bleed, renal stones, renal failure, deafness, coagulopathy and polycystic disease. In girls during the peri-pubertal period, a history of menarche is useful. In a sexually active teenager, the social history should take into account any recent sexual activity and any known exposure to sexually transmitted diseases since cystitis and urethritis can present with hematuria.

Physical Examination

The presence or absence of hypertension and edema suggestive of acute nephritic syndrome, determines how urgent and extensive the diagnostic evaluation should be. Associated rashes or arthritis may indicate hematuria due to systemic lupus erythematosus or Henoch Schönlein

nephritis. The presence of fever or loin pain may point to pyelonephritis. A palpable and ballotable renal mass will require radiological investigations to exclude hydronephrosis, polycystic kidney or renal tumor. Screening for eye abnormalities may be useful if there is a suggestive family history of familial hematuric syndromes associated with progression to end-stage kidney disease.

Investigations

Investigations to look for the cause of hematuria can be extensive. Tailoring the evaluation according to the type of clinical presentation reduce unnecessary laboratory and radiological investigations (Fig. 14.1). The first step is to confirm hematuria with urine microscopic examination. If the child has associated fever or irritative urinary symptoms, urine culture should be sent to rule out urinary tract infection. For children with an incidental finding of microscopic hematuria during illness or after exertion, further evaluation is required only if there is persistent microscopic hematuria on at least two of three consecutive samples.

The next step in the evaluation is to determine the site of bleeding. Two investigations that

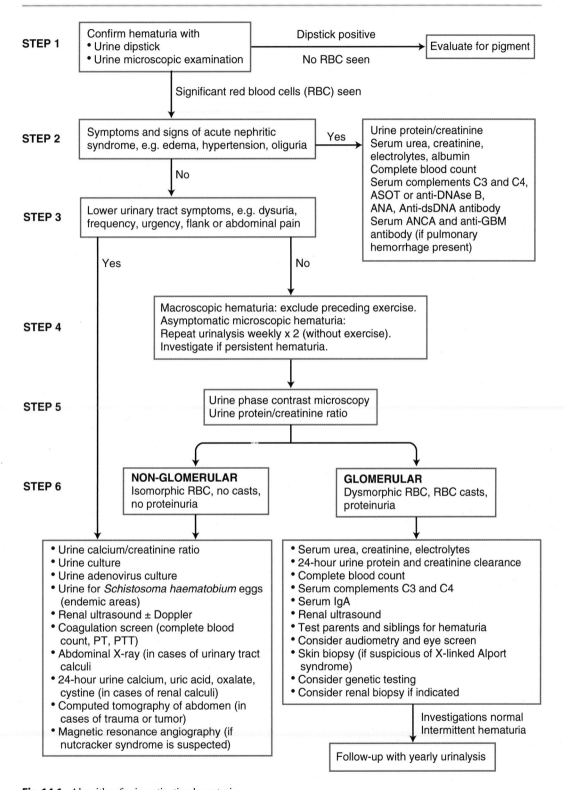

Fig. 14.1 Algorithm for investigating hematuria

should be done once hematuria is confirmed are urine tests for protein and urine phase contrast microscopic examination to look at the red blood cell morphology. Hematuria (gross or microscopic) associated with significant dysmorphic red blood cells, in particular acanthocytes (ring forms with vesicle-shaped protrusions) [39], and proteinuria indicate glomerular bleeding. It is important to remember that some proteinuria may also be present in non-glomerular causes of macroscopic hematuria. However, the proteinuria usually does not exceed 2+ (1 g/L) on dipstick examination if the only source of protein is from extra- glomerular bleed. Therefore, a child with proteinuria 2+ or more should be investigated for glomerulonephritis. Similarly, red blood cell casts, if present, are highly specific for glomerulonephritis.

Renal function needs to be determined in children with glomerular pathology. If there is significant proteinuria, the serum albumin should be measured. In addition, laboratory investigations to look for the cause should be done. These include serum complements C3 and C4, anti-streptolysin O titers (ASOT) or anti-DNAse B, anti-nuclear antibodies (ANA), anti-double-stranded DNA (dsDNA) antibody, anti-neutrophil cytoplasmic antibodies (ANCA), IgA levels, hepatitis B surface antigen and viral titers if appropriate. Serum IgA levels are increased in 30–50 % of adult patients, but in only 8–16 % of children with IgA nephropathy [40]. In countries where IgA nephropathy is an important cause of glomerulo-nephritis, 10–35 % of children undergoing renal biopsy for isolated hematuria were found to have IgA nephropathy [40, 41].

The clinical presentation is important in deciding the type of investigations required. For example, a preceding sore throat, pyoderma or impetigo and the presence of edema, hypertension and proteinuria are suggestive of post- streptococcal glomerulonephritis. Serum ASOT and complement C3 levels would suffice in this case. If these tests are not informative, then further investigations are warranted to rule out other causes of glomerulonephritis. If a familial hematuria syndrome is suspected, an audiological examination may be useful to detect high frequency sensorineural hearing deficit in Alport syndrome. If suspicion of X-linked Alport syndrome is high, skin biopsy with immuno-staining for the α5(IV) chain can be useful. The presence of macrothrombocytopenia with or without basophilic cytoplasmic leukocyte inclusion bodies (Döhle-like bodies) suggests *MYH9* syndromes [20]. The yield of renal ultrasonography for evaluation of the asymptomatic child with microscopic hematuria of glomerular origin remains unproven [42]. However, it may be useful to determine the size of the kidneys as a guide to chronicity in patients with evidence of progressive renal disease, and also to diagnose polycystic kidneys in the presence of a suggestive family history.

Hematuria associated with mainly isomorphic red blood cells, together with absence of red blood cell casts and proteinuria indicate a non-glomerular cause. Urine calcium over creatinine ratio is done to rule out hypercalciuria. In endemic areas, urine should be examined after sedimentation for *Schistosoma haematobium* eggs, especially during the day when excretion is highest. Ultrasound of the kidneys and bladder is indicated to exclude hydronephrosis, renal calculi, malignancy or cystic renal disease. A plain abdominal X-ray may be necessary to exclude ureteric stones. If a urinary tract calculus is identified, a complete assessment of the urinary constituents associated with stone risk is needed (see Chap. 44 on "Renal Calculi"). If the investigations reveal the presence of tumor, structural urogenital abnormality or urinary calculus, a urological referral is required. A coagulation screen may be necessary when there is a family history of bleeding diathesis. Computed tomography scan of the abdomen and pelvis may be required if there is a history of abdominal trauma followed by gross hematuria. If the nutcracker syndrome is suspected in a child with recurrent gross hematuria, Doppler sonography is a useful diagnostic tool, followed by magnetic resonance angiography for confirmation.

Cystoscopy may also be required in cases of children with recurrent nonglomerular macroscopic hematuria of unknown cause. Cystoscopy in children seldom reveals the cause of hematuria, but should be done when preliminary investigations have failed to find a cause, and bladder or urethral pathology is a consideration because of accompanying voiding symptoms. Initial hematuria suggests a urethral origin for the hematuria, whereas terminal hematuria is indicative of a bladder cause. Vascular malformations in the bladder have been detected via cystoscopy. In the rare instance when a bladder mass is noted on ultrasound, cystoscopy is also indicated. Cystoscopy to lateralize the source of bleeding is performed best during active bleeding.

An asymptomatic child with an incidental finding of persistent microscopic hematuria often poses the greatest dilemma regarding the extent of investigations and subsequent follow-up. The most common diagnoses in children with persistent microscopic hematuria without proteinuria and hypertension are TBMN, idiopathic hypercalciuria, IgA nephropathy and Alport syndrome. It is therefore worthwhile to screen family members for microscopic hematuria. If the parents are found to have incidental asymptomatic microscopic hematuria without proteinuria and renal failure, TBMN is the most likely cause. More extensive evaluation is then not necessary. However, it is important that these patients are followed up yearly to detect proteinuria which is an indication of a familial hematuria syndrome associated with progressive renal disease. In communities where post-infectious GN is common, subclinical disease is also a common cause of persistent microscopic hematuria.

Indications for Renal Biopsy

Renal biopsy is usually not indicated in isolated glomerular hematuria. Renal biopsy should be considered in the following cases of hematuria associated with:

- Significant proteinuria, except in poststreptococcal glomerulonephritis
- Persistent low serum complement C3
- Unexplained azotemia
- Systemic diseases such as systemic lupus erythematosus or ANCA-positive vasculitis
- Family history of significant renal disease suggestive of progressive forms of familial hematuria syndromes including Alport syndrome
- Recurrent gross hematuria of unknown etiology where investigations are suggestive of a glomerular pathology
- Persistent glomerular hematuria where the parents are anxious about the diagnosis and prognosis.

With recent improvements in understanding the molecular genetics of the hereditary nephritis syndromes, genetic testing, if available and affordable, can sometimes contribute useful diagnostic and prognostic information and may even obviate the need for an invasive kidney biopsy [43].

Proteinuria

It is well-established that proteinuria is a mediator of progressive renal insufficiency in both adults and children [44–46] as well as a risk factor for cardiovascular disease [47–49]. On the other hand, proteinuria can also be a transient finding in children, occurring during times of stress including exercise, fever and dehydration, and does not denote renal disease.

Renal Handling of Proteins

Plasma proteins can cross the normal glomerular barrier. The ability of these proteins to cross the glomerular barrier is related primarily to the molecular size and charge. The larger plasma proteins, such as globulins, are virtually excluded from the normal glomerular filtrate. Smaller proteins like albumin are filtered in low concentrations. Molecular charge plays an important role in determining glomerular permeability to macromolecules. This is due to the presence of negatively charged sialoproteins that line the surfaces of both the glomerular endothelial and epithelial cells, and glycosaminoglycans present in the glomerular basement membrane. Hence, negatively charged molecules are less able to cross the glomerulus than neutral molecules of identical size. On the other hand, positively charged molecules have enhanced clearances.

After crossing the glomerular barrier, 71 % of the filtered proteins are reabsorbed by the proximal tubule, 23 % by the loop of Henle and 3 % by the collecting duct. Under normal conditions, approximately 60 % of protein in normal urine is derived from plasma protein. Albumin predominates and constitutes about 40 % of the filtered urinary protein. The rest of the urinary proteins are globulins, peptides, enzymes, hormones and partially degraded plasma proteins. The proteins are degraded in the tubular cells by lysosomal enzymes to low molecular weight fragments and amino acids. Excretion of these low molecular weight proteins result from a balance between the amount of these proteins filtered and the amount reabsorbed.

Forty percent of normal urinary protein is of tissue rather than plasma origin. This consists of a heterogeneous group of numerous proteins, many of which are glycoproteins. Some of these are derived from cells lining the urinary tract and have the potential of being important diagnostic indicators. The major protein in this group is Tamm-Horsfall protein or uromodulin, which is a major constituent of urinary casts [50]. It is excreted in amounts of 30–60 mg/day in the adult. It is secreted into the urine mainly at the thick ascending limb of the loop of Henle.

Excess urinary protein losses can be due to either increased permeability of the glomeruli to the passage of serum proteins (glomerular proteinuria), decreased reabsorption of proteins by the renal tubules (tubular proteinuria), or increased secretion of tissue protein into the urine (secretory proteinuria). Additionally, increased excretion of low molecular weight proteins, such as beta-2 microglobulin and amino acids, may be due to marked overproduction of the protein resulting in the filtered load exceeding the normal proximal reabsorptive capacity (overflow proteinuria).

Albuminuria

Albuminuria refers to abnormal loss of albumin in the urine. Albumin is found in the urine in normal subjects and in larger quantities in patients with kidney disease. Recent recommendations for measurement of urine protein emphasize quantification of albuminuria rather than urinary total protein, as epidemiologic data worldwide have demonstrated a strong graded relationship between the quantity of urine albumin with both kidney and cardiovascular disease risk in adults. KDIGO (Kidney Disease Improving Global Outcomes) 2012 Clinical Practice Guideline for the Evaluation and Management of Chronic Kidney Disease has incorporated albuminuria in the criteria and classification of chronic kidney disease in the adults [51]. A urinary albumin excretion rate of 30 mg/24 h or more sustained for longer than 3 months is used to indicate chronic kidney disease in adults. This value is considered to be approximately equivalent to an albumin-to-creatinine ratio in a random untimed urine sample of 30 mg/g or 3 mg/mmol. On the other hand, urinary albumin excretion rates in children and adolescents vary with age. Urinary albumin excretion is estimated to be lowest in children age less than 6 years, followed by an increase through the adolescent years with a peak at age 15–16 years [52].

Microalbuminuria is a relative misnomer. It implies "small size" but actually refers to the presence of a relatively small quantity of protein in the urine, which is below the detection threshold of a standard urine dipstick test. Albuminuria in children and adolescents has been defined as urinary albumin excretion rate of 30–300 mg/24 h urine collection, 20–200 µg/min in a night time collection and 3–30 mg/mmol creatinine (30–300 mg/g creatinine) in a first morning spot urine sample [53]. This range of urinary albumin excretion, although used in the pediatric population, is derived from population studies in adults.

The prevalence of albuminuria in children and adolescents is estimated to be about 5.7–7.3 % in boys and 12.7–15.1 % in girls from the National Health and Nutrition Examination Survey III (NHANES III) in the United States [53]. The higher prevalence of albuminuria in girls than boys could be due to the bigger muscle mass and urinary creatinine excretion of the boys resulting in their smaller albumin:creatinine ratio values. There is a positive association between albumin:creatinine ratios and pubertal development stage [54]. Girls appear to have a peak albumin:creatinine ratio at Tanner stage 4 (14 years old), whereas in boys, there is no increase in albumin:creatinine ratio till they reach full maturity at Tanner 5 (18 years old) [54]. Estimation of the prevalence of actual albuminuria in children and adolescents can be difficult because a great percentage of children (30–50 %) may have transient non-repetitive albuminuria because of strenuous exercise [55] or during febrile illnesses.

The significance of albuminuria in diabetic children and adolescents is well established and urinary albumin excretion rate has been used as a screening test for the presence of diabetic nephropathy [56]. The significance of using albuminuria for other conditions in the pediatric population is less well defined. A cross-sectional study analyzing the NHANES data for 12–19-year old adolescents [57] showed that despite the presence of cardiovascular risk factors, overweight teenagers had a lower prevalence rate of albuminuria compared to healthy controls. The reason for this lower prevalence of albuminuria in obese teenagers is uncertain but one explanation is that lower exercise levels in obese teenagers leads to less confounding influence by orthostatic proteinuria. On the other hand, another study has shown that obese children (body mass index 30.4 kg/m^2) compared to normal weight children (body mass index 18.2 kg/m^2) were found to have a significantly higher albumin:creatinine ratio determined in a random spot urine sample [58], indicating early renal dysfunction as a consequence of obesity. The albumin:creatinine ratio in these obese children was also associated with impaired glucose tolerance and hypercholesterolemia, two of the most important features of the metabolic syndrome [58]. The relationship between albuminuria and cardiovascular disease in the pediatric population is not as well studied as in adults [52]. Further longitudinal research is required to evaluate the significance of increased urinary albumin excretion rate in obese children with regards to the future development of cardiovascular morbidity in adulthood.

Definition of Abnormal Urinary Protein Excretion in Children

Normal urinary protein excretion varies across age, sex, puberty and/or body size. Neonates and young infants are expected and allowed to have higher urinary losses of both glomerular and tubular proteinuria due to lack of maturation in the proximal tubular reabsorption of proteins. In infants less than 6 months of age, at least one study has suggested that as much as 6–8 mg/m^2/h or up to 300 mg/1.73 m^2/day of proteinuria is acceptable [59]. The normal rate of protein excretion in the urine for children 6–24 months of age is less than 4 mg/m^2/h or 150 mg/1.73 m^2/day [60]. The first morning spot urine protein-to-creatinine ratio is defined as normal when it is less than 50 mg/mmol (or 500 mg/g).

Children older than 24 months of age are expected to achieve normal adult urinary protein values with the caveat of an exaggerated postural loss of glomerular protein (albumin) which can be seen in 2–5 % of the adolescent population (i.e., orthostatic proteinuria) [55]. Hence, in children older than 24 months, the normal rate of protein excretion in the urine is still less than 4 mg/m^2/h or less than 150 mg/1.73 m^2/day. However, the first morning spot urine protein-to-creatinine ratio is defined as normal at less than 20 mg/mmol (or 200 mg/g) and spot urine albumin-to-creatinine ratio normal at less than 3 mg/mmol (or 30 mg/g) [60].

At all ages, urinary protein excretion of greater than 40 mg/m^2/h or 3 g/1.73 m^2/day is defined as nephrotic range proteinuria (Table 14.4) [60]. If albumin excretion is measured, nephrotic range proteinuria is defined as urine albumin greater than 2,200 mg/1.73 m^2/day or albumin-to-creatinine ratio greater than 220 mg/mmol or 2,200 mg/g [51].

With regards to using urinary albumin or protein excretion in the classification of children with chronic kidney disease, variations in the definition of abnormal urinary albumin or protein excretion based on age must be taken into account. Abnormal urinary protein excretion in children should also take into account the possibility of tubular versus glomerular proteinuria

Table 14.4 Quantification of urinary protein excretion in children

Method	Abnormal proteinuria	Precautions
Urine dipstick	≥1+ in an urine specimen of specific gravity ≥1.002	False-positive if urine pH >8.0 or specific gravity >1.025 or tested within 24 h of radiocontrast study
Sulfosalicylic acid test	≥1+	False-positive with iodinated radiocontrast agents
Urine protein:creatinine ratio (PCR) in spot urine	>20 mg/mmol (>0.020 g/mmol) or >200 mg/g *in children >2 years old* [46]	Protein excretion varies with child's age
	>50 mg/mmol (>0.05 g/mmol) or >500 mg/g *in children 6 months to 2 years old*	
	Nephrotic range: >220 mg/mmol (>0.22 g/mmol) or >2,200 mg/g [51]	
Timed urine protein excretion rate (PER)	>4 mg/m^2/h or >150 mg/1.73 m^2/24 h *in children >6 months old*	In an accurately collected 24-h urine specimen, the urine creatinine should be in the range of 0.13–0.20 mmol/kg or 16–24 mg/kg ideal body weight for females, and 0.18–0.23 mmol/kg or 21–27 mg/kg ideal body weight for males
	>8 mg/m^2/h or >300 mg/1.73 m^2/24 h *in children <6 months old*	
	Nephrotic range: >40 mg/m^2/h or >3 g/1.73 m^2/24 h [55]	
Urine albumin:creatinine ratio (ACR) in spot urine	>3 mg/mmol (>0.003 g/mmol) or	
	>30 mg/g in children >2 years	
Timed urine albumin excretion rate (AER)	>30 mg/1.73 m^2/24 h	

dominance depending on the underlying disease. Urinary albumin excretion rate may be normal in tubular proteinuria. Hence, in children, the quantification of total protein, as compared to the albumin only fraction, may be the preferred method of assigning risk in relation to the presence of urinary protein.

The KDIGO 2012 guidelines recommended a urinary total protein or albumin excretion rate above the normal value for age to be used for children and adolescents from birth to 18 years [51]. Table 14.5 shows the categories of persistent albuminuria with corresponding measurement of proteinuria to be used in the classification of chronic kidney disease. Albuminuria is classified into normal to mildly elevated, moderately increased and severely increased. However, in children, urine protein to creatinine ratio is still the preferred test, followed by albuminuria, and lastly by automated reagent strips for detection of proteinuria. This is because the vast majority of children have underlying congenital anomalies of

the kidney and urinary tract, unlike in adults where the etiology of chronic kidney disease is attributed to an underlying glomerular disease, diabetic nephropathy or hypertensive damage. The use of albumin excretion may therefore be less sensitive for diagnostic purposes in children as those with underlying tubular conditions will tend to excrete more Tamm-Horsfall protein and other low molecular-weight proteins.

Urine Dipstick

The urine dipstick is an excellent screening test for the presence of proteinuria [60]. The dipstick is impregnated with the dye tetrabromophenol blue buffered to pH 3.5. At a constant pH, the binding of protein to this dye results in the development of a blue colour in proportion to the amount of protein present. If urine is protein-free, the dipstick is yellow. The color of the dipstick changes through yellow-green, to green, to a green-blue with increasing concentrations of protein. The dipstick can be read as negative,

Table 14.5 Categories of albuminuria in chronic kidney disease

Measure	Categories		
	Normal to mildly increased (A1)	Moderately increased (A2)	Severely increased (A3)
Albumin excretion rate (mg/1.73 m^2/24 h)	<30	30–300	>300
Protein excretion rate (mg/1.73 m^2/24 h)	<150	150–500	>500
Albumin:creatinine ratio (ACR)			
(g/mmol)	<0.003	0.003–0.030	>0.030
(mg/mmol)	<3	3–30	>30
(mg/g)	<30	30–300	>300
Protein:creatinine ratio (PCR)			
(g/mmol)	<0.015	0.015–0.050	>0.050
(mg/mmol)	<15	15–50	>50
(mg/g)	<150	150–500	>500
Protein reagent strip	Negative to trace	Trace to +	+ or greater

For an exact conversion from mg/g of creatinine to mg/mmol of creatinine, multiply by 0.113. The relationships between albumin excretion rate and albumin:creatinine ratio and between protein excretion rate and protein:creatinine ratio are based on the assumption that average creatinine excretion rate is approximately 1 g/day or 10 mmol/day

Used with permission of the Nature Publishing Group from Kidney Disease: Improving Global Outcomes (KDIGO) CKD Work Group [51]

trace, 1+, 2+, 3+ and 4+ which corresponds to insignificant, less than 0.2 g/L, 0.3 g/L, 1 g/L, 3 g/L and greater than 20 g/L concentrations respectively.

The dipstick test has a few limitations. Observer error can occur during interpretation of the color of the dipstick. False positive and false negative tests for protein can occur. If the dipstick is kept in the urine too long, the buffer may leach out and a false positive test may result. False positive tests for protein can also occur in the presence of gross hematuria, pyuria and bacteriuria or if the urine is contaminated with antiseptics such as chlorhexidine or benzalkonium which are often used for skin cleansing prior to clean catch of the urine. False positive results may result with urine specimens after the administration of radiographic contrast such as after an intravenous urogram, penicillin or cephalosporin therapy, tolbutamide or sulfonamides.

The result of the dipstick test can be affected by the concentration and the pH of the urine. If the urine is very dilute, the urinary protein concentration may be reduced to a level below the sensitivity of the dipstick (0.1–0.15 g/L) even in patients excreting up to 1 g of protein per day. Hence, we should interpret with caution any negative dipstick result for protein in urine with a specific gravity of less than 1.002. On the other hand, if the urine is highly concentrated with urine specific gravity greater than 1.025, a healthy child can register trace of protein on the dipstick, resulting in a false positive result. The dipstick test for protein can be affected by pH of urine. Very alkaline urine (pH greater than 8.0) can cause a false positive result while very acid urine (pH less than 4.5) can cause a false negative result.

False negative results occur in non-albumin proteinuria. Albumin binds better to the dye than other proteins. Hence, the urine dipstick primarily detects albumin, leaving low molecular weight proteins undetected. The dipstick results correlate better with the level of albuminuria than with total proteinuria. Hence the dipstick is highly specific for albuminuria, but relatively insensitive, and is unable to detect microalbuminuria associated with early glomerular injury seen in diabetic nephropathy or cardiovascular disease. A negative dipstick test for protein does not exclude the presence in the urine of low concentrations of globulins, mucoproteins or Bence-Jones protein.

Sulfosalicylic Acid Test

An alternative method to measure urine protein in patients with questionable proteinuria by dipstick in the office is the sulfosalicylic precipitation of protein in urine. This technique provides a more quantitative estimate of all the proteins present in the urine, including both albumin and the low molecular weight proteins. This test is performed by mixing one part urine supernatant with three parts 3 % sulfosalicylic acid, and the resultant turbidity is then graded as shown in Table 14.6 [61]. As with the urine dipstick, iodinated radiocontrast agents can cause a false positive result, hence the urine should not be tested for at least 24 h after a contrast study.

Quantification of Proteinuria: 24-Hour Urine Specimen Versus Spot Urine Specimen

The results obtained with urine dipstick and with quantitative 24-h protein excretion methods correlate fairly well in most situations. As mentioned earlier, the dipstick is sensitive to albumin, whereas quantitative methods detect all kinds of proteins including globulin and low molecular weight protein. For example, in multiple myeloma, large amounts of protein are excreted and yet the urine dipstick for protein is negative. Hence quantitative urinary protein measurement is necessary in this case. A more important rea-

son why quantitative measurement of protein loss in the urine should be done is to determine whether the patient requires a more extensive evaluation. Very often, urine with a dipstick reading of protein 1+, when sent for quantitative measurement, was found to contain protein within the normal acceptable range.

Quantification of proteinuria has traditionally demanded timed urine collection. Urinary protein excretion in adults is usually measured in a 24-h urine collection. This is more accurate than spot urine protein analysis. However, 24-h urine collection poses logistical problems with timing and volume measurements, especially in young children who have yet to achieve continence at night. In this case, a 12-h urine collection can be done, and the protein excretion rate is then extrapolated to a 24-h value by using the appropriate correction factor.

The other method is to obtain a single voided urine sample. The concentrations of both protein and creatinine are measured in the urine sample and protein levels are expressed per unit of creatinine. The advantages of this method include not requiring timed urine samples and not having to correct for body size. The assumption is creatinine excretion is directly related to body mass and is relatively constant throughout the day.

Many studies have found that the amount of protein excreted in a 24-h urine correlates extremely well with the protein to creatinine ratio measured in random urine samples [62, 63].

What remains debatable is whether early morning urine samples or random urine samples obtained during normal activities in the day are better in reflecting renal disease. The urine protein to creatinine ratio is higher in urine samples obtained in a person in an upright position than in a recumbent position, a phenomenon known as orthostatic proteinuria [55]. Studies that included subjects with normal renal function as well as those with renal failure have shown that urine protein to creatinine ratios from daytime samples correlated better with 24-h urine protein excretion values than did values from early morning samples [55]. On the other hand, early morning samples had the better correlation when data were evaluated from normal subjects and from

Table 14.6 Sulfosalicylic acid test

Grade	Appearance	Protein concentration (g/L)
0	No turbidity	0
Trace	Slight turbidity	0.01–0.1
1+	Turbidity through which print can be read	0.15–0.3
2+	White cloud without precipitate through which heavy black lines on a white background can be seen	0.4–1
3+	White cloud with precipitate through which heavy black lines cannot be seen	1.5–3.5
4+	Flocculent precipitate	>5

those with renal disease that were associated with normal glomerular filtration rates [64]. In subjects with renal disease and orthostatic proteinuria, daytime urine protein to creatinine ratios can be misleading. Hence in the evaluation of children with possible renal disease, the first morning urine specimen is recommended for urine protein to creatinine ratio quantification, so as to eliminate the effect of posture. In general, the 24-h urine collection for protein excretion is ideal as the initial diagnostic investigation, with the exception of children who have yet to achieve continence, whereas the first morning spot urine protein to creatinine ratio is useful to monitor progress of proteinuria.

The dipstick, Multistix® PRO (Bayer, Elkhart, Ind., USA), is able to analyze concentrations of both urinary protein and creatinine semi-quantitatively in only 60 s and has become commercially available. The semi-quantitative urine protein to creatinine ratio by Multistix® PRO correlated well with both quantitative urine protein to creatinine ratio and daily urinary protein excretion [65, 66], and use of the Multistix® PRO would avoid errors and difficulties associated with timed urine collection. It may become a useful tool to monitor the urinary protein excretion in children with renal diseases at the outpatient setting.

Clinical Scenarios

Child with Intermittent Proteinuria

In intermittent proteinuria, protein is detectable in only some of the urine samples collected. This may be related to posture or occur at random. Orthostatic (postural) proteinuria is defined as elevated protein excretion when the subject is upright but normal protein excretion during recumbency. This occurs commonly in adolescents with a prevalence of 2–5 % [67]. Total urine protein excretion rarely exceeds $1 \text{ g}/1.73 \text{ m}^2/\text{day}$ in orthostatic proteinuria. The first step in patients who present with persistent proteinuria is to do a spot urine protein to creatinine ratio on a first morning urine specimen after overnight recumbency. Orthostatic proteinuria is suggested by a normal first morning urine protein to creatinine ratio.

The postulated causes of orthostatic proteinuria are alterations in renal or glomerular hemodynamics, circulating immune complexes and partial renal vein entrapment [68]. Long- term studies where patients have been followed-up for up to 50 years have documented the benign nature of orthostatic proteinuria, although rare cases of glomerulosclerosis have been identified later in life in patients who were initially diagnosed to have orthostatic proteinuria [69, 70].

No treatment is required for children with orthostatic proteinuria. It is important to remember that patients with glomerular disease may have an orthostatic component to their proteinuria. Protein excretion in these patients is greater when they are active or upright than when they are resting. Hence, orthostatic proteinuria should not be diagnosed unless the urine collected when the subject at rest has no detectable protein.

Frequently, intermittent proteinuria is not related to posture. It may be found after exercise or in association with stress, dehydration or fever. It may occur on a random basis for which there is no obvious cause. A large proportion of healthy children may have an occasional urine sample, which contains protein in detectable concentrations. Although such proteinuria can be indicative of serious disease of the urinary tract, this is the exception rather than the rule. The vast majority of observations have indicated that the intermittent occurrence of protein in the urine, as an isolated finding, does not indicate the presence of such disease.

Child with Persistent Proteinuria

Persistent proteinuria is defined as proteinuria of 1+ or more by dipstick on multiple occasions. This is abnormal and should be further investigated. Subjects who have persistent proteinuria, especially if this is associated with additional evidence of renal disease such as microscopic hematuria, are the ones most likely to have significant pathology in the urinary tract. In the Japanese school screening study, which looked at almost five million children, the prevalence of persistent isolated proteinuria was 0.07 % in the 6–11-year age group, and this rose to 0.37 % in the 12–14-year olds [28].

Table 14.7 Causes of proteinuria in children

Intermittent proteinuria	Persistent proteinuria	
	Glomerular	Tubular
Non-postural	Primary glomerulopathies	Hereditary
Fever	Minimal change disease	Proximal renal tubular acidosis
Exercise	Focal segmental glomerulosclerosis	Cystinosis
Emotional stress	Mesangiocapillary glomerulonephritis	Galactosemia
No known cause	Membranous nephropathy	Tyrosinemia type
Postural (Orthostatic)	Rapidly progressive glomerulonephritis	Hereditary fructose intolerance
	Congenital nephrotic syndrome	Wilson disease
	Secondary glomerulonephritis	Lowe syndrome
	Post-infectious glomerulonephritis	Dent's disease
	Lupus nephritis	Acquired
	IgA nephropathy	Pyelonephritis
	Henoch-Schönlein nephritis	Interstitial nephritis
	Alport syndrome	Acute tubular necrosis
	Hepatitis B nephropathy	Analgesic abuse
	Hepatitis C nephropathy	Drugs such as penicillamine
	Human immunodeficiency virus (HIV) nephropathy	Heavy metal poisoning (e.g., lead, cadmium, gold, mercury)
	Amyloidosis	Vitamin D intoxication
	Hemolytic uremic syndrome	
	Diabetes mellitus	
	Hypertension	
	Hyperfiltration following nephron loss	
	Reflux nephropathy	

The majority of cases of persistent proteinuria are of glomerular origin though non-glomerular mechanisms can also cause marked proteinuria (Table 14.7). Glomerular proteinuria may be due to the following factors:

- Increase in glomerular permeability to plasma proteins in residual nephrons in cases where there is reduction in nephron mass. This mechanism probably explains the increased proteinuria seen in patients with progressive renal disease reaching end- stage and the increased proteinuria observed in renal transplant donors [71].
- Loss of negative charge in the glomerular filtration barrier [72, 73]. This results in albuminuria mainly. There is little increase in glomerular permeability to globulins; hence, the proteinuria is highly selective. A typical example is minimal change disease.
- Direct injury to the glomerular filtration barrier. The glomerular capillary wall consists of three structural components that form the permselectivity barrier, the endothelial cells, glomerular basement membrane and podo-

cytes. It is now realized that the podocyte is crucial for maintenance of the glomerular filter, and disruption of the epithelial slit diaphragm finally leads to proteinuria [74]. These changes have been demonstrated in patients with nephrotic syndrome irrespective of the primary disease. Such injury increases the "effective pore size" in the glomeruli, resulting in increase in the permeability of the mechanical barriers to the filtration of proteins. Hence, there is increase in filtration of albumin and also the larger proteins such as globulins. The clearance of globulins is relatively high and the proteinuria is described as non-selective.

- Mutations of key podocyte genes. Recent advances have revealed that mutations of genes involved in regulation of the slit diaphragm proteins and their interaction with the actin cytoskeleton, also result in proteinuria.
- Changes in glomerular capillary pressure due to disease and resulting in increased filtration fraction [44, 45, 75]. Examples are increased filtration fraction in hyper-reninemia and hyperfiltration of nephrons in the early stages of diabetic nephropathy.

The resulting increased filtered load of protein overwhelms the tubular reabsorptive mechanisms; hence, the excess protein appears in the urine. Glomerular proteinuria can be classified as selective or nonselective. In selective proteinuria, there is a predominance of low molecular weight proteins such as albumin or transferrin, as compared to higher molecular weight proteins characterized by IgG. The selectivity index is expressed as the clearance ratio of IgG over albumin or transferrin. An index less than 0.1 is indicative of highly selective proteinuria [76, 77], and this is seen in steroid-sensitive nephrotic syndrome and Finnish-type congenital nephrotic syndrome. More recent studies have shown that there is a significant relationship between selectivity of proteinuria and tubulointerstitial damage in renal disease [78]. When proteinuria is highly selective, tubulointerstitial damage is less frequently seen on histology.

Non-glomerular mechanisms include tubular proteinuria, overflow proteinuria and secretory proteinuria. Tubular proteinuria results when there is damage to the proximal convoluted tubule, which normally reabsorbs most of the filtered protein. The amount of protein in the urine due to tubular damage is usually not large and does not exceed more than 1 g/1.73 m^2/day. Glomerular and tubular proteinuria can be distinguished by protein electrophoresis of the urine. The primary protein in glomerular proteinuria is albumin, whereas in tubular proteinuria the low molecular weight proteins (LMWp) migrate primarily in the α and β regions. β_2-microglobulin (b2M), α_1-microglobulin (a1M) and retinol-binding protein (RBP) are the markers commonly used as the index for tubular proteinuria [79]. Children with proximal tubulopathies such as Lowe syndrome and Dent's disease present with tubular proteinuria. Albuminuria can be seen in the long-term course of many tubulopathies as a marker of late glomerular involvement.

Overflow proteinuria results when the concentration of filterable proteins in the glomerular filtrate exceeds the maximal tubular reabsorption capability for that protein. This can occur even with normal renal function. Examples include monoclonal gammopathy of undetermined sig-

nificance or multiple myeloma in adults (immunoglobulin light chains or Bence-Jones protein), hemoglobinuria, myoglobinuria, β_2- microglobulinemia, myelomonocytic leukemia and even following transfusions. After multiple transfusions of either albumin or whole blood, plasma albumin concentration may increase sufficiently to cause albuminuria.

In secretory proteinuria, the increased excretion of tissue proteins into the urine may result in proteinuria. The typical example is excretion of Tamm-Horsfall protein in the neonatal period accounting for the higher levels of protein excretion typically seen at this age. In urinary tract infections, mild proteinuria may be detected due to irritation of the urinary tract and increased secretion of tissue proteins into the urine. Secretory proteinuria also occurs in analgesic nephropathy and inflammation of the accessory sex glands.

Child with Nephrotic Syndrome

Nephrotic syndrome is defined as heavy proteinuria that is severe enough to cause hypoalbuminemia, edema and hypercholesterolemia. Nephrotic range proteinuria is defined as greater than 40 mg/m^2/h or greater than 3 g/1.73 m^2/day for timed urine collection, or random urine protein to creatinine ratio of greater than 0.2 g/mmol (200 mg/mmol) or 2,000 mg/g [60]. The evaluation and management of a child presenting with nephrotic syndrome is different from that of a child with proteinuria of non-nephrotic range. Nephrotic syndrome will be discussed elsewhere in the book.

Clinical Approach to Proteinuria

The finding of proteinuria in a single urine specimen in children and adolescents is relatively common. In large school screening programs, the prevalence of isolated proteinuria on a single urine screen ranged from 1.2 to 15 % of children [30, 80, 81]. The finding of persistent proteinuria on repeated urine testing is much less common. When proteinuria is detected, it is important to determine whether it is intermittent, especially orthostatic, or persistent in type. It is also important to exclude acute nephritic or nephrotic syndrome because these conditions demand urgent investigations and treatment.

History

Inquire about symptoms of renal failure or glomerulonephritis (edema, hematuria, polyuria, nocturia), and connective tissue disorders (including rashes and joint pain). A past history of recurrent urinary tract infections may suggest reflux nephropathy. Enquire about intake of drugs that may be associated with proteinuria such as nonsteroidal anti-inflammatory medications. A family history of polycystic kidney disease, hematuria/proteinuria, nephrotic syndrome, renal failure or deafness should be obtained.

Physical Examination

Examination may reveal evidence of renal failure such as growth failure, anemia and renal osteodystrophy. Blood pressure must be measured as hypertension is an important prognostic indicator in chronic kidney disease. Presence of raised jugular venous pressure, hepatomegaly and edema suggest that child may be fluid overloaded due to acute nephritic syndrome or renal impairment, requiring urgent diuresis. Look for signs of nephrotic syndrome such as generalized edema, ascites, pleural effusion and scrotal edema (in a male). Associated signs of systemic illnesses, such as palpable purpuric rash on the lower limbs suggesting Henoch Schönlein purpura and joint swelling suggesting connective tissue disorders, should be sought. Palpable flank masses may suggest hydronephrosis or polycystic kidney disease.

Investigations

Isolated proteinuria is benign in the vast majority of children and can be transient and postural; hence, it is inappropriate to extensively investigate all children found to have proteinuria. A step-by-step approach is recommended to evaluate isolated proteinuria in an asymptomatic child. However, if the child has signs and symptoms suggestive of renal disease, a detailed investigation should start early. Similarly, if the initial urine dipstick shows the presence of hematuria besides proteinuria, detailed evaluation for renal disease should be performed. Microscopic hematuria is the most common indicator of a glomerular lesion in a proteinuric patient. The existence of hematuria with proteinuria carries a more serious connotation than just proteinuria alone. Investigations including renal biopsy of school children with persistent hematuria and proteinuria have found that 25–60 % had evidence of a glomerulopathy [31, 82], especially in those with heavy proteinuria of greater than 1 g/L [31].

In an asymptomatic child, the first step is to determine whether the proteinuria is persistent (Fig. 14.2). Most children who are found to have proteinuria on screening urine dipstick do not have renal disease, and the proteinuria will resolve on repeat testing [28]. If proteinuria of 1+ or more persists on two subsequent dipstick tests at weekly intervals, further investigations are required. If proteinuria is absent on subsequent testing, the initial proteinuria may be transient and related to fever, severe exercise or emotional stress, and no further investigations are required. The parents and patient should be reassured and as a precaution, a urine dipstick test for protein can be repeated in 3–6 months. If proteinuria on dipstick recurs or is persistent, the next step is to quantify the amount of proteinuria.

There are two methods to quantify proteinuria, spot urine protein to creatinine ratio and 24-h urinary total protein collection. An early morning spot urine protein to creatinine ratio is recommended to exclude orthostatic proteinuria. In orthostatic proteinuria, the first morning urine sample is negative for protein and the later urine samples may contain varying concentrations of protein, whereas the 24-h urinary total protein is normal or mildly elevated. If orthostatic proteinuria is strongly suspected, one way to prove this is to provide the family with urine dipsticks and instruct them on their use. The child's urine is tested twice a day for 1 week. The two urine samples to be checked daily are the first urine sample voided in the morning as soon as the child wakes up and the last urine sample voided in the evening before the child sleeps. It is important that the child remains supine in bed throughout the

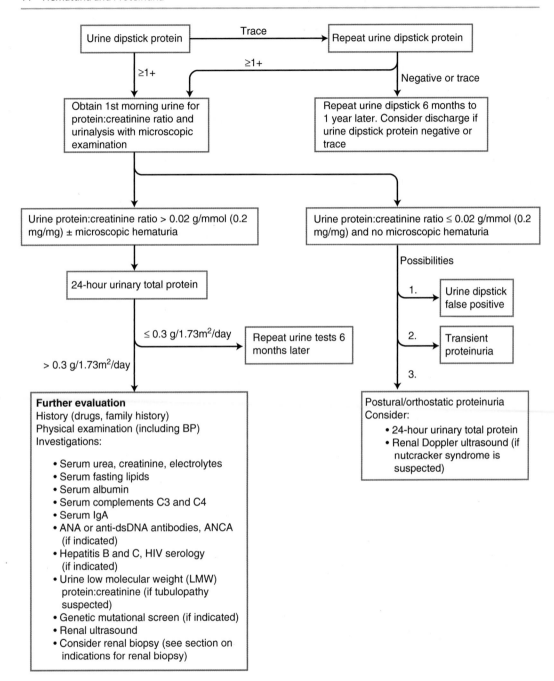

Fig. 14.2 Algorithm for investigating proteinuria

night so that the early morning urine sample consists of urine formed in the recumbent position. The evening urine sample consists of urine formed in the upright position. If the urine dipstick is persistently negative in the morning and positive in the evening, orthostatic proteinuria is

likely. No further investigations are required, and the urine should be rechecked for proteinuria in 1 year as a precaution.

If spot urine protein to creatinine ratio is more than 0.02 g/mmol (20 mg/mmol) or 0.2 mg/mg, it is advisable to confirm the presence of significant proteinuria with a 24-h urinary total protein collection. After excluding transient and orthostatic proteinuria, and if the 24-h urinary total protein is greater than 0.3 g/1.73 m^2/day, it is useful to evaluate for renal disease.

Urinary protein excretion less than 0.3 g/1.73 m^2/day is associated with regression of proteinuric chronic nephropathies [83], suggesting that investigations are only necessary above this level. The suggested work-up includes the following:

1. *Urine examination*: Microscopic examination of the fresh urine sample for blood, casts and crystals is required. A clean catch urine sample for culture may be necessary to rule out occult urinary tract infection, especially if there is a history of recurrent fevers in infancy. If a tubular disorder or interstitial nephritis is suggested from the history or urinary findings of eosinophils, measurement of the urinary excretion of β_2-microglobulin, α_1-microglobulin and retinol-binding protein, markers of tubular proteinuria, can be helpful. Tubular proteinuria is suspected if the urinary excretion of β_2-microglobulin, α_1-microglobulin and retinol-binding protein exceeds 0.04, 2.2 and 0.024 mg/mmol creatinine or 4×10^{-4}, 0.022 and 2.4×10^{-4} mg/mg creatinine respectively [79].

2. *Blood examination*. Assess the renal function with serum urea, creatinine and electrolytes. Creatinine clearance or application of an estimating formula such as the revised Schwartz formula [84] gives a more accurate picture of renal function than serum creatinine alone. A reduction in renal function is one of the most important indications for a renal biopsy. Serum total protein and albumin should be checked. Most proteinuric patients do not have decreased levels of proteins or albumin in their blood unless they have nephrotic syndrome or they have heavy proteinuria for a significant period of time. Hypoproteinemia may be an indication for renal biopsy. In addition, serum cholesterol is measured as an indicator of the presence or absence of hyperlipidemia and nephrotic syndrome.

Serum levels of the third and fourth components of the complement pathway (C3 and C4) should be checked routinely as this may provide evidence of glomerulonephritis. Decreased C3 and C4 levels are seen in systemic lupus erythematosus, while decreased C3 with normal C4 levels are seen in post-infectious glomerulonephritis or C3 glomerulopathies including mesangiocapillary (membranoproliferative) glomerulonephritis. Anti-nuclear antibodies, anti-dsDNA antibodies, IgA levels, anti-streptolysin O titers (ASOT) or anti-DNAse B titers, anti-neutrophil cytoplasmic antibodies (ANCA), hepatitis B, hepatitis C and human immunodeficiency virus (HIV) serology should be considered if the clinical setting and preliminary investigations are suggestive, as these may give a clue to the underlying etiology of the proteinuria. In addition, appropriate mutational screening should be considered if a hereditary disorder for the proteinuria or nephrotic syndrome is suspected.

3. *Renal imaging*. Renal ultrasonography is done routinely in the evaluation of isolated proteinuria to identify anatomical abnormalities of the kidneys or urinary tract as these can result in reduction of nephron mass. A significant difference in the sizes of the kidneys may suggest underlying reflux nephropathy or renal dysplasia. If reflux nephropathy is suspected, a DMSA scan is useful to demonstrate the existence of renal scars. Renal Doppler sonography is helpful if the patient has co-existing hypertension as proteinuria can occur in hypertensive nephropathy due to renal artery stenosis. In patients with orthostatic proteinuria, Doppler sonography of the left renal vein may be a useful screening tool to exclude the nutcracker syndrome [85].

4. *Audiometry*. Audiometry is indicated when there is a family history of nephritis, renal failure or deafness. Deafness may be detected during later childhood in Alport syndrome, and is generally associated with progressive renal disease.

If these urine and blood tests as well as the initial renal ultrasound are normal, and if the proteinuria is less than 1 g/1.73 m²/day, it is unlikely that the child has a serious renal disease. The family should therefore be reassured that the proteinuria may disappear or it may persist without any evidence of progressive renal failure developing. As the level of proteinuria is associated with outcome in chronic nephropathies [44, 83, 86], it is also important to emphasize to the family that follow-up urine tests are necessary. The child should be reviewed in 3–6 months. If the repeat test shows that the proteinuria is not marked (i.e., less than 1 g/1.73 m²/day), the child's urine is then monitored twice during the subsequent year and yearly thereafter. If there is persistent significant proteinuria on follow-up, a renal biopsy may be indicated.

Indications for Renal Biopsy

Renal biopsy is indicated in the following situations:

- Persistent significant proteinuria of more than 1 g/1.73 m²/day [87] or random urine protein to creatinine ratio of >0.05 g/mmol (>50 mg/mmol, >0.5 g/g) [88]. The heavier the proteinuria, the more likely a tissue diagnosis will be obtained from the renal biopsy. A study on renal biopsies in Japanese children with asymptomatic persistent isolated proteinuria showed that a considerably high ratio (41.4 %) of significant glomerular changes, such as focal segmental glomerulosclerosis, could be detected when using a urine protein to creatinine ratio >0.5 g/g as a biopsy criterion [88]. The exception here is the child who presents with typical steroid sensitive nephrotic syndrome suggestive of minimal change disease, where renal biopsy is not indicated at presentation.
- Proteinuria associated with urinary sediment abnormalities. Renal biopsy is more likely to be diagnostic when proteinuria is associated with urinary sediment abnormalities than when either proteinuria or hematuria is isolated abnormalities.
- Decreased glomerular filtration rate (GFR). A GFR of less than 60 ml/1.73 m²/min is an indication for renal biopsy. The exception is a child who is recovering from an acute glomerulonephritis, e.g., post-infectious glomerulonephritis. In this case, the GFR should be re-measured in a month's time, and if the GFR remains low, a renal biopsy is required.
- Persistent low C3 levels for more than 3 months. A low C3 level during the acute phase of post-infectious glomerulonephritis is not an indication for biopsy. If the C3 level remains low after 3 months, a renal biopsy is indicated.
- Evidence of a vasculitis (such as systemic lupus erythematosus, Henoch Schönlein purpura, ANCA-positive vasculitis) either clinically or serologically.

Treatment Options for Significant Proteinuria in the Non-nephrotic Range

It is well-recognized that glomerular proteinuria may play a role in the progression of kidney disease [89]. Proteinuria has also been identified as a risk factor for cardiovascular disease in adults and children [47–49]. Moreover, as the severity of proteinuria increases, it is associated with metabolic disturbances such as hypercholesterolemia, hypertriglyceridemia and hypercoagulability that contribute to cardiovascular disease. Does proteinuria result in decreased levels of plasma proteins? The liver has considerable reserve capacity for increased production of new proteins and often can compensate for urinary losses. Only when proteinuria is heavy and chronic, exceeding the patient's ability to make new protein, hypoproteinemia may ensue such as in nephrotic syndrome.

The following are postulated mechanisms whereby proteinuria may induce renal injury: [60].

- Filtration of lipoproteins and absorption by proximal tubules may activate inflammatory pathways causing cell injury.
- Filtration of cytokines or chemokines may provoke cell proliferation, inflammatory cell infiltration, and activation of infiltrating cells.

- Filtration or generation of novel antigens may function as antigen-presenting cells and initiate a cellular immune response.
- Iron that is filtered into tubular fluid and bound to transferrin may be directly toxic or may have indirect effects due to iron-catalyzed synthesis of reactive oxygen metabolites.
- Activation of the alternative complement pathway by proximal tubules may be harmful.
- The release of lysosomal enzymes into the cytoplasm of protein-reabsorbing tubules may cause damage.
- The release of vasoconstricting molecules may cause ischemic tubular injury.
- Interstitial fibrosis may result from the release of fibrosis-promoting factors from renal cells activated or injured by proteinuria.
- The proteinaceous casts can obstruct renal tubules.

Persistent significant proteinuria should be regarded seriously. Besides finding out the exact cause and targeting specific therapy if possible, other treatment options include dietary protein recommendations and use of anti-proteinuric medications.

Dietary Protein Recommendations

Dietary protein restrictions have been proposed in adults with chronic kidney disease to stabilize renal function [83, 90]. In a small series of children with chronic renal insufficiency, some benefit from dietary protein restriction has been described [91]. However, another controlled study has not demonstrated a significant impact of protein restriction on the rate of progression of renal disease [46]. High dietary protein intake may indeed worsen proteinuria in some patients with nephrotic syndrome. Moreover, it does not result in a higher serum albumin. Hence, it is best to avoid an excess of dietary protein in children with proteinuric renal diseases. It is recommended that children with proteinuria receive the recommended daily allowance of protein for age and should not be protein-restricted [92].

Drugs with Anti-proteinuric Effects

Certain classes of antihypertensive agents, such as the angiotensin converting enzyme inhibitors (ACEI) and the angiotensin II receptor blockers (ARB) can reduce systemic blood pressure and exert other beneficial effects, such as decreasing urinary protein excretion and decreasing the risk of renal fibrosis. In addition, renal function is better preserved in children with chronic kidney disease when lower systolic blood pressures are achieved [93]. However, the long-term benefit of ACEIs and ARBs in children and adolescents with proteinuria remains to be established Intensive blood pressure control with ACEI effectively delays the progression of renal disease among children with an underlying glomerulopathy or renal hypoplasia or dysplasia, but not among children with other congenital or hereditary nephropathies. In addition, it has been shown that there is gradual rebound of proteinuria during ongoing ACEI inhibition in children after an initial 50% decrease, despite persistently good blood pressure control in the ESCAPE Trial [94].

There are reports of infants born to mothers taking ACEI during the second and third trimesters of pregnancy who developed oligohydramnios, pulmonary hypoplasia and postnatal hypertension. Postmortem examination of these neonates who died showed severe glomerular and tubular malformations in the kidneys. Hence, ACEI are contraindicated during pregnancy [95]. The safety of ACEI and angiotensin II receptor blockers in young infants is still unknown. Cases of ACEI-induced nephrotoxicity had been reported in premature infants with cardiac failure due to congenital heart disease [96] and young infants after cardiac surgery [97]. There was no underlying renal disease found in these infants and acute renal failure was reversible upon discontinuation of the ACEI. Another concern of ACEIs in premature infants is that they may impair the final stages of renal maturation, and therefore should be avoided before a corrected post-conceptual age of 44 weeks [98].

Aliskiren, the first orally active direct renin inhibitor, has shown promising results in proteinuria reduction in adult patients with chronic kidney disease [99]. In a case series of four children treated with aliskiren for refractory proteinuria, three children experienced clinically significant adverse effects, including symptomatic hypotension, hyperkalemia and accelerated loss of kidney function [100]. Hence, clinicians should exercise caution when prescribing aliskiren until appropriate pediatric trials establish dosing, efficacy and safety.

Conclusion

Hematuria or proteinuria in children is a frequently encountered problem. Many investigations have been recommended in the workup for a child presenting with hematuria or proteinuria. Many of the cases of hematuria or proteinuria are normal transient findings. Hence, a stepwise evaluation is recommended to avoid unnecessary and expensive investigations and yet not to miss serious conditions. Early detection and treatment of serious conditions would hopefully delay or prevent the onset of renal insufficiency. Screening programs for hematuria and proteinuria may be able to identify children at an earlier stage; however, the major disadvantage is the cost effectiveness, as well as the anxiety that will be created in parents and children where the finding is spurious or transient. Screening for albuminuria is currently recommended for a child with diabetes mellitus and chronic kidney disease. The significance of detecting albuminuria for other conditions in the pediatric population is yet to be determined.

References

1. Vehaskari VM, Rapola J, Koskimies O, Savilahti E, Vilska J, Hallman N. Microscopic hematuria in schoolchildren: epidemiology and clinicopathologic evaluation. J Pediatr. 1979;95:676–84.
2. Shaw Jr ST, Poon SY, Wong ET. Routine urinalysis: is the dipstick enough? JAMA. 1985;253: 1596–600.
3. Dodge WF. Cost effectiveness of renal disease screening. Am J Dis Child. 1977;131:1274–80.
4. Fairley KF, Birch DF. Microscopic urinalysis in glomerulonephritis. Kidney Int Suppl. 1993;42:S9–12.
5. Pollock C, Pei-Ling L, Gÿory AZ, Grigg R, Gallery ED, Caterson R, Ibels L, Mahony J, Waugh
6. Schramek P, Moritsch A, Haschkowitz H, Binder BR, Maier M. In vitro generation of dysmorphic erythrocytes. Kidney Int. 1989;36:72–7.
7. Shichiri M, Hosoda K, Nishio Y, Ogura M, Suenaga M, Saito H, Tomura S, Shiigai T. Red-cell-volume distribution curves in diagnosis of glomerular and non- glomerular hematuria. Lancet. 1988;1:908–11.
8. Ito CA, Pecoits-Filho R, Bail L, Wosiack MA, Afinovicz D, Hauser AB. Comparative analysis of two methodologies for the identification of urinary red blood cell casts. J Bras Nefrol. 2011;33(4):402–7.
9. Pham PT, Pham PC, Wilkinson AH, Lew SQ. Renal abnormalities in sickle cell anemia. Kidney Int. 2000;57:1–8.
10. Hohenfellner M, Steinbach F, Schultz-Lampel D, Lampel A, Steinbach F, Cramer BM, Thuroff JW. The nutcracker syndrome: new aspects of pathophysiology, diagnosis and treatment. J Urol. 1991;146:685–8.
11. Mazzoni MB, Kottanatu L, Simonetti GD, Ragazzi M, Bianchetti MG, Fossali EF, Milani GP. Renal vein obstruction and orthostatic proteinuria: a review. Nephrol Dial Transplant. 2011;26(2):562–5.
12. Okada M, Tsuzuki K, Ito S. Diagnosis of the nutcracker phenomenon using two- dimensional ultrasonography. Clin Nephrol. 1998;49:35–40.
13. Cho BS, Suh JS, Hahn WH, Kim SD, Lim JW. Multidetector computed tomography findings and correlations with proteinuria in nutcracker syndrome. Pediatr Nephrol. 2010;25(3):469–75.
14. Tanaka H, Waga S. Spontaneous remission of persistent severe hematuria in an adolescent with nutcracker syndrome: seven years' observation. Clin Exp Nephrol. 2004;8:68–70.
15. Shin JL, Park JM, Lee SM, Shin YH, Kim JH, Lee JS, Kim MJ. Factors affecting spontaneous resolution of hematuria in childhood nutcracker syndrome. Pediatr Nephrol. 2005;20:609–13.
16. Venkatachalam S, Bumpus K, Kapadia SR, Gray B, Lyden S, Shishehbor MH. The nutcracker syndrome. Ann Vasc Surg. 2011;25(8):1154–64.
17. Athanasiou Y, Voskarides K, Gale DP, Damianou L, Patsias C, Zavros M, Maxwell PH, Cook HT, Demosthenous P, Hadjisavvas A, Kyriacou K, Zouvani I, Pierides A, Deltas C. Familial C3 glomerulopathy associated with CFHR5 mutations: clinical characteristics of 91 patients in 16 pedigrees. Clin J Am Soc Nephrol. 2011;6:1436–46.
18. Deltas C, Pierides A, Voskarides K. Molecular genetics of familial hematuric diseases. Nephrol Dial Transplant. 2013;28(12):2946–60.
19. Seri M, Pecci A, Di Bari F, Cusano R, Savino M, Panza E, Nigro N, Noris P, Gangarossa S, Rocca B, Gresele P, Bizzaro N, Malatesta P, Koivisto PA, Longo I, Musso R, Pecoraro C, Iolascon A, Magrini U, Soriano JR, Renieri A, Ghiggeri GM, Ravazzolo R, Balduini CL, Savoia A. MYH9-related disease.

D. Dysmorphism of urinary red blood cells – value in diagnosis. Kidney Int. 1989;36:1045–9.

May-Hegglin anomaly, Sebastian syndrome, Fechtner syndrome, and Epstein syndrome are not distinct entities but represent a variable expression of a single illness. Medicine. 2003;82:203–15.

20. Han KH, Lee HK, Kang HG, Moon KC, Lee JH, Park YS, Ha IS, Ahn HS, Choi Y, Cheong HI. Renal manifestations of patients with MYH9-related disorders. Pediatr Nephrol. 2011;26:549–55.

21. Plaisier E, Gribouval O, Alamowitch S, Mougenot B, Prost C, Verpont MCX, Marro B, Desmettre T, Cohen SY, Roullet E, Dracon M, Fardeau M, Van Agtmael T, Kerjaschki D, Antignac C, Ronco P. COL4A1 mutations and hereditary angiopathy, nephropathy, aneurysms, and muscle cramps. N Engl J Med. 2007;357:2687–95.

22. Mufson MA, Belshe RB, Horrigan TJ, Zollar LM. Causes of acute hemorrhagic cystitis in children. Am J Dis Child. 1973;126:605–9.

23. Summer AP, Stauffer W, Maroushek SR, Nevins TE. Hematuria in children due to schistosomiasis in a nonendemic setting. Clin Pediatr (Phila). 2006;45:177–81.

24. Altintepe L, Tonbul HZ, Ozbey I, Guney I, Odabas AR, Cetinkaya R, Piskin MM, Selcuk Y. Urinary tuberculosis: ten years' experience. Ren Fail. 2005;27:657–61.

25. Polinsky MS, Kaiser BA, Baluarte HJ, Gruskin AB. Renal stones and hypercalciuria. Adv Pediatr. 1993;40:353–84.

26. Stapleton FB, Roy SIII, Noe HN, Jerkins G. Hypercalciuria in children with hematuria. N Engl J Med. 1984;310:1345–8.

27. Shaw NJ, Wheeldon J, Brocklehurst JT. Indices of intact serum parathyroid hormone and renal excretion of calcium, phosphate and magnesium. Arch Dis Child. 1990;65:1208–12.

28. Murakami M, Yamamoto H, Ueda Y, Murakami K, Yamauchi K. Urinary screening of elementary and junior high-school children over a 13-year period in Tokyo. Pediatr Nephrol. 1991;5:50–3.

29. Zainal D, Baba A, Mustaffa BE. Screening proteinuria and hematuria in Malaysian children. Southeast Asian J Trop Med Public Health. 1995;26:785–8.

30. Yap HK, Quek CM, Shen Q, Joshi V, Chia KS. Role of urinary screening programmes in children in the prevention of chronic kidney disease. Ann Acad Med Singapore. 2005;34:3–7.

31. Lin CY, Hsieh CC, Chen WP, Yang LY, Wang HH. The underlying diseases and follow-up in Taiwanese children screened by urinalysis. Pediatr Nephrol. 2001;16:232–7.

32. Cho BS, Kim SD, Choi YM, Kang HH. School urinalysis screening in Korea: prevalence of chronic renal disease. Pediatr Nephrol. 2001;16:1126–8.

33. Vivante A, Afek A, Frenkel-Nir Y, Tzur D, Farfel A, Golan E, Chaiter Y, Shohat T, Skorecki K, Calderon-Margalit R. Persistent asymptomatic isolated microscopic hematuria in Israeli adolescents and young adults and risk for end-stage renal disease. JAMA. 2011;306:729–36.

34. Diven SC, Travis LB. A practical primary care approach to hematuria in children. Pediatr Nephrol. 2000;14:65–72.

35. Buzza M, Wilson D, Savige J. Segregation of hematuria in thin basement membrane disease with haplotypes at the loci for Alport syndrome. Kidney Int. 2001;59:1670–6.

36. Carasi C, Van't Hoff WG, Rees L, Risdon RA, Trompeter RS, Dillon MJ. Childhood thin GBM disease: review of 22 children with family studies and long-term follow-up. Pediatr Nephrol. 2005;20:1098–105.

37. Strøm EH, Banfi G, Krapf R, Abt AB, Mazzucco G, Monga G, Gloor F, Neuweiler J, Riess R, Stosiek P, et al. Glomerulopathy associated with predominant fibronectin deposits: a newly recognized hereditary disease. Kidney Int. 1995;48:163–70.

38. Castelletti F, Donadelli R, Banterla F, Hildebrandt F, Zipfel PF, Bresin E, Otto E, Skerka C, Renieri A, Todeschini M, Caprioli J, Caruso RM, Artuso R, Remuzzi G, Noris M. Mutations in FN1 cause glomerulopathy with fibronectin deposits. Proc Natl Acad Sci U S A. 2008;105:2538–43.

39. Köhler H, Wandel E, Brunck B. Acanthocyturia – a characteristic marker for glomerular bleeding. Kidney Int. 1991;40:115–20.

40. Yoshikawa N, Iijima K, Ito H. IgA nephropathy in children. Nephron. 1999;83:1–12.

41. Coppo R, Gianoglio B, Porcellini G, Maringhini S. Frequency of renal diseases and clinical indication for renal biopsy in children (Report of the Italian National Registry for Renal biopsies in children). Nephrol Dial Transplant. 1998;13:293–7.

42. Feld LG, Meyers KE, Kaplan BS, et al. Limited evaluation of microscopic hematuria in pediatrics. Pediatrics. 1998;102:E42.

43. Gale DP. How benign is hematuria? Using genetics to predict prognosis. Pediatr Nephrol. 2013;28:1183–93.

44. Ruggenenti P, Perna A, Mosconi L, Pisoni R, Remuzzi G. Urinary protein excretion rate is the best independent predictor of ESRF in non-diabetic proteinuric chronic nephropathies. Kidney Int. 1998;53:1209–16.

45. Remuzzi G, Ruggenenti P, Benigni A. Understanding the nature of renal disease progression. Kidney Int. 1997;51:2–15.

46. Wingen AM, Fabian-Bach C, Schaefer F, Mehls O. Randomised, multicenter study of a low-protein diet on the progression of renal failure in children. Lancet. 1997;349:1117–23.

47. Grimm RH, Svendsen KH, Kasiske B, Keane WF, Wahi MM. Proteinuria is a risk factor for mortality over 10 years of follow-up: MRFIT Research Group, Multiple Risk Factor Intervention Trial. Kidney Int Suppl. 1997;63:S10–4.

48. Kannel WB, Stampfer MJ, Castelli WP, Verter J. The prognostic significance of proteinuria: the Framingham Study. Am Heart J. 1984;108:1347–52.

49. Portman RJ, Hawkins E, Verani R. Premature atherosclerosis in pediatric renal patients: report of the Southwest Pediatric Nephrology Study Group. Pediatr Res. 1991;29:349A.

50. Kumar S, Muchmore A. Tamm-Horsfall protein-uromodulin (1950–1990). Kidney Int. 1990;37:1395–401.

51. Kidney Disease: Improving Global Outcomes (KDIGO) CKD Work Group. KDIGO 2012 clinical practice guideline for the evaluation and management of chronic kidney disease. Kidney Int Suppl. 2013;3:1–150.

52. Rademacher ER, Sinaiko AR. Albuminuria in children. Curr Opin Nephrol Hypertens. 2009;18:246–51.

53. Jones CA, Francis ME, Eberhardt MS, Chavers B, Coresh J, Engelgau M, et al. Microalbuminuria in the US population: Third National Health and Nutrition Examination Survey. Am J Kidney Dis. 2002;39:445–59.

54. Bangstad HJ, Jorgensen KD, Kjaersgaard P, Mevold K, Hanssen KF. Urinary albumin excretion rate and puberty in non-diabetic children and adolescents. Acta Paediatr. 1993;82:857–62.

55. Houser MT, Jahn MF, Kobayashi A, Walburn J. Assessment of urinary protein excretion in the adolescent: effect of body position and exercise. J Pediatr. 1986;109:556–61.

56. Amin R, Turner C, van Aken S, Bahu TK, Watts A, Lindsell DR, et al. The relationship between microalbuminuria and glomerular filtration rate in young type 1 diabetic subjects: the Oxford Regional Prospective Study. Kidney Int. 2005;68:1740–9.

57. Nguyen S, McCulloch C, Brakeman P, Portale A, Hsu CY. Being overweight modifies the association between cardiovascular risk factors and microalbuminuria in adolescents. Pediatrics. 2008;121:37–45.

58. Csernus K, Lanyi E, Erhardt E, Molnar D. Effect of childhood obesity and obesity-related cardiovascular risk factors on glomerular and tubular protein excretion. Eur J Pediatr. 2005;164:44–9.

59. Brem AS. Neonatal hematuria and proteinuria. Clin Perinatol. 1981;8:321–32.

60. Hogg RJ, Portman RJ, Milliner D, Lemley KV, Eddy A, Ingelfinger J. Evaluation and management of proteinuria and nephrotic syndrome in children: recommendations from a pediatric nephrology panel established at the National Kidney Foundation Conference on Proteinuria, Albuminuria, Risk, Assessment, Detection, and Elimination (PARADE). Pediatrics. 2000;105:1242–9.

61. Rose BD. Pathophysiology of renal disease. 2nd ed. New York: McGraw-Hill; 1987. p. 11–6.

62. Elises JS, Griffiths PD, Hocking MD, Taylor CM, White RH. Simplified quantification of urinary protein excretion in children. Clin Nephrol. 1988;30:225–9.

63. Ginsberg JM, Chang BS, Matarese RA, Garella S. Use of single voided urine samples to estimate quantitative proteinuria. N Engl J Med. 1983;309:1543–6.

64. Yoshimoto M, Tsukahara H, Saito M, Hayashi S, Haruki S, Fujisawa S, Sudo M. Evaluation of variability of proteinuria indices. Pediatr Nephrol. 1990;4:136–9.

65. Kaneko K, Someya T, Nishizaki N, Shimojima T, Ohtaki R, Kaneko KI. Simplified quantification of urinary protein excretion using a novel dipstick in children. Pediatr Nephrol. 2005;20:834–6.

66. Guy M, Newall R, Borzomato J, Kalra PA, Price C. Use of a first-line urine protein-to-creatinine ratio strip test on random urines to rule out proteinuria in patients with chronic kidney disease. Nephrol Dial Transplant. 2009;24(4):1189–93.

67. Sebestyen JF, Alon US. The teenager with asymptomatic proteinuria: think orthostatic first. Clin Pediatr. 2011;50(3):179–82.

68. Vehaskari VM. Mechanism of orthostatic proteinuria. Pediatr Nephrol. 1990;4:328–30.

69. Berns JS, McDonald B, Gaudio KM, Siegel NJ. Progression of orthostatic proteinuria to focal and segmental glomerulosclerosis. Clin Pediatr. 1986;25:165–6.

70. Springberg PD, Garrett Jr LE, Thompson Jr AL, Collins NF, Lordon RE, Robinson RR. Fixed and reproducible orthostatic proteinuria: results of a 20-year follow-up study. Ann Intern Med. 1982;97:516–9.

71. Rizvi SA, Naqvi SA, Jawad F, Ahmed E, Asghar A, Zafar MN, Akhtar F. Living kidney donor follow-up in a dedicated clinic. Transplantation. 2005;79:1247–51.

72. Chang RL, Deen WM, Robertson CR, Brenner BM. Permselectivity of the glomerular capillary wall: III. Restricted transport of polyanions. Kidney Int. 1975;8:212–8.

73. Takahashi S, Watanabe S, Wada N, Murakami H, Funaki S, Yan K, Kondo Y, Harada K, Nagata M. Charge selective function in childhood glomerular diseases. Pediatr Res. 2006;59:336–40.

74. Kriz W, Kretzler M, Provoost AP, Shirato I. Stability and leakiness: opposing challenges to the glomerulus. Kidney Int. 1996;49:1570–4.

75. Ruggenenti P, Remuzzi G. The role of protein traffic in the progression of renal diseases. Annu Rev Med. 2000;51:315–27.

76. Joachim GR, Cameron JS, Schwartz M, Becker EL. Selectivity of protein excretion in patients with the nephrotic syndrome. J Clin Invest. 1964;43:2332–46.

77. Cameron JS, White RHR. Selectivity of proteinuria in children with the nephrotic syndrome. Lancet. 1965;1:463–8.

78. Bazzi C, Petrini C, Rizza V, Arrigo G, D'Amico G. A modern approach to selectivity of proteinuria and tubulointerstitial damage in nephrotic syndrome. Kidney Int. 2000;58:1732–41.

79. Bergon E, Granados R, Fernandez-Segoviano P, Miravalles E, Bergon M. Classification of renal pro-

teinuria: a simple algorithm. Clin Chem Lab Med. 2002;40:1143–50.

80. Dodge WF, West EF, Smith EH, Bunce HIII. Proteinuria and hematuria in school-age children: epidemiology and early natural history. J Pediatr. 1976;88:327–47.

81. Vehaskari VM, Rapola J. Isolated proteinuria: analysis of a school-age population. J Pediatr. 1982;101: 661–8.

82. Hisano S, Ueda K. Asymptomatic hematuria and proteinuria: renal pathology and clinical outcome in 54 children. Pediatr Nephrol. 1989;3:229–34.

83. Ruggenenti P, Schieppati A, Remuzzi G. Progression, remission, regression of chronic renal diseases. Lancet. 2001;357:1601–8.

84. Schwartz GJ, Munoz A, Schneider MF, Mak RH, Kaskel F, Warady BA, Furth SL. New equations to estimate GFR inchildren with CKD. J Am Soc Nephrol. 2009;20:629–37.

85. Park SJ, Lim JW, Cho BS, Yoon TY, Oh JH. Nutcracker syndrome in children with orthostatic proteinuria: diagnosis on the basis of Doppler sonography. J Ultrasound Med. 2002;21:39–45.

86. Perna A, Remuzzi G. Abnormal permeability to proteins and glomerular lesions: a meta-analysis of experimental and human studies. Am J Kidney Dis. 1996;27:34–41.

87. Bergstein JM. A practical approach to proteinuria. Pediatr Nephrol. 1999;13:697–700.

88. Hama T, Nakanishi K, Shima Y, Mukaiyama H, Togawa H, Tanaka R, Hamahira K, Kaito H, Iijima K, Yoshikawa N. Renal biopsy criterion in children with asymptomatic constant isolated proteinuria. Nephrol Dial Transplant. 2012;27:3186–90.

89. Williams JD, Coles GA. Proteinuria – a direct cause of renal morbidity. Kidney Int. 1994;45:443–50.

90. Kasiske BL, Lakatua JD, Ma JZ, Louis TA. A meta-analysis of the effects of dietary protein restriction on the rate of decline in renal function. Am J Kidney Dis. 1998;31:954–61.

91. Jureidini KF, Hogg RJ, van Renen MJ, Southwood TR, Henning PH, Cobiac L, Daniels L, Harris S. Evaluation of long-term aggressive dietary management of chronic renal failure in children. Pediatr Nephrol. 1990;4:1–10.

92. Uauy RD, Hogg RJ, Brewer ED, Reisch JS, Cunningham C, Holliday MA. Dietary protein and growth in infants with chronic renal insufficiency: a report from the Southwest Pediatric Nephrology Study Group and the University of California San Francisco. Pediatr Nephrol. 1994;8:45–50.

93. Ellis D, Vats A, Moritz ML, Reitz S, Grosso MJ, Janosky JE. Long-term antiproteinuric and renoprotective efficacy and safety of losartan in children with proteinuria. J Pediatr. 2003;143:89–97.

94. The ESCAPE Trial Group. Strict blood-pressure control and progression of renal failure in children. N Engl J Med. 2009;361:1639–1650.95.

95. Tabacova S. Mode of action: angiotensin-converting enzyme inhibition – developmental effects associated with exposure to ACE inhibitors. Crit Rev Toxicol. 2005;35:747–55.

96. Lee GJ, Cohen R, Chang AC, Cleary JP. Angiotensin converting enzyme inhibitor (ACEI)-induced acute renal failure in premature newborns with congenital heart disease. J Pediatr Pharmacol Ther. 2010;15(4):290–6.

97. Gantenbein MH, Bauersfeld U, Baenziger O, Frey B, Neuhaus T, Sennhauser F, Bernet V. Side effects of angiotensin converting enzyme inhibitor (captopril) in newborns and young infants. J Perinat Med. 2008;36(5):448–52.

98. Dionne JM, Abitbol CL, Flynn JT. Hypertension in infancy: diagnosis, management and outcome. Pediatr Nephrol. 2012;27:17–32.

99. Persson F, Rossing P, Reinhard H, Juhl T, Stehouwer CD, Schalkwijk C, Danser AH, Boomsma F, Frandsen E, Parving HH. Renal effects of aliskiren compared with and in combination with irbesartan in patients with type 2 diabetes, hypertension and albuminuria. Diabetes Care. 2009;32:1873–9.

100. Kelland EE, McAuley LM, Filler G. Are we ready to use aliskiren in children? Pediatr Nephrol. 2011;26: 473–7.

Steroid Sensitive Nephrotic Syndrome

15

Elisabeth M. Hodson, Stephen I. Alexander, and Nicole Graf

Abbreviations

APN	Arbeitsgemeinschaft für Pädiatrische Nephrologie
BMC	Bone mineral content
BMD	Bone mineral density
BMI	Body mass index
CI	Confidence intervals
CNI	Calcineurin inhibitor
DXA	Dual energy x-ray absorptiometry
ESRD	End stage renal disease
FRNS	Frequently relapsing steroid sensitive nephrotic syndrome
FSGS	Focal and segmental glomerulosclerosis
GFR	Glomerular filtration rate
HR	Hazard ratio
ISKDC	International Study of Kidney Disease in Children
KDIGO	Kidney Disease. Improving Global Outcomes
MCD	Minimal change disease
MesPGN	Mesangial proliferative glomerulonephritis
MMF	Mycophenolate mofetil
MPA	Mycophenolic acid
RCT	Randomized controlled trial
RR	Relative risk
SDNS	Steroid dependent steroid sensitive nephrotic syndrome
SDS	Standard deviation score
SIRS	Soluble immune response suppressor
SLE	Systemic lupus erythematosus
SRNS	Steroid resistant nephrotic syndrome
SSNS	Steroid sensitive nephrotic syndrome
VEGF	Vascular endothelial growth factor
VPF	Vascular permeability factor

E.M. Hodson (✉) • S.I. Alexander • N. Graf
Children's Hospital at West, Locked Bag 4001,
Westmead, NSW 2145, Australia
e-mail: elisabeth.hodson@health.nws.gov.au;
stephen.alexander@health.nws.gov.au;
nicola.graf@health.nws.gov.au

Introduction

Nephrotic syndrome is characterized by massive proteinuria, hypoalbuminaemia and generalized oedema. Clinically childhood nephrotic syndrome has been classified into steroid sensitive nephrotic syndrome (SSNS), steroid resistant nephrotic syndrome (SRNS), congenital and infantile nephrotic syndrome (0–12 months) and nephrotic syndrome secondary to other diseases including Henoch Schönlein nephritis, systemic lupus erythematosus (SLE) and hepatitis B nephropathy. Between 1967 and 1974, the International Study of Kidney Disease in Childhood (ISKDC) enrolled 521 children aged 12 weeks to 16 years with idiopathic nephrotic syndrome to evaluate the histopathological, clinical and laboratory characteristics of nephrotic syndrome in children. The kidney biopsy studies demonstrated that about 80 % of children had

© Springer-Verlag Berlin Heidelberg 2016
D.F. Geary, F. Schaefer (eds.), *Pediatric Kidney Disease*, DOI 10.1007/978-3-662-52972-0_15

either minimal change disease (MCD; 76.4 %), focal and segmental glomerulosclerosis (FSGS; 6.9 %) or mesangioproliferative glomerulonephritis (MesPGN: 2.3 %) [1]. Subsequently the ISKDC demonstrated that the response to corticosteroids was highly predictive of renal histology with 93 % of children with MCD achieving complete remission following an 8 week course of prednisone [2]. However, between 25 and 50 % of children with MesPGN or FSGS on biopsy also responded to prednisone [2]. Now kidney biopsies are generally limited to children with unusual clinical features at presentation or to children who fail to respond to corticosteroids. Since most children do not undergo kidney biopsy at diagnosis, children with idiopathic nephrotic syndrome are now classified according to their initial response to corticosteroids into SSNS or SRNS. Although many children with SSNS have one or more relapses, the majority continues to respond to corticosteroids throughout their subsequent course [3–5] and the long term prognosis for complete resolution with normal kidney function is good. This chapter is devoted to SSNS. Commonly used definitions for SSNS and SRNS are shown in Table 15.1.

Epidemiology

Prospective studies of children with newly diagnosed idiopathic nephrotic syndrome identified through Pediatric Surveillance Units in the Netherlands, Australia and New Zealand reported incidences of idiopathic nephrotic syndrome of 1.12–1.9 per 100,000 children aged below 16 years [11–13]. In retrospective studies, the reported incidence of idiopathic nephrotic syndrome varied between 1.8 and 11.6 per 100,000 children aged below 16 years [11, 14–16] with a cumulative prevalence of 16 per 100,000 children [15]. The incidence is higher in Asian [14], African American [16] and Arab [17] children. In children in northern England, the overall rates were 7.4 (95 % confidence intervals [CI] 5.3–9.5) for south Asian children compared with 1.6 (95 % CI 1.3–1.8) per 100,000 children/year for non-south Asian children [14] with 88 % responsive to corticosteroids.

Table 15.1 Definitions used in idiopathic nephrotic syndrome

Classification	Definition
Nephrotic syndrome	Oedema, uPCR[a] ≥200 mg/mmol (≥2000 mg/g) or ≥50 mg/kg/day or ≥3+ on urine dipstick, hypoalbuminaemia ≤25 g/L (≤2.5 mg/dl)
Complete remission	uPCR ≤20 mg/mmol (≤200 mg/g) or ≤1+ protein on urine dipstick for 3 consecutive days
Initial responder	Attainment of complete remission within initial 4 weeks of corticosteroid therapy
Initial non-responder/ steroid resistance	Failure to achieve remission during initial 8 weeks of corticosteroid therapy
Relapse	uPCR ≥200 mg/mmol (≥2000 mg/g) or ≥3+ protein or more on urine dipstick for 3 consecutive days
Infrequent relapse	One relapse within 6 months of initial response or 1–3 relapses in any 12 month period
Frequent relapse	Two or more relapses within 6 months of initial response or 4 or more relapses in any 12 month period
Steroid dependence	Two consecutive relapses during corticosteroid therapy or within 14 days of ceasing therapy
Late non-responder	Persistent proteinuria during ≥4 weeks of corticosteroids following one or more remissions

Data from References [6–10]
[a]*uPCR* urine protein-creatinine ratio

SSNS is more common in boys than girls with a male: female ratio of around 2:1 and a peak incidence between 1 and 4 years [1, 14, 15]. There is a decreasing trend with increasing age in the incidence of idiopathic nephrotic syndrome overall and of the proportion with SSNS (Table 15.2). SSNS is less common in African [18] and African-American children [16]. In the past three decades there is evidence for an increase in the proportion of children with biopsy documented FSGS suggesting an increase in steroid resistant nephrotic syndrome [19]. A review of retrospective studies from tertiary services comparing the prevalence of FSGS over

Table 15.2 Nephrotic syndrome in Yorkshire, UK, 1987–1998

Age group	Steroid sensitive nephrotic syndrome		Steroid resistant nephrotic syndrome		All primary nephrotic syndrome	
	Incidence[a]	95 % CI[b]	Incidence	95 % CI	Incidence	95 % CI
0–<1 year	0.5	0.0–1.1	0.2	0.0–0.5	0.5	0.0–1.1
1–4 years	4.1	3.3–5.0	0.5	0.2–0.8	4.6	3.7–5.5
5–9 years	1.7	1.2–2.3	0.2	0.0–0.4	1.9	1.4–2.5
10–15 years	0.9	0.6–1.2	0.2	0.1–0.4	1.1	0.7–1.5
Total	2.0	1.7–2.3	0.3	0.2–0.4	2.3	2.0–2.6

Used with permission of Springer Science + Business Media from McKinney et al. [14]
[a]Incidence per 100,000 patient years in children aged 0–15 years
[b]Confidence intervals

two time periods found that the odds of FSGS increased twofold. However, the analyses involved fewer than 1000 children, there was significant heterogeneity in the results and bias related to selective referral to tertiary centres could not be excluded.

Aetiology and Pathogenesis

A T Cell Disease But New Thoughts on B Cells

A series of clinical observations led Dr Shaloub in 1974 to propose that SSNS was due to an abnormality of function in T cells [20]. Nephrotic syndrome had been observed in patients with Hodgkins lymphoma, and cases of thymoma [21, 22]. The disease was noted to remit in children who had measles, which led some people to propose using measles as a therapeutic strategy [23–25]. A major effect of measles is to inhibit cell mediated immunity thereby shutting down T cell function. Further the response of nephrotic syndrome to T cell suppressive agents such as steroids or calcineurin inhibitors (CNI) also supported their role in nephrotic syndrome [20]. These features all suggested that lymphocytes are key cells in SSNS. Recent success in treating recurrent FSGS and SSNS with the CD20 B cell depleting antibody rituximab raises the possibility of either B cells influencing T cells or B cells themselves being primary players in nephrotic syndrome. However, current data on the role of B cells are limited.

A Circulating Factor

MCD appears to exist in a spectrum with FSGS. A proportion of children with MCD on clinical and histological grounds evolve into FSGS [26]. In both there appears to be a circulating factor with the children with FSGS being less responsive to therapeutic agents. Within this group is a subset of children where the disease resides in structural changes in the glomeruli with genetic mutations in key glomerular slit process proteins including nephrin, podocin, Actinin4 and WT-1. These are described elsewhere but in brief are associated with no response to steroids and progression to end-stage renal failure, and do not show evidence of a circulating factor as demonstrated by rapid recurrence of disease in a transplanted kidney. The timing of response with the return to normal function taking days to weeks is also supportive of slow podocyte recovery from an injurious cytokine. The higher rates of recurrence in children with FSGS receiving living related kidneys suggests that there may be a degree of HLA restriction of response and this is also supported by HLA linkage studies showing that increased incidence of disease is tied to certain alleles such as HLA B8, B13, DWQ2, DQB10301 and DR7 [27–30].

Various growth factors and cytokines have been proposed as pathogenic in SSNS over the years. The initial identification of the factor, vascular permeability factor (VPF) now called vascular endothelial growth factor (VEGF), was thought to have identified the key protein leading to nephrotic syndrome [31–33]. However, the identification of this protein in normal urine delayed further investigation of its role. More recently it has been noted to be increased in urine during relapses of nephrotic syndrome though circulating levels are unchanged suggesting that VEGF levels reflect the concomitant proteinuria [34, 35]. Recent tissue-specific knock-outs of VEGF in mice restricted to podocytes have demonstrated a key role for local VEGF in maintaining glomerular endothelial integrity and again reinforced its importance though perhaps more locally in maintaining permeability [36, 37]. Soluble immune response suppressor (SIRS) was also identified as a potential protein mediating nephrotic syndrome but again the inability to characterize this protein despite many mechanistic observations led to its exclusion as the likely factor [32, 33, 38]. Other circulating factors have been proposed and the development of functional assay of glomerular permeability by Dr Savin in the late 1990s identified a proteinuric factor that was small, highly glycosylated, and hydrophobic [39]. This appeared to be likely to allow fractionation of nephrotic sera and identification of the factor. Other observations that protein A columns could remove the nephrotic factor post-transplant also seemed to point to identifying features [40]. More recently induction of proteinuria in rats with transfer of serum may allow models that can identify this factor as has the demonstration that overexpression of the Th2 cytokine IL-13 induces proteinuria in rats [41]. Recently podocyte-secreted angiopoietin-like-4 was found to mediate proteinuria in SSNS using overexpression in the podocyte in rat models though further confirmatory studies are awaited [42].

The central role of T cells in disease has led to a number of strategies to identify the underlying defect. The thought that the disease was caused by a low frequency pathogenic clone has given way to a view that there is a generalized alteration in the lymphocytes that is triggered in these individuals and then can be switched off by treatment. This has been studied in several ways including assessment of T cell derived cytokine responses either directly in plasma or by measurement of supernatants from activated mononuclear cells or measurement of RNA, assessment of T cell subsets by immuno-phenotyping or finally by functional assays of cell mediated immunity. More recently the identification of a role for micro-RNAs in FSGS suggested this may be a fruitful area of study [43].

Phenotypes of Cytokine Secreting T Cells: Th1, Th2, Treg, Th17

Naïve T cells on activation become polarized into different subsets defined by their cytokine production and driven by the cytokine milieu in which they are activated. The initial division of T cells was into CD4 (originally helper) T cells, that respond to exogenous antigen presented by antigen presenting cells in the context of MHC Class II, and CD8 (originally effector) T cells that respond to internal antigens presented by all cells. CD4 T cells were further divided into Th1 and Th2 cells based on the cytokines they produced [44]. This was initially observed in mice but human Th1 cells also produce cytokines such as IFN-gamma and TNF, which are used in cell mediated immune responses. Th2 cells produce IL-4, IL-5 and IL-13 which are key to humoral immunity and are used by B cells to class switch and act as growth factors for eosinophils [45, 46]. It is now apparent that CD8 T cells can produce cytokines and can be polarized to Tc1 and Tc2 expressing similar cytokines to those in CD4 Th cell subsets [47]. The observation that allergy is more common in children with nephrotic syndrome suggested that this might be a Th2 disease [27]. A subset of T cells thought to suppress activity in other T cells was originally described as suppressor T cells and these have recently been reclassified as regulatory T cells. These are thymically derived and express regulatory cytokines such as TGF-β and IL-10 and express regulatory molecules such as CTLA-4. A key marker of these cells is the expression of the transcription factor foxp3 [48–50]. Interestingly there is now another T cell subset that is an alternative to regulatory T cells called the Th17 cell because it expresses the cytokine IL-17. Th17 cells are induced by IL-23 but can be generated by IL-6 and TGF-β thus acting as an alternate pathway of development to regulatory T cells [50, 51].

In general, studies of cytokines have been disappointing. No clear up-regulation of Th2 type cytokines has been demonstrated. Studies of serum of patients in remission show IL-1 unchanged, IL-2 normal or undetected in four of five studies, sIL-2R increased in four of six studies, IFN-gamma normal or not detected in three and increased in two studies, IL-4 normal or decreased, IL-8 normal, increased and decreased in four studies, IL-10, IL-12 and IL-13 either normal or not detected and TNF-α normal in three of four studies [52]. Studies of culture supernatants of stimulated mononuclear cells from children with active SSNS are also highly variable though four studies suggest elevated IL-4, two studies elevated IL-12, and five studies elevated TNF-α. RNA measurements for specific cytokines in blood have been equally unrewarding as have those using intracellular cytokine staining [52]. Urinary reports are confounded by concurrent proteinuria but there has been a recent report of IL-17 increased in the urine of patients with SSNS [31, 53]. Other non-T cell inflammatory proteins associated with SSNS include neopterin which is produced by activated macrophages and is increased in SSNS [54].

Molecular Studies

Other molecular strategies have been used. These include comparisons of the RNA expressed in CD2 positive cells during relapse and remission. This showed limited Th1 and Th2 like profiles but rather the expression of early thymic type genes suggesting that the lymphocytes involved may be recent emigrants from the thymus. Other comparative arrays have shown an upregulation of TRAIL RNA but no increase in secreted TRAIL, a T cell death effector molecule [55, 56]. Other studies in FSGS kidney tissue show upregulation of CD8 T cell effector molecules [57]. While a role for the signaling molecule NFkB has been suggested studies find differences in expression of its components only in SRNS [58–60]. Gene linkage other than HLA linkage has shown

that in familial SSNS a locus exists at 2p12-p13.2 with a LOD score of >3.0 [61]. Though a number of candidate genes exist in this region none have yet been identified in these families as causing disease.

Role of the Thymus

The expression data above, the association of nephrotic syndrome with T cell lymphomas and thymomas, and the timing of thymic involution occurring around puberty at the same time as the resolution of relapses for the majority of children with uncomplicated SSNS and the exquisite sensitivity of thymocytes to steroids all suggest a role for early T cells or other thymically derived cells in SSNS. However, clear evidence for this is not yet available.

Role of Infection

While there has been no clear infectious agent identified as inducing nephrotic syndrome, there is an identifiable viral prodrome in around 50 % of cases of relapse. Whether this merely reflects cytokine release with the initiation of nephrotic syndrome or whether this is initiation of the disease by a viral trigger is not clear. Some groups have postulated that inflammation through TLRs may upregulate CD80 on podocytes leading to activation though CD80 and nephrosis [62].

Summary

While the evidence supports a role for T cells activated to secrete a permeability factor, identifying the specific T cell changes or characterization of the factor remains a major challenge in SSNS. The clinical results with rituximab in depleting B cells, and the data on CD80 expression on podocytes raise other alternatives as potential causes of SSNS including circulating cells other than T cells and specific podocyte responses, but there are limited data so far on these pathways.

Histopathology

Steroid sensitive nephrotic syndrome comprises a spectrum of disease that includes MCD, MesPGN (also known as "diffuse mesangial hypercellularity"), IgM nephropathy and FSGS. Although these are readily distinguished on biopsy, the clinical significance of this distinction remains controversial with significant overlap in behaviour and variation in morphological diagnosis over time in a small proportion of cases. This confusion is reflected in the literature. Some studies suggest a difference in behaviour between those with and without mesangial hypercellularity in the absence of immune deposits [63]. Some studies suggest an increased risk of steroid resistance and/or development of focal sclerosing lesions with MesPGN/IgM nephropathy [64, 65] with some studies documenting transition of MCD, MesPGN and IgM nephropathy to FSGS in frequently relapsing patients over time [26, 66]. In addition some studies suggest that the response to therapy in cases with immune deposition is "unpredictable" [67] or variable [68], and finally a number of studies have failed to find any significant difference in outcomes between these categories [69, 70]. Histological overlap also exists with MCD, MesPGN and FSGS in patients with predominant mesangial deposition of C1q (C1q nephropathy), although representing a small minority of patients with initial presentation of clinical nephrotic syndrome [71–73]. Similarly, mesangial IgA deposition in association with nephrotic syndrome has also been described in a defined subset of IgA nephropathy patients, with either MCD like changes or MesPGN on biopsy. IgA with MCD-like changes is generally responsive to steroid therapy, although with a significant rate of relapse [74]. Regardless of histopathology, children with disease resistant to steroids generally have a poorer outcome compared with those with responsive disease [75]. The ultimate prognosis for children with primary nephrotic syndrome and frequently relapsing disease associated with mesangial hypercellularity and/or positive immunofluorescence remains difficult to predict.

Minimal Change Disease (MCD)

The defining histological feature of minimal change disease (MCD) is normal appearing glomeruli on light microscopic examination (Fig. 15.1). This assumes that the specimen has an adequate sample of glomeruli, including deep glomeruli from the juxtamedullary region of the renal cortex. Glomeruli of normal young children are generally smaller compared with adults so appear relatively hypercellular. There is no significant expansion of mesangial matrix, and no increase in mesangial cellularity (either by increased numbers of mesangial cells or infiltration by inflammatory cells). The cytoplasm of the podocytes may appear to be mildly swollen or vacuolated. Glomerular capillary loops remain patent, and in many cases may appear mildly dilated. The glomerular capillary walls are thin with no evidence of basement membrane thickening. No basement membrane reduplication or epithelial spike formation are evident on examination of silver stained sections. The presence of an occasional glomerular "tip" lesion, defined as adhesion of the tuft to the Bowman's capsule at the site of opening of the proximal convoluted tubule, may be seen in MCD provided the glomerulus is otherwise normal in size and cellularity [76, 77]. The interstitium is normal without significant inflammation,

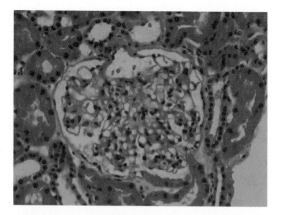

Fig. 15.1 The glomerulus appears normal to light microscopic examination, with normal mesangial matrix and cellularity. Capillary loops are dilated with normal thin capillary walls (H&E stain, ×400)

fibrosis or tubular atrophy. Proximal tubule epithelial cells may contain hyaline droplets consistent with protein loss.

The immunofluoresence in MCD is negative. Very small amounts of IgM or C3 are considered by some to be compatible with MCD; however, any significant immune reactant even in the setting of histologically normal glomeruli effectively excludes this diagnosis [67, 70, 75]. However, the clinical significance of these immune positive cases with normal histology is still controversial, and many now consider that these cases represent a spectrum of disease rather than distinct entities. Electron microscopic examination of untreated MCD shows uniform abnormality of the podocytes, with marked effacement of the foot processes over at least 50 % of the glomerular capillary surface resulting in a smooth homogenous layer of epithelial cell cytoplasm which lacks the normal interdigitation. The cytoplasm of the cells may be enlarged with clear vacuoles and prominence of organelles. This is accompanied by microvillus transformation along the urinary surface of the podocytes (Fig. 15.2). The glomerular basement membrane otherwise appears normal, as do the mesangial cells and matrix. Immune deposits are absent. These changes are commonly modified with steroid treatment, and the degree of foot process effacement may be incomplete if the biopsy is taken from a partially treated patient.

Mesangial Proliferative Glomerulopathy (MesPGN)

Light microscopic examination of MesPGN shows generalized, diffuse mesangial cell hyperplasia, involving over 80 % of the glomeruli. Increased numbers of mesangial cell nuclei are clearly present within mesangial matrix which is either normal or only mildly increased in amount (Fig. 15.3). There is generally no obvious lobulation of the glomerulus, and segmental sclerosis is absent. As in MCD, glomerular basement membranes remain thin and capillary loops clearly patent. By definition, spikes are not seen in silver stained sections. There is no significant interstitial change (either tubular atrophy or fibrosis) to suggest glomerular loss. Glomerular immaturity, characterized by hypercellularity and a layer of cuboidal epithelium along the surface of the glomerular tuft, may be seen in some cases, particularly in younger children. Recent studies have suggested that these cases may have a less favourable clinical course [78].

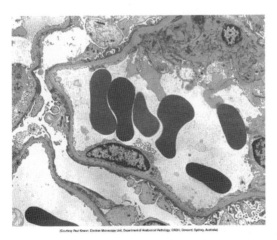

Fig. 15.2 Low power electron photomicrograph includes a capillary loop with extensive effacement of foot processes accompanied by swelling and microvillarisation of podocytes. Glomerular basement membranes are of normal appearance and no dense deposits are seen (Courtesy of Paul Kirwan, Electron Microscopy Unit, Department of Anatomical Pathology, CRGH, Concord, Sydney, Australia)

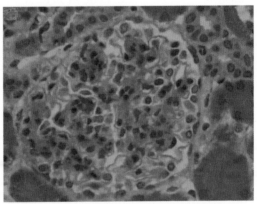

Fig. 15.3 The glomerulus shows increased numbers of mesangial cells with mildly increased matrix. The capillary loops appear normal (H&E stain, ×400)

Many cases of MesPGN show positive granular mesangial IgM +/− C3 and very occasionally small amounts of C1q or IgG, although a proportion of cases have negative immunofluorescence. Some have considered these immune-positive cases as MesPGN, while others separate the positive cases into further distinct categories, most commonly IgM nephropathy. As noted earlier, these three "entities" (MCD, MesPGN, IgM Nephropathy) probably represent a spectrum rather than separate diseases. On electron microscopy there is mesangial cell hyperplasia with effacement of epithelial cell foot processes and microvillus transformation of epithelial cells. Dense deposits are not typically found, and the glomerular capillary basement membrane is normal.

IgM Nephropathy

IgM Nephropathy shows light microscopic features that may mimic those of either MCD or MesPGN. The sampled glomeruli may appear completely normal on routine stains, or may show diffuse mesangial hypercellularity. Some cases will show a combination of features, with some but not all glomeruli appearing hypercellular. As with MCD and MesPGN, segmental sclerosing lesions are not seen in an adequately sampled specimen, glomerular capillary loops remain thin walled and patent, and there is no basement membrane thickening or evidence of spike formation. Interstitial changes are absent. Granular deposits of IgM are confined to the mesangium and are generally seen in all glomeruli regardless of their histological appearance. Lesser amounts of C3 are common, and some cases may also show small amounts of C1q or IgG. In these cases, the IgM should remain as the dominant reactant. On electron microscopy there may be a mild increase in mesangial matrix. Immune deposits are often absent though some cases will show occasional small dense deposits that are located in paramesangial regions. Effacement of epithelial cell foot processes is usually seen to a varying degree, usually with microvillus transformation.

IgA Nephropathy with Nephrotic Syndrome

IgA nephropathy may present with clinical nephrotic syndrome indistinguishable from MCD in approximately 8–10 % of cases. Nephrotic IgA nephropathy may show light microscopic features of MCD, MesPGN, or a focal GN (proliferative or sclerosing); however, it is defined by the presence of dominant mesangial IgA deposition (frequently with some associated C3, and in approximately 50 % of cases with lesser amounts of IgG and/or IgM), usually with electron microscopic evidence of immune deposits.

C1q Nephropathy

C1q nephropathy is an uncommon disorder that may also present with clinical nephrotic syndrome. Histology of these cases most commonly shows an MCD-like picture (70–75 % of cases), with MesPGN (20 %) and FSGS (7–13 %) seen in some cases. Distinction is made with immunofluorescence finding of predominant C1q deposition in the mesangium and electron dense deposits on electron microscopic examination. Although many of these cases are clinically steroid resistant or steroid dependent, being more likely to require chronic immunosuppression and combined therapy, overall prognosis is good in particular for those with minimal changes on light microscopy. Of note, a number of studies have shown disappearance of the C1q deposits following therapy [71, 73].

Focal Segmental Glomerulosclerosis

Although FSGS more commonly results in steroid resistant disease, a proportion of cases will respond, at least initially, to steroid therapy [79, 80], and thus brief mention of the pathological features is made here. In FSGS, segmental (involving only a portion of the tuft) and focal (involving some but not all glomeruli) sclerosis of glomeruli is present. The light microscopic changes are not specific for primary idiopathic

FSGS and other causes of segmental sclerosing lesions need to be excluded [81]. The sclerosed segments show collapse of the glomerular capillary with increase in matrix material though with variable patterns of glomerular involvement [82]. The uninvolved portion of the glomerular tuft should appear essentially normal. Idiopathic FSGS typically shows early preferential involvement of the deep juxtamedullary glomeruli so that adequate sampling of this region is needed to reduce the risk of missing a focal lesion. (This risk is estimated at 35 % if only 10 glomeruli are examined, falling to a 12 % risk if 20 glomeruli are examined [79]). Even a single segmental sclerosing lesion away from the glomerular tip is sufficient to exclude a diagnosis of MCD. Clues to the presence of possible FSGS without diagnostic sclerosing lesions include abnormal glomerular enlargement, which appears to be an early indicator of the sclerotic process, and focal interstitial fibrosis and tubular atrophy (above that expected for age), which suggest glomerular loss [79]. Typically idiopathic primary FSGS shows negative immunofluorescence though non-specific uptake of IgM may be seen, commonly within sclerosed segments. Deposits similar to that of IgM nephropathy may also be present. On electron microscopy non-sclerosed glomeruli show epithelial cell foot process fusion though this may not be complete or as widespread as in typical untreated MCD. However, this is often not helpful in making this distinction as steroid therapy may partially restore foot processes in MCD.

Clinico-pathological Correlations at Presentation of Nephrotic Syndrome

Children with MCD cannot be separated on clinical features from those with FSGS or MesPGN though children with MCD are generally younger and less likely to have haematuria, hypertension and kidney dysfunction at presentation [1]. The ISKDC found that 80 % of children with MCD were aged 6 years and under compared with 50 % of children with FSGS. Systolic and diastolic blood pressures were elevated at presentation in 21 % and 14 % of children with MCD and 49 % and 33 % of children with FSGS. Haematuria occurred in 23 % of children with MCD and 48 % of children with FSGS.

Clinical and Laboratory Features at Onset of Nephrotic Syndrome

In 30–50 % cases the onset of SSNS is preceded by an upper respiratory tract infection [83, 84]. Atopy is more common in children with SSNS compared with children without SSNS [84] and more common in SSNS than SRNS [85] but an acute allergic reaction rarely precipitates a relapse. The most common initial symptom in SSNS is periorbital oedema though the significance of this finding may not be realized till the child develops generalized oedema and ascites [86]. Frequently the periorbital oedema is misdiagnosed as an allergy or as conjunctivitis. Symptoms may be present for as long as a year before diagnosis though 78 % present within a month of the first symptom. The degree of oedema is variable with some children having only mild periorbital and ankle oedema while others have pleural effusions and gross ascites with scrotal and penile oedema in boys and labial oedema in girls. The rapid formation of oedema with reduction in plasma volume may be associated with abdominal pain and malaise. Some children have serious infections at presentation including peritonitis [87]. Elevated systolic and diastolic blood pressures are present in 5–20 % at presentation in children but generally hypertension does not persist [1, 83]. Urinalysis shows ≥3–4 + protein on urinalysis with a urine protein-creatinine ratio (uPCR) ≥200 mg/mmol (≥2000 mg/g). Microscopic haematuria is present at diagnosis in 20–30 % of children but rarely persists and macroscopic haematuria is rare occurring in less than 1 % of children with SSNS [1, 83]. Serum albumin levels usually fall below 20 g/L and may be less than 10 g/L with a concomitant reduction in total protein levels. Kidney function is generally normal though serum creatinine may be elevated at presentation in association with intravascular volume depletion and rarely acute kidney failure. Children have elevated cholesterol and triglycerides at presentation and these continue to be abnormal while the child remains nephrotic. However, measurements of lipids at presentation do not provide useful additional information contributing to diagnosis or management of these children. Serum electrolytes are usually within the normal range. Total serum calcium levels are low associated with hypoalbuminaemia but ionized calcium is usually normal. Haemoglobin and haematocrit levels may be elevated at presentation in patients with reduced plasma volumes.

Outcome of Children with SSNS

Relapse

Despite a relapsing course, the long-term prognosis for most children with SSNS is for resolution of their disease and maintenance of normal kidney function. Follow up studies of children with SSNS and MCD [3, 5] indicate that 80–90 % children relapse one or more times. Among children, who relapse, 35–50 % relapse frequently or become steroid dependent [3, 5]. Although numerous predictors for a frequently relapsing or steroid dependent course have been identified, there is considerable variation in significant predictors between studies. Most studies of predictors have been retrospective studies from tertiary paediatric nephrology services. Predictors include young age at presentation [88], male sex [88, 89], a longer time to first remission after commencing prednisone [90–94], a shorter time between first remission and first relapse [5, 93, 95], the number of relapses in the first 6 months after presentation [90, 92, 95], infection at presentation or relapse [90, 95], the need for pulse methylprednisolone to achieve remission [94, 96] and low birth weight [97].

Five series involving 463 patients provide information on the likelihood of relapses persisting into adult life [4, 89, 98–100]. The duration of follow up varied from 10 to 44 years. The proportion of patients still having relapses of nephrotic syndrome as adults varied between 7 % and 42 %. Lahdenkari and colleagues [98] reported the 30 year follow up of children with SSNS first reported by Koskimies and co-workers in 1982 [3]. Of 104 patients, 10 % experienced episodes of SSNS as adults. The period between childhood and adult episodes was 2–17 years with an average of 4.6 years (range 1–11 years) between adulthood episodes. Two other studies with follow up periods of 20 years reported relapse rates of 33 % and 42 % in adult patients [4, 99]. The higher relapse rates probably reflect patient selection in these studies with high proportions of frequently relapsing or steroid dependent patients as evidenced by the need for corticosteroid sparing therapy. In both studies adult patients with relapses had had significantly higher numbers of relapses per year in childhood with childhood rates per year being 0.95–1.3 in adults with relapses compared with 0.3–0.42 per year among adults without relapses. Some studies [4, 100] but not others [99] suggest that younger age at onset predicts a higher likelihood of continuing to relapse in adult life.

Kidney Function and Development of Late Steroid Resistance

Development of late steroid resistance is well recognised but it has not been extensively studied. In European studies, the majority of children with SSNS and biopsy proven or presumed MCD do not develop late steroid resistance and have a good prognosis for kidney function. In the ISKDC series of 334 children with SSNS and MCD, 15 (4.5 %) children became transiently non-responsive to steroids but only one child (0.3 %) became persistently non-responsive to therapy and developed ESRD [5]. Similarly in the five series of 463 patients [4, 89, 98–100], only 1 patient (0.2 %) developed late steroid resistance and progressed to end stage kidney failure (ESRD) [4]. However, studies from the USA have identified higher risks of late steroid resistance and ESRD [101, 102]. In a retrospective analysis of 115 children with SSNS, 19 (17 %) developed late steroid resistance with its development being associated with a shorter interval to first relapse and with relapse during the initial steroid therapy [102]. Although more African American children had initial steroid resistance, ethnicity did not predict for late steroid resistance [102]. A retrospective study from the USA Midwest Pediatric Nephrology Consortium investigated the outcomes in 29 children with late steroid resistance [103]. The median time to late steroid resistance was 19 months (range 2–170 months). After a mean follow up of 85 ± 47 months, 20 (70 %) children were in complete or partial remission following treatment with CNI, mycophenolate mofetil (MMF) or alkylating agents. Six (21 %) had persistent nephrotic range proteinuria and three (10 %) had reached ESRD. Fewer African-American children responded to treatment compared with other children. These data suggest that children with late steroid resistance are more likely to respond to non-corticosteroid immunosuppressive agents and to have a better prognosis for kidney function compared with children with initial steroid resistance. Although initial steroid resistance is commonly associated with FSGS on kidney biopsy, the authors found no consistent relationship between initial or later kidney histology and late steroid resistance. Previous studies [104–107] have emphasized that progression to chronic kidney failure is not seen or is uncommon in children with FSGS if they continue to be steroid sensitive during follow up periods averaging about 10 years.

Other Complications of Steroid Sensitive Nephrotic Syndrome

Compared with earlier data, death is now uncommon in children with nephrotic syndrome. One study reported only one death (0.7 %) associated with disease among 138 children with SSNS presenting between 1970 and 2003 [99]. The death rate before corticosteroids and antibiotics were available was 40 %, of whom half died from infection [86]. In the 1960s, 1970s and 1980s death rates of around 7 % were reported among children with SSNS [83, 100, 108]. Infection,

particularly pneumonia and urinary tract infections, remains the most important cause of hospital admissions in children with nephrotic syndrome [109, 110]. Routine screening for latent tuberculosis infection before treatment is indicated in areas with a high prevalence of tuberculosis but this is not cost effective in areas with a low prevalence [111]. Thromboembolism, most commonly venous, is a rare but potentially life threatening complication of SSNS though it is more common in children with congenital nephrotic syndrome or SRNS and in children aged over 12 years [112]. The majority of clinically evident venous thromboembolic episodes present in the first 3 months after nephrotic syndrome diagnosis [113]. Admissions for nephrotic syndrome complicated by acute kidney injury increased significantly between 2000 and 2009 while admission rates for infection and thromboembolism were unchanged [109]. Admissions complicated by infection, hypertension, thromboembolism and acute kidney injury result in longer hospital stays and increased costs [109, 110, 114].

Indications for Kidney Biopsy

Following the studies of the ISKDC, routine kidney biopsy at presentation and before corticosteroid administration has been abandoned. Biopsy is reserved for nephrotic children aged below 1 year and for older children, for children with unusual clinical and laboratory features (macroscopic haematuria, hypertension, persistent kidney insufficiency and low C3 component of complement), for those with initial or secondary steroid resistance and for those with frequent relapses before administering second line therapy. Rarely SSNS presents in the first year of life and may prove difficult to differentiate at presentation from other forms of nephrotic syndrome occurring in this age group. Most paediatric nephrologists would consider biopsy necessary before using corticosteroids in children aged less than 1 year. Originally biopsies at presentation were recommended for children aged above 8–10 years based on the ISKDC studies [115].

Now many paediatric nephrologists do not have a rigid upper age limit for treating children with idiopathic nephrotic syndrome without prior kidney biopsy and will give corticosteroids to children and adolescents if kidney function and complements are normal, persistent hypertension absent and microscopic haematuria transitory. This management is supported by retrospective studies of clinicopathological correlations in Indian children and adolescents, in which children without two or more abnormal clinical features generally demonstrated steroid sensitivity regardless of histology [116, 117]. However, these data may not apply to African-American adolescent populations where the incidence of MCD at 20–30% [118] is much lower than the 40–50% seen in Indian or Northern European adolescents [14, 116]; kidney biopsy is recommended for children aged 12 years or above in the USA [119].

Opinions differ as to whether children with SSNS should have kidney biopsies before commencing corticosteroid sparing therapies. In some centres particularly in North America, kidney biopsies are commonly carried out before using alternative therapy while this practice has been largely abandoned in Europe and India. Three surveys of North American paediatric nephrologists in 1994, 2009 and 2013 found that 33%, 23% and 19% of respondents would biopsy children with frequently relapsing SSNS (FRNS) while 49%, 33% and 40% would biopsy children with steroid dependent SSNS (SDNS) [120–122]. Respondents reported that biopsies before commencing alternative therapy provided them with prognostic information or would influence therapy with the choice of steroid sparing agent varying according to histology [120–122]. Studies from North America have demonstrated that kidney pathology (FSGS, MesPGN and IgM nephropathy) with less favourable prognoses are common in children with FRNS or SDNS [123, 124], that steroid dependent patients with MesPGN, IgM nephropathy or FSGS are more likely to have one or more relapses after cyclophosphamide therapy compared with children with MCD [66, 104] and that African American children with FSGS are more likely to progress to chronic kidney failure [125]. In contrast studies from Europe and India [105, 117, 126] have demonstrated no relationship between kidney histology and the pre-biopsy or post cyclophosphamide course even though MesPGN and FSGS are more common in selected series of children with FRNS or SDNS compared with ISKDC data. It could be argued that kidney biopsies should be obtained before commencing treatment with CNIs to provide a baseline for interstitial and tubular damage due to the underlying disease particularly in children with FSGS, where CNIs are considered the treatment of choice [120, 122]. However, there are no data to support or refute this argument.

Before the clinician biopsies a child with FRNS or SDNS, he or she should consider whether the benefits of this procedure outweigh the potential risk of significant haemorrhage (1%) [127]. In particular the clinician needs to know whether the kidney pathology will influence the specific therapy administered and/or whether it will provide information on the likelihood of the child developing end stage renal failure. Studies show that, even if the kidney biopsy shows FSGS, the most important predictor for end stage renal failure in idiopathic nephrotic syndrome is not the kidney pathology but the achievement and maintenance of remission following any therapy [128]. Thus kidney biopsy before commencing corticosteroid sparing therapy is not indicated in children who continue to achieve complete remission with corticosteroids.

Management of Steroid Sensitive Nephrotic Syndrome

Treatment of the First Episode of Nephrotic Syndrome with Corticosteroids

Corticosteroids have been used to treat idiopathic nephrotic syndrome since the early 1950s [129]. Because of the clear net benefits of corticosteroids, no placebo-controlled trials were performed in children with nephrotic syndrome. The ISKDC agreed on a standard corticosteroid regimen for the first episode of SSNS [130] and this has provided the control group against which to test other regimens of prednisone or prednisolone therapy. At presentation children received prednisone 60 mg/m²/day (maximum dose 80 mg) in divided doses for 4 weeks followed by 40 mg/m²/day (maximum 60 mg/day) in divided doses on three consecutive days out of 7 days for 4 weeks. Subsequently a randomized controlled trial (RCT) carried out by the Arbeitsgemeinschaft für Pädiatrische Nephrologie (APN) [131] demonstrated that alternate day prednisone was more effective in maintaining remission than prednisone given on three consecutive days out of 7 days so alternate day prednisone dosing is generally used now. Since no significant differences in the time to remission or risk for subsequent relapse between single and divided doses of prednisone have been demonstrated [132], a single daily dose is now the preferred option during daily therapy to achieve greater compliance. No RCTs have examined lower daily doses of prednisone in the initial episode of nephrotic syndrome though in a small case series, doses of 30 mg/m²/day led to remission durations of similar lengths to the 60 mg/m²/day dose used by the ISKDC [133]. For ease of clinical use, a dose of 2 mg/kg has commonly been substituted for 60 mg/m²/day. However, dosing per kilogram results in lower dosing for patients with weights below 30 kg [134] and two retrospective studies have suggested that relative underdosing may increase the likelihood of FRNS [135, 136]. RCTs are required to determine if significant differences in outcomes exist if prednisone dose is calculated using weight rather than surface area.

Though demonstrated to be more effective than shorter durations of treatment (1 trial; 60 patients; relative risk [RR] 1.46, 95 % CI 1.01–2.12) [137, 138], the ISDKC/APN regimen is associated with a high relapse rate so RCTs investigated longer durations of prednisone compared with the ISKDC/APN regimen to determine if longer durations of prednisone reduced the risk of relapse and reduced the number of children, who developed FRNS or SDNS. In a meta-analysis of six trials [138], which compared 2 months of prednisone with periods of 3 months or more, prednisone administration for 3–7 months (daily for 4–8 weeks at 60 mg/m²/day and then on alternate days) reduced the risk of relapse by 30 % and of FRNS by 37 % at 12–24 months (6 trials [139–144]; 452 patients; RR 0.63, 95 % CI 0.58–0.84). There were no significant differences in the risks of adverse effects (Table 15.3). Similarly in a meta-analysis of five trials, which compared 3 months of prednisone with 6 months, prednisone administration for 6 months reduced the risk of relapse by 43 % and of FRNS by 46 % (4 trials; 424 patients; RR 0.57, 95 % CI 0.43–0.77) [143, 146–148].

Regression analysis suggested that duration of prednisone therapy was more important than total dose in determining the risk of relapse and of FRNS [138]. However, only three studies included in these meta-analyses were considered at low risk of bias for sequence generation and

Table 15.3 Adverse effects of corticosteroids

Adverse effects	No. of trials	No. of patients	% harms in high dose group	% harms in standard group	Risk difference (95 % confidence intervals)
Hypertension	7	526	11	6.2	0.05 (−0.03 to 0.06)
Ophthalmological disorders	6	460	4.9	5.1	0.00 (−0.04 to 0.12)
Growth retardation	4	354	5.1	11.2	−0.02 (−0.08 to 0.04)
Psychological disorders	4	293	4.6	2.1	0.01 (−0.03 to 0.06)
Cushing's syndrome	4	292	37.3	30.6	0.15 (−0.06 to 0.36)
Osteoporosis	3	233	0.81	4.5	−0.02 (−0.09 to 0.05)
Severe infections	2	172	32.7	40.8	−0.08 (−0.23 to 0.06)

Adverse effects of corticosteroids by 12–24 months following treatment of the first episode of steroid sensitive nephrotic syndrome for 3–7 months (total prednisone induction dose 2922–5235 mg/m²) compared with 2 months (total induction dose 2240 mg/m²). Data from seven randomised controlled trials [139–145]

allocation concealment and no studies were blinded. It is well known that trials with inadequate allocation concealment and lack of blinding can exaggerate the efficacy of therapy [149, 150]. Three new well designed RCTs (two placebo-controlled) have challenged the results of this systematic review [138]. A placebo controlled RCT [151] compared 3 months of prednisone (median cumulative dose 3360 mg/m^2) given over 3 months with the same median cumulative dose (3390 mg/m^2) given over 6 months and found no significant difference between durations in the number of children, who developed FRNS and SDNS (hazard ratio [HR] 0.97; 95 % CI 0.60–1.56) suggesting that total dose rather than duration was more important in reducing the risk of FRNS. Two further large trials suggest that there is no benefit on the risk of relapse or of FRNS of increasing the duration of prednisone therapy in the initial episode of SSNS beyond 8–12 weeks. A Japanese open label trial [152] compared 2 months of prednisone (total dose 2240 mg/m^2) with 6 months (total dose 3885 mg/m^2) in 255 children with their initial episode of SSNS. They found that the FRNS-free intervals at 24 months did not differ significantly being 56.2 % (95 % CI 47.0–64.4 %) in the 2 month treatment group and 50.8 % (95 % CI 41.4–59.4 %) in the 6 month group. An Indian placebo-controlled trial [153] compared 3 months of prednisone (total dose 3072 ± 580 mg/m^2) with 6 months (total dose 3683 ± 465 mg/m^2) in 180 children. There were no significant differences between groups in the numbers with FRNS (39 % prednisone group versus 40 % placebo group) or with sustained remission (48 % versus 36 %). The results of a fourth well designed placebo controlled RCT, comparing 2 months with 4 months of prednisone therapy with an emphasis on the documentation of harms, are awaited (ISRCTN16645249).

Surveys published in 2000, 2009 and 2013 of pediatric nephrologists in North America demonstrated considerable variation among respondents in their approach to the first episode of idiopathic nephrotic syndrome though the majority used total durations of therapy exceeding the ISKDC's 8 week regimen [120, 122, 154]. Paediatric

nephrologists have been reluctant to increase the duration of prednisone therapy possibly because data on benefits and harms come from relatively small trials of variable quality [138]. Current international and national guidelines suggest 12 weeks or more of prednisone in the initial episode of SSNS [6, 7, 119, 155].

Treatment of Relapsing SSNS with Corticosteroids

The ISKDC defined relapse as recurrence of proteinuria for three consecutive days without reference to the presence or absence of oedema (Table 15.1). Opinions differ on whether prednisone should be recommenced immediately when proteinuria has persisted for 3 days to avoid the associated complications of an oedematous relapse [156] or whether treatment should be deferred for several days [8] to determine whether proteinuria will resolve spontaneously. Proteinuria may remit spontaneously in 15–30 % relapses without commencing prednisone or increasing the dose [157, 158]. Spontaneous remissions may occur after 10–14 days of proteinuria [157]. Narchi has argued that defining and treating relapse only on the basis of proteinuria for 3 days could lead to children being erroneously labelled as having FRNS and given long term corticosteroid therapy or corticosteroid sparing agents unnecessarily [158]. There is no evidence that delaying treatment increases the time to subsequent remission so that it is reasonable to wait for some days of proteinuria before commencing corticosteroids provided the child remains well and without significant oedema. Compliance with prednisone therapy in a child with multiple relapses should be considered since poor compliance could be misinterpreted as steroid dependence. If available, triamcinolone acetonide, a long acting steroid for intramuscular injection, may be used instead of oral prednisone treatment if non-compliance is suspected [159].

The ISKDC proposed that relapses should be treated with daily prednisone (60 mg/m^2/day) till the child had been in remission for 3 days followed by prednisone on three consecutive days out of seven for 4 weeks. In the absence of data from RCTs, paediatric nephrologists have generally continued to treat relapses with daily prednisone (60 mg/m^2/day) till the child achieves remission and then continued alternate day therapy for 4 weeks or more depending on the frequency of relapses. In FRNS observational studies have demonstrated that low-dose alternate-day prednisone (mean dose 0.48 mg/kg on alternate days) or low-dose daily prednisone (0.25 mg/kg/day) reduced the risk of relapse in FRNS compared with historical controls with maintenance of growth rates [160, 161]. Recent guidelines recommend low dose alternate day prednisone in children with FRNS and SDNS [162]. Three RCTs have demonstrated that, in children with FRNS on low dose alternate day prednisone, increasing the frequency to daily administration at the onset of an intercurrent infection significantly reduces the risk of relapse [163–165] although cumulative prednisone dose/year was not significantly different between treatment groups [164]. The results of a fourth RCT evaluating this regimen in European children are awaited (ISRCTN10900733).

Adverse Effects of Corticosteroids

The most frequent adverse effects of prednisone reported in the experimental and control groups of RCTs are shown in Table 15.3. The three recent RCTs reported no differences in adverse effects between treatment groups [151, 153] except that significantly more children developed central obesity after 6 months of therapy in the Japanese study [152]. These numbers taken from short-term trials underestimate the true burden of adverse effects of corticosteroids in children with SSNS. Behavioural changes are common and include anxiety, depression, emotional lability, aggressive behaviour, inattention, hyperactivity and sleep disturbance [166, 167]. In addition nephrotic syndrome causes significant mental and economic stress on families [168]. Two studies of 43 and 15 patients have reported the rate of long term complications of the disease and its treatment in adults with continuing relapses [4,

169]. Complications included osteoporosis (63 %; 27 %), short stature (16 %; 20 %), obesity (5 %; 13 %), hypertension (7 %; 46 %) and oligozoospermia or decreased sperm motility (50 %). The risk for cardiovascular disease in adults, who had SSNS in childhood, does not appear to differ from rates in the normal population but only 62 patients were followed up [170].

The current practice of using alternate day rather than daily prednisone to maintain remission results from early reports that growth was less affected by alternate day prednisone. An RCT demonstrated that children given alternate day prednisone after kidney transplantation grow better than those given daily prednisone [171]. Recent studies of children with FRNS or SDNS, which have evaluated the adverse effects of corticosteroids on linear growth, have shown variable results. In a study of 56 children with FRNS or SDNS, children lost 0.49 ± 0.6 of height standard deviation score (SDS) during pre-pubertal growth [172]. Prednisone therapy was the only significant variable associated with the negative delta SDS. In a second study, growth rates remained normal if prednisone doses were maintained below 1.5 mg/kg on alternate days in 41 prepubertal children [173]. A third study of 64 boys found that growth rates remained stable from diagnosis for 5 years and then deteriorated [174]. In two studies final height was significantly below target in children, who required prednisone during puberty [172, 174] though partial catch up growth occurred in pubertal children permanently withdrawn from prednisone [172]. However, a third study of 60 children with SSNS found that final height SDS did not differ significantly from initial height SDS (−0.60 ± 1.0 versus −0.64 ± 0.92) though the mean final height SDS differed significantly from that expected in healthy children [175].

Derangements of bone mineral metabolism may occur in patients with nephrotic syndrome and normal kidney function. Vitamin D-binding protein and 25-hydroxyvitamin D levels are reduced in nephrotic children [176] while generally levels of calcium, 1,25-dihydroxyvitamin D and parathyroid hormone levels are normal [176–178]. 25-hydroxyvitamin D levels increase in remission but remain low compared with healthy children [178]. Abnormalities of bone mineral metabolism are aggravated by treatment with corticosteroids. Corticosteroids reduce bone formation by inhibiting osteoblast activity and inhibiting bone matrix formation. In addition they increase bone resorption directly and by reducing calcium absorption via inhibition of Vitamin D activity with a secondary increased release of parathyroid hormone [179, 180]. Low bone area and trabecular thickness with focal areas of osteoid accumulation consistent with osteopenia and abnormal mineralisation have been found in children with steroid dependent SSNS [180]; bone formation rate correlated inversely with the daily prednisone dose. Serum osteocalcin and alkaline phosphatase levels fall during corticosteroid therapy consistent with reduced bone formation [178].

Corticosteroid therapy is associated with osteopenia (decrease in quantity of bone tissue) and osteoporosis (osteopenia with bone fragility). Trabecular bone is affected more severely than cortical bone. Dual energy x-ray absorptiometry (DXA) is widely used to assess bone mass in children with SSNS. DXA measures the mass of bone mineral per projection area (grams/cm^2), which is a size dependent measure [181]. Thus results must be corrected for height in short children to prevent underestimation of bone mineral density (BMD) in comparison with age matched controls. A North American cross-sectional study of 60 children with SSNS, who had received an average of 23 g of prednisone, demonstrated that whole body bone mineral content (BMC) was increased and lumbar spine BMC was normal in children with SSNS compared with age matched local controls when adjusted for bone area, height, age, sex, pubertal stage and race [182]. Nephrotic children had significantly lower z-scores for height and higher z-scores for weight and body mass index (BMI) compared with controls. The authors concluded that corticosteroid induced increases in BMI were associated with increased whole body BMC and maintenance of BMC of spine. In contrast in 100 non obese Indian children with SSNS, who had received 5.6–18 g of prednisone, 61 %

had low BMD levels compared to normal values from North American controls [177]. No children developed fractures. These data indicate that differences in growth and body composition in different study populations need to be considered when interpreting studies of bone mass in children with SSNS. In a prospective Canadian study, lumbar spine BMD was studied at baseline (median 18 days from prednisone initiation), 3, 6, 9 and 12 months after the onset of nephrotic syndrome [183]. Only 51 % of children were receiving prednisone by 12 months. Mean lumbar spine BMD was significantly reduced at baseline and 3 months but subsequently mean values did not differ significantly from values in healthy children. Cross sectional and longitudinal studies using peripheral quantitative computed tomography (pQCT) in children with nephrotic syndrome have confirmed differential effects of corticosteroids on cortical and trabecular bone mineral densities with evidence of reduced bone formation [184, 185].

Corticosteroid associated fractures are rare in children with SSNS unlike children with chronic inflammatory disorders such as juvenile rheumatoid arthritis. In the Canadian study, only 3 children (6 %) of 65 children had asymptomatic vertebral fractures by 12 months after commencing prednisone [183]. In chronic inflammatory disorders, it is difficult to differentiate between the effects of corticosteroids and the effects of increased inflammatory cytokines, malnutrition and reduced mobility on bone mass. Children with SSNS, who do not have these additional disease effects, appear to be at less risk of osteoporosis [181]. Bone mineral density improves in children with SSNS, who are given vitamin D and calcium supplements, and many clinicians routinely prescribe supplements during prednisone therapy [186, 187]. The Committee on Nutrition of the French Society of Paediatrics recommend that children with nephrotic syndrome should receive daily vitamin D supplements particularly in winter months [188]. It is important to ensure optimum bone health in all children with SSNS by ensuring adequate intakes of calcium and vitamin D for age, regular exercise and normal pubertal progression [181].

Corticosteroid Sparing Agents in Frequently Relapsing and Steroid Dependent SSNS

Corticosteroid sparing agents are indicated in children, who have frequent relapses despite low dose alternate day prednisone and/or who have significant adverse effects of prednisone therapy. Commonly used corticosteroid sparing agents include alkylating agents (cyclophosphamide, chlorambucil), levamisole, CNI (cyclosporin, tacrolimus) and MMF. In addition mizoribine is often used in Japan. Recently rituximab has been increasingly used in children with prednisone and CNI dependent nephrotic syndrome.

Alkylating Agents

The use of cyclophosphamide and chlorambucil in childhood nephrotic syndrome was first described in 1963 [189] and 1966 respectively [190]. In RCTs alkylating agents (oral cyclophosphamide 2–3 mg/kg/day or chlorambucil 0.2 mg/kg/day administered for 8 weeks) reduced the risk of relapse by 60 % in frequently relapsing SSNS at 6–12 months after treatment (six trials [191–196]; 198 children; RR 0.43; 95 % CI 0.31–0.60) (Fig. 15.4) [197]. No significant difference in efficacy between cyclophosphamide and chlorambucil could be demonstrated in a single comparison trial [198]. In an RCT, there was no significant difference in efficacy between 8 and 12 weeks of cyclophosphamide [199] though a study comparing treated patients with historical controls had suggested a benefit of treating for 12 weeks [200]. Two studies have shown that intravenous cyclophosphamide (500 mg/m^2/dose for six monthly doses) was more effective than oral cyclophosphamide (2 mg/kg/day for 12 weeks) in reducing the risk for relapse at 6 months (RR 0.56; 95 % CI 0.33–0.92) but not at 2 years [197, 201, 202]; in both studies the cumulative dose of cyclophosphamide was lower in the intravenous treated groups. There are few data on the efficacy of second courses of alkylating agents though disease-free survival may be better than following the first course [203].

Many children will relapse after a course of an alkylating agent. In a systematic review of 26

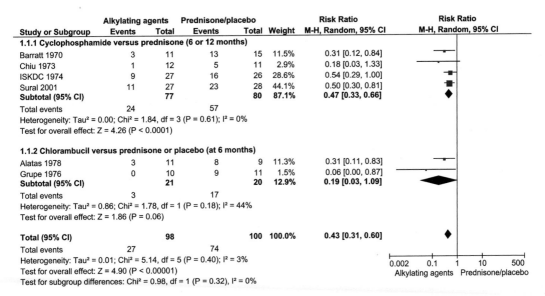

Fig. 15.4 Meta-analyses of the relative risk (95 % confidence intervals) for relapse of nephrotic syndrome by 6–12 months in six trials comparing alkylating agents (cyclophosphamide [CPA] or chlorambucil [CHL]) with prednisone alone or placebo in children with relapsing steroid sensitive nephrotic syndrome. Results are shown ordered by trial weights. The test statistic Z indicates that alkylating agents were significantly more effective in reducing the number of children who relapse compared with prednisone or placebo (Used with permission of John Wiley and Sons from Pravitsitthikul et al. [197])

studies of cyclophosphamide and chlorambucil usage in SSNS, overall relapse-free survival after 5 years was below 40% [203]. For FRNS, relapse-free survivals were 72% and 36% after 2 and 5 years respectively. For steroid dependent children, relapse-free survivals were 40% and 24% after 2 and 5 years respectively. More recent single centre studies have found similar results [204–207]. Children were more likely to relapse following alkylating agents if they had relapsed on prednisone doses above 1.4 mg/kg [205] and if they were aged below 6 years at cyclophosphamide initiation [206, 207]. Based on the differential response to alkylating agents, the Children's Nephrotic Syndrome Consensus Conference (USA) recommended that alkylating agents be the first steroid sparing agent used in FRNS but that cyclosporin should be the first line agent in SDNS [119].

Adverse effects with alkylating agents are frequent and may be severe. Latta and co-workers identified adverse effects from 38 reports involving 866 children, who received 906 courses of cyclophosphamide and 638 children, who received 671 courses of chlorambucil, for FRNS or SSNS (Table 15.4) [203]. They concluded that chlorambucil in the recommended dosage was potentially more toxic than cyclophosphamide based on a higher risk of infections, malignancies and seizures. However, this conclusion was not based on comparative data from RCTs so differences in patient populations between cyclophosphamide and chlorambucil studies cannot be excluded. Alkylating agents may reduce male fertility and cause abnormal gonadal function in men. In SSNS there is a dose dependent relationship between the number of patients with sperm counts below 10^6/ml and the cumulative dose of cyclophosphamide [203]. The threshold cumulative dose for safe use of cyclophosphamide remains uncertain because of individual reports of oligospermia in boys receiving less than 200 mg/kg. These data suggest that single courses of cyclophosphamide at a dose of 2 mg/kg/day should not exceed 12 weeks (cumulative dose 168 mg/kg). There are few data on gonadal toxicity with chlorambucil in SSNS. In male patients treated for lymphoma, total doses of 10–17 mg/kg led to azoospermia [208]; similar total doses are used in SSNS. Gonadal toxicity is less severe in women with most reports observing little or no toxicity with alkylating agents in SSNS [203]. The KDIGO guidelines suggest that second courses of alkylating agents should not be given because of their potential long term toxicity [6].

Calcineurin Inhibitors

Cyclosporin has been used to treat children with frequently relapsing or steroid dependent SSNS since 1985 [209]. Two small trials have demonstrated no significant difference in the risk of relapse during treatment between alkylating agents given for 6 or 8 weeks and cyclosporin given for 6 or 9 months (Two studies; 95 children; RR 0.91; 95% CI 0.55–1.48) [197, 210, 211]. However, most children treated with cyclosporin relapsed when therapy was ceased so the risk of relapse with alkylating agents was

Table 15.4 Adverse effects of alkylating agents in children with steroid sensitive nephrotic syndrome

Adverse effect		Cyclophosphamide		Chlorambucil	
		Total assessed	N (%) with outcome	Total assessed	N (%) with outcome
Deaths	Patients	866	7 (0.8%)	625	7 (1.1%)
Malignancies	Patients	866	2 (0.2%)	534	3 (0.6%)
Seizures	Patients	866	0 (0%)	266	9 (3.4%)
Infections	Courses	609	9 (1.5%)	552	35 (6.3%)
Haemorrhagic cystitis	Courses	762	22 (2.2%)	552	0 (0%)
Leucopenia	Courses	619	210 (32.4%)	456	151 (33%)
Thrombocytopenia	Courses	214	5 (2.1%)	408	24 (5.9%)
Hair loss	Courses	736	131 (17.8%)	237	5 (2.1%)

Used with permission Springer Science + Business Media from Latta et al. [203]

significantly lower compared with cyclosporin (RR 0.51; 95 % CI 0.35–0.74) after cyclosporin had been ceased for 12–15 months. In a prospective 2 year follow up of 44 children, in whom cyclosporin was discontinued after completion of an RCT, 37 (84 %) experienced a relapse [212]. Relapses occurred in 81 % (26/32), without relapse during cyclosporin therapy, and in 92 % (11/12) children, who had one or more relapses during cyclosporin therapy. The probability that children would re-develop FRNS or SDNS by 2 years was 75 % and 53 % respectively in children with or without relapse during their previous cyclosporin therapy. Adverse effects of cyclosporin reported in four trials were common with 13 % of children developing hypertension, 10 % reduced kidney function, 23 % gum hypertrophy and 27 % hirsutism [197]. A potentially serious adverse effect of CNI is posterior reversible encephalopathy syndrome (PRES) [213]. Nephrotic syndrome per se and hypertension also are predisposing factors for PRES.

Cyclosporin (microemulsified) is usually commenced at 4–5 mg/kg/day in two divided doses with subsequent dosing altered to achieve 12 h trough whole blood levels (C_0) of 80–150 ng/ml (67–125 nmol/L) initially. In an RCT the sustained remission rate at 2 years was significantly higher in children with C_0 levels maintained between 80 and 100 ng/ml (50–67 nmol/L) [mean dose 4.8 mg/kg/day] compared with children treated with a fixed dose of 2.5 mg/kg/day (sustained remission rates 50 % versus 15 %) [214]. Hypertension and mild arteriolar hyalinosis were less common in the fixed dose group. The cyclosporin dose, required to maintain trough levels, may be reduced by one third by administering ketoconazole as a cyclosporin sparing agent with reduction in drug costs [215]. Studies in children with SSNS have demonstrated better correlations between area under the curve concentrations of cyclosporin and 2 h post dose levels (C_2) than with trough levels [216]. A Japanese RCT compared the effect of two different C_2 levels on the relapse rate in children with FRNS or SDNS [217]. Children were randomised to receive cyclosporin to achieve whole blood C_2 levels of 600–700 ng/ml (499–582 nmol/L) for 6 months

followed by 450–550 ng/ml (374–457 nmol/L) for 18 months or to achieve C_2 levels of 450–550 ng/ml (374–457 nmol/L) for 6 months and then 300–400 ng/ml (250–333 nmol/L). The sustained remission rate was slightly but not significantly higher in the high C_2 level group compared with the lower C_2 level group but the relapse rate was significantly lower in the high level group; adverse effects did not differ between groups. RCTs are now required to compare C_0 compared with C_2 monitoring to determine which cyclosporin regimen is the most effective and safe in children with FRNS and SDNS.

Tacrolimus has not been studied in RCTs in children with SSNS. It is increasingly used because of the cosmetic effects of cyclosporin. Its efficacy appears to be similar to cyclosporin. In a prospective uncontrolled study of 74 children (50 on tacrolimus; 24 on cyclosporin), relapse frequency during 2 years follow-up did not differ significantly between treatments [218]. Nephrotoxicity defined as an increase in creatinine >25 % of baseline was less common in tacrolimus treated children and diabetes mellitus was not reported. The starting dose of tacrolimus was 0.5–1.5 mg/kg/day in two divided doses; subsequently the dose was adjusted to 12 h trough levels of 5–12 ng/ml (6–14 nmol/L). In a retrospective study of 13 children treated with tacrolimus (0.1–0.2 mg/kg/day), relapse rate was reduced from 3.5 ± 1.6 relapses per year before tacrolimus to 0.9 ± 1.1 relapses per year after 12 months of tacrolimus (P < 0.001) [219].

Cyclosporin toxicity is well documented in children receiving this therapy outside the transplant setting [220] though few studies have correlated clinical toxicity with morphologic features [221, 222]. The toxic effects are essentially the same in transplant and non transplant settings. Cyclosporin toxicity may be characterized by reduction in glomerular filtration rate with no discernible histological abnormality or by acute and chronic tubular and/or vascular changes in the kidney. Acute changes of toxic tubulopathy are classically described as "isometric" vacuolation of proximal tubular epithelial cells. However, this is often a focal phenomenon, and may only be seen in a small number of tubules in a biopsy sample. The vacuoles are of similar size (hence "isometric"), and occur on the basis of dilatation of the smooth endoplasmic reticulum of the cells. Non-specific changes of acute tubular necrosis may be seen in some cases, with intraluminal desquamation of epithelial cells, dilatation of the tubules and regenerative nuclear changes. Acute vascular changes may result in microvascular thrombosis, endothelial and myocyte necrosis. Chronic vascular changes include nodular hyaline arteriopathy, which arises on the basis of individual myocyte necrosis of arteriolar smooth muscle, and "striped" interstitial fibrosis and tubular atrophy that reflect focal ischaemic damage. Ultimately, chronic cyclosporin nephrotoxicity can result in glomerular changes of chronic ischaemia and/or focal and segmental glomerulosclerosis. The morphological nephrotoxic effects of tacrolimus are essentially the same as those seen with cyclosporin and include acute tubular necrosis, acute and chronic vascular changes, and interstitial fibrosis.

Cyclosporin-induced tubulointerstitial lesions on kidney biopsy are reported in 30–40 % of children, who have received cyclosporin for 12 months or more [223–225]. Cyclosporin associated arteriopathy is uncommon. Risk factors for fibrosis are total duration of cyclosporin therapy, having heavy proteinuria for more than 30 days during therapy [223] and higher trough cyclosporin levels [226], higher 2 h peak cyclosporin levels and concurrent use of angiotensin-converting enzyme inhibitors or angiotensin II receptor blockers [225]. Arteriopathy but not interstitial fibrosis improves after cyclosporin has been ceased for 12 months or more [227]. The duration of administration of cyclosporin is controversial with some authors suggesting that cyclosporin duration should not exceed 2 years [223]. However, other authors have suggested that longer periods of cyclosporin may be well tolerated [228]. There are few data on kidney histology in children with SSNS who have received tacrolimus but increases in interstitial fibrosis correlated with trough tacrolimus levels [229]. These few data suggest that as with cyclosporin, the lowest possible dose of tacrolimus should be used to maintain remission.

Levamisole

Levamisole is an antihelminthic agent with immunomodulatory properties [230]. Its use in childhood nephrotic syndrome was first described by Tanphaichitr and co-workers in 1980 [231] and since then many studies have described its benefits [230]. Levamisole is usually administered in a dose of 2.5 mg/kg on alternate days. Levamisole given for 4 months to 1 year reduced the risk of relapse by 50 % in comparison with prednisone alone in six trials (327 patients; RR 0.41; 95 % CI 0.27–0.61) [194, 232–236] but was ineffective in a seventh trial, in which a lower total dose of levamisole was given [197, 237]. The results of a double-blind trial evaluating levamisole compared with placebo in 103 children with FRNS or SDNS are expected in 2014 (ISRCTN23853712). A retrospective study of 304 children with FRNS or SDNS on alternate day prednisone found that levamisole therapy (mean duration 18 months) resulted in a significant reduction in relapse rate and in prednisone dosage [238]. Poor response to levamisole was associated with the need for previous treatment with alkylating agents and cyclosporin. In two RCTs the efficacy of levamisole in frequently relapsing and steroid dependent SSNS appears similar to cyclophosphamide given intravenously [239] or orally [194]. Adverse effects of levamisole are uncommon but include leucopenia, gastrointestinal effects and occasionally vasculitis [240, 241]. These data suggest that levamisole is a useful additional corticosteroid sparing agent. However, levamisole is currently unavailable in many countries.

Mycophenolate Mofetil

MMF is an inhibitor of the de novo purine pathway with inhibitory effects on T and B lymphocyte proliferation [242]. It has become an important corticosteroid sparing agent in children with FRNS or SDNS. Three prospective studies involving 76 children, who were treated for 6–12 months, reported a reduction in relapse rate of 50–75 % during treatment [242–244]. Prednisone dose could be ceased in about half the patients [242, 244]. Most children relapsed when MMF was ceased. No RCT has compared MMF with prednisone alone. However, three RCTs have assessed the relative efficacies of MMF and cyclosporin [245, 246] and of MMF and levamisole [247]. In a parallel group trial, 31 children with FRNS or SDNS were randomised to receive MMF 1200 mg/m^2/day or cyclosporin at a starting dose of 4–5 mg/kg/day for 12 months [245]. The relapse rate was significantly higher with MMF compared with cyclosporin (mean difference 0.75; 95 % CI 0.01–1.49) [197]. Sixty children with FRNS or SDNS entered a cross over trial [246]; group A received MMF (1000–1200 mg/m^2/day) with the dose adjusted to pre-dose mycophenolic acid [MPA] levels of 1.5–2.5 μg/ml for 12 months followed by cyclosporin (150 mg/m^2/day in two doses adjusted to trough levels of 80–100 ng/ml (66–83 nmol/L) for 12 months while group B received cyclosporin first followed by MMF. Relapses occurred in 21 children (82 relapses) treated with MMF and 9 patients (13 relapses) treated with cyclosporin; time to relapse was significantly longer in cyclosporin treated children in the first but not the second 12 months of the study. In both studies GFR increased during MMF treatment compared with cyclosporin treatment. In the third RCT, 112 children were randomised to receive MMF (1200 mg/m^2/day) or levamisole 2.5 mg/kg on alternate days. MMF was significantly more effective in reducing the relapse rate and prednisone dose at 12 months compared with levamisole in children with SDNS; in children with FRNS relapse rates did not differ between treatments but prednisone dose was lower in the MMF treated group [247]. Thus MMF appears to be an effective corticosteroid sparing agent in children with FRNS or SDNS.

In the cross over study [246], post hoc analysis showed that children with high MPA exposure (median MPA area under the curve [AUC] >50 μg·hr/ml) had significantly fewer relapses compared with low MPA exposure (median MPA-AUC ≤50 μg·hr/ml). Although predose MPA levels did not predict for relapse, a level of >3.5 μg/ml predicted for an MPA-AUC of >50 μg·hr/ml. In an earlier study trough levels of MPA below 2.5 μg/ml were associated with a greater risk of relapse [244]. The main adverse effects of MMF are abdominal pain, diarrhoea, anaemia, leucopenia and thrombocytopenia although to date MMF has been well tolerated in children with SSNS with only mild abdominal pain reported [242, 244]. In children, who relapse on MMF alone, a combination of cyclosporin and MMF may maintain remission with the potential for using lower cyclosporin doses [244].

Choice of First Corticosteroid Sparing Agent for Children with FRNS or SDNS

RCTs to date have not provided sufficient data on the comparative efficacy and adverse effects of corticosteroid sparing agents to allow definitive recommendations on which medication should be the first agent used in FRNS or SDNS. Although the Children's Nephrotic Syndrome Consensus Conference (USA) [119] recommended that alkylating agents be the first steroid sparing agent used in FRNS while cyclosporin should be the first line agent in SDNS, other international [6] and national guidelines [7, 155] have not provided recommendations on which medication should be preferred. Table 15.5, adapted from the KDIGO Clinical Practice Guidelines for Glomerulonephritis, lists the advantages and disadvantages of each corticosteroid sparing medication, which currently might be considered as the first agent [6]. The choice of first agent will depend on clinician and family preferences based on an assessment of the benefits and harms as well as the cost and availability of medications.

Rituximab

Rituximab is a mouse-human chimeric monoclonal antibody which binds to the CD20 antigen expressed on B cells. It was initially developed for the treatment of B-cell lymphomas. In 2004, resolution of FRNS occurred in a child treated with rituximab for idiopathic thrombocytopenic purpura [248]. There are limited data from RCTs on the efficacy of rituximab in SDNS. One RCT compared one dose of rituximab (375 mg/m^2) together with cyclosporin and prednisone with cyclosporin and prednisone alone in 54 children; at 3 months five (18 %) children receiving rituximab had relapsed compared with 13 (48 %) not receiving rituximab [249]. Preliminary data from two other RCTs (one placebo controlled) enrolling 30 and 48 children, respectively, also reported prolonged time to relapse and reduced relapse rates with rituximab [250, 251]. A further placebo controlled trial is in progress (Clinicaltrials. gov identifier NCT 01268033).

Several observational studies show that rituximab reduces the risk of relapse in SDNS and allows prednisone and other immunosuppressive agents to be ceased or the doses to be significantly reduced in the majority of children with follow up periods up to 3 years [252–258]. There is no consistent dosing regimen reported with studies using one to four weekly doses of 375 mg/m^2. Relapse rates tend to be higher when only single doses of rituximab are used. Duration of remission following a single dose of rituximab may be prolonged by continuing MMF or cyclosporin [259, 260]. Treatment leads to a suppression of CD19 cells to below 1 % and relapse generally occurs when levels of CD19 cells recover. In France repeated doses of rituximab have been used to maintain levels of CD19 cells below 1 % [255, 257]. In 18 children with SDNS followed for a mean of 3.2 years, re-treatment when CD19 cell levels rose led to a mean time to relapse of 24.5 months with 44.5 % of children off other immunosuppressive medications at last follow up (2–5.2 years); mean time to relapse without re-treatment was 9 months [257].

Because of the uncertainty about long term adverse effects and its cost, rituximab use has generally been restricted to children with steroid and cyclosporin dependent SSNS. However, in a retrospective study, Sinha and coworkers [219] compared the efficacy of two to three doses of rituximab (to achieve CD19 cell levels <1 %) with tacrolimus (0.1–0.2 mg/kg/day) given for 12 months in 23 children with SDNS, who had not received a calcineurin inhibitor previously. There were no significant differences in the relapse rates at 12 months. Prednisone dose could be reduced with both medications.

The main adverse effects reported with rituximab have been acute episodes of bronchospasm, hypotension, fever and arthralgias occurring during or immediately after intravenous infusion. Premedication with anti-histamine and anti-pyretic agents is recommended. However, more serious adverse effects reported in children with nephrotic syndrome include fatal pulmonary fibrosis [261], *Pneumocystis jiroveci* pneumonia with respiratory failure [262, 263], bacterial pneumonia including *Pseuodomonas aeroginosa* pneumonia [253] and severe myocarditis requiring heart transplantation [264]. Also existing hypogammaglobulinaemia may be prolonged by rituximab [265]. Though not yet reported in children with SSNS, a survey of patients with SLE treated with rituximab identified 57 patients with multifocal leucoencephalopathy caused by JC polyomavirus [266].

Further RCTs of rituximab therapy are required to evaluate the efficacy and safety of rituximab in SDNS before the place of rituximab in the management of SSNS can be determined. As emphasised by Boyer and Niaudet in a recent editorial, children with SDNS are not cured by rituximab but shift from dependence on calcineurin inhibitors and prednisone to dependency on rituximab [267]. Until further data are available, rituximab use should be restricted to children with steroid and CNI dependence who continue to have frequent relapses and/or have serious adverse effects of these medications [6].

Other Agents

In RCTs, no significant reduction in the risk of relapse has been demonstrated with azathioprine [197]. Mizoribine blocks purine biosynthesis pathways and is used in Japan for children with SSNS. In an RCT involving 197 children, who received 4 mg/kg/day of mizoribine or placebo, there was no significant difference in relapse rates and 16 % of treated patients developed hyperuricaemia [268]. However, mizoribine continues to be used with reports that higher dose mizoribine (5 mg/kg/day) can significantly reduce relapse rate and prednisone dose required [269]. A pilot study of the HIV antiprotease drug, saquinavir, in six children with SDNS poorly responsive to other medications, resulted in reduced relapse rates and lower prednisone dose in five children [270].

Table 15.5 Advantages and disadvantages of corticosteroid-sparing agents as first agent for use in frequently relapsing or steroid dependent steroid sensitive nephrotic syndrome

Medication	Advantages	Disadvantages
Cyclophosphamide	Prolonged remission off therapy	Less effective in SDNS
	Inexpensive	Monitoring of blood count during therapy
		Potential serious short- and long-term adverse effects
		Only one course should be given
Chlorambucil	Prolonged remission off therapy	Less effective in SDNS
	Inexpensive	Monitoring of blood count during therapy
		Potential serious adverse effects
		Only one course should be given
		Not approved in some countries
Levamisole	Few adverse effects	Continued treatment required to maintain remission
	Generally inexpensive	Limited availability
		Not approved for SSNS in some countries
Mycophenolate mofetil	Prolonged remissions in some children with FRNS and SDNS	Continued treatment required to maintain remission
	Few adverse effects	Less effective than CNIs
		Expensive
		Not approved for SSNS in some countries
Cyclosporine	Prolonged remissions in some children with SDNS	Continued treatment required to maintain remission
		Expensive
		Nephrotoxic
		Cosmetic side-effects
Tacrolimus	Prolonged remissions in some children with SDNS	Continued treatment required to maintain remission
		Expensive
		Nephrotoxic
		Risk of diabetes mellitus
		Not approved for SSNS in some countries

Used with permission from Kidney Disease: Improving Global Outcomes (KDIGO) Glomerulonephritis Work Group [6]
FRNS frequently relapsing steroid- sensitive nephrotic syndrome, *SDNS* steroid dependent steroid-sensitive nephrotic syndrome

Vaccinations in Children with SSNS

Physicians should encourage families to complete routine childhood vaccination programmes though the timing of administration of live vaccines (varicella or measles, mumps, rubella [MMR]) may need to be altered if the child is receiving high dose corticosteroids or corticosteroid sparing agents. *Steptococcus pneumoniae* and *Haemophilis influenza* are important causes of invasive infections in children with SSNS. Vaccines against both organisms are included in the routine vaccination schedules of many countries. The safety and efficacy of the 7-valent pneumococcal conjugate vaccine (PCV7) and the 23-valent pneumococcal polysaccharide vaccine (PPSV23) have been demonstrated in children with SSNS [271–273]. In 33 children with nephrotic syndrome, who received PCV7, sero-type specific antibodies increased in all children on low dose prednisone (<1 mg/kg on alternate days) and remained elevated for 12–14 months; the response was inferior in some children receiving CNI or MMF [271]. Response to PPSV23 was similar in 30 nephrotic children, who received PPSV23 while on prednisone 60 mg/m²/day, to that seen in 13 children on low dose alternate day prednisone

[272]. Similar rises in anti-pneumococcal antibody levels were detected in both groups for up to 36 months. Response was not affected by non-corticosteroid immunosuppressive agents. Relapse rates did not increase following vaccination compared with the pre-vaccination period [271] or compared with historical controls [272]. The Centre for Disease Control and Prevention's Advisory Committee on Immunization Practices now recommends that the newer 13-valent pneumococcal conjugate vaccine (PCV13) be given routinely to all children aged below 60 months and to children with immunocompromising conditions including nephrotic syndrome to 18 years [274, 275]. The Committee advises that PCV13 should be administered whether or not the child has previously received PCV7 and/or PPSV23. To broaden protection against serotypes not in PCV13, PPSV23 is also recommended for all children aged 2 years and over with immunocompromising conditions. In addition to the routine vaccinations, influenza vaccine should be given annually to children with nephrotic syndrome, who are receiving corticosteroids and/or other immunosuppressive agents [276]. Contacts of these children should also receive influenza vaccine. Hepatitis B vaccination should be administered to at risk children. Seroprotection rates were higher in SSNS than SRNS and higher in those who had received prednisone compared with those receiving prednisone with corticosteroid sparing agents [277]. Live vaccines are contraindicated in children on high dose prednisone or on other immunosuppressive agents. Most national recommendations on the administration of live vaccines in children do not specifically address children with SSNS. Based on a study of the South West Pediatric Nephrology Group [278], which demonstrated the safety and efficacy of varicella vaccine in children with SSNS, the KDIGO guidelines suggest that children not be given varicella vaccines until their prednisone dose is below 1 mg/kg/day (maximum 20 mg daily) or below 2 mg/kg on alternate days (maximum 40 mg on alternate days) and that live vaccines should not be given until children have been off cytotoxic agents for more than 3 months and off

other immunosuppressive agents (CNIs, levamisole, MMF) for at least 1 month [6]. Individual clinicians may decide that children should be off such medications for longer periods. Varicella vaccination of household contacts is also recommended [276].

Conclusions

Though the long-term outlook in most children with SSNS is for resolution of nephrotic syndrome and continuing normal kidney function, approximately half of these children will suffer multiple relapses requiring corticosteroids and one or more corticosteroid sparing agents during the course of their disease and are at risk of multiple disease and treatment related complications. In summary:

- SSNS is more common in Asian but less common in African and African-American children compared with Caucasian children. The proportion of children with idiopathic nephrotic syndrome, who respond to corticosteroids, may be decreasing.
- The aetiology and pathogenesis of SSNS remains largely unknown.
- The outcome of SSNS is for resolution of disease and normal kidney function in the majority of patients.
- The prognosis for long-term kidney function in SSNS depends on complete remission of proteinuria rather than histology so that kidney biopsies are usually not required at presentation or before commencing corticosteroid sparing therapy in children with SSNS.
- New data from large well-designed RCTs challenge previous data from six trials combined in a meta-analysis and indicate that the risk of relapse and the risk of developing FRNS are not significantly reduced by increasing the duration of corticosteroid therapy beyond 8–12 weeks in the first episode of SSNS.
- Further data from RCTs are required to determine the most effective way of using low dose corticosteroids in children with FRNS and SDNS.

- Data from RCTs have demonstrated the efficacy of alkylating agents and levamisole compared with prednisone alone. However, in RCTs there is no significant difference in the risk of relapse between azathioprine or mizoribine when compared with prednisone or placebo.
- RCTs have evaluated the relative efficacies of alkylating agents and cyclosporin or levamisole and of mycophenolate mofetil and cyclosporin or levamisole. However, these data are insufficient to provide definitive recommendations on which corticosteroid sparing agent should be preferred as the first agent in a child with FRNS or SDNS.

Further information on the underlying cause of SSNS is needed to guide therapy. New randomised controlled trials are required both to compare new therapies with existing therapies and to determine the optimal regimens for using corticosteroid therapy in SSNS. In particular further studies are required to determine the optimum total dose of corticosteroid therapy required in the initial episode of SSNS and the place of tacrolimus and rituximab in the management of children with SDNS.

References

1. Nephrotic syndrome in children: prediction of histopathology from clinical and laboratory characteristics at time of diagnosis. A report of the International Study of Kidney Disease in Children. Kidney Int. 1978;13(2):159–65.
2. The primary nephrotic syndrome in children. Identification of patients with minimal change nephrotic syndrome from initial response to prednisone. A report of the International Study of Kidney Disease in Children. J Pediatr. 1981;98(4):561–4.
3. Koskimies O, Vilska J, Rapola J, Hallman N. Long-term outcome of primary nephrotic syndrome. Arch Dis Child. 1982;57(7):544–8.
4. Fakhouri F, Bocquet N, Taupin P, Presne C, Gagnadoux M-F, Landais P, et al. Steroid-sensitive nephrotic syndrome: from childhood to adulthood. Am J Kidney Dis. 2003;41(3):550–7.
5. Tarshish P, Tobin JN, Bernstein J, Edelmann Jr CM. Prognostic significance of the early course of minimal change nephrotic syndrome: report of the International Study of Kidney Disease in Children. J Am Soc Nephrol. 1997;8(5):769–76.
6. Kidney Disease: Improving Global Outcomes (KDIGO) Glomerulonephritis Work Group. KDIGO clinical practice guideline for glomerulonephritis. Kidney Int. 2012;2(Supplement 2):139–274.
7. Indian Pediatric Nephrology Group IAoP, Bagga A, Ali U, Banerjee S, Kanitkar M, Phadke KD, et al. Management of steroid sensitive nephrotic syndrome: revised guidelines. Indian Pediatr. 2008; 45(3):203–14.
8. Consensus statement on management and audit potential for steroid responsive nephrotic syndrome. Report of a Workshop by the British Association for Paediatric Nephrology and Research Unit, Royal College of Physicians. Arch Dis Child. 1994; 70(2):151–7.
9. Abramowicz M, Barnett HL, Edelmann Jr CM, Greifer I, Kobayashi O, Arneil GC, et al. Controlled trial of azathioprine in children with nephrotic syndrome. A report for the international study of kidney disease in children. Lancet. 1970;1(7654):959–61.
10. Hogg RJ, Portman RJ, Milliner D, Lemley KV, Eddy A, Ingelfinger J. Evaluation and management of proteinuria and nephrotic syndrome in children: recommendations from a pediatric nephrology panel established at the National Kidney Foundation conference on proteinuria, albuminuria, risk, assessment, detection, and elimination (PARADE). Pediatrics. 2000;105(6):1242–9.
11. El Bakkali L, Rodrigues Pereira R, Kuik DJ, Ket JCF, van Wijk JAE. Nephrotic syndrome in The Netherlands: a population-based cohort study and a review of the literature. Pediatr Nephrol. 2011;26(8): 1241–6.
12. Wong W. Idiopathic nephrotic syndrome in New Zealand children, demographic, clinical features, initial management and outcome after twelve-month follow-up: results of a three-year national surveillance study. J Paediatr Child Health. 2007;43(5):337–41.
13. Fletcher JT, Hodson EM, Willis NS, Puckeridge S, Craig JC. Population-based study of nephrotic syndrome: incidence, demographics, clinical presentation and risk factors [Abstract]. Pediatr Nephrol. 2004;19:C96.
14. McKinney PA, Feltbower RG, Brocklebank JT, Fitzpatrick MM. Time trends and ethnic patterns of childhood nephrotic syndrome in Yorkshire, UK. Pediatr Nephrol. 2001;16(12):1040–4.
15. Schlesinger ER, Sultz HA, Mosher WE, Feldman JG. The nephrotic syndrome. Its incidence and implications for the community. Am J Dis Child. 1968;116(6):623–32.
16. Srivastava T, Simon SD, Alon US. High incidence of focal segmental glomerulosclerosis in nephrotic syndrome of childhood. Pediatr Nephrol. 1999;13(1):13–8.
17. Elzouki AY, Amin F, Jaiswal OP. Primary nephrotic syndrome in Arab children. Arch Dis Child. 1984;59(3):253–5.
18. Bhimma R, Coovadia HM, Adhikari M. Nephrotic syndrome in South African children: changing per-

spectives over 20 years. Pediatr Nephrol. 1997;11(4):429–34.

19. Borges FF, Shiraichi L, da Silva MPH, Nishimoto EI, Nogueira PCK. Is focal segmental glomerulosclerosis increasing in patients with nephrotic syndrome? Pediatr Nephrol. 2007;22(9):1309–13.

20. Shalhoub RJ. Pathogenesis of lipoid nephrosis: a disorder of T-cell function. Lancet. 1974;2(7880): 556–60.

21. Routledge RC, Hann IM, Jones PH. Hodgkin's disease complicated by the nephrotic syndrome. Cancer. 1976;38(4):1735–40.

22. Yum MN, Edwards JL, Kleit S. Glomerular lesions in Hodgkin disease. Arch Pathol Lab Med. 1975;99(12):645–9.

23. Keng KL, Kuipers F. Inoculation with measles virus in therapy of nephrotic syndrome. Ned Tijdschr Geneeskd. 1951;95(25):1806–14. Besmetting met mazelenvirus als therapie bij een nephrotisch syndroom.

24. Lander HB. Effects of measles on nephrotic syndrome. AMA Am J Dis Child. 1949;78(5):813–5.

25. Rosenblum AH, Lander HB, Fisher RM. Measles in the nephrotic syndrome. J Pediatr. 1949;35(5): 574–84.

26. Tejani A. Morphological transition in minimal change nephrotic syndrome. Nephron. 1985;39(3): 157–9.

27. Cambon-Thomsen A, Bouissou F, Abbal M, Duprat MP, Barthe P, Calot M, et al. [HLA and Bf in idiopathic nephrotic syndrome in children: differences between corticosensitive and corticoresistant forms] HLA et Bf dans le syndrome nephrotique idiopathique de l'enfant: differences entre les formes corticosensibles et corticoresistantes. Pathol Biol. 1986;34(6):725–30.

28. Kobayashi T, Ogawa A, Takahashi K, Uchiyama M. HLA-DQB1 allele associates with idiopathic nephrotic syndrome in Japanese children. Acta Paediatr Jpn. 1995;37(3):293–6.

29. Lagueruela CC, Buettner TL, Cole BR, Kissane JM, Robson AM. HLA extended haplotypes in steroid-sensitive nephrotic syndrome of childhood. Kidney Int. 1990;38(1):145–50.

30. Noss G, Bachmann HJ, Olbing H. Association of minimal change nephrotic syndrome (MCNS) with HLA-B8 an B13. Clin Nephrol. 1981;15(4):172–4.

31. Brenchley PEC. Vascular permeability factors in steroid-sensitive nephrotic syndrome and focal segmental glomerulosclerosis. Nephrol Dial Transplant. 2003;18 Suppl 6:vi21–5.

32. Eddy AA, Schnaper HW. The nephrotic syndrome: from the simple to the complex. Semin Nephrol. 1998;18(3):304–16.

33. Schnaper HW, Aune TM. Identification of the lymphokine soluble immune response suppressor in urine of nephrotic children. J Clin Invest. 1985;76(1):341–9.

34. Matsumoto K, Kanmatsuse K. Elevated vascular endothelial growth factor levels in the urine of patients with minimal-change nephrotic syndrome. Clin Nephrol. 2001;55(4):269–74.

35. Webb NJ, Watson CJ, Roberts IS, Bottomley MJ, Jones CA, Lewis MA, et al. Circulating vascular endothelial growth factor is not increased during relapses of steroid-sensitive nephrotic syndrome. Kidney Int. 1999;55(3):1063–71.

36. Eremina V, Cui S, Gerber H, Ferrara N, Haigh J, Nagy A, et al. Vascular endothelial growth factor a signaling in the podocyte-endothelial compartment is required for mesangial cell migration and survival. J Am Soc Nephrol. 2006;17(3):724–35.

37. Eremina V, Sood M, Haigh J, Nagy A, Lajoie G, Ferrara N, et al. Glomerular-specific alterations of VEGF-A expression lead to distinct congenital and acquired renal diseases. J Clin Invest. 2003;111(5):707–16.

38. Schnaper HW, Aune TM. Steroid-sensitive mechanism of soluble immune response suppressor production in steroid-responsive nephrotic syndrome. J Clin Invest. 1987;79(1):257–64.

39. Savin VJ, Sharma R, Sharma M, McCarthy ET, Swan SK, Ellis E, et al. Circulating factor associated with increased glomerular permeability to albumin in recurrent focal segmental glomerulosclerosis. N Engl J Med. 1996;334(14):878–83.

40. Dantal J, Bigot E, Bogers W, Testa A, Kriaa F, Jacques Y, et al. Effect of plasma protein adsorption on protein excretion in kidney-transplant recipients with recurrent nephrotic syndrome. N Engl J Med. 1994;330(1):7–14.

41. Garin EH, Laflam PF, Muffly K. Proteinuria and fusion of podocyte foot processes in rats after infusion of cytokine from patients with idiopathic minimal lesion nephrotic syndrome. Nephron Exp Nephrol. 2006;102(3–4):e105–12.

42. Clement LC, Avila-Casado C, Mace C, Soria E, Bakker WW, Kersten S, et al. Podocyte-secreted angiopoietin-like-4 mediates proteinuria in glucocorticoid-sensitive nephrotic syndrome. Nat Med. 2011;17(1):117–22.

43. Gebeshuber CA, Kornauth C, Dong L, Sierig R, Seibler J, Reiss M, et al. Focal segmental glomerulosclerosis is induced by microRNA-193a and its downregulation of WT1. Nat Med. 2013;19(4):481–7.

44. Abbas AK, Murphy KM, Sher A. Functional diversity of helper T lymphocytes. Nature. 1996;383(6603):787–93.

45. Mosmann TR, Cherwinski H, Bond MW, Giedlin MA, Coffman RL. Two types of murine helper T cell clone. I. Definition according to profiles of lymphokine activities and secreted proteins. J Immunol. 1986;136(7):2348–57.

46. Street NE, Mosmann TR. Functional diversity of T lymphocytes due to secretion of different cytokine patterns. FASEB J. 1991;5(2):171–7.

47. Sad S, Marcotte R, Mosmann TR. Cytokine-induced differentiation of precursor mouse CD8+ T cells into cytotoxic CD8+ T cells secreting Th1 or Th2 cytokines. Immunity. 1995;2(3):271–9.

48. Fehervari Z, Sakaguchi S. Development and function of CD25+CD4+ regulatory T cells. Curr Opin Immunol. 2004;16(2):203–8.

49. Hori S, Nomura T, Sakaguchi S. Control of regulatory T cell development by the transcription factor Foxp3. Science. 2003;299(5609):1057–61.

50. Iwakura Y, Ishigame H. The IL-23/IL-17 axis in inflammation. J Clin Invest. 2006;116(5):1218–22.

51. Weaver CT, Harrington LE, Mangan PR, Gavrieli M, Murphy KM. Th17: an effector CD4 T cell lineage with regulatory T cell ties. Immunity. 2006; 24(6):677–88.

52. Araya CE, Wasserfall CH, Brusko TM, Mu W, Segal MS, Johnson RJ, et al. A case of unfulfilled expectations. Cytokines in idiopathic minimal lesion nephrotic syndrome. Pediatr Nephrol. 2006;21(5):603–10.

53. Matsumoto K, Kanmatsuse K. Increased urinary excretion of interleukin-17 in nephrotic patients. Nephron. 2002;91(2):243–9.

54. Bakr A, Rageh I, el-Azouny M, Deyab S, Lotfy H. Serum neopterin levels in children with primary nephrotic syndrome. Acta Paediatr. 2006;95(7): 854–6.

55. Mansour H, Cheval L, Elalouf J-M, Aude J-C, Alyanakian M-A, Mougenot B, et al. T-cell transcriptome analysis points up a thymic disorder in idiopathic nephrotic syndrome. Kidney Int. 2005;67(6):2168–77.

56. Okuyama S, Komatsuda A, Wakui H, Aiba N, Fujishima N, Iwamoto K, et al. Up-regulation of TRAIL mRNA expression in peripheral blood mononuclear cells from patients with minimal-change nephrotic syndrome. Nephrol Dial Transplant. 2005;20(3):539–44.

57. Strehlau J, Schachter AD, Pavlakis M, Singh A, Tejani A, Strom TB. Activated intrarenal transcription of CTL-effectors and TGF-beta1 in children with focal segmental glomerulosclerosis. Kidney Int. 2002;61(1):90–5.

58. Schachter AD. The pediatric nephrotic syndrome spectrum: clinical homogeneity and molecular heterogeneity. Pediatr Transplant. 2004;8(4):344–8.

59. Aviles DH, Matti Vehaskari V, Manning J, Ochoa AC, Zea AH. Decreased expression of T-cell NF-kappaB p65 subunit in steroid-resistant nephrotic syndrome. Kidney Int. 2004;66(1):60–7.

60. Valanciute A, le Gouvello S, Solhonne B, Pawlak A, Grimbert P, Lyonnet L, et al. NF-kappa B p65 antagonizes IL-4 induction by c-maf in minimal change nephrotic syndrome. J Immunol. 2004;172(1):688–98.

61. Ruf RG, Fuchshuber A, Karle SM, Lemainque A, Huck K, Wienker T, et al. Identification of the first gene locus (SSNS1) for steroid-sensitive nephrotic syndrome on chromosome 2p. J Am Soc Nephrol. 2003;14(7):1897–900.

62. Ishimoto T, Shimada M, Gabriela G, Kosugi T, Sato W, Lee PY, et al. Toll-like receptor 3 ligand, polyIC, induces proteinuria and glomerular CD80, and increases urinary CD80 in mice. Nephrol Dial Transplant. 2013;28(6):1439–46.

63. Murphy WM, Jukkola AF, Roy 3rd S. Nephrotic syndrome with mesangial-cell proliferation in children – a distinct entity? Am J Clin Pathol. 1979;72(1):42–7.

64. Waldherr R, Gubler MC, Levy M, Broyer M, Habib R. The significance of pure diffuse mesangial proliferation in idiopathic nephrotic syndrome. Clin Nephrol. 1978;10(5):171–9.

65. Zeis PM, Kavazarakis E, Nakopoulou L, Moustaki M, Messaritaki A, Zeis MP, et al. Glomerulopathy with mesangial IgM deposits: long-term follow up of 64 children. Pediatr Int. 2001;43(3):287–92.

66. Tejani A, Phadke K, Nicastri A, Adamson O, Chen CK, Trachtman H, et al. Efficacy of cyclophosphamide in steroid-sensitive childhood nephrotic syndrome with different morphological lesions. Nephron. 1985;41(2):170–3.

67. Kopolovic J, Shvil Y, Pomeranz A, Ron N, Rubinger D, Oren R. IgM nephropathy: morphological study related to clinical findings. Am J Nephrol. 1987;7(4):275–80.

68. Hsu HC, Chen WY, Lin GJ, Chen L, Kao SL, Huang CC, et al. Clinical and immunopathologic study of mesangial IgM nephropathy: report of 41 cases. Histopathology. 1984;8(3):435–46.

69. Habib R, Girardin E, Gagnadoux MF, Hinglais N, Levy M, Broyer M. Immunopathological findings in idiopathic nephrosis: clinical significance of glomerular "immune deposits.". Pediatr Nephrol. 1988;2(4):402–8.

70. Al-Eisa A, Carter JE, Lirenman DS, Magil AB. Childhood IgM nephropathy: comparison with minimal change disease. Nephron. 1996;72(1):37–43.

71. Fukuma Y, Hisano S, Segawa Y, Niimi K, Tsuru N, Kaku Y, et al. Clinicopathologic correlation of C1q nephropathy in children. Am J Kidney Dis. 2006;47(3):412–8.

72. Wong CS, Fink CA, Baechle J, Harris AA, Staples AO, Brandt JR. C1q nephropathy and minimal change nephrotic syndrome. Pediatr Nephrol. 2009;24(4):761–7.

73. Hisano S, Fukuma Y, Segawa Y, Niimi K, Kaku Y, Hatae K, et al. Clinicopathologic correlation and outcome of C1q nephropathy. Clin J Am Soc Nephrol CJASN. 2008;3(6):1637–43.

74. Qin J, Yang Q, Tang X, Chen W, Li Z, Mao H, et al. Clinicopathologic features and treatment response in nephrotic IgA nephropathy with minimal change disease. Clin Nephrol. 2013;79(1):37–44.

75. Myllymaki J, Saha H, Mustonen J, Helin H, Pasternack A. IgM nephropathy: clinical picture and long-term prognosis. Am J Kidney Dis. 2003;41(2):343–50.

76. Haas M, Yousefzadeh N. Glomerular tip lesion in minimal change nephropathy: a study of autopsies before 1950. Am J Kidney Dis. 2002;39(6): 1168–75.

77. Howie AJ. Pathology of minimal change nephropathy and segmental sclerosing glomerular disorders. Nephrol Dial Transplant. 2003;18 Suppl 6:vi33–8.

78. Ostalska-Nowicka D, Zachwieja J, Maciejewski J, Wozniak A, Salwa-Urawska W. The prognostic value of glomerular immaturity in the nephrotic syndrome in children. Pediatr Nephrol. 2004;19(6): 633–7.

79. Ichikawa I, Fogo A. Focal segmental glomerulosclerosis. Pediatr Nephrol. 1996;10(3):374–91.

80. Schnaper HW. Idiopathic focal segmental glomerulosclerosis. Semin Nephrol. 2003;23(2):183–93.

81. McAdams AJ, Valentini RP, Welch TR. The non-specificity of focal segmental glomerulosclerosis. The defining characteristics of primary focal glomerulosclerosis, mesangial proliferation, and minimal change. Medicine (Baltimore). 1997;76(1): 42–52.

82. D'Agati V. Pathologic classification of focal segmental glomerulosclerosis. Semin Nephrol. 2003; 23(2):117–34.

83. Habib R, Kleinknecht C. The primary nephrotic syndrome of childhood. Classification and clinicopathologic study of 406 cases. Pathol Annu. 1971;6: 417–74.

84. Meadow SR, Sarsfield JK. Steroid-responsive and nephrotic syndrome and allergy: clinical studies. Arch Dis Child. 1981;56(7):509–16.

85. Salsano ME, Graziano L, Luongo I, Pilla P, Giordano M, Lama G. Atopy in childhood idiopathic nephrotic syndrome. Acta Paediatr. 2007;96(4):561–6.

86. Arneil GC. 164 children with nephrosis. Lancet. 1961;2:1103–10.

87. Alwadhi RK, Mathew JL, Rath B. Clinical profile of children with nephrotic syndrome not on glucorticoid therapy, but presenting with infection. J Paediatr Child Health. 2004;40(1–2):28–32.

88. Andersen RF, Thrane N, Noergaard K, Rytter L, Jespersen B, Rittig S. Early age at debut is a predictor of steroid-dependent and frequent relapsing nephrotic syndrome. Pediatr Nephrol. 2010;25(7): 1299–304.

89. Lewis MA, Baildom EM, Davis N, Houston IB, Postlethwaite RJ. Nephrotic syndrome: from toddlers to twenties. Lancet. 1989;1(8632):255–9.

90. Yap HK, Han EJ, Heng CK, Gong WK. Risk factors for steroid dependency in children with idiopathic nephrotic syndrome. Pediatr Nephrol. 2001;16(12): 1049–52.

91. Vivarelli M, Moscaritolo E, Tsalkidis A, Massella L, Emma F. Time for initial response to steroids is a major prognostic factor in idiopathic nephrotic syndrome. J Pediatr. 2010;156(6):965–71.

92. Fujinaga S, Hirano D, Nishizaki N. Early identification of steroid dependency in Japanese children with steroid-sensitive nephrotic syndrome undergoing short-term initial steroid therapy. Pediatr Nephrol. 2011;26(3):485–6.

93. Nakanishi K, Iijima K, Ishikura K, Hataya H, Sasaki S, Honda M, et al. Two-year outcome of the ISKDC regimen and frequently relapsing risk in children with idiopathic nephrotic syndrome. Clin J Am Soc Nephrol. 2013;8:787–96.

94. Harambat J, Godron A, Ernould S, Rigothier C, Llanas B, Leroy S. Prediction of steroid-sparing agent use in childhood idiopathic nephrotic syndrome. Pediatr Nephrol. 2013;28(4):631–8.

95. Noer MS. Predictors of relapse in steroid-sensitive nephrotic syndrome. Southeast Asian J Trop Med Public Health. 2005;36(5):1313–20.

96. Letavernier B, Letavernier E, Leroy S, Baudet-Bonneville V, Bensman A, Ulinski T. Prediction of high-degree steroid dependency in pediatric idiopathic nephrotic syndrome. Pediatr Nephrol. 2008;23(12):2221–6.

97. Teeninga N, Schreuder MF, Bokenkamp A, Delemarre-van de Waal HA, van Wijk JAE. Influence of low birth weight on minimal change nephrotic syndrome in children, including a meta-analysis. Nephrol Dial Transplant. 2008;23(5):1615–20.

98. Lahdenkari A-T, Suvanto M, Kajantie E, Koskimies O, Kestila M, Jalanko H. Clinical features and outcome of childhood minimal change nephrotic syndrome: is genetics involved? Pediatr Nephrol. 2005;20(8):1073–80.

99. Ruth E-M, Kemper MJ, Leumann EP, Laube GF, Neuhaus TJ. Children with steroid-sensitive nephrotic syndrome come of age: long-term outcome. J Pediatr. 2005;147(2):202–7.

100. Trompeter RS, Lloyd BW, Hicks J, White RH, Cameron JS. Long-term outcome for children with minimal-change nephrotic syndrome. Lancet. 1985;1(8425):368–70.

101. Siegel NJ, Goldberg B, Krassner LS, Hayslett JP. Long-term follow-up of children with steroid-responsive nephrotic syndrome. J Pediatr. 1972;81(2):251–8.

102. Kim JS, Bellew CA, Silverstein DM, Aviles DH, Boineau FG, Vehaskari VM. High incidence of initial and late steroid resistance in childhood nephrotic syndrome. Kidney Int. 2005;68(3):1275–81.

103. Straatmann C, Ayoob R, Gbadegesin R, Gibson K, Rheault MN, Srivastava T, et al. Treatment outcome of late steroid-resistant nephrotic syndrome: a study by the Midwest Pediatric Nephrology Consortium. Pediatr Nephrol. 2013;28(8):1235–41.

104. Berns JS, Gaudio KM, Krassner LS, Anderson FP, Durante D, McDonald BM, et al. Steroid-responsive nephrotic syndrome of childhood: a long-term study of clinical course, histopathology, efficacy of cyclophosphamide therapy, and effects on growth. Am J Kidney Dis. 1987;9(2):108–14.

105. Webb NJ, Lewis MA, Iqbal J, Smart PJ, Lendon M, Postlethwaite RJ. Childhood steroid-sensitive nephrotic syndrome: does the histology matter? Am J Kidney Dis. 1996;27(4):484–8.

106. Cattran DC, Rao P. Long-term outcome in children and adults with classic focal segmental glomerulosclerosis. Am J Kidney Dis. 1998;32(1):72–9.

107. Abrantes MM, Cardoso LSB, Lima EM, Silva JMP, Diniz JS, Bambirra EA, et al. Clinical course of 110

children and adolescents with primary focal segmental glomerulosclerosis. Pediatr Nephrol. 2006;21(4): 482–9.

108. Minimal change nephrotic syndrome in children: deaths during the first 5 to 15 years' observation. Report of the International Study of Kidney Disease in Children. Pediatrics. 1984;73(4):497–501.

109. Rheault MN, Wei C-C, Hains DS, Wang W, Kerlin BA, Smoyer WE. Increased frequency of acute kidney injury among children hospitalized with nephrotic syndrome. Pediatr Nephrol. 2014. doi:10.1007/s00467-013-2607-4.

110. Wei C-C, Yu IW, Lin H-W, Tsai AC. Occurrence of infection among children with nephrotic syndrome during hospitalizations. Nephrology. 2012;17(8): 681–8.

111. Laskin BL, Goebel J, Starke JR, Schauer DP, Eckman MH. Cost-effectiveness of latent tuberculosis screening before steroid therapy for idiopathic nephrotic syndrome in children. Am J Kidney Dis. 2013;61(1):22–32.

112. Kerlin BA, Ayoob R, Smoyer WE. Epidemiology and pathophysiology of nephrotic syndrome-associated thromboembolic disease. Clin J Am Soc Nephrol CJASN. 2012;7(3):513–20.

113. Kerlin BA, Haworth K, Smoyer WE. Venous thromboembolism in pediatric nephrotic syndrome. Pediatr Nephrol. 2013. doi:10.1007/s00467-013-2525-5.

114. Gipson DS, Messer KL, Tran CL, Herreshoff EG, Samuel JP, Massengill SF, et al. Inpatient health care utilization in the United States among children, adolescents, and young adults with nephrotic syndrome. Am J Kidney Dis. 2013;61(6):910–7.

115. Broyer M, Meyrier A, Niaudet P, Habib R. Minimal changes and focal and segmental glomerulosclerosis. In: Cameron JS, Davison AM, Grunfeld J-P, Kerr D, Ritz E, editors. Oxford textbook of clinical nephrology. Oxford: Oxford University Press; 1992. p. 298–339.

116. Gulati S, Sural S, Sharma RK, Gupta A, Gupta RK. Spectrum of adolescent-onset nephrotic syndrome in Indian children. Pediatr Nephrol. 2001;16(12):1045–8.

117. Gulati S, Sharma AP, Sharma RK, Gupta A, Gupta RK. Do current recommendations for kidney biopsy in nephrotic syndrome need modifications? Pediatr Nephrol. 2002;17(6):404–8.

118. Baqi N, Singh A, Balachandra S, Ahmad H, Nicastri A, Kytinski S, et al. The paucity of minimal change disease in adolescents with primary nephrotic syndrome. Pediatr Nephrol. 1998;12(2):105–7.

119. Gipson DS, Massengill SF, Yao L, Nagaraj S, Smoyer WE, Mahan JD, et al. Management of childhood onset nephrotic syndrome. Pediatrics. 2009;124(2):747–57.

120. Samuel S, Morgan CJ, Bitzan N, Mammen C, Dart AB, Manns BJ, et al. Substantial practice variation exists in the management of childhood nephrotic syndrome. Pediatr Nephrol. 2013;29(12):2289–98.

121. Primack WA, Schulman SL, Kaplan BS. An analysis of the approach to management of childhood nephrotic syndrome by pediatric nephrologists. Am J Kidney Dis. 1994;23(4):524–7.

122. MacHardy N, Miles PV, Massengill SF, Smoyer WE, Mahan JD, Greenbaum L, et al. Management patterns of childhood-onset nephrotic syndrome. Pediatr Nephrol. 2009;24(11):2193–201.

123. Siegel NJ, Gaudio KM, Krassner LS, McDonald BM, Anderson FP, Kashgarian M. Steroid-dependent nephrotic syndrome in children: histopathology and relapses after cyclophosphamide treatment. Kidney Int. 1981;19(3):454–9.

124. Trachtman H, Carroll F, Phadke K, Khawar M, Nicastri A, Chen CK, et al. Paucity of minimal-change lesion in children with early frequently relapsing steroid-responsive nephrotic syndrome. Am J Nephrol. 1987;7(1):13–7.

125. Sorof JM, Hawkins EP, Brewer ED, Boydstun II, Kale AS, Powell DR. Age and ethnicity affect the risk and outcome of focal segmental glomerulosclerosis. Pediatr Nephrol. 1998;12(9):764–8.

126. Stadermann MB, Lilien MR, van de Kar NCAJ, Monnens LAH, Schroder CH. Is biopsy required prior to cyclophosphamide in steroid-sensitive nephrotic syndrome? Clin Nephrol. 2003;60(5):315–7.

127. White RH, Poole C. Day care renal biopsy. Pediatr Nephrol. 1996;10(4):408–11.

128. Gipson DS, Chin H, Presler TP, Jennette C, Ferris ME, Massengill S, et al. Differential risk of remission and ESRD in childhood FSGS. Pediatr Nephrol. 2006;21(3):344–9.

129. Arneil GC. Treatment of nephrosis with prednisolone. Lancet. 1956;270(6920):409–11.

130. Arneil GC. The nephrotic syndrome. Pediatr Clin N Am. 1971;18(2):547–59.

131. Alternate-day versus intermittent prednisone in frequently relapsing nephrotic syndrome. A report of "Arbetsgemeinschaft für Pädiatrische Nephrologie." Lancet. 1979;1(8113):401–3.

132. Ekka BK, Bagga A, Srivastava RN. Single- versus divided-dose prednisolone therapy for relapses of nephrotic syndrome. Pediatr Nephrol. 1997;11(5): 597–9.

133. Choonara IA, Heney D, Meadow SR. Low dose prednisolone in nephrotic syndrome. Arch Dis Child. 1989;64(4):610–1.

134. Feber J, Al-Matrafi J, Farhadi E, Vaillancourt R, Wolfish N. Prednisone dosing per body weight or body surface area in children with nephrotic syndrome: is it equivalent? Pediatr Nephrol. 2009;24(5): 1027–31.

135. Saadeh SA, Baracco R, Jain A, Kapur G, Mattoo TK, Valentini RP. Weight or body surface area dosing of steroids in nephrotic syndrome: is there an outcome difference? Pediatr Nephrol. 2011;26(12): 2167–71.

136. Hirano D, Fujimaru T. Two dosing regimens for steroid therapy in nephrotic syndrome [Letter]. Pediatr Nephrol. 2013. doi:10.1007/s00467-013-2417-8.

137. Short versus standard prednisone therapy for initial treatment of idiopathic nephrotic syndrome in children. Arbeitsgemeinschaft für Pädiatrische Nephrologie. Lancet. 1988;1(8582):380–3.

138. Hodson EM, Willis NS, Craig JC. Corticosteroid therapy for nephrotic syndrome in children. Cochrane Database Syst Rev. 2007;4, CD001533.

139. Bagga A, Hari P, Srivastava RN. Prolonged versus standard prednisolone therapy for initial episode of nephrotic syndrome. Pediatr Nephrol. 1999;13(9): 824–7.

140. Ueda N, Chihara M, Kawaguchi S, Niinomi Y, Nonoda T, Matsumoto J, et al. Intermittent versus long-term tapering prednisolone for initial therapy in children with idiopathic nephrotic syndrome. J Pediatr. 1988;112(1):122–6.

141. Norero C, Delucchi A, Lagos E, Rosati P. [Initial therapy of primary nephrotic syndrome in children: evaluation in a period of 18 months of two prednisone treatment schedules. Chilean Co-operative Group of Study of Nephrotic Syndrome in Children] Cuadro inicial del sindrome nefrosico primario del nino: evaluacion a 18 meses de dos esquemas de tratamiento con prednisona. Rev Med Chil. 1996;124(5):567–72.

142. Ehrich JH, Brodehl J. Long versus standard prednisone therapy for initial treatment of idiopathic nephrotic syndrome in children. Arbeitsgemeinschaft für Pädiatrische Nephrologie. Eur J Pediatr. 1993;152(4):357–61.

143. Ksiazek J, Wyszynska T. Short versus long initial prednisone treatment in steroid-sensitive nephrotic syndrome in children. Acta Paediatr. 1995;84(8): 889–93.

144. Jayantha U. Comparison of ISKDC regime with a 7 months regime in the first attack of nephrotic syndrome [Abstract]. Pediatr Nephrol. 2004;19:C81.

145. Hiraoka M, Tsukahara H, Haruki S, Hayashi S, Takeda N, Miyagawa K, et al. Older boys benefit from higher initial prednisolone therapy for nephrotic syndrome. The West Japan Cooperative Study of Kidney Disease in Children. Kidney Int. 2000;58(3):1247–52.

146. Hiraoka M, Tsukahara H, Matsubara K, Tsurusawa M, Takeda N, Haruki S, et al. A randomized study of two long-course prednisolone regimens for nephrotic syndrome in children. Am J Kidney Dis. 2003;41(6): 1155–62.

147. Sharma RK, Ahmed M, Gupta A, Gulati S, Sharma AP. Comparison of abrupt withdrawal versus slow tapering regimens of prednisolone therapy in the management of the first episode of steroid responsive childhood idiopathic nephrotic syndrome [Abstract]. J Am Soc Nephrol. 2000;11(97A).

148. Mishra OP, Thakur N, Mishra RN, Prasad R. Prolonged versus standard prednisolone therapy for initial episode of idiopathic nephrotic syndrome. J Nephrol. 2012;25(3):394–400.

149. Schulz KF, Chalmers I, Hayes RJ, Altman DG. Empirical evidence of bias. Dimensions of methodological quality associated with estimates of treatment effects in controlled trials. JAMA. 1995;273(5):408–12.

150. Moher D, Pham B, Jones A, Cook DJ, Jadad AR, Moher M, et al. Does quality of reports of randomised trials affect estimates of intervention efficacy reported in meta-analyses? Lancet. 1998; 352(9128):609–13.

151. Teeninga N, Kist-van Holthe J, van Rijskwijk N, de Mos N, Wetzels JF, Nauta J. Extending prednisolone therapy does not reduce relapse in childhood nephrotic syndrome. J Am Soc Nephrol. 2013;24(1): 149–59.

152. Yoshikawa N, Nakanishi K, Oba MS, Ohashi Y, Iijima K. Increased duration and dose of prednisolone (PSL) treatment does not reduce relapses in childhood nephrotic syndrome [Abstract]. American Society of Nephrology Kidney Week 2013; 5–10 Nov 2013; Atlanta.

153. Sinha A, Bagga A, Sharma S, Saha A, Kumar M, Afzal K, et al. Randomized double blind, placebo controlled trial to compare the efficacy of 3-months versus 6-months therapy with prednisolone for the first episode of idiopathic nephrotic syndrome [Abstract]. Pediatr Nephrol. 2013;28:1361.

154. Lande MB, Leonard MB. Variability among pediatric nephrologists in the initial therapy of nephrotic syndrome. Pediatr Nephrol. 2000;14(8–9):766–9.

155. Syndrome néphrotique idiopathique de l'enfant. Haute Autorité de Santé. 2008:1–22.

156. Brodehl J. The treatment of minimal change nephrotic syndrome: lessons learned from multicentre co-operative studies. Eur J Pediatr. 1991; 150(6):380–7.

157. Wingen AM, Muller-Wiefel DE, Scharer K. Spontaneous remissions in frequently relapsing and steroid dependent idiopathic nephrotic syndrome. Clin Nephrol. 1985;23(1):35–40.

158. Narchi H. Nephrotic syndrome relapse: need for a better evidence based definition. Arch Dis Child. 2004;89(4):395.

159. Ulinski T, Aoun B. New treatment strategies in idiopathic nephrotic syndrome. Minerva Pediatr. 2012;64(2):135–43.

160. Srivastava RN, Vasudev AS, Bagga A, Sunderam KR. Long-term, low-dose prednisolone therapy in frequently relapsing nephrotic syndrome. Pediatr Nephrol. 1992;6(3):247–50.

161. Elzouki AY, Jaiswal OP. Long-term, small dose prednisone therapy in frequently relapsing nephrotic syndrome of childhood. Effect on remission, statural growth, obesity, and infection rate. Clin Pediatr (Phila). 1988;27(8):387–92.

162. Lombel RM, Gipson DS, Hodson EM. Treatment of steroid-sensitive nephrotic syndrome: new guidelines from KDIGO. Pediatr Nephrol. 2013;28(3): 415–26.

163. Abeyagunawardena AS, Trompeter RS. Increasing the dose of prednisolone during viral infections reduces the risk of relapse in nephrotic syndrome: a

randomised controlled trial. Arch Dis Child. 2008;93(3):226–8.

164. Gulati A, Sinha A, Sreenivas V, Math A, Hari P, Bagga A. Daily corticosteroids reduce infection-associated relapses in frequently relapsing nephrotic syndrome: a randomized controlled trial. Clin J Am Soc Nephrol CJASN. 2011;6(1):63–9.

165. Mattoo TK, Mahmoud MA. Increased maintenance corticosteroids during upper respiratory infection decrease the risk of relapse in nephrotic syndrome. Nephron. 2000;85(4):343–5.

166. Mishra OP, Basu B, Upadhyay SK, Prasad R, Schaefer F. Behavioural abnormalities in children with nephrotic syndrome. Nephrol Dial Transplant. 2010;25(8):2537–41.

167. Neuhaus TJ, Langlois V, Licht C. Behavioural abnormalities in children with nephrotic syndrome – an underappreciated complication of a standard treatment? Nephrol Dial Transplant. 2010;25(8):2397–9.

168. Mitra S, Banerjee S. The impact of pediatric nephrotic syndrome on families. Pediatr Nephrol. 2011;26(8):1235–40.

169. Kyrieleis HAC, Lowik MM, Pronk I, Cruysberg HRM, Kremer JAM, Oyen WJG, et al. Long-term outcome of biopsy-proven, frequently relapsing minimal-change nephrotic syndrome in children. Clin J Am Soc Nephrol CJASN. 2009;4(10):1593–600.

170. Lechner BL, Bockenhauer D, Iragorri S, Kennedy TL, Siegel NJ. The risk of cardiovascular disease in adults who have had childhood nephrotic syndrome. Pediatr Nephrol. 2004;19(7):744–8.

171. Broyer M, Guest G, Gagnadoux MF. Growth rate in children receiving alternate-day corticosteroid treatment after kidney transplantation. J Pediatr. 1992;120(5):721–5.

172. Emma F, Sesto A, Rizzoni G. Long-term linear growth of children with severe steroid-responsive nephrotic syndrome. Pediatr Nephrol. 2003;18(8):783–8.

173. Simmonds J, Grundy N, Trompeter R, Tullus K. Long-term steroid treatment and growth: a study in steroid-dependent nephrotic syndrome. Arch Dis Child. 2010;95(2):146–9.

174. Leroy V, Baudouin V, Alberti C, Guest G, Niaudet P, Loirat C, et al. Growth in boys with idiopathic nephrotic syndrome on long-term cyclosporin and steroid treatment. Pediatr Nephrol. 2009;24(12):2393–400.

175. Donatti TL, Koch VH. Final height of adults with childhood-onset steroid-responsive idiopathic nephrotic syndrome. Pediatr Nephrol. 2009;24(12):2401–8.

176. Grymonprez A, Proesmans W, Van Dyck M, Jans I, Goos G, Bouillon R. Vitamin D metabolites in childhood nephrotic syndrome. Pediatr Nephrol. 1995;9(3):278–81.

177. Gulati S, Godbole M, Singh U, Gulati K, Srivastava A. Are children with idiopathic nephrotic syndrome at risk for metabolic bone disease? Am J Kidney Dis. 2003;41(6):1163–9.

178. Biyikli NK, Emre S, Sirin A, Bilge I. Biochemical bone markers in nephrotic children. Pediatr Nephrol. 2004;19(8):869–73.

179. Bachrach LK. Bare-bones fact – children are not small adults. N Engl J Med. 2004;351(9):924–6.

180. Freundlich M, Jofe M, Goodman WG, Salusky IB. Bone histology in steroid-treated children with non-azotemic nephrotic syndrome. Pediatr Nephrol. 2004;19(4):400–7.

181. Munns CF, Cowell CT. Prevention and treatment of osteoporosis in chronically ill children. J Musculoskelet Neuronal Interact. 2005;5(3):262–72.

182. Leonard MB, Feldman HI, Shults J, Zemel BS, Foster BJ, Stallings VA. Long-term, high-dose glucocorticoids and bone mineral content in childhood glucocorticoid-sensitive nephrotic syndrome. N Engl J Med. 2004;351(9):868–75.

183. Phan V, Blydt-Hansen T, Feber J, Alos N, Arora S, Atkinson S, et al. Skeletal findings in the first twelve months following initiation of glucocorticoid therapy for pediatric nephrotic syndrome. Osteoporos Int. 2013. doi:10.1007/s00198-013-2466-7.

184. Tsampalieros A, Gupta P, Denburg MR, Shults J, Zemel BS, Mostoufi-Moab S, et al. Glucocorticoid effects on changes in bone mineral density and cortical structure in childhood nephrotic syndrome. J Bone Miner Res. 2013;28(3):480–8.

185. Wetzsteon RJ, Shults J, Zemel BS, Gupta PU, Burnham JM, Herskovitz RM, et al. Divergent effects of glucocorticoids on cortical and trabecular compartment BMD in childhood nephrotic syndrome. J Bone Miner Res. 2009;24(3):503–13.

186. Gulati S, Sharma RK, Gulati K, Singh U, Srivastava A. Longitudinal follow-up of bone mineral density in children with nephrotic syndrome and the role of calcium and vitamin D supplements. Nephrol Dial Transplant. 2005;20(8):1598–603.

187. Bak M, Serdaroglu E, Guclu R. Prophylactic calcium and vitamin D treatments in steroid-treated children with nephrotic syndrome. Pediatr Nephrol. 2006;21(3):350–4.

188. Vidailhet M, Mallet E, Bocquet A, Bresson JL, Briend A, Chouraqui JP, et al. Vitamin D: still a topical matter in children and adolescents. A position paper by the Committee on Nutrition of the French Society of Paediatrics. Arch Pediatr. 2012;19(3):316–28.

189. Coldbeck JH. Experience with Alkylating agents in the treatment of children with the nephrotic syndrome. Med J Aust. 1963;2:987–9.

190. Grupe WE, Heymann W. Cytotoxic drugs in steroid-resistant renal disease. Alkylating and antimetabolic agents in the treatment of nephrotic syndrome, lupus nephritis, chronic glomerulonephritis, and purpura nephritis in children. Am J Dis Child. 1966;112(5):448–58.

191. Chiu J, McLaine PN, Drummond KN. A controlled prospective study of cyclophosphamide in relapsing,

corticosteroid-responsive, minimal-lesion nephrotic syndrome in childhood. J Pediatr. 1973;82(4):607–13.

192. Barratt TM, Soothill JF. Controlled trial of cyclophosphamide in steroid-sensitive relapsing nephrotic syndrome of childhood. Lancet. 1970;2(7671): 479–82.

193. Prospective, controlled trial of cyclophosphamide therapy in children with nephrotic syndrome. Report of the International study of Kidney Disease in Children. Lancet. 1974;2(7878):423–7.

194. Sural S, Pahari DK, Mitra K, Bhattacharya S, Mondal S, Taraphder A. Efficacy of levamisole compared to cyclophosphamide and steroid in frequently relapsing (FR) minimal change nephrotic syndrome (MCNS) [abstract]. J Am Soc Nephrol. 2001; 12:126A.

195. Grupe WE, Makker SP, Ingelfinger JR. Chlorambucil treatment of frequently relapsing nephrotic syndrome. N Engl J Med. 1976;295(14):746–9.

196. Alatas H, Wirya IG, Tambunan T, Himawan S. Controlled trial of chlorambucil in frequently relapsing nephrotic syndrome in children (a preliminary report). J Med Assoc Thai. 1978;61 Suppl 1:222–8.

197. Pravitsitthikul N, Willis NS, Hodson EM, Craig JC. Non-corticosteroid immunosuppressive medications for steroid-sensitive nephrotic syndrome in children. Cochrane Database Syst Rev. 2013; CD002290 DOI: 10.1002/14651858.

198. Effect of cytotoxic drugs in frequently relapsing nephrotic syndrome with and without steroid dependence. A report of the "Arbetsgemeinschaft für Pädiatrische Nephrologie." N Engl J Med. 1982;306(8):451–4.

199. Ueda N, Kuno K, Ito S. Eight and 12 week courses of cyclophosphamide in nephrotic syndrome. Arch Dis Child. 1990;65(10):1147–50.

200. Cyclophosphamide treatment of steroid dependent nephrotic syndrome: comparison of eight week with 12 week course. Report of Arbeitsgemeinschaft für Pädiatrische Nephrologie. Arch Dis Child. 1987; 62(11):1102–6.

201. Prasad N, Gulati S, Sharma RK, Singh U, Ahmed M. Pulse cyclophosphamide therapy in steroid-dependent nephrotic syndrome. Pediatr Nephrol. 2004;19(5):494–8.

202. Abeyagunawardena AS, Trompeter RS. Intravenous pulsed vs oral cyclophosphamide therapy in steroid dependant nephrotic syndrome [abstract]. Pediatr Nephrol. 2006;21(10):1535.

203. Latta K, von Schnakenburg C, Ehrich JH. A meta-analysis of cytotoxic treatment for frequently relapsing nephrotic syndrome in children. Pediatr Nephrol. 2001;16(3):271–82.

204. Vester U, Kranz B, Zimmermann S, Hoyer PF. Cyclophosphamide in steroid-sensitive nephrotic syndrome: outcome and outlook. Pediatr Nephrol. 2003;18(7):661–4.

205. Zagury A, De Oliveira AL, De Moraes CAP, De Araujo Montalvao JA, Novaes RHLL, De Sa VM,

et al. Long-term follow-up after cyclophosphamide therapy in steroid-dependent nephrotic syndrome. Pediatr Nephrol. 2011;26(6):915–20.

206. Azib S, Macher MA, Kwon T, Dechartres A, Alberti C, Loirat C, et al. Cyclophosphamide in steroid-dependent nephrotic syndrome. Pediatr Nephrol. 2011;26(6):927–32.

207. Cammas B, Harambat J, Bertholet-Thomas A, Bouissou F, Morin D, Guigonis V, et al. Long-term effects of cyclophosphamide therapy in steroid-dependent or frequently relapsing idiopathic nephrotic syndrome. Nephrol Dial Transplant. 2011; 26(1):178–84.

208. Miller DG. Alkylating agents and human spermatogenesis. JAMA. 1971;217(12):1662–5.

209. Tejani A, Butt K, Khawar R, Suthabthuran M, Rosenthal CJ, Trachtman H, et al. Cyclosporine (Cy) induced remission of relapsing nephrotic syndrome (RNS) in children [Abstract]. Kidney Int. 1985;29:206.

210. Ponticelli C, Edefonti A, Ghio L, Rizzoni G, Rinaldi S, Gusmano R, et al. Cyclosporin versus cyclophosphamide for patients with steroid-dependent and frequently relapsing idiopathic nephrotic syndrome: a multicentre randomized controlled trial. Nephrol Dial Transplant. 1993;8(12):1326–32.

211. Niaudet P. Comparison of cyclosporin and chlorambucil in the treatment of steroid-dependent idiopathic nephrotic syndrome: a multicentre randomized controlled trial. The French Society of Paediatric Nephrology. Pediatr Nephrol. 1992;6(1):1–3.

212. Ishikura K, Yoshikawa N, Nakazato H, Sasaki S, Iijima K, Nakanishi K, et al. Two-year follow-up of a prospective clinical trial of cyclosporine for frequently relapsing nephrotic syndrome in children. Clin J Am Soc Nephrol CJASN. 2012;7(10): 1576–83.

213. Ishikura K, Hamasaki Y, Sakai T, Hataya H, Mak RH, Honda M. Posterior reversible encephalopathy syndrome in children with kidney diseases. Pediatr Nephrol. 2012;27(3):375–84.

214. Ishikura K, Ikeda M, Hattori S, Yoshikawa N, Sasaki S, Iijima K, et al. Effective and safe treatment with cyclosporine in nephrotic children: a prospective, randomized multicenter trial. Kidney Int. 2008; 73(10):1167–73.

215. el-Husseini A, el-Basuony F, Mahmoud I, Donia A, Hassan N, Sayed-Ahmad N, et al. Co-administration of cyclosporine and ketoconazole in idiopathic childhood nephrosis. Pediatr Nephrol. 2004;19(9): 976–81.

216. Filler G. How should microemulsified Cyclosporine A (Neoral) therapy in patients with nephrotic syndrome be monitored? Nephrol Dial Transplant. 2005;20(6):1032–4.

217. Iijima K, Sako M, Oba MS, Ito S, Hataya H, Tanaka R, et al. Cyclosporine C_2 monitoring for the treatment of frequently relapsing nephrotic syndrome in children: a multicenter randomized Phase II trial. Clin J Am Soc Nephrol. 2014;9(2):271–8.

218. Wang W, Xia Y, Mao J, Chen Y, Wang D, Shen H, et al. Treatment of tacrolimus or cyclosporine A in children with idiopathic nephrotic syndrome. Pediatr Nephrol. 2012;27(11):2073–9.

219. Sinha A, Bagga A, Gulati A, Hari P. Short-term efficacy of rituximab versus tacrolimus in steroid-dependent nephrotic syndrome. Pediatr Nephrol. 2012;27(2):235–41.

220. Tirelli AS, Paterlini G, Ghio L, Edefonti A, Assael BM, Bettinelli A, et al. Renal effects of cyclosporin A in children treated for idiopathic nephrotic syndrome. Acta Paediatr. 1993;82(5):463–8.

221. D'Agati VD. Morphologic features of cyclosporin nephrotoxicity. Contrib Nephrol. 1995;114:84–110.

222. Mihatsch MJ, Thiel G, Ryffel B. Morphologic diagnosis of cyclosporine nephrotoxicity. Semin Diagn Pathol. 1988;5(1):104–21.

223. Iijima K, Hamahira K, Tanaka R, Kobayashi A, Nozu K, Nakamura H, et al. Risk factors for cyclosporine-induced tubulointerstitial lesions in children with minimal change nephrotic syndrome. Kidney Int. 2002;61(5):1801–5.

224. Niaudet P, Habib R, Tete MJ, Hinglais N, Broyer M. Cyclosporin in the treatment of idiopathic nephrotic syndrome in children. Pediatr Nephrol. 1987;1(4):566–73.

225. Kengne-Wafo S, Massella L, Diomedi-Camassei F, Gianviti A, Vivarelli M, Greco M, et al. Risk factors for cyclosporin A nephrotoxicity in children with steroid-dependant nephrotic syndrome. Clin J Am Soc Nephrol CJASN. 2009;4(9):1409–16.

226. Kim JH, Park SJ, Yoon SJ, Lim BJ, Jeong HJ, Lee JS, et al. Predictive factors for ciclosporin-associated nephrotoxicity in children with minimal change nephrotic syndrome. J Clin Pathol. 2011;64(6):516–9.

227. Hamahira K, Iijima K, Tanaka R, Nakamura H, Yoshikawa N. Recovery from cyclosporine-associated arteriolopathy in childhood nephrotic syndrome. Pediatr Nephrol. 2001;16(9):723–7.

228. Kranz B, Vester U, Buscher R, Wingen A-M, Hoyer PF. Cyclosporine-A-induced nephrotoxicity in children with minimal-change nephrotic syndrome: long-term treatment up to 10 years. Pediatr Nephrol. 2008;23(4):581–6.

229. Morgan C, Sis B, Pinsk M, Yiu V. Renal interstitial fibrosis in children treated with FK506 for nephrotic syndrome. Nephrol Dial Transplant. 2011;26(9):2860–5.

230. Davin JC, Merkus MP. Levamisole in steroid-sensitive nephrotic syndrome of childhood: the lost paradise? Pediatr Nephrol. 2005;20(1):10–4.

231. Tanphaichitr P, Tanphaichitr D, Sureeratanan J, Chatasingh S. Treatment of nephrotic syndrome with levamisole. J Pediatr. 1980;96(3 Pt 1):490–3.

232. Dayal U, Dayal AK, Shastry JC, Raghupathy P. Use of levamisole in maintaining remission in steroid-sensitive nephrotic syndrome in children. Nephron. 1994;66(4):408–12. Erratum appears in Nephron 1994;67(4):507.

233. Levamisole for corticosteroid-dependent nephrotic syndrome in childhood. British Association for Paediatric Nephrology. Lancet. 1991;337(8757):1555–7.

234. Rashid HU, Ahmed S, Fatima N, Khanam A. Levamisole in the treatment of steroid dependent or frequently relapsing nephrotic syndrome in children. Bangladesh Ren J. 1996;15(1):6–8.

235. Abeyagunawardena AS, Trompeter RS. Efficacy of levamisole as a single agent in maintaining remission in steroid dependant nephrotic syndrome [abstract]. Pediatr Nephrol. 2006;21(10):1503.

236. Al-Saran K, Mirza K, Al-Ghanam G, Abdelkarim M. Experience with levamisole in frequently relapsing, steroid-dependent nephrotic syndrome. Pediatr Nephrol. 2006;21(2):201–5.

237. Weiss R. Randomized double-blind placebo controlled, multi-center trial of levamisole for children with frequently relapsing/steroid dependent nephrotic syndrome [Abstract]. J Am Soc Nephrol. 1993;4:289.

238. Madani A, Isfahani S-T, Rahimzadeh N, Fereshtehnejad S-M, Hoseini R, Moghtaderi M, et al. Effect of levamisole in steroid-dependent nephrotic syndrome. Iran J Kidney Dis. 2010;4(4):292–6.

239. Donia AF, Ammar HM, El-Agroudy AE-B, Moustafa FE-H, Sobh MA-K. Long-term results of two unconventional agents in steroid-dependent nephrotic children. Pediatr Nephrol. 2005;20(10):1420–5.

240. Palcoux JB, Niaudet P, Goumy P. Side effects of levamisole in children with nephrosis. Pediatr Nephrol. 1994;8(2):263–4.

241. Barbano G, Ginevri F, Ghiggeri GM, Gusmano R. Disseminated autoimmune disease during levamisole treatment of nephrotic syndrome. Pediatr Nephrol. 1999;13(7):602–3.

242. Bagga A, Hari P, Moudgil A, Jordan SC. Mycophenolate mofetil and prednisolone therapy in children with steroid-dependent nephrotic syndrome. Am J Kidney Dis. 2003;42(6):1114–20.

243. Hogg RJ, Fitzgibbons L, Bruick J, Bunke M, Ault B, Baqi N, et al. Mycophenolate mofetil in children with frequently relapsing nephrotic syndrome: a report from the Southwest Pediatric Nephrology Study Group. Clin J Am Soc Nephrol CJASN. 2006;1(6):1173–8.

244. Mendizabal S, Zamora I, Berbel O, Sanahuja MJ, Fuentes J, Simon J. Mycophenolate mofetil in steroid/cyclosporine-dependent/resistant nephrotic syndrome. Pediatr Nephrol. 2005;20(7):914–9.

245. Dorresteijn EM, Kist-van Holthe JE, Levtchenko EN, Nauta J, Hop WCJ, van der Heijden AJ. Mycophenolate mofetil versus cyclosporine for remission maintenance in nephrotic syndrome. Pediatr Nephrol. 2008;23(11):2013–20.

246. Gellermann J, Weber L, Pape L, Tonshoff B, Hoyer PF, Querfeld U, et al. Mycophenolate mofetil vs cyclosporin A in children with frequently relapsing

nephrotic syndrome. J Am Soc Nephrol. 2013;24: 1689–97.

247. Basu B, Pandey CM, Mishra OP. Randomized controlled trial to compare the efficacy & safety of mycophenolate mofetil vs. levamisole in children with frequently relapsing and steroid dependent nephrotic syndrome [Abstract]. Pediatr Nephrol. 2013;28:1353.

248. Benz K, Dotsch J, Rascher W, Stachel D. Change of the course of steroid-dependent nephrotic syndrome after rituximab therapy. Pediatr Nephrol. 2004;19(7):794–7.

249. Ravani P, Magnasco A, Edefonti A, Murer L, Rossi R, Ghio L, et al. Short-term effects of rituximab in children with steroid- and calcineurin-dependent nephrotic syndrome: a randomized controlled trial. Clin J Am Soc Nephrol CJASN. 2011;6(6): 1308–15.

250. Anh YH, Kim SH, Han KH, Cho HY, Shin JI, Cho MH, et al. Efficacy and safety of rituximab in children with refractory nephrotic syndrome: a multicenter clinical trial [Abstract]. Pediatr Nephrol. 2013;28:1361.

251. Iijima K, Sako M, Nozu K, Tsuchida N, Tanaka R, Ishikura K, et al. Multicenter, double-blind, placebo-controlled, randomized trial of rituximab for the treatment of childhood-onset refractory nephrotic syndrome [Abstract]. Pediatr Nephrol. 2013; 28(1362).

252. Guigonis V, Dallocchio A, Baudouin V, Dehennault M, Hachon-Le Camus C, Afanetti M, et al. Rituximab treatment for severe steroid- or cyclosporine-dependent nephrotic syndrome: a multicentric series of 22 cases. Pediatr Nephrol. 2008;23(8):1269–79.

253. Prytula A, Iijima K, Kamei K, Geary D, Gottlich E, Majeed A, et al. Rituximab in refractory nephrotic syndrome. Pediatr Nephrol. 2010;25(3):461–8.

254. Kemper MJ, Gellermann J, Habbig S, Krmar RT, Dittrich K, Jungraithmayr T, et al. Long-term follow-up after rituximab for steroid-dependent idiopathic nephrotic syndrome. Nephrol Dial Transplant. 2012;27(5):1910–5.

255. Sellier-Leclerc A-L, Baudouin V, Kwon T, Macher M-A, Guerin V, Lapillonne H, et al. Rituximab in steroid-dependent idiopathic nephrotic syndrome in childhood – follow-up after CD19 recovery. Nephrol Dial Transplant. 2012;27(3):1083–9.

256. Ito S, Kamei K, Ogura M, Udagawa T, Fujinaga S, Saito M, et al. Survey of rituximab treatment for childhood-onset refractory nephrotic syndrome. Pediatr Nephrol. 2013;28(2):257–64.

257. Tellier S, Brochard K, Garnier A, Bandin F, Llanas B, Guigonis V, et al. Long-term outcome of children treated with rituximab for idiopathic nephrotic syndrome. Pediatr Nephrol. 2013;28(6):911–8.

258. Ravani P, Ponticelli A, Siciliano C, Fornoni A, Magnasco A, Sica F, et al. Rituximab is a safe and effective long-term treatment for children with steroid and calcineurin inhibitor-dependent idiopathic nephrotic syndrome. Kidney Int. 2013;84: 1025–33.

259. Ito S, Kamei K, Ogura M, Sato M, Fujimaru T, Ishikawa T, et al. Maintenance therapy with mycophenolate mofetil after rituximab in pediatric patients with steroid-dependent nephrotic syndrome. Pediatr Nephrol. 2011;26(10):1823–8.

260. Fujinaga S, Someya T, Watanabe T, Ito A, Ohtomo Y, Shimizu T, et al. Cyclosporine versus mycophenolate mofetil for maintenance of remission of steroid-dependent nephrotic syndrome after a single infusion of rituximab. Eur J Pediatr. 2013;172(4): 513–8.

261. Chaumais M-C, Garnier A, Chalard F, Peuchmaur M, Dauger S, Jacqz-Agrain E, et al. Fatal pulmonary fibrosis after rituximab administration. Pediatr Nephrol. 2009;24(9):1753–5.

262. Czarniak P, Zaluska-Lesniewska I, Zagozdzon I, Zurowska A. Difficulties in diagnosing severe *Pneumocystis jiroveci* pneumonia after rituximab therapy in steroid-dependent nephrotic syndrome. Pediatr Nephrol. 2013;29:987–8.

263. Sato M, Ito S, Ogura M, Kamei K, Miyairi I, Miyata I, et al. Atypical Pneumocystis jiroveci pneumonia with multiple nodular granulomas after rituximab for refractory nephrotic syndrome. Pediatr Nephrol. 2013;28(1):145–9.

264. Sellier-Leclerc A-L, Belli E, Guerin V, Dorfmuller P, Deschenes G. Fulminant viral myocarditis after rituximab in pediatric nephrotic syndrome. Pediatr Nephrol. 2013;28:1875–9.

265. Delbe-Bertin L, Aoun B, Tudorache E, Lapillone H, Ulinski T. Does rituximab induce hypogammaglobulinemia in patients with pediatric idiopathic nephrotic syndrome? Pediatr Nephrol. 2013;28(3): 447–51.

266. Carson KR, Evens AM, Richey EA, Habermann TM, Focosi D, Seymour JF, et al. Progressive multifocal leukoencephalopathy after rituximab therapy in HIV-negative patients: a report of 57 cases from the Research on Adverse Drug Events and Reports project. Blood. 2009;113(20):4834–40.

267. Boyer O, Niaudet P. Rituximab in childhood steroid-dependent nephrotic syndrome. Nat Rev Nephrol. 2013;9:562–3.

268. Yoshioka K, Ohashi Y, Sakai T, Ito H, Yoshikawa N, Nakamura H, et al. A multicenter trial of mizoribine compared with placebo in children with frequently relapsing nephrotic syndrome. Kidney Int. 2000;58(1):317–24.

269. Fujinaga S, Hirano D, Nishizaki N, Someya T, Ohtomo Y, Ohtsuka Y, et al. Single daily high-dose mizoribine therapy for children with steroid-dependent nephrotic syndrome prior to cyclosporine administration. Pediatr Nephrol. 2011;26(3):479–83.

270. Coppo R, Camilla R, Porcellini MG, Peruzzi L, Gianoglio B, Amore A, et al. Saquinavir in steroid-dependent and -resistant nephrotic syndrome: a pilot study. Nephrol Dial Transplant. 2012;27(5):1902–10.

271. Liakou CD, Askiti V, Mitsioni A, Stefanidis CJ, Theodoridou MC, Spoulou VI. Safety, immunogenicity and kinetics of immune response to 7-valent pneumococcal conjugate vaccine in children with idiopathic nephrotic syndrome. Vaccine. 2011;29(40):6834–7.
272. Ulinski T, Leroy S, Dubrel M, Danon S, Bensman A. High serological response to pneumococcal vaccine in nephrotic children at disease onset on high-dose prednisone. Pediatr Nephrol. 2008;23(7):1107–13.
273. Aoun B, Wannous H, Azema C, Ulinski T. Polysaccharide pneumococcal vaccination of nephrotic children at disease onset-long-term data. Pediatr Nephrol. 2010;25(9):1773–4.
274. Centers for Disease C. Use of 13-valent pneumococcal conjugate vaccine and 23-valent pneumococcal polysaccharide vaccine among children aged 6–18 years with immunocompromising conditions: recommendations of the Advisory Committee on Immunization Practices (ACIP). MMWR Morb Mortal Wkly Rep. 2013;62(25):521–4.
275. Centers for Disease C, Prevention. Licensure of a 13-valent pneumococcal conjugate vaccine (PCV13) and recommendations for use among children – Advisory Committee on Immunization Practices (ACIP), 2010. MMWR Morb Mortal Wkly Rep. 2010;59(9):258–61.
276. Australian immunisation handbook. 2013. http://www.health.gov.au/internet/immunise/publishing.nsf/Content/Handbook-home.
277. Mantan M, Pandharikar N, Yadav S, Chakravati A, Sethi CR. Seroprotection for hepatitis B in children with nephrotic syndrome. Pediatr Nephrol. 2013. doi:10.1007/s00467-013-2538-0.
278. Furth SL, Arbus GS, Hogg R, Tarver J, Chan C, Fivush BA, et al. Varicella vaccination in children with nephrotic syndrome: a report of the Southwest Pediatric Nephrology Study Group. J Pediatr. 2003;142(2):145–8.

Steroid Resistant Nephrotic Syndrome

16

Rasheed Gbadegesin, Keisha L. Gibson, and William E. Smoyer

Abbreviations

ACE	Angiotensin converting enzyme
ACEI	Angiotensin converting enzyme inhibitor
ACTH	Adrenocorticotropic hormone
ACTN4	Actinin-alpha 4
ANA	Antinuclear antibody
anti-dsDNA	Anti–double stranded DNA
APOL1	Apolipoprotein L1
ARB	Angiotensin receptor blocker
CKD	Chronic kidney disease
CLC-1	Cardiotrophin like cytokine-1
CSA	Cyclosporine
eGFR	Estimated glomerular filtration rate
ESKD	End stage kidney disease
FRNS	Frequent relapsing nephrotic syndrome
FSGS	Focal segmental glomerulosclerosis
GBM	Glomerular basement membrane
GFB	Glomerular filtration barrier
GPC5	Glypican type 5
HDL	High density lipoprotein
HMG CoA	Hydroxymethylglutaryl CoA
INF2	Inverted formin 2
LDL	Low density lipoprotein
MCNS	Minimal change nephrotic syndrome
MMF	Mycophenolate mofetil
MPGN	Membrano proliferative glomerulonephritis
MYH9	Non-muscle myosin heavy chain IIA type 9
NPHS1	Nephrin
NPHS2	Podocin
PLCE1	Phospholipase C Epsilon 1gene
PLCε1	Phospholipase C epsilon 1 protein
RDA	Recommended daily allowance
RVT	Renal vein thrombosis
SDNS	Steroid dependent nephrotic syndrome
SRNS	Steroid resistant nephrotic syndrome
SSNS	Steroid sensitive nephrotic syndrome
sUPAR	Soluble form of urokinase-type plasminogen activator receptor

R. Gbadegesin (✉)
Department of Pediatrics, Division of Nephrology, Children's Health Center, Duke University Medical Center, T-Level, Rm 0909, 3959, Durham, NC 27710, USA
e-mail: rasheed.gbadegesin@duke.edu

K.L. Gibson
Department of Medicine, UNC Kidney Center, University of North Carolina at Chapel Hill, 7024 Burnett-Womack Bldg, Chapel Hill, NC 27599, USA
e-mail: kgibson@med.unc.eduand

W.E. Smoyer
Center for Clinical and Translational Research, Nationwide Children's Hospital, 700 Children's Drive, Rm W 303, Columbus, OH 43205, USA
e-mail: william.smoyer@nationwidechildrens.org

© Springer-Verlag Berlin Heidelberg 2016
D.F. Geary, F. Schaefer (eds.), *Pediatric Kidney Disease*, DOI 10.1007/978-3-662-52972-0_16

TNF-α	Tumor Necrosis Factor-alpha
TRPC6	Transient receptor potential cation channel protein type C6
UPAR	Urokinase-type plasminogen activator receptor
VLDL	Very low density lipoprotein

Introduction

Nephrotic syndrome is among the most common forms of kidney disease seen in children. The first clinical description of nephrotic syndrome is credited to Roelans in the late fifteenth century, although Zuinger later provided a detailed description of the clinical disease course and identified it as an important cause of chronic renal failure prior to the introduction of glucocorticoids [1]. Nephrotic syndrome is characterized by massive proteinuria, hypoalbuminemia, and edema, although additional clinical features such as hyperlipidemia are also typically present. Children usually present with nephrotic syndrome in the first several years of life, often with periorbital swelling with or without generalized edema. Clinical disease is believed to result from the development of structural and functional defects in the glomerular filtration barrier, resulting in the urinary loss of massive amounts of serum proteins. Physiologically, the liver attempts to compensate for this excessive loss of protein, presumably due to the decreased serum oncotic pressure, by dramatically increasing the synthesis of proteins and lipoproteins. Clinical manifestations of nephrotic syndrome develop when the urinary protein loss exceeds the capacity of the liver to synthesize albumin (and other proteins), resulting in hypoalbuminemia and edema. In children, idiopathic nephrotic syndrome is the most common cause of disease, although less commonly it can be secondary to a variety of glomerular and systemic diseases.

Prior to the introduction of antibiotics, corticosteroids and other immunosuppressive medications, nephrotic syndrome was associated with extremely high mortality rates. Indeed, almost two-thirds of children died from complications of disease, most commonly due to infection. Dramatic improvement in mortality was first noted in 1939 after the introduction of sulfonamides, and shortly thereafter penicillin. By the 1950s, the introduction of adrenocorticotropic hormone (ACTH) and cortisone further reduced mortality to ~9%, and was noted to occur in direct association with resolution of proteinuria [2]. Only after the introduction of such "effective" therapy, however, was it discovered that ~20% of children diagnosed with nephrotic syndrome failed to have resolution of proteinuria after treatment with corticosteroids. These children came to be labeled as having "steroid resistant nephrotic syndrome" (SRNS). While details related to steroid sensitive forms of nephrotic syndrome are discussed elsewhere in this text, the remainder of this chapter will focus on the epidemiology, diagnosis, treatment and clinical outcomes of those children who fail to enter clinical remission after treatment with glucocorticoids.

Definitions

One of the initial challenges of discussing the multiple issues related to children with steroid resistant nephrotic syndrome (SRNS) is that its very definition has never been standardized within the pediatric nephrology community. This has created significant challenges to our efforts to better understand the disease process as well as to interpret research publications. In this light, an important challenge for the pediatric nephrology community in the future is to establish and utilize clinically relevant definitions that are able to clearly distinguish steroid sensitive and steroid resistant nephrotic syndrome. Below are two of the most commonly used definitions:

Steroid Sensitive Nephrotic Syndrome (SSNS): Children who enter complete clinical remission in response to corticosteroid treatment alone are referred to as having steroid-sensitive nephrotic syndrome (SSNS).

Steroid Resistant Nephrotic Syndrome (SRNS): Children who fail to enter complete clinical remission after 8 weeks of corticosteroid treatment are referred to as having SRNS [3, 4].

It should be noted, however, that significant discrepancies exist in the literature about the definition for SRNS. While some authors define this state as a failure to enter remission after 4 weeks of prednisone at a dose of 60 mg/m^2/d, (see Chap. 15), others define it as failure to enter remission after 4 weeks of prednisone at a dose of 60 mg/m^2/d followed by 4 weeks of alternate-day prednisone at a dose of 40 mg/m^2/dose, or as 4 weeks of prednisone at a dose of 60 mg/m^2/d followed by three intravenous pulses of methylprednisolone at a dose of 1000 mg/1.73 m^2/dose [5, 6]. While these discrepancies make direct comparison of published reports comparing the efficacy of newer treatments for nephrotic syndrome more difficult, the most important implication for a child given the label of SRNS is that he or she is at significantly higher risk for both the development of complications of the disease (discussed later in this chapter) as well as progression of the disease to chronic kidney disease (CKD) or end stage kidney disease (ESKD).

Development of SRNS may occur either at the onset of disease or later in the clinical course. If a child never enters complete remission after initial presentation, he or she is referred to as having primary SRNS, whereas if he or she initially enters into complete remission early in the course and later develops steroid resistance he or she is referred to as having secondary or late SRNS [7].

Epidemiology

The annual incidence of nephrotic syndrome in most countries studied to date is ~2–7 new cases per 100,000 children [4, 8–11], and the prevalence is ~16 cases per 100,000 children [4]. In young children there is a male preponderance, with a male to female ratio of 2:1, although this gender disparity completely disappears by adolescence [9, 12–15].

The incidence of nephrotic syndrome has been largely unchanged over the last 35 years, but the histopathologic lesions associated with nephrotic syndrome appear to be evolving. Some reports from various countries suggest that the incidence of focal segmental glomerulosclerosis (FSGS) is increasing, even after correction for variations in renal biopsy practices, and also assuming that children who did not undergo a renal biopsy had minimal change nephrotic syndrome (MCNS) [9, 12–15].

The histologic patterns and incidence of nephrotic syndrome are also affected by ethnicity and geographic location. For instance, idiopathic nephrotic syndrome in the United Kingdom was found to be six times more common among Asian children living in the UK compared to European children [16]. In contrast, in Sub-Saharan Africa, idiopathic nephrotic syndrome occurs less commonly and disease is more commonly due to infection-associated glomerular lesions [17–19]. In the US, nephrotic syndrome has a relatively proportionate incidence among children of various ethnic backgrounds. A review of children with nephrotic syndrome in Texas reported that the distribution of children closely resembled the ethnic composition of the surrounding community [12]. These data in conjunction with the data from African countries suggest that the interaction of environmental and genetic factors plays an important role in the pathogenesis of nephrotic syndrome. Despite this, race alone seems to have a clear correlation with the histologic lesion associated with nephrotic syndrome. Indeed, 47 % of African American children with nephrotic syndrome in the above study were found to have FSGS, while only 11 % of Hispanic and 18 % of Caucasian children had this unfavorable lesion [12].

The age at presentation with nephrotic syndrome also has strong correlations with the frequency of presentation, as well as the associated renal histology. The most common age for presentation with nephrotic syndrome is 2 years, and 70–80 % of all cases of nephrotic syndrome develop in children <6 years of age [4, 8]. In addition, children diagnosed prior to 6 years of age comprised 80 % of those with MCNS, compared to 50 % of those with FSGS, and only 2.6 % of those with MPGN [20]. When analyzed based on renal histology, the median age at presentation was 3 years for MCNS, 6 years for FSGS, and 10 years for MPGN [20]. Therefore, excluding presentation in the first 12 months of life, these data suggest that the likelihood of having MCNS as a cause for nephrotic syndrome decreases with increasing age, while the likelihood for having the less favorable diagnoses of FSGS or MPGN increases [20, 21].

The renal histology associated with nephrotic syndrome additionally has important implications regarding the likelihood of a clinical response to steroid treatment. Although ~80 % of children diagnosed with nephrotic syndrome in the multi-center International Study of Kidney Diseases in Children (ISKDC) study entered clinical remission following an initial 8-week course of prednisone, analysis of these children based on histology identified steroid responsiveness in 93 % of those with MCNS, but only 30 % of those with FSGS and 7 % of those with MPGN [5, 20]. Additional variables associated with clinical steroid responsiveness include ethnicity and geographic location. While 80 % of children in western countries have steroid sensitive nephrotic syndrome, studies from South Africa, Nigeria, and Ghana reported steroid responsiveness in only 10–50 % of children with nephrotic syndrome [19, 22, 23].

Failure to enter into complete remission following steroid treatment (SRNS) has important implications regarding the risk for development of progressive chronic kidney disease (CKD) or ESKD later in life. A multi-center study of 75 children with FSGS reported that within 5 years from the diagnosis of FSGS, 21 % of children had developed ESKD, 23 % had developed CKD, and 37 % had developed persistent proteinuria, while only 11 % remained in remission [24]. Together, these data suggest that once a child is given the diagnosis of FSGS, his risk for the development of CKD or ESKD is almost 50 % within the following 5 years.

Etiology

Based on the variability in the definitions of SRNS described above, it is not surprising that SRNS is a heterogeneous clinical condition with multiple etiologies. The histopathologic entities that may cause SRNS vary in different series depending on the age group and the population being studied. However, in different series focusing on children presenting after the first year of life, the common pathologic variants associated with SRNS include focal segmental glomerulosclerosis (FSGS), membranous glomerulopathy, membranoproliferative glomerulopathy (MPGN), and minimal change disease (MCD) [9, 12, 25–28]. The majority of cases are due to disease on the continuum between MCD and FSGS (Table 16.1). Since the MCD/FSGS spectrum represents the most common pathologic variants of SRNS, and since other chapters are devoted to each of the other histologic variants, the rest of this chapter will focus mainly on FSGS.

Focal Segmental Glomerulosclerosis (FSGS)

Focal segmental glomerulosclerosis (FSGS) is a pathologic finding that is characterized by focal glomerulosclerosis or tuft collapse, segmental hyalinosis, IgM deposits on immunofluorescence staining, and podocyte foot process effacement on electron microscopy [29]. In the majority of children it is characterized by SRNS and progression to end-stage kidney disease (ESKD) within 5–10 years of diagnosis [24]. It was first described in kidney biopsies of adults with nephrotic syndrome by Fahr in 1925, although it was Rich who later made the observation that the lesion of

Table 16.1 Pathologic findings in steroid resistant nephrotic syndrome

Histology	South-Asia[a] [25, 26] n=326	South-Africa [28] n=183	Poland [27] n=34	USA[b] [9, 12] n=253
MCD	38.4	36.1	5.9	45.4
FSGS	41.5	36.1	32.4	26.5
MESGN	14.1	8.1	55.8	10.3
MEMB	4.0	–	–	1.2
MPGN	1.0	–	5.9	7.5
OTHERS	1.0	19.7	–	9.1

[a]Two studies one each from Pakistan and India [25, 26]
[b]Summary of two studies. Some of the patients were diagnosed with frequent relapsing and steroid dependent NS [9, 12]

FSGS in children with nephrotic syndrome classically starts from the corticomedullary junction before involving other parts of the renal cortex [30, 31]. The observation of Rich is probably the explanation for why many cases of FSGS are initially misdiagnosed as MCD since early disease may be confined to the corticomedullary junction. The incidence of FSGS is estimated at seven per million people, and the incidence is higher in blacks than whites and the rate of decline in kidney function is also worse in blacks [32]. The incidence of FSGS is increasing in all populations. In a predominant adult cohort, Kitiyakara et al., reported an 11-fold increase among dialysis patients over a 21 year period, and a similar pattern was reported in a population-based study in the USA [33, 34]. The most compelling pediatric data to date are contained in a metanalysis that examined over 1100 nephrotic patients over two time points. This study demonstrated a twofold increase in the incidence of nephrotic syndrome in children [35]. The reason for the increasing incidence is unknown, but possible explanations include changing criteria in the selection of patients for kidney biopsy, better diagnostic instruments, or changing environmental factors such as infection-driven disease.

Clinical and Pathologic Classification of FSGS

Until recently, FSGS was classified based on presumed causes, and it is recognized that the etiology is unknown in more than 80% of cases of so called primary or idiopathic FSGS. The rest may be secondary to other disease processes such as infectious agents like hepatitis, HIV, toxic agents, ischemia, obesity and other glomerulonephritides. A list of causes of FSGS is shown in Table 16.2. Familial or hereditary cases of FSGS are increasingly being recognized with advances in genomic science. Although this group is estimated to be responsible for <5% of all cases, detailed studies of hereditary FSGS have shed more light on the molecular pathogenesis of the disease [36]. It has been recognized by pathologists that the morphological changes in kidney biopsies of patients with

FSGS are heterogeneous; however, until recently there was no standard classification of FSGS. In order to standardize the pathological diagnosis of FSGS and relate histologic findings to clinical course, the Columbia classification of FSGS was proposed [37]. In this classification schema, five patterns of FSGS have been proposed including: (1) FSGS not otherwise specified (NOS), (2) Perihilar variant, (3) Cellular variant, (4) Tip variant, and (5) Collapsing variant (Table 16.3 and Fig. 16.1a–j). The clinical significance of the variants is still being studied. In a cohort of adults with FSGS, it was reported that collapsing FSGS had the highest rate of renal insufficiency at presentation and worst long term outcome [38].

Table 16.2 Etiology of FSGS

Primary/idiopathic FSGS (80% of all cases)
Familial FSGS (See Tables 16.4 and 16.5)
Infections
HIV infection
Hepatitis B and C
Cytomegalovirus
Epstein-Barr virus
Parvovirus B19
Drugs/toxic agents
Captopril
Non-steroidal anti-inflammatory drugs (NSAIDS)
Gold
Interferon-α
Lithium
Pamidronate
Mercury
Heroin
Hyperfiltration
Obesity
Bilateral or unilateral renal dysplasia
Reflux nephropathy
Other causes of glomerulonephritis associated with nephron loss
Aging
Ischemia
Renal artery stenosis
Hypertensive kidney disease
Calcineurin inhibitor nephrotoxicity
Acute and chronic renal allograft rejection
Cholesterol crystal embolism
Cyanotic congenital heart disease

Table 16.3 Outcome of FSGS histologic subtypes in the NIH-sponsored FSGS trial

FSGS subtypes	Frequency (%) n = 138	% with ESKD at 3 years
NOS	68	20
Collapsing	12	47
Tip	10	7
Perihilar	7	Number too small
Cellular	3	Number too small

Data from Sorof et al. [21]

The most comprehensive prospective report of the clinical significance of the classification in children comes from the analysis of the kidney biopsies from the patient cohort in the recently-completed FSGS trial [39]. In this study FSGS NOS was the most common variant, being responsible for 68 % of all cases, with collapsing, tip, perihilar and cellular variants responsible for 12 %, 10 %, 7 % and 3 %, respectively. Patients with collapsing FSGS were more likely to be black and to have nephrotic syndrome with renal impairment at presentation, compared to patients with NOS and tip variants [39]. Furthermore, globally sclerotic changes were found more commonly in the NOS variant while segmental sclerosis, tubular atrophy and interstitial fibrosis were found more commonly in collapsing FSGS [39]. At the end of 3 years follow up, 47 % of patients with collapsing FSGS were in ESKD compared with 20 % and 7 % for the NOS and tip variants, respectively [39]. Thus, in this study collapsing FSGS appeared to have the worst prognosis, while the tip variant had the most favorable prognosis (Table 16.3).

Pathogenesis

The Glomerular Filtration Barrier and the Podocyte

The central abnormality in all cases of nephrotic syndrome is the development of massive proteinuria. Although the molecular basis for this is still speculative, there is evidence that nephrotic syndrome due to FSGS is due to a defect in the glomerular filtration barrier (GFB). The glomerular filtration barrier is made up of specialized fenestrated endothelial cells, the glomerular basement membrane (GBM), and glomerular epithelial cells (podocytes) whose distal foot processes are attached to the GBM (Fig. 16.2) [40]. Maintenance of the functional integrity of the GFB depends on structural and functional interactions among the three components of the GFB [41–45]. Recent evidence from the study of familial FSGS suggests that the podocyte is the most important component of the GFB in that virtually all the genes mutated in hereditary FSGS localize to the podocyte and its slit diaphragm [46–62]. These observations have given rise to the concept of FSGS being a podocytopathy [63]. Podocytes are terminally differentiated glomerular visceral epithelial cells, consisting of a cell body, major and primary processes, and foot processes that interdigitate with neighboring podocytes to form a highly specialized gap junction, the slit diaphragm. The mechanisms by which podocyte damage evolves into the pathological appearance seen in FSGS have been studied extensively by Kriz and colleagues in a series of experiments in murine models of FSGS [64]. The initial defect appears to be a reduction in podocyte number and the inability of podocytes to completely cover the glomerular tufts. The reduction in podocyte density causes the loss of separation between the glomerular tuft and Bowman's capsule, leading to the formation of synechiae or adhesions between the tuft and the Bowman's capsule [64]. The perfused capillaries lacking podocytes at the site of tuft adhesion then deliver their filtrate into the interstitium instead of Bowman's space (Fig. 16.3) [64]. This misdirected filtration through capillaries lacking podocytes leads to progression of segmental injury, tubular degeneration and interstitial fibrosis [64]. Further evidence for the role of podocytopenia in the pathogenesis of FSGS was shown by Wiggins' group using a rat model of diphtheria toxin-induced podocyte depletion in which the extent of podocyte loss is regulated [65]. In this model, mild podocyte loss resulted in hypertrophy of the remaining podocytes to cover the glomerular basement membrane. However, with moderate to severe depletion, FSGS and global sclerosis developed [65].

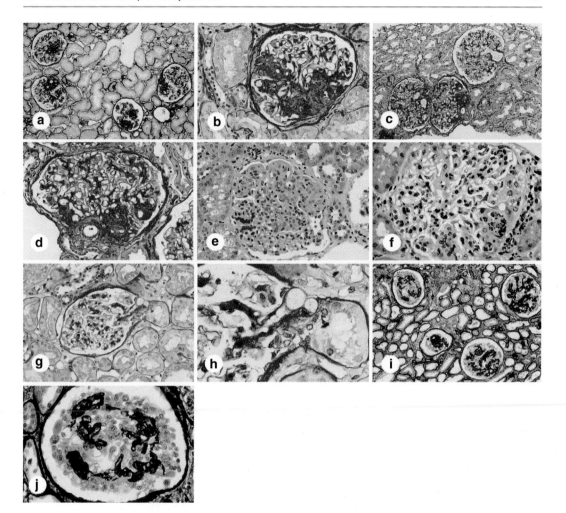

Fig. 16.1 (a-j). Columbia classification of FSGS. *FSGS NOS*: (**a**) *Low* power magnification showing segmental sclerosis in two glomeruli. Lesions are characterized by increased matrix and obliteration of the capillary lumen. Distribution of lesions within the tuft is variable. (**b**) PAS staining at higher magnification showing obliteration of glomerular tuft by increased matrix and hyaline deposit. Sclerosed segments form adhesions to Bowman's capsule, note that there is no podocyte hypertrophy or hyperplasia. *FSGS perihilar variant*: (**c**) *Low* power examination showing segmental sclerosis affecting the vascular pole in one of three glomeruli. The lesion shows increased sclerosis and hyalinosis and there is adhesion of the sclerotic segment to the Bowman's capsule in the vascular pole region. (**d**) *Higher* magnification of C showing increased sclerosis and glassy hyalinosis deposited in the vascular pole segment of the tuft. *FSGS cellular variant*: (**e**) The glomerulus in this image shows endocapillary hypercellularity. The involved segments are engorged with endocapillary cells including mononuclear leukocytes. (**f**) Further

demonstration of numerous endocapillary leukocytes mimicking endocapillary glomerulonephritis. In addition there is hypertrophy and hyperplasia of overlying podocytes. *FSGS tip variant*: (**g**) *Low* power view shows a segmental lesion involving the tip domain at the origin of the tubular pole. (**h**) *Higher* magnification of the lesion in G showing endocapillary foam cells and adhesion of the sclerotic segment to Bowman's capsule at the mouth of the proximal tubule. *FSGS collapsing variant*: (**i**) *Low* power magnification shows four glomeruli with global collapse of the tuft and podocyte hypertrophy and hyperplasia with tubular degenerative changes. (**j**) *High* power magnification shows global occlusion of capillary lumina by implosive collapse of the glomerular basement membranes. There is no significant increase in intracapillary cells or matrix. Overlying podocytes form a cellular corona over the collapsed tuft. Some of the enlarged podocytes appear binucleated and have lost their cohesion to the tuft (Used with permission of Elsevier from D'Agati et al. [37])

The Role of Circulating Factors

There are experimental data to support the existence of soluble mediators that may alter capillary wall permeability in nephrotic syndrome; most of these observations came from the work of Savin et al. [66–69]. Evidence for this includes:

1. Development of nephrotic syndrome in newborn babies born to mothers with nephrotic syndrome who apparently transferred a soluble factor to their fetuses in utero [68],
2. Marked reduction of proteinuria following treatment with Protein A immunoadsorption in various types of primary nephrotic syndrome [70],
3. Recurrence of FSGS in transplanted kidneys in patients with primary FSGS, with remission of recurrent disease induced by treatment with Protein A immunoadsorption, due to presumed removal of circulating factors, [71], and

4. Induction of enhanced glomerular permeability in experimental animals injected with serum from patients with FSGS recurrence in transplanted kidneys [72].

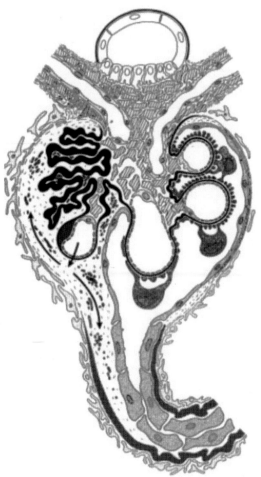

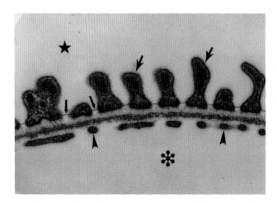

Fig. 16.2 Electron Micrograph of the Components of the Glomerular Filtration Barrier. During normal glomerular filtration, plasma water is filtered from the glomerular capillary lumen (*asterisk*) through the fenestrated endothelial cell layer (*arrowheads*), then across the glomerular basement membrane (*GBM*) and through the slit diaphragms (*small arrows*) which bridge the filtration slits between adjacent podocyte foot processes (*large arrows*) and finally into the urinary space (*star*) where it enters the lumen of the proximal tubule. These podocyte foot processes are normally tall and evenly-spaced along the GBM, but during nephrotic syndrome they become spread out along the GBM, with apical displacement of the slit diaphragms. The layer of negatively-charged glycocalyx can be seen in this image as a blurry coating on the apical surfaces of the podocyte foot processes (Used with permission from Smoyer et al. [40])

Fig. 16.3 Kriz's misdirected filtration hypothesis of evolving FSGS lesion. The glomerular basement membrane (*GBM*) is shown in black, podocytes are densely stippled, parietal epithelial cells are less densely stippled and interstitial as well as endothelial cells are loosely stippled, mesangial cells are hatched. The tuft adhesion contains several collapsed capillary loops. It also contains a perfused loop, which is partially hyalinized. The filtrate of this loop is delivered into a paraglomerular space that is separated from the interstitium by a layer of fibroblasts. This newly created space extends onto the outer aspect of the tubule by expanding and/or separating the tubular basement membrane from its epithelium (Used with permission of Oxford University Press from Kriz [64])

Furthermore, inhibitors of glomerular permeability have also been isolated from the serum of children with FSGS, and identified as components of apolipoproteins, suggesting that an imbalance between serum permeability factors and permeability inhibitors may have a pathogenic role in FSGS [73]. The physicochemical properties of the circulating factors have been subjects of intense research in the past. In the last 5 years, candidate molecules have been reported both from human and experimental animal studies. Using a galactose affinity purification method to enrich serum/plasma from patients with FSGS and FSGS recurrence, Savin et al. showed by mass spectrometry that cardiotrophin like cytokine-1 (CLC-1), a member of the IL-6 cytokine family, is a candidate FSGS permeability factor [74, 75]. In this study, they found that CLC-1 was present in the plasma of patients with FSGS and in patients with recurrent FSGS in their renal allografts, its concentration may be up to 100 times that of normal subjects. In addition, they showed that CLC-1 decreases nephrin expression in podocyte culture [75]. Based on the affinity of CLC-1 for galactose, there have been several case reports in the literature on the use of galactose in the treatment of de-novo FSGS and recurrence, albeit with mixed results [76–78]. These studies are discussed later in this chapter. More recently, a soluble form of urokinase-type plasminogen activator receptor (sUPAR) has been proposed as another candidate FSGS permeability factor [79]. Urokinase-type plasminogen activator receptor (UPAR) is a glycosylphosphatidylinositol (GPI)-anchored membrane glycoprotein. It is cleaved from the membrane at different domains to produce different soluble (sUPAR) isoforms [80, 81]. sUPAR has been suggested as a FSGS permeability factor based on the observation of Wei and his colleagues that podocyte specific overexpression of UPAR in mice can cause proteinuria and that injection of mice with sUPAR can also induce proteinuria [79]. This effect is thought to be mediated through activation of podocyte β3-integrin. Following these findings there have been multiple reports on the diagnostic value of sUPAR in FSGS and FSGS recurrence. In a study of the cohort from the NIH sponsored FSGS clinical trial and the European consortium for the study of SRNS (PodoNet), Wei et al reported elevated sUPAR levels (serum level (>3000 pg/ml) in 84.3 % of patients in the US FSGS cohort and 55.3 % in the PodoNet cohort compared with 6 % in controls. In addition, they found an inverse correlation between eGFR and sUPAR levels, suggesting that reduced GFR may lead to reduced excretion of sUPAR [82]. A similar pattern was reported by Huan et al.; however, they did not find any difference in sUPAR levels between children with primary and secondary FSGS [83]. In contrast, Bock et al. did not find any differences in sUPAR levels in children with FSGS, non-FSGS kidney disease and healthy controls, similar to the pattern reported by Maas et al. in a limited cohort of adult patients with FSGS [84, 85]. A summary of the different studies has been the subject of multiple recent reviews [86–88]. Based on these conflicting reports, the value of measuring sUPAR for clinical decision making is still uncertain for both primary FSGS and recurrent FSGS in kidney allograft and there is a need for further studies. In addition, since not all FSGS patients have elevated sUPAR levels, it is logical to speculate that there are probably additional isoforms of sUPAR as well as other permeability factors that are important in the pathogenesis of FSGS.

Hereditary FSGS

Familial and hereditary FSGS constitute less than 5 % of all cases of FSGS; however, they have shed significant light on the pathogenesis of the disease since the discovery by Kestila et al. of nephrin (NPHS1) as the gene mutated in congenital nephrotic syndrome more than 15 years ago [46]. Since then many FSGS genes have been reported by different groups, and virtually all of these genes are either important components of the podocyte slit diaphragm or they are important in maintaining the functional integrity of the podocyte actin cytoskeleton [46–62] (Fig. 16.4). With recent advances in genomic technology and ready availability of high throughput sequencing platforms, many more FSGS genes will almost certainly be discovered. Below is a description of several of the key FSGS and nephrotic syndrome genes:

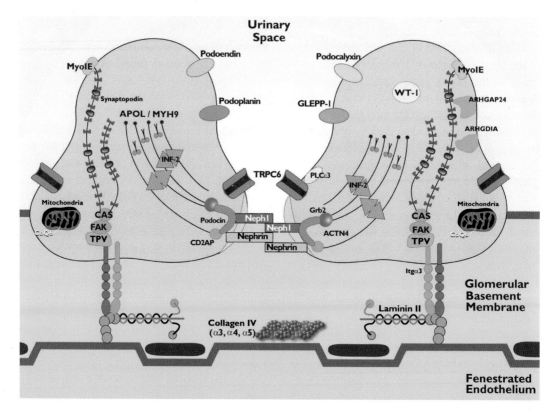

Fig. 16.4 Schematic of the podocyte and the glomerular filtration barrier (*GFB*). The GFB is composed of the podocytes, the glomerular basement membrane and the fenestrated endothelial cells. The podocyte has a unique actin cytoskeleton made up of F-actin and non-muscle myosin such as MYH9 and MYO1E. Its other structural components include; actin-binding proteins such as synaptopodin and α-actinin4 (ACTN4) and actin polymerization regulatory protein inverted formin 2 (INF2). Mutations in *ACTN4*, *INF2*, *MYO1E* genes are causes of hereditary FSGS and *MYH9/APOL1* locus is a genetic risk factor for FSGS in African Americans. Wilms' tumor 1 (*WT1*) gene is a nuclear transcription factor that is expressed in the podocyte, mutations in *WT1* is a cause of syndromic and non-syndromic DMS and FSGS. The cell-cell junction of the podocyte (the slit diaphragm) is formed by nephrin, podocin, CD2 associated protein (CD2AP) and NEPH1. Podocin associates with lipid rafts, a signaling domain of the slit diaphragm. It recruits nephrin and NEPH1 to form a signaling complex with other molecules such as Transient Receptor Potential Cation Channel, Type 6 (TRPC6), growth factor receptor-bound protein 2 (Grb2) and Phospholipase C epsilon-1 (PLCE1) at the slit diaphragm. Mutations in *nephrin* (*NPHS1*), *podocin* (*NPHS2*), *TRPC6, PLCE1 and CD2AP* are causes of familial FSGS in humans. The apical membrane of the podocyte is formed by negatively charged molecules such as podocalyxin, podoplanin, podoendin and glomerular epithelial protein-1 (GLEPP-1). Mutations in *GLEPP-1* gene are a cause of early onset steroid resistant nephrotic syndrome. RhoA-activated Rac1 GTPase-activating protein (Rac1-GAP), (ARHGAP24) and its regulator RhoGDIα (ARHGDIA) are critical for maintaining podocyte cell shape and membrane dynamics. Mutations in ARHGAP24 and ARHGDIA genes are associated with autosomal dominant FSGS and early onset SRNA respectively. *COQ6* is a mitochondrial gene and mutations in it can cause syndromic congenital nephrotic syndrome. The basal part of the podocyte contains α3β1 integrin and α and β dystroglycans that anchors the podocyte to the glomerular basement membrane (GBM). Talin, Paxillin and Vincullin (TPV) interact with different laminins in the GBM, especially laminin β2. Mutations in *laminin β2 and ITGA3 genes* can cause early onset nephrotic syndrome

Autosomal Recessive Genes

Autosomal recessive (AR) gene defects are highly penetrant, and they are often early-onset, therapy-resistant and rapidly progressive, with most children reaching ESKD within 5 years of diagnosis [48]. Nephrin (*NPHS1*) was cloned and identified as the first genetic cause of nephrotic syndrome in 1998 [46]. Nephrin localizes to the podocyte slit diaphragm and forms the zipper-like structure that is discernible by transmission electron microscopy of the slit diaphragm. Shortly after this, podocin was positionally cloned by Antignac group in children with AR FSGS. Disease due to podocin mutations is characterized by early onset, SRNS and rapid progression to ESKD [48]. Like nephrin, podocin is expressed in podocytes and localizes to the intercellular junction of the podocyte foot processes [48]. Podocin mutations have been reported to be responsible for up to 20 % of all cases of childhood-onset FSGS in Europe and other populations with significant founder effects [89]. Mutations in *PLCE1/NPHS3* have also been reported as a cause of early-onset nephrotic syndrome that is characterized by diffuse mesangial sclerosis (DMS) and FSGS [54]. In one limited series, mutations in *PLCE1* were found to be responsible for about 28 % of all cases of isolated

DMS [90]. PLCε1 is a member of the phospholipase family of proteins that catalyze the hydrolysis of polyphosphoinositides such as phosphatdylinositol-4,5-bisphosphate (PtdIns(4,5)P2) to generate the second messengers Ins(1,4,5)P3 and diacylglycerol [91]. The products of this reaction initiate a cascade of intracellular responses that result in cell growth and differentiation and gene expression. The mechanisms by which *PLCE1* mutations cause disease are unknown. However, PLCε1 is expressed in developing and mature podocytes and defects in *PLCE1* gene can cause glomerular developmental arrest and may reduce nephrin/podocin expression [54]. Other AR genes and their resulting phenotypes that have been reported are listed in Table 16.4.

Autosomal Dominant FSGS

Autosomal dominant (AD) causes of FSGS that have been reported in the last 10 years include mutations in actinin-alpha 4 (*ACTN4*), transient receptor potential cation channel protein, type C6 (*TRPC6*) and inverted formin 2 (*INF2*) [49, 52, 56]. Unlike autosomal recessive conditions, most AD diseases are characterized by onset in late childhood and adulthood and incomplete penetrance. However, similar to AR disease, they are

Table 16.4 Autosomal recessive FSGS and SRNS

Genes	Protein localization	Locus	Phenotype
NPHS1/Nephrin	Podocyte and slit diaphragm	19q13.1	Congenital nephrotic syndrome
NPHS2/Podocin	Podocyte and slit diaphragm	1q25-q31	Early onset FSGS
PLCE1 (AR)	Podocyte	10q23-q24	Non syndromic DMS, FSGS
SMARCAL1 (AR)	Podocyte	2q34-q36	Syndromic immune complex nephritis and skeletal defect
LAMB2 (AR)	Glomerular basement membrane	3p21	Syndromic DMS, isolated FSGS
SCARB2 (AR)	Lysosome	4q21.1	Syndromic FSGS
COQ6	Mitochondrial protein	14q24	Syndromic FSGS/DMS
ITGA3	Glomerular basement membrane	17q21	Syndromic SRNS
PTPRO/GLEPP1	Podocyte	12p12	FSGS/MCD
MYO1E	Podocyte	15q21	FSGS
ARHGDIA	Podocyte	17q25	DMS

Table 16.5 Autosomal dominant FSGS and SRNS

Genes	Protein localization	Locus	Phenotype
CD2AP	Podocyte and slit diaphragm	6p12.3	FSGS
WT1	Podocyte	11p13	Syndromic DMS, syndromic and isolated FSGS
α-actinin 4	Podocyte	19q13	FSGS
TRPC6	Podocyte and slit diaphragm	11q21-q22	FSGS
LMX1B	Podocyte	9q34.1	Syndromic NS and skeletal dysplasia
INF2	Podocyte	14q32	FSGS Charcot-Marie-Tooth disease
ARHGAP24	Podocyte	4q21	FSGS

often therapy-resistant. Out of all the AD genes reported so far, *INF2* mutations seem to be the most common, as they are reported to be responsible for about 16 % of all AD FSGS in three independent studies [56, 92–94]. The mechanisms by which mutations in the genes cause FSGS are still being uncovered. It appears, however, that most of the mutations have significant effects on the podocyte actin cytoskeleton, causing disruption of normal actin assembly and polymerization [49, 52, 56]. Table 16.5 shows a list of AD genes reported so far, and further discussion of these genes can be found in Chap. 17.

Polygenic

Genetic risk factors for FSGS have also been reported in population based study. Using the strategy of mapping by admixture linkage disequilibrium, two studies reported sequence variation in non-muscle myosin heavy chain IIA (*MYH9*) as a risk factor for FSGS and ESKD in African Americans [95, 96]. *MYH9* is a non-muscle myosin type IIA which is an important component of the podocyte cytoskeleton and presumably contributes to its contractile function. Further refinement of the *MYH9* locus showed that it is in linkage disequilibrium with the locus for *APOL1*, the gene encoding apolipoprotein L1 [97]. Variants in the coding regions of *APOL1* have been associated with FSGS in African Americans. In another Japanese study, variants in glypican-5 (*GPC5*) were also found to be associated with different proteinuric kidney diseases including FSGS and MCD [98]. The mechanisms by which different variants predispose to SRNS and FSGS are the subjects of ongoing studies.

Treatment of Steroid Resistant Nephrotic Syndrome

Diagnostic Evaluation

Basic chemistries including serum creatinine, serum albumin, and a complete blood count are important for estimating renal function and confirming the presence or absence of overt nephrosis in the initial work-up of nephrotic syndrome. Renal biopsy is indicated in patients where steroid resistance has been established or features not typical of minimal change disease (MCD) are present (e.g., hypertension, age >12, or active urinary sediment). If not already completed, SRNS patients require a diligent effort to rule out secondary disease processes. Ideally tuberculosis status by Mantoux tuberculin skin test or quantiferron gold should be established prior to committing to corticosteroid therapy. Tests for hepatitis B and C, HIV, and even syphilis may be useful. Tests for lupus nephritis, including antinuclear antibody (ANA), anti–double stranded DNA (anti-dsDNA) antibodies, and serum complement levels may also be indicated.

Specific Therapy

Immunomodulatory Therapy

The initial treatment for new-onset nephrotic syndrome generally includes 60 mg/m^2/day or 2 mg/kg/day (maximum 60 mg/day) of prednisone for 6 weeks followed by 40 mg/m^2/day or 1.5 mg/kg/day every other day for 6 weeks and then discontinuation of prednisone without a taper. This practice guideline established by the Kidney Disease: Improving Global Outcomes (KDIGO) Glomerulonephritis Work Group modifies previous practice standards of a maximum dose of 80 mg/day of prednisone, extends the initial high dose exposure, and abolishes the need for a taper. A direct correlation between a longer duration of steroid therapy and a longer duration of remission, and an indirect correlation with the frequency of relapses has been reported in a recent Cochrane review for patients that are steroid sensitive. Steroid resistance is defined as a lack of entry into full remission after 6 weeks of daily therapy. Treatment decisions regarding the implementation of additional immunosuppressive agents are largely weighted by steroid responsiveness patterns [99].

Secondary Therapies

In patients with frequent relapsing NS (FRNS) and steroid dependent NS (SDNS), alternative agents with potential steroid-sparing effects are often used, including alkylating agents such as cyclophosphamide, levamisole, and chlorambucil, calcineurin inhibitors such as cyclosporine (CSA) and tacrolimus, and purine analogs such as mycophenolate mofetil (MMF) (Table 16.6). In patients with SRNS, however, the most commonly used agents include cyclosporine, tacrolimus, high dose intravenous methylprednisolone, and MMF, although the efficacy of almost all of these agents is lower in these patients compared to those with either FRNS or SDNS [100, 101]. Several randomized trials have suggested improved remission rates in patients with SRNS when treated with cyclosporine with or without corticosteroids. These data supported

the design of the National Institutes of Health (NIH)-sponsored multicenter randomized trial of 192 children and young adults with steroid resistant FSGS comparing CSA as the control arm to a combination of mycophenolate mofetil (MMF) and pulse dexamethasone. In this study, no difference in remission rate between the two groups was found, possibly due to underpowered recruitment, and the rates of adverse events were noted to be similar [102]. Differences in efficacy between CSA versus tacrolimus have not been found, yet the body of literature for CSA is more extensive [100, 103]. The side effect profiles in regards to nephrotoxicity are similar between the agents, but gingival hyperplasia and hypertrichosis are more prevalent with CSA and glucose intolerance occurs more frequently with tacrolimus (Table 16.6). In addition to immunomodulation, anti-proteinuric effects of CSA may be mediated by hemodynamic effects which reduce renal blood flow. Also calcineurin inhibitors may induce remission by inhibition of calcineurin-mediated degradation of synaptopodin and stabilization of the podocyte actin cytoskeleton [104–106].

Rituximab is a chimeric monoclonal antibody directed against CD20. Studies suggest rituximab may act by inducing regulatory T lymphocytes, as has been observed in patients with lupus nephritis [107]. Rituximab may also directly protect podocytes by stabilizing the podocyte cytoskeleton and preventing apoptosis through an interaction with the sphingomyelin phosphodiesterase acid-like 3b protein that is expressed in podocytes [108]. In a retrospective review of 33 patients with SRNS treated with two to four doses of intravenous rituximab, and followed for ≥12 months, 9 (27.2 %) patients with SRNS showed complete remission, 7 (21.2 %) had partial remission, and 17 (51.5 %) had no response after 6 months of observation [109]. In an open-labeled, controlled trial that randomized 31 children with SRNS to either receive rituximab or continue their prednisone and calcineurin inhibitors, no subjects in either arm achieved significant reduction of proteinuria [110].

Table 16.6 Treatment options for steroid resistant nephrotic syndrome

Drug	Efficacy evidence	Toxicity	Benefit
IV corticosteroids	Good	Weight gain	May potentiate effects of concurrent second line agents like calcineurin inhibitors
		Hypertension	
		Glucose intolerance	
		Hyperlipidemia	
		Striae	
Cyclosporine	Good	Nephrotoxicity	May only require low dose
		Hypertension	
		Gingival hyperplasia	
Tacrolimus	Good	Nephrotoxicity	May only require low dose
		Hypertension	
		Glucose Intolerance	
Mycophenolate mofetil	Mixed	GI intolerance	No nephrotoxicity
		Teratogenicity	
Cyclophosphamide	Poor	Infertility	May induce remission without need for continued immunosuppression
		Hemorrhagic cystitis	
		Increased malignancy risk	
Rituximab	Mixed	Infections	May enable discontinuation of daily immunosuppressive medications
		Long-term effects unknown	
ACE inhibitors/ARBs	Good	May lower eGFR	Slowed progression of CKD
		Teratogencity	
ACTH	Sparse	Similar to corticosteroids	May spare additional immunosuppression if responsive

ACTH adrenocorticotropic hormone

General Therapy

Anti-proteinuric Agents

Several controlled and non-controlled clinical studies have confirmed the antiproteinuric effect of angiotensin-converting enzyme (ACE) inhibitors in adults and children with glomerular diseases [111–115]. Similar effects have also been well-reported with angiotensin-receptor blockers (ARBs) [116]. The anti-proteinuric effects of ACEIs and ARBs are due to their ability to reduce glomerular capillary plasma flow rate, decrease transcapillary hydraulic pressure, and alter the permselectivity of the glomerular filtration barrier. In patients exposed to ACE inhibitors, a phenomenon known as "aldosterone escape" has been identified with the observation of subsequent long-term increase in plasma aldosterone levels noted in many patients enrolled in ACE inhibitor clinical trials. The addition of aldoste-

rone blockade with ACE inhibition has been shown to reduce urine protein excretion from 30 to 58 % in patients with both diabetic and non-diabetic proteinuria [117]. The mechanism of action is postulated to be related to blockage of pro-fibrotic effects aldosterone appears to have in several organs including the kidney [118].

Novel Therapies: Galactose, Anti-fibrotics, ACTH

The FONT2 study (Novel Therapies in the Treatment of Resistant FSGS) aimed to compare novel therapies in patients with FSGS that have failed standard immunosuppressive therapies with conservative management [119]. In vitro studies have documented decreases in glomerular permeability when isolated glomeruli were incubated with galactose-containing sera [74]. The proposed mechanism suggests galactose may bind a glomerular permeability factor thus rendering it ineffective. Another proposed mechanism for proteinuria in patients with SRNS implicate Tumor Necrosis Factor-alpha (TNF-α), a proinflammatory cytokine that is important in the recruitment of leukocytes to the site of glomerular injury, induction of cytokines and growth factors, generation of oxygen radicals with increased glomerular endothelial cell permeability, cytotoxicity, and induction of apoptosis. These data formed the scientific basis for the FONT 2 which randomized patients with resistant FSGS to conservative management (ACE inhibition), adalimumab (TNF-α antibody) or oral galactose. Results from this trial are expected in 2014.

ACTH (Adrenocorticotropic Hormone) was the therapy of choice for children with nephrotic syndrome in the 1950s before corticosteroids became widely available [120, 121]. The development of an ACTH analog has made this therapy available once again for physicians to use as a second line agent in the treatment of SRNS. The largest published series to date by Hogan et al. reports a cumulative remission rate of 29 % in 24 patients with SRNS and SDNS treated with subcutaneous ACTH [122].

Treatment of Complications of Nephrotic Syndrome

Hyperlipidemia

Hyperlipidemia is a common clinical finding in children with nephrotic syndrome. The characteristic lipid profile includes elevations in total plasma cholesterol, very low-density lipoprotein (VLDL), and low-density lipoprotein (LDL) cholesterol, triglyceride, lipoprotein A, as well as variable alterations (more typically decreased) in high-density lipoprotein (HDL) cholesterol [123, 124]. While the hyperlipidemia in children with SSNS is often transient and usually returns to normal after remission, children with SRNS refractory to therapy often have sustained hyperlipidemia. Such chronic hyperlipidemia has been associated with an increased risk for cardiovascular complications and progressive glomerular damage in adults [125–129]. Based on this, pharmacologic treatment of hyperlipidemia in children with refractory nephrotic syndrome may both reduce the risk for cardiovascular complications later in life and reduce the risk of disease progression.

The potential usefulness of hydroxymethylglutaryl CoA (HMG CoA) reductase inhibitors (statins) in children with SRNS has been reported in a few uncontrolled trials. One study reported a 41 % reduction in cholesterol and 44 % reduction in triglyceride levels within 6 months of treatment [130]. A second study found significant reductions within 2–4 months in total cholesterol (40 %), LDL cholesterol (44 %), and triglyceride (33 %) levels, but no significant changes in HDL cholesterol levels [131]. Treatment was found to be very safe in these studies, with no associated adverse clinical or laboratory events. Although the long-term safety of statins in children has not yet been established, these medications appear to be generally well-tolerated in adults with nephrotic syndrome, with only minor side effects such as asymptomatic increases in liver enzymes, creatine kinase, and rarely diarrhea [132].

Thrombosis

The risk of thromboembolic phenomenon in children with nephrotic syndrome is estimated to be 1.8–5 % with higher risk reported in children with SRNS compared with those with SSNS [133, 134]. Factors contributing to an increased risk of thrombosis during nephrotic syndrome include abnormalities of the coagulation cascade, such as increased clotting factor synthesis in the liver (factors I, II, V, VII, VIII, X, and XIII) and loss of coagulation inhibitors such as antithrombin III in the urine. Other prothrombotic risks present in these children include increased platelet aggregability (and sometimes thrombocytosis), hyperviscosity resulting from increased fibrinogen levels, hyperlipidemia, prolonged immobilization, and the use of diuretics. In one series, the use of diuretics was found to be the major iatrogenic risk factor for thrombosis [134].

The majority of episodes of thrombosis are venous in origin. The most common sites for thrombosis are the deep leg veins, ileofemoral veins, and the inferior vena cava. In addition, use of central venous catheters can further increase the risk of thrombosis. Renal vein thrombosis (RVT) can also occur and may manifest as gross hematuria with or without acute renal failure. Development of these features should prompt either renal Doppler ultrasonography or magnetic resonance angiography to rule out RVT. Pulmonary embolism is another important complication that may be fatal if not recognized early. Rarely, cerebral venous thrombosis, most commonly in the sagittal sinus, has also been reported [135]. In addition to imaging studies, development of thrombosis should prompt an evaluation for possible inherited hypercoagulable states. The typical acute management of thrombosis in children with nephrotic syndrome includes initial heparin infusion or low molecular weight heparin, followed by transition to warfarin for 6 months. Children with a history of prior thrombosis should also receive prophylactic anticoagulation therapy during future relapses.

Nutrition

Several recommendations supported by observational data exist regarding nutrition in pediatric patients with nephrotic syndrome. Specifically, children with nephrotic syndrome and edema should be evaluated for malabsorption and subsequent malnutrition due to bowel wall edema. In edematous patients long-term sodium restriction is appropriate with a goal of approximately 1–2 meq/kg/day to a maximum of 2000 mg/day. In patients with persistent hyperlipidemia due to inability to control nephrosis, a low saturated fat diet should be instituted with their HMG CoA-reductase inhibitor. Protein intake should only be supplemented at the Recommended Daily Allowance (RDA) [136]. Although it would appear intuitive that states of excess urinary protein loss should warrant increase dietary protein intake, several studies have successfully chal-

lenged this notion. In nephrotic rats, augmentation of dietary protein was found to stimulate albumin synthesis by increasing albumin mRNA content in the liver, but there was also a notable increase in glomerular permeability and subsequent increased urinary excretion of albumin [137]. No change in albumin synthesis was noted with dietary protein restriction in this model or in nephrotic patients.

Infections and Immunizations

Children with nephrotic syndrome are at increased risk for infections, including but not limited to streptococcus and staphylococcal species due to urinary losses of IgG, loss of factors crucial for regulation of the alternative complement pathway, and large fluid collections prone to breeding bacteria. Common infections reported in children regardless of concurrent glucocorticoid therapy include peritonitis, pneumonia, empyemas, and urinary tract infections. A retrospective review (1970 through 1980) revealed 24 episodes of peritonitis in 19 of 351 children with idiopathic nephrotic syndrome [138]. Infections overwhelmingly contributed to the high mortality in children with nephrotic syndrome prior to the wide availability of corticosteroids and antibiotics.

Since the mid-1990s, vaccination using the 23-valent polysaccharide pneumococcal vaccine (PPSV23) has been recommended for children with nephrotic syndrome or CKD by the Advisory Committee on Immunization Practices (ACIP) [139]. Due to the low immunogenicity of this vaccine in children less than 2 years of age, the 13-valent polysaccharide pneumococcal vaccine (PCV13) which recently replaced the PCV7 is recommended at ages 2, 4, 6, and 12–15 months. The ACIP further recommends that children with CKD and nephrotic syndrome should receive supplemental immunization with PPSV23 over the age of 2 years at least 8 weeks after the final dose of PCV13. A second dose of PPSV23 should be repeated in 5 years.

Live-viral vaccines (rotavirus vaccine, varicella vaccine, measles, mumps, and rubella vaccine, and the live-attenuated influenza vaccine) are generally recommended to be avoided in CKD patients who are immunosuppressed and therefore should be avoided in patients that are frankly nephrotic and/or currently receiving immunosuppressive therapy including daily high-dose corticosteroids. Risk of serious adverse events related to live attenuated vaccination in children with nephrotic syndrome who are in remission off therapy or only on low dose alternate day therapy has been largely unsubstantiated in retrospective observational and prospective open label studies. An open-label study of pediatric patients with steroid sensitive NS in remission either off therapy or well-controlled on low-dose alternate day therapy revealed successful seroconversion with detectable antibody titers in 28 of 28 patients at 1 year post and 21 of 23 at 2 years post receiving two doses of an attenuated live varicella vaccination. In this trial six patients experienced a NS relapse within 2 weeks of vaccination, but there were no serious adverse events seen in the 2 year follow-up period [140]. Other studies endorse the safety of attenuated varicella vaccine in patients with nephrotic syndrome who are in remission [141].

Kidney Transplantation

Recurrence of nephrotic syndrome may occur in up to 30 % in the first kidney allograft of patients with ESKD due to FSGS and approach 100 % in those who have a history of prior allograft loss due to FSGS. Young age, mesangial proliferation in the native kidneys, a rapid progression to ESKD, a pre-transplant bilateral nephrectomy, and white ethnicity are clinical factors that have been reported to be associated with increased risk of recurrence post-transplant [142, 143]. In addition the risk of recurrence in patients with genetic forms of FSGS appears to be significantly reduced compared with the idiopathic form. The histologic variant type of FSGS does not appear to be predictive of disease recurrence. There is a higher risk of recurrence in living donor transplant pediatric recipients;

however, the reduced risk of rejection and a lower immunosuppression in living-related transplants may overcome the deleterious effect of recurrent glomerulonephritis [144]. The management of recurrent FSGS disease remains controversial and results from observational reports vary. The implementation of plasma exchange is supported in part by the idea of a circulating permeability factor. Up to 70 % of children with recurrent FSGS treated with repeated plasma exchanges may achieve at least a partial remission.

Future Directions

Genetic Testing

The clinical value of genetic testing in SRNS is not in doubt as it can help with making decisions on the intensity and duration of immunosuppression, as well as with pre and post-transplant management. What is controversial is the role of routine genetic testing in all children with SRNS. Depending on the population being studied, the prevalence of monogenic SRNS/FSGS varies between <1 and 25 % [89, 145–148]. The prevalence seems to be highest in Europe where there are clear founder effects for *NPHS2* and *NPHS1* mutations. On the other hand, the prevalence seems to be lower in the United States, especially among African Americans [89, 145–149]. Evidence from different studies in the literature seems to suggest that genetic testing is warranted in the following group of patients as they are more likely to have single gene defects: (1) All children presenting with nephrotic syndrome in the first year of life, (2) All patients in whom SRNS is part of a syndrome and (3) All patients with a family history of NS or chronic kidney disease [36]. We propose the use of the algorithm shown in Fig. 16.5 to determine which SRNS patients should receive genetic testing, and which specific tests should be ordered. The hope is that the rapid technological advances in genome science will be translated to the bedside in the near future such that whole exome/

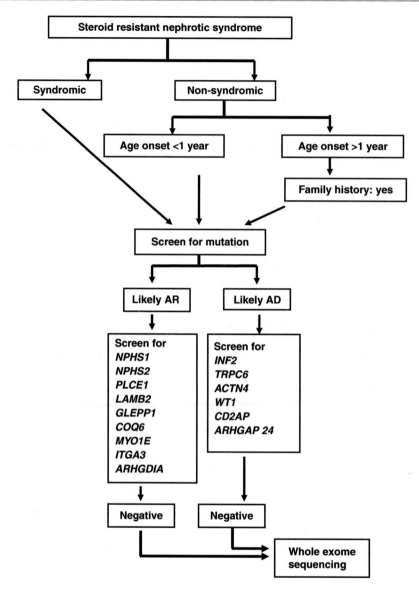

Fig. 16.5 Algorithm to determine which SRNS patients should receive genetic testing, and which specific tests should be ordered

whole genome sequencing will be readily available, affordable and the bioinformatics pipeline necessary for meaningful interpretation of the results will be developed. With this method, more novel genes for SRNS/FSGS will be identified and these discoveries will hopefully improve our understanding of the molecular mechanisms of SRNS, as well as identify novel therapeutic targets.

References

1. Arneil GC. The nephrotic syndrome. Pediatr Clin North Am. 1971;18(2):547–59.
2. Arneil GC, Lam CN. Long-term assessment of steroid therapy in childhood nephrosis. Lancet. 1966;2(7468):819–21.
3. ISKDC. The primary nephrotic syndrome in children. Identification of patients with minimal change nephrotic syndrome from initial response to prednisone. J Pediatr. 1981;98(4):561–4.

4. Niaudet P. Steroid-resistant idiopathic nephrotic syndrome in children. In: Avner ED, Harmon WE, Niaudet P, editors. Pediatric nephrology. Philadelphia: Lippincott Williams & Wilkins; 2004. p. 557–73.

5. ISKDC. Primary nephrotic syndrome in children: clinical significances of histopathologic variants of minimal change and of diffuse mesangial hypercellularity. Kidney Int. 1981;20(6):765–71.

6. Niaudet P, Gagnadoux MF, Broyer M. Treatment of childhood steroid-resistant idiopathic nephrotic syndrome. Adv Nephrol Necker Hosp. 1998;28:43–61.

7. Straatmann C, Ayoob R, Gbadegesin R, et al. Treatment outcome of late steroid-resistant nephrotic syndrome: a study by the Midwest Pediatric Nephrology Consortium. Pediatr Nephrol. 2013;28(8):1235–41.

8. Nash MA, et al. In: Edelmann CMJ, editor. The nephrotic syndrome, in pediatric kidney disease. Boston: Little, Brown, and Company; 1992. p. 1247–66.

9. Srivastava T, Simon SD, Alon US. High incidence of focal segmental glomerulosclerosis in nephrotic syndrome of childhood. Pediatr Nephrol. 1999;13(1):13–8.

10. Hogg RJ, et al. Evaluation and management of proteinuria and nephrotic syndrome in children: recommendations from a pediatric nephrology panel established at the national kidney foundation conference on Proteinuria, Albuminuria, Risk, Assessment, Detection, and Elimination (PARADE). Pediatrics. 2000;105(6):1242–9.

11. McEnery PT, Strife CF. Nephrotic syndrome in childhood. Management and treatment in patients with minimal change disease, mesangial proliferation, or focal glomerulosclerosis. Pediatr Clin North Am. 1982;29(4):875–94.

12. Bonilla-Felix M, et al. Changing patterns in the histopathology of idiopathic nephrotic syndrome in children. Kidney Int. 1999;55(5):1885–90.

13. Eddy AA, Symons JM. Nephrotic syndrome in childhood. Lancet. 2003;362(9384):629–39.

14. Filler G, et al. Is there really an increase in nonminimal change nephrotic syndrome in children? Am J Kidney Disease. 2003;42(6):1107–13.

15. Kari JA. Changing trends of histopathology in childhood nephrotic syndrome in western Saudi Arabia. Saudi Med J. 2002;23(3):317–21.

16. Sharples PM, Poulton J, White RH. Steroid responsive nephrotic syndrome is more common in Asians. Arch Dis Child. 1985;60(11):1014–7.

17. Coovadia HM, Adhikari M, Morel-Maroger L. Clinico-pathological features of the nephrotic syndrome in South African children. Q J Med. 1979;48(189):77–91.

18. Hendrickse RG, et al. Quartan malarial nephrotic syndrome. Collaborative clinicopathological study in Nigerian children. Lancet. 1972;1(1761):1143–9.

19. Abdurrahman MB. Clinicopathological features of childhood nephrotic syndrome in northern Nigeria. Q J Med. 1990;75(278):563–76.

20. Children, T.I.S.o.K.D.i. Nephrotic syndrome in children: prediction of histopathology from clinical and laboratory characteristics at time of diagnosis. Kidney Int. 1978;13:159–65.

21. Sorof JM, et al. Age and ethnicity affect the risk and outcome of focal segmental glomerulosclerosis. Pediatr Nephrol. 1998;12(9):764–8.

22. Bhimma R, Coovadia HM, Adhikari M. Nephrotic syndrome in South African children: changing perspectives over 20 years. Pediatr Nephrol. 1997;11(4):429–34.

23. Doe JY, et al. Nephrotic syndrome in African children: lack of evidence for "tropical nephrotic syndrome"? Nephrol Dialysis Trans. 2006;21(3):672–6.

24. The Southwest Pediatric Nephrology Study Group. Focal segmental glomerulosclerosis in children with idiopathic nephrotic syndrome: a report of the Southwest Pediatric Nephrology Study Group. Kidney Int. 1985;27:442–9.

25. Mubarak M, Lanewala A, Kazi JI, Akhter F, Sher A, Fayyaz A, Bhatti S. Histopathological spectrum of childhood nephrotic syndrome in Pakistan. Clin Exp Nephrol. 2009;13:589–93.

26. Nammalwar BR, Vijayakumar M, Prahlad N. Experience of renal biopsy in children with nephrotic syndrome. Pediatr Nephrol. 2006;21(2):286–8.

27. Banaszak B, Banaszak P. The increasing incidence of initial steroid resistance in childhood nephrotic syndrome. Pediatr Nephrol. 2012;27(6):927–32.

28. Bhimma R, Adhikari M, Asharam K. Steroid-resistant nephrotic syndrome: the influence of race on cyclophosphamide sensitivity. Pediatr Nephrol. 2006;21(12):1847–53.

29. Churg J, Habib R, White RH. Pathology of the nephrotic syndrome in children: a report for the International Study of Kidney Disease in Children. Lancet. 1970;760:1299–302.

30. Cameron JS. Focal segmental glomerulosclerosis in adults. Nephrol Dial Transplant. 2003;18:vi45–51.

31. Rich AR. A hitherto undescribed vulnerability of the juxtamedullary glomeruli in lipoid nephrosis. Bull Johns Hopkins Hosp. 1957;100:173–86.

32. Kitiyakara C, Kopp JB, Eggers P. Trends in the epidemiology of focal segmental glomerulosclerosis. Semin Nephrol. 2003;23:172–82.

33. Kitiyakara C, Eggers P, Kopp JB. Twenty-one-year trend in ESRD due to focal segmental glomerulosclerosis in the United States. Am J Kidney Dis. 2004;44:815–25.

34. Swaminathan S, Leung N, Lager DJ, Melton 3rd LJ, Bergstralh EJ, Rohlinger A, Fervenza FC. Changing incidence of glomerular disease in Olmsted County, Minnesota: a 30-year renal biopsy study. Clin J Am Soc Nephrol. 2006;1:483–7.

35. Borges FF, Shiraichi L, da Silva MP, Nishimoto EI, Nogueira PC. Is focal segmental glomerulosclerosis increasing in patients with nephrotic syndrome? Pediatr Nephrol. 2007;22:1309–13.

36. Gbadegesin RA, Winn MP, Smoyer WE. Genetic testing in nephrotic syndrome – challenges and opportunities. Nat Rev Nephrol. 2013;9:179–84.

37. D'Agati VD, Fogo AB, Bruijn JA, Jennette JC. Pathologic classification of focal segmental glomerulosclerosis: a working proposal. Am J Kidney Dis. 2004;43:368–82.

38. Stokes MB, Valeri AM, Markowitz GS, D'Agati VD. Cellular focal segmental glomerulosclerosis: clinical and pathologic features. Kidney Int. 2006;70:1783–92.

39. D'Agati VD, Alster JM, Jennette JC, Thomas DB, Pullman J, Savino DA, Cohen AH, Gipson DS, Gassman JJ, Radeva MK, Moxey-Mims MM, Friedman AL, Kaskel FJ, Trachtman H, Alpers CE, Fogo AB, Greene TH, Nast CC. Association of histologic variants in FSGS clinical trial with presenting features and outcomes. Clin J Am Soc Nephrol. 2013;8:399–406.

40. Smoyer WE, Mundel P. Regulation of podocyte structure during the development of nephrotic syndrome. J Mol Med. 1998;76:172–83.

41. Partanen TA, Arola J, Saaristo A, Jussila L, Ora A, Miettinen M, Stacker SA, Achen MG, Alitalo K. VEGF-C and VEGF-D expression in neuroendocrine cells and their receptor, VEGFR-3, in fenestrated blood vessels in human tissues. FASEB J. 2000;14:2087–96.

42. Rostgaard J, Qvortrup K. Sieve plugs in fenestrae of glomerular capillaries – site of the filtration barrier? Cells Tissues Organs. 2002;170:132–8.

43. Weinbaum S, Tarbell JM, Damiano ER. The structure and function of the endothelial glycocalyx layer. Annu Rev Plant Physiol Plant Mol Biol. 2007;9:121–67.

44. Ballermann BJ, Stan RV. Resolved: capillary endothelium is a major contributor to the glomerular filtration barrier. J Am Soc Nephrol. 2007;18:2432–8.

45. Vaughan MR, Quaggin SE. How do mesangial and endothelial cells form the glomerular tuft? J Am Soc Nephrol. 2008;19:24–33.

46. Kestilä M, Lenkkeri U, Männikkö M, Lamerdin J, McCready P, Putaala H, Ruotsalainen V, Morita T, Nissinen M, Herva R, Kashtan CE, Peltonen L, Holmberg C, Olsen A, Tryggvason K. Positionally cloned gene for a novel glomerular protein – nephrin – is mutated in congenital nephrotic syndrome. Mol Cell. 1998;1:575–82.

47. Shih NY, et al. Congenital nephrotic syndrome in mice lacking CD2-associated protein. Science. 1999;286(5438):312–5.

48. Boute N, Gribouval O, Roselli S, Benessy F, Lee H, Fuchshuber A, Dahan K, Gubler MC, Niaudet P, Antignac C. NPHS2, encoding the glomerular protein podocin, is mutated in autosomal recessive steroid-resistant nephrotic syndrome. Nat Genet. 2000;24:349–54.

49. Kaplan JM, et al. Mutations in ACTN4, encoding alpha-actinin-4, cause familial focal segmental glomerulosclerosis. Nat Genet. 2000;24(3):251–6.

50. Boerkoel CF, Takashima H, John J, Yan J, Stankiewicz P, Rosenbarker L, André JL, Bogdanovic R, Burguet A, Cockfield S, Cordeiro I, Fründ S, Illies F, Joseph M, Kaitila I, Lama G, Loirat C, McLeod DR, Milford DV, Petty EM, Rodrigo F, Saraiva JM, Schmidt B, Smith GC, Spranger J, Stein A, Thiele H, Tizard J, Weksberg R, Lupski JR, Stockton DW. Mutant chromatin remodeling protein SMARCAL1 causes Schimke immuno-osseous dysplasia. Nat Genet. 2002;30:215–20.

51. Zenker M, Aigner T, Wendler O, Tralau T, Müntefering H, Fenski R, Pitz S, Schumacher V, Royer-Pokora B, Wühl E, Cochat P, Bouvier R, Kraus C, Mark K, Madlon H, Dötsch J, Rascher W, Maruniak-Chudek I, Lennert T, Neumann LM, Reis A. Human laminin beta2 deficiency causes congenital nephrosis with mesangial sclerosis and distinct eye abnormalities. Hum Mol Genet. 2004;13:2625–32.

52. Winn MP, et al. A mutation in the TRPC6 cation channel causes familial focal segmental glomerulosclerosis. Science. 2005;308(5729):1801–4.

53. Niaudet P, Gubler MC. WT1 and glomerular diseases. Pediatr Nephrol. 2006;21:1653–60.

54. Hinkes B, Wiggins RC, Gbadegesin R, Vlangos CN, Seelow D, Nurnberg G, Garg P, Verma R, Chaib H, Hoskins BE, Ashraf S, Becker C, Hennies HC, Goyal M, Wharram BL, Schachter AD, Mudumana S, Drummond I, Kerjaschki D, Waldherr R, Dietrich A, Ozaltin F, Bakkaloglu A, Cleper R, Basel-Vanagaite L, Pohl M, Griebel M, Tsygin AN, Soylu A, Muller D, Sorli CS, Bunney TD, Katan M, Liu J, Attanasio M, O'Toole JF, Hasselbacher K, Mucha B, Otto EA, Airik R, Kispert A, Kelley GG, Smrcka AV, Gudermann T, Holzman LB, Nurnberg P, Hildebrandt F. Positional cloning uncovers mutations in plce1 responsible for a nephrotic syndrome variant that may be reversible. Nat Genet. 2006;38:1397–405.

55. Berkovic SF, et al. Array-based gene discovery with three unrelated subjects shows SCARB2/LIMP-2 deficiency causes myoclonus epilepsy and glomerulosclerosis. Am J Hum Genet. 2008;82:673–84.

56. Brown EJ, et al. Mutations in the formin gene INF2 cause focal segmental glomerulosclerosis. Nat Genet. 2010;42:72–6.

57. Heeringa SF, et al. COQ6 mutations in human patients produce nephrotic syndrome with sensorineural deafness. J Clin Invest. 2011;121:2013–24.

58. Akilesh S, et al. Arhgap24 inactivates Rac1 in mouse podocytes, and a mutant form is associated with familial focal segmental glomerulosclerosis. J Clin Invest. 2011;121:4127–37.

59. Mele C, et al. MYO1E mutations and childhood familial focal segmental glomerulosclerosis. N Engl J Med. 2011;365:295–306.

60. Ozaltin F, et al. Disruption of PTPRO causes childhood-onset nephrotic syndrome. Am J Hum Genet. 2011;89:139–47.

61. Has C, Spartà G, Kiritsi D, Weibel L, Moeller A, Vega-Warner V, Waters A, He Y, Anikster Y, Esser P,

Straub BK, Hausser I, Bockenhauer D, Dekel B, Hildebrandt F, Bruckner-Tuderman L, Laube GF. Integrin α3 mutations with kidney, lung, and skin disease. N Engl J Med. 2012;366(16):1508–14.

62. Gupta IR, Baldwin C, Auguste D, Ha KC, El Andalousi J, Fahiminiya S, Bitzan M, Bernard C, Akbari MR, Narod SA, Rosenblatt DS, Majewski J, Takano T. ARHGDIA: a novel gene implicated in nephrotic syndrome. J Med Genet. 2013;50(5):330–8.

63. Wiggins RC. The spectrum of podocytopathies: a unifying view of glomerular diseases. Kidney Int. 2007;71:1205–14.

64. Kriz W. The pathogenesis of 'classic' focal segmental glomerulosclerosis-lessons from rat models. Nephrol Dial Transplant. 2003;6:vi39–44.

65. Wharram BL, Goyal M, Wiggins JE, Sanden SK, Hussain S, Filipiak WE, Saunders TL, Dysko RC, Kohno K, Holzman LB, Wiggins RC. Podocyte depletion causes glomerulosclerosis: diphtheria toxin-induced podocyte depletion in rats expressing human diphtheria toxin receptor transgene. J Am Soc Nephrol. 2005;16:2941–52.

66. Carrie BJ, Salyer WR, Myers BD. Minimal change nephropathy: an electrochemical disorder of the glomerular membrane. Am J Med. 1981;70(2):262–8.

67. Shalhoub RJ. Pathogenesis of lipoid nephrosis: a disorder of T-cell function. Lancet. 1974;2(7880):556–60.

68. Kemper MJ, Wolf G, Muller-Wiefel DE. Transmission of glomerular permeability factor from a mother to her child. New Engl J Med. 2001;344(5):386–7.

69. Meyrier A. Mechanisms of disease: focal segmental glomerulosclerosis. Nat Clin Pract Nephrol. 2005;1(1):44–54.

70. Sasdelli M, et al. Cell mediated immunity in idiopathic glomerulonephritis. Clin Exp Immunol. 1984;46(1):27–34.

71. Dantal J, et al. Effect of plasma protein adsorption on protein excretion in kidney-transplant recipients with recurrent nephrotic syndrome. New Engl J Med. 1994;330(1):7–14.

72. Savin VJ, et al. Circulating factor associated with increased glomerular permeability to albumin in recurrent focal segmental glomerulosclerosis. New Engl J Med. 1996;334(14):878–83.

73. Candiano G, et al. Inhibition of renal permeability towards albumin: a new function of apolipoproteins with possible pathogenetic relevance in focal glomerulosclerosis. Electrophoresis. 2001;22(9):1819–25.

74. Savin VJ, McCarthy ET, Sharma R, Charba D, Sharma M. Galactose binds to focal segmental glomerulosclerosis permeability factor and inhibits its activity. Transl Res. 2008;151(6):288–92.

75. Savin VJ, McCarthy ET, Sharma R, Reddy S, Dong J, Hess S, Kopp J. Cardiotrophin-like cytokine-1: candidate for the focal segmental glomerulosclerosis permeability factor. J Am Soc Nephrol. 2008;19.

76. De Smet E, Rioux JP, Ammann H, Déziel C, Quérin S. FSGS permeability factor-associated nephrotic syndrome: remission after oral galactose therapy. Nephrol Dial Transplant. 2009;24(9):2938–40.

77. Kopač M, Meglič A, Rus RR. Partial remission of resistant nephrotic syndrome after oral galactose therapy. Ther Apher Dial. 2011;15(3):269–72.

78. Sgambat K, Banks M, Moudgil A. Effect of galactose on glomerular permeability and proteinuria in steroid-resistant nephrotic syndrome. Pediatr Nephrol. 2013;28(11):2131–5.

79. Wei C, El Hindi S, Li J, Fornoni A, Goes N, Sageshima J, Maiguel D, Karumanchi SA, Yap HK, Saleem M, Zhang Q, Nikolic B, Chaudhuri A, Daftarian P, Salido E, Torres A, Salifu M, Sarwal MM, Schaefer F, Morath C, Schwenger V, Zeier M, Gupta V, Roth D, Rastaldi MP, Burke G, Ruiz P, Reiser J. Circulating urokinase receptor as a cause of focal segmental glomerulosclerosis. Nat Med. 2011;17(8):952–60.

80. Behrendt N, Rønne E, Ploug M, Petri T, Løber D, Nielsen LS, Schleuning WD, Blasi F, Appella E, Danø K. The human receptor for urokinase plasminogen activator. NH2-terminal amino acid sequence and glycosylation variants. J Biol Chem. 1990;265(11):6453–60.

81. Sidenius N, Sier CF, Blasi F. Shedding and cleavage of the urokinase receptor (uPAR): identification and characterisation of uPAR fragments in vitro and in vivo. FEBS Lett. 2000;475(1):52–6.

82. Wei C, Trachtman H, Li J, Dong C, Friedman AL, Gassman JJ, McMahan JL, Radeva M, Heil KM, Trautmann A, Anarat A, Emre S, Ghiggeri GM, Ozaltin F, Haffner D, Gipson DS, Kaskel F, Fischer DC, Schaefer F, Reiser J, PodoNet and FSGS CT Study Consortia. Circulating suPAR in two cohorts of primary FSGS. J Am Soc Nephrol. 2012;23(12):2051–9.

83. Huang J, Liu G, Zhang YM, Cui Z, Wang F, Liu XJ, Chu R, Chen Y, Zhao MH. Plasma soluble urokinase receptor levels are increased but do not distinguish primary from secondary focal segmental glomerulosclerosis. Kidney Int. 2013;84(2):366–72.

84. Maas RJ, Wetzels JF, Deegens JK. Serum-soluble urokinase receptor concentration in primary FSGS. Kidney Int. 2012;81(10):1043–4.

85. Bock ME, Price HE, Gallon L, Langman CB. Serum soluble urokinase-type plasminogen activator receptor levels and idiopathic FSGS in children: a single-center report. Clin J Am Soc Nephrol. 2013;8(8):1304–11.

86. Maas RJ, Deegens JK, Wetzels JF. Serum suPAR in patients with FSGS: trash or treasure? Pediatr Nephrol. 2013;28(7):1041–8.

87. Sever S, Trachtman H, Wei C, Reiser J. Is there clinical value in measuring suPAR levels in FSGS? Clin J Am Soc Nephrol. 2013;8(8):1273–5.

88. Reiser J. Circulating permeability factor suPAR: from concept to discovery to clinic. Trans Am Clin Climatol Assoc. 2013;124:133–8.

89. Ruf RG, Lichtenberger A, Karle SM, Haas JP, Anacleto FE, Schultheiss M, Zalewski I, Imm A, Ruf EM, Mucha B, Bagga A, Neuhaus T, Fuchshuber A, Bakkaloglu A, Hildebrandt F, Arbeitsgemeinschaft Für Pädiatrische Nephrologie Study Group. Patients with mutations in NPHS2 (podocin) do not respond to standard steroid treatment of nephrotic syndrome. J Am Soc Nephrol. 2004;15:722–32.

90. Gbadegesin R, Hinkes BG, Hoskins BE, Vlangos CN, Heeringa SF, Liu J, Loirat C, Ozaltin F, Hashmi S, Ulmer F, Cleper R, Ettenger R, Antignac C, Wiggins RC, Zenker M, Hildebrandt F. Mutations in PLCE1 are a major cause of isolated diffuse mesangial sclerosis (IDMS). Nephrol Dial Transplant. 2008;23:1291–7.

91. Wing MR, Bourdon DM, Harden TK. PLC-epsilon: a shared effector protein in Ras-, Rho-, and G alpha beta gamma-mediated signaling. Mol Interv. 2003;3:273–80.

92. Boyer O, Benoit G, Gribouval O, Nevo F, Tête MJ, Dantal J, Gilbert-Dussardier B, Touchard G, Karras A, Presne C, Grunfeld JP, Legendre C, Joly D, Rieu P, Mohsin N, Hannedouche T, Moal V, Gubler MC, Broutin I, Mollet G, Antignac C. Mutations in INF2 are a major cause of autosomal dominant focal segmental glomerulosclerosis. J Am Soc Nephrol. 2011;22(2):239–45.

93. Gbadegesin RA, Lavin PJ, Hall G, Bartkowiak B, Homstad A, Jiang R, Wu G, Byrd A, Lynn K, Wolfish N, Ottati C, Stevens P, Howell D, Conlon P, Winn MP. Inverted formin 2 mutations with variable expression in patients with sporadic and hereditary focal and segmental glomerulosclerosis. Kidney Int. 2012;81(1):94–9.

94. Barua M, Brown EJ, Charoonratana VT, Genovese G, Sun H, Pollak MR. Mutations in the INF2 gene account for a significant proportion of familial but not sporadic focal and segmental glomerulosclerosis. Kidney Int. 2013;83(2):316–22.

95. Kopp JB, Smith MW, Nelson GW, Johnson RC, Freedman BI, Bowden DW, Oleksyk T, McKenzie LM, Kajiyama H, Ahuja TS, Berns JS, Briggs W, Cho ME, Dart RA, Kimmel PL, Korbet SM, Michel DM, Mokrzycki MH, Schelling JR, Simon E, Trachtman H, Vlahov D, Winkler CA. MYH9 is a major-effect risk gene for focal segmental glomerulosclerosis. Nat Genet. 2008;40:1175–84.

96. Kao WH, Klag MJ, Meoni LA, Reich D, Berthier-Schaad Y, Li M, Coresh J, Patterson N, Tandon A, Powe NR, Fink NE, Sadler JH, Weir MR, Abboud HE, Adler SG, Divers J, Iyengar SK, Freedman BI, Kimmel PL, Knowler WC, Kohn OF, Kramp K, Leehey DJ, Nicholas SB, Pahl MV, Schelling JR, Sedor JR, Thornley-Brown D, Winkler CA, Smith MW, Parekh RS, Family Investigation of Nephropathy and Diabetes Research Group. MYH9 is associated with nondiabetic end-stage renal disease in African Americans. Nat Genet. 2008;40:1185–92.

97. Genovese G, Friedman DJ, Ross MD, Lecordier L, Uzureau P, Freedman BI, Bowden DW, Langefeld CD, Oleksyk TK, Uscinski Knob AL, Bernhardy AJ, Hicks PJ, Nelson GW, Vanhollebeke B, Winkler CA, Kopp JB, Pays E, Pollak MR. Association of trypanolytic ApoL1 variants with kidney disease in African Americans. Science. 2010;329:841–5.

98. Okamoto K, Tokunaga K, Doi K, Fujita T, Suzuki H, Katoh T, Watanabe T, Nishida N, Mabuchi A, Takahashi A, Kubo M, Maeda S, Nakamura Y, Noiri E. Common variation in GPC5 is associated with acquired nephrotic syndrome. Nat Genet. 2011;43:459–63.

99. Lombel RM, Hodson EM, Gipson DS. Kidney disease: improving global outcomes. Treatment of steroid-resistant nephrotic syndrome in children: new guidelines from KDIGO. Pediatr Nephrol. 2013;28(3):409–14.

100. Cattran DC, Appel GB, Hebert LA, Hunsicker LG, Pohl MA, Hoy WE, Maxwell DR, Kunis CL. A randomized trial of cyclosporine in patients with steroid-resistant focal segmental glomerulosclerosis. North America Nephrotic Syndrome Study Group. Kidney Int. 1999;56(6):2220–6.

101. Tune BM, Mendoza SA. Treatment of the idiopathic nephrotic syndrome: regimens and outcomes in children and adults. J Am Soc Nephrol. 1997;8(5):824–32.

102. Gipson DS, Trachtman H, Kaskel FJ, Greene TH, Radeva MK, Gassman JJ, Moxey-Mims MM, Hogg RJ, Watkins SL, Fine RN, Hogan SL, Middleton JP, Vehaskari VM, Flynn PA, Powell LM, Vento SM, McMahan JL, Siegel N, D'Agati VD, Friedman AL. Clinical trial of focal segmental glomerulosclerosis in children and young adults. Kidney Int. 2011;80(8):868–78.

103. Lieberman KV, Tejani A. A randomized double-blind placebo-controlled trial of cyclosporine in steroid-resistant idiopathic focal segmental glomerulosclerosis in children. J Am Soc Nephrol. 1996;7(1):56–63.

104. Bensman A, Niaudet P. Non-immunologic mechanisms of calcineurin inhibitors explain its antiproteinuric effects in genetic glomerulopathies. Pediatr Nephrol. 2010;25(7):1197–9.

105. Faul C, Donnelly M, Merscher-Gomez S, Chang YH, Franz S, Delfgaauw J, Chang JM, Choi HY, Campbell KN, Kim K, Reiser J, Mundel P. The actin cytoskeleton of kidney podocytes is a direct target of the antiproteinuric effect of cyclosporine A. Nat Med. 2008;14(9):931–8.

106. Murray BM, Paller MS, Ferris TF. Effect of cyclosporine administration on renal hemodynamics in conscious rats. Kidney Int. 1985;28(5):767–74.

107. Sfikakis PP, Souliotis VL, Fragiadaki KG, Moutsopoulos HM, Boletis JN, Theofilopoulos AN. Increased expression of the FoxP3 functional marker of regulatory T cells following B cell

depletion with rituximab in patients with lupus nephritis. Clin Immunol. 2007;123(1):66–73.

108. AFornoni A, Sageshima J, Wei C, Merscher-Gomez S, Aguillon-Prada R, Jauregui AN, Li J, Mattiazzi A, Ciancio G, Chen L, Zilleruelo G, Abitbol C, Chandar J, Seeherunvong W, Ricordi C, Ikehata M, Rastaldi MP, Reiser J, Burke GW. Rituximab targets podocytes in recurrent focal segmental glomerulosclerosis. Sci Transl Med. 2011;3(85):85ra46.

109. Gulati A, Sinha A, Jordan SC, Hari P, Dinda AK, Sharma S, Srivastava RN, Moudgil A, Bagga A. Efficacy and safety of treatment with rituximab for difficult steroid-resistant and -dependent nephrotic syndrome: multicentric report. Clin J Am Soc Nephrol. 2010;5(12):2207–12.

110. Magnasco A, Ravani P, Edefonti A, Murer L, Ghio L, Belingheri M, Benetti E, Murtas C, Messina G, Massella L, Porcellini MG, Montagna M, Regazzi M, Scolari F, Ghiggeri GM. Rituximab in children with resistant idiopathic nephrotic syndrome. J Am Soc Nephrol. 2012;23(6):1117–24.

111. Delucchi A, Cano F, Rodriguez E, Wolff E, Gonzalez X, Cumsille MA. Enalapril and prednisone in children with nephrotic-range proteinuria. Pediatr Nephrol. 2000;14(12):1088–91.

112. Lama G, Luongo I, Piscitelli A, Salsano ME. Enalapril: antiproteinuric effect in children with nephrotic syndrome. Clin Nephrol. 2000;53(6):432–6.

113. Milliner DS, Morgenstern BZ. Angiotensin converting enzyme inhibitors for reduction of proteinuria in children with steroid-resistant nephrotic syndrome. Pediatr Nephrol. 1991;5(5):587–90.

114. Prasher PK, Varma PP, Baliga KV. Efficacy of enalapril in the treatment of steroid resistant idiopathic nephrotic syndrome. J Assoc Physicians India. 1999;47(2):180–2.

115. Trachtman H, Gauthier B. Effect of angiotensin-converting enzyme inhibitor therapy on proteinuria in children with renal disease. J Pediatr. 1988;112(2):295–8.

116. Ellis D, Vats A, Moritz ML, Reitz S, Grosso MJ, Janosky JE. Long-term antiproteinuric and renoprotective efficacy and safety of losartan in children with proteinuria. J Pediatr. 2003;143(1):89–97.

117. Boesby L, Elung-Jensen T, Klausen TW, Strandgaard S, Kamper AL, Boesby L, Elung-Jensen T, Klausen TW, Strandgaard S, Kamper AL. Moderate antiproteinuric effect of add-on aldosterone blockade with eplerenone in non-diabetic chronic kidney disease. A randomized cross-over study. PLoS One. 2011;6(11):e26904.

118. Bomback AS, Kshirsagar AV, Amamoo MA, Klemmer PJ. Change in proteinuria after adding aldosterone blockers to ACE inhibitors or angiotensin receptor blockers in CKD: a systematic review. Am J Kidney Dis. 2008;51(2):199–211.

119. Trachtman H, Vento S, Gipson D, Wickman L, Gassman J, Joy M, Savin V, Somers M, Pinsk M, Greene T. Novel therapies for resistant focal seg-

mental glomerulosclerosis (FONT) phase II clinical trial: study design. BMC Nephrol. 2011;12:8.

120. Rapoport M, McCrory WW, Michie AJ, Barbero G, Barnett HL, Forman CW, McNamara H. Effects of corticotrophin on children with nephrotic syndrome: clinical observations on 34 children; the effect of cortisone in 4. Am J Dis Child. 1951;82(2):248–53.

121. Barnett HL. Effect of ACTH in children with the nephrotic syndrome. Pediatrics. 1952;9(3):341.

122. Hogan J, Bomback AS, Mehta K, Canetta PA, Rao MK, Appel GB, Radhakrishnan J, Lafayette RA. Treatment of idiopathic FSGS with adrenocorticotropic hormone gel. Clin J Am Soc Nephrol. 2013;8(12):2072–81.

123. Querfeld U. Should hyperlipidemia in children with the nephrotic syndrome be treated? Pediatr Nephrol. 1999;13(1):77–84.

124. Querfeld U, Lang M, Friedrich JB, Kohl B, Fiehn W, Schärer K. Lipoprotein(a) serum levels and apolipoprotein(a) phenotypes in children with chronic renal disease. Pediatr Res. 1993;34(6):772–6.

125. Keane WF. Lipids and the kidney. Kidney Int. 1994;46(3):910–20.

126. Moorhead JF, Wheeler DC, Varghese Z. Glomerular structures and lipids in progressive renal disease. Am J Med. 1989;87(5N):12N–20.

127. Samuelsson O, Mulec H, Knight-Gibson C, Attman PO, Kron B, Larsson R, Weiss L, Wedel H, Alaupovic P. Lipoprotein abnormalities are associated with increased rate of progression of human chronic renal insufficiency. Nephrol Dial Transplant. 1997;12(9):1908–15.

128. Taal MW. Slowing the progression of adult chronic kidney disease: therapeutic advances. Drugs. 2004;64(20):2273–89.

129. Veverka A, Jolly JL. Recent advances in the secondary prevention of coronary heart disease. Expert Rev Cardiovasc Ther. 2004;2(6):877–89.

130. Coleman JE, Watson AR. Hyperlipidaemia, diet and simvastatin therapy in steroid-resistant nephrotic syndrome of childhood. Pediatr Nephrol. 1996;10(2):171–4.

131. Sanjad SA, Al-Abbad A, Al-Shorafa S. Management of hyperlipidemia in children with refractory nephrotic syndrome: the effect of statin therapy. J Pediatr. 1997;130(3):470–4.

132. Olbricht CJ, Wanner C, Thiery J, Basten A. Simvastatin in nephrotic syndrome. Simvastatin in Nephrotic Syndrome Study Group. Kidney Int Suppl. 1999;71:S113–6.

133. Citak A, Emre S, Sâirin A, Bilge I, Nayir A. Hemostatic problems and thromboembolic complications in nephrotic children. Pediatr Nephrol. 2000;14(2):138–42.

134. Lilova MI, Velkovski IG, Topalov IB. Thromboembolic complications in children with nephrotic syndrome in Bulgaria (1974–1996). Pediatr Nephrol. 2000;15(1–2):74–8.

135. Gangakhedkar A, Wong W, Pitcher LA. Cerebral thrombosis in childhood nephrosis. J Paediatr Child Health. 2005;41(4):221–4.

136. Sedman A, Friedman A, Boineau F, Strife CF, Fine R. Nutritional management of the child with mild to moderate chronic renal failure. J Pediatr. 1996;129(2):s13–8.

137. Kaysen GA. Albumin metabolism in the nephrotic syndrome: the effect of dietary protein intake. Am J Kidney Dis. 1988;12(6):461–80.

138. Krensky AM, Ingelfinger JR, Grupe WE. Peritonitis in childhood nephrotic syndrome: 1970–1980. Am J Dis Child. 1982;136(8):732–6.

139. American Academy of Pediatrics Committee on Infectious Diseases. Recommendations for the prevention of Streptococcus pneumoniae infections in infants and children: use of 13-valent pneumococcal conjugate vaccine (PCV13) and pneumococcal polysaccharide vaccine (PPSV23). Pediatrics. 2010;126(1):186–90.

140. Furth SL, Arbus GS, Hogg R, Tarver J, Chan C, Fivush BA, Southwest Pediatric Nephrology Study Group. Varicella vaccination in children with nephrotic syndrome: a report of the Southwest Pediatric Nephrology Study Group. J Pediatr. 2003;142(2):145–8.

141. Quien RM, Kaiser BA, Deforest A, Polinsky MS, Fisher M, Baluarte HJ. Response to the varicella vaccine in children with nephrotic syndrome. J Pediatr. 1997;131(5):688–90.

142. Banfi G, Colturi C, Montagnino G, Ponticelli C. The recurrence of focal segmental glomerulosclerosis in kidney transplant patients treated with cyclosporine. Transplantation. 1990;50(4):594–6.

143. Canaud G, Dion D, Zuber J, Gubler MC, Sberro R, Thervet E, Snanoudj R, Charbit M, Salomon R, Martinez F, Legendre C, Noel LH, Niaudet P. Recurrence of nephrotic syndrome after transplantation in a mixed population of children and adults: course of glomerular lesions and value of the Columbia classification of histological variants of focal and segmental glomerulosclerosis (FSGS). Nephrol Dial Transplant. 2010;25(4): 1321–8.

144. Baum MA, Stablein DM, Panzarino VM, Tejani A, Harmon WE, Alexander SR. Loss of living donor renal allograft survival advantage in children with focal segmental glomerulosclerosis. Kidney Int. 2001;59(1):328–33.

145. Hinkes B, et al. Specific podocin mutations correlate with age of onset in steroid-resistant nephrotic syndrome. J Am Soc Nephrol. 2008;19:365–71.

146. Hinkes BG, et al. Nephrotic syndrome in the first year of life: two thirds of cases are caused by mutations in 4 genes (NPHS1, NPHS2, WT1, and LAMB2). Pediatrics. 2007;119:e907–19.

147. Santín S, et al. Clinical utility of genetic testing in children and adults with steroid-resistant nephrotic syndrome. Clin J Am Soc Nephrol. 2011;6: 1139–48.

148. Büscher AK, et al. Mutations in podocyte genes are a rare cause of primary FSGS associated with ESRD in adult patients. Clin Nephrol. 2012;78:47–53.

149. Chernin G, Heeringa SF, Gbadegesin R, Liu J, Hinkes BG, Vlangos CN, Vega-Warner V, Hildebrandt F. Low prevalence of NPHS2 mutations in African American children with steroid-resistant nephrotic syndrome. Pediatr Nephrol. 2008;23(9):1455–60.

Stefanie Weber

Introduction

During the past two decades defects in various genes have been associated with the development of steroid resistant nephrotic syndrome (SRNS) in children and adults. These genes encode for proteins that participate in the development and structural architecture of glomerular visceral epithelial cells (podocytes). These insights moved the podocyte with its interdigitating foot processes and slit diaphragm (SD) into the center of interest regarding the pathophysiology of proteinuria.

While light microscopy shows variable aspects ranging from minimal change nephropathy to diffuse mesangial sclerosis or focal-segmental glomerulosclerosis (Fig. 17.1a, b), all hereditary proteinuria syndromes share a common phenotype when evaluated by electron microscopy, which uniformly demonstrates the typical flattening of the foot processes and loss of the SD. With respect to the clinical course, different entities can be distinguished, especially referring to the onset of the disease and modi of inheritance. Disorders of early glomerular development most often manifest prenatally, directly after birth or in early infancy. Disorders with late-onset nephrotic

syndrome typically manifest as FSGS in adolescence or adulthood, frequently following an autosomal-dominant mode of inheritance with incomplete penetrance and variable expression. In rare cases, extrarenal symptoms are associated with hereditary nephrotic syndrome, e.g., in Denys-Drash, Frasier, Schimke and Pierson syndrome. In the following, important genes involved in hereditary nephrotic syndrome will be discussed. Given the rapid development in the field, this list is comprehensive, though may not be complete.

Hereditary Disorders of Early Glomerular Development

Podocytes develop from the nephrogenic blastema in a chain of events in conjunction with the development of the renal glomeruli. First, local condensation of the mesenchyme leads to the formation of the nephron anlage, i.e., the comma-shaped and the S-shaped bodies and eventually the formation of the mature glomerulus. Podocytes are the first cells that can clearly be distinguished in this process, forming a disk-like layer of epithelial cells. The subsequent differentiation to mature podocytes with interdigitating primary and secondary foot processes is associated with a general loss of the ability for further proliferation. At this stage, early cell-cell contacts (adherens junctions) have developed into a specialized structure, the SD, spanning the intercellular space. The final

S. Weber
Pediatric Nephrology/Pediatrics II, University
Children's Hospital Marburg, Baldingerstrasse 35033,
Marburg, Germany
e-mail: stefanie.weber@med.uni-marburg.de

© Springer-Verlag Berlin Heidelberg 2016
D.F. Geary, F. Schaefer (eds.), *Pediatric Kidney Disease*, DOI 10.1007/978-3-662-52972-0_17

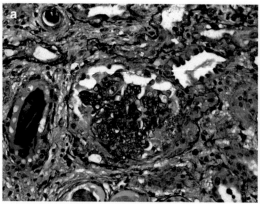

Fig. 17.1 (**a, b**). Kidney histology of a patient with diffuse mesangial sclerosis (**a**) and focal-segmental glomerulosclerosis (**b**), respectively. PAS staining; magnification 40× (Courtesy of Kerstin Amann, Institut of Pathology, Department of Nephropathology, University Hospital Erlangen, Germany)

glomerular filtration barrier is constituted by the fenestrated endothelium, the glomerular basement membrane (GBM) and interdigitating podocytes.

A number of genes are involved in these processes (Table 17.1 and Fig. 17.2), and *WT1* is one of the major mediators of podocyte differentiation. *NPHS1* and *NPHS2* code for nephrin and podocin, respectively, two proteins that have important roles for the organization of the SD. *LAMB2* encodes laminin ß2, one component of the heterotrimeric laminins that link the podocyte to the GBM. *LMX1b* encodes the transcription factor Lmx1b that in the kidney is exclusively expressed in podocytes. It is one of the crucial genes regulating gene expression during early steps of podocyte development. The most recently identified gene involved in early-onset nephrotic syndrome (NPHS3), *PLCE1*, encodes for phospholipase C epsilon-1, involved in podocyte signaling processes.

WT1 Gene Mutations

The *Wilms tumor* is one of the most common solid tumors of childhood, occurring in 1 of 10,000 children and accounting for 8 % of childhood cancers. The Wilms' tumor suppressor gene (*WT1*) was first identified in 1990 [1]. *WT1* locates on chromosome 11p13 and encodes a zinc finger transcription factor that regulates the expression of many genes during kidney and urogenital development. Mutations in *WT1* were first identified in pediatric patients affected by Wilms' tumor, aniridia, genitourinary malformations and mental retardation (WAGR syndrome) [2]. These were truncating mutations, associated with complete loss-of-function of WT1. *WT1* mutations were also identified in patients with isolated Wilms' tumor [3]. In tumor material of isolated cases both germline and somatic mutations have been detected. Familial Wilms tumor forms seem to follow a dominant pattern of inheritance, with dominant germline mutations. However, in a number of these cases the classical two-hit inactivation model, with loss of heterozygosity due to a second somatic event, has been described as the underlying cause of tumor development [4].

Subsequently, *WT1* mutations were also associated with Denys-Drash syndrome (DDS) [5], Frasier syndrome (FS) [6], and diffuse mesangial sclerosis (DMS) with isolated nephrotic syndrome (NS) [7]. The full picture of autosomal dominant *Denys-Drash syndrome* is characterized by early onset NS, male pseudohermaphroditism, gonadal dysgenesis and the development of Wilms tumor (in more than 90 % of patients). The Wilms tumor may precede or develop after the manifestation of NS. Age at onset of NS is generally within the first months of life [8]. In rare cases enlarged and hyperechogenic kidneys were already demonstrated by prenatal ultrasound [9]. Renal histology typically presents with DMS [10] and electron

Table 17.1 Overview on important disorders causing hereditary nephrotic syndromes

	Inheritance	Locus	Gene	Protein	OMIM accession no.
Early-onset nephrotic syndrome					
Isolated DMS	AR	11p13	*WT1*	WT1	256370
Denys-Drash syndrome (typically DMS)	AD	11p13	*WT1*	WT1	194080
Frasier syndrome (typically FSGS)	AD	11p13	*WT1*	WT1	136680
Congenital nephrotic syndrome/Finnish type	AR	19q13	*NPHS1*	Nephrin	602716
Recessive familial SRNS (MC/FSGS)	AR	1q25	*NPHS2*	Podocin	600995
Pierson syndrome	AR	3p21	*LAMB2*	Laminin β2	609049
Nail-patella syndrome	AD	9q34.1	*LMX1B*	LMX1B	161200
Recessive nephrotic syndrome (DMS/FSGS)	AR	10q23-q24	*NPHS3/PLCE1*	PLCE1	608414
Recessive nephrotic syndrome (FSGS)	AR	12p12.3	*PTPRO*	PTPRO	614196
Recessive congenital nephrotic syndrome (DMS)	AR	17q25.3	*ARHGDIA*	ARHGDIA	615244
Recessive childhood-onset nephrotic syndrome	AR	16p13.13	*EMP2*	EMP2	602334
Late-onset nephrotic syndrome/FSGS					
FSGS1	AD	19q13	*ACTN4*	α-Actinin 4	603278
FSGS2	AD	11q21-22	*TRPC6*	TRPC6	603965
FSGS3 (*CD2AP*-associated disease susceptibility)	AR/AD	6	*CD2AP*	CD2AP	607832
FSGS4 (*MYH9*-associated disease susceptibility)	AD	22q12.3	*MYH9/APOE1*	MYH9/APO1	612551
FSGS5	AD	14q32.33	*INF2*	INF2	613237
FSGS6	AR	15q22.2	*MYO1E*	MYO1E	614131
Mitochondrial disease					
Early-onset SRNS with variable extrarenal symptoms	AR	4q21-q22	*COQ2*	COQ2	609825
Early-onset SRNS with sensorineural deafness	AR	14q24.3	*COQ6*	Q10 mono-oxigenase 6	614647
SRNS/FSGS	AR	19q13.2	*ADCK4*	ADCK4	615573
Syndromal disease					
Schimke immuno-osseous dysplasia	AR	2q34-q36	*SMARCAL1*	SMARCAL1	242900

microscopy reveals foot process effacement. The NS is resistant to steroid treatment and renal function is deteriorating rapidly to end-stage renal disease (ESRD) already during infancy. Bilateral nephrectomy is generally advised in ESRD in order to prevent the development of Wilms tumor [11]. Recurrence of NS after kidney transplantation has not been observed so far [12].

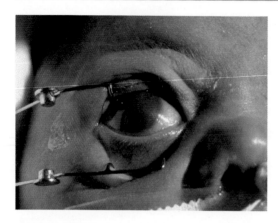

Fig. 17.2 Typical aspect of a patient with Pierson syndrome and microcoria (Courtesy of Kveta Blahova, Pediatric Clinic, Charles University, Prague, Czech Republic)

Dominant *WT1* mutations are identified in the vast majority of DDS patients. These mutations predominantly affect exons 8 and 9 of the *WT1* gene and most of them are de novo mutations not observed in the parents. Most *WT1* mutations associated with DDS are missense mutations affecting conserved amino acids of the zinc finger domains, with p.R394W being the most frequent mutation observed. These alterations of the zinc finger structure reduce the DNA binding capacity of the *WT1* protein [13]. A heterozygous knock-in mouse model has been created for the p.R394W missense mutation, presenting with DMS and male genital anomalies [14] supporting the dominant nature of the disease.

Of note, some of the patients affected by *WT1* mutations in exons 8 and 9 do not present with the full picture of DDS but with isolated DMS. *WT1* analysis should therefore be performed in all children with isolated DMS and early-onset NS because of the high risk of Wilms tumor development in case of a positive mutation analysis result. Close monitoring by renal ultrasound (e.g., every 6 months) is important in all children with *WT1* mutation and early-onset NS. In addition, karyotype analysis is recommended in all girls with isolated DMS to detect a possible male pseudohermaphroditism. Some patients with isolated DMS present with recessive mutations in *WT1* with both the maternal and paternal allele being affected [7].

Frasier syndrome is also characterized by a progressive glomerulopathy and male pseudoher-maphroditism [15]; however, there are specific differences to DDS: the onset of proteinuria occurs later in childhood and the deterioration of renal function is slower. ESRD develops only in the second or third decade of life. As in DDS, proteinuria and NS are steroid-resistant. Renal histology in FS patients typically shows focal and segmental glomerulosclerosis (FSGS) [16]; in a minority of patients only minimal change lesions are observed. In female patients, the genitourinary tract is normally developed, whereas a complete sex reversal with gonadal dysgenesis is observed in 46,XY patients. Primary amenorrhoea in conjunction with NS is a typical feature of these 46,XY patients and should prompt molecular analysis of *WT1*. While the risk to develop a Wilms tumor is low in patients with FS, gonadoblastomata, developing from gonadal dysgenesis, are frequently observed. After the diagnosis of FS, gonadectomy is highly recommended in 46,XY patients.

In 1997, it was first demonstrated that mutations in the *WT1* gene also underly the pathogenesis of FS [6]. Notably, the class of mutations in FS differs from DDS: whereas mutations affecting the coding sequence of exons 8 and 9 cause DDS, mutations associated with FS represent donor splice-site mutations located in intron 9. Similar to DDS, these mutations occur in a heterozygous state and, frequently, they are de novo mutations not observed in the parents. The donor splice-site of intron 9 plays an important role for the generation of the KTS isoform of the WT1 protein. This isoform contains three additional amino acids (lysine-threonine-serine; KTS). It has been demonstrated that the (+) KTS/(−) KTS protein dose ratio is of high relevance for WT1 action during genitourinary and kidney development. In FS patients, this ratio is markedly reduced due to the splice-site mutations [6].

Large genotype-phenotype studies confirm these associations based on the nature of the underlying mutation [17]. Still, there is some overlap and phenotypic heterogeneity in selected cases: splice-site mutations typical for FS may in some cases be found in patients with DDS [5] or isolated DMS [18], and patients with typical DDS mutations may display with isolated FSGS

[19] or Wilms' tumor without NS [20]. As a conclusion, analysis of *WT1* should be included in the routine genetic testing in patients with SRNS.

NPHS1 Gene Mutations Associated with Autosomal Recessive CNS of the Finnish Type (CNF)

CNS of the Finnish type is characterized by autosomal recessive inheritance and the development of proteinuria in utero [21]. The responsible gene was mapped in 1994 to chromosome 19q13 [22] and mutations in *NPHS1* have been subsequently identified in affected children [23]. *NPHS1* encodes for nephrin, a zipper-like protein of the glomerular SD. Typically, severe NS manifests before 3 months of age and renal biopsy specimens show immature glomeruli, mesangial cell hypercellularity, glomerular foot process effacement and microcystic dilatations of the proximal tubules. NS is steroid-resistant in these patients and treatment options comprise albumin infusions, pharmacological interventions with ACE inhibitors and indomethacin and ultimately uni- or bilateral nephrectomy [24–27].

Nephrin is exclusively expressed in podocytes, at the level of the SD once full differentiation has occurred [28]. Nephrin belongs to the immunoglobulin superfamily with a single putative transmembrane domain, a short intracellular N-terminus and long extracellular C-terminus [23]. The extracellular C-terminus is predicted to bridge the intercellular space between the interdigitating foot processes, rendering nephrin a key component of the SD. Nephrin strands contribute to the porous structure of the SD, forming pores of approximately 40 nm in size [29]. These pores are currently believed to be in part responsible for the size selectivity of the SD and the glomerular filtration barrier.

Apart from its role as a structural protein, nephrin also appears to participate in intracellular signaling pathways maintaining the functional integrity of the podocyte [30–32]. The SD is discussed to constitute a highly dynamic protein complex that recruits signal transduction components and initiates signaling to regulate complex biologic programs in the podocyte. A number of proteins within this signaling platform were identified to interact with nephrin, among these podocin, CD2AP and TRPC6, all of which are also associated with the development of NS when altered by gene mutations (see below). It is suggested that the plasma membrane of the filtration slit has a special lipid composition comparable to lipid rafts [33]. Lipid rafts are specialized microdomains of the plasma membrane with a unique lipid content and a concentrated assembly of signal transduction molecules [34]. It was shown that nephrin is a lipid raft-associated protein at the SD and that podocin serves to recruit nephrin into these microdomains. Disease-causing podocin mutations fail to target nephrin into rafts, altering nephrin-induced signal transduction [32]. In summary, these studies confirm the extraordinary role of SD proteins for the maintenance of the glomerular filtration barrier.

Mutations in *NPHS1* were first identified in the Finnish population, leading to the classification of "Finnish type" CNS. Two truncating mutations were found with high frequency in affected Finnish children suggesting an underlying founder effect in the Finnish population: p.L41fsX90 (Fin major, truncating the majority of the protein) and p.R1109X (Fin minor, truncating only a short C-terminal part). In subsequent studies, *NPHS1* mutations were also identified in non-Finnish patients throughout the world. The Fin major and Fin minor mutations are only rarely observed in non-Finnish patients. Several mutational hot spots were identified affecting the immunoglobulin domains of the nephrin protein [35]. The immunoglobulin domains 2, 4 and 7 appear particularly important for gene function. In addition to the high prevalence in Finland, *NPHS1* mutations are also common among Mennonites in Pennsylvania, 8 % of this population is carrier of a heterozygous mutant allele [36].

Recent studies pointed out that congenital nephrotic syndrome can also be caused by recessive mutations in *NPHS2* (see below), particularly involving nonsense-, frameshift or the homozygous missense mutation p.R138Q [37–39]. In rare cases a triallelic digenic mode of inheritance was observed in patients with CNS/SRNS: in these patients, sequence variations in both *NPHS1* and *NPHS2* were identified with a total of three affected alleles (two *NPHS1* mutations and one *NPHS2* sequence variation or vice versa) [35]. It is speculated that the additional sequence variation of the second gene plays a role as a genetic modifier, possibly aggravating the clinical phenotype.

NPHS2 Gene Mutations Associated with Autosomal Recessive Steroid-Resistant Nephrotic Syndrome

The *NPHS2* gene was mapped by linkage analysis in eight families with autosomal recessive SRNS to chromosome 1q25-q31 [40] and recessive mutations in *NPHS2* were identified subsequently [41]. NS in these families was characterized by steroid-resistance, age at onset between 3 and 5 years and no recurrence of proteinuria after renal transplantation. *NPHS2* mutations have never been reported in patients with SSNS. Renal histology typically shows FSGS; however, some patients present with only minimal change lesions. In some cases progression from minimal change lesions to FSGS has been demonstrated in repeat biopsies.

NPHS2 encodes for podocin, a 42 kD integral membrane protein expressed in both fetal and mature glomeruli [41]. By electron microscopy and immunogold labeling it was demonstrated that the site of expression is the SD of the podocytes. As both protein termini are located in the cytosol and podocin is predicted to have only one membrane domain, a hair-pin like structure of the protein was proposed. Interacting with both nephrin and CD2AP, podocin appears to link nephrin to the podocyte cytoskeleton. In patients affected by recessive mutations in *NPHS2*, SD formation is impaired and the typical foot process effacement is visible. These observations suggest that podocin has an important function for maintaining the glomerular filtration barrier. The knockout of *Nphs2* in mice is associated with a phenotype highly reminiscent of the human disease with podocyte foot process effacement, nephrotic range proteinuria and chronic renal insufficiency [42]. As nephrin, podocin is localized in lipid rafts [33] and is important for recruiting nephrin to these microdomains of the plasma membrane [32]. Some mutations in *NPHS2* impair the ability of podocin to target nephrin to the rafts, especially the most frequent mutation identified in European patients (p.R138Q) [32].

Up to now, more than 125 pathogenic mutations have been described in *NPHS2* [43]; most mutations affect the stomatin domain located in the C-terminal part of the protein [37, 44]. Mutations in *NPHS2* were first identified in infants with SRNS and rapid progression to ESRD [41]. Subsequently, however, it became evident that defects in podocin can be responsible for SRNS manifesting at any age from birth to adulthood [45–47]. A partial genotype-phenotype correlation is apparent: while frameshift-, nonsense- and the p.R138Q mutation in homozygosity are typically associated with early-onset NS, other missense mutations (e.g., p.V180M, p.R238S) are predominantly found in patients with a later onset of SRNS [37]. A single nucleotide polymorphism in *NPHS2* (p.R229Q) has been identified to be a common cause of adulthood-onset of hereditary nephrotic syndrome when present in compound heterozygosity with specific pathogenic *NPHS2* mutations [48–50]. In the study of Machuca et al., among 119 patients diagnosed with NS presenting after 18 years of age, 18 patients were found to have one pathogenic mutation and p.R229Q, but none with two pathogenic mutations in *NPHS2* [50]. Screening for the p.R229Q variant seems therefore recommended in adolescent or adult patients. Recent data demonstrated that the pathogenicity of p.R229Q depends on the *trans*-associated mutation. It was shown that the association of *NPHS2*-p.R229Q with specific exon 7 or exon 8 mutations in *NPHS2* altered heterodimerization and mislocalization of the encoded p.Arg229Gln podocin protein [51]. Following this study, homozygosity of *NPHS2*-p.R229Q alone is not disease causing. This observation is important as the p.R229Q variant is prevalent in heterozygous state in approximately 3 % of the normal population (range 0.5–7 %, depending on the genetic background) [51], resulting in a frequency of homozygous carriers of up to 1 %.

Still, the p.R229Q variant is discussed to be a non-neutral PM with an enhanced frequency in FSGS patient cohorts of different ethnical origins [52]. In vitro studies have demonstrated that p.R229Q podocin shows decreased binding to its interacting protein partner nephrin [48] and in a large study of more than 1,500 individuals of the general population p.R229Q was significantly associated with the prevalence of microalbuminuria, a risk factor for developing chronic renal insufficiency and cardiovascular events [53].

LAMB2 Gene Mutations Associated with Pierson Syndrome

Pierson syndrome is characterized by CNS and peculiar eye abnormalities including a typical non-reactive narrowing of the pupils (microcoria, Fig. 17.3) but also additional lens and corneal abnormalities [54]. Recessive mutations in *LAMB2* on chromosome 3p21 were identified as underlying genetic defect [55]. *LAMB2* encodes for the protein laminin β2, one component of the trimeric laminins in the kidney that crosslink the basolateral membrane of the podocyte to the GBM. Most disease-associated alleles identified in Pierson patients were truncating mutations leading to loss of laminin β2 expression in the kidney [55]. Ocular laminin β2 expression in unaffected controls was strongest in the intraocular muscles, corresponding well to the characteristic hypoplasia of ciliary and pupillary muscles observed in affected patients. Subsequent genotype-phenotype studies revealed that some mutations in *LAMB2*, especially hypomorphic missense mutations, can be associated with a phenotypic spectrum that is much broader than previously anticipated including isolated CNS or CNS with minor ocular changes different from those observed in Pierson syndrome [56]. Fetal ultrasound in four consecutive fetuses of a family with Pierson syndrome and positive *LAMB2* mutation analysis consistently revealed marked hyperechogenicity of the kidneys and variable degrees of pyelectasis by 15 weeks of gestation [57]. Placentas were significantly enlarged. Hydrops fetalis due to severe hypalbuminemia demonstrated by chordocentesis occurred

in one fetus and anencephaly was detected in another fetus. Development of oligohydramnios indicated a prenatal decline of renal excretory function. From these studies it can be concluded that mutational analysis in *LAMB2* should also be considered in isolated CNS if no mutations were found in *NPHS1*, *NPHS2*, or *WT1*, and in cases with prenatal onset of nephrotic disease with typical sonomorphologic findings of the kidneys and the development of oligohydramnios.

The *LAMB2* missense mutation p.C321R, for example, has been identified in congenital nephrotic syndrome with only mild extrarenal symptoms. Functional studies in cell culture and mice suggested defective intracellular trafficking of the mutant protein, associated with endoplasmatic reticulum stress [58]. Another missense mutation (p.S80R) has been identified in homozygous state a teenage girl with severe myopia since early infancy and nephrotic range proteinuria first detected at the age of 6 but normal renal function. Renal biopsy revealed mild DMS and a residual expression of laminin β2 [59]. Summarizing these reports, it becomes obvious that the phenotype associated with pathogenic *LAMB2* mutations can be very variable and that genetic testing for *LAMB2* mutations should be considered in all patients with either early-onset proteinuria or glomerular proteinuria with an abnormal ocular phenotype.

LMX1b Gene Mutations Associated with Autosomal Dominant Nail-Patella Syndrome

Nail-patella syndrome (NPS) or onychoosteodysplasia is caused by dominant mutations in the *LMX1b* gene, located on chromosome 9q34.1 and encoding the LIM-homeodomain protein Lmx1b. Lmx1b plays a central role in dorsal/ventral patterning of the vertebrate limb and targeted disruption of Lmx1b results in skeletal defects, including hypoplastic nails, absent patellae, and a unique form of renal dysplasia [60]. Prominent features of affected children are dysplasia of nails and absent or hypodysplastic patellae. In many patients, also iliac horns, dysplasia of the elbows, glaucoma and/or hearing impairment are detected.

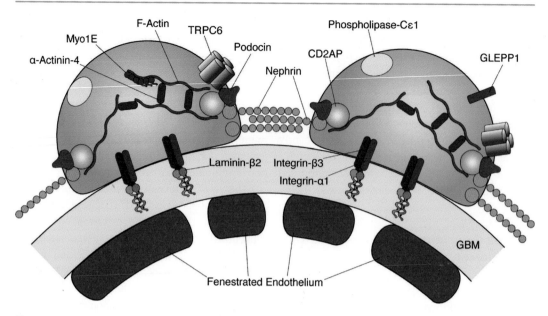

Fig. 17.3 Schema of a podocyte foot process cross-section, depicting important components involved in hereditary nephrotic syndrome

LMX1b is highly expressed in podocytes and patients can also present with an involvement of the kidney comprising proteinuria, nephrotic syndrome or renal insufficiency. Overall, nephropathy is reported in approximately 40% of affected patients (microalbuminuria or overt proteinuria) [61] but ESRD in less than 10% [62]. Interestingly, renal involvement appears significantly more frequent in females and in patients with a positive family history of NPS nephropathy [61]. In NPS patients with renal involvement, electron microscopy shows collagen fibril-like deposition in the GBM with typical lucent areas [63]. These characteristic ultrastructural changes can even be present in patients without apparent nephropathy [64]. Large genotype-phenotype studies demonstrated that individuals with an *LMX1B* mutation located in the homeodomain showed a significantly higher frequency of renal protein loss and higher values of proteinuria than subjects with mutations in the LIM domains [61]. Recent studies identified *LMX1B* missense mutations affecting residue p.R246 also in a subset of patients with isolated FSGS without extrarenal symptoms, expending the spectrum of FGSG-related genes to *LMX1B* [65, 66]. Insight into Lmx1b function was further obtained by the generation of *Lmx1b* knockout animals [67]. In *Lmx1b*(−/−) mice the

expression of GBM collagens is reduced and podocytes have a reduced number of foot processes, are dysplastic, and lack typical SD structures. Interestingly, mRNA and protein levels for CD2AP and podocin are greatly reduced in these kidneys and several *LMX1B* binding sites were identified in the putative regulatory regions of both *CD2AP* and *NPHS2* (encoding podocin) [67]. These observations support a cooperative role for Lmx1b, CD2AP and podocin in foot process and slit diaphragm formation.

PLCE1 Gene Mutations Associated with Autosomal Recessive Nephrotic Syndrome

Following positional cloning, a gene locus for nephrotic syndrome (*NPHS3*) was mapped to chromosome 10q23-q24 and homozygous truncating mutations were identified in the gene *PLCE1*, encoding the enzyme phospholipase C-ε1 which is involved in intracellular signal transduction [68]. Onset of nephrotic syndrome was generally early in affected children and renal histology revealed DMS in most cases. In subsequent studies, mutations in *PLCE1* were identified in a relevant percentage of patients with DMS

(28–33 %) [69, 70] and with a lower frequency in hereditary FSGS (8 %) [70]. Interestingly, two of the individuals with truncating *PLCE1* mutations entered sustained remission following steroid or cyclosporin A treatment [69]. The observation of a possible responsiveness to immunosuppression in *PLCE1* mutation carriers awaits confirmation in a larger number of affected patients.

PLCE1 is widely expressed in many tissues including also the podocytes. The knock-down of *pcle1* in zebrafish is associated with the development of podocyte foot process effacement and edematous outer appearance of the fish [68] confirming a specific role of phospholipase C epsilon-1 for the maintanance of the glomerular filtration barrier. Still, the pathogenesis of isolated podocyte damage and the development of proteinuria in patients lacking phospholipase C epsilon-1 remains to be elucidated.

PTPRO Gene Mutations Associated with Autosomal Recessive Nephrotic Syndrome

Homozygous *PTPRO* splice-site mutations were identified in two families of Turkish origin with childhood-onset nephrotic syndrome and minimal change nephropathy or FSGS on renal biopsy [71]. Nephrotic syndrome was resistent to oral prednisone therapy but a partial response to an intensified immunosppressive regimen including pulse methylprednisolone and cyclosporin A was observed in some cases. PTPRO, identical to glomerular epithelial protein-1 (GLEPP1), is a receptor-like membrane protein tyrosine phosphatase expressed at the apical membrane of the podocyte foot processes in the kidney. Disruption of *Ptpro* in mice results in alterations of the podocyte structure and a reduction of the glomerular filtration rate indicating a role of PTPRO for proper podocyte function.

ARHGDIA Gene Mutations in Autosomal Recessive DMS

A recessive mutation in *ARHGDIA*, encoding a regulator of Rho-GTPases, was detected in two

female siblings born to consanguineous parents. Both girls presented with congenital nephrotic syndrome and DMS on renal histology [72]. The homozygous 3-bp in-frame deletion mutation in *ARHGDIA* seems to be implicated in the hyperactivation of Rho-GTPases, causing a derangement of the podocyte actin cytoskeleton. *Arghdia* knock-out mice develop podocyte damage, severe proteinuria and progressive renal failure, suporting a role of human *ARHGDIA* in the pathogenesis of proteinuric disease.

EMP2 Gene Mutations Associated with Autosomal Recessive Childhood-Onset Nephrotic Syndrome

Mutations in podocyte genes have only exceptionally been identified in children with steroid-sensitive nephrotic syndrome (SSNS) [44, 73]. However, by homozygosity mapping and whole exome sequencing in 67 families biallelic mutations in *EMP2* were identified in one pair of siblings of Turkish origin, affected by frequently relapsing nephrotic syndrome with remission after cyclophosphamide treatment. In both, onset of the disease was below 3 years of age. Subsequently, more than 1,600 individuals with nephrotic syndrome were screened for recessive mutations in *EMP2* and two more patients with SRNS (of Turkish and of African origin) were identified [74]. *EMP2* encodes epithelial membrane protein 2, discussed to be involved in cell proliferation and cell-cell interactions. The knock-down of *emp2* in the zebrafish resulted in pericardial effusions, consistent with a role of epithelial membrane protein 2 in keeping-up glomerular filtration [74].

Hereditary Disorders with Late-Onset Nephrotic Syndrome

Hereditary late-onset FSGS is a heterogeneous condition generally transmitted in an autosomal dominant fashion (with the exception of autosomal recessive FSGS6). Different disease loci have been mapped in affected families (FGSG1-FSGS6) and responsible genetic defects have been identified in many podocyte-associated genes, frequently involving actin cytoskeleton architecture and dynamics.

ACTN4 Gene Mutations Associated with Adulthood FSGS (FSGS1)

In 1998, a locus for autosomal dominant late-onset FSGS was mapped to chromosome 19q13 (FSGS1) [75] and mutations in *ACTN4* were identified as the underlying pathogenic cause [76]. *ACTN4* encodes for α-actinin-4, an actin-bundling protein of the cytoskeleton highly expressed in podocytes. Both a knock-down and an overexpression transgenic mouse model have been established for *Actn4*, demonstrating proteinuria and podocyte alterations. It was therefore discussed that α-actinin-4 plays an important role for the cytoskeletal function of the podocyte. Young knock-out mice present with focal areas of foot process effacement and older animals with diffuse effacement and globally disrupted podocyte morphology [77]. Moreover, *Actn4* was shown to be upregulated in the kidneys of different animal models of proteinuria. Human *ACTN4* mutations were identified in three different families with FSGS [76]. The clinical course in affected family members was characterized by progressively increasing proteinuria starting in adolescence and developing into FSGS and chronic renal insufficiency later in adult life. ESRD was observed in a number of affected individuals. All *ACTN4* mutations identified so far represent non-conservative amino acid substitutions affecting the actin-binding domain of α-actinin-4. In vitro studies demonstrated that mutant α-actinin-4 binds filamentous actin more strongly than wild-type protein. Based on this observation it was proposed that dominant mutations in *ACTN4* interfere with the maintenance of podocyte architecture: a proper organisation of the cytoskeleton seems to be important for normal functioning of podocyte foot processes. Interestingly, however, not all mutation carriers of the families reported by Kaplan et al. presented with a renal phenotype. The observed incomplete penetrance suggests that additional (genetic or non-genetic) factors are involved in the pathogenesis that in conjunction with a mutation in *ACTN4* lead to the manifestation of FSGS. *ACTN4* mutations may confer *disease susceptibility*, as also discussed for mutations in *CD2AP* and *TRPC6*. However, mutations in *ACTN4* represent a rare cause of hereditary FSGS, accounting for approximately 0–4 % of familial FSGS, depending on the study cohort [45, 78, 79].

TRPC6 Gene Mutations Associated with Late-Onset FSGS (FSGS2)

In 1999, a second gene locus for autosomal dominant FSGS was mapped to chromosome 11q21-q22 using a 399-member Caucasian kindred of British heritage dating back seven generations [80]. Fourteen deceased family members had suffered from ESRD, 14 living family members were on dialysis or had undergone renal transplantation, and 3 individuals were proteinuric. Six years later, the responsible gene *TRPC6* was identified [81, 82]. *TRPC6* encodes the transient receptor potential cation channel TRPC6 that is thought to mediate capacitative calcium entry into cells. Expression analysis revealed that TRPC6 is highly expressed in the kidney and also in podocytes at the site of the SD. A dominant missense mutation was identified in the original family of Winn et al., and five additional families with mutations in *TRPC6* were characterized by Reiser et al. Two of the missense mutations in the latter study were shown to increase the current amplitudes of TRPC6, consistent with a gain-of-function effect of the mutations. Interestingly, however, both studies describe carrier individuals with a normal renal phenotype, pointing to an incomplete penetrance of the mutations. *TRPC6* mutations have been identified in very few children; early disease onset seems to be exceptional. So far, it is unknown how the dysfunction of a cation channel is related to the development of podocyte damage and loss of the glomerular filtration barrier. One hypothesis is related to the observation that MEC-2, a *C. elegans* homologue of podocin, participates in the mechanosensation of the worm. MEC-2 is physically and functionally linked to ion channels, transducing the signals of mechanosensation. Since TRPC6 interacts with podocin and nephrin at the SD, it was proposed that podocin takes part in mechanosensation processes at the glomerular filtration barrier, transducing signals to TRPC6 which in turn modulates intracellular calcium concentrations in the podocyte. Nephrin, on the other hand, is thought to stimulate different pathways of the intracellular signaling machinery. Therefore, a complex protein network involving nephrin, podocin, CD2AP and the cation channel TRPC6 is established to maintain the SD structure of the foot process. Mutations in TRPC6 likely affect this functional network by altering the intracellular calcium concentration of the podocyte.

CD2AP Gene Mutations Associated with Adulthood FSGS (FSGS3)

In 1999, FSGS3 was shown to map to chromosome 6 and reported to be caused by haploinsufficiency for *CD2AP* [83]. *CD2AP* encodes for the CD2-associated protein CD2AP, an actin-binding protein that was originally identified as a cytoplasmic ligand of the CD2 receptor on T and natural killer cells. *CD2AP* knock-out mice presented not only with impaired immune functions but also with severe NS and FSGS, accompanied by mesangial hypercellularity and extracellular matrix deposition [84]. Electron microscopy showed the typical loss of podocyte foot process integrity with process effacement and loss of the SD structure. Screening in FSGS patients led to the identification of a dominant *CD2AP* mutation (a 2-bp substitution altering the exon 7 splice acceptor site) in two adult patients with late-onset FSGS [83]. An enhanced disease susceptibility for FSGS conferred by the change in CD2AP expression was postulated as the underlying pathogenic mechanism. CD2AP interacts with nephrin and both proteins localize to lipid rafts in the plasma membrane [33], suggesting that CD2AP is required to connect nephrin (and thus the SD) to the cytoskeleton of the podocyte. An impairment of CD2AP function might be associated with enhanced cytoskeletal fragility, predisposing to podocyte damage.

Susceptibility to Genetic Locus 22q12.3 (FSGS4), Including the Genes MYH9 and APOE1

Multiple single nucleotide polymorphisms (SNP) in the gene *MYH9* were recessively associated with idiopathic and HIV-associated FSGS and hypertensive end-stage renal disease (ESRD) in African American adult patients [85]. However, subsequent genomewide analyses in large patient cohorts suggested that a positively selected risk variant could be in a larger interval containing the *APOL* genes rather than be confined to *MYH9*. Two *APOL1* risks variants for FSGS were identified to be common in African but absent in European chromosomes. As APOL1 is a serum factor that lyses trypanosomes and in vitro assays revealed that only the kidney disease-associated APOL1 variants lysed Trypanosoma brucei rhodesiense it was speculated that evolution of a critical survival factor in Africa may have contributed to the high rates of renal disease in African Americans [86].

INF2 Gene Mutations Associated with Autosomal Dominant FSGS (FSGS5) and Charcot-Marie-Tooth Disease

Mutations in *INF2*, encoding inverted formin-2, were first identified in 11 FSGS families with onset of proteinuria in adolescence or adulthood [87]. Proteinuria was typically moderate, accompanied by microscopic hematuria and hypertension in some cases. Proteinuria was progressive, often leading to ESRD. Renal biopsies showed the presence of FSGS and unusually prominent actin bundles within the foot processes, on electron microscopy. Being part of the actin cytoskeleton Inf2/inverted formin-2 interacts with actin and is involved in both polymerization and depolymerization of actin filaments. Interestingly, mutations in *INF2* were also identified in patients with dominant intermediate Charcot-Marie-Tooth (CMT) disease and FSGS-associated proteinuria [88], localizing to a disctinct area of the *INF2* gene. Mutant INF2 protein was abnormally distributed in the cytoplasm and the actin cytoskeleton and microtubule network were disorganized, not only in podoctes but also in peripheral Schwann cells, leading to disturbed myelin formation and CMT.

Mutations in MYO1E in Autosomal Recessive FSGS (FSGS6)

Recessive homozygous mutations in *MYOE1*, encoding a nonmuscle membrane-associated class I myosin, were reported in children and adolescent patients of consanguineous union affected by nephrotic-range proteinuria, microhematuria, hypoalbuminemia, and edema [89]. Renal biopsy demonstrated FSGS, tubular atrophy and interstitial fibrosis. *Myoe1*-knockout mice show a similar phenoytpe with proteinuria, hematuria and progessive renal failure, indicating a defect in the glomerular filtration barrier. Impaired intracellular trafficking of the mutant protein seems to be implicated in the pathogenesis of *MYO1E*-associated disease.

Mitochondrial Disorders Associated with Nephrotic Syndrome

Several gene mutations in different components of the coenzyme Q_{10} (CoQ_{10}) biosynthesis pathway have recently been identified to be involved in hereditary nephrotic syndrome, frequently associated with extrarenal symptoms. Recessive mutations in *COQ2* were first identified in 2006 in a pair of siblings with early-onset glomerular lesions, steroid resistant nephrotic syndrome and CoQ_{10} deficiency [90]. The gene *COQ2* encodes for the para-hydroxybenzoate-polyprenyl transferase enzyme of the CoQ_{10} synthesis pathway. An increased number of abnormal mitochondria in podocytes and other glomerular cells was demonstrated by electron microscopy. Following this initial study, more patients were identified with a similar clinical course and loss-of-function mutations in *COQ2* [91, 92]. Extrarenal symptoms of mitochondrial disease are not obligatory but developed in a subset of affected patients to a varying degree, including

encephalopathy, lactacidosis, myoclonic epilepsy and hypertrophic cardiomyopathy.

Early-onset SRNS associated with sensorineural deafness has subsequently been attributed to recessive mutations in *COQ6* encoding for CoQ_{10} biosynthesis monooxygenase 6 [93]. Renal histology revealed FSGS lesions in most cases with COQ6 mutations but DMS has also been observed.

Most recently, mutations in *ADCK4* were associated with disturbed CoQ_{10} biosynthesis and identified by homozygosity mapping and whole exome sequencing in children with SRNS and school age onset of nephrotic syndrome [94]. *ADCK4* encodes the aarF domain containing kinase 4, a protein partially expressed in podocyte foot processes but also in podocyte mitochondria. ADCK4 colocalizes with COQ6 and COQ7 and CoQ_{10} serum levels are reduced in affected patients.

Of note, *COQ2*, *COQ6* and *ADCK4* are all nuclear genes encoding mitochondrial proteins. Therefore, the inheritance of associated disorders follows the Mendelian rules of autosomal recessive disease.

These findings indicate that the podocyte reacts very sensitively to disturbances of energy supply and it can be expected that mutations in other genes encoding mitochondrial proteins will be discovered in patients with SRNS in the future.

Most importantly and in contrast to all other hereditary disorders of the podocyte, these mitochondriopathies offer for a first time a potential causal treatment option by supplementation of CoQ_{10}. In several patients affected by mutations in *COQ2*, *COQ6* and *ADCK4*, beneficial antiproteinuric effects were induced by oral medication with CoQ_{10} - opening a new therapeutic avenue for these patients with otherwise steroid resistant NS [93–95].

Syndromal Disorders Associated with Nephrotic Syndrome

A large number of syndromes have been described on clinical grounds in patients presenting with (steroid-resistant) proteinuria in addition to various extrarenal manifestations. A genetic basis has been identified only in a minority of these syndromes.

Here, we discuss two important syndromes that invariably present with SRNS, Schimke syndrome and Galloway-Mowat syndrome.

Schimke Syndrome

Schimke immuno-osseous dysplasia maps to chromosome 2q34-36 and is caused by recessive mutations in the *SMARCAL1* gene [96]. *SMARCAL1* encodes the SWI/SNF-related, matrix-associated, actin-dependent regulator of chromatin subfamily a-like protein 1, a protein involved in the remodeling of chromatin to change nucleosome compaction for gene regulation, replication, recombination, and DNA repair. The clinical phenotype of Schimke immuno-osseous dysplasia is characterized by growth retardation due to spondyloepiphyseal dysplasia, a slowly progressive immune defect, cerebral infarcts, skin pigmentation and SRNS beginning in childhood. FSGS lesions are frequently observed in kidney biopsy specimen and the majority of patients progress to ESRD. However, disease severity and age at onset follow a continuum from early onset and severe symptoms with death early in life to later onset and mild symptoms with survival into adulthood. Genotype-phenotype studies suggest that recessive loss-of-function mutations (frameshift, stop and splice-site mutations) are generally associated with a more severe course of the disease while some missense mutations allow a retention of partial *SMARCAL1* function and thus cause milder disease [96].

Galloway-Mowat Syndrome

The Galloway-Mowat syndrome (GMS) is characterized by microcephaly and other brain anomalies, severe mental retardation and early-onset NS (CNS) [97]. Both FSGS and DMS were observed in kidney biopsies of affected individuals [97, 98]. An important number of patients also presents with hiatus hernia. Both males and females are affected and an occurence in siblings of the same family has been reported. These observations point to a possible autosomal recessive mode of inheritance but no gene locus has been identified so far. However, as different genetic research groups work hard to map the causative gene locus, new insights into the pathology of GMS can be awaited soon.

Clinical Aspects

Clinical aspects of NS are discussed in all detail in former chapters. Here, we want to focus on some issues specific for genetic forms of SRNS.

Therapeutic Implications

The therapy of SRNS in general is demanding. Numerous immunosuppressive agents have shown some efficacy in a fraction of the SRNS population, including cyclophosphamide, azathioprine, cyclosporine and mycophenolate mofetil, mostly in combination with glucocorticoids. However, genetically determined forms of SRNS have proven insensitive to immunosuppressive interventions, which is pathophysiologically explained by the presence of intrinsic defects in podocyte architecture and function [99]. Hence, it is suggested to spare children with hereditary SRNS, especially with *NPHS2* mutations, from any form of immunosppressive treatment. Conversely, *NPHS2* mutations have never been reported in patients with steroid sensitive NS [44], so screening for this mutation seems not indicated even in patients with reduced steroid sensitivity (such as frequent relapsers or steroid dependency).

Antiproteinuric pharmacological treatment with ACE inhibitors, AT1 receptor blockers or dual blockage with coadministration of both is probably effective in slowing down the progression of renal insufficiency also in genetic SRNS, although efficacy has not been formally proven in carriers of individual mutations.

Living Related Donor Transplantation

Living-related kidney transplantation is generally considered the therapy of first choice in pediatric patients with ESRD. However, in patients affected by SRNS due to germline mutations in podocyte genes several aspects need to be considered. First, it is unknown as yet how kidneys of a heterozygous donor behave and develop in a recipient with recessive SRNS: The parents of affected children with recessive SRNS carry one mutant allele each that is also present in the transplanted kidney. It could be speculated that these kidneys are more easily prone to develop proteinuria if other proproteinuric factors (e.g., arterial hypertension, salt-rich diet) are superposed. While animal models of SRNS do not support this hypothesis so far, comprehensive human data adressing this question are lacking. Consequences for the donor should also be considered. It is as yet unknown whether the prognosis of the remaining single kidney in the heterozygous parental donor is impaired by the gene mutation. Again, the remaining heterozygous kidney might be more susceptible to proteinuric disease than single kidneys of individuals without mutations. Up to know our experience with living-related donor transplantation in hereditary SRNS is very limited and does not support a restriction in affected children. Still, careful surveillance of both donor and recipient seems advisable.

In families of patients affected by autosomal dominant late-onset SRNS, only one of the parents is carrier of the pathogenic sequence variation. Genetic testing of family members will be helpful to delineate mutation carriers in the family. If the mutation occurred as a de novo mutation in the patient, both parents are equally suitable for living donor transplantation from a genetic point of view.

Recurrence of Nephrotic Syndrome After Renal Transplantation

Many investigators have studied the pathogenesis of increased glomerular permeability and recurrence of proteinuria after transplantation in FSGS. In general, recurrence of proteinuria after renal transplantation is observed in approximately 30% of FSGS patients [100]. This risk appears higher in children than in adult patients [101]. Affected patients present with proteinuria, which is often in the nephrotic range. Frequently proteinuria recurs within few days after renal transplantation. In children, the mean time to recurrent proteinuria is 14 days post-transplant [102]. Recurrence of proteinuria/FSGS following renal transplantation negatively impacts graft survival in both children and adult patients. Risk factors are an age less than 15 years, rapid progression of renal insufficiency and diffuse mesangial proliferation in the initial biopsy of the native kidney [103]. In non-hereditary FSGS/SRNS, the recurrence of proteinuria is discussed to follow a T cell dysfunction and production of proteinuric circulating factors, including soluble urokinase receptor, hemopexin, and cardiotrophin-like cytokine-1 [104, 105].

In *NPHS2*-associated SRNS/FSGS recurrence of post-transplant proteinuria is a rare phenomenon, observed in less than 10% of transplanted patients [37, 44, 106]. The identification of a homozygous truncating *NPHS2* mutation in one patient with post-transplant NS prompted the search for anti-podocin antibodies but all results were negative excluding a de novo glomerulonephitis as underlying cause [37]. Anti-podocin antibodies were also not identifiable in a study including patients with *NPHS2* missense mutations and post-transplant NS [107].

In CNF, the risk of a recurrence of proteinuria after transplantation seems to be important: it was demonstrated that especially patients affected by the Fin major mutation have a risk of approximately 25% of post-transplant NS. Subsequent studies revealed that the pathogenesis of this recurrence is related to the development of anti-nephrin antibodies directed against the wildtype nephrin protein residing in the transplanted kidney [107], analogous to the anti-GBM antibodies against type IV collagen causing post-transplant de novo glomerulonephritis in patients with Alport syndrome. Treatment options of post-transplant NS in these patients are scarce; a subset of patients seems to respond to cyclophosphamide [108].

Genetic Testing

Following the rapid technological development in human genetics and genome research, different approaches can be applied in order to identify gene mutations in patients with SRNS and/or

FSGS. Conventional Sanger sequencing can be performed in patients with specific phenotypes, e.g., sequencing of *WT1* in Denys-Drash or *LAMB2* in Pierson syndrome. Sanger sequencing is also useful in patients with congenital NS (*NPHS1*) or school-aged patients with SRNS (*NPHS2*), where the likelihood of a positive result is relatively high. In adolescents and young adults, a different screening rationale should be applied. The *NPHS2*-p.R229Q sequence variation in compound heterozygosity with specific pathogenic *NPHS2* mutations is frequently found in late-onset SRNS [45, 50, 51]. In addition, autosomal dominant disease due to mutations in *WT1, TRPC6, INF2* and *ACTN4* can be identified in adolescents and young adults, particularly in case of dominant transmission but to a minor extent also in sporadic cases [45, 109, 110].

However, panels of podocytopathy-associated genes have recently been developed by many commercial and non-commercial laboratories, which allow simultaneous sequencing of more than 20 genes in one experimental run by next generation sequencing techniques. Given the diversity of genes involved in SRNS or FSGS and the continuous reduction in costs, this technology is rapidly gaining acceptance. Moreover, whole exome sequencing is now available at low cost and is currently being developed for clinical diagnostic application. Advantages of this approach, besides low cost and processing times compared to conventional Sanger sequencing, include the identification of gene mutations in novel genes and the unraveling of gene mutations in phenotypically complex cases. Still, the interpretation of huge data sets can be challenging and necessitates biostatistical expertise. Furthermore, numerous ethical issues still need to be adressed, especially with respect to the possible incidental identification of mutations in SRNS-unrelated genes associated with severe disorders and high phenoytpic penetrance, e.g. in cancer genes. In these cases genetic counseling will be demanding.

Genetic Counseling

Positive results of mutational analysis in pediatric patients with SRNS should be followed by adequate genetic counseling. This demands close collaboration between pediatric nephrologists and human geneticists. Parents of children affected by recessive disease will have a chance of 25 % to give birth to another affected child. In parents of children with dominant disease, this risk amounts to 50 % (with the exception of patients with de novo mutations, in these families, the risk of recurrence is very low). Parents of affected children need to be informed that treatment options are limited in hereditary SRNS and that renal function may deteriorate rapidly. Close monitoring of renal function and early teratment of complications of chronic renal insufficiency are advised. In autosomal dominant FSGS, genetic counseling might be difficult due to the fact of incomplete penetrance and variable expressivity. It seems that individual mutation carriers can be affected to a differing degree with an obvious mild phenotype in some family members and ESRD in others. Genetic counseling is not only important for the parents but also for the affected child. Children with recessive disease will transmit a heterozygous mutation to their own children in the future. As long as the other parent is not mutation carrier, all offspring will be healthy. Patients affected by dominant FSGS will transmit the pathogenic mutation in 50 % of cases but offspring carrying the mutation might be affected by FSGS.

In some cases, established genotype-phenotype correlations might be helpful to estimate the risk of a more severe clinical course. In *NPHS2*-associated SRNS, for example, some mutations have been associated with early-onset and aggravated clinical course while other mutations weres shown to be less pathogenic [40]. For other disease entities, the analysis of clinical symptoms of other affected family members can be of help to predict the severity of the disease: in NPS, the risk of having a child with NPS nephropathy is about 1:4 and the risk of having a child in whom renal failure will develop is about 1:10 if NPS nephropathy occurs in other family members [53]. Genetic counseling is especially important in families affected by NS with serious prognosis. In children affected by CNS with female outer appearance, mutation analysis in *WT1* is mandatory in order to rule out a risk for Wilms tumor development.

Due to the implementation of next generation sequencing techniques in the clinical routine setting, many patients are identified to carry a significant number of sequence variations of unknown relevance in different podocyte genes, not following simple Medelian inheritance. Whether these gene variants act as modifiers, accumulate to confer a susceptibility for the develoment of NS or are just polymorphisms without biological function remains difficult to be designated in many cases. Genetic counseling will have to make allowance for this in the future.

Acknowledgement I would like to thank Martin Zenker (Institute of Human Genetics, University of Erlangen-Nuremberg) for his reflections on Pierson syndrome.

References

1. Rose EA, Glaser T, Jones C, et al. Complete physical map of the WAGR region of 11p13 localizes a candidate Wilms' tumor gene. Cell. 1990;60:405–508.
2. Gessler M, Poustka A, Cavenee W, et al. Homozygous deletion in Wilms tumours of a zinc-finger gene identified by chromosome jumping. Nature. 1990; 343:774–8.
3. Haber DA, Buckler AJ, Glaser T, et al. An internal deletion within an 11p13 zinc finger gene contributes to the development of Wilms' tumor. Cell. 1990;61:1257–69.
4. Schumacher V, Schneider S, Figge A, et al. Correlation of germ-line mutations and two-hit inactivation of the WT1 gene with Wilms tumors of stromal-predominant histology. Proc Natl Acad Sci U S A. 1997;94:3972–7.
5. Pelletier J, Bruening W, Kashtan CE, et al. Germline mutations in the Wilms' tumor suppressor gene are associated with abnormal urogenital development in Denys-Drash syndrome. Cell. 1991;67(2):437–47.
6. Barbaux S, Niaudet P, Gubler MC, et al. Donor splice-site mutations in WT1 are responsible for Frasier syndrome. Nat Genet. 1997;17(4):467–70.
7. Jeanpierre C, Denamur E, Henry I, et al. Identification of constitutional WT1 mutations, in patients with isolated diffuse mesangial sclerosis, and analysis of genotype/phenotype correlations by use of a computerized mutation database. Am J Hum Genet. 1998;62(4):824–33.
8. Habib R, Gubler MC, Antignac C, et al. Diffuse mesangial sclerosis: a congenital glomerulopathy with nephrotic syndrome. Adv Nephrol Necker Hosp. 1993;22:43–57.
9. Maalouf EF, Ferguson J, van Heyningen V, et al. In utero nephropathy, Denys-Drash syndrome and Potter phenotype. Pediatr Nephrol. 1998;12(6): 449–51.
10. Habib R, Loirat C, Gubler MC, et al. The nephropathy associated with male pseudohermaphroditism and Wilms' tumor (Drash syndrome): a distinctive glomerular lesion – report of 10 cases. Clin Nephrol. 1985;24(6):269–78.
11. Hu M, Zhang GY, Arbuckle S, et al. Prophylactic bilateral nephrectomies in two paediatric patients with missense mutations in the WT1 gene. Nephrol Dial Transplant. 2004;19(1):223–6.
12. Niaudet P, Gubler MC. WT1 and glomerular diseases. Pediatr Nephrol. 2006;21(11):1653–60.
13. Little M, Wells C. A clinical overview of WT1 gene mutations. Hum Mutat. 1997;9(3):209–25.
14. Gao F, Maiti S, Sun G, et al. The Wt1+/R394W mouse displays glomerulosclerosis and early-onset renal failure characteristic of human Denys-Drash syndrome. Mol Cell Biol. 2004;24(22):9899–910.
15. Frasier SD, Bashore RA, Mosier HD. Gonadoblastoma associated with pure gonadal dysgenesis in monozygous twins. J Pediatr. 1964; 64:740–5.
16. Gubler MC, Yang Y, Jeanpierre C, et al. WT1, renal development, and glomerulopathies. Adv Nephrol Necker Hosp. 1999;29:299–315.
17. Lipska BS, Ranchin B, Iatropoulos P, et al. Genotype-phenotype associations in WT1 glomerulopathy. Kidney Int. 2014;85(5):1169–78. doi:10.1038/ki.2013.519.
18. Denamur E, Bocquet N, Baudouin V, et al. WT1 splice-site mutations are rarely associated with primary steroid-resistant focal and segmental glomerulosclerosis. Kidney Int. 2000;57(5):1868–72.
19. Koziell AB, Grundy R, Barratt TM, et al. Evidence for the genetic heterogeneity of nephropathic phenotypes associated with Denys-Drash and Frasier syndromes. Am J Hum Genet. 1999;64(6): 1778–81.
20. Kaplinsky C, Ghahremani M, Frishberg Y, et al. Familial Wilms' tumor associated with a WT1 zinc finger mutation. Genomics. 1996;38(3):451–3.
21. Rapola J. Congenital nephrotic syndrome. Pediatr Nephrol. 1987;1(3):441–6.
22. Kestila M, Mannikko M, Holmberg C, et al. Congenital nephrotic syndrome of the Finnish type maps to the long arm of chromosome 19. Am J Hum Genet. 1994;54:757–64.
23. Kestila M, Lenkkeri U, Mannikko M, et al. Positionally cloned gene for a novel glomerular protein – nephrin – is mutated in congenital nephrotic syndrome. Mol Cell. 1998;1(4):575–82.
24. Coulthard MG. Management of Finnish congenital nephrotic syndrome by unilateral nephrectomy. Pediatr Nephrol. 1989;3(4):451–3.
25. Holmberg C, Antikainen M, Ronnholm K, et al. Management of congenital nephrotic syndrome of the Finnish type. Pediatr Nephrol. 1995;9(1):87–93.
26. Pomeranz A, Wolach B, Bernheim J, et al. Successful treatment of Finnish congenital nephrotic syndrome

with captopril and indomethacin. J Pediatr. 1995; 126(1):140–2.

27. Kovacevic L, Reid CJ, Rigden SP. Management of congenital nephrotic syndrome. Pediatr Nephrol. 2003;18(5):426–30.

28. Ruotsalainen V, Ljungberg P, Wartiovaara J, et al. Nephrin is specifically located at the slit diaphragm of glomerular podocytes. Proc Natl Acad Sci U S A. 1999;96(14):7962–7.

29. Wartiovaara J, Ofverstedt LG, Khoshnoodi J, et al. Nephrin strands contribute to a porous slit diaphragm scaffold as revealed by electron tomography. J Clin Invest. 2004;114(10):1475–83.

30. Huber TB, Kottgen M, Schilling B, et al. Interaction with podocin facilitates nephrin signaling. J Biol Chem. 2001;276:41543–6.

31. Huber TB, Hartleben B, Kim J, et al. Nephrin and CD2AP associate with phosphoinositide 3-OH kinase and stimulate AKT-dependent signaling. Mol Cell Biol. 2003;23:4917–28.

32. Huber TB, Simons M, Hartleben B, et al. Molecular basis of the functional podocin-nephrin complex: mutations in the NPHS2 gene disrupt nephrin targeting to lipid raft microdomains. Hum Mol Genet. 2003;12:3397–405.

33. Schwarz K, Simons M, Reiser J, et al. Podocin, a raft-associated component of the glomerular slit diaphragm, interacts with CD2AP and nephrin. J Clin Invest. 2001;108:1621–9.

34. Simons K, Toomre D. Lipid rafts and signal transduction. Nat Rev Mol Cell Biol. 2000;1:31–9.

35. Koziell A, Grech V, Hussain S, et al. Genotype/phenotype correlations of NPHS1 and NPHS2 mutations in nephrotic syndrome advocate a functional inter-relationship in glomerular filtration. Hum Mol Genet. 2002;11(4):379–88.

36. Bolk S, Puffenberger EG, Hudson J, et al. Elevated frequency and allelic heterogeneity of congenital nephrotic syndrome, Finnish type, in the old order Mennonites. Am J Hum Genet. 1999;65(6):1785–90.

37. Weber S, Gribouval O, Esquivel EL, et al. NPHS2 mutation analysis shows genetic heterogeneity of steroid-resistant nephrotic syndrome and low posttransplant recurrence. Kidney Int. 2004;66(2):571–9.

38. Hinkes B, Vlangos C, Heeringa S, Mucha B, Gbadegesin R, Liu J, Hasselbacher K, Ozaltin F, Hildebrandt F, APN Study Group. Specific podocin mutations correlate with age of onset in steroid-resistant nephrotic syndrome. J Am Soc Nephrol. 2008;19(2):365–71.

39. Santín S, Tazón-Vega B, Silva I, Cobo MÁ, Giménez I, Ruíz P, García-Maset R, Ballarín J, Torra R, Ars E, FSGS Spanish Study Group. Clinical value of NPHS2 analysis in early- and adult-onset steroid-resistant nephrotic syndrome. Clin J Am Soc Nephrol. 2011;6(2):344–54.

40. Fuchshuber A, Jean G, Gribouval O, et al. Mapping a gene (SRN1) to chromosome 1q25-q31 in idiopathic nephrotic syndrome confirms a distinct entity of autosomal recessive nephrosis. Hum Molec Genet. 1995;4:2155–8.

41. Boute N, Gribouval O, Roselli S, et al. NPHS2, encoding the glomerular protein podocin, is mutated in autosomal recessive steroid-resistant nephrotic syndrome. Nat Genet. 2000;24(4):349–54.

42. Roselli S, Heidet L, Sich M, et al. Early glomerular filtration defect and severe renal disease in podocin-deficient mice. Mol Cell Biol. 2004;24:550–60.

43. Bouchireb K, Boyer O, Gribouval O, Nevo F, Huynh-Cong E, Morinière V, Campait R, Ars E, Brackman D, Dantal J, Eckart P, Gigante M, Lipska BS, Liutkus A, Megarbane A, Mohsin N, Ozaltin F, Saleem MA, Schaefer F, Soulami K, Torra R, Garcelon N, Mollet G, Dahan K, Antignac C. NPHS2 mutations in steroid-resistant nephrotic syndrome: a mutation update and the associated phenotypic spectrum. Hum Mutat. 2014;35(2):178–86.

44. Ruf RG, Lichtenberger A, Karle SM, et al. Patients with mutations in NPHS2 (podocin) do not respond to standard steroid treatment of nephrotic syndrome. J Am Soc Nephrol. 2004;15(3):722–32.

45. Lipska BS, Iatropoulos P, Maranta R, et al. Genetic screening in adolescents with steroid-resistant nephrotic syndrome. Kidney Int. 2013;84(1):206–13.

46. Caridi G, Bertelli R, Di Duca M, et al. Broadening the spectrum of diseases related to podocin mutations. J Am Soc Nephrol. 2003;14(5):1278–86.

47. Caridi G, Bertelli R, Scolari F, et al. Podocin mutations in sporadic focal-segmental glomerulosclerosis occurring in adulthood. Kidney Int. 2003;64(1):365.

48. Schultheiss M, Ruf RG, Mucha BE, et al. No evidence for genotype/phenotype correlation in NPHS1 and NPHS2 mutations. Pediatr Nephrol. 2004;19(12):1340–8.

49. Tsukaguchi H, Sudhakar A, Le TC, et al. NPHS2 mutations in late-onset focal segmental glomerulosclerosis: R229Q is a common disease-associated allele. J Clin Invest. 2002;110(11):1659–66.

50. Machuca E, Hummel A, Nevo F, Dantal J, Martinez F, Al-Sabban E, Baudouin V, Abel L, Grünfeld JP, Antignac C. Clinical and epidemiological assessment of steroid-resistant nephrotic syndrome associated with the NPHS2 R229Q variant. Kidney Int. 2009;75(7):727–35.

51. Tory K, Menyhárd DK, Woerner S, Nevo F, Gribouval O, Kerti A, Stráner P, Arrondel C, Cong EH, Tulassay T, Mollet G, Perczel A, Antignac C. Mutation-dependent recessive inheritance of NPHS2-associated steroid-resistant nephrotic syndrome. Nat Genet. 2014;46(3):299–304. doi:10.1038/ng.2898.

52. Franceschini N, North KE, Kopp JB, et al. NPHS2 gene, nephrotic syndrome and focal segmental glomerulosclerosis: a HuGE review. Genet Med. 2006;8(2):63–75.

53. Pereira AC, Pereira AB, Mota GF, et al. NPHS2 R229Q functional variant is associated with microalbuminuria in the general population. Kidney Int. 2004;65(3):1026–30.

54. Pierson M, Cordier J, Hervouuet F, et al. An unusual congenital and familial congenital malformative combination involving the eye and the kidney. J Genet Hum. 1963;12:184–213.

55. Zenker M, Aigner T, Wendler O, et al. Human laminin beta2 deficiency causes congenital nephrosis with mesangial sclerosis and distinct eye abnormalities. Hum Mol Genet. 2004;13(21):2625–32.

56. Hasselbacher K, Wiggins RC, Matejas V, et al. Recessive missense mutations in LAMB2 expand the clinical spectrum of LAMB2-associated disorders. Kidney Int. 2006;70(6):1008–12.

57. Mark K, Reis A, Zenker M. Prenatal findings in four consecutive pregnancies with fetal Pierson syndrome, a newly defined congenital nephrosis syndrome. Prenat Diagn. 2006;26(3):262–6.

58. Chen YM, Zhou Y, Go G, Marmerstein JT, Kikkawa Y, Miner JH. Laminin β2 gene missense mutation produces endoplasmic reticulum stress in podocytes. J Am Soc Nephrol. 2013;24(8):1223–33.

59. Lehnhardt A, Lama A, Amann K, Matejas V, Zenker M, Kemper MJ. Pierson syndromein an adolescent girl with nephrotic range proteinuria but a normal GFR. Pediatr Nephrol. 2012;27(5):865–8.

60. Chen H, Lun Y, Ovchinnikov D, et al. Limb and kidney defects in Lmx1b mutant mice suggest an involvement of LMX1B in human nail patella syndrome. Nat Genet. 1998;19(1):51–5.

61. Bongers EM, Huysmans FT, Levtchenko E, et al. Genotype-phenotype studies in nail-patella syndrome show that LMX1B mutation location is involved in the risk of developing nephropathy. Eur J Hum Genet. 2005;13(8):935–46.

62. Looij Jr BJ, te Slaa RL, Hogewind BL, et al. Genetic counselling in hereditary osteo-onychodysplasia (HOOD, nail-patella syndrome) with nephropathy. J Med Genet. 1988;25(10):682–6.

63. Browning MC, Weidner N, Lorentz Jr WB. Renal histopathology of the nail-patella syndrome in a two-year-old boy. Clin Nephrol. 1988;29(4):210–3.

64. Taguchi T, Takebayashi S, Nishimura M, et al. Nephropathy of nail-patella syndrome. Ultrastruct Pathol. 1988;12(2):175–83.

65. Boyer O, Woerner S, Yang F, Oakeley EJ, Linghu B, Gribouval O, Tête MJ, Duca JS, Klickstein L, Damask AJ, Szustakowski JD, Heibel F, Matignon M, Baudouin V, Chantrel F, Champigneulle J, Martin L, Nitschké P, Gubler MC, Johnson KJ, Chibout SD, Antignac C. LMX1B mutations cause hereditary FSGS without extrarenal involvement. J Am Soc Nephrol. 2013;24(8):1216–22.

66. Isojima T, Harita Y, Furuyama M, Sugawara N, Ishizuka K, Horita S, Kajiho Y, Miura K, Igarashi T, Hattori M, Kitanaka S. LMX1B mutation with residual transcriptional activity as a cause of isolated glomerulopathy. Nephrol Dial Transplant. 2014;29(1):81–8.

67. Miner JH, Morello R, Andrews KL, et al. Transcriptional induction of slit diaphragm genes by Lmx1b is required in podocyte differentiation. J Clin Invest. 2002;109(8):1065–72.

68. Hinkes B, Wiggins RC, Gbadegesin R, et al. Positional cloning uncovers mutations in PLCE1 responsible for a nephrotic syndrome variant that may be reversible. Nat Genet. 2006;38(12):1397–405.

69. Gbadegesin R, Hinkes BG, Hoskins BE, Vlangos CN, Heeringa SF, Liu J, Loirat C, Ozaltin F, Hashmi S, Ulmer F, Cleper R, Ettenger R, Antignac C, Wiggins RC, Zenker M, Hildebrandt F. Mutations in PLCE1 are a major cause of isolated diffuse mesangial sclerosis (IDMS). Nephrol Dial Transplant. 2008;23(4):1291–7.

70. Boyer O, Benoit G, Gribouval O, Nevo F, Pawtowski A, Bilge I, Bircan Z, Deschênes G, Guay-Woodford LM, Hall M, Macher MA, Soulami K, Stefanidis CJ, Weiss R, Loirat C, Gubler MC, Antignac C. Mutational analysis of the PLCE1 gene in steroid resistant nephrotic syndrome. J Med Genet. 2010;47(7):445–52.

71. Ozaltin F, Ibsirlioglu T, Taskiran EZ, Baydar DE, Kaymaz F, Buyukcelik M, Kilic BD, Balat A, Iatropoulos P, Asan E, Akarsu NA, Schaefer F, Yilmaz E, Bakkaloglu A, PodoNet Consortium. Disruption of PTPRO causes childhood-onset nephrotic syndrome. Am J Hum Genet. 2011;89(1):139–47.

72. Gupta IR, Baldwin C, Auguste D, Ha KC, El Andalousi J, Fahiminiya S, Bitzan M, Bernard C, Akbari MR, Narod SA, Rosenblatt DS, Majewski J, Takano T. ARHGDIA: a novel gene implicated in nephrotic syndrome. J Med Genet. 2013;50(5):330–8.

73. Giglio S, Provenzano A, Mazzinghi B, et al. Heterogeneous genetic alterations in sporadic nephrotic syndrome associate with resistance to immunosuppression. J Am Soc Nephrol. 2014;26(1):230–6.

74. Gee HY, Ashraf S, Wan X, et al. Mutations in EMP2 cause childhood-onset nephrotic syndrome. Am J Hum Genet. 2014;94(6):884–90.

75. Mathis BJ, Kim SH, Calabrese K, et al. A locus for inherited focal segmental glomerulosclerosis maps to chromosome 19q13. Kidney Int. 1998;53(2):282–6.

76. Kaplan JM, Kim SH, North KN, et al. Mutations in ACTN4, encoding alpha-actinin-4, cause familial focal segmental glomerulosclerosis. Nat Genet. 2000;24(3):251–6.

77. Kos CH, Le TC, Sinha S, et al. Mice deficient in alpha-actinin-4 have severe glomerular disease. J Clin Invest. 2003;111(11):1683–90.

78. Weins A, Kenlan P, Herbert S, et al. Mutational and biological analysis of alpha-actinin-4 in focal segmental glomerulosclerosis. J Am Soc Nephrol. 2005;16(12):3694–701.

79. McCarthy HJ, Bierzynska A, Wherlock M, Ognjanovic M, Kerecuk L, Hegde S, Feather S, Gilbert RD, Krischock L, Jones C, Sinha MD, Webb NJ, Christian M, Williams MM, Marks S, Koziell A, Welsh GI, Saleem MA, RADAR the UK SRNS Study Group. Simultaneous sequencing of 24 genes associated with steroid-resistant nephrotic syndrome. Clin J Am Soc Nephrol. 2013;8(4):637–48.

80. Winn MP, Conlon PJ, Lynn KL, et al. Linkage of a gene causing familial focal segmental glomerulosclerosis to chromosome 11 and further evidence of genetic heterogeneity. Genomics. 1999;58(2):113–20.

81. Winn MP, Conlon PJ, Lynn KL, et al. A mutation in the TRPC6 cation channel causes familial focal segmental glomerulosclerosis. Science. 2005;308(5729):1801–4.

82. Reiser J, Polu KR, Moller CC, et al. TRPC6 is a glomerular slit diaphragm-associated channel required for normal renal function. Nat Genet. 2005;37(7):739–44.

83. Kim JM, Wu H, Green G, et al. CD2-associated protein haploinsufficiency is linked to glomerular disease susceptibility. Science. 2003;300:1298–300.

84. Shih NY, Li J, Karpitskii V, et al. Congenital nephrotic syndrome in mice lacking CD2-associated protein. Science. 1999;286:312–5.

85. Kopp JB, Smith MW, Nelson GW, Johnson RC, Freedman BI, Bowden DW, Oleksyk T, McKenzie LM, Kajiyama H, Ahuja TS, Berns JS, Briggs W, Cho ME, Dart RA, Kimmel PL, Korbet SM, Michel DM, Mokrzycki MH, Schelling JR, Simon E, Trachtman H, Vlahov D, Winkler CA. MYH9 is a major-effect risk gene for focal segmental glomerulosclerosis. Nat Genet. 2008;40(10):1175–84.

86. Genovese G, Friedman DJ, Ross MD, Lecordier L, Uzureau P, Freedman BI, Bowden DW, Langefeld CD, Oleksyk TK, Uscinski Knob AL, Bernhardy AJ, Hicks PJ, Nelson GW, Vanhollebeke B, Winkler CA, Kopp JB, Pays E, Pollak MR. Association of trypanolytic ApoL1 variants with kidney disease in African Americans. Science. 2010;329(5993):841–5.

87. Brown EJ, Schlöndorff JS, Becker DJ, Tsukaguchi H, Tonna SJ, Uscinski AL, Higgs HN, Henderson JM, Pollak MR. Mutations in the formin gene INF2 cause focal segmental glomerulosclerosis. Nat Genet. 2010;42(1):72–6.

88. Boyer O, Nevo F, Plaisier E, Funalot B, Gribouval O, Benoit G, Cong EH, Arrondel C, Tête MJ, Montjean R, Richard L, Karras A, Pouteil-Noble C, Balafrej L, Bonnardeaux A, Canaud G, Charasse C, Dantal J, Deschenes G, Deteix P, Dubourg O, Petiot P, Pouthier D, Leguern E, Guiochon-Mantel A, Broutin I, Gubler MC, Saunier S, Ronco P, Vallat JM, Alonso MA, Antignac C, Mollet G. INF2 mutations in Charcot-Marie-Tooth disease with glomerulopathy. N Engl J Med. 2011;365(25):2377–88.

89. Mele C, Iatropoulos P, Donadelli R, Calabria A, Maranta R, Cassis P, Buelli S, Tomasoni S, Piras R, Krendel M, Bettoni S, Morigi M, Delledonne M, Pecoraro C, Abbate I, Capobianchi MR, Hildebrandt F, Otto E, Schaefer F, Macciardi F, Ozaltin F, Emre S, Ibsirlioglu T, Benigni A, Remuzzi G, Noris M, PodoNet Consortium. MYO1E mutations and childhood familial focal segmental glomerulosclerosis. N Engl J Med. 2011;365(4):295–306.

90. Quinzii C, Naini A, Salviati L, Trevisson E, Navas P, Dimauro S, Hirano M. A mutation in para-hydroxybenzoate-polyprenyl transferase (COQ2) causes primary coenzyme Q10 deficiency. Am J Hum Genet. 2006;78(2):345–9.

91. Diomedi-Camassei F, Di Giandomenico S, Santorelli FM, Caridi G, Piemonte F, Montini G, Ghiggeri GM, Murer L, Barisoni L, Pastore A, Muda AO, Valente ML, Bertini E, Emma F. COQ2 nephropathy: a newly described inherited mitochondriopathy with primary renal involvement. J Am Soc Nephrol. 2007;18(10):2773–80.

92. Scalais E, Chafai R, Van Coster R, Bindl L, Nuttin C, Panagiotaraki C, Seneca S, Lissens W, Ribes A, Geers C, Smet J, De Meirleir L. Early myoclonic epilepsy, hypertrophic cardiomyopathy and subsequently a nephrotic syndrome in a patient with CoQ10 deficiency caused by mutations in para-hydroxybenzoate-polyprenyl transferase (COQ2). Eur J Paediatr Neurol. 2013;17(6):625–30.

93. Heeringa SF, Chernin G, Chaki M, Zhou W, Sloan AJ, Ji Z, Xie LX, Salviati L, Hurd TW, Vega-Warner V, Killen PD, Raphael Y, Ashraf S, Ovunc B, Schoeb DS, McLaughlin HM, Airik R, Vlangos CN, Gbadegesin R, Hinkes B, Saisawat P, Trevisson E, Doimo M, Casarin A, Pertegato V, Giorgi G, Prokisch H, Rötig A, Nürnberg G, Becker C, Wang S, Ozaltin F, Topaloglu R, Bakkaloglu A, Bakkaloglu SA, Müller D, Beissert A, Mir S, Berdeli A, Varpizen S, Zenker M, Matejas V, Santos-Ocaña C, Navas P, Kusakabe T, Kispert A, Akman S, Soliman NA, Krick S, Mundel P, Reiser J, Nürnberg P, Clarke CF, Wiggins RC, Faul C, Hildebrandt F. COQ6 mutations in human patients produce nephrotic syndrome with sensorineural deafness. J Clin Invest. 2011;121(5):2013–24.

94. Ashraf S, Gee HY, Woerner S, Xie LX, Vega-Warner V, Lovric S, Fang H, Song X, Cattran DC, Avila-Casado C, Paterson AD, Nitschké P, Bole-Feysot C, Cochat P, Esteve-Rudd J, Haberberger B, Allen SJ, Zhou W, Airik R, Otto EA, Barua M, Al-Hamed MH, Kari JA, Evans J, Bierzynska A, Saleem MA, Böckenhauer D, Kleta R, El Desoky S, Hacihamdioglu DO, Gok F, Washburn J, Wiggins RC, Choi M, Lifton RP, Levy S, Han Z, Salviati L, Prokisch H, Williams DS, Pollak M, Clarke CF, Pei Y, Antignac C, Hildebrandt F. ADCK4 mutations promote steroid-resistant nephrotic syndrome through CoQ10 biosynthesis disruption. J Clin Invest. 2013;123(12):5179–89.

95. Montini G, Malaventura C, Salviati L. Early coenzyme Q10 supplementation in primary coenzyme Q10 deficiency. N Engl J Med. 2008;358(26):2849–50.

96. Boerkoel CF, Takashima H, John J, et al. Mutant chromatin remodeling protein SMARCAL1 causes Schimke immuno-osseous dysplasia. Nat Genet. 2002;30(2):215–20.

97. Galloway WH, Mowat AP. Congenital microcephaly with hiatus hernia and nephrotic syndrome in two sibs. J Med Genet. 1968;5(4):319–21.

98. Garty BZ, Eisenstein B, Sandbank J, et al. Microcephaly and congenital nephrotic syndrome

owing to diffuse mesangial sclerosis: an autosomal recessive syndrome. J Med Genet. 1994;31(2): 121–5.

99. Büscher AK, Kranz B, Büscher R, Hildebrandt F, Dworniczak B, Pennekamp P, Kuwertz-Bröking E, Wingen AM, John U, Kemper M, Monnens L, Hoyer PF, Weber S, Konrad M. Immunosuppression and renal outcome in congenital and pediatric steroid-resistant nephrotic syndrome. Clin J Am Soc Nephrol. 2010;5(11):2075–84.

100. Artero M, Biava C, Amend W, et al. Recurrent focal glomerulosclerosis: natural history and response to therapy. Am J Med. 1992;92(4):375–83.

101. Senggutuvan P, Cameron JS, Hartley RB, et al. Recurrence of focal segmental glomerulosclerosis in transplanted kidneys: analysis of incidence and risk factors in 59 allografts. Pediatr Nephrol. 1990;4(1): 21–8.

102. Tejani A, Stablein DH. Recurrence of focal segmental glomerulosclerosis posttransplantation: a special report of the North American Pediatric Renal Transplant Cooperative Study. J Am Soc Nephrol. 1992;2(12 Suppl):S258–63.

103. Habib R, Hebert D, Gagnadoux MF, et al. Transplantation in idiopathic nephrosis. Transplant Proc. 1982;14(3):489–95.

104. McCarthy ET, Sharma M, Savin VJ. Circulating permeability factors in idiopathic nephrotic syndrome and focal segmental glomerulosclerosis. Clin J Am Soc Nephrol. 2010;5(11):2115–21.

105. Coppo R. Different targets for treating focal segmental glomerular sclerosis. Contrib Nephrol. 2013;181: 84–90.

106. Höcker B, Knüppel T, Waldherr R, et al. Recurrence of proteinuria 10 years post-transplant in NPHS2-associated focal segmental glomerulosclerosis after conversion from cyclosporin A to sirolimus. Pediatr Nephrol. 2006;21(10):1476–9.

107. Bertelli R, Ginevri F, Caridi G, et al. Recurrence of focal segmental glomerulosclerosis after renal transplantation in patients with mutations of podocin. Am J Kidney Dis. 2003;41(6):1314–21.

108. Patrakka J, Ruotsalainen V, Reponen P, et al. Recurrence of nephrotic syndrome in kidney grafts of patients with congenital nephrotic syndrome of the Finnish type: role of nephrin. Transplantation. 2002;73(3):394–403.

109. Santín S, Bullich G, Tazón-Vega B, García-Maset R, Giménez I, Silva I, Ruíz P, Ballarín J, Torra R, Ars E. Clinical utility of genetic testing in children and adults with steroid-resistant nephrotic syndrome. Clin J Am Soc Nephrol. 2011;6(5):1139–48.

110. Büscher AK, Konrad M, Nagel M, et al. Mutations in podocyte genes are a rare cause of primary FSGS associated with ESRD in adult patients. Clin Nephrol. 2012;78(1):47–53.

Alport Syndrome and Thin Basement Membrane Nephropathy

Michelle N. Rheault and Clifford E. Kashtan

Introduction

Several forms of familial glomerular hematuria result from mutations that affect type IV collagen, the major collagenous constituent of glomerular basement membranes (GBM): Alport syndrome (AS), thin basement membrane nephropathy (TBMN) and HANAC syndrome. Persistent hematuria is a cardinal feature of each of these disorders. Mutations in any of three type IV collagen genes, COL4A3, COL4A4 or COL4A5 can cause AS, which is characterized clinically by progressive deterioration of kidney function with associated hearing and ocular involvement in many affected individuals. A majority of affected individuals demonstrate X-linked inheritance; however, autosomal recessive and autosomal dominant transmission is also observed. TBMN, previously known as "benign familial hematuria," generally is non-progressive and does not have associated extra-renal findings. About 40% of cases of TBMN exhibit mutations in COL4A3 or COL4A4 or linkage to one of these genes. Together, AS and TBMN account for about 30–50% of children with isolated glomerular hematuria seen in pediatric nephrology clinics

[1–5]. Hereditary angiopathy with nephropathy, aneurysms and cramps (HANAC syndrome) arises from mutations in the COL4A1 gene.

Alport Syndrome

Introduction

The first description of a family with inherited hematuria appeared in 1902 in a report by Guthrie [6]. Subsequent monographs about this family by Hurst in 1923 [7] and Alport in 1927 [8] established that affected individuals in this family, particularly males, developed deafness and uremia. The advent of electron microscopy led to the discovery of unique glomerular basement membrane (GBM) abnormalities in patients with AS [9–11], setting the stage for the histochemical [12–14] and genetic [15, 16] studies that resulted in the identification of type IV collagen genes as the sites of disease-causing mutations. AS occurs in approximately 1:50,000 live births and accounts for 1.3% and 0.4% of pediatric and adult end-stage renal disease (ESRD) patients in the United States, respectively [17].

M.N. Rheault • C.E. Kashtan (✉)
Department of Pediatrics, Division of Pediatric
Nephrology, University of Minnesota Masonic
Children's Hospital, 2450 Riverside Ave, MB 680,
Minneapolis, MN 55454, USA
e-mail: rheau002@umn.edu; kasht001@umn.edu

© Springer-Verlag Berlin Heidelberg 2016
D.F. Geary, F. Schaefer (eds.), Pediatric Kidney Disease, DOI 10.1007/978-3-662-52972-0_18

Etiology and Pathogenesis

Type IV Collagen Proteins, Tissue Distribution, and Genes

Six isoforms of type IV collagen, $\alpha1(IV)$-$\alpha6(IV)$, are encoded by six genes, COL4A1-COL4A6. The type IV collagen genes are arranged in pairs on three chromosomes: COL4A1-COL4A2 on chromosome 13, COL4A3-COL4A4 on chromosome 2, and COL4A5-COL4A6 on the X chromosome. The paired genes are arranged in a 5'-5' fashion, separated by sequences of varying length containing regulatory elements [18, 19]. All type IV collagen isoforms share several basic structural features: a major collagenous domain of approximately 1,400 residues containing the repetitive triplet sequence glycine (Gly)-X-Y, in which X and Y represent a variety of other amino acids; a C-terminal noncollagenous (NC1) domain of approximately 230 residues; and a noncollagenous N-terminal sequence of 15–20 residues. The collagenous domains each contain approximately 20 interruptions of the collagenous triplet sequence, while each NC1 domain contains 12 conserved cysteine residues. Type IV collagen chains self associate to form triple helical structures or "trimers." The specificity of chain association is determined by amino acid sequences within the NC1 domains and results in only three trimeric species that are found in nature: $\alpha1_2\alpha2(IV)$, $\alpha3\alpha4\alpha5(IV)$ and $\alpha5_2\alpha6(IV)$ [20]. Unlike interstitial collagens, which lose their NC1 domains and form fibrillar networks, type IV collagen trimers form open, nonfibrillar networks through NC1-NC1 and N-terminal interactions [21].

$\alpha1_2\alpha2(IV)$ trimers are found in all basement membranes, whereas $\alpha3\alpha4\alpha5(IV)$ and $\alpha5_2\alpha6(IV)$ trimers have a more restricted distribution. In normal human kidneys, $\alpha3\alpha4\alpha5(IV)$ trimers are found in GBM, Bowman's capsules, and the basement membranes of distal tubules, while $\alpha5_2\alpha6(IV)$ trimers are detectable in Bowman's capsules, basement membranes of distal tubules and collecting ducts, but not GBM [22, 23]. $\alpha5_2\alpha6(IV)$ trimers are also present in normal epidermal basement membranes as well as some alimentary canal, ocular, and vascular basement membranes. $\alpha3\alpha4\alpha5(IV)$ trimers also occur in several basement membranes of the eye and of the cochlea [24–26].

Mutations in any of the COL4A3, COL4A4, or COL4A5 genes will affect the formation and composition of affected basement membranes. If any of the $\alpha3(IV)$, $\alpha4(IV)$, or $\alpha5(IV)$ chains are absent due to severe mutations (deletions, frame shift mutations, premature stop codons), then the other collagen chains are degraded and no $\alpha3\alpha4\alpha5(IV)$ trimers are deposited in basement membranes [27]. In this case, the embryonal $\alpha1_2\alpha2(IV)$ network persists. Missense mutations, particularly those that affect the glycine residues involved in triple helix formation, may lead to the formation of abnormally folded trimers that are either degraded or deposited into the basement membrane with formation of an abnormal type IV collagen network. Due to a greater number of disulfide bonds, the $\alpha3\alpha4\alpha5(IV)$ network is more highly cross-linked and is more resistant to proteases than the $\alpha1_2\alpha2(IV)$ network [27, 28]. Absence of the $\alpha3\alpha4\alpha5(IV)$ network leads to increased distensibility in the lens capsule when tested in experimental models of AS [29]. The glomerular capillary walls of AS patients may also be mechanically weak and provoke pathologic stretch-related responses in glomerular cells [30].

Genetics

AS occurs in three genetic forms: X-linked (XLAS), autosomal recessive (ARAS) and autosomal dominant (ADAS) (Table 18.1). XLAS, caused by mutations in COL4A5, was classically thought to account for approximately 80 % of AS patients while ARAS, caused by mutations in both alleles of COL4A3 or COL4A4, accounted for about 15 % of the AS population. Affected males with XLAS are hemizygotes who carry a single mutant COL4A5 allele, while affected females are heterozygotes carrying normal and mutant alleles. Individuals with ARAS may be homozygotes, with identical mutations in both alleles of the affected gene or they may be compound heterozygotes, with different mutations in the two alleles [31]. With the advent of next generation sequencing, recent studies are suggesting a higher percentage of patients with AS who

Table 18.1 Familial glomerular hematuria due to type IV collagen mutations

	Genetic locus	Protein product	Renal symptoms	ESRD	GBM ultrastructure	Extrarenal manifestations
Alport syndrome						
X-linked	COL4A5	α5(IV)	Hematuria	All males, some females	Thinning (early)	Deafness
			Proteinuria		Lamellation (late)	Lenticonus
			Hypertension			Perimacular flecks
Autosomal recessive	COL4A3	α3(IV)	Hematuria	All males and females	Thinning (early)	Deafness
	COL4A4 (biallelic)	α4(IV)	Proteinuria		Lamellation (late)	Lenticonus
			Hypertension			Perimacular flecks
Autosomal dominant	COL4A3	α3(IV)	Hematuria	Males and females (late)	Thinning (early)	Deafness
	COL4A4 (heterozygous)	α4(IV)	Proteinuria		Lamellation (late)	
			Hypertension			
Thin basement Membrane Nephropathy	COL4A3 COL4A4 (heterozygous)	α3(IV) α4(IV)	Hematuria	Rare	Thinning	Rare
HANAC syndrome						
Autosomal dominant	COL4A1	α1(IV)	Hematuria	?	Normal	Arterial aneurysms
			Cysts			Muscle cramps
			CKD			

CKD chronic kidney disease, *ESRD* end-stage renal disease, *GBM* glomerular basement membrane

demonstrate autosomal dominant inheritance than was previously recognized, up to 31 % in one report [32]. ADAS is caused by heterozygous mutations in *COL4A3* or *COL4A4* [33]. Heterozygous mutations in either *COL4A3* or *COL4A4* have been associated with both ADAS and TBMN; however, it is not clear why some individuals develop a progressive nephropathy while others have a benign clinical course [34].

Over 700 pathogenic mutations have been identified in the *COL4A5* gene in patients and families with XLAS [35]. Mutations can be found along the entire 51 exons of the gene without identified hot spots. About 10–15 % of *COL4A5* mutations occur as spontaneous events, therefore a family history of renal disease is not required for a diagnosis of XLAS. A variety of mutation types have been described: large rearrangements (~20 %), small deletions and insertions (~20 %), missense mutations altering a glycine residue in the collagenous domain of α5(IV) (30 %), other missense mutations (~8 %), nonsense mutations (~5 %) and splice-site mutations (~15 %) [36]. The type of *COL4A5* mutation, or *COL4A5* genotype, has a significant impact on the course of XLAS in affected males [36, 37]. In males with a large deletion, nonsense mutation or a small mutation changing the mRNA reading frame, the risk of developing ESRD before age 30 is 90 %. In contrast, 70 % of patients with a splice-site and 50 % of patients with a missense mutation progress to ESRD before age 30 [36]. In addition, the position of a glycine substitution within the gene may also impact the rate of disease progression as those with 5′ glycine missense mutations demonstrate a more severe phenotype than those with 3′ glycine mutations [37]. In contrast to males with XLAS, a statistical relationship between *COL4A5* genotype and renal phenotype cannot be demonstrated in females with XLAS [38].

Clinical Manifestations

Males with XLAS and ARAS inevitably develop end-stage renal disease (ESRD) at a rate that is influenced by genotype [31, 36]. While most females with XLAS have non-progressive or slowly progressive renal disease, a significant minority demonstrates progression to ESRD. The course of AS is similar in females and males with ARAS [31]. In general, patients with ADAS progress less rapidly than patients with XLAS or ARAS and are less likely to have extra-renal manifestations [39].

Renal Symptoms

Persistent microscopic hematuria (MH) occurs in all males with AS, regardless of genetic type, and is probably present from early in infancy. Approximately 95 % of heterozygous females with XLAS have persistent or intermittent MH [38], and 100 % of females with ARAS have persistent MH. Gross hematuria is not unusual in affected boys and girls with Alport syndrome, occurring at least once in approximately 60 % of affected males [36, 40].

In males with XLAS, and in males and females with ARAS, proteinuria typically becomes detectable in late childhood or early adolescence and is progressive. Affected children first demonstrate microalbuminuria that progresses to overt proteinuria with time [41]. In one large cohort of females with XLAS, 75 % were found to have proteinuria, although the timing of onset was not investigated [38].

Blood pressure is typically normal in childhood but, like proteinuria, hypertension is common in adolescent males with XLAS or ARAS, and in females with ARAS. Most females with XLAS have normal blood pressure, but hypertension may develop, particularly in those with proteinuria.

All males with XLAS eventually require renal replacement therapy, with 50 % of untreated males reaching ESRD by age 25, 80 % by age 40 and 100 % by age 60 [36]. The timing of ESRD in patients with ARAS is probably similar to XLAS males, although ARAS patients with normal renal function in their 30s and 40s have been reported [31]. In patients with ADAS, the age at

which 50 % of patients have progressed to ESRD is approximately 50 years, or twice as long as XLAS males [39].

Females who are heterozygous for *COL4A5* mutations ("carriers" of XLAS) demonstrate widely variable disease outcomes with some women demonstrating only lifelong asymptomatic hematuria while others develop chronic progressive kidney disease including ESRD [42]. The risk of ESRD is lower in XLAS females than in XLAS males, but it is by no means trivial. About 12 % of XLAS females reach ESRD by age 45, 30 % by age 60 and 40 % by age 80 [38]. The explanation for the wide variability in outcomes for XLAS females is uncertain, but likely multifactorial. Risk factors for ESRD in XLAS females include proteinuria and sensorineural deafness [38, 43]. X-inactivation, the process by which one X chromosome in females is silenced to adjust for gene dosage differences between males and females, may play a role in renal disease progression in XLAS females [44, 45]. In a mouse model of female XLAS, modest skewing of X-inactivation to favor expression of the wild type $\alpha5(IV)$ was associated with a survival advantage [46]. Further studies are required to determine how to accurately predict the risk of progressive renal disease in women who are affected with XLAS.

The Alport nephropathy progresses predictably through a series of clinical phases. Phase I typically lasts from birth until late childhood or early adolescence, and is characterized by isolated hematuria, with normal protein excretion and renal function. In Phase II, initially microalbuminuria followed by overt proteinuria is superimposed on hematuria, but renal function remains normal. Patients in Phase III exhibit declining renal function in addition to hematuria and proteinuria, and those in Phase IV have end-stage renal disease. These phases have histological correlates, as described in the next section. The rate of passage through these phases is primarily a function of the causative mutation, at least in males with XLAS. Patients with *COL4A5* mutations that prevent production of any functional protein (deletions, nonsense mutations) proceed through these phases more rapidly than those whose mutations allow synthesis of a functional, albeit abnormal, protein (some missense mutations). Females with XLAS can be viewed as passing through the same phases as males, although the rate of progression is typically so slow that the journey to ESRD may not be completed during the individual's lifetime.

Hearing

Newborn hearing screening is normal in males with XLAS, and in males and females with ARAS, but bilateral impairment of perception of high frequency sounds frequently becomes detectable in late childhood. The hearing deficit is progressive, and extends into the range of conversational speech with advancing age. The deficit usually does not exceed 60–70 dB and speech discrimination is preserved, so that affected individuals benefit from hearing aids. Sensorineural hearing loss (SNHL) is present in 50 % of XLAS males by approximately age 15, 75 % by age 25, and 90 % by age 40 [36]. Like the effect on renal disease progression, missense mutations in COL4A5 are associated with an attenuated risk of hearing loss. The risk of SNHL before age 30 is 60 % in patients with misssense mutations, while the risk of SNHL before age 30 is 90 % in those with other types of mutations [36]. SNHL is less frequent in females with XLAS. About 10 % of XLAS females have SNHL by 40 years of age, and about 20 % by age 60 [38]. SNHL is common in ARAS as well with approximately 66 % of individuals affected [31].

The SNHL in AS has been localized to the cochlea [47]. In control cochleae, the α3(IV), α4(IV) and α5(IV) chains are expressed in the spiral limbus, the spiral ligament, stria vascularis and in the basement membrane situated between the Organ of Corti and the basilar membrane [48–50]. However, these chains are not expressed in the cochleae of ARAS mice [49], XLAS dogs [50] or men with XLAS [26]. Examination of well-preserved cochleae from men with XLAS revealed a unique zone of separation between the organ of Corti and the underlying basilar membrane, as well as cellular infiltration of the tunnel of Corti and the spaces of Nuel [51]. These changes may be associated with abnormal tuning of basilar membrane motion and hair cell stimu-

lation, resulting in defective hearing. An alternative hypothesis is that hearing is impaired by changes in potassium concentration in the scala media induced by abnormalities of type IV collagen in the stria vascularis [52].

Ocular Anomalies

Abnormalities of the lens and the retina are common in individuals with AS, typically becoming apparent in the second to third decade of life in XLAS males and in both males and females with ARAS. The α3(IV), α4(IV) and α5(IV) chains are normal components of the anterior lens capsule and other ocular basement membranes, and mutations that interfere with the formation or deposition of α3α4α5(IV) trimers prevent expression of these chains in the eye [24, 48]. Anterior lenticonus, which is considered virtually pathognomonic for AS [53], is absent at birth and manifests during the second and third decades of life in ~13–25 % of affected individuals [36, 54]. In this disorder, the anterior lens capsule is markedly attenuated, especially over the central region of the lens, and exhibits focal areas of dehiscence leading to refractive errors and, in some cases, cataracts [55, 56]. Anterior lenticonus has been described only rarely in heterozygous females with COL4A5 mutations [38]. Dot-fleck retinopathy, a characteristic alteration of retinal pigmentation concentrated in the perimacular region [57], is also common in AS patients and does not appear to be associated with any abnormality in vision [36]. Recurrent corneal erosions [58, 59] and posterior polymorphous dystrophy, manifested by clear vesicles on the posterior surface of the cornea [60], have also been described in AS.

Leiomyomatosis

Several dozen families in which AS is transmitted in association with leiomyomas of the esophagus and tracheobronchial tree have been described [61]. Affected individuals carry X-chromosomal deletions that involve the COL4A5 gene and terminate within the second intron of the adjacent COL4A6 gene [62–64]. Those affected tend to become symptomatic in late childhood, and may exhibit dysphagia, postprandial vomiting, epigastric or retrosternal pain, recurrent bronchitis, dyspnea, cough or stridor. Females with the AS-leiomyomatosis complex typically have genital leiomyomas, with clitoral hypertrophy and variable involvement of the labia majora and uterus.

Other Findings

AS associated with mental retardation, mid-face hypoplasia and elliptocytosis has been described in association with large $COL4A5$ deletions that extend beyond the 5′ terminus of the gene [65]. Early development of aortic root dilatation and aneurysms of the thoracic and abdominal aorta, as well as other arterial vessels, have been described in AS males, perhaps due to abnormalities in the $\alpha5_2\alpha6$(IV) network in arterial smooth muscle basement membranes [66].

Renal Histopathology

Children with AS typically show little in the way of renal parenchymal changes by light microscopy before about 5 years of age. In older patients, mesangial hypercellularity and matrix expansion may be observed. As the disease progresses, focal segmental glomerulosclerosis, tubular atrophy and interstitial fibrosis become the predominant light microscopic abnormalities. Although some patients exhibit increased numbers of immature glomeruli or interstitial foam cells, these changes are not specific for AS.

Electron microscopy of renal biopsy specimens is frequently diagnostic, although the expression of the pathognomonic lesion is age-dependent and, for those with XLAS, gender-dependent. In early childhood, the predominant ultrastructural lesion in males is diffuse attenuation of the GBM. This may be identical in appearance to patients with TBMN. The classic ultrastructural lesion is diffuse thickening of the glomerular capillary wall, accompanied by "basket-weave" transformation of the lamina densa, intramembranous vesicles, scalloping of the epithelial surface of the GBM and effacement of podocyte foot-processes (Fig. 18.1). These changes are more prevalent in affected males, typically becoming prominent in late childhood

and adolescence. Affected females can display a spectrum of lesions, demonstrating either predominantly normal-appearing GBM, focal GBM attenuation, diffuse GBM attenuation, thickening/basket-weaving, or diffuse basket-weaving. The extent of the GBM lesion progresses inexorably in males, although the rate of progression may be influenced by $COL4A5$ genotype. Females may have static or progressive GBM lesions. X-chromosome inactivation pattern, age and $COL4A5$ genotype could all contribute to the dynamics of GBM change in affected females.

The classic GBM lesion is not found in all kindreds with AS. Adult patients who demonstrate only GBM thinning, yet have $COL4A5$ mutations, have been described. Although these represent a minority of Alport patients and families, they highlight the somewhat vague histological distinction between AS and TBMN. This issue is discussed further in the section on TBMN.

Routine immunofluorescence microscopy is normal, or shows nonspecific deposition of immunoproteins, in patients with AS. In contrast, specific immunostaining for type IV collagen α chains is frequently diagnostic, and can distinguish the X-linked and autosomal recessive forms of the disease (Fig. 18.1). The utility of this approach derives from the fact that most disease-causing mutations in AS alter the expression of the $\alpha3\alpha4\alpha5$(IV) and $\alpha5_2\alpha6$(IV) trimers in renal basement membranes. Most $COL4A5$ mutations prevent expression of both trimer forms in the kidney, so that in about 80 % of XLAS males immunostaining of renal biopsy specimens for $\alpha3$(IV), $\alpha4$(IV) and $\alpha5$(IV) chains is completely negative [67]. About 60–70 % of XLAS females exhibit mosaic expression of these chains, while in the remainder immunostaining for these chains is normal. The biallelic mutations in $COL4A3$ and $COL4A4$ that cause ARAS often prevent expression of $\alpha3\alpha4\alpha5$(IV) trimers but have no effect on expression of $\alpha5_2\alpha6$(IV) trimers. In renal biopsy specimens from patients with ARAS, immunostaining for $\alpha3$(IV) and $\alpha4$(IV) chains is negative in the GBM. However, while immunostaining of GBM for the $\alpha5$(IV) chain is negative due to the absence of $\alpha3\alpha4\alpha5$(IV) trimers, Bowman's capsules, distal tubular basement membranes and

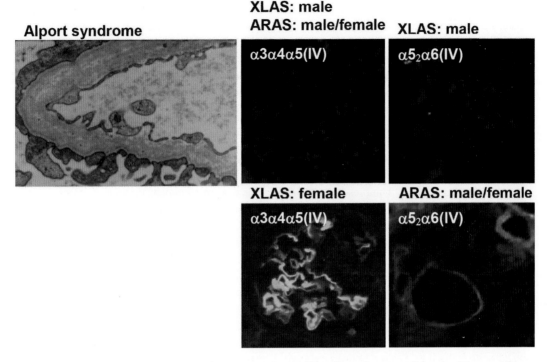

Fig. 18.1 Typical findings on electron microscopy and type IV collagen immunostaining in Alport syndrome. Abbreviations – *XLAS* X-linked Alport syndrome, *ARAS* autosomal recessive Alport syndrome

collecting duct basement membranes are positive for α5(IV), due to the unimpaired expression of α5₂α6(IV) trimers. Heterozygous carriers of a single *COL4A3* or *COL4A4* mutation have exhibited normal renal basement membrane immunostaining for α3(IV), α4(IV) and α5(IV) chains when studied.

The α5₂α6(IV) trimer is a normal component of epidermal basement membranes (EBM). Consequently, about 80 % of males with XLAS can be diagnosed by skin biopsy on the basis of absence of α5(IV) expression in EBM. In 60–70 % of XLAS females there is a mosaic pattern of immunostaining for α5(IV). EBM expression of α5(IV) is normal in patients with ARAS and in subjects with heterozygous mutations in *COL4A3* or *COL4A4*.

Diagnosis and Differential Diagnosis

AS is just one potential cause of familial and sporadic glomerular hematuria. Accurate diagnosis rests on careful clinical evaluation, a precise family history, selective application of invasive diagnostic techniques and, in appropriate patients, molecular diagnosis.

The presence of isolated microscopic hematuria in a child with a positive family history for hematuria, an autosomal dominant pattern of inheritance, and a negative family history for ESRD strongly suggests a diagnosis of TBMN. Less common conditions associated with familial glomerular hematuria include the autosomal dominant *MYH9* disorders (Epstein and Fechtner syndromes), in which macrothrombocytopenia is a constant feature; familial IgA nephropathy and X-linked membranoproliferative glomerulonephritis.

When family history for hematuria is negative, the differential diagnosis of isolated glomerular hematuria, or hematuria associated with proteinuria, includes IgA nephropathy, the various forms of C3 nephropathy, membranous nephropathy, lupus nephritis, postinfectious glomerulonephritis and Henoch-Schönlein nephritis, among others, in addition to AS and TBMN. Some of these conditions will be strongly suspected on the basis of clinical findings (e.g., rash and joint complaints) while others will be suggested by laboratory findings, such as hypocomplementemia.

Formal audiometric and ophthalmological examinations should be considered as part of the diagnostic evaluation in children with persistent microscopic hematuria. Audiometry may be very helpful in children over age 6–8 years, especially boys, since high-frequency SNHL would point toward a diagnosis of AS. The presence of anterior lenticonus or the dot-fleck retinopathy may be diagnostic. However, these lesions are more prevalent in patients with advanced disease, and less likely to be present in the young patients in whom diagnostic ambiguity tends to be the greatest.

Tissue studies are appropriate when clinical and pedigree information does not allow a diagnosis of thin basement membrane nephropathy and when AS cannot be ruled out by symptoms and laboratory findings. Several options are available for confirming a diagnosis of AS including skin biopsy, kidney biopsy and mutation analysis. Skin biopsy is often utilized as the initial invasive diagnostic procedure in patients suspected of AS as it is less invasive and expensive than a renal biopsy. On skin biopsy, the majority of subjects with XLAS will display abnormal expression of the α5(IV) chain in epidermal basement membranes (EBM), as described above. Normal EBM α5(IV) expression in a patient with hematuria has several possible explanations: (1) the patient has XLAS, but his or her *COL4A5* mutation allows EBM expression of α5(IV); (2) the patient has ARAS, or ADAS, in which α5(IV) expression is expected to be preserved; or (3) the patient has a disease other than AS. Renal biopsy would then provide the opportunity to diagnose other diseases, to examine type IV collagen α chain expression in renal basement membranes, and to evaluate GBM at the ultrastructural level.

Mutation analysis using conventional Sanger sequencing is capable of identifying *COL4A5* mutations in 80–90 % of males with XLAS [68]. High mutations detection rates in *COL4A3* and *COL4A4* in patients with ARAS are also possible, particularly if there is parental consanguin-

ity. Commercially available genetic testing for mutations in *COL4A3*, *COL4A4*, and *COL4A5* is available in the United States and around the world. Next generation sequencing, which allows simultaneous analysis of *COL4A3*, *COL4A4* and *COL4A5*, appears likely to eventually supplant Sanger sequencing as the preferred approach.

Treatment

The goal of treatment in AS is to slow the progression of kidney disease and delay the need for renal replacement therapy. Several therapeutic approaches have demonstrated efficacy in murine ARAS, including angiotensin blockade [69–71], inhibition of TGFβ-1 [72], chemokine receptor 1 blockade [73], administration of bone morphogenic protein-7 [74], suppression of matrix metalloproteinases [28] and bone marrow transplantation [75]. Cyclosporine therapy slowed progression of kidney disease in a canine model of AS; however, human studies have demonstrated significant nephrotoxicity and adverse effects and this treatment is not recommended [76–78]. Angiotensin converting enzyme (ACE) inhibition also prolonged survival in a canine XLAS model [79]. Uncontrolled studies in human AS subjects have shown that ACE inhibition can reduce proteinuria, at least transiently [80, 81]. A multicenter, randomized, double-blind study comparing losartan with placebo or amlodipine in 30 children with AS demonstrated a significant reduction in proteinuria in the losartan treated group [82]. An extension of this study showed comparable efficacy of either enalapril or losartan in reducing proteinuria in children with AS [83]. A report from the European Alport Registry, which includes 283 patients over 20 years, compared renal outcomes in AS patients treated with ACE inhibition at various time points: at onset of microalbuminuria, at onset of proteinuria, or in CKD stage III-IV [84]. This retrospective review demonstrated a delay in renal replacement therapy by 3 years in the treated CKD group and by 18 years in the treated proteinuric group [84]. Side effects of ACE inhibition were rare and included hyperkalemia (<2 %), cough (<1 %), and hypotension (<1 %). Based on these findings a prospective, double-blind, randomized, placebo controlled trial is underway to compare outcomes in AS patients treated with ramipril vs. placebo at an early time point (microalbuminuria or isolated hematuria) [85].

Current clinical practice guidelines recommend treatment with an ACE inhibitor for affected individuals with proteinuria, including heterozygous females (Table 18.2) [41]. Treatment should be considered for those with microalbuminuria and a family history of ESRD <30 years of age or a severe *COL4A5* mutation (deletion, splice site, or nonsense mutation) [41, 86]. There are insufficient data to recommend treatment for individuals with microscopic hematuria only; however, the ongoing clinical trial in this population hopefully will shed light on the utility of treatment at this early stage of disease. Treatment of hypertension and other manifestations of advancing disease is of course an important component of therapy for AS. Similar to other children with chronic kidney disease, blood pressures should be controlled to the 50 % for age, gender, and height in children with AS in order to slow the progression of kidney disease [87].

Renal Transplantation

In general, outcomes following renal transplantation in patients with AS are excellent [88]. Clinicians involved in transplantation of AS patients must address two important aspects of the disease. First, the donor selection process must avoid nephrectomy in relatives at risk for end-stage renal disease. Second, post-transplant management should provide surveillance for post-transplant anti-GBM nephritis, a complication unique to AS.

Informed donor evaluation requires familiarity with the genetics of AS and the signs and symptoms of the disease. In families with XLAS, 100 % of affected males and ~95 % of affected females exhibit hematuria. Consequently, males who do not have hematuria are not affected, and a female without hematuria has only about a 5 % risk of being affected. Given an estimated 30 % risk of end-stage renal disease in women with AS [38], these women should generally be discouraged from kidney donation, even if hematuria is their only symptom. A report from Germany described five women with XLAS and one ARAS carrier who served as kidney donors [89]. One donor had proteinuria prior to transplant and all had microscopic hematuria. Three donors developed new onset hypertension and two developed new proteinuria while renal function declined by 25–60 % over 2–14 years after donation in four of the donors, highlighting the increased donor risk in this population [89].

Overt anti-GBM nephritis occurs in 3–5 % of transplanted AS males [90]. Onset is typically within the first post-transplant year, and the disease usually results in irreversible graft failure within weeks to months of diagnosis. The risk of

Table 18.2 Recommendations for intervention based on urinary findings and anticipated disease course

| | Family history of early ESRD (<30 years) or severe[a] *COL4A5* mutation | | Family history of late ESRD (>30 years) or less severe[b] *COL4A5* mutation | |
	Males	Females	Males	Females
Hematuria	Intervention prior to onset of microalbuminuria is not recommended at this time	No	No	No
Hematuria + microalbuminuria	Consider intervention	Consider intervention	No	No
Hematuria + proteinuria	Yes	Yes	Yes	Yes

Used with permission of Springer Science + Business Media from Kashtan et al. [41]
ESRD end stage renal disease
[a]Deletion, nonsense, or splice site mutation
[b]Missense mutation

recurrence in subsequent allografts is high. In males with XLAS, the primary target of anti-GBM antibodies is the α5(IV) chain [91, 92]. Both males and females with ARAS can develop post-transplant anti-GBM nephritis, and in these cases the primary antibody target is the α3(IV) chain [91, 93]. The α3(IV) chain is also the target of Goodpasture autoantibodies, but the epitope identified by these antibodies differs from the α3(IV) epitope recognized by ARAS anti-GBM alloantibodies [94].

Thin Basement Membrane Nephropathy

Introduction

The term "benign familial hematuria" (BFH) was historically used to describe kindreds displaying autosomal dominant transmission of isolated, nonprogressive glomerular hematuria [95–97]. Renal biopsy findings in these families are typically limited to GBM attenuation by electron microscopy. In 1996, Lemmink and colleagues were the first to report a heterozygous *COL4A3* mutation in a family with BFH [34]. "Thin basement membrane nephropathy" (TBMN) has gradually become the preferred term for hematuria associated with GBM attenuation and a nonprogressive course (Table 18.1). TBMN generally has a good prognosis; however, there is an increased risk of hypertension, proteinuria, and renal impairment in affected individuals [98]. The prevalence of TBMN is estimated at 1–2 % of the population [99].

In discussing TBMN, it is important to recall that GBM thinning is a pathological description rather than a distinct, homogeneous entity. GBM attenuation can result from hemizygous or heterozygous mutations in *COL4A5* (XLAS), biallelic mutations in *COL4A3* or *COL4A4* (ARAS), heterozygous mutations in *COL4A3* or *COL4A4* (the carrier state for ARAS) or mutations at other unknown genetic loci.

It is the underlying cause of GBM attenuation that determines prognosis, perhaps in combination with remote modifier loci, rather than the GBM thinning itself. Hemizygous mutations in *COL4A5*, and biallelic mutations in *COL4A3* or *COL4A4*, lead to progressive GBM thickening and renal failure, while heterozygous mutations in *COL4A3* or *COL4A4* may be associated with persistent GBM attenuation and a benign outcome (TBMN) or slowly progressive disease (ADAS). Women with heterozygous mutations in *COL4A5* are arrayed across the middle of the prognostic spectrum. The range of outcomes likely reflects differences between cellular responses to complete absence of α3α4α5 trimers (ARAS and hemizygous XLAS), mixed α3α4α5-positive and α3α4α5-negative GBM (heterozygous XLAS) and homogeneous reduction in α3α4α5 content (heterozygous *COL4A3* or *COL4A4* mutations).

Etiology and Pathogenesis

The essential features of the type IV collagen protein family are discussed in the preceding section on AS. It is possible that heterozygous mutations in *COL4A3* or *COL4A4* result in reduction of α3α4α5(IV) trimers in GBM; however, this has not been assessed using quantitative methodologies. Identification of mutations in *COL4A3* or *COL4A4*, or demonstration of genetic linkage to these loci, has been achieved in about 40 % of TBMN families. About 20 mutations in *COL4A3* and *COL4A4*, predominantly single nucleotide substitutions, have been described in TBMN families [5]. Other loci for TBMN have yet to be identified.

It is assumed that the attenuated GBM of TBMN and early AS is mechanically fragile and that, as a result, the glomerular capillary wall has an increased potential for rupture at physiologic levels of intracapillary pressure. This mechanism remains theoretical, since it has never been tested in vivo or in the laboratory. There is indirect evidence in support of this hypothesis. Persistent microscopic hematuria is more common in women, who have relatively thin GBM [100]. Macroscopic hematuria, intermittent or persistent, is fairly common in children with Alport syndrome, but tends to disappear with age, perhaps because the GBM thickens and becomes less susceptible to rupture [40].

Clinical Manifestations

TBMN is the most common cause of persistent microscopic hematuria in children and adults [101]. Children with TBMN typically exhibit persistent microscopic hematuria, although intermittent microhematuria may be observed. Episodic gross hematuria may occur in association with acute infection. Proteinuria is rare in childhood but can be observed in a significant proportion of adult patients [102]. Chronic kidney disease (CKD) or ESRD is observed in <5% of affected adults [102–105]. Extrarenal abnormalities, such as hearing loss or ocular defects, are unusual and probably unrelated.

Histopathology

Light and routine immunofluorescence microscopy typically shows no abnormalities, especially in children. Adult TBMN patients with renal dysfunction or hypertension may exhibit premature glomerular obsolescence [104]. Type IV collagen staining demonstrates no abnormalities in the renal basement membrane expression of the $\alpha 3$-$\alpha 6$(IV) chains, in contrast to patients with AS [14, 106]. Characteristic thinning of the GBM can be identified on electron microscopy. Patients with TBMD typically exhibit diffuse thinning of the lamina densa and, perhaps as a result, of the GBM as a whole. The thickness of normal GBM is age- and gender-dependent. Both the lamina densa and the GBM increase rapidly in thickness between birth and age 2 years, followed by gradual thickening throughout childhood and adolescence [107]. GBM thickness of adult men exceeds that of adult women [108]. Because a variety of techniques have been used to measure GBM width, there is no standard definition of "thin" GBM (Fig. 18.2). The cut-off value in adults ranges from 250 to 330 nm, depending upon technique [109, 110]. For children, the cut-off is in the range of 200–250 nm (250 nm is within 2SD of the mean at age 11) [2, 3, 111].

Diagnosis and Differential Diagnosis

IgA nephropathy, TBMN and Alport syndrome comprise the most common causes of glomerular hematuria in the pediatric population. Careful clinical evaluation and thorough pedigree analysis can help segregate children with glomerular hematuria into those who require renal biopsy or other tissue studies, and those who can be followed prospectively without the need for tissue studies. Since adults with familial hematuria may not be aware that they are affected [112], obtaining urinalyses on the parents of children with hematuria may be very helpful.

In a child with isolated microscopic hematuria, a strong family history of dominantly-transmitted hematuria, and a negative family history for renal failure, a clinical diagnosis of TBMN can be made, and renal biopsy withheld. These children should be monitored every 1–2 years for the development of proteinuria or hypertension, and to update the family history [86].

In the child with GBM attenuation and a negative or limited family history, the challenge for the clinician is to distinguish TBMN and AS. Audiometry and ophthalmologic examination may be helpful if abnormal, but the younger the child, the less useful these tests are, given the usual natural history of hearing loss and ocular changes in AS (see preceding section). Renal biopsy with immunostaining for type IV collagen $\alpha 3$(IV), $\alpha 4$(IV) and $\alpha 5$(IV) chains can be particularly helpful in these situations, as discussed in the section on AS. While molecular analysis of type IV collagen genes is available in a number of research and commercial laboratories, it is often unnecessary to obtain genetic confirmation in patients with TBMN unless the course is atypical. Genetic testing for mutations in *COL4A3-COL4A5* should be considered in individuals with proteinuria, renal impairment, or when AS cannot be excluded based on family history.

Treatment

Treatment is not necessary for the great majority of TBMN patients, especially children, since the course of the disorder is typically benign. Adult patients with proteinuria are theoretically candidates for angiotensin blockade, although there are no specific studies in this area.

Thin basement membrane nephropathy

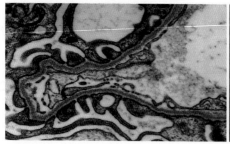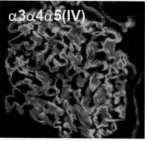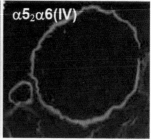

Fig. 18.2 Typical findings on electron microscopy and type IV collagen immunostaining in thin basement membrane nephropathy

Hereditary Angiopathy with Nephropathy, Aneurysms, and Cramps (Hanac Syndrome)

Introduction

This autosomal dominant disorder results from mutations in the *COL4A1* gene (Table 18.1) [113–115]. Complete absence of *COL4A1* is embryonic lethal in mice [116]. Missense mutations that allow for expression of an abnormal α1(IV) chain lead to the development of HANAC syndrome. Renal findings include gross and microscopic hematuria, cysts and chronic kidney disease. Vascular anomalies include cerebral artery aneurysms and retinal arteriolar tortuosity. Affected individuals may have recurrent muscle cramps and elevated creatine kinase levels.

Pathology

No abnormalities of GBM ultrastructure or basement membrane expression of type IV collagen chains have been observed in renal biopsy specimens from affected individuals with hematuria. Irregular thickening, lamellation and focal interruptions of Bowman's capsules, tubular basement membranes and interstitial capillary basement membranes have been described, as well as abnormalities of epidermal basement membranes and dermal arterial basement membranes.

Genetics

The reported mutations in HANAC syndrome families affect highly conserved glycine residues in the collagenous domain of the α1(IV) chain, potentially affecting integrin binding sites.

References

1. Trachtman H, Weiss R, Bennett B, Griefer I. Isolated hematuria in children: indications for a renal biopsy. Kidney Int. 1984;25:94–9.
2. Schroder CH, Bontemps CM, Assmann KJM, Schuurmans-Stekhoven JH, Foidart JM, Monnens LAH, et al. Renal biopsy and family studies in 65 children with isolated hematuria. Acta Paediatr Scand. 1990;79:630–6.
3. Lang S, Stevenson B, Risdon RA. Thin basement membrane nephropathy as a cause of recurrent haematuria in childhood. Histopathology. 1990;16:331–7.
4. Piqueras AI, White RH, Raafat F, Moghal N, Milford DV. Renal biopsy diagnosis in children presenting with hematuria. Pediatr Nephrol. 1998;12:386–91.
5. Rana K, Wang YY, Buzza M, Tonna S, Zhang KW, Lin T, et al. The genetics of thin basement membrane nephropathy. Semin Nephrol. 2005;25:163–70.
6. Guthrie LG. "Idiopathic", or congenital, hereditary and familial hematuria. Lancet. 1902;1:1243–6.
7. Hurst AF. Hereditary familial congenital haemorrhagic nephritis occurring in sixteen individuals in three generations. Guy's Hosp Rec. 1923;3:368–70.
8. Alport AC. Hereditary familial congenital haemorrhagic nephritis. Br Med J. 1927;1:504–6.
9. Hinglais N, Grunfeld J-P, Bois LE. Characteristic ultrastructural lesion of the glomerular basement

membrane in progressive hereditary nephritis (Alport's syndrome). Lab Invest. 1972;27:473–87.

10. Spear GS, Slusser RJ. Alport's syndrome: emphasizing electron microscopic studies of the glomerulus. Am J Pathol. 1972;69:213–22.

11. Churg J, Sherman RL. Pathologic characteristics of hereditary nephritis. Arch Pathol. 1973;95:374–9.

12. Olson DL, Anand SK, Landing BH, Heuser E, Grushkin CM, Lieberman E. Diagnosis of hereditary nephritis by failure of glomeruli to bind antiglomerular basement membrane antibodies. J Pediatr. 1980;96:697–9.

13. McCoy RC, Johnson HK, Stone WJ, Wilson CB. Absence of nephritogenic GBM antigen(s) in some patients with hereditary nephritis. Kidney Int. 1982;21:642–52.

14. Kashtan C, Fish AJ, Kleppel M, Yoshioka K, Michael AF. Nephritogenic antigen determinants in epidermal and renal basement membranes of kindreds with Alport-type familial nephritis. J Clin Invest. 1986;78:1035–44.

15. Atkin CL, Hasstedt SJ, Menlove L, Cannon L, Kirschner N, Schwartz C, et al. Mapping of Alport syndrome to the long arm of the X chromosome. Am J Hum Genet. 1988;42:249–55.

16. Barker DF, Hostikka SL, Zhou J, Chow LT, Oliphant AR, Gerken SC, et al. Identification of mutations in the COL4A5 collagen gene in Alport syndrome. Science. 1990;248:1224–7.

17. USRDS. USRDS 2013 Annual data report: Altas of Chronic Kidney Disease and End-Stage Renal Disease in the United States. Bethesda, National Institutes of Health NIoDaDaKD; 2013.

18. Poschl E, Pollner R, Kuhn K. The genes for the alpha 1(IV) and alpha 2(IV) chains of human basement membrane collagen type IV are arranged head-to-head and separated by a bidirectional promoter of unique structure. EMBO J. 1988;7(9):2687–95.

19. Segal Y, Zhuang L, Rondeau E, Sraer JD, Zhou J. Regulation of the paired type IV collagen genes COL4A5 and COL4A6. Role of the proximal promoter region. J Biol Chem. 2001;276(15):11791–7.

20. Khoshnoodi J, Cartailler JP, Alvares K, Veis A, Hudson BG. Molecular recognition in the assembly of collagens: terminal noncollagenous domains are key recognition modules in the formation of triple helical protomers. J Biol Chem. 2006;281(50):38117–21.

21. Hudson BG. The molecular basis of Goodpasture and Alport syndromes: beacons for the discovery of the collagen IV family. J Am Soc Nephrol. 2004;15(10):2514–27.

22. Yoshioka K, Hino S, Takemura T, Maki S, Wieslander J, Takekoshi Y, et al. Type IV Collagen a5 chain: normal distribution and abnormalities in X-linked Alport syndrome revealed by monoclonal antibody. Am J Pathol. 1994;144:986–96.

23. Peissel B, Geng L, Kalluri R, Kashtan C, Rennke HG, Gallo GR, et al. Comparative distribution of the a1(IV), a5(IV) and a6(IV) collagen chains in normal human adult and fetal tissues and in kidneys from X-linked Alport syndrome patients. J Clin Invest. 1995;96:1948–57.

24. Cheong HI, Kashtan CE, Kim Y, Kleppel MM, Michael AF. Immunohistologic studies of type IV collagen in anterior lens capsules of patients with Alport syndrome. Lab Invest. 1994;70:553–7.

25. Cosgrove D, Kornak JM, Samuelson G. Expression of basement membrane type IV collagen chains during postnatal development in the murine cochlea. Hear Res. 1996;100:21–32.

26. Zehnder AF, Adams JC, Santi PA, Kristiansen AG, Wacharasindhu C, Mann S, et al. Distribution of type IV collagen in the cochlea in Alport syndrome. Arch Otolaryngol Head Neck Surg. 2005;131:1007–13.

27. Gunwar S, Ballester F, Noelken ME, Sado Y, Ninomiya Y, Hudson BG. Glomerular basement membrane. Identification of a novel disulfide-cross-linked network of alpha3, alpha4, and alpha5 chains of type IV collagen and its implications for the pathogenesis of Alport syndrome. J Biol Chem. 1998;273(15):8767–75.

28. Zeisberg M, Khurana M, Rao VH, Cosgrove D, Rougier JP, Werner MC, et al. Stage-specific action of matrix metalloproteinases influences progressive hereditary kidney disease. PLoS Med. 2006;3(4):e100.

29. Gyoneva L, Segal Y, Dorfman KD, Barocas VH. Mechanical response of wild-type and Alport murine lens capsules during osmotic swelling. Exp Eye Res. 2013;113:87–91.

30. Meehan DT, Delimont D, Cheung L, Zallocchi M, Sansom SC, Holzclaw JD, et al. Biomechanical strain causes maladaptive gene regulation, contributing to Alport glomerular disease. Kidney Int. 2009;76(9):968–76.

31. Storey H, Savige J, Sivakumar V, Abbs S, Flinter FA. COL4A3/COL4A4 mutations and features in individuals with autosomal recessive Alport syndrome. J Am Soc Nephrol. 2013;24(12):1945–54.

32. Chiara F, Laura D, Rossella T, Dorella DP, Sandro F, Giorgia G, et al. Unbiased next generation sequencing analysis confirms the existence of autosomal dominant Alport syndrome in a relevant fraction of cases. Clin Genet. 2014;86(3):252–7.

33. Pescucci C, Mari F, Longo I, Vogiatzi P, Caselli R, Scala E, et al. Autosomal-dominant Alport syndrome: natural history of a disease due to COL4A3 or COL4A4 gene. Kidney Int. 2004;65(5):1598–603.

34. Lemmink HH, Nillesen WN, Mochizuki T, Schroder CH, Brunner HG, van Oost BA, et al. Benign familial hematuria due to mutation of the type IV collagen alpha4 gene. J Clin Invest. 1996;98(5):1114–8.

35. Crockett DK, Pont-Kingdon G, Gedge F, Sumner K, Seamons R, Lyon E. The Alport syndrome COL4A5 variant database. Hum Mutat. 2010;31(8):E1652–7.

36. Jais JP, Knebelmann B, Giatras I, De Marchi M, Rizzoni G, Renieri A, et al. X-linked Alport syndrome: natural history in 195 families and genotype-phenotype

correlations in males. J Am Soc Nephrol. 2000;11: 649–57.

37. Gross O, Netzer KO, Lambrecht R, Seibold S, Weber M. Meta-analysis of genotype-phenotype correlation in X-linked Alport syndrome: impact on clinical counseling. Nephrol Dial Transplant. 2002;17:1218–27.

38. Jais JP, Knebelmann B, Giatras I, De Marchi M, Rizzoni G, Renieri A, et al. X-linked Alport syndrome: natural history and genotype-phenotype correlations in girls and women belonging to 195 families: a "European Community Alport Syndrome Concerted Action" study. J Am Soc Nephrol. 2003; 14:2603–10.

39. Marcocci E, Uliana V, Bruttini M, Artuso R, Silengo MC, Zerial M, et al. Autosomal dominant Alport syndrome: molecular analysis of the COL4A4 gene and clinical outcome. Nephrol Dial Transplant. 2009;24(5):1464–71.

40. Gubler M, Levy M, Broyer M, Naizot C, Gonzales G, Perrin D, et al. Alport's syndrome: a report of 58 cases and a review of the literature. Am J Med. 1981;70:493–505.

41. Kashtan CE, Ding J, Gregory M, Gross O, Heidet L, Knebelmann B, et al. Clinical practice recommendations for the treatment of Alport syndrome: a statement of the Alport Syndrome Research Collaborative. Pediatr Nephrol. 2013;28(1):5–11.

42. Rheault MN. Women and Alport syndrome. Pediatr Nephrol. 2012;27(1):41–6.

43. Grunfeld J-P, Noel LH, Hafez S, Droz D. Renal prognosis in women with hereditary nephritis. Clin Nephrol. 1985;23:267–71.

44. Guo C, Van Damme B, Vanrenterghem Y, Devriendt K, Cassiman JJ, Marynen P. Severe alport phenotype in a woman with two missense mutations in the same COL4A5 gene and preponderant inactivation of the X chromosome carrying the normal allele. J Clin Invest. 1995;95(4):1832–7.

45. Iijima K, Nozu K, Kamei K, Nakayama M, Ito S, Matsuoka K, et al. Severe Alport syndrome in a young woman caused by a t(X;1)(q22.3;p36.32) balanced translocation. Pediatr Nephrol. 2010;25(10):2165–70.

46. Rheault MN, Kren SM, Hartich LA, Wall M, Thomas W, Mesa HA, et al. X-inactivation modifies disease severity in female carriers of murine X-linked Alport syndrome. Nephrol Dial Transplant. 2010;25(3):764–9.

47. Wester DC, Atkin CL, Gregory MC. Alport syndrome: clinical update. J Am Acad Audiol. 1995;6:73–9.

48. Kleppel MM, Santi PA, Cameron JD, Wieslander J, Michael AF. Human tissue distribution of novel basement membrane collagen. Am J Pathol. 1989;134:813–25.

49. Cosgrove D, Samuelson G, Meehan DT, Miller C, McGee J, Walsh EJ, et al. Ultrastructural, physiological, and molecular defects in the inner ear of a geneknockout mouse model of autosomal Alport syndrome. Hear Res. 1998;121:84–98.

50. Harvey SJ, Mount R, Sado Y, Naito I, Ninomiya Y, Harrison R, et al. The inner ear of dogs with X-linked

nephritis provides clues to the pathogenesis of hearing loss in X-linked Alport syndrome. Am J Pathol. 2001;159(3):1097–104.

51. Merchant SN, Burgess BJ, Adams JC, Kashtan CE, Gregory MC, Santi PA, et al. Temporal bone histopathology in alport syndrome. Laryngoscope. 2004; 114(9):1609–18.

52. Gratton MA, Rao VH, Meehan DT, Askew C, Cosgrove D. Matrix metalloproteinase dysregulation in the stria vascularis of mice with Alport syndrome: implications for capillary basement membrane pathology. Am J Pathol. 2005;166(5):1465–74.

53. Nielsen CE. Lenticonus anterior and Alport's syndrome. Arch Ophthalmol. 1978;56:518–30.

54. Colville DJ, Savige J. Alport syndrome. A review of the ocular manifestations. Ophthalmic Genet. 1997;18(4):161–73.

55. Streeten BW, Robinson MR, Wallace R, Jones DB. Lens capsule abnormalities in Alport's syndrome. Arch Ophthalmol. 1987;105:1693–7.

56. Kato T, Watanabe Y, Nakayasu K, Kanai A, Yajima Y. The ultrastructure of the lens capsule abnormalities in Alport's syndrome. Jpn J Ophthalmol. 1998;42:401–5.

57. Perrin D, Jungers P, Grunfeld JP, Delons S, Noel LH, Zenatti C. Perimacular changes in Alport's syndrome. Clin Nephrol. 1980;13:163–7.

58. Rhys C, Snyers B, Pirson Y. Recurrent corneal erosion associated with Alport's syndrome. Kidney Int. 1997;52:208–11.

59. Burke JP, Clearkin LG, Talbot JF. Recurrent corneal epithelial erosions in Alport's syndrome. Acta Ophthalmol. 1991;69:555–7.

60. Teekhasaenee C, Nimmanit S, Wutthiphan S, Vareesangthip K, Laohapand T, Malasitr P, et al. Posterior polymorphous dystrophy and Alport syndrome. Ophthalmology. 1991;98:1207–15.

61. Antignac C, Heidet L. Mutations in Alport syndrome associated with diffuse esophageal leiomyomatosis. Contrib Nephrol. 1996;117:172–82.

62. Antignac C, Knebelmann B, Druout L, Gros F, Deschenes G, Hors-Cayla M-C, et al. Deletions in the COL4A5 collagen gene in X-linked Alport syndrome: characterization of the pathological transcripts in non-renal cells and correlation with disease expression. J Clin Invest. 1994;93:1195–207.

63. Zhou J, Mochizuki T, Smeets H, Antignac C, Laurila P, de Paepe A, et al. Deletion of the paired a5(IV) and a6(IV) collagen genes in inherited smooth muscle tumors. Science. 1993;261:1167–9.

64. Segal Y, Peissel B, Renieri A, de Marchi M, Ballabio A, Pei Y, et al. LINE-1 elements at the sites of molecular rearrangements in Alport syndromediffuse leiomyomatosis. Am J Hum Genet. 1999;64:62–9.

65. Jonsson JJ, Renieri A, Gallagher PG, Kashtan CE, Cherniske EM, Bruttini M, et al. Alport syndrome, mental retardation, midface hypoplasia, and elliptocytosis: a new X linked contiguous gene deletion syndrome? J Med Genet. 1998;35(4):273–8.

66. Kashtan CE, Segal Y, Flinter F, Makanjuola D, Gan JS, Watnick T. Aortic abnormalities in males with Alport syndrome. Nephrol Dial Transplant. 2010; 25(11):3554–60.
67. Kashtan CE, Kleppel MM, Gubler MC. Immunohistologic findings in Alport syndrome. Contrib Nephrol. 1996;117:142–53.
68. Martin P, Heiskari N, Zhou J, Leinonen A, Tumelius T, Hertz JM, et al. High mutation detection rate in the COL4A5 collagen gene in suspected Alport syndrome using PCR and direct DNA sequencing. J Am Soc Nephrol. 1998;9:2291–301.
69. Gross O, Schulze-Lohoff E, Koepke ML, Beirowski B, Addicks K, Bloch W, et al. Antifibrotic, nephroprotective potential of ACE inhibitor vs AT1 antagonist in a murine model of renal fibrosis. Nephrol Dial Transplant. 2004;19(7):1716–23.
70. Gross O, Beirowski B, Koepke ML, Kuck J, Reiner M, Addicks K, et al. Preemptive ramipril therapy delays renal failure and reduces renal fibrosis in COL4A3-knockout mice with Alport syndrome. Kidney Int. 2003;63(2):438–46.
71. Gross O, Koepke ML, Beirowski B, Schulze-Lohoff E, Segerer S, Weber M. Nephroprotection by antifibrotic and anti-inflammatory effects of the vasopeptidase inhibitor AVE7688. Kidney Int. 2005;68: 456–63.
72. Sayers R, Kalluri R, Rodgers KD, Shield CF, Meehan DT, Cosgrove D. Role for transforming growth factor-beta 1 in Alport renal disease progression. Kidney Int. 1999;56:1662–73.
73. Ninichuk V, Gross O, Reichel C, Kandoga A, Pawar RD, Ciubar R, et al. Delayed chemokine receptor 1 blockade prolongs survival in collagen 4A3-deficient miche with Alport disease. J Am Soc Nephrol. 2005;16:977–85.
74. Zeisberg M, Bottiglio C, Kumar N, Maeshima Y, Strutz F, Muller GA, et al. Bone morphogenic protein-7 inhibits progression of chronic renal fibrosis associated with two genetic mouse models. Am J Physiol Renal Physiol. 2003;285(6):F1060–7.
75. Sugimoto H, Mundel TM, Sund M, Xie L, Cosgrove D, Kalluri R. Bone-marrow-derived stem cells repair basement membrane collagen defects and reverse genetic kidney disease. Proc Natl Acad Sci U S A. 2006;103(19):7321–6.
76. Chen D, Jefferson B, Harvey SJ, Zheng K, Gartley CJ, Jacobs RM, et al. Cyclosporine a slows the progressive renal disease of alport syndrome (X-linked hereditary nephritis): results from a canine model. J Am Soc Nephrol. 2003;14(3):690–8.
77. Charbit M, Gubler MC, Dechaux M, Gagnadoux MF, Grunfeld JP, Niaudet P. Cyclosporin therapy in patients with Alport syndrome. Pediatr Nephrol (Berlin, Germany). 2007;22(1):57–63.
78. Massella L, Muda AO, Legato A, Di Zazzo G, Giannakakis K, Emma F. Cyclosporine A treatment in patients with Alport syndrome: a single-center experience. Pediatr Nephrol (Berlin, Germany). 2010;25(7):1269–75.
79. Grodecki KM, Gains MJ, Baumal R, Osmond DH, Cotter B, Valli VE, Jacobs RM. Treatment of X-linked hereditary nephritis in Samoyed dogs with angiotensin converting enzyme inhibitor. J Comp Pathol. 1997;117:209–25.
80. Cohen EP, Lemann J. In hereditary nephritis angiotensin-converting enzyme inhibition decreases proteinuria and may slow the rate of progression. Am J Kidney Dis. 1996;27:199–203.
81. Proesmans W, Van Dyck M. Enalapril in children with Alport syndrome. Pediatr Nephrol. 2004;19(3): 271–5.
82. Webb NJ, Lam C, Shahinfar S, Strehlau J, Wells TG, Gleim GW, et al. Efficacy and safety of losartan in children with Alport syndrome – results from a subgroup analysis of a prospective, randomized, placebo- or amlodipine-controlled trial. Nephrol Dial Transplant. 2011;26(8):2521–6.
83. Webb NJ, Shahinfar S, Wells TG, Massaad R, Gleim GW, McCrary Sisk C, et al. Losartan and enalapril are comparable in reducing proteinuria in children with Alport syndrome. Pediatr Nephrol. 2013;28(5): 737–43.
84. Gross O, Licht C, Anders HJ, Hoppe B, Beck B, Tonshoff B, et al. Early angiotensin-converting enzyme inhibition in Alport syndrome delays renal failure and improves life expectancy. Kidney Int. 2012;81(5):494–501.
85. Gross O, Friede T, Hilgers R, Gorlitz A, Gavenis K, Ahmed R, et al. Safety and efficacy of the ACE-inhibitor Ramipril in Alport syndrome: the double-blind, randomized, placebo-controlled, multicenter phase III EARLY PRO-TECT Alport trial in pediatric patients. ISRN Pediatr. 2012;2012:436046.
86. Savige J, Gregory M, Gross O, Kashtan C, Ding J, Flinter F. Expert guidelines for the management of Alport syndrome and thin basement membrane nephropathy. J Am Soc Nephrol. 2013;24(3):364–75.
87. Wuhl E, Trivelli A, Picca S, Litwin M, Peco-Antic A, Zurowska A, et al. Strict blood-pressure control and progression of renal failure in children. N Engl J Med. 2009;361(17):1639–50.
88. Temme J, Kramer A, Jager KJ, Lange K, Peters F, Muller GA, et al. Outcomes of male patients with Alport syndrome undergoing renal replacement therapy. Clin J Am Soc Nephrol. 2012;7(12):1969–76.
89. Gross O, Weber M, Fries JW, Muller GA. Living donor kidney transplantation from relatives with mild urinary abnormalities in Alport syndrome: long-term risk, benefit and outcome. Nephrol Dial Transplant. 2009;24(5):1626–30.
90. Kashtan CE. Renal transplantation in patients with Alport syndrome. Pediatr Transplant. 2006;10: 651–7.
91. Brainwood D, Kashtan C, Gubler MC, Turner AN. Targets of alloantibodies in Alport antiglomerular basement membrane disease after renal transplantation. Kidney Int. 1998;53:762–6.
92. Dehan P, Van Den Heuvel LPWJ, Smeets HJM, Tryggvason K, Foidart J-M. Identification of

post-transplant anti-a5(IV) collagen alloantibodies in X-linked Alport syndrome. Nephrol Dial Transplant. 1996;11:1983–8.

93. Kalluri R, van den Heuvel LP, Smeets HJM, Schroder CH, Lemmink HH, Boutaud A, et al. A COL4A3 gene mutation and post-transplant anti-a3(IV) collagen alloantibodies in Alport syndrome. Kidney Int. 1995;47:1199–204.

94. Wang XP, Fogo AB, Colon S, Giannico G, Abul-Ezz SR, Miner JH, et al. Distinct epitopes for anti-glomerular basement membrane Alport alloantibodies and goodpasture autoantibodies within the noncollagenous domain of {alpha}3(IV) collagen: a janus-faced antigen. J Am Soc Nephrol. 2005;16: 3563–71.

95. Marks MI, Drummond KN. Benign familial hematuria. Pediatrics. 1969;44:590–3.

96. McConville JM, West CD, McAdams AJ. Familial and nonfamilial benign hematuria. J Pediatr. 1966; 69:207–14.

97. Pardo V, Berian MG, Levi DF, Strauss J. Benign primary hematuria: clinicopathologic study of 65 patients. Am J Med. 1979;67:817–22.

98. Savige J, Rana K, Tonna S, Buzza M, Dagher H, Wang YY. Thin basement membrane nephropathy. Kidney Int. 2003;64(4):1169–78.

99. Haas M. Thin glomerular basement membrane nephropathy: incidence in 3471 consecutive renal biopsies examined by electron microscopy. Arch Pathol Lab Med. 2006;130(5):699–706.

100. Dische FE, Anderson VER, Keane SJ, Taube D, Bewick M, Parsons V. Incidence of thin membrane nephropathy: morphometric investigation of a population sample. J Clin Pathol. 1990;43:457–60.

101. Tryggvason K, Patrakka J. Thin basement membrane nephropathy. J Am Soc Nephrol. 2006;17(3):813–22.

102. Gregory MC. The clinical features of thin basement membrane nephropathy. Semin Nephrol. 2005;25(3): 140–5.

103. Auwardt R, Savige J, Wilson D. A comparison of the clinical and laboratory features of thin basement membrane disease (TBMD) and IgA glomerulonephritis (IgA GN). Clin Nephrol. 1999;52(1):1–4.

104. Nieuwhof CM, de Heer F, de Leeuw P, van Breda Vriesman PJ. Thin GBM nephropathy: premature glomerular obsolescence is associated with hypertension and late onset renal failure. Kidney Int. 1997;51(5):1596–601.

105. van Paassen P, van Breda Vriesman PJ, van Rie H, Tervaert JW. Signs and symptoms of thin basement membrane nephropathy: a prospective regional study on primary glomerular disease-The Limburg Renal Registry. Kidney Int. 2004;66(3):909–13.

106. Pettersson E, Tornroth T, Wieslander J. Abnormally thin glomerular basement membrane and the Goodpasture epitope. Clin Nephrol. 1990;33:105–9.

107. Vogler C, McAdams AJ, Homan SM. Glomerular basement membrane and lamina densa in infants and children: an ultrastructural evaluation. Pediatr Pathol. 1987;7:527–34.

108. Steffes MW, Barbosa J, Basgen JM, Sutherland DER, Najarian JS, Mauer SM. Quantitative glomerular morphology of the normal human kidney. Kidney Int. 1983;49:82–6.

109. Dische FE. Measurement of glomerular basement membrane thickness and its application to the diagnosis of thin-membrane nephropathy. Arch Pathol Lab Med. 1992;116:43–9.

110. Tiebosch ATMG, Frederik PM, van Breda Vriesman PJC, Mooy JMV, van Rie H, van de Wiel TWM, et al. Thin-basement-membrane nephropathy in adults with persistent hematuria. N Engl J Med. 1989;320:14–8.

111. Milanesi C, Rizzoni G, Braggion F, Galdiolo D. Electron microscopy for measurement of glomerular basement membrane width in children with benign familial hematuria. Appl Pathol. 1984;2:199–204.

112. Blumenthal SS, Fritsche C, Lemann J. Establishing the diagnosis of benign familial hematuria: the importance of examining the urine sediment of family members. JAMA. 1988;259:2263–6.

113. Plaisier E, Gribouval O, Alamowitch S, Mougenot B, Prost C, Verpont MC, et al. COL4A1 mutations and hereditary angiopathy, nephropathy, aneurysms, and muscle cramps. N Engl J Med. 2007;357(26): 2687–95.

114. Plaisier E, Chen Z, Gekeler F, Benhassine S, Dahan K, Marro B, et al. Novel COL4A1 mutations associated with HANAC syndrome: a role for the triple helical CB3[IV] domain. Am J Med Genet A. 2010;152A(10):2550–5.

115. Alamowitch S, Plaisier E, Favrole P, Prost C, Chen Z, Van Agtmael T, et al. Cerebrovascular disease related to COL4A1 mutations in HANAC syndrome. Neurology. 2009;73(22):1873–82.

116. Poschl E, Schlotzer-Schrehardt U, Brachvogel B, Saito K, Ninomiya Y, Mayer U. Collagen IV is essential for basement membrane stability but dispensable for initiation of its assembly during early development. Development. 2004;131(7):1619–28.

IgA Nephropathy

19

Rosanna Coppo and Alessandro Amore

Introduction

Primary IgA nephropathy (IgAN) is the commonest glomerular disease in children and adolescents who undergo renal biopsy because of isolated microscopic hematuria or hematuria associated with non-nephrotic proteinuria [1]. Its prevalence varies in different reports, mostly due to the variable criteria for performing renal biopsy in young subjects, ranging from routine practice after detection of urine anomalies by school screening programs to watchful waiting attitude, limiting renal biopsy to cases having developed proteinuria. It is likely that several cases of IgAN originating in the pediatric age group are missed because most of them are asymptomatic and not detectable because the worldwide majority of children do not undergo regular screening programs.

IgAN had been considered a benign renal disease in adults and even more so in children; however, this belief was found not to be true in both age groups. The interest in IgAN in children has increased since recognition that most subjects with IgAN entering a chronic dialysis program are young adults [2] and, since the decline of

R. Coppo (✉) • A. Amore
Department of Nephrology, Dialysis, and Transplantation, Regina Margherita Children's Hospital, Piazza Polonia 94, Torino 10126, Italy
e-mail: rosanna.coppo@unito.it;
alessandro.amore@unito.it

renal function in these patients is slow [about 25 % of the cases need dialysis in 20 years] [3], it is clear that several progressive IgAN begin in childhood. Hence, detecting IgAN at the beginning of its natural history in childhood may offer an important opportunity for early treatment of the nephritis and/or its complications, with benefits for these patients in the pediatric age group but even more in adult life.

Epidemiology and Genetic Background

Primary IgAN is detected more frequently in males [4]. Its prevalence in children varies mostly in accordance with the policy for indication to renal biopsy in various Countries. In Asia, particularly in Japan and Korea, where urine screening programs are active in scholars, the prevalence of IgAN is up to 50 % of all glomerular diseases detected at renal biopsy [5–7]. In Europe and North America, where no mandatory urine screening testing in children is active, IgAN in children represents 20 % of renal biopsies [8–11].

Genetic factors may also account for the frequency of IgAN which is common in Asians, moderately prevalent in Europeans, and rare in Africans [12]. It is not known if these differences represent variation in genes, environment, or ascertainment.

Recent data indicate that genetic factors can contribute to the risk of developing IgAN. In a

© Springer-Verlag Berlin Heidelberg 2016
D.F. Geary, F. Schaefer (eds.), *Pediatric Kidney Disease*, DOI 10.1007/978-3-662-52972-0_19

genome wide associated study (GWAS) seven IgAN susceptibility loci have been identified. The strongest signal was detected for genes in the MHC region on chromosome 6 (Chr.6p21: *HLA-DQB1/DRB1*, *PSMB9/TAP1*, and *DPA1/DPB2* loci). Other relevant signals were related to regulation of the complement cascade on Chr.1q32 (*CFHR3/R1* and *CFHR3* loci), and to mucosal immunity on Chr.22q12 (*HORMAD2*, *DEFA* and *TNFSF13* loci) [13, 14]. These IgAN loci are associated with risk of other immune-mediated disorders such as type I diabetes, multiple sclerosis, or inflammatory bowel disease. GWAS indicated an East–West and South–North gradient in disease risk, and it has been suggested that differences in disease prevalence among world populations correlate with different prevalence of IgAN. These studies, however, explained only 4.7 % of overall IgAN risk [14], and indicate that additional factors contribute to the development of this renal disease.

Recent studies suggest a role for post-transcriptional regulation of gene expression due to the modulatory effect of micro-RNAs, small molecules which can impair the transcription of RNAs. Serum levels of miRNA-148b have been found to be increased in patients with IgAN, and this may be of relevance, since this miRNA modulates expression of the enzyme gactosyltrasferase which is active in the galactosylation of IgA1, deficient in patients with IgAN [15].

Pathogenesis

The deposition of IgA containing immune complexes and complement factors in the glomeruli is considered the clue to the pathogenesis of IgAN. These immune complexes are formed because of a dysregulated mucosal immunity. A role for mucosal immunity in IgAN has been hypothesized for decades, because of the typical manifestation of gross hematuria in coincidence with upper respiratory tract infections [16]. Experimental models with pathogen administration including intranasal administration of Sendai virus, a common respiratory pathogen [17, 18], Haemophilus parainfluenzae antigens, Coxsackie

B4 or Staphylococcus Aureus cell envelope. reproduced IgA mesangial deposits. IgAN was also reproduced in experimental animals by oral immunization with alimentary antigens, mostly gliadin [19, 20]. High levels of circulating IgA containing immune complexes (IgAIC), theoretically formed after contact with mucosal pathogens or alimentary antigens have been detected in 30–70 % of patients, and polymeric IgA1 subclass is the predominant subtype of IgA present [21, 22]. However, no specific viral or alimentary antigens have been found in renal mesangial deposits, and a dysregulated IgA immune response more than an increased exposure to antigens, seems to play the major pathogenic role. Patients with IgAN present with an increased intestinal permeability [23], which likely leads to increased antigenic exposure in association with altered mucosal immune response [16].

The most relevant abnormality of IgA molecules, which is observed in 80 % of patients with IgAN, is an altered glycosylation of the IgA1 subclass of IgA [22, 24–27]. Aberrantly glycosylated IgA1 is prevalent in mesangial deposits of these patients [24]. An insertion of 18 amino acids in the hinge region between CH1 and CH2 domains represents the major structural difference between IgA1 and IgA2, which is lacking it [24] (Fig. 19.1a,b). The amino acid sequence shows three threonine and three serine residues bound to five short O-linked oligosaccharide chains. The O-glycosylation consists of a core N-acetyl galactosamine (GalNAc) which occurs alone or extended with β1,3 linked Gal or further with sialic acid in α2, 3 and/or α2, 6 linkage [25].

In healthy subjects serum IgA1 consists of a mixture of molecules with different O-glycoforms, whereas in patients with IgAN there is a presence of abnormal IgA1 O-glycoform, a high frequency of O-glycans consisting of GalNAc alone [26, 27] or with premature sialylation of GalNac due to a hyperactive sialyltransferase gene [28]. Such aberrantly glycosylated IgA1 can circulate in monomeric form or participate in macromolecular self-aggregates; but they can elicit an IgG autoimmune response [26]. IgG antibodies were found to recognize GalNAc-containing epitopes on the galactose-deficient hinge region of IgA1,

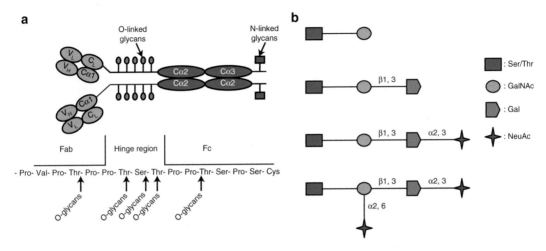

Fig. 19.1 (**a**) The IgA molecule, with particular magnification of the hinge region. (**b**) Different *O*-glycoforms of circulating IgA1 molecules in IgAN

forming IgG/IgA1IC or to react with antigens and form true IgAIC. IgAIC or IgG/IgA1IC IC constituted by aberrantly glycosylated IgA1 escape clearance by hepatic receptors and have a preferential renal deposition due to reactivity with mesangial matrix components fibronectin, laminin and collagen [22]. Serum levels of IgG/IgA1IC were found to correlate with disease activity in adults and in children with IgAN [29, 30]. It is of interest that these IgG may cross react with bacterial or viral cell-surface GalNAc- containing glycoproteins present on pathogens and with Gal deficient O-linked glycans expressed on the IgA1 molecule [31].

The extension of Gal to the GalNAc core of carbohydrates chains of IgA1 is under the effect of a β1,3 Gal transferase (C1GALT1) working with its chaperone Cosmc (core 1 GALT specific molecular chaperone). No convincing report of association with single nucleotide polymorphisms of the C1GALT1 gene has been published; however, the recent report of increased serum levels of miRNA-148b, which can interact with the transcription of C1GALT1 gene, is of interest [15].

Studies of familial cases of IgA nephropathy families by whole-genome scanning revealed a close association with the trait 6q 22-23 by linkage analysis in 60 % of familial IgAN [32]. High levels of aberrantly glycosylated IgA1 is inherited in familial and sporadic IgAN as they are

detected in 45 % of relatives of familial cases and in 25 % of relatives of sporadic cases. However, since these relatives are healthy, additional co-factors must exist. These findings support the hypothesis that IgA nephropathy is a multifactorial or "complex" disease in which one or more genes, probably in combination with environmental factors, may be responsible for the onset of the disease.

Systemic oxidative stress is triggered by circulating IgAIC containing degalactosylated IgA1 [33]. Elevated levels of advanced oxidation protein products (AOPP) have been detected in sera of patients with IgAN and found to be correlated with the amount of proteinuria and with the decrease in renal function during follow-up. The association of high levels of aberrantly glycosylated IgA1 and AOPPs represents a risk factor for progression of IgAN.

Acquired factors which modulate the immune response are likely to be activated in some patients, with increased production of IL-4 and IL-5 by Th2 lymphocytes in IgAN leading to synthesis of abnormally glycosylated IgA1 which is eventually deposited in the glomeruli [34].

The interaction with Fcα receptors on mesangial cells results in cellular activation and flogistic mediator synthesis including a variety of cytokines (IL6, PDGF, IL1, TNF-α, TGFβ), vasoactive factors (prostaglandins, thromboxane, leukotrienes, endothelin, PAF, NO) or chemokines (MCP-1,

IL-8, MIP-1, RANTES). The influx of monocytes and lymphocytes into the mesangium is enhanced by the C3 co-deposition.

The immune activation of mesangial cells leads to cell contraction, hemodynamic modifications and activation of the Renin-Angiotensin System (RAS) [35]. Angiotensin II enhances the release of cytokines and chemokines and potentiates the actions of PDGF and TGFβ as growth factors for mesangial cells, further favouring proliferation and accumulation of extracellular matrix, and ultimately promoting sclerosis. In IgAN, there is no definite evidence of altered ACE genotype frequency, even though some reports associated one genotype (DD) with a greater rate of progression in IgAN and a better response to ACE-I treatment [36].

The recent development of proteomics has allowed the identification of uromodulin as a urinary marker distinguishing IgAN from healthy controls and other glomerular diseases [37].

Renal Pathology of Children with IgAN

Primary IgAN typically presents with focal or diffuse proliferation of mesangial cells and expansion of the extracellular matrix. In both adults and children endocapillary hypercellularity or extracapillary proliferation with crescent formation can be detected in active cases, while glomerular hyalinosis and segmental or global sclerosis or tubulo-interstitial fibrosis are most prominent in patients with long lasting disease. The histological features in children are usually moderate, and the rapidly progressive forms with crescents involving more than 50 % of glomeruli are exceptional. Interstitial and arteriolar changes are infrequently found.

Several Authors have proposed histological classifications of IgAN based on individual lesion intensity or extension [38]. A new classification has recently been produced by a Consensus of Pathologists and Nephrologists, the Oxford clinicopathological classification [39, 40]. It consists of a combined score of four lesions [mesangial and endocapillary hypercellularity, segmental glomerulosclerosis and tubular atrophy/interstitial fibrosis], MEST, which were found to be predictive of outcome independent of clinical assessment (Fig. 19.2a–d). Although children with IgAN displayed more proliferative lesions and fewer chronic changes than adults, the predictive value of each lesion in the Oxford IgAN clinicopathological classification on renal survival was similar in children and adults [41].

In a recent Japanese study [42] the Oxford criteria were validated, and attention was focused on a small subgroup of children with crescents. A significant effect of crescents on progression of IgAN was found at univariate analysis; however, it was not confirmed at multivariate analysis when MEST data were included.

By definition, IgA is the dominant immunoglobulin present in all glomeruli (Fig. 19.3), almost exclusively polymeric IgA1 with λ light chain. C3 is detectable in up to 70 % of renal biopsies with the same distribution as IgA. IgG is present in 50–70 % of the renal biopsies, often intense as IgA, a feature that explains why this disease was initially called IgA–IgG nephropathy. IgM deposits are also found, but less commonly [31–66 %]. The early complement components, such as C1q and C4, are rarely detected, but when present they are invariably associated with IgG and/or IgM.

The spatial distribution of IgA and C3 in mesangial deposits, studied by confocal laser microscopy, shows IgA and C3 coated by IgA in milder cases. A stronger deposition of C3c than C3d has been reported in IgAN with endocapillary proliferation and active disease.

The most characteristic change on electron microscopy is the presence of electron-dense deposits in mesangial and paramesangial areas.

Clinical Features of IgAn in Children

IgAN is not common in children under the age of 3 years, while it is most frequent in adolescents. Even though in several children the diagnosis follows a chance finding of microscopic haematuria and/or proteinuria [6], the most

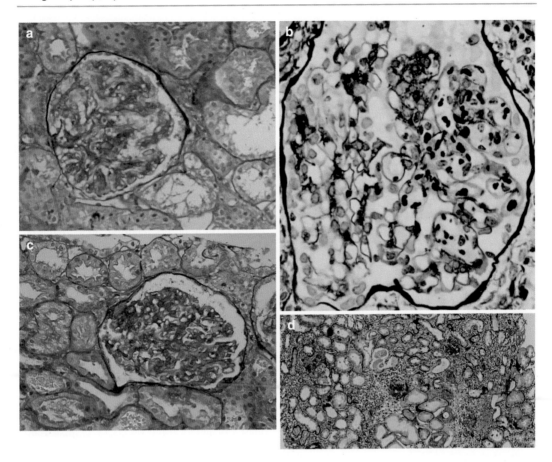

Fig. 19.2 Pathology features in IgA nephropathy. (**a**) Mesangial hypercellularity. (**b**) Endocapillary hypercellularity. (**c**) Segmental glomerulosclerosis. (**d**) Tubular atro-phy/interstitial fibrosis (Courtesy of Professor Sandrine Florquin, Academic Medical Center, Amsterdam)

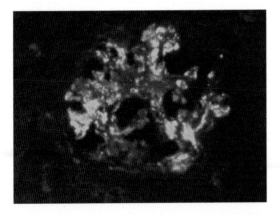

Fig. 19.3 Renal biopsy of a child with IgA nephropathy. Immunofluorescence with anti IgA antibody. Mesangial distribution of IgA staining

typical feature of IgAN is gross hematuria coincident with upper respiratory tract infections or other mucosal inflammatory processes (in 30–40 % of children) [7, 8, 10, 11]. Macroscopic hematuria rarely occurs after vaccination or heavy physical exercise. The interval between the precipitating event and the appearance of macrohaematuria is usually very short (12–72 h). The macroscopic hematuria persists for few days sometimes with flank and loin pain and fever. Some children have recurrent episodes without relevant urinary abnormalities in between. A transient increase in proteinuria occurs in coincidence with episodes of gross hematuria. In asymptomatic patients, as those detected at routine medical examination, proteinuria may be found in 3–13 % of cases [7, 8, 10, 11]. In some children the clinical onset can be a classic nephrotic syndrome, and only the renal biopsy allows a correct diagnosis of IgAN.

In some children gross hematuria is associated with increased serum creatinine and hypertension [7, 8, 11] seldom with acute oliguric renal failure due to tubular obstruction by packed red blood cells and in rare cases the disease progresses to chronic renal failure due to extensive crescentic lesions [7]. Hypertension usually develops during along term follow-up or in particularly severe cases [7, 8].

Risk Factors for Progression

The prognosis of IgAN was initially considered to be more benign in children than in adults, but long-term studies have failed to confirm this assessment. The natural history of IgAN in children represents, with few exceptions, the early phase of the overall natural history of the disease. Severe clinical signs usually develop after 5–15 years indicating the need for long follow-up including adult life, to define the history and the progression of IgAN in children [43].

In the first report by Levy et al. [10], a follow-up of 13 years in 91 French children demonstrated that only eight children [9 %] developed renal failure. However, persistent signs of active renal disease develop at long-term follow-up as reported in 47 % of Swedish children [44] after 10 years, including proteinuria in 35 %, hypertension in 9 %, and decreased GFR in 3 %. In Japan Yoshikawa et al. [7] found urinary abnormalities in 38 % of patients, persistent heavy proteinuria in 10 %, and progression to chronic renal failure in 5 % of 200 children who were followed for a mean period of 5 years. A Finnish study from Ronkainen et al. [45] more recently reported that subjects with IgAN originating in childhood, after two decades may have no signs of urinary disease in one third of the cases, and minor urinary abnormalities in another third, but the last third had CKD and 10 % had ESRF. At last follow-up some 40 % of subjects were receiving medications for hypertension, proteinuria or both

and this had been started a mean of 10 years after the initial diagnosis.

In short term follow-up studies children seem to have a better prognosis than adults, while a 20 year survival analysis showed that IgAN in children was as progressive as in adults [6, 9, 46]. The recent report in Finnish patients diagnosed with IgAN prior to age of 18 years, predicted renal survival rates from time of onset of symptoms of 93 % and 87 % at 10 and 20 years respectively [45]. A recent investigation from Japan on 181 pediatric IgAN, followed after a mean of 7 years from onset, reported 50 % in clinical remission and a predicted survival rate of 92 % at 10 years and 89 % at 20 years [47]. Children with IgAN can have spontaneous remission of the urinary symptoms, as observed in 96 Japanese children with IgAN and minor renal damage who did not receive medication after diagnosis [48]. Spontaneous remission could be observed after 5–8 years, but also recurrences of urinary symptoms were detected in 20 % at 5 years and 42 % at 10 years after remission. Hence IgAN in children has to be considered as a chronic disease with phases of activity and others of clinical remission, rendering difficult the establishment of a long term prognosis on the basis of a short initial follow-up after renal biopsy.

Some children, usually those presenting with moderate microscopic hematuria without proteinuria and displaying the mildest lesions, do not progress to end-stage renal failure over decades of observation. In children with progressive IgAN, the clinical course is often slow and indolent. The most relevant factors which trigger IgAN progression in adults, such as chronically reduced renal function at onset and persistent hypertension, are uncommon in children [2, 44, 49].

In the ongoing European validation study of the Oxford classification of IgA nephropathy (VALIGA), which enrolled 1147 patients, data on children with primary IgAN, reported by 20 centers from 11 European countries showed that clinical data, including proteinuria or blood pressure at renal biopsy are not significantly associated with the final outcome, indicating a possibility of spontaneous or [as it is in most of the cases] drug-induced remission. Conversely, the most relevant risk for progression in children is the persistence of proteinuria during follow-up, the so called time-average proteinuria. The threshold for follow-up of proteinuria in children is probably lower than what is accepted for adults. In adults with IgAN, only proteinuria values >1 g/day are considered a significant risk for progression, which deserve treatment, according to KDIGO recommendations [50]. For children, KDIGO suggests that also proteinuria >0.5 and <1 g/1.73 m^2/day has to be considered as a risk factor to be targeted for treatment. From data on long term follow-up studies in children with IgAN, a residual proteinuria <0.2 g/1.73 m^2/day after a treatment represents for children with IgAN a marker of favourable outcome [51, 52].

Treatment

Tonsillectomy

One of the first treatments considered for IgAN, particularly in children with recurrent gross hematuria has been tonsillectomy, aimed at interrupting the pathogenic sequences initiated by upper-respiratory tract infection leading to hematuria. B cells from bone marrow are likely to be the major source of aberrantly glycosylated IgA in patients with IgAN, but these cells have previously encountered the antigen at mucosal sites and are then relocated to bone marrow [53]. Tonsillectomy can remove a relevant source of pathogens which multiply in tonsils and remove macrophages and T cells in lymphoid tonsil follicles; hence, a source of aberrantly glycosylated IgA1 may theoretically be removed as well. In children it remains controversial whether adenotonsillectomy ultimately results in decreased serum immunoglobulins levels or, if so, whether such a decrease is associated with increased susceptibility to upper respiratory tract infections. In a randomized trial in non IgAN children [54] the IgA levels were significantly decreased after 1 year of follow-up; however, no relation was found between immunoglobulins levels and frequency of subsequent respiratory infections. Moreover, in children with repeated infections in spite of tonsillectomy, IgA levels increased again, indicating that the remaining mucosa-associated lymphoid tissue can compensate for the loss of tonsils and adenoid tissue [54]. Even though tonsillectomy can reduce the frequency of gross hematuria and produce some benefits, this intervention does not reach levels of sufficient evidence and KDIGO recommendations suggest tonsillectomy not be performed in patients with IgAN without a clinical indication [50].

However, tonsillectomy is supported by two large retrospective studies from Japan, which reported that the benefit on renal function decline are demonstrated after a follow-up longer than 10 years [55–58]. Tonsillectomy has a clear indication when tonsils are a true infectious focus, in case of recurrent tonsillitis (>3 per year), otherwise the efficacy of the procedure is often supported only in association with other therapy and the benefit is unclear [59].

Inhibition of the Renin-Angiotensin System (RAS Inhibition)

In all children with IgAN blood pressure [BP] control should be strict, (<90th percentile for height, sex and age) particularly when proteinuria is present, in which cases BP control has to be targeted to the 50th percentile, which corresponds to the target recommended in adults by KDIGO [50]. The drugs of choice for BP control in IgAN are RAS inhibitors either Angiotensin Converting Enzyme Inhibitors (ACE-Is) or Angiotensin Receptor Blockers (ARBs).

Current therapeutic strategies for IgAN in children and in adults have been directed towards modulating the glomerular response to immune deposits, in order to decrease the resultant tissue damage and progression towards sclerosis. Children with IgAN and heavy proteinuria are at risk for progressive disease. RAS inhibition has a strong rationale for use in IgAN, not only because it improves two principal progression factors (hypertension and proteinuria) but because it can inhibits the long series of potentially negative effects caused by Angiotensin II on mesangial cells particularly in presence of mesangial immune deposits.

We performed a European multicenter randomized controlled trial including children and young patients (3–35 years old) with a constant level of proteinuria (>1 <3.5 g/day/1.73 m^2 over the 3 months before enrolment) and normal or moderately reduced renal function. Fifty-seven patients, randomized to receive Benazepril 0.2 mg/kg/day or placebo, completed the trial (median follow-up 42 months). The primary outcome of renal disease progression, defined as >30% decrease in baseline glomerular filtration rate and/or worsening of proteinuria to nephrotic range, was significantly different between the two groups. A stable remission of proteinuria (<0.5 g/day/1.73 m^2) was observed in 56% of ACE-I patients versus 8% of placebo patients. The multivariate analysis showed that treatment with ACE-I was the independent predictor of prognosis, while no influence on the progression of renal damage was found for gender, age, baseline glomerular filtration rate, systolic or diastolic blood pressure, mean arterial pressure, and proteinuria [60].

Based on the evidence of the harmful effects of proteinuria in children with IgAN, KDIGO suggests to treat children with IgAN and persistent proteinuria >0.5 and <1 g/1.73 m^2/day, with RAS inhibition. There are no data to indicate a preference of ACE-Is over ARBs or vice versa, except in terms of lesser side-effects with ARBs in respect to ACE-Is. A small study in children with IgAN supports some benefits for reduction of proteinuria after combination of ACE-Is and ARBs [61], but this matter is still controversial in adults.

Glucocorticoids

KDIGO suggests that, if proteinuria persists unchanged after 3–6 months of RAS inhibition, glucocorticoids have to be considered for treatment of IgAN in children as well as in adults [50, 62]. There is presently little evidence that glucocorticoids provide additional benefits to supportive care with RAS inhibition; however, RCTs are ongoing in Europe and in China to address this important issue.

A US randomized, placebo-controlled, double-blind trial using prednisone (60 mg/m^2 every other day for 3 months, then 40 mg/m^2 every other day for 9 months, then 30 mg/m^2 every other day for

12 month) or fish oil (4 g/day for 2 years) failed to find significant benefit of treatment [63]. However, the relatively short follow-up period, inequality of baseline proteinuria, and small numbers of patients precludes a valid conclusion.

Yoshikawa et al. used a rather aggressive treatment for children with IgAN and severe histologic lesions, identified as severe mesangial proliferation. The children were randomized into two groups, one receiving prednisone, azathioprine, heparin-warfarin and dipyridamole and the other heparin-warfarin and dipyridamole. The trial lasted for 2 years and reported a significant reduction in proteinuria, serum IgA concentration, mesangial deposition, and prevention of increased number of sclerosed glomeruli [64]. After a follow-up of 10 years of free treatment, the children who had the immunosuppressive combination therapy showed a better survival to the end point of glomerular filtration rate <60 ml/min/1.73 m^2 [97% vs 84.8% in the anticoagulation treatment arm].

In another study in children with the same entry criterium of severe mesangial proliferation, a similar combination therapy produced a disappearance of IgA mesangial deposits after 2 years of treatment [65]. Ten years after the completion of the trial, patients in whom IgA deposits had disappeared had a significantly higher frequency of proteinuria-free survival. These reports suggest that early aggressive treatment in children with modifiable histologic risk factors for progression can in the long term protect the kidneys from a sclerotic evolution of renal changes.

These studies did not address the issue of any advantage of prednisone alone versus association of prednisone with azathioprine. In adults, no additional benefits of azathioprine were detected in patients treated with three series of methylprednisone pulses over 6 months [66].

KDIGO guidelines do not support the use of mycophenolate mofetil in IgAN, even though some uncontrolled study claims some benefits.

Rapidly Progressive Crescentic IgAN

The role of crescents in the progression of IgAN is considered as certain on the basis of experimental animal models, even though not proved by RCTs and not clearly detected in retrospective studies, based on cohort examination. According to KDIGO, IgAN with crescents involving more than 50% of glomeruli and with rapidly progressive renal deterioration may benefit from steroids and cyclophosphamide, analogous to the treatment of ANCA vasculitis [50]. Prompt use of aggressive immunosuppressive treatment, sometimes in association with plasmapheresis, has showed some benefits in slowing the relentless progression of these difficult cases [67].

Nephrotic Syndrome Associated with IgAN

These cases have features of idiopathic nephrotic syndrome associated with IgA mesangial deposits. The recommended treatment is the same as for minimal change disease and the outcome generally favourable.

Other Treatments

Even though evidence is moderate, KDIGO suggests using fish oil in the treatment of IgAN with persistent proteinuria despite 3–6 months of optimized supportive care (including ACE-Is or ARBs and blood pressure control).

Vitamin E, used as an anti-oxidant drug, was given for 1–2 years in a double-blind placebo-CT in 62 children and showed significant reduction in proteinuria, with a trend towards better preservation of renal function, hence missing a definite conclusion of its benefit on reno-protection [68].

No consistent benefits have been reported for anti-coagulants.

New Perspective in the Approach to the Treatment of IgAN in Children

The treatment of IgAN in children seems to be promising for long-term outcome, since children are more likely than adults to be treated in early stages, when mesangial proliferative lesions/endocapillary proliferations are more prominent than sclerosis, and when proteinuria is not massive. On the other hand, we have to take into consideration toxicity and side effects of these treatments, which are particularly undesired in patients with mild disease, and the possibility of spontaneous remission in mild cases [57].

According to KDIGO 2012 recommendations, the treatment of IgAN in adults and in children is mostly driven by the level of proteinuria at renal biopsy, advanced renal failure, beyond a "point of no return" being the only limitation. These recommendations originate from the available evidence in the literature. However, proteinuria can be associated with active lesions but also be the clinical manifestation of sclerotic lesions. The recent identification of pathologic features which represent risk factors independent from proteinuria, blood pressure and level of glomerular filtration rate at renal biopsy, strongly suggests there should be an integrated approach to treatment as indicated in Fig. 19.4.

For all children with IgAN a general approach is to carefully control BP and use RAS inhibition to target blood pressure <90th centile for high, sex and age or <50th centile if proteinuria is present. Tonsillectomy is performed only in cases with recurrent tonsillitis [>3 episodes/year] and repeated macroscopic hematuria.

For children with mild IgAN disease, presenting with normal glomerular filtration rate urinary protein/creatinine ratio (Up/Ucr) <0.5, normal BP and with all MEST (see legend for Fig. 19.4) negative [0], a watchful waiting attitude is suggested, prescribing RAS-inhibition if Up/Ucr increases above 0.5.

For children with IgAN and moderate/severe IgAN (Up/Ucr >0.5), any positive MEST, without severe irreversible sclerotic changes, glucocorticoids should be added to RAS inhibition. Methylprednisolone pulses [62] or oral steroids over at least 6 months can be adopted.

In cases with severe endocapillary proliferation or with crescents formations involving >30% of the glomeruli, with a rapidly progressive course, there are some possibilities of improvement with cyclophosphamide.

Fig. 19.4 Treatment of children with primary IgA nephropathy (*IgAN*). – *e-GFR* estimated glomerular filtration rate in children calculated with Swartz formula; – up/Ucr urinary protein/creatinine ratio; – normal blood pressure <90th percentile corrected for high, sex and age; – MEST: scores derived from Oxford classification of IgAN [39, 40]. *M* mesangial hypercellularity, *E* endocapillary hypercellularity, *S* segmental sclerosis, *T* tubular atrophy/interstitial fibrosis

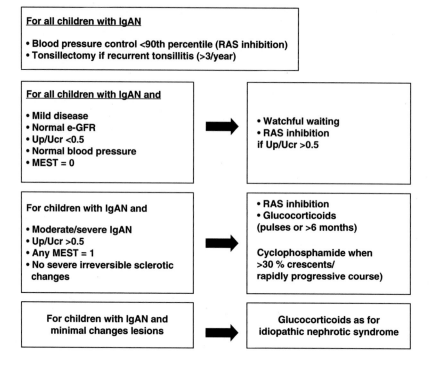

In children with IgAN, minimal change lesions and nephrotic syndrome, a protocol similar to that recommended for idiopathic nephritic syndrome is a suitable choice.

References

1. Berger J, Hinglais N. Les depots intercapillaires d'IgAIgG. J Urol Nephrol. 1968;74(9):694–5.
2. Coppo R, Amore A, Hogg R, Emancipator S. Idiopathic nephropathy with IgA deposits. Pediatr Nephrol. 2000;15(1–2):139–50.
3. Davin JC, Ten Berge IJ, Weening JJ. What is the difference between IgA nephropathy and Henoch-Schönlein purpura nephritis? Kidney Int. 2001;59(3):823–34.
4. D'Amico G, Imbasciati E, Barbiano Di Belgioioso G, Bertoli S, Fogazzi G, Ferrario F, Fellin G, Ragni A, Colasanti G, Minetti L, et al. Idiopathic IgA mesangial nephropathy. Clinical and histological study of 374 patients. Medicine (Baltimore). 1985;64(1):49–60.
5. Koyama A, Igarashi M, Kobayashi M. Natural history and risk factors for immunoglobulin A nephropathy in Japan. Research Group on Progressive Renal Diseases. Am J Kidney Dis. 1997;29(4):526–32.
6. Kusumoto Y, Takebayashi S, Taguchi T, Harada T, Naito S. Long-term prognosis and prognostic indices of IgA nephropathy in juvenile and in adult Japanese. Clin Nephrol. 1987;28(3):118–24.

7. Yoshikawa N, Iijima K, Ito H. IgA nephropathy in children. Nephron. 1999;83(1):1–12.
8. Coppo R, Gianoglio B, Porcellini MG, Maringhini S. Frequency of renal diseases and clinical indications for renal biopsy in children (report of the Italian National Registry of Renal Biopsies in Children). Group of Renal Immunopathology of the Italian Society of Pediatric Nephrology and Group of Renal Immunopathology of the Italian Society of Nephrology. Nephrol Dial Transplant. 1998;13(2):293–7.
9. Wyatt RJ, Julian BA, Bhathena DB, Mitchell BL, Holland NH, Malluche HH. Iga nephropathy: presentation, clinical course, and prognosis in children and adults. Am J Kidney Dis. 1984;4(2):192–200.
10. Lévy M, Gonzalez-Burchard G, Broyer M, Dommergues JP, Foulard M, Sorez JP, Habib R. Berger's disease in children. Natural history and outcome. Medicine (Baltimore). 1985;64(3):157–80.
11. Schena FP. A retrospective analysis of the natural history of primary IgA nephropathy worldwide. Am J Med. 1990;89(2):209–15.
12. McGrogan A, Franssen CF, de Vries CS. The incidence of primary glomerulonephritis worldwide: a systematic review of the literature. Nephrol Dial Transplant. 2011;26(2):414–30.
13. Gharavi AG, Kiryluk K, Choi M, Li Y, Hou P, Xie J, Sanna-Cherchi S, Men CJ, Julian BA, Wyatt RJ, Novak J, He JC, Wang H, Lv J, Zhu L, Wang W, Wang Z, Yasuno K, Gunel M, Mane S, Umlauf S, Tikhonova I, Beerman I, Savoldi S, Magistroni R, Ghiggeri GM, Bodria M, Lugani F, Ravani P, Ponticelli C, Allegri L, Boscutti G, Frasca G, Amore A, Peruzzi L, Coppo R,

Izzi C, Viola BF, Prati E, Salvadori M, Mignani R, Gesualdo L, Bertinetto F, Mesiano P, Amoroso A, Scolari F, Chen N, Zhang H, Lifton RP. Genome-wide association study identifies susceptibility loci for IgA nephropathy. Nat Genet. 2011;43(4):321–7.

14. Kiryluk K, Li Y, Sanna-Cherchi S, Rohanizadegan M, Suzuki H, Eitner F, Snyder HJ, Choi M, Hou P, Scolari F, Izzi C, Gigante M, Gesualdo L, Savoldi S, Amoroso A, Cusi D, Zamboli P, Julian BA, Novak J, Wyatt RJ, Mucha K, Perola M, Kristiansson K, Viktorin A, Magnusson PK, Thorleifsson G, Thorsteinsdottir U, Stefansson K, Boland A, Metzger M, Thibaudin L, Wanner C, Jager KJ, Goto S, Maixnerova D, Karnib HH, Nagy J, Panzer U, Xie J, Chen N, Tesar V, Narita I, Berthoux F, Floege J, Stengel B, Zhang H, Lifton RP, Gharavi AG. Geographic differences in genetic susceptibility to IgA nephropathy: GWAS replication study and geospatial risk analysis. PLoS Genet. 2012;8(6):e1002765.

15. Serino G, Sallustio F, Cox SN, Pesce F, Schena FP. Abnormal miR-148b expression promotes aberrant glycosylation of IgA1 in IgA nephropathy. J Am Soc Nephrol. 2012;23(5):814–24.

16. Emancipator SN. Immunoregulatory factors in the pathogenesis of IgA nephropathy. Kidney Int. 1990; 38(6):1216–29.

17. Yamashita M, Chintalacharuvu SR, Kobayashi N, Nedrud JG, Lamm ME, Tomino Y, Emancipator SN. Analysis of innate immune responses in a model of IgA nephropathy induced by Sendai virus. Contrib Nephrol. 2007;157:159–63.

18. Amore A, Coppo R, Nedrud JG, Sigmund N, Lamm ME, Emancipator SN. The role of nasal tolerance in a model of IgA nephropathy induced in mice by Sendai virus. Clin Immunol. 2004;113(1):101–8.

19. Coppo R, Roccatello D, Amore A, Quattrocchio G, Molino A, Gianoglio B, Amoroso A, Bajardi P, Piccoli G. Effects of a gluten-free diet in primary IgA nephropathy. Clin Nephrol. 1990;33(2):72–86.

20. Smerud HK, Fellström B, Hällgren R, Osagie S, Venge P, Kristjánsson G. Gluten sensitivity in patients with IgA nephropathy. Nephrol Dial Transplant. 2009;24(8):2476–81.

21. Schena FP, Pastore A, Ludovico N, Sinico RA, Benuzzi S, Montinaro V. Increased serum levels of IgA1-IgG immune complexes and anti-F(ab′)2 antibodies in patients with primary IgA nephropathy. Clin Exp Immunol. 1989;77(1):15–20.

22. Coppo R, Amore A, Gianoglio B, Porcellini MG, Peruzzi L, Gusmano R, Giani M, Sereni F, Gianviti A, Rizzoni G, et al. Macromolecular IgA and abnormal IgA reactivity in sera from children with IgA nephropathy. Italian Collaborative Paediatric IgA Nephropathy Study. Clin Nephrol. 1995;43(1):1–13.

23. Kloster Smerud H, Fellström B, Hällgren R, Osagie S, Venge P, Kristjánsson G. Gastrointestinal sensitivity to soy and milk proteins in patients with IgA nephropathy. Clin Nephrol. 2010;74(5):364–71.

24. Hiki Y, Tanaka A, Kokubo T, Iwase H, Nishikido J, Hotta K, Kobayashi Y. Analyses of IgA1 hinge glycopeptides in IgA nephropathy by matrix-assisted laser desorption/ionization time-of-flight mass spectrometry. J Am Soc Nephrol. 1998;9(4):577–82.

25. Allen AC, Bailey EM, Barratt J, Buck KS, Feehally J. Analysis of IgA1 O-glycans in IgA nephropathy by fluorophore-assisted carbohydrate electrophoresis. J Am Soc Nephrol. 1999;10(8):1763–71.

26. Suzuki H, Moldoveanu Z, Hall S, Brown R, Julian BA, Wyatt RJ, Tomana M, Tomino Y, Novak J, Mestecky J. IgA nephropathy: characterization of IgG antibodies specific for galactose-deficient IgA1. Contrib Nephrol. 2007;157:129–33.

27. Mestecky J, Tomana M, Moldoveanu Z, Julian BA, Suzuki H, Matousovic K, Renfrow MB, Novak L, Wyatt RJ, Novak J. Role of aberrant glycosylation of IgA1 molecules in the pathogenesis of IgA nephropathy. Kidney Blood Press Res. 2008;31(1): 29–37.

28. Raska M, Moldoveanu Z, Suzuki H, Brown R, Kulhavy R, Andrasi J, Hall S, Vu HL, Carlsson F, Lindahl G, Tomana M, Julian BA, Wyatt RJ, Mestecky J, Novak J. Identification and characterization of CMP-NeuAc:GalNAc-IgA1 alpha2,6-sialyltransferase in IgA1-producing cells. J Mol Biol. 2007;369(1): 69–78.

29. Berthoux F, Suzuki H, Thibaudin L, Yanagawa H, Maillard N, Mariat C, Tomino Y, Julian BA, Novak J. Autoantibodies targeting galactose-deficient IgA1 associate with progression of IgA nephropathy. J Am Soc Nephrol. 2012;23(9):1579–87.

30. Mestecky J, Raska M, Julian BA, Gharavi AG, Renfrow MB, Moldoveanu Z, Novak L, Matousovic K, Novak J. IgA nephropathy: molecular mechanisms of the disease. Annu Rev Pathol. 2013;8:217–40.

31. Suzuki H, Kiryluk K, Novak J, Moldoveanu Z, Herr AB, Renfrow MB, Wyatt RJ, Scolari F, Mestecky J, Gharavi AG, Julian BA. The pathophysiology of IgA nephropathy. J Am Soc Nephrol. 2011;22(10): 1795–803.

32. Gharavi AG, Yan Y, Scolari F, Schena FP, Frasca GM, Ghiggeri GM, Cooper K, Amoroso A, Viola BF, Battini G, Caridi G, Canova C, Farhi A, Subramanian V, Nelson-Williams C, Woodford S, Julian BA, Wyatt RJ, Lifton RP. IgA nephropathy, the most common cause of glomerulonephritis, is linked to 6q22-23. Nat Genet. 2000;26(3):354–7.

33. Camilla R, Suzuki H, Daprà V, Loiacono E, Peruzzi L, Amore A, Ghiggeri GM, Mazzucco G, Scolari F, Gharavi AG, Appel GB, Troyanov S, Novak J, Julian BA, Coppo R. Oxidative stress and galactose-deficient IgA1 as markers of progression in IgA nephropathy. Clin J Am Soc Nephrol. 2011;6(8):1903–11.

34. Chintalacharuvu SR, Nagy NU, Sigmund N, Nedrud JG, Amm ME, Emancipator SN. T cell cytokines determine the severity of experimental IgA nephropathy by regulating IgA glycosylation. Clin Exp Immunol. 2001;126(2):326–33.

35. Coppo R, Amore A, Gianoglio B, Cacace G, Picciotto G, Roccatello D, Peruzzi L, Piccoli G, De Filippi PG. Angiotensin II local hyperreactivity in the progression of IgA nephropathy. Am J Kidney Dis. 1993;21(6):593–602.

36. Schena FP, D'Altri C, Cerullo G, Manno C, Gesualdo L. ACE gene polymorphism and IgA nephropathy: an ethnically homogeneous study and a meta-analysis. Kidney Int. 2001;60(2):732–40.

37. Graterol F, Navarro-Muñoz M, Ibernon M, López D, Troya MI, Pérez V, Bonet J, Romero R. Poor histological lesions in IgA nephropathy may be reflected in blood and urine peptide profiling. BMC Nephrol. 2013;14(1):82.

38. Haas M. Histologic subclassification of IgA nephropathy: a clinicopathologic study of 244 cases. Am J Kidney Dis. 1997;29(6):829–42.

39. Working Group of the International IgA Nephropathy Network and the Renal Pathology Society, Cattran DC, Coppo R, Cook HT, Feehally J, Roberts IS, Troyanov S, Alpers CE, Amore A, Barratt J, Berthoux F, Bonsib S, Bruijn JA, D'Agati V, D'Amico G, Emancipator S, Emma F, Ferrario F, Fervenza FC, Florquin S, Fogo A, Geddes CC, Groene HJ, Haas M, Herzenberg AM, Hill PA, Hogg RJ, Hsu SI, Jennette JC, Joh K, Julian BA, Kawamura T, Lai FM, Leung CB, Li LS, Li PK, Liu ZH, Mackinnon B, Mezzano S, Schena FP, Tomino Y, Walker PD, Wang H, Weening JJ, Yoshikawa N, Zhang H. The Oxford classification of IgA nephropathy: rationale, clinicopathological correlations, and classification. Kidney Int. 2009; 76(5):534–45.

40. Working Group of the International IgA Nephropathy Network and the Renal Pathology Society, Roberts IS, Cook HT, Troyanov S, Alpers CE, Amore A, Barratt J, Berthoux F, Bonsib S, Bruijn JA, Cattran DC, Coppo R, D'Agati V, D'Amico G, Emancipator S, Emma F, Feehally J, Ferrario F, Fervenza FC, Florquin S, Fogo A, Geddes CC, Groene HJ, Haas M, Herzenberg AM, Hill PA, Hogg RJ, Hsu SI, Jennette JC, Joh K, Julian BA, Kawamura T, Lai FM, Li LS, Li PK, Liu ZH, Mackinnon B, Mezzano S, Schena FP, Tomino Y, Walker PD, Wang H, Weening JJ, Yoshikawa N, Zhang H. The Oxford classification of IgA nephropathy: pathology definitions, correlations, and reproducibility. Kidney Int. 2009;76(5):546–56.

41. Working Group of the International IgA Nephropathy Network and the Renal Pathology Society, Coppo R, Troyanov S, Camilla R, Hogg RJ, Cattran DC, Cook HT, Feehally J, Roberts IS, Amore A, Alpers CE, Barratt J, Berthoux F, Bonsib S, Bruijn JA, D'Agati V, D'Amico G, Emancipator SN, Emma F, Ferrario F, Fervenza FC, Florquin S, Fogo AB, Geddes CC, Groene HJ, Haas M, Herzenberg AM, Hill PA, Hsu SI, Jennette JC, Joh K, Julian BA, Kawamura T, Lai FM, Li LS, Li PK, Liu ZH, Mezzano S, Schena FP, Tomino Y, Walker PD, Wang H, Weening JJ, Yoshikawa N, Zhang H. The Oxford IgA nephropathy clinicopathological classification is valid for children as well as adults. Kidney Int. 2010;77(10):921–7.

42. Shima Y, Nakanishi K, Hama T, Mukaiyama H, Togawa H, Hashimura Y, Kaito H, Sako M, Iijima K, Yoshikawa N. Validity of the Oxford classification of IgA nephropathy in children. Pediatr Nephrol. 2012; 27(5):783–92.

43. Coppo R, D'Amico G. Factors predicting progression of IgA nephropathies. J Nephrol. 2005;18(5):503–12.

44. Linné T, Berg U, Bohman SO, Sigström L. Course and long-term outcome of idiopathic IgA nephropathy in children. Pediatr Nephrol. 1991;5(4):383–6.

45. Ronkainen J, Ala-Houhala M, Autio-Harmainen H, Jahnukainen T, Koskimies O, Merenmies J, Mustonen J, Ormälä T, Turtinen J, Nuutinen M. Long-term outcome 19 years after childhood IgA nephritis: a retrospective cohort study. Pediatr Nephrol. 2006;21(9): 1266–73.

46. Wyatt RJ, Kritchevsky SB, Woodford SY, Miller PM, Roy 3rd S, Holland NH, Jackson E, Bishof NA. IgA nephropathy: long-term prognosis for pediatric patients. J Pediatr. 1995;127(6):913–9.

47. Nozawa R, Suzuki J, Takahashi A, Isome M, Kawasaki Y, Suzuki S, Suzuki H. Clinicopathological features and the prognosis of IgA nephropathy in Japanese children on long-term observation. Clin Nephrol. 2005;64(3):171–9.

48. Shima Y, Nakanishi K, Hama T, Mukaiyama H, Togawa H, Sako M, Kaito H, Nozu K, Tanaka R, Iijima K, Yoshikawa N. Spontaneous remission in children with IgA nephropathy. Pediatr Nephrol. 2013;28(1):71–6.

49. Hogg RJ, Silva FG, Wyatt RJ, Reisch JS, Argyle JC, Savino DA. Prognostic indicators in children with IgA nephropathy – report of the Southwest Pediatric Nephrology Study Group. Pediatr Nephrol. 1994;8(1): 15–20.

50. Radhakrishnan J, Cattran DC. The KDIGO practice guideline on glomerulonephritis: reading between the (guide)lines – application to the individual patient. Kidney Int. 2012;82(8):840–56.

51. Kamei K, Nakanishi K, Ito S, Saito M, Sako M, Ishikura K, Hataya H, Honda M, Iijima K, Yoshikawa N, Japanese Pediatric IgA Nephropathy Treatment Study Group. Long-term results of a randomized controlled trial in childhood IgA nephropathy. Clin J Am Soc Nephrol. 2011;6(6):1301–7.

52. Shima Y, Nakanishi K, Kamei K, Togawa H, Nozu K, Tanaka R, Sasaki S, Iijima K, Yoshikawa N. Disappearance of glomerular IgA deposits in childhood IgA nephropathy showing diffuse mesangial proliferation after 2 years of combination/prednisolone therapy. Nephrol Dial Transplant. 2011;26(1):163–9.

53. Harper SJ, Allen AC, Layward L, Hattersley J, Veitch PS, Feehally J. Increased immunoglobulin A and immunoglobulin A1 cells in bone marrow trephine biopsy specimens in immunoglobulin A nephropathy. Am J Kidney Dis. 1994;24(6):888–92.

54. van den Akker EH, Sanders EA, van Staaij BK, Rijkers GT, Rovers MM, Hoes AW, Schilder AG. Long-term effects of pediatric adenotonsillectomy on serum immunoglobulin levels: results of a randomized controlled trial. Ann Allergy Asthma Immunol. 2006 ;97(2):251–6.

55. Xie Y, Nishi S, Ueno M, Imai N, Sakatsume M, Narita I, Suzuki Y, Akazawa K, Shimada H, Arakawa M, Gejyo F. The efficacy of tonsillectomy on long-term

renal survival in patients with IgA nephropathy. Kidney Int. 2003;63(5):1861–7.

56. Akagi H, Kosaka M, Hattori K, Doi A, Fukushima K, Okano M, Kariya S, Nishizaki K, Sugiyama N, Shikata K, Makino H, Masuda Y. Long-term results of tonsillectomy as a treatment for IgA nephropathy. Acta Otolaryngol Suppl. 2004;555:38–42.

57. Sato M, Hotta O, Tomioka S, Horigome I, Chiba S, Miyazaki M, Noshiro H, Taguma Y. Cohort study of advanced IgA nephropathy: efficacy and limitations of corticosteroids with tonsillectomy. Nephron Clin Pract. 2003;93(4):c137–45.

58. Miyazaki M, Hotta O, Komatsuda A, Nakai S, Shoji T, Yasunaga C, Taguma Y, Japanese Multicenter Study Group on Treatment of IgA Nephropathy (JST-IgAN). A multicenter prospective cohort study of tonsillectomy and steroid therapy in Japanese patients with IgA nephropathy: a 5-year report. Contrib Nephrol. 2007;157:94–8.

59. Kawasaki Y, Takano K, Suyama K, Isome M, Suzuki H, Sakuma H, Fujiki T, Suzuki H, Hosoya M. Efficacy of tonsillectomy pulse therapy versus multiple-drug therapy for IgA nephropathy. Pediatr Nephrol. 2006;21(11):1701–6.

60. Coppo R, Peruzzi L, Amore A, Piccoli A, Cochat P, Stone R, Kirschstein M, Linné T. IgACE: a placebo-controlled, randomized trial of angiotensin-converting enzyme inhibitors in children and young people with IgA nephropathy and moderate proteinuria. J Am Soc Nephrol. 2007;18(6):1880–8.

61. Yang Y, Ohta K, Shimizu M, Nakai A, Kasahara Y, Yachie A, Koizumi S. Treatment with low-dose angiotensin-converting enzyme inhibitor (ACEI) plus angiotensin II receptor blocker (ARB) in pediatric patients with IgA nephropathy. Clin Nephrol. 2005;64(1):35–40.

62. Pozzi C, Andrulli S, Del Vecchio L, Melis P, Fogazzi GB, Altieri P, Ponticelli C, Locatelli F. Corticosteroid effectiveness in IgA nephropathy: long-term results of a randomized, controlled trial. J Am Soc Nephrol. 2004;15(1):157–63.

63. Hogg RJ, Lee J, Nardelli N, Julian BA, Cattran D, Waldo B, Wyatt R, Jennette JC, Sibley R, Hyland K, Fitzgibbons L, Hirschman G, Donadio Jr JV, Holub BJ, Southwest Pediatric Nephrology Study Group. Clinical trial to evaluate omega-3 fatty acids and alternate day prednisone in patients with IgA nephropathy: report from the Southwest Pediatric Nephrology Study Group. Clin J Am Soc Nephrol. 2006;1(3):467–74.

64. Yoshikawa N, Ito H, Sakai T, Takekoshi Y, Honda M, Awazu M, Ito K, Iitaka K, Koitabashi Y, Yamaoka K, Nakagawa K, Nakamura H, Matsuyama S, Seino Y, Takeda N, Hattori S, Ninomiya M. A controlled trial of combined therapy for newly diagnosed severe childhood IgA nephropathy. The Japanese Pediatric IgA Nephropathy Treatment Study Group. J Am Soc Nephrol. 1999;10(1):101–9.

65. Yoshikawa N, Honda M, Iijima K, Awazu M, Hattori S, Nakanishi K, Ito H, Japanese Pediatric IgA Nephropathy Treatment Study Group. Steroid treatment for severe childhood IgA nephropathy: a randomized, controlled trial. Clin J Am Soc Nephrol. 2006;1(3):511–7.

66. Pozzi C, Andrulli S, Pani A, Scaini P, Del Vecchio L, Fogazzi G, Vogt B, De Cristofaro V, Allegri L, Cirami L, Procaccini AD, Locatelli F. Addition of azathioprine to corticosteroids does not benefit patients with IgA nephropathy. J Am Soc Nephrol. 2010;21(10):1783–90.

67. Shenoy M, Ognjanovic MV, Coulthard MG. Treating severe Henoch-Schönlein and IgA nephritis with plasmapheresis alone. Pediatr Nephrol. 2007;22(8):1167–71.

68. Chan JC, Mahan JD, Trachtman H, Scheinman J, Flynn JT, Alon US, Lande MB, Weiss RA, Norkus EP. Vitamin E therapy in IgA nephropathy: a double-blind, placebo-controlled study. Pediatr Nephrol. 2003;18(10):1015–9.

Membranous Nephropathy

20

Pierre Ronco, Hanna Debiec, and Sanjeev Gulati

Incidence

Nephrotic syndrome is one of the most common kidney disorders encountered in day to day nephrology practice. In children it occurs at a reported incidence of 2 per 100,000 per year and a cumulative prevalence of 16 per 100,000 children.

Membranous nephropathy (MN) is an uncommon cause of nephrotic syndrome in children [1, 2]. In pediatric cohorts, idiopathic MN accounted for 1.5–1.7% of cases in children with idiopathic nephrotic syndrome biopsied at disease onset [3–7], and for 4–7% of children with steroid resistant nephrotic syndrome [8] (Table 20.1 [9]). Because many children with steroid-sensitive nephrotic syndrome will never be biopsied, the relative prevalence of MN versus minimal change disease and focal segmental glomerular sclerosis is unclear. Another bias is the age range of the population. In a series from Pakistan that investigated 538 children who underwent biopsy for idiopathic nephrotic syndrome, there was a significant difference between the 3% rate of MN in children aged <13 years and the 18.5% rate found in adolescents aged 13–18 years [10]. Similar rates were found in adolescents in two different cohorts [11, 12].

MN has been reported to account for only 0.6% of pediatric chronic and end-stage kidney disease cases, with a median age at onset of ESRD being 16 years [3, 13]. This is in contrast to adults, in whom MN is one of the more common forms of nephrotic syndrome and a leading cause of end stage renal disease [14, 15]. A notable exception is nephrotic syndrome in South-African children, 40% of whom show MN on biopsy, associated with hepatitis B virus antigen in 86% of cases [16]. MN has a 2:1 predilection for males over females although this sex ratio is variable from a series to another.

Etiology

MN occurs in idiopathic and secondary forms which can be distinguished by clinical, laboratory, and histological features. In secondary MN related to lupus or hepatitis, concomitant mesangial or subendothelial deposits may be present [17]. Children have a higher frequency of secondary MN compared to adults. The principal causes of the secondary variety in children appear to be infections and autoimmune diseases (Table 20.2). Drugs and

P. Ronco (✉) • H. Debiec
Department of Nephrology and Dialysis, Tenon Hospital, UMR_S 1155, 4 rue de la Chine, Paris 75020, France
e-mail: pierreronco@yahoo.fr; hanna.debiec@upmc.fr

S. Gulati
Department of Nephrology, Fortis Institute of Renal Sciences and Transplantation, 474, Sector A, Pocket C, Vasant Kunj, New Delhi 110070, India
e-mail: sgulatipedneph@yahoo.com

© Springer-Verlag Berlin Heidelberg 2016
D.F. Geary, F. Schaefer (eds.), *Pediatric Kidney Disease*, DOI 10.1007/978-3-662-52972-0_20

Table 20.1 Differences between pediatric and adult membranous nephropathy

Disease type and demographic and clinical features	Pediatric MN	Adult MN
Disease type/subtype		
Proportion of primary nephrotic syndrome cases that are MN	<5% (children) 5–20% (adolescents)	15–30%
MN that is primary ("idiopathic")	Minority	Majority
Proportion of primary MN that is PLA2R-associated	45% (more common in adolescents)	70–80%
Demographic and clinical features		
Male predominance	Variable	Yes
Full nephrotic syndrome	40–75%	75%
Microscopic hematuria	70–90% (can be macroscopic)	50%
Hypertension	<10%	30%
Thromboembolic events	<5%	10–20%
Spontaneous remission	Common	30%
Progressive renal impairment	<25%	30–40%
Pathologic features		
Mesangial deposits	Up to 50%	30%
Segmental distribution of deposits	Occasional	Very rare

Used with permission of Springer Science + Business Media from Ayalon and Beck [9]
MN membranous nephropathy

neoplasms are rare causes of MN in children. Hepatitis B is an important factor in etiology of disease in the parts of world, where hepatitis B is endemic [16, 18–20]. The incidence of hepatitis B-related MN significantly decreased in the two decades after implementation of the universal HBV vaccination program in Taiwan, possibly as a result of the significant reduction in HBV carriers via horizontal transmission [21]. Similar observations were made in South Africa [22]. Other infections like schistosomiasis, filariasis, malaria and syphilis are also important conditions linked to development of MN in the prevalent area [23, 24]. Rarely secondary MN has also been seen following a hematopoietic cell transplant and as a de novo glomerulopathy following renal transplantation [25].

Pathophysiology

MN is characterized by an apparent thickening of glomerular capillary walls by light microscopy [26]. This thickening is actually mostly due to immune complex deposition or formation in the subepithelial space on the outer aspect of the glomerular basement membrane (GBM). These subepithelial immune deposits consist of several components, including IgG, antigens that have long eluded identification, and the membrane attack complex of complement which is assembled from complement components to form C5b-9. IgG4 is usually the most prominent IgG subclass deposited in idiopathic MN, although variable amounts of IgG1 are usually associated with immune deposits. By contrast, deposition of IgG1, IgG2 and IgG3 exceeds that of IgG4 in secondary MN [27–29]. The formation of subepithelial immune deposits and complement activation is responsible for the functional impairment of the glomerular capillary wall which causes proteinuria. Idiopathic MN is usually considered an autoimmune disease, whereas exogenous antigens such as viral and tumoral antigens are thought to be involved in secondary forms of the disease. In recent years, great progress has been achieved in the understanding of the molecular pathomechanisms of human MN with the identification of several antigens and predisposing gene variants in adult and childhood MN (Fig. 20.1a–c). These major breakthroughs have opened up a new era

Table 20.2 Secondary causes of membranous nephropathy

A. Autoimmune diseases
1. Systemic lupus erythematosus
2. Enteropathy/diabetes mellitus
3. Pemphigus
4. Ulcerative colitis
5. Ankylosing spondylitis
6. Dermatomyositis
7. Graves disease
8. Hashimoto disease
9. Mixed connective-tissue disease
10. Rheumatoid arthritis
11. Sjögren syndrome
12. Systemic sclerosis
B. Infectious diseases
1. Hepatitis B: this occurs in children in endemic areas
2. Hepatitis C
3. Quartan malaria
4. Leprosy
5. Hydatid cyst
6. Schistosomiasis
7. Congenital syphilis
8. Enterococcal endocarditis
9. Filariasis
C. Drugs and heavy metals
1. Penicillamine
2. Gold
3. Captopril
4. Non-steroidal anti-inflammatory agents
5. Recombinant enzyme used in enzyme replacement therapy
D. Neoplastic
1. Neuroblastoma
2. Ovarian tumours
3. Wilm's tumour
4. Gonadoblastoma
E. Other conditions
1. IgA deficiency
2. Kidney transplant (de novo)
3. Fanconi syndrome
4. Sickle cell disease
5. Stem cell transplant
6. Anti-tubular basement membrane
7. Anti-alveolar basement membrane antibodies
8. Anti-bovine serum albumin antibodies
9. Idiopathic thrombocytopenia
10. Juvenile cirrhosis
11. Familial truncating mutation in metallomembrane endopeptidase

for the diagnosis and monitoring of MN from early infancy to adulthood [30].

Brief Review of Heymann Nephritis, the First Experimental Model of MN

In 1959, Heymann, a pediatrician from Cleveland (Ohio, USA), and his collaborators described a rat model of MN, referred to as active Heymann nephritis, which was induced by the immunization of Lewis rats with crude kidney extracts and was reminiscent of the disease in humans [31]. Because the subepithelial deposits were induced by fractions of renal brush-border membrane rather than by glomerular extracts, the deposits were initially believed to result from glomerular trapping of circulating immune complexes composed of brush-border-related antigens and the corresponding antibodies. Subsequently, however, the development of passive Heymann nephritis in rats injected with rabbit anti-rat brush-border antibodies, argued against a role for circulating immune complexes. With the use of ex vivo and isolated perfused kidney systems, Van Damme et al. and Couser et al. [32, 33] demonstrated that anti-brush border antibodies bound to an antigenic target located on podocytes, which indicated that the disease was caused by the in situ formation of immune complexes.

The autoantigenic target in the rat disease was identified by Kerjaschki and Farquhar in the early 1980s [34, 35] as the podocyte membrane protein now called megalin. The polyspecific receptor megalin, a member of the low density lipoprotein-receptor superfamily, is expressed with clathrin at the sole of podocyte foot processes (where immune complexes are formed). The continued growth of immune deposits seems to require the de novo synthesis by the podocytes of new molecules of megalin, which are assumed to be delivered via vesicles that eventually fuse with the cell membrane at the base of the foot processes [36]. These findings provided the first evidence that podocytes actively contribute to the formation of glomerular immune deposits in MN.

Although considerable insight in the mechanisms of immune complex formation and their

a Endogenous antigen and maternal alloantibodies

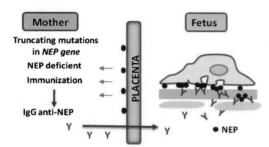

b Exogenous antigen and allo- or xenoantibodies

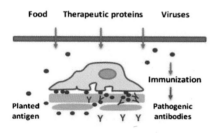

c Endogenous antigen and autoantibodies

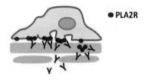

Fig. 20.1 Schematic representation of membranous nephropathy etiologies in children. (**a**) NEP-related alloimmune glomerulopathy. Neutral endopeptidase (*NEP*, *blue dots*) serves as a pathogenic antigen in the podocyte cell membrane. Antibodies to this protein originate in women who genetically lack NEP because of truncating mutations in the *MME* gene (gene for NEP). Immunization occurs during pregnancy when the mother's immune system is first exposed to NEP which is strongly expressed by placental cells and by fetal cells entering the mother's blood. From about the 18th week of gestation, maternal antibodies are actively transported across the placenta to the fetus, where they bind to the NEP antigen expressed on podocytes. (**b**) Exogenous antigen-induced membranous nephropathy. Foreign, exogenous proteins commonly induce the production of antibodies. Owing to unusual physicochemical properties, these antigens can be trapped in the glomerular basement membrane where they can serve as a target for circulating antibodies, leading to the formation of in situ immune complexes. *Green dots*, cationic bovine serumalbumin (*cBSA*) from the diet, infused enzymes used in enzyme replacement therapy (*ERT*), Hepatitis B antigens. (**c**) PLA2R-related autoimmune membranous nephropathy. The phospholipase A2 receptor (*red dots*), an integral membrane glycoprotein of podocytes, is a target antigen for circulating autoantibodies

nephritogenic potential has been provided by studies of Heymann nephritis, megalin cannot be taken responsible for human MN. As recently shown, megalin is weakly expressed in human podocytes [37]. However, megalin has neither been detected in subepithelial immune deposits, nor have circulating anti-megalin antibodies been found in patients with MN.

Allommune Neonatal MN: Neutral Endopeptidase as the Target Antigen

A human counterpart to passive Heymann nephritis was identified in a neonate with MN [38] (Fig. 20.1a). Because of the early occurrence of the disease during antenatal life, it was tempting to speculate that the mother became immunized during pregnancy and the nephritogenic antibodies were transferred to the fetus. Interspecies differences observed when human, rat and rabbit kidneys were incubated with sera from the mother and infant were suggestive of reactivity with NEP, which was confirmed by immunoprecipitation of rat brush-border extracts [38, 39]. Colocalization of NEP, IgG and C5-b9 within the human immune deposits and transfer experiments, in which a pregnant rabbit was injected with the IgG fraction from the mother, established that the disease was caused by anti-NEP antibodies [38, 40]. NEP is an enzyme responsible for the degradation of biologically active peptides such as enkephalin, natriuretic peptides, endothelin, bradykinin and substance P in the vicinity of their receptors. In the kidney, NEP is detected at the podocyte surface, in the brush border and in vessel walls. It is found in numerous organs but in very specific localizations, and in the granulocytes as well. NEP is identical to the common acute lymphoblastic leukaemia antigen (CALLA) and to CD10.

Because the mother did not show any renal manifestation even though she had persistently high titers of anti-NEP antibody, it was hypothesized that she might be deficient in NEP. This hypothesis was supported by the lack of reactivity of her granulocyte extracts with a panel of anti-NEP antibodies [38]. Four additional families with maternofetal alloimmune MN were identified. All immunized mothers were NEP deficient as a result of truncating mutations in exon 7 and exon 15 of the NEP gene [39, 41].

Alloimmunization can be triggered by previous spontaneous miscarriages or by the ongoing pregnancy during which the mother's immune system is first exposed to the NEP of paternal origin on syncytiotrophoblastic cells. The NEP-deficient individuals had normal blood pressure, renal functional tests, and lymphocyte phenotype and function [39], which is in contrast with the observations made in NEP null mice that show hypotension, greater sensitivity to septic shock, early onset Alzheimer's disease and prostatic tumours [42]. Because mutations in the NEP gene are asymptomatic, one can expect a high prevalence in selected populations such as those from which the cases originated.

After birth, all infants showed a rapid improvement of renal failure and the nephrotic syndrome owing to the short lifespan of maternal IgG. There were, however, two exceptions. The first one is a newborn who had persisting renal failure requiring dialysis despite exchange transfusions. Because the mother had high titers of anti-NEP IgG1 contrasting with very low titer of anti-NEP IgG4, we concluded that the IgG1 was responsible for the disease. This finding is in keeping with the capacity of IgG1 to activate complement whereas IgG4 usually fail to do so. The second exception, the oldest patient, is of particular clinical interest because of the late development of severe chronic renal failure with nephrotic range proteinuria leading to end-stage renal disease. Although a repeat kidney biopsy was not available, the delayed renal manifestations are likely to result from an aged MN combined with the postponed consequences of immunologically mediated antenatal nephron loss. Deposition of IgG produced by the infant to idiotypes or allotypes on the maternal IgG might also have contributed to further progression of the disease. These observations suggest that anti-NEP-induced antenatal renal disease might account for "idiopathic" MN or chronic renal failure detected during adolescence or early adulthood.

NEP-related alloimmune glomerulopathy defines a novel organ-specific disease caused by maternofetal incompatibility where a genetic defect in the mother leads to development of MN in her fetus. Although this disease appears to be rare, analysis of its pathogenic mechanisms provided the proof of concept that a podocyte antigen could be responsible for human MN, as is the case for megalin in the rat, and laid the foundation for the identification of M-type phospholipase A2 receptor (PLA2R) mostly involved in MN in the adult.

Role of Anti-PLA2R-Related MN in Childhood

In the context of the studies exploring neonatal alloimmune MN, another podocyte antigen, the type-M receptor of phospholipase A2 (PLA2R), was identified as a potential target antigen in about 70 % of adult patients with idiopathic MN [43] (Fig. 20.1c). Irrespective of the role of this antigen in the pathogenesis of MN, anti-PLA2R antibody appears to be a very good biomarker for this disease. Assays of circulating anti-PLA2R antibodies based on immunofluorescence (IFA) of PLA2R1 transfected cells and on ELISA are now commercially available in most countries. They have induced a paradigm shift in the diagnosis and monitoring of adult patients with MN. Specificity of anti-PLA2R for MN is close to 100 %. Patients with other causes of the nephrotic syndrome or healthy individuals have no detectable level of anti-PLA2R antibody. The specificity is such that in elderly patients, in those with poor clinical condition or with life-threatening complications of the nephrotic syndrome such as lung emboli, the kidney biopsy can be postponed or even omitted. Sensitivity of the test for idiopathic MN is about 70–80 % in all studied populations so far, except in Japan where the prevalence seems much lower [44]. However, a fraction of the antibody-negative patients might have a secondary cause undiagnosed at the time of kidney biopsy.

A low prevalence of anti-PLA2R antibodies was observed in secondary forms of MN associated with SLE, infectious disease, drug intoxication, graft-versus-host disease or malignancy taken as a whole [45–49] although in those cases, coincidental occurrence of the PLA2R-related MN and underlying disorder cannot be excluded. There may be exceptions: indeed, patients with MN associated with active sarcoidosis or replicating hepatitis B appear to have a high prevalence of PLA2R-related disease, which suggests that the immunologic setting of sarcoidosis and hepatitis B might trigger or enhance immunization against PLA2R [47, 50, 51]. Because therapeutic strategies are different for patients with idiopathic and secondary MN, discriminating between these two groups of patients is of utmost clinical importance.

Detection of PLA2R antigen in glomerular immune deposits is even more sensitive than that of anti-PLA2R antibodies since this antigen can be detected in antibody-negative patients [52], which could be explained by rapid clearance of circulating antibodies, immunological remission, or delayed biopsy after disease onset. This test enables the retrospective diagnosis of MN in archival, paraffin-embedded biopsy specimens, which is crucial for the monitoring of patients who will benefit from a kidney graft. Its positivity also is a strong clue to primary MN [50, 53]. Conversely, circulating antibodies are not always associated with deposits of PLA2R antigen, which suggests that not all antibodies to PLA2R are pathogenic [52]. Combined assessment of circulating anti-PLA2R antibodies and PLA2R antigen in biopsy specimens might help to better select the patients for appropriate therapy.

Several studies indicate that anti-PLA2R antibodies are correlated with proteinuria and disease activity since they usually disappear during a spontaneous or treatment-induced remission and reappear at relapse [45, 54–56] although there are outliers. Anti-PLA2R antibodies are also prognostic markers because high level is associated with a lower chance of spontaneous [54] or immunosuppressive therapy- induced [57] remission, with a lower rate of response to Rituximab [58] and with a higher risk of deterioration of renal function [59].

Although these data can probably be extrapolated to children, the prevalence of anti-PLA2R antibodies has not been studied systematically in cohorts of children with MN but preliminary observations suggest that it is lower than in adult patients and that these antibodies are not observed in children below 10 years. Based on differences in the prevalence of MN in adolescence versus childhood, the associations with primary PLA2R-asssociated MN are also likely to differ in these two age groups. PLA2R antigen staining was observed in kidney biopsies of 10 out of 41 adolescents with idiopathic MN [60]. Morphologic findings associated with negative PLA2R staining included segmental membranous lesions, mesangial and subendothelial deposits, C1q and "full-house" staining, although at >3 years average follow up, all patients were still considered as having primary MN. These findings suggest a more diverse and currently incompletely explained set of etiologies in pediatric MN.

Food Antigen-Related MN

In the wake of studies devoted to childhood MN, high levels of anti-bovine serum albumin (BSA) antibodies were detected in four of five children, all aged less than 5 years, and 7 of 41 adults with "idiopathic" MN analyzed consecutively [61]. These 11 patients also had elevated levels of circulating BSA; however, isoelectric focusing showed that affinity-purified BSA from the blood turned out to be cationic only in the four children, whereas in the adults, BSA had the same slightly anionic isoelectric point as native BSA. BSA was detected in subepithelial immune deposits only in children with both anti-BSA antibodies and high levels of circulating cationic BSA, and it colocalized with IgG, in the absence of PLA2R. Ig eluted from kidney biopsy samples of children with BSA deposits belonged to IgG1 and IgG4 subclasses and specifically reacted with BSA, but not with human serum albumin.

Cow's milk is the major source of BSA in young children. Although it is unknown why cationic BSA was formed, differences in food processing and intestinal microbiota might be responsible for modifications of BSA. Whatever the chemical modifications involved, MN related to cationic BSA seems to be the human counterpart of the rabbit experimental model established in the early 1980s where cationized, but not anionized, BSA induced MN [62, 63], (Fig. 20.1b). These clinical findings strongly support the scenario of "planted" antigen in the human disease.

Identification of a food antigen as a cause of childhood MN is a major breakthrough in the field of kidney diseases. Other food antigens might be involved, particularly during early childhood, because of increased permeability of the intestinal barrier at this age and frequent gastroenteritis episodes. The implication of non-dietary antigens from the environment should also be considered.

Enzyme Replacement Therapy as a Cause of Alloimmune MN

Alloimmune reactions can occur during enzyme replacement therapy (ERT) [64–66]. Because of the absence or very low levels of enzyme in many patients, therapeutic proteins are potential alloantigens that commonly trigger immunization. Alloantibodies may be without clinical significance or may lead to hypersensitivity reactions, decreased bioavailability, and efficacy of the therapeutic proteins. Only two cases have been reported so far but the prevalence of ERT-induced renal complications is probably underestimated.

A first case of nephrotic syndrome with mesangial and subepithelial Ig deposits was reported in a highly sensitized patient with Pompe disease treated with recombinant human alpha-glucosidase (rhGAA) [67]. The nephrotic syndrome developed while the patient was undergoing an experimental immune tolerance regimen based on escalating doses of rhGAA. Subepithelial immune deposits were associated with mesangium expansion, numerous mesangial deposits by IF and electron microscopy, and presence of rhGAA antigen in the mesangium. These findings recapitulate the immune complex glomerulonephritis observed in early chronic serum sickness induced by repeated injections of exogenous protein (Fig. 20.1b). The nephrotic syndrome resolved after ERT was decreased.

The second case was a patient with mucopolysaccharidosis type VI treated with recommended doses of human recombinant arylsulfatase B (rhASB) [68] (Fig. 20.1b). The clinical circumstances in this case, particularly the resolution of proteinuria when ERT was suspended, and the finding that IgG eluted from the biopsy specimen reacted specifically with rhASB strongly suggested that the alloimmune response to the recombinant enzyme was the cause of the disease.

The Case of Secondary MN

Hepatitis B, hepatitis C and Helicobacter pylori antigens, tumor antigens, thyroglobulin, and DNA containing material were detected in subepithelial deposits in patients with secondary MN [69–73]. These antigens may have been trapped in the glomerular basement membrane owing to unusual physicochemical properties as is the case for cationic albumin. Alternatively, small-sized circulating non-precipitating IgG4 complexes containing these antigens could become deposited in the glomerular basement membrane as in the chronic serum sickness model although there is no experimental evidence yet supporting this hypothesis in humans.

Genetic Factors

Irrespective of the target antigens involved in primary and secondary MN, genetic factors most likely play an important role. The influence of genetic factors is well established both in rodents [74, 75] and in European Caucasians, who show a strong association of MN with the HLA-B8DR3 haplotype and other HLA class II immune response genes [76–81]. Genome-wide association studies (GWAS) have described significant associations of the HLA-DQA1 and PLA2R1 loci with idiopathic MN in white adult patients [82]. Interestingly, carrying the risk alleles of the two genes had an additive effect. Patients with all four risk alleles had an odds ratio of 78 for the disease compared with individuals who had only the protective alleles. These genetic data were confirmed in ethnically distant populations from Europe [59, 83] and Asia [84–86]. The finding of common predisposing variants of PLA2R1 conserved across these populations and the observation that anti-PLA2R antibodies were detected in 73 % of the patients with the high-risk variants whereas they were absent in all carriers of protective genotypes [86], support the role of PLA2R1 as a major predisposing gene in adults. Robust genetic data are lacking in children where the prevalence of PLA2R-related MN is much lower although it increases with age. A strong association with HLA-DQA1 alleles has also been reported in two HLA identical brothers [87].

Because of the strong association of PLA2R1 SNPs with MN in adult Caucasians and the likelihood that PLA2R like its mannose receptor family undergoes conformational changes, it has been tempting to speculate that rare gene variants of the coding sequence could induce an unusual conformation of the antigen/epitopes, thus triggering autoimmunity. This hypothesis could not be verified by sequencing studies [88] which, however, do not exclude a role for non-coding variants or epigenetic events possibly increasing expression of PLA2R target antigen on podocyte membrane.

Other non-HLA alleles also predispose individuals towards the development or progression of MN such as the tumor necrosis factor (TNF) allele G308A, polymorphisms in genes encoding IL-6 and STAT4, nephrin (NPHS1) and the plasminogen activator inhibitor type-1 (PAI1) [44]. Overall, these data suggest that a combination of gene variants initiates disease and that modifier genes controlling glomerular permeability, inflammation and fibrosis might be involved in the pathogenesis of MN.

Clinical Features

The children exhibit the typical clinical signs and symptoms of idiopathic nephrotic syndrome and also may present with anasarca, microhematuria, and hypertension [5, 7], (Table 20.1). The onset of the edema in MN is typically more gradual than that seen in minimal change disease or primary focal glomerular sclerosis. Children are usually nonresponsive to a standard 4-week course of oral prednisone therapy [8]. On the other hand, asymptomatic, nephrotic range proteinuria has been reported in 16–38 % [6, 7]. Acute renal failure is unusual and should direct investigation towards other diagnoses or related conditions, such as bilateral renal vein thrombosis, excessive diuresis, or the use of nephrotoxic medications. Hence, the diagnosis of MN is most often made when children with steroid resistant nephrotic syndrome (SRNS) are biopsied. In children, MN differs in several important aspects from the adult phenotype: an apparent associated cause is more common, macroscopic hematuria occurs in up to 40 % of the patients [20, 89], a relapsing course is more often noted, renal venous thrombosis is rarely observed and evolution to renal failure is less frequent (Table 20.1).

The clinical manifestations of HBV associated nephropathy usually differ from primary MN. These children either present with nephrotic syndrome or they are detected by routine urine and serological testing. Microscopic hematuria even without proteinuria has been reported anecdotally. The mean age at presentation for HBV related MN is 5–7 years in cases of horizontal transmission, whereas children who acquire infection vertically present in infancy. The incidence of hypertension in HBV associated disease is less than 25 % [72].

Due to the decreasing prevalence of HBV-associated MN, SLE now takes the lead in pediatric MN. Among nine series of children and adolescents with any type of lupus nephritis, class V MN accounted for 9 % [90]. However, a retrospective study from the U.S. including 82 % of African Americans, showed a 30 % prevalence and all these cases were females [91]; this huge female predominance was also observed in China [92]. Very importantly, class V lupus nephritis can be the initial presentation of SLE in the absence of extra-renal manifestations and of serological manifestations of SLE such as hypocomplementemia or anti-double stranded DNA antibodies which will often appear later.

Maternofetal alloimmune glomerulopathy should be suspected if renal manifestations are present at birth, if they improve or disappear within the first weeks of life even though they can reappear later, and if they increase in severity with the reiteration of pregnancies.

A diagnosis of *BSA-related MN* should be considered in young children with MN, less than 5 years of age.

Laboratory Investigations

The initial diagnostic workup of MN will encompass the standard biochemical and hematological workup of idiopathic nephrotic syndrome. In case of suspected or histopathologically confirmed diagnosis of MN, serum should be screened for anti-PLA2R antibodies, complement levels, antinuclear and ds-DNA antibodies, hepatitis B early and surface antigen and hepatitis B surface antibodies.

Children with *HBV related MN* show positivity of hepatitis B surface antigen (HbsAg) and usually hepatitis B surface antibody is not detected. The hepatitis B early antigen (HbcAg) can be detected in serum of 90 % of patients. Hypocomplementemia (low C3 and C4) is observed at disease onset but titres of C3, C4 return to normal in later course of disease. Circulatory immune complexes are detected in 80 % of patients. Serum levels of transaminases may be raised on presentation [18, 72]. Liver biopsy shows evidence of chronic persistent hepatitis mainly in children but chronic active hepatitis is seen in adults.

In families with suspected *maternofetal alloimmune glomerulopathy,* circulating anti-NEP antibodies should be screened for in the mother and the child. Mother's urine and granulocytes can be evaluated by Western blot analysis for the absence of NEP. Anti-NEP antibodies fail to detect any reactivity in the mothers' samples whereas a specific band appears in the corresponding samples from their children who are heterozygous for the mutation. The last step should be the search for a gene mutation starting with exon 7 sequencing [41].

Histopathology

Light microscopy shows involvement of all glomeruli. The histological hallmark under light microscopy is diffuse global capillary wall thickening [44] (Fig. 20.2a). The size of the glomerulus appears normal or slightly increased with normal cell content. Overt mesangial hypercellularity is suggestive of secondary MN. The epithelial cells appear normal but rarely may be enlarged or prominent. Epithelial cell crescents are seen rarely in the clinical setting of rapidly progressive glomerulonephritis. The mesangial matrix is not increased and capillary loops are usually patent. The diffuse capillary wall thickening is best appreciated in the periodic acid methenamine silver stained sections in which subepithelial deposits are not stained and glomerular basement membrane (GBM) is stained black (Fig. 20.2b). The unstained deposits are surrounded by newly synthesized black staining GBM that appears as small spikes projecting from the GBM towards the urinary space (Fig. 20.2b). The light microscopic features may vary with the stage of disease. As the disease progresses, glomeruli become segmentally and globally sclerosed and develop adhesions to Bowman's capsule. Tubular atrophy, interstitial fibrosis, and mononuclear cell infiltration ensue and herald a poor functional prognosis.

The hallmark of *immunofluorescence microscopy* is uniform, granular capillary wall staining for IgG and C3 (Fig. 20.3a, b). However, some biopsy specimens show segmental deposits with distinct features of complement activation [93]. The most intense staining is seen for IgG, which is universal and of the IgG4 subclass. If mesangial deposits of IgG or a "full-house" fluorescence with staining for IgG, IgA, IgM, C3 and C1q are seen, then a secondary cause, e.g., SLE, should be suspected. C3 deposition is also found in more than 95 % cases but it is weaker in intensity. Staining for C1q and C4 has been described but intense staining for C1q should raise suspicion of SLE. C4d and C4bp have been identified in 92 % cases [94]. Membrane attack complex (C5b-9) is present in a location similar to IgG. Complement deposition correlates quantitatively with the rate

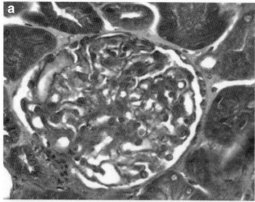

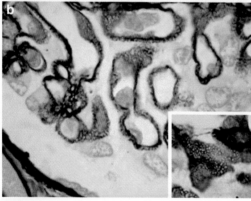

Fig. 20.2 Light microscopy (Massson's trichrome). Masson's trichrome staining of a glomerulus from a patient with idiopathic membranous nephropathy. Glomerular basement membranes are thickened by diffuse epimembranous deposits (**a**). Johns silver stain of a glomerulus from a patient with idiopathic membranous nephropathy shows "spikes" corresponding to newly synthesized basement membrane surrounding immune complexes. *Inset*: tangential section of the GBM (**b**) (Both: Courtesy of Professor Patrice Callard)

of progression of renal dysfunction [95]. CD20 positive cellular infiltrates have recently been demonstrated in human MN [96].

The characteristic *electron microscopy* finding in MN is the presence of subepithelial electron-dense, immune complex deposits. These correspond to the granular IgG deposits seen by immunofluorescence (Fig. 20.4). Epithelial foot process effacement and microvillous transformation occur in all stages of MN in association with heavy proteinuria. No electron dense deposits are observed in the subendothelial space or in the mesangium. The presence of mesangial and/or subendothelial complement or immunoglobulin

deposits or of endothelial tubuloreticular structures is suggestive of secondary MN, e.g., due to SLE.

Specific Diagnostic Approaches

In families with suspected *maternofetal alloimmune glomerulopathy*, a kidney biopsy should be performed to establish the diagnosis of MN in the absence of family history and serological evidence. Anti-NEP antibodies can be searched by indirect immunofluorescence on kidney sections from rat, rabbit, and human because of phylogenetic variations of NEP expression. The absence of NEP reactivity with rat podocytes contrasting with the strong reactivity with rabbit and human podocytes is very suggestive of anti-NEP antibodies [41].

In children with suspected *BSA-related MN*, BSA should be searched in immune deposits in cryostat kidney sections by immunofluorescence [61].

Disease Staging

Five morphological stages of MN are recognized [97]. The stages based on combination of light and electron microscopic features are as follows:

- Stage I. The light microscopy shows normal GBM in thickness and appearance. The electron dense deposits are small, flat but discrete. The smaller deposits are located at the site of slit diaphragm while moderate size deposits are located adjacent to the fused foot process.
- Stage II. Thickening of glomerular basement membrane is discernible by light microscopy. The electron dense deposits are increased in number and size. These deposits are flanked by prominent spikes in almost every capillary loop.
- Stage III. The basement membrane material (spikes) completely surrounds the deposits. These are larger and acquire intramembranous position. The capillary wall is irregular and has a moth eaten appearance. A few synechiae can be seen.
- Stage IV. The GBM is severely altered, irregularly thickened. The deposits are only a few in number or completely absent. The vacuolated appearance of GBM is discernible. The loss of

deposits is seen as electrolucent areas in the basement membrane.

- Stage V. The stage is characterized by return of GBM to normal. The only residual membrane disturbance is seen in the inner aspect of the basement membrane. The GBM appears very delicate and only partially thickened.

The most common lesion seen in children is stage II, followed by stage III and mixed stage [98, 99]. While a relationship between histological stage and clinical outcome has been shown in adults, there is paucity of data to determine correlation between the histological stages and clinical outcome in children [100].

Prognosis and Predictors

The course of idiopathic MN is variable. As a rule of thirds in adults with MN, approximately one third of patients undergoes spontaneous remission and maintains normal renal function with or without occasional relapses [15, 101]. Another third of patients display persistent proteinuria of variable degree, with normal or mildly impaired but stable GFR. The remaining patients develop progressive chronic kidney disease (CKD) eventually leading to end-stage renal disease (ESRD). In a review of natural history studies in untreated adults with *idiopathic MN*, 50 % of these patients either died or developed end stage renal disease within 10 years of disease onset [15].

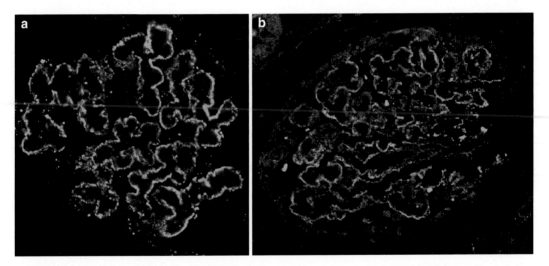

Fig. 20.3 Immunofluorescence. Glomerulus with diffuse, finely granular deposition of IgG (**a**) and C3 (**b**) along the outer surface of all capillary walls

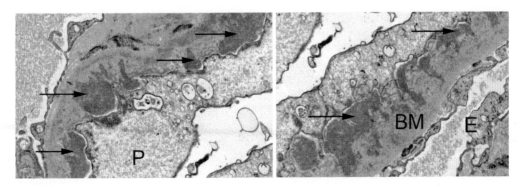

Fig. 20.4 Electron microscopy. Electron-dense deposits (*arrows*) are seen in the sub-epithelial space between the glomerular basement membrane (*BM*) and the podocyte (*P*); *E* endothelial cell (Courtesy of Professor Patrice Callard)

Children seem to have a relatively better over-all outcome than adults [2, 102], with some of the more recent series reporting overall remission rates of 75 % [20, 103] (Table 20.1); however, most studies still show decreased kidney function in about 20 % of patients at final follow-up [7, 20]. It should be emphasized that the existing information about natural history and treatment outcomes of idiopathic MN in children is not only uncontrolled but also there is considerable variability regarding the therapeutic protocols used and the definition of remission. Individually based decisions are therefore of paramount importance to minimize the risk of progression to renal failure.

Unfortunately, predictors of outcome are still poorly defined in children. The prevailing degree of proteinuria seems to be a valuable predictor of outcome, which is excellent in children with asymptomatic non-nephrotic proteinuria whereas approximately 25 % of those with nephrotic syndrome will develop renal failure within 1–17 years. Of note in Makker's series, all patients who developed CKD presented with nephrotic syndrome [104]. Hypertension and interstitial fibrosis on biopsy might be further predictors of adverse outcome [7, 103].

In the adult, there is no difference in response to treatment between anti-PLA2R positive and anti-PLA2R negative patients although the response rate to rituximab appears to be lower in patients with a high titer of antibodies [58]. Persistence of onti-PLA2R antibodies at the end of the immunosuppressive treatment predicts relapse [105]. Further studies are required to confirm the anti-PLA2R antibody predictive value in children.

The natural history of *HBV associated MN* is incompletely understood. Approximately 30–60 % of patients may experience spontaneous regression of nephrotic syndrome. The duration of nephrotic syndrome tends to be 12 months or longer in these patients.

Treatment

The first and foremost step is to investigate for any secondary causes like Hepatitis B, Hepatitis C and SLE. Successful treatment of the underly-ing is usually curative in secondary forms. In the absence of any large series and controlled trials, guidelines for treatment of idiopathic MN are largely extrapolated from studies in adult patients. The latest treatment recommendations have recently been detailed in the KDIGO Glomerulonephritis Guidelines which contain a section on the treatment of pediatric disease [106]. The consensus of this committee and of many pediatric nephrologists is that treatment of idiopathic MN in children should follow the recommendations for treatment of idiopathic MN in adults.

Patients with histologically confirmed MN and *asymptomatic non-nephrotic proteinuria* should be monitored on conservative therapy since they may undergo spontaneous remission. During this period supportive management should be instituted. Such measures include a low-salt diet, RAS antagonists and diuretics to reduce edema. Hypertension should be treated consequently, preferentially with RAS antagonists taking advantage of their dual antihypertensive and antiproteinuric action. These patients will not be treated with immunosuppressive therapy unless proteinuria increases despite maximum conservative therapy or renal function deteriorates.

The management of *children with nephrotic syndrome* is often empiric and mirrors the treatment of adult patients with idiopathic MN, with the difference that children have often received 4–8 weeks of oral corticosteroids before the biopsy was performed (as they were initially considered to have minimal change disease). The role of immunosuppressive therapy in children is controversial [104]. According to the KDIGO Glomerulonephritis Guidelines [106], immunosuppressive therapy is recommended when at least one of the following conditions is met:

- Persistent nephrotic syndrome without progressive decline of urinary protein excretion despite anti-proteinuric therapy during an observation period of at least 6 months;
- Progressive decline in renal function: increase of serum creatinine level by 30 % or more within 6–12 months from the time of diagnosis,

provided that eGFR is not less than 25–30 ml/min/1.73 m^2 and this change is not explained by superimposed complications;

• Presence of severe, disabling, or life-threatening (thromboembolism) symptoms related to nephrotic syndrome.

It is recommended to avoid immunosuppressive therapy in patients with a serum creatinine level persistently >3.5 mg/dl or an eGFR <30 ml/min/1.73 m^2, with reduction of kidney size on ultrasound, and with diffuse glomerular sclerosis and interstitial fibrosis at kidney biopsy.

The initial recommended therapy consists of a *6-month course of alternating monthly cycles of oral and i.v. corticosteroids and oral alkylating agents,* that is the Ponticelli's protocol [107], with cyclophosphamide being preferred to chlorambucil to reduce side effects notably azoospermia. Even with cyclophosphamide, there is always the added concern of inducing infertility. One option that provides a relatively low exposure to cyclophosphamide (total dose of <200 mg/kg) involves a 12-week regimen using daily cyclophosphamide (2 mg/kg/day) with alternate-day steroids, as used successfully in a small uncontrolled study [6]. We have successfully used monthly intravenous cyclophosphamide infusions (500 mg/m^2) (along with alternate monthly prednisone), which results in a 40 % lower cumulative dose. Peripheral blood counts should be monitored and the cytotoxic agents withheld at a total leukocyte count <3,000/mm^3 or in the presence of an active infection. It is recommended that patients be managed for at least 6 months following the completion of the immunosuppressive regimen before considering a treatment failure if there is no remission, unless kidney function is deteriorating or severe, disabling, or potentially life-threatening complications related to the nephrotic syndrome are present.

Calcineurin inhibitors (cyclosporine or tacrolimus) may also be effective but, based on experience in adults, they require at least 6–12 months of therapy with a slow taper to avoid relapse. It is suggested that cyclosporine or tacrolimus be used as second-line therapy in children resistant to alkylating agent/steroid-based initial therapy. [106]. Cyclosporine is usually administered at a dose of 3.5 mg/kg/day for 1 year in combination with oral prednisone (2 mg/kg/day) which is gradually tapered off over 3–6 months. It is suggested that calcineurin inhibitors be discontinued in patients who do not achieve complete or partial remission after 6 months of treatment and that blood levels be monitored regularly during the initial treatment period, and whenever there is an unexplained rise in serum creatinine level (>20 %) during therapy [106].

Other agents, such *as the B-cell depleting agent rituximab, mycophenolate and adrenocorticotrophic hormone (ACTH),* have been used in small and/or non-randomized studies in adults, but no evidence exists as to their use or appropriateness in children. Of note, rituximab is associated with high remission rates and only mild adverse effects have been reported in adults [108–110]. Until the eagerly awaited results of two upcoming randomized controlled trials, rituximab is usually prescribed as a second-line or third-line treatment only.

In patients with PLA2R-related MN, quantification of anti-PLA2R antibodies will most likely become an invaluable tool for the monitoring of disease immunological activity and the titration of immunosuppressive treatments. Antibodies disappear before proteinuria in patients treated with rituximab [55, 58], which leads to consider withdrawal of immunosuppressive treatment at the time of immunological remission before renal remission is achieved. The time-lag between immunological and renal remission most likely corresponds to the time required for restoration of the glomerular capillary wall. Anti-PLA2R antibody levels at the end of therapy may also predict the subsequent course. In a small series of 48 patients treated with immunosuppressive agents, 58 % of antibody-negative patients were in persistent remission after 5 years compared with none of antibody-positive patients [105]. However, further prospective studies on large cohorts of patients are needed before drawing definitive conclusions and extrapolating them to children. They will also enable to establish the meaning and therapeutic implication of the persistence of

PLA2R antigen in immune deposits in repeat biopsies.

Secondary Membranous Nephropathy

A meta-analysis demonstrated a beneficial effect of *interferon-α* (IFN) therapy in adult patients with *hepatitis B associated MN* who were treated for 3–6 months. In the only prospective trial in children, all 20 patients treated with IFN achieved remission, while 50% of patients in the control group had persistent nephrotic syndrome and 50% had mild proteinuria [111, 112]. In the group on IFN, 18 patients had HbsAg and HbeAg seroconversion to negative status and 4 patients had HbeAg seroconversion only. There was no seroconversion in patients on conservative treatment. *Lamivudine* has a role in patients with persistent proteinuria. A recent study compared the renal outcome of adults with MN related to chronic HBV infection with lamivudine vs. conservative treatment [113]. The ten patients on Lamivudine had a 100% 3-year survival, as compared to 58% in the 12 patients on conservative treatment. Anecdotal reports have shown reversal of MN by Lamivudine also in children with Hepatitis B associated MN [114]. National vaccination programs for HBV in Taiwan, China and South Africa have induced a major decline of the incidence of HBV-associated MN [21, 115, 116].

MN is the histopathological phenotype in 10–20% of children with *lupus nephritis*. Children with MN secondary to lupus nephritis are usually treated with Ponticelli's protocol [103, 104]. In case of superimposed features of Class IV nephritis they are treated with intravenous cyclophosphamide and oral prednisone.

In *MN induced by anti-NEP alloimmunization*, spontaneous outcome is usually favorable owing to the short half-life of maternal antibodies. In more severe forms with AKI, exchange transfusion is advocated. Neonates born after a second pregnancy are at major risk because of dramatically increased levels of anti-NEP antibodies on re-exposure of the mother to placental NEP antigen. Monitoring of pregnancies in NEP deficient mothers relies on ELISA of anti-NEP antibodies with determination of IgG1 and IgG4 subclasses. Immunosuppressive treatments should be adapted to evolution and subclass of antibodies [117].

In *BSA-induced MN*, eliminating this protein from the diet could be beneficial. Circulating anti-BSA antibodies and BSA antigen should be monitored during follow-up because they were shown to correlate with disease activity [61].

Conclusion

Membranous nephropathy is an uncommon cause of nephrotic syndrome in children. The diagnosis is usually established when the children are biopsied after being labeled as steroid resistant. It is imperative to rule out secondary disease entities as these may respond to treatment of the underlying condition. The initial management of idiopathic MN should be conservative. Immunosuppressive therapy should be considered for those children who develop nephrotic-range proteinuria and/or progressive renal dysfunction.

References

1. Eddy AA, Symons JM. Nephrotic syndrome in childhood. Lancet. 2003;362(9384):629–39.
2. Cameron JS. Membranous nephropathy in childhood and its treatment. Pediatr Nephrol. 1990;4(2): 193–8.
3. North American Pediatric Renal Trials and Collaborative Studies (NAPRTCS). Annual report 2007. Available at www.naprtcs.org. Accessed 12 Jul 2008.
4. International Study of Kidney Disease in Children. Nephrotic syndrome: prediction of histopathology from clinical and laboratory characteristics at time of diagnosis. Kidney Int. 1978;13:159–65.
5. Kumar J, Gulati S, Sharma AP, Sharma RK, Gupta RK. Histopathological spectrum of childhood nephrotic syndrome in Indian children. Pediatr Nephrol. 2003;18(7):657–60.
6. Valentini RP, Mattoo TK, Kapur G, Imam A. Membranous glomerulonephritis: treatment response and outcome in children. Pediatr Nephrol. 2009;24(2):301–8.
7. Chen A, Frank R, Vento S, et al. Idiopathic membranous nephropathy in pediatric patients: presentation, response to therapy, and long-term outcome. BMC Nephrol. 2007;6:8–11.

8. Gulati S, Sengupta A, Sharma RK, Gupta RK, Sharma AP, Gupta A. Steroid resistant nephrotic syndrome. Indian Pediatr. 2006;43(4):373–4.

9. Ayalon R, Beck Jr LH. Membranous nephropathy: not just a disease for adults. Pediatr Nephrol. 2015;30(1):31–9.

10. Mubarak M, Kazi JI, Lanewala A, Hashmi S, Akhter F. Pathology of idiopathic nephrotic syndrome in children: are the adolescents different from young children? Nephrol Dial Transplant. 2012;27(2):722–6.

11. Hogg RJ, Silva FG, Berry PL, Wenz JE. Glomerular lesions in adolescents with gross hematuria or the nephrotic syndrome. Report of the Southwest Pediatric Nephrology Study Group. Pediatr Nephrol. 1993;7(1):27–31.

12. Moxey-Mims MM, Stapleton FB, Feld LG. Applying decision analysis to management of adolescent idiopathic nephrotic syndrome. Pediatr Nephrol. 1994;8(6):660–4.

13. US Renal Data System (2012) U.S. Renal Data System, USRDS 2012 annual data report: atlas of end-stage renal disease in the United States. National Institutes of Health, National Institute for Diabetes and Digestive and Kidney Diseases, Bethesda. Available at http://www.usrds.org/archive.aspx.

14. Simon P, Ramée MP, Autuly V, Laruelle E, Charasse C, Cam G, Ang KS. Epidemiology of primary glomerular diseases in a French region. Variations according to period and age. Kidney Int. 1994;46:1192–8.

15. Glassock RJ. Diagnosis and natural course of membranous nephropathy. Semin Nephrol. 2003;23:324–32.

16. Bhimma R, Coovadia HM, Adhikari M. Nephrotic syndrome in South African children: changing perspectives over 20 years. Pediatr Nephrol. 1997;11(4):429–34.

17. Glassock RJ. Secondary membranous glomerulonephritis. Nephrol Dial Transplant. 1992;7 Suppl 1:64–71.

18. Lin CY. Hepatitis B, virus associated membranous nephropathy: clinical features, immunological profiles and outcome. Nephron. 1990;55:37–44.

19. Hu HC, Wu CY, Lin CY, et al. Membranous nephropathy in 52 hepatitis B surface antigen (HBsAg) carrier children in Taiwan. Kidney Int. 1989;36:1103–7.

20. Lee BH, Cho HY, Kang HG, Ha IS, Cheong HI, Moon KC, Lim IS, Choy Y. Idiopathic membranous nephropathy in children. Pediatr Nephrol. 2006;21:1707–15.

21. Liao MT, Chang MH, Lin FG, Tsai IJ, Chang YW, Tsau YK. Universal hepatitis B vaccination reduces childhood hepatitis B virus-associated membranous nephropathy. Pediatrics. 2011;128(3):e600–6044.

22. Burnett RJ, Kramvis A, Dochez C, Meheus A. An update after 16 years of hepatitis B vaccination in South Africa. Vaccine. 2012;30 Suppl 3:C45–51.

23. Hendrickise RG, Adeniyi A. Quartan malarial nephrotic syndrome in children. Kidney Int. 1979;16:67–74.

24. Ngu JL, Chatelanet F, Leke R, et al. Nephropathy in Cameroon: evidence for filarial derived immune complex pathogenesis in some cases. Clin Nephrol. 1985;24:128–34.

25. Ponticelli C, Moroni G, Glassock RJ. De Novo glomerular diseases after renal transplantation. Clin J Am Soc Nephrol. 2014;9:1479–87.

26. Jones DB. Nephrotic glomerulonephritis. Am J Pathol. 1957;33:313–29.

27. Imai H, Hamai K, Komatsuda A, Ohtani H, Miura AB. IgG subclasses in patients with membranoproliferative glomerulonephritis, membranous nephropathy, and lupus nephritis. Kidney Int. 1997;51:270–6.

28. Kuroki A, Shibata T, Honda H, Totsuka D, Kobayashi K, Sugisaki T. Glomerular and serum IgG subclasses in diffuse proliferative lupus nephritis, membranous lupus nephritis, and idiopathic membranous nephropathy. Intern Med. 2002;41:936–42.

29. Ohtani H, Wakui H, Komatsuda A, et al. Distribution of glomerular IgG subclass deposits in malignancy-associated membranous nephropathy. Nephrol Dial Transplant. 2004;19:574–9.

30. Debiec H, Ronco P. Immunopathogenesis of membranous nephropathy: an update. Semin Immunopathol. 2014;36(4):381–97.

31. Heymann W, Hackel DB, Harwood S, Wilson SGF, Hunter JL. Production of nephrotic syndrome in rats by Freund's adjuvants and rat kidney suspension. Proc Soc Exp Biol Med. 1959;100:660–4.

32. Van Damme BJ, Fleuren GJ, Bakker WW, Vernier RL, Hoedemaeker PJ. Experimental glomerulonephritis in the rat induced by antibodies directed against tubular antigens. V. Fixed glomerular antigens in the pathogenesis of heterologous immune complex glomerulonephritis. Lab Invest. 1978;38:502–10.

33. Couser WG, Steinmuller DR, Stilmant MM, Salant DJ, Lowenstein LM. Experimental glomerulonephritis in the isolated perfused rat kidney. J Clin Invest. 1978;62:1275–87.

34. Kerjaschki D, Farquhar MG. The pathogenic antigen of Heymann nephritis is a membrane glycoprotein of the renal proximal tubule brush border. Proc Natl Acad Sci. 1982;79:5557–61.

35. Kerjaschki D, Farquhar MG. Immunocytochemical localization of the Heymann nephritis antigen (gp330) in glomerular epithelial cells of normal Lewis rats. J Exp Med. 1983;157:667–86.

36. Allegri L, Brianti E, Chatelet F, Manara GC, Ronco P, Verroust P. Polyvalent antigen-antibody interactions are required for the formation of electron-dense immune deposits in passive Heymann's nephritis. Am J Pathol. 1986;125:1–6.

37. Prabakaran T, Nielsen R, Larsen JV, et al. Receptor-mediated endocytosis of α-galactosidase A in human podocytes in Fabry disease. PLoS One. 2011;6:e25065.

38. Debiec H, Guigonis V, Mougenot B, et al. Antenatal membranous glomerulonephritis due to anti-neutral

endopeptidase antibodies. N Engl J Med. 2002;346:2053–60.

39. Debiec H, Nauta J, Coulet F, et al. Role of truncating mutations in MME gene in feto-maternal alloimmunization and neonatal glomerulopathies. Lancet. 2004;364:1252–9.

40. Ronco P, Debiec H. Molecular pathomechanisms of membranous nephropathy: from Heymann nephritis to alloimmunization. J Am Soc Nephrol. 2005;16: 1205–13.

41. Vivarelli M, Emma F, Pelle T, et al. Genetic homogeneity but IgG subclass-dependent clinical variability of alloimmune membranous nephropathy with anti-neutral endopeptidase antibodies. Kidney Int. 2015;87(3):602–9. doi: 10.1038/ki.2015.381. Epub 2015 Jan 7.

42. Lu B, Figini M, Emanueli C, et al. The control of microvascular permeability and blood pressure by neutral endopeptidase. Nat Med. 1997;3:904–7.

43. Beck Jr LH, Bonegio RG, Lambeau G, et al. M-type phospholipase A2 receptor as target antigen in idiopathic MN. N Engl J Med. 2009;361:11–21.

44. Ronco P, Debiec H. Pathogenesis of membranous nephropathy: recent advances and future challenges. Nat Rev Nephrol. 2012;8:203–13.

45. Qin W, Beck Jr LH, Zeng C, et al. Anti-phospholipase A2 receptor antibody in membranous nephropathy. J Am Soc Nephrol. 2011;22:1137–43.

46. Hoxha E, Harendza S, Zahner G, et al. An immuno-fluorescence test for phospholipase-A_2-receptor antibodies and its clinical usefulness in patients with membranous glomerulonephritis. Nephrol Dial Transplant. 2011;26:2526–32.

47. Knehtl M, Debiec H, Kamgang P, et al. A case of phospholipase A_2 receptor-positive membranous nephropathy preceding sarcoid-associated granulomatous tubulointerstitial nephritis. Am J Kidney Dis. 2011;57:140–3.

48. Nawaz FA, Larsen CP, Troxell ML. Membranous nephropathy and nonsteroidal anti-inflammatory agents. Am J Kidney Dis. 2013;62:1012–7.

49. Huang X, Qin W, Zhang M, Zheng C, Zeng C, Liu Z. Detection of anti-PLA2R autoantibodies and IgG subclasses in post-allogeneic hematopoietic stem cell transplantation membranous nephropathy. Am J Med Sci. 2013;346:32–7.

50. Larsen CP, Messias NC, Silva FG, Messias E, Walker PD. Determination of primary versus secondary membranous glomerulopathy utilizing phospholipase A2 receptor staining in renal biopsies. Mod Pathol. 2013;26:709–15.

51. Svobodova B, Honsova E, Ronco P, Tesar V, Debiec H. Kidney biopsy is a sensitive tool for retrospective diagnosis of PLA2R-related membranous nephropathy. Nephrol Dial Transplant. 2013;28:1839–44.

52. Debiec H, Ronco P. PLA2R autoantibodies and PLA2R glomerular deposits in membranous nephropathy. N Engl J Med. 2011;364:689–90.

53. Hoxha E, Kneißler U, Stege G, Zahner G, Thiele I, Panzer U, Harendza S, Helmchen UM, Stahl RA. Enhanced expression of the M-type phospholipase A2 receptor in glomeruli correlates with serum receptor antibodies in primary membranous nephropathy. Kidney Int. 2012;82:797–804.

54. Hofstra JM, Debiec H, Short CD, Pellé T, Kleta R, Mathieson PW, Ronco P, Brenchley PE, Wetzels JF. Antiphospholipase A2 receptor antibody titer and subclass in idiopathic membranous nephropathy. J Am Soc Nephrol. 2012;23:1735–43.

55. Beck Jr LH, Fervenza FC, Beck DM, Bonegio RG, Malik FA, Erickson SB, Cosio FG, Cattran DC, Salant DJ. Rituximab-induced depletion of anti-PLA2R autoantibodies predicts response in membranous nephropathy. J Am Soc Nephrol. 2011;22: 1543–50.

56. Oh YJ, Yang SH, Kim DK, Kang SW, Kim YS. Autoantibodies against phospholipase A2 receptor in Korean patients with membranous nephropathy. PLoS One. 2013;8:e62151.

57. Hoxha E, Thiele I, Zahner G, Panzer U, Harendza S, Stahl RA. Phospholipase A2 receptor autoantibodies and clinical outcome in patients with primary membranous nephropathy. J Am Soc Nephrol. 2014;25(6):1357–66.

58. Ruggenenti P, Debiec H, Ruggiero B, et al. Anti-phospholipase A2 receptor antibody titer predicts post-rituximab outcome of membranous nephropathy. J Am Soc Nephrol. 2015;26(10):2545–58. doi: 10.1681/ASN.201407060. Epub 2015.

59. Kanigicherla D, Gummadova J, McKenzie EA, et al. Anti-PLA2R antibodies measured by ELISA predict long-term outcome in a prevalent population of patients with idiopathic membranous nephropathy. Kidney Int. 2013;83:940–8.

60. Cossey LN, Walker PD, Larsen CP. Phospholipase A2 receptor staining in pediatric idiopathic membranous glomerulopathy. Pediatr Nephrol. 2013;28: 2307–11.

61. Debiec H, Lefeu F, Kemper MJ, et al. Early childhood membranous nephropathy due to cationic bovine serum albumin. N Engl J Med. 2011;364: 2101–10.

62. Border WA, Ward HJ, Kamil ES, Cohen AH. Induction of membranous nephropathy in rabbits by administration of an exogenous cationic antigen. J Clin Invest. 1982;69:451–61.

63. Adler SG, Wang H, Ward HJ, Cohen AH, Border WA. Electrical charge. Its role in the pathogenesis and prevention of experimental membranous nephropathy in the rabbit. J Clin Invest. 1983;71:487–99.

64. Richards SM. Immunologic considerations for enzyme replacement therapy in the treatment of lysosomal storage disorders. Clin Appl Immunol Rev. 2002;2:241–53.

65. Brooks DA. Immune response to enzyme replacement therapy in lysosomal storage disorder patients and animal models. Mol Genet Metab. 1999;68:268–75.

66. Koren E, Zuckerman LA, Mire-Sluis AR. Immune responses to therapeutic proteins in humans – clini-

cal significance, assessment and prediction. Curr Pharm Biotechnol. 2002;3:349–60.

67. Hunley TE, Corzo D, Dudek M, Kishnani P, Amalfitano A, Chen YT, Richards SM, Phillips 3rd JA, Fogo AB, Tiller GE. Nephrotic syndrome complicating alpha-glucosidase replacement therapy for Pompe disease. Pediatrics. 2004;114:e532–5.

68. Debiec H, Valayannopoulos V, Boyer O, Nöel LH, Callard P, Sarda H, de Lonlay P, Niaudet P, Ronco P. Allo-immune membranous nephropathy and recombinant aryl sulfatase replacement therapy: a need for tolerance induction therapy. J Am Soc Nephrol. 2014;25(4):675–80.

69. Jordan SC, Buckingham B, Sakai R, Olson D. Studies of immune-complex glomerulonephritis mediated by human thyroglobulin. N Engl J Med. 1981;304:1212–5.

70. Takekoshi Y, Tanaka M, Miyakawa Y, Yoshizawa H, Takahashi K, Mayumi M. Free "small" and IgG-associated "large" hepatitis B e antigen in the serum and glomerular capillary walls of two patients with membranous glomerulonephritis. N Engl J Med. 1979;300:814–9.

71. Hörl WH, Kerjaschki D. Membranous glomerulonephritis (MGN). J Nephrol. 2000;13:291–316.

72. Bhimma R, Coovadia HM. Hepatitis B virus-associated nephropathy. Am J Nephrol. 2004;24:198–211.

73. Nakahara K, Takahashi H, Okuse C, Shigefuku R, Yamada N, Murao M, Matsunaga K, Koike J, Yotsuyanagi H, Suzuki M, Kimura K, Itoh F. Membranous nephropathy associated with chronic hepatitis B occurring in a short period after acute hepatitis B virus infection. Intern Med. 2010;49:383–8.

74. Bagchus WM, Hoedemaeker PJ, Vos JT, Bakker WW. Thymocytes reacting with heterologous antibodies against GP 330 in autologous immune complex glomerulopathy (AICG) in the rat. The relation between susceptibility for AICG and anti-GP 330-binding thymocytes. Immunobiology. 1989;179:432–44.

75. Chen JS, Chen A, Chang LC, et al. Mouse model of membranous nephropathy induced by cationic bovine serum albumin: antigen dose-response relations and strain differences. Nephrol Dial Transplant. 2004;19:2721–8.

76. Vaughan RW, Demaine AG, Welsh KI. A DQA1 allele is strongly associated with idiopathic membranous nephropathy. Tissue Antigens. 1989;34:261–9.

77. Chevrier D, Giral M, Perrichot R, et al. Idiopathic and secondary membranous nephropathy and polymorphism at TAP1 and HLA-DMA loci. Tissue Antigens. 1997;50:164–9.

78. Le Petit JC, Laurent B, Berthoux FC. HLA-DR3 and idiopathic membranous nephritis (IMN) association. Tissue Antigens. 1982;20:227–8.

79. Dyer PA, Short CD, Clarke EA, Mallick NP. HLA antigen and gene polymorphisms and haplotypes established by family studies in membranous nephropathy. Nephrol Dial Transplant. 1992;1(7 Suppl):42–7.

80. Berthoux FC, Laurent B, le Petit JC, et al. Immunogenetics and immunopathology of human primary membranous glomerulonephritis: HLA-A, B, DR antigens; functional activity of splenic macrophage Fc-receptors and peripheral blood T-lymphocyte subpopulations. Clin Nephrol. 1984;22:15–20.

81. Sacks SH, Warner C, Campbell RD, Dunham I. Molecular mapping of the HLA class II region in HLA-DR3 associated idiopathic membranous nephropathy. Kidney Int Suppl. 1993;39:S13–9.

82. Stanescu HC, Arcos-Burgos M, Medlar A, et al. Risk HLA-DQA1 and PLA(2)R1 alleles in idiopathic membranous nephropathy. N Engl J Med. 2011;364:616–26.

83. Bullich G, Ballarín J, Oliver A, Ayasreh N, Silva I, Santín S, Díaz-Encarnación MM, Torra R, Ars E. HLA-DQA1 and PLA2R1 polymorphisms and risk of idiopathic membranous nephropathy. Clin J Am Soc Nephrol. 2014;9:335–43.

84. Liu YH, Chen CH, Chen SY, et al. Association of phospholipase A2 receptor 1 polymorphisms with idiopathic membranous nephropathy in Chinese patients in Taiwan. J Biomed Sci. 2010;17:81–8.

85. Kim S, Chin HJ, Na KY, et al. Single nucleotide polymorphisms in the phospholipase A2 receptor gene are associated with genetic susceptibility to idiopathic membranous nephropathy. Nephron Clin Pract. 2011;117:c253–8.

86. Lv J, Hou W, Zhou X, et al. Interaction between PLA2R1 and HLA-DQA1 variants associates with anti-PLA2R antibodies and membranous nephropathy. J Am Soc Nephrol. 2013;24:1323–9.

87. Vangelista A, Tazzari R, Bonomini V. Idiopathic membranous nephropathy in 2twin brothers. Nephron. 1988;50:79–80.

88. Coenen MJ, Hofstra JM, Debiec H, et al. Phospholipase A2 receptor (PLA2R1) sequence variants in idiopathic membranous nephropathy. J Am Soc Nephrol. 2013;24:677–83.

89. Tsukahara H, Takahashi Y, Yoshimoto M, Hayashi S, Fujisawa S, Suehiro F, Akaishi K, Nomura Y, Morikawa K, Sudo M. Clinical course and outcome of idiopathic membranous nephropathy in Japanese children. Pediatr Nephrol. 1993;7(4):387–91.

90. Cameron JS. Lupus and lupus nephritis in children. Adv Nephrol Necker Hosp. 1993;22:59–119.

91. Lau KK, Jones DP, Hastings MC, Gaber LW, Ault BH. Short- term outcomes of severe lupus nephritis in a cohort of predominantly African-American children. Pediatr Nephrol. 2006;21:655–62.

92. Wong SN, Chan WK, Hui J, Chim S, Lee TL, Lee KP, Leung LC, Tse NK, Yuen SF. Membranous lupus nephritis in Chinese children–a case series and review of the literature. Pediatr Nephrol. 2009;24:1989–96.

93. Segawa Y, Hisano S, Matsushita M, et al. IgG subclasses and complement pathway in segmental and

global membranous nephropathy. Pediatr Nephrol. 2010;25:1091–9.

94. Kusonoki Y, Itami N, Tochimarn H, Takekoshi Y, Nagasawa S, Yoshiki T. Glomerular deposition of C4 cleavage fragment (C4d) and C4 binding protein in idiopathic membranous glomerulonephritis. Nephron. 1989;51:17–9.

95. Troyanov S, Roasio L, Pandes M, Herzenberg AM, Cattran DC. Renal pathology in idiopathic membranous nephropathy: a new perspective. Kidney Int. 2006;69(9):1641–8.

96. Cohen CD, Calvaresi N, Armelloni S, Armelloni S, Schindt H, Herger A, et al. CD20 + ve infiltrates in human membranous glomerulonephritis. J Nephrol. 2005;18(3):328–33.

97. Ehrenreich T, Churg J. Pathology of membranous nephropathy. In: Scommers SC, editor. Pathology annual. New York: Appleton-Century-Crofts; 1968. p. 145–86.

98. Habib R, Kleinknecht C, Gubler MC. Extramembranous glomerulonephritis in children: report of 50 cases. J Pediatr. 1973;82:754–66.

99. Latham P, Poucell S, Koresaar A, et al. Idiopathic membranous glomerulopathy in Canadian children: a clinicopathologic study. J Pediatr. 1982;101:682–5.

100. Southwest Pediatric Nephrology Study Group. Comparison of idiopathic and systemic lupus erythematosus associated membranous glomerulonephritis in children. Am J Kidney Dis. 1986;7:115–24.

101. Polanco N, Gutiérrez E, Covarsí A, Ariza F, Carreño A, Vigil A, Baltar J, Fernández-Fresnedo G, Martín C, Pons S, Lorenzo D, Bernis C, Arrizabalaga P, Fernández-Juárez G, Barrio V, Sierra M, Castellanos I, Espinosa M, Rivera F, Oliet A, Fernández-Vega F, Praga M. Spontaneous remission of nephrotic syndrome in idiopathic membranous nephropathy. J Am Soc Nephrol. 2010;21:697–704.

102. Kleinknecht C, Levy M, Gagnadoux MF, Habib R. Membranous glomerulonephritis with extra-renal disorders in children. Medicine (Baltimore). 1979;58(3):219–28.

103. Menon S, Valentini RP. Membranous nephropathy in children: clinical presentation and therapeutic approach. Pediatr Nephrol. 2010;2:1419–28.

104. Makker SP. Treatment of membranous nephropathy in children. Semin Nephrol. 2003;23(4):379–85.

105. Bech AP, Hofstra JM, Brenchley PE, Wetzels JF. Association of anti-PLA2R antibodies with outcomes after immunosuppressive therapy in idiopathic membranous nephropathy. Clin J Am Soc Nephrol. 2014;9(8):1386–92.

106. KDIGO. Glomerulonephritis guideline. Kidney Int Suppl. 2012;2:139.

107. Ponticelli C, Zucchelli P, Passerini P, et al. A 10-year follow-up of a randomized study with methylprednisolone and chlorambucil in membranous nephropathy. Kidney Int. 1995;48(5):1600–4.

108. Remuzzi G, Chiurchiu C, Abbate M, Brusegan V, Bontempelli M, Ruggenenti P. Rituximab for idiopathic membranous nephropathy. Lancet. 2002;360(9337):923–4.

109. Fervenza FC, Abraham RS, Erickson SB, Irazabal MV, Eirin A, Specks U, Nachman PH, Bergstralh EJ, Leung N, Cosio FG, Hogan MC, Dillon JJ, Hickson LJ, Li X, Cattran DC, Mayo Nephrology Collaborative Group. Rituximab therapy in idiopathic membranous nephropathy: a 2-year study. Clin J Am Soc Nephrol. 2010;5(12):2188–98.

110. Ruggenenti P, Cravedi P, Chianca A, Perna A, Ruggiero B, Gaspari F, Rambaldi A, Marasà M, Remuzzi G. Rituximab in idiopathic membranous nephropathy. J Am Soc Nephrol. 2012;23(8):1416–25.

111. Lin CY. Treatment of hepatitis B virus associated membranous nephropathy with recombinant alfa interferon. Kidney Int. 1991;47:225–30.

112. Bhimma R, Coovadia HM, Kramvis A, Adhikari M, Kew MC. Treatment of hepatitis B virus associated nephropathy in black children. Pediatr Nephrol. 2002;17:393–9.

113. Tang S, Lai FM, Lui YH, Tang CS, Kung NN, Ho YW, Chan KW, Leung JC, Lai KN. Lamivudine in hepatitis B associated M N. Kidney Int. 2005;68:1750–8.

114. Filler G, Feber J, Weiler G, Le Saux S. Another case of HBV associated membranous glomerulonephritis resolving on Lamivudine. Arch Dis Child. 2003;8:460.

115. Fang ZL, Harrison TJ, Yang JY, Chen QY, Wang XY, Mo JJ. Prevalence of hepatitis B virus infection in a highly endemic area of southern China after catch-up immunization. J Med Virol. 2012;84:878–84.

116. Xu H, Sun L, Zhou LJ, Fang LJ, Sheng FY, Guo YQ. The effect of hepatitis B vaccination on the incidence of childhood HBV-associated nephritis. Pediatr Nephrol. 2003;18:1216–9.

117. Nortier JL, Debiec H, Tournay Y, Mougenot B, Nöel JC, Deschodt-Lanckman MM, Janssen F, Ronco P. Neonatal disease in neutral endopeptidase alloimmunization: lessons for immunological monitoring. Pediatr Nephrol. 2006;21:1399–405.

Velibor Tasic

Introduction

There is confusion about the terminology describing the infection related glomerulopathies. In order to better understand the pathogenesis and management of infection-related glomerulonephritis (GN) Nadasdy and Hebert suggest further classification as either post-infectious GN or the GN of active infection [1]. Acute post-infectious glomerulonephritis (APIG) is the most common pathology in underdeveloped countries and is due to a wide spectrum of infective agents which may produce acute glomerular injury. The prototype of APIG is acute post-streptococcal glomerulonephritis. In post-infectious glomerulonephritis the infection is mild and has usually resolved spontaneously or with antibiotics at the onset of glomerulonephritis, 1–3 weeks later. In GN due to active infection the scenario is different; the patient develops infection which does not resolve spontaneously and very often antibiotics are not administered since the infection is not recognized or considered to be serious. Several weeks after infection, the patient develops glomerulonephritis, which manifests with hematuria, proteinuria, acute nephritic syndrome or renal failure. The crucial difference is in the antimicrobial treat-

ment, while its administration in post-infectious GN has no effect on progression of GN, in the GN of active infection systemic administration of antibiotics leads to cure of the infection which is the source of antigen production and this treatment ultimately leads to resolution of the glomerulonephritis.

The clinical presentation of infection-related GN varies from subclinical disease to severe acute kidney injury. In the majority of cases the disease has a mild clinical course. There is a growing list of infective agents which may cause infection related GN (bacteria, viruses, fungi and parasites), Table 21.1.

Pathogenesis of infection related GN is related to: (i) formation and deposition of circulating immune-complexes in glomeruli; (ii) implantation of the antigen in glomerular structures initiating immunologic reactions and formation immune-complexes in situ; or (iii) modifications of native glomerular structures which become autoantigens [2]. The end result is activation of the complement system and coagulation cascade, production of various proinflamatory cytokines, adhesion molecules and chemoattractant factors. This leads to various degree of proliferation of glomerular cells and infiltration with polymorphonucelar cells.

The most common histological presentation of infection related GN is diffuse endocapillary or proliferative glomerulonephritis (group A Streptococcus, Streptococcus viridans, Staphylococcus aureus, Diplococcus, Brucella melitensis,

V. Tasic
Department of Pediatric Nephrology, University Children's Hospital, 17 Vodnjanska, Skopje 1000, Macedonia
e-mail: vtasic2003@gmail.com

© Springer-Verlag Berlin Heidelberg 2016
D.F. Geary, F. Schaefer (eds.), *Pediatric Kidney Disease*, DOI 10.1007/978-3-662-52972-0_21

Table 21.1 Etiological agents associated with infection related glomerulonephritis

Bacterial	Viral	Fungal	Parasites
Streptococcus group A, C, G	Coxsackievirus	Coccidioides immitis	Plasmodium malariae
Streptococcus viridans	Echovirus	Candida	Plasmodium falciparum
Staphylococcus (auresus, albus)	Cytomegalovirus	Histoplasma	Schistosoma mansoni
Pneumococcus	Epstein Barr virus		Leischmania
Hemophilus	Hepatitis B, C		Toxoplasma gondii
Neisseria meningitis	HIV		Filariasis
Mycobacteria	Rubella		Trichinosis
Salmonella typhosa	Measles		Trypanosomes
Klebsiella pneumoniae	Varicella		Echinococcus
E.coli	Vaccinia		
Yersinia enterocolitica	Parvovirus		
Legionella	Influenza		
Brucella melitensis	Adenovirus		
Listeria	Rickettsial scrub typhus		
Leptospira	Mumps		
Treponema pallidum	Hantavirus		
Corynebacterium bovis	Rotavirus		
Actinobacilli			
Cat-scratch bacillus			

Measles, Mumps, Varicella, Cat scratch etc) but it may present as diffuse crescentic glomerulonephritis (Streptococcus, Staphylococcus, Varicella, Treponema pallidum) or focal crescentic nephritis (Streptococcus). Mesangiocapillary glomerulonephritis is associated with infections caused with Hepatitis C virus and Streptococcus viridans. Infections with Hepatitis B virus, Syphilis, Filaria, Schistosoma, Mycobacterium, Plasmodium falciparum give the picture of membranous glomerulonephritis. Mesangioproliferative glomerulonephritis (focal or diffuse) is associated with Diplococcus, Salmonella, Hepatitis B virus, Influenza virus and Adenovirus infections. Focal segmental, necrotizing and sclerosing glomerulonephritis is seen in bacterial endocarditis and mesangiolytic glomerulonephritis with ECHO virus infections.

The initial infection may have a mild or severe clinical course. The children may present signs of pneumonia, meningitis, sepsis, infective endocarditis or infected shunt for hydrocephalus [3–6]. The signs of glomerulonephritis may be very mild (proteinuria and hematuria), but more severe clinical picture may develop with presence of hypertension, circulatory congestion, nephrotic syndrome and acute kidney injury. Usually there is transitory hypocomplementemia.

As already mentioned renal biopsy shows various types of glomerular lesions, of which the most common is acute endocapillary and proliferative glomerulonephritis, but tubulointersitial injury also may be present [7]. Immunofluorescent studies show granular deposits of immunoglobulins and complement. The treatment consists of vigorous antibiotic administration (particularly in patients with infective endocarditis), surgery and other supportive measures.

In developed countries the incidence of post-streptococcal glomerulonephritis has declined over the past five decades, but Staphylococcus, including methicillin-resistant strain, emerged as a more frequent underlying infection particularly in older adults and diabetics who often have worse clinical features and outcome [1, 8–10]. Renal biopsy shows diffuse glomerular endocapillary hypercellularity with neutrophil infiltration on light microscopy, dominant IgA depositis and the presence of subepithelial humps on electron microscopy. This entity was entitled IgA dominant postinfectious glomerulonephritis and should be differentiated from classic IgA nephropathy because of different treatment strategies. Kimata et al. [11] have recently described the youngest patient – a 6 year old girl with methicillin-resistant Staphylococcus aureus-associated glomerulonephritis (MRSA-GN) who initially presented with pneumonia. Vigorous antibiotic treatment resulted in resolution of the glomerulonephritis; in contrast, corticosteroid treatment failed.

It is believed that the outcome of infectious related GN is benign, but in the case of acute renal failure and crescents on biopsy, corticosteroids, methylprednisolone pulses and cyclophosphamide may be benefitial [6]. The literature is sparse with studies dealing with long term prognosis of non-streptococcal GN. In a study from Milan 50 adult patients with infection associated GN have been followed for 90 ± 78 months; at the last observation 37 % had renal insufficiency or were on hemodyalisis [12]. The unfavourable outcome was due to the underlying disease and presence of interstitial infiltration on renal biopsy.

Post-streptococcal Glomerulonephritis

Post-streptococcal glomerulonephritis (PSGN) is still the most common glomerulopathy in underdeveloped countries. The disease is characterized by sudden onset of nephritic signs-hematuria, edema, hypertension, oliguria and azotemia [2, 13]. The disease was recognized as a complication of scarlet fever in eighteenth century. As a result of antibiotic therapy and improved social, economic, educational status and health care PSGN is rarely seen in western countries, mainly as sporadic cases [14–16].

Epidemiology

PSGN is a worldwide disease [17–22]. It is a complication of pyoderma due to hot climate and high humidity in tropics. Skin injuries, insect bites, bad hygiene and sanitation predispose to infection with group A beta hemolytic streptococcus (GABHS) [23]. In countries with moderate and cold climates PSGN is usually a complication of upper respiratory tract infections (pharyngitis) during the winter months. Streptococcal M types 2, 47, 49, 55, 57, 60 are associated with PSGN following pyoderma, while M types 1, 2, 3, 4, 12, 25 and 45 are associated with PSGN following pharyingitis. Typically the disease has seasonal character, but isolated cases may be seen throughout the whole year. In the past great epidemics of PSGN following impetigo were reported. In some areas (Trinidad,

Maracaibo) epidemics appear cyclically every 5–7 years; there is no satisfactory explanation for this phenomenon [13]. Populations at risk include children and soldiers, due to intimate contact, overcrowded living conditions, bad hygiene and sanitation. The ratio male: female is up to 2:1, but when subclinical cases are included than there is no male predominance. The disease is most common in children aged 3–12 years, although PSGN has been reported in infants [24, 25]. The risk for developing PSGN after infection with a nephritogenic strain of GABHS is about 15 %; for M type 49 it is 5 % after pharyngeal infection and 25 % after pyderma [26]. Rarely, PSGN is reported as a complication of piercing [27], circumcision [28], in transplanted kidney [29] and as a manifestation of immune reconstitution inflammatory syndrome in pediatric HIV infected patient [30]. Besides GABHS, streptococci from group C and G can also cause acute glomerulonephritis [31–33] but the concept of a common nephritogenic antigen is questionable [34].

Pathogenesis

There is clear evidence that PSGN is an immune complex disease, but it is still a matter of controversy, debate and research efforts to identify which antigen is really nephritogenic [35, 36]. The proposed mechanisms are:

1. deposition of circulating immune complexes containing nephritogenic antigen in glomeruli
2. implantation of the nephritogenic antigen into glomerular structures and in situ formation of immune complexes
3. molecular mimicry between streptococcal antigens and normal glomerular antigens which react with antibodies against streptococcal antigens
4. direct activation of the complement system by implanted streptococcal antigens. Many proteins such as endostreptosin, preabsorbing antigen, nephritis strain–associated protein, streptococcal pyrogenic exotoxin B (SPEB), nephritis-associated plasmin receptor (NaPlr) have been considered as potent nephritogenic antigens in PSGN [37–45].

One should document a nephritogenic antigen in renal biopsy specimen from patients with PSGN; the same antigen should be extracted from streptococci obtained from PSGN patients, but not from streptococci cultured from patients with rheumatic fever, and finally sera from PSGN patients in convalescent phase should contain significant titer of antibodies against the nephritogenic antigen. Lange and his group [39, 40] considered that endostreptosin (ESS) was an ideal nephrotogenic antigen because it fulfilled the three abovementioned criteria. Interestingly, ESS was identified in early biopsy specimens, but not in late ones. The authors proved in animal experiments that ESS implanted very early in the course of the disease on the glomerular basement membrane and was identified with fluorescent technique using anti-ESS antibodies. In the late course of the disease the organism produced anti-ESS antibodies which coupled with ESS and thus enabled detection of the ESS. The two main disadvantages of this theory are: (i) endostreptosin is an anionic antigen and this cannot explain its implantation on the GBM; (ii) injections of ESS has never induced histological changes and clinical features compatible with PSGN.

Vogt et al. pointed that cationic antigens were responsible for immunopathogenesis of PSGN; they identified cationic antigens in 8 out of 18 biopsy specimens from PSGN patients and confirmed that streptococci cultured from PSGN patients produced cationic antigens [42]. Later this antigen was confirmed to be streptococcal pyrogenic exotoxin B (zymogen, SPEB). Besides SPEB, a plasmin binding membrane receptor, the glyceraldehyde phosphate dehydrogenase (NAPlr/Plr, GAPDH) has been considered as a serious candidate to be a nephritogenic antigen [36, 44, 46, 47]. Both antigens induce long lasting antibody response and antibodies against NaPlr can be detected 10 years after an acute episode; this explains why second attacks of PSGN are extremely rare. Nephritogenic potential is not limited only to GABHS, but extends to groups C and G with sporadic and epidemic cases of PSGN reported after infection with these streptococcal groups too. The common pathway for both antigens is binding to the plasmin, which activates

complement, promotes chemotaxis and degradation of GBM components. Bound plasmin can cause tissue destruction by direct action on the GBM, or by indirect activation of procollagenases and other matrix metalloproteinases. In this way the circulating immune complexes can easily pass through the altered GBM and accumulate in the subepithelial space as humps.

NAPlr has been isolated from both groups A and C streptococci, and was considered as a putative antigen in the Japanese population with serum antibodies detected in 92 % of convalescing PSGN patients and in 60 % of patients with uncomplicated streptococcal infections [44]. In a recent study glomerular deposits and serum antibodies against these two putative antigens have been examined concurrently in biopsies and sera from same PSGN patients [45]. The results from this study pointed that SPEB is the most likely major antigen involved in pathogenesis of PSGN in patients from Latin America, US and Europe. Recently, researchers extensively studied the genome of *S. equi* subsp. *Zooepidemicus* strain MGCS10565, a Lancefield group C organism that caused an epidemic of nephritis in Brazil and found that this organism lacked a gene related to *speB* and seriously questioned the concept that SpeB or antibodies reacting with it singularly cause PSGN [34].

Immune complexes deposited from the circulation or formed in situ activate the complement cascade that leads to production of various cytokines and other cellular immune factors which initiate an inflammatory response manifested by cellular proliferation and edema of the glomerular tuft [48, 49].

In some PSGN patients, rheumatoid factor, cryoglobulins, and antineutrophil cytoplasmic antibodies are present [50–54]. The significance of these autoimmune (epi) phenomena is not defined.

Pathology

The typical pathohistologic picture on light microscopy is diffuse enlargement of all glomeruli due to hypercellularity (Fig. 21.1). There is swelling of the endothelial cells that leads to the obliteration of

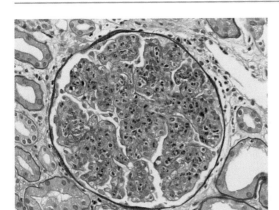

Fig. 21.1 Acute post-streptococcal glomerulonephritis. The glomerulus is enlarged and hypercellular, capillary loops obliterated and there is infiltration with polymorphonuclear leukocytes (hematoxylin and eosin, ×400) (Courtesy of Prof. N. Kambham, MD, Dept. of Pathology, Stanford University)

the capillary loops. The number of mesangial cells is increased. There is recruitment of numerous inflammatory cells in the glomeruli, mainly polymorphonuclear leukocytes and monocytes; thus this pathological picture is termed exudative proliferative glomerulonephritis. Polymorphonuclear leukocytes may be seen in the tubular lumen. If the mesangial proliferation is axial, than the glomerulus has lobular appearance. Capillary walls are not thickened. Arterioles and tubules are not affected. Edema of the interestitium and infiltration with inflammatory cells may be found. Rarely, proliferation of parietal cells of Bowman's capsule may result in formation of crescents; if their percentage is high, the disease may run a rapidly progressive course.

By immunofluorescence, the common finding in the acute phase is an irregular granular capillary and mesangial staining for complement alone, or complement and immunoglobulins, while in the resolving phase there is only mesangial staining (Fig. 21.2a–c). The predominant finding is the presence of C3 and IgG, but C4, C1q, IgM, fibrinogen and factor B may be also found. Sorger et al. described three types of immune deposits in PSGN [55]. Starry sky is the fine granular deposition of C3 and IgG along the capillary walls in the first week of the disease (Fig. 21.2a). Mesangial pattern is found between

the fourth and sixth week after the disease onset; the only immune reactant is C3 which is found in a mesangial location (Fig. 21.2b). Garland type is characterized by dense, confluent deposits along the capillary loops, while mesangial and endocapillary locations are preserved (Fig. 21.2c). Subepithelial location of the deposits correlates with the humps seen on electron microscopy. Garland type is associated with massive proteinuria and does not correlate with the time of renal biopsy [56].

In clinically atypical cases with acute kidney injury and nephrotic syndrome NAPlr staining of the glomeruli is a useful tool for confirmation of the diagnosis of PSGN [57].

The typical finding on electron microscopy in the acute phase of the disease is that of deposits on the subepithelial side of the GBM (humps), Fig. 21.3. These deposits disappear after the sixth week from the disease onset [58].

Parallel to the clinical resolution of the disease there is marked improvement of the histological picture with resolution of exudative and endocapillary changes; in the convalescent phase there is still mesangial proliferation (resolving mesangioproliferative glomerulonephritis). Subepithelial deposits disappear or their number significantly diminishes after the sixth week; the same happens with immune deposits. It takes usually 1 year for complete normalization of the histological finding.

Clinical Features

The latent period between the upper respiratory infection (pharyngitis) and nephritis is usually 10–14 days or 2–4 weeks after pyoderma. One third of PSGN patients develop discrete microscopic hematuria and/or proteinuria in the latent period. Usually the disease has sudden onset with development of nephritic syndrome (edema, oliguria, azotemia hematuria, hypertension). If a child with an upper respiratory tract infection develops nephritic signs after 2–3 days one should be suspicious of other pathology than PSGN (i.e., IgA nephropathy, or Alport syndrome). At the onset of the disease non-specific

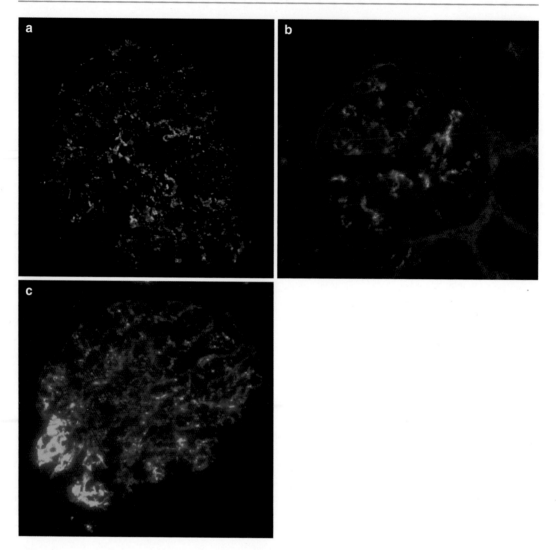

Fig. 21.2 Immunofluorescent study in acute post-streptococcal glomerulonephritis showing intensive immune deposit of C3. (**a**) Starry sky pattern (×400). (**b**) Mesangial pattern (×400). (**c**) Garland pattern (×400) (Courtesy of Prof. N. Kambham, MD, Dept. of Pathology, Stanford University)

symptoms may be present, such as pallor, malaise, low grade fever, lethargy, anorexia and headache.

Gross hematuria is present in 30–70 % patients with PSGN, while microscopic hematuria is present in all patients. Microscopic examination of the urine reveals the presence of dysmorphic red blood cells and casts. The urine is described as being smoky, cola colored, tea colored or rusty. Gross hematuria may last few hours during the day. Usually it resolves after 1–2 weeks and transforms into microscopic hematuria. Once gross hematuria has resolved, relapses may appear after physical exercise or intercurrent infections. Anecdotally few patients have minimal urinary finding (few red blood cells/per high power field) with severe clinical presentation of the disease [59, 60].

Edema in PSGN results from retention of salt and water. Despite the sodium retention, the increased level of atrial natriuretic peptide in plasma of PSGN patients indicates unresponsiveness of the kidneys to its action [61]. Very often edema is not recognized by parents, it becomes

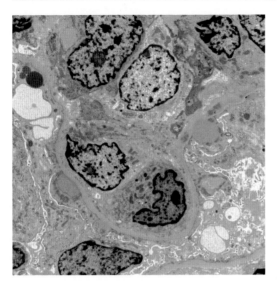

Fig. 21.3 Acute poststreptococcal glomerulonephritis. Typical electron dense deposits (humps) located on the subepithelial side of the glomerular basement membrane (electron micrograph, ×8000) (Courtesy of Prof. N. Kambham, MD, Dept. of Pathology, Stanford University)

obvious that a child had significant edema in the diuretic phase when there is a marked weight loss. Most children have mild morning periorbital edema. That is predilectional place due to reduced tissue resistance. Also edema may be located in the pretibial area and may be generalized (anasarca) with presence of pleural effusion and ascites. In the case careful restriction of water and salt is undertaken early, edema may be prevented as well as the consequences-circulatory congestion and hypertension.

Hypertension is the third cardinal sign in PSGN and is found in up to 70% of hospitalized children. Hypertension in PSGN is low renin type due to retention of water and salt which leads to expansion of the extracellular fluid volume with consequent suppression of the renin-angiotensin-aldosteron axis. Usually it is mild and has a biphasic character. If hypertension is severe and associated with retinal changes one should be suspicious of pre-existing renal disease. Normalization of the blood pressure correlates with increased diuresis and recovery of the renal function. If elevated blood pressure persists 4 weeks after disease onset one should raise suspicion for rapidly progressive disease or chronic glomerulonephritis.

Complications

Circulatory congestion is the most common complication in hospitalized children with PSGN. If severe, it can lead to pulmonary edema which represents an emergency state and requires prompt and appropriate therapy. The signs of circulatory congestions are tachycardia, dyspnoea, ortopnea and cough. On auscultation pulmonary rales may be audible. Sometimes clinical signs may be subtle, but chest radiograph shows signs of congestion. Since children and young individuals have healthy cardiovascular systems, cardiac failure is rarely seen.

Hypertensive encephalopathy is another serious complication found in 0.5–10% of hospitalized patients [13]. The most common clinical signs are nausea, vomiting, headache and impairment of consciousness that varies from somnolence to coma. The children may manifest seizures, hemiparesis, amaurosis and aphasia. These symptoms are a consequence of sudden elevation of the blood pressure that impairs cerebral autoregulation leading to vasogenic edema. EEG record shows non-specific changes, which resolves in parallel with resolution of the neurological symptoms. Analysis of the cerebrospinal fluid may reveal the presence of protein but no cellular elements. On magnetic resonance imaging scan there is typical alteration of the posterior white matter which is termed reversible posterior leukoencephalopathy syndrome [62, 63]. The images show edematous lesions primarily involving the posterior supratentorial white matter and corticomedullary junction. Neurological complications in PSGN can not be attributed exclusively to hypertensive encephalopathy or abnormal serum biochemistry, particularly in those patients with normal blood pressure during the incident (i.e., seizures). With advances in neuroimaging techniques there is clear evidence that some children develop cerebral vasculitis [64, 65]. This has practical implication because it may require different treatment modalities.

The third serious complication in PSGN is acute renal failure characterized by oliguria to anuria, severe azotemia, acid-base and electrolyte disturbances. Hyperkalemia may be a fatal complication due to cardiovascular effects and requires urgent conservative treatment and dialysis.

Clinical Variants

Clinical PSGN represents only 10% of all cases, while 90% of cases develop subclinical disease, which, due to absence of symptoms, escapes medical attention [13]. Rarely patients may present the features of nephrotic syndrome (0.4%) or rapidly progressive disease (0.1%). The incidence of subclinical disease (expressed as ratio subclinical: clinical disease) varies from 0.03 to 19.0 [66, 67]. This difference is most likely due to the applied methodology and the type of the studied population: epidemic contacts [26], family contacts [66, 68, 69] or patients with well documented streptococcal infections [67, 70]. The population at risk has been tested for urinary abnormalities and hypocomplementemia once or sequentially, the latter increased chance to detect urinary abnormalities and hypocomplementemia which may be transitory and normalize within a week.

Sagel et al. had followed 248 children from various areas of New York 4–6 weeks after well documented streptococcal infection [67]. Abnormal urinalysis with hypocomplementemia was detected in 20 children, but only one had symptomatic disease. The incidence of nephritis after streptococcal infection in this report was 8.08% and the ratio subclinical/clinical nephritis 19.0. Renal biopsy was performed in all 20 children and showed histological lesions varying from mild focal cellular proliferation to classical exudative and proliferative glomerulonephritis. Only one child had normal histology and lack of immune deposits. The authors concluded that in clinical practice only a minority of PSGN cases (clinical) are detected ("the tip of the iceberg").

Yoshizawa et al. performed a similar study in Japan; 12 out of 49 patients with well documented streptococcal infection developed subclinical nephritis (24%) and all 12 patients had abnormal renal biopsies [70].

In a study of family contacts from Macedonia, the incidence of nephritis in parents and siblings was 0% and 9.4% respectively [69]. It seems that parents are "protected" from developing PSGN. The ratio of subclinical/clinical nephritis in contacts was 1.28. An additional number of family contacts had glomerular type microhematuria and elevated ASO titre; thus one may speculate that they also had subclinical PSGN and that their complement levels normalized before occurrence of nephritis in index cases. Lange et al. pointed that the finding of significant titers of endostreptosin antibodies in patients with chronic glomerulonephritis or on hemodialysis suggested the possibility of previous undetected subclinical PSGN [39, 71].

Nephrotic syndrome may be seen in 4–25% of hospitalized children with PSGN. It usually resolves within 2–3 weeks; in cases where it persists beyond this period it is associated with an unfavourable outcome of the disease. Less than 1% of hospitalized children develop rapidly progressive disease which is characterized by prolonged oligo-anuria, uremia, hypertension, anemia and persistent nephrotic syndrome. On renal biopsy crescentic nephritis is found, and the percentage of crescents correlates with the severity of the disease and final outcome.

As already mentioned a few patient may develop cerebral vasculitis; cutaneous and gastrointestinal vasculitis have also been reported in PSGN patients and may mimic Heonoch-Schonlein purpura [72]. In very few cases PSGN may be associated with rheumatic fever [73, 74]. An unusual or atypical course of the disease is reported in patients with concurrent IgA nephropathy, diabetes mellitus, hemolytic uremic syndrome, reflux nephropathy and bilateral renal hypoplasia [75–78]. Simultaneous occurrence of acute thrombocytopenic purpura has also been reported in few PSGN patients [79–81]. The most likely mechanism is production of autoantiboidies cross-reactive against GABHS and against platelets [80].

Laboratory Findings

Proteinuria and hematuria are found in almost all patients with PSGN. The presence of red blood cell casts and dysmorphyc erythrocytes points to the glomerular origin of hematuria. In a few patients minimal urinary findings are in contrast with severe clinical presentation.

A mild dilutional anemia may be seen at the onset of the disease and is due to expansion of the extracellular fluid volume. Thrombocytopenia is extremely rare; its presence suggests the possibility of systemic lupus erythematosis or hemolytic uremic syndrome. If there is no significant impairment of glomerular filtration rate blood chemistry is almost normal; severe reduction of renal function leads to hyperkalemia, uremia and acidosis. Hypoprotreinemia, hypoalbuminema and hyperlipidemia are evident if there is associated nephrotic syndrome.

Evidence for previous streptococcal infection should be looked in all patients. Cultures from the throat or skin should be obtained depending on the site of the initial infection. Antibodies against streptococcal antigens (antistreptolysin O, antihialuronidase, antiDNA-se B titer), or combination of antigens (streptozyme) should be measured serially during the course of the disease. Of note, in post-pyodermic disease there is an insignificant rise in antistreptolysin titres. Testing antizymogen titres is very sensitive and specific for diagnosing streptococcal infection in PSGN patients but this test is not available for routine practice. Also a high titre of antibodies against glyceraldehydes phosphate dehydrogenase is found in PSGN patients.

Complement studies: There is marked depression of serum hemolytic component CH50 and C3 due to activation of the alternative pathway. In some patients there is also depression of C2 and C4 fraction suggesting activation of both classical and alternative pathways [82]. Usually complement levels normalize within 6–8 weeks, if hypocomplementemia persists more than 3 months one should strongly consider an alternative diagnosis (membranoproliferative glomerulonephritis).

Kozyro et al. tested children with PSGN for the presence of antibodies against C1q and found that 8 of 24 were positive for anti-C1q [83]. They found that anti-C1q positive children had more severe clinical presentation of the disease (hypertension, proteinuria) and unfavourable resolution of the disease.

Renal Biopsy and Differential Diagnosis

Usually children with PSGN have a favourable disease course and outcome, thus renal biopsy is not necessary. In cases of severe or atypical clinical presentation and/or delayed recovery then renal biopsy is mandatory. Indications for renal biopsy are given in Table 21.2.

PSGN should be differentiated from the following diseases: IgA nephritis (short latent period), hereditary nephritis (family history, short latent period), MPGN (persistent hypocomplementemia and unresolving nephritic syndrome), lupus nephritis (persistent hypocomplementemia, systemic manifestation), glomerulonephritis in acute and chronic infections (evidence for other non-streptococcal infection), vasculitides (polyarteritis nodosa, Hoenoch Schonlein purpura), haemolytic-uremic syndrome (hemolysis, thrombocytopenia).

Vernon et al. presented a girl who developed chronic kidney disease and persistent hypocomplementemia after streptococcal throat infection. Kidney biopsy 1 year after presentation revealed features of C3 glomerulopathy while complement studies detected heterozygous mutation in the

Table 21.2 Indications for renal biopsy

Early stage	Recovery phase
Age <2 years	Depressed GFR >4 weeks
Short latent period	Hypocomplementemia >12 weeks
Severe anuria	Persistent proteinuria >6 months
Rapidoprogressive course	Persistent microhematuria >18 months
Hypertension >2 weeks	
Depressed GFR >2 weeks	
Normal complement levels	
Non significant titres of antistreptococcal antibodies	
Extrarenal manifestation	

complement factor H-related protein 5 gene (CFHR5) [84]. A group from the Mayo Clinic presented a series of 11 patients who had atypical postinfectious glomerulonephritis [85]. Renal biopsy was performed due to persistent proteinuria/hematuria and C3 hypocomplementemia. On light microscopy there were exudative and proliferative changes; immunofluorescent studies revealed dominant C3 mesangial deposits while electronomicroscopy revealed subepithelial humps. In 10 of 11 patients they detected underlying defect in the alternative pathway of the complement regulation either as a presence of autoantibodies against C3 convertase or mutation in complement regulatory genes.

Treatment

Bed rest and limited activity are indicated in the early stage of the disease, particularly if circulatory overload and hypertension are present. There is no evidence that prolonged bed rest hastens the recovery.

In most cases fluid and salt restriction are sufficient to prevent edema and hypertension. Salt intake should be limited to less than 1.0 g/day. Usually protein intake should be limited to 1.0 g/kg/day. In case of marked azotemia calories should be provided from carbohydrates and fats. It is essential to create the diet according to individual clinical and biochemical indices. Diuresis and body weight should be monitored every day. Loop diuretic (furosemide 1–2 mg/kg/day) is indicated if there is moderate circulatory congestion. Higher doses up to 5 mg/kg per dose I.V. are indicated if there is pulmonary edema. Particular caution should be paid to patients with severe azotemia because of potential ototoxicity.

Moderate hypertension should be treated with diuretics and oral antihypertensive drugs (nifedipine, hydralasine, prazosin). Although short treatment with captopril is promising in controlling hypertension there is concern for worsening hyperkalemia [86]. In a hypertensive emergency the drug of choice is Labetalol 0.5–1.0 mg/kg/h I.V. As an alternative emergency drug one may administer diazoxide 2–3 mg/kg I.V. slowly over 30 min or nitroprusside 0.5–2 mcg/kg/min I.V. Short acting nifedipine (0.25–0.5 mg/kg/dose) administered by oral/sublingual route has been very popular for hypertensive emergencies without encephalopathy. Since serious and fatal adverse effects were reported in adults, it should be administered in children with great caution [87].

Hyperkalemia should be prevented with restricted potassium intake. If present, conservative treatment should be started immediately to prevent fatal complication. Severe hyperkalemia, azotemia, acidosis, uncontrolled hypertension, cardiovascular insufficiency and pulmonary edema are indications for urgent dialysis.

Digitalis is not indicated in patients with cardiovascular insufficiency since it accumulates in renal failure. Children with pre-existing cardiac disease should continue digitalization with adjustment of the dose according to the level of the renal function impairment.

There is no clear evidence that immunosuppressive therapy has a beneficial effect in children with crescentic PSGN. In those with >30 % crescents one may attempt pulse methylpredinoslone 0.5–1.0 g/1.73 m [2] for 3–5 days. Roy et al. analyzed ten children with crescentic PSGN; five were given quintuple therapy (including immunosuppressive drugs) and five were given only supportive treatment [88]. At the end of the follow up there was no advantage of any treatment options; the benefit of quintuple treatment was faster normalization of serum creatinine and shortening of the hospital stay.

Antibiotic therapy is indicated if there are still signs of streptococcal infection (pharyngitis, pyoderma) or patients have positive throat or skin culture. Oral penicillin V (or erythromycin for allergic patients) is preferred over parenteral treatment. Antibiotic treatment does not alter the course of the disease, but from the epidemiological aspect it is very important to prevent spread of nephritogenic strains of GABHS to the close contacts. Long term antibiotic prophylaxis is not justified since second attacks of PSGN are very rare [89].

Prognosis

There is general agreement that prognosis of PSGN in children in the acute phase is excellent, with mortality less than 1 % due to improved conservative management and availability of dialysis techniques. Concerning the medium and long term outcome there is wide range of different data; from those suggesting unfavourable outcome in the series of Baldwin et al. [90, 91], to excellent outcomes reported by Potter et al. [92]. This is mainly due to different criteria for selection of patients for prognostic studies, excellently reviewed in detail by Cameron [93]. When comparing the results, one should have in mind that only clinical cases (10 %) are included in the analysis, while those with subclinical and mild disease may escape medical attention. From those who present to the doctor only a minority with severe clinical presentation are referred to the nephrologist for biopsy. The series differ in respect to following parameters: pediatric/adult, sporadic/epidemic, evidence/ no evidence for previous streptococcal infection, with/without renal biopsy, with/without crescents on renal biopsy etc.

In a study by Vogl et al. [94], 36 children and 101 adults had biopsy and serological confirmation of PSGN and had been followed for 2–13 years; none of children reached end stage renal disease, but 10 % had elevated serum creatinine between 1 and 2 mg/dl. Clark et al. provided excellent information concerning long term outcome of PSGN in children [95]. Although their series was small, it was exclusively pediatric with adequate documentation of streptococcal infection and initial biopsy in all children and rebiopsies in some of them. Thirty children had been followed up from 14.6 to 22 years (mean 19 years). Urinary abnormalities were registered in 20 % of patients during the follow up, but none had reduced GFR, assessed with creatinine clearance. Clark et al. questioned the role of renal biopsy for diagnosis and follow up of children with typical PSGN.

As already mentioned Baldwin et al. reported unfavourable data on long term prognosis of PSGN [90, 91]. In their series 37 out of 126 patients were children; 11 patients progressed to terminal uremia, 9 in the first 6 months. During the follow up of 2–15 years proteinuria, hypertension and reduced GFR were registered in half of the patients. A total of 174 renal biopsies were performed in this patient series; in the first years after the acute episode there was a prevalence of proliferative changes, while in two-third of the late biopsies there were sclerosing lesions, which Baldwin considered as an indicator of chronicity. The results of this study were seriously criticized; this was a highly selected patient population; even 20 % presented with nephrotic syndrome. Patients who died or rapidly progressed to uremia had crescentic nephritis at biopsy, a substantial number of patients was lost during the follow up with selection of those who had more severe disease. Furthermore, GFR in this study was not corrected for sex, age and body surface area. The same group reported six patients with PSGN who progressed to terminal uremia 2–12 years after resolution of acute nephritis and normalization of the GFR [96]. Of note, five of six patients had nephrotic syndrome at the disease onset. In addition Gallo et al. presented data on the morphologic alteration in renal biopsies from patients who recovered from PSGN and found that the incidence of glomerular and vascular sclerosis increased with time [97]. The clinical consequence of this healing process is reduced renal functional reserve after a protein loading test [98, 99].

The two studies from Maracaibo, Venezuela also pointed to the progressive character of PSGN [100, 101]. One hundred and twenty patients (101 children) who had survived the epidemics in 1968 had been evaluated between 1973 and 1975. Proteinuria, microhematuria, hypertension or reduced GFR were found in 36.7 % adult patients compared with 8.7 % pediatric patients. Renal biopsies showed advanced glomerulosclerosis in all patients with abnormal findings. Mild to moderate mesangial proliferation and glomerulosclerosis were evidenced even in those patients who had not any clinical abnormality.

Herrera and Rodríguez-Iturbe investigated the inidence of ESRD among Goajiros Indians a semi-nomad tribe that live on the Goajiro peninsula, in the northwestern part of Venezuela [102]. The incidence of ESRD was 1.7 times higher than the incidence for the country. Also, the attack rate of PSGN was double compared with the general population in the neighboring Maracaibo city. Low birth weight was common among Goajiros Indians (23 % of newborns weight less than 1000 g). The authors concluded that high attack rate of PSGN and low nephron endowment were responsible for the increased risk of ESRD in this population.

Contrary to these reports Dodge et al. [103] and Travis et al. [104] reported excellent clinical and histological healing of the disease in their pediatric series. Dodge et al. found that the presence of proteinuria was in contrast to histological healing; it had an orthostatic character before definitively cleared [103]. In a study from Macedonia 40 postnephritic children were investigated 3 months to 10 years after the acute episode, but no increase in proteinuria was found after moderate to strenuous physical activity [105]. Perlman et al. reevaluated 61 children 10 years after the original epidemics in 1963 [106]. All children had normal GFR, three had proteinuria >100 mg/24, but all had normal morphology on renal biopsy. A total of 16 children had renal biopsy, 4 patients had minimal focal proliferation, but no sclerosing lesions were seen.

Three studies from Trinidad evaluated medium and long term prognosis of PSGN. These are the largest studies, predominantly pediatric, with excellent results concerning presence of urinary abnormalities, hypertension or impaired renal function [92, 107, 108]. Renal biopsy was not performed in many studies for diagnosis and follow up of PSGN in children, but the diagnosis was based on firm clinical and serological documentation of previous streptococcal infection and transitory hypocomplementemia. Results of these studies unquestionably confirmed the benign course of PSGN in children with very low percent of those with urinary abnormalities, hypertension or reduced GFR [109–111]. Besides clinical healing there was complete functional recovery in almost all patients; Drukker et al. found that natriuretic response was excellent in postnephritic children after I.V. saline loading [112].

In some communities of Australia and New Zealand inhabited by the indigenous population there is still high attack rate of PSGN [113, 114]. Repeated episodes of PSGN and low number of nephrons due to higher rate of prematurity contribute to higher prevalence of chronic kidney disease in the Aboriginal population [115, 116].

From analysis of different studies the following risk factors for unfavourable outcome were identified: older age, high serum creatinine at presentation, nephrotic syndrome and crescents on renal biopsy. Even after initial normalization of the renal function, definite impairment of the GFR may ensue many years after disease onset; thus children who present with crescents need indefinite follow up [117].

Prognosis of PSGN caused by group C *Streptococcus Zooepidemicus* is not so good; after a mean time of 5.4 years after epidemics in Brazil, a relatively high percent of patients had increased microalbuminuria, hypertension and reduced GFR [118]. Since only a few children were evaluated in this study conclusions could not be drawn for this age group.

Shunt Nephritis

Immune complex glomerulonephritis associated with infection of a ventriculoatrial shunts was first reported in 1965 by Black et al. [119]. Shunt infections are common event but only few patients develop glomerulonephritis (2%). The ventriculoperitoneal shunts are now preferred over ventriculoatrial shunts because of lower rates of complications including shunt infections. The clinical features of shunt nephritis are variable and include proteinuria, hematuria, hypertension, nephrotic syndrome, anemia and compromised renal function [10, 120]. Symptoms of shunt infections may be present and include fever, anemia, malaise, hepatosplenomegaly and cerebral symptoms. Colonization of the shunt may persist for months and years in otherwise asymptomatic patients. Low grade fever may be the only sign of active shunt infection and this may result in delay of correct diagnosis. Staphylococcus epidermidis is the most common pathogen in 75% of all shunt infections. This is a skin contaminant most likely introduced during the surgical procedure. Other isolated pathogens are S. Aureus, Corynebacterium, Listeria, Pseudomonas, Propionibacterium acnes and Bacillus species [10, 121].

Laboratory investigations reveal hypocomplementemia (C3 complement depressed in 90%), elevated erythrocyte sedimentation rate, cryoglobulinemia and positive blood or cerebrospinal fluid cultures. Patients with ventriculoatrial shunt who manifest unexplained hematuria or proteinuria, compromised renal function should undergo promptly diagnostic work up for subacute shunt infection, even in the absence of fever and leukocytosis [10]. Renal biopsy shows membranoproliferative pattern on light microscopy in majority of patients [120]. Immunofluorescence studies demonstrate granular deposits of C3, IgM and IgG in subendothelial and mesangial location. Persistent antigenemia is responsible for immune complex formation, but it is unclear whether the immune complexes are formed in the circulation or in situ. Their presence induces complement activation trough the classical pathway, which further mediates injury to glomerular cells (trough the C5–9 complex) and generates chemotactic peptides (C3a, C5a) that perpetuate local inflammation.

The prognosis of shunt nephritis is excellent in respect of renal function and proteinuria if the infected shunt is removed and aggressive and appropriate antibiotic treatment is administered. Renal function normalizes within a few weeks and hypocomplementemia also resolves [10, 120]. Delayed removal of the infected shunt may result in progressive worsening of the renal function and leads to end stage renal disease.

Endocarditis-Associated Glomerulonephritis

Infective endocarditis (IE) is mainly a complication of congenital or rheumatic heart disease in children and still has high mortality despite appropriate antibiotic therapy. Renal involvement occurs in about 25 % of the patients with IE and manifests as renal infarcts, glomerulonephritis and interstitial nephritis [10]. The most common pathogen is still Streptococcus viridians whose indolent clinical course enables prolonged antibody response and formation of circulating immune complexes which predispose to development of glomerulonephritis. Besides low virulent Stretoccoccus viridians other causative pathogens are S. epidermidis, Enterococcus, Hemophilus influenza, Actinobacillus, Chlamydia, Bartonella henselae, Coxiella burnetti, etc.

Children with acute IE present with severe illness including fever, anemia, heart murmur, hepatosplenomegaly, skin purpura and retinal hemorrhages (Roth spots) while in those with a subacute course the symptoms may be subtle and recognizable during the work up of glomerulonephritis. Glomerulonephritis usually ensues within 7–10 days of clinical illness. Duration of endocarditis does not increase the risk of developing glomerulonephritis. The symptoms may be variable from mild proteinuria/hematuria to severe rapidly progressive course. The commonest presentation is acute nephritic syndrome. Laboratory investigation reveals hypocomplementemia which correlates with severity of renal disease and infection. Rheumatoid factor may be positive and some patients may have circulating antineutrophil cytoplasmic antibody (ANCA), specifically the PR3 type.

The kidney biopsy findings are diverse, with most frequently reported focal segmental proliferation followed by diffuse endocapillary proliferation. Exudative features are similar to those seen in PSGN. Crescents and glomerular necrosis may also be present and in some patients may affect >50 % of glomeruli [6]. The tubular atrophy and fibrosis correlates with the extent of glomerular necrosis and crescents. Rarely, membranoproliferative GN resembling MPGN type I may be present and the biopsy shows diffuse mesangial and endocapillary proliferation, lobular accentuation, and GBM reduplication. During resolution of the glomerulonephritis mesangial proliferation is the dominant histological pattern. Immunofluorescence studies show dominant deposits of C3 and less intense of IgG and IgM in mesangisl areas and in capillary walls. Electronomicroscopy detects subepithelial deposits in the early phase while in the latter course of the disease they are located in subendothelial and mesangial areas.

Endocarditis-associated GN represents an immune complex disease with deposition of circulating immune complexes in the glomeruli but also there is evidence for in situ formation of complexes. The nephritogenic bacterial antigens were identified within the affected glomeruli in S. aureus and streptococcal infections. Treatment consists of antibiotic therapy and surgery in order to remove valvular vegetations and eradicate the infection. Most infective and non-infective complications of IE resolve on treatment with appropriate antibiotics. In few patients with proliferative lesions and no improvement with antibiotics, corticosteroids and cyclophosphamide may be useful [6, 122]. Patients with crescentic GN may benefit from plasmapheresis.

HIV Related Kidney Disease

Highly active antiretroviral therapy (HAART) has significantly decreased the mortality rate in children with perinatal HIV infection. The increased survival and the treatment itself has resulted in number of non-infectious complications among which renal disorders are within the first ten. Chronic kidney disease in children with perinatal HIV infection is the consequence of primary HIV infection, antiretroviral therapy and other nehrotoxic drugs. The spectrum of kidney disease includes chronic glomerular disorders, such as HIV associated nephropathy (HIVAN), HIV immune complex kidney disease (HIVICK), the thrombotic microangiopathies (atypical haemolytic uremic syndrome and thrombotic thrombocytopenic purpura), disorders of proximal tubular function and acute kidney injury [123].

The histological feature of HIVAN in children is classical focal segmental glomerulosclerosis (FSGS) with or without mesangial hyperplasia in combination with microcystic tubular dilatation and interstitial inflammation. This is in contrast with adults where collapsing FSGS is the typical histological finding. Two pediatric studies have reported collapsing FSGS in 14 and 32.5 % [124, 125]. This has important prognostic implications in children since collapsing FSGS has more rapid and progressive course towards ESRD compared with the classical form.

In the pathogenesis of HIVAN the initial event is infection of the kidney epithelial cells by HIV-1, but it is still enigmatic how the virus enters the epithelial cells since podocytes and renal tubular cells do not express CD4 or other co-receptors. The injured podocytes undergo proliferation and apoptosis and then the remaining podocytes hypertrophy and leave bare segments of basement membrane that promotes the development of the sclerotic lesions that characterize HIVAN. HIV nef and tat genes are incriminated for glomerular pathology while vpr genes are responsible for tubular lesions. Host genetic factors predispose to development of HIVAN and progression to ESRD [123]. In favor of this are data that African-Americans have a higher incidence of HIVAN with a rapid and unfavorable course. Polymorphisms G1 and G2 in the APOL-1 gene adjacent to the MYH9 gene were found to be highly associated with FSGS and HIVAN. These risk polymorphisms were found with increased frequencies in African population.

HIVICK occurs as the result of deposition of circulating immune complexes in the glomeruli or their formation in situ. Immune complexes contain viral core and envelope antigens. In addition HIV patients may have other immune complex mediated diseases (IgA nephropathy, membranous glomerulonephritis or membranoproliferative glomerulonephritis very often associated with hepatitis A, B and C coinfection). Lupus like glomerulonephritis may be also found by immunofluorescent and electronomicroscopy studies in the absence of clinical and serological features of systemic lupus erythematosus.

In blacks and in Hispanic populations, FSGS with or without collapsing glomeruli and microcystic tubular dilatation are common while mesangial hyperplasia and immune complex-type disease predominates in Caucasians. Other glomerular pathologies may be also detected in HIV infected children and adults such as postinfectious glomerulonephritis, minimal change disease, diabetic nephropathy, amiloidosis, thrombotic microangiopathy etc.

Persistent proteinuria ($\geq$1+; urinary protein/creatinine ratio >2.0) and microhematuria point to HIVAN [123, 126–128]. Additional suggestive features are finding of microcysts (shed epithelial cells) in the urinary sediment, highly echogenic kidneys, black race and nephrotic range proteinuria with or without edema or hypertension. These criteria are suggestive but not confirmatory, definitive diagnosis of HIVAN should be established by renal biopsy [123].

Children with perinatal HIV infection can suffer from tubulointeriticial nephritis and may present with non specific symptoms of acute kidney injury. The common incriminated agents are non steroidal antiinflamatory drugs (NSAID), trimetoprim-sulfamethoxazole, indinavir, ritonavir and others. Various electrolyte and acid base disturbances may be found in children with perinatal HIV infections as a consequence of malnutrition, gastroenteritis, pneumonia, intracranial infections and SIADH. Antiretroviral agents such as tenofovir can cause proximal tubular dysfunction, nephrogenic diabetes insipidus and acute kidney injury.

Treatment of HIVAN-High active antriretroviral therapy should be immediately instituted in children who show proteinuria, hematuria or acute kidney injury. If already on HAART, it may point to inadequate disease control evidenced by CD4 depletion and/or a high viral load. Resistance testing enables choice of optimal HAART regimen. Since many antiretroviral drugs are excreted unchanged into the urine, modification of the dosage should be done according to the level of the glomerular filtration rate. Nephrotoxic drugs should be avoided.

Although there are no controlled randomized trials ACE inhibitors and ARB blocking have been used in addition to HAART therapy in many centers in order to decrease proteinuria. Steroids and immunosuppressive agents are not recommended for treatment of children with HIVAN [123].

Both dialysis modalities are used in HIV infected children with ESRD. Those on peritoneal dialysis have increased risk of recurrent peritonitis and aggravation of malnutrition, while those on hemodialysis with central venous lines have high risk of tunnel infections and thrombosis. In the pre-HAART era, there were huge concerns about transplantation in otherwise immunocompromised patients. With better control of the disease with HAART, improved prophylaxis and treatment of opportunistic infections, transplantation is now the optimal treatment modality for these children if one adheres to very stringent criteria.

References

1. Nadasdy T, Hebert LA. Infection-related glomerulonephritis: understanding mechanisms. Semin Nephrol. 2011;31:369–75.
2. Sulyok E. Acute proliferative glomerulonephritis. In: Avner ED, Harmon WE, Niaudet P, editors. Pediatric nephrology. 5th ed. Philadelphia: Lippincott Williams and Wilkins; 2004. p. 601–13.
3. Forrest JW, John F, Mills LR, et al. Immune complex glomerulonephritis associated with Klebsiella pneumonia infection. Clin Nephrol. 1977;7:76–80.
4. Rainford DJ, Woodrow DF, Sloper JC, et al. Post meningococcal acute glomerulo-nephritis. Clin Nephrol. 1978;9:249–53.
5. Doregatti C, Volpi A, Torri Tarelli L, et al. Acute glomerulonephritis in human brucellosis. Nephron. 1983;41:365–6.
6. Sadikoglu B, Bilge I, Kilicaslan I, Gokce MG, Emre S, Ertugrul T. Crescentic glomerulonephritis in a child with infective endocarditis. Pediatr Nephrol. 2006;21:867–9.
7. Ferrario F, Kourilsky O, Morel-Maroger L. Acute endocapillary glomerulonephritis: a histologic and clinical comparison between patients with and without acute renal failure. Clin Nephrol. 1983;19:17–23.
8. Nasr SH, Radhakrishnan J, D'Agati VD. Bacterial infection-related glomerulonephritis in adults. Kidney Int. 2013;83:792–803.
9. Nast CC. Infection-related glomerulonephritis: changing demographics and outcomes. Adv Chronic Kidney Dis. 2012;19:68–75.
10. Kambham N. Postinfectious glomerulonephritis. Adv Anat Pathol. 2012;19:338–47.
11. Kimata T, Tsuji S, Yoshimura K, Tsukaguchi H, Kaneko K. Methicillin-resistant Staphylococcus aureus-related glomerulonephritis in a child. Pediatr Nephrol. 2012;27:2149–52.
12. Moroni G, Pozzi C, Quaglini S, et al. Long-term prognosis of diffuse proliferative glomerulonephritis associated with infection in adults. Nephrol Dial Transplant. 2002;17:1204–11.
13. Rodriguez-Iturbe B. Acute poststreptococcal glomerulonephritis. In: Schrier RW, Gottschalk CW, editors. Disease of the kidney. Boston: Little Brown; 1988. p. 1929–47.
14. Meadow SR. Poststreptococcal glomerulonephtis-a rare disease? Arch Dis Child. 1975;50:379–82.
15. Yap H, Chia K, Murugasu B, et al. Acute glomerulonephritis-changing patterns in Singapore children. Pediatr Nephrol. 1990;4:482–4.
16. Eison TM, Ault BH, Jones DP, Chesney RW, Wyatt RJ. Post-streptococcal acute glomerulonephritis in children: clinical features and pathogenesis. Pediatr Nephrol. 2011;26:165–80.
17. Knuffash FA, Sharda DC, Majeed HA. Sporadic pharyngitis-associated acute poststreptococcal glomerulonephritis. Clin Pediatr. 1986;25:181–4.

18. Sarkissian A, Papazian M, Azatian G, Arikiants N, Babloyan A, Leumann E. An epidemic of acute postinfectious glomerulonephritis in Armenia. Arch Dis Child. 1997;77:342–4.

19. Majeed HA, Khuffash FA, Sharda DC, Farwana SS, el-Sherbiny AF, Ghafour SY. Children with acute rheumatic fever and acute poststreptococcal glomerulonephritis and their families in a subtropical zone: a three-year prospective comparative epidemiological study. Int J Epidemiol. 1987;16:561–8.

20. Streeton CL, Hanna JN, Messer RD, Merianos A. An epidemic of acute post-streptococcal glomerulonephritis among aboriginal children. J Paediatr Child Health. 1995;31:245–8.

21. Leung DTY, Tseng RYM, Go SH, et al. Poststreptococcal glomerulonephritis in Hong Kong. Arch Dis Child. 1987;62:1075–6.

22. Margolis HS, Lum MKW, Bender TR, et al. Acute glomerulonephritis and streptococcal skin lesions in Eskimo children. Am J Dis Child. 1980;134:681–5.

23. Svartman M, Potter EV, Poon-King T, Earle DP. Streptococcal infection of scabetic lesions related to acute glomerulonephritis in Trinidad. J Lab Clin Med. 1973;81:182–93.

24. Li Volti S, Furnari ML, Garozzo R, et al. Acute poststreptococcal glomerulonephritis in an 8-month old girl. Pediatr Nephrol. 1993;7:737–9.

25. Kari JA, Bamagai A, Jalalah SM. Severe acute poststreptococcal glomerulonephritis in an infant. Saudi J Kidney Dis Transplant. 2013;24:546–8.

26. Anthony BF, Kaplan EL, Wannamaker LW, et al. Attack rates of acute nephritis after type 49 streptococcal infection of the skin and of the respiratory tract. J Clin Invest. 1969;48:1697–702.

27. Ahmed-Jushuf IH, Selby PL, Brownjohn AM. Acute post-streptococcal glomerulonephritis following ear piercing. Postgrad Med J. 1984;60(699):73–4.

28. Tasic V, Polenakovic M. Acute poststreptococcal glomerulonephritis following circumcision. Pediatr Nephrol. 2000;15:274–5.

29. Sorof JM, Weidner N, Potter D, Portale AA. Acute poststreptococcal glomerulonephritis in a renal allograft. Pediatr Nephrol. 1995;9:317–20.

30. Martin J, Kaul A, Schacht R. Acute poststreptococcal glomerulonephritis: a manifestation of immune reconstitution inflammatory syndrome. Pediatrics. 2012;130:e710–3.

31. Gnann JW, Gray BM, Griffin FM, Dismukes WE. Acute glomerulonephritis following group G streptococcal infection. J Infect Dis. 1987;156:411–2.

32. Barnham M, Thornton T, Lange K. Nephritis caused by streptococcus zooepidemicus (Lancefield group C). Lancet. 1983;1:945–8.

33. Francis AJ, Nimmo GR, Efstratiou A, Galanis V, Nuttall N. Investigation of milk-borne Streptococcus zooepidemicus infection associated with glomerulonephritis in Australia. J Infect. 1993;27:317–23.

34. Beres SB, Sesso R, Pinto SW, Hoe NP, Porcella SF, Deleo FR, Musser JM. Genome sequence of a Lancefield group C Streptococcus zooepidemicus strain causing epidemic nephritis: new information about an old disease. PLoS One. 2008;3:e3026.

35. Yoshizawa N. Acute glomerulonephritis. Intern Med. 2000;39:687–94.

36. Rodriguez Iturbe B. Nephritis-associated streptococcal antigens: where are we now? J Am Soc Nephrol. 2004;15:1961–2.

37. Cronin W, Deol H, Azadegan A, Lange K. Endostreptosin: isolation of the probable immunogen of acute poststreptococcal glomerulonephritis (PSGN). Clin Exp Immunol. 1989;76:198–203.

38. Cronin WJ, Lange K. Immunologic evidence for the in situ deposition of a cytoplasmatic streptococcal antigen (endostreptosin) on the glomerular basement memebrane in rats. Clin Nephrol. 1990;31:143–6.

39. Lange K, Selingson G, Cronin W. Evidence for the in situ origin of poststreptococcal glomerulonephritis: glomerular localization of endostreptosin and the clinical significance of the subsequent antibody responce. Clin Nephrol. 1983;19:3–10.

40. Lange K, Ahmed U, Kleinberger H, Treser G. A hitherto unknown streptococcal antigen and its probable relation to acute poststreptococcal glomerulonephritis. Clin Nephrol. 1976;5:207–15.

41. Rodriguez-Iturbe B, Rabideau D, Garcia R, et al. Characterization of the glomerular antibody in acute poststreptococcal glomerulonephritis. Ann Intern Med. 1980;92:478–81.

42. Vogt A, Batsford S, Rodriguez-Iturbe B, Garcia R. Cationic antigens in poststreptococcal glomerulonephritis. Clin Nephrol. 1983;20:271–9.

43. Parra G, Rodriguez-Iturbe B, Batsford S, Vogt A, Mezzano S, Olavarria F, Exeni R, Laso M, Orta N. Antibody to streptococcal zymogen in the serum of patients with acute glomerulonephritis: a multicentric study. Kidney Int. 1998;54:509–17.

44. Yoshizawa N, Yamakami K, Fujino M, Oda T, Tamura K, Matsumoto K, Sugisaki T, Boule MDP. Nephritis-associated plasmin receptor and acute glomerulonephritis: characterization of the antigen and associated immune response. J Am Soc Nephrol. 2004;15:1785–93.

45. Batsford SR, Mezzano S, Mihatsch M, Schiltz E, Rodriguez Iturbe B. Is the nephritogenic antigen in post-streptococcal glomerulonephritis pyrogenic exotoxin B (SPE B) or GAPDH? Kidney Int. 2005;68:1120–9.

46. Oda T, Yoshizawa N, Yamakami K, Tamura K, Kuroki A, Sugisaki T, Sawanobori E, Higashida K, Ohtomo Y, Hotta O, Kumagai H, Miura S. Localization of nephritis-associated plasmin receptor in acute poststreptococcal glomerulonephritis. Hum Pathol. 2010;41:1276–85.

47. Oda T, Yoshizawa N, Yamakami K, Sakurai Y, Takechi H, Yamamoto K, Oshima N, Kumagai H. The role of nephritis-associated plasmin receptor (NAPlr) in glomerulonephritis associated with streptococcal infection. J Biomed Biotechnol. 2012;2012:417675.

48. Soto HM, Parra G, Rodriguez-Itrube B. Circulating levels of cytokines in poststreptococcal glomerulonephritis. Clin Nephrol. 1997;47:6–12.

49. Matsell DG, Wayatt RJ, Gaber LW. Terminal complement complexes in acute poststreptococcal glomerulonephritis. Pediatr Nephrol. 1994;8:671–7.

50. Garin E, Fenell R, Shulman S, et al. Clinical significance of the presence of cryoglobulins in patients with glomerulonephritis not associated with systemic disease. Clin Nephrol. 1980;13:5–11.

51. Mezzano S, Olavarria F, Ardiles L, Lopez MI. Incidence of circulating immune complexes in patients with acute poststreptococcal glomerulonephritis and in patients with streptococcal impetigo. Clin Nephrol. 1986;26:61–5.

52. Sesso RC, Ramos OL, Pereira AB. Detection of IgG-rheumatoid factor in sera of patients with acute poststreptococcal glomerulonephritis and its relationship with circulating immunocomplexes. Clin Nephrol. 1986;25:55–60.

53. Villches AR, Williams DG. Persistent anti-DNA antibodies and DNA-anti-DNA complexes in poststreptococcal glomerulonephritis. Clin Nephrol. 1984;22:97–101.

54. Ardiles LG, Valderrama G, Moya P, Mezzano SA. Incidence and studies on antigenic specificities of antineutrophil-cytoplasmic autoantibodies (ANCA) in poststreptococcal glomerulonephritis. Clin Nephrol. 1997;47:1–5.

55. Sorger K, Gessler U, Hubner FK, et al. Subtypes of acute postinfectious glomerulo-nephritis. Synopsis of clinical and pathological features. Clin Nephrol. 1982;17:114–28.

56. Sorger K, Balun J, Hubner FK, et al. The garland type of acute postinfectious glomerulonephritis: morphological characteristics and follow-up studies. Clin Nephrol. 1983;20:17–26.

57. Kokuzawa A, Morishita Y, Yoshizawa H, Iwazu K, Komada T, Akimoto T, Saito O, Oda T, Takemoto F, Ando Y, Muto S, Yumura W, Kusano E. Acute poststreptococcal glomerulonephritis with acute kidney injury in nephrotic syndrome with the glomerular deposition of nephritis-associated plasmin receptor antigen. Intern Med. 2013;52:2087–91.

58. Tornroth T. The fate of subepithelial deposits in acute poststreptococcal glomerulonephritis. Lab Invest. 1976;35:461–74.

59. Cohen JA, Levitt MF. Acute glomerulonephritis with few urinary abnormalities. Report of two cases proved by renal biopsy. N Engl J Med. 1963;268:749–53.

60. Robson WL, Leung AK. Post-streptococcal glomerulonephritis with minimal abnormalities in the urinary sediment. J Singap Paediatr Soc. 1992;34:232–4.

61. Ozdemir S, Saatçi U, Beşbaş N, Bakkaloglu A, Ozen S, Koray Z. Plasma atrial natriuretic peptide and endothelin levels in acute poststreptococcal glomerulonephritis. Pediatr Nephrol. 1992;6:519–22.

62. Fux CA, Bianchetti MG, Jakob SM, Remonda L. Reversible encephalopathy complicating poststreptococcal glomerulonephritis. Pediatr Infect Dis J. 2006;25:85–7.

63. Endo A, Fuchigami T, Hasegawa M, Hashimoto K, Fujita Y, Inamo Y, Mugishima H. Posterior reversible encephalopathy syndrome in childhood: report of four cases and review of the literature. Pediatr Emerg Care. 2012;28:153–7.

64. Kaplan RA, Zwick DL, Hellerstein S, et al. Cerebral vasculitis in acute poststreptococcal glomerulonephritis. Pediatr Nephrol. 1993;7:194–6.

65. Rovang RD, Zawada Jr ET, Santella RN, Jaqua RA, Boice JL, Welter RL. Cerebral vasculitis associated with acute post-streptococcal glomerulonephritis. Am J Nephrol. 1997;17:89–92.

66. Sharrett AR, Poon-King T, Potter EV, et al. Subclinical nephritis in South Trinidad. Am J Epidemiol. 1971;91:231–45.

67. Sagel I, Treser G, Ty A, et al. Occurrence and nature of glomerular lesions after group A streptococci infections in children. Ann Intern Med. 1973;79:492–9.

68. Rodriguez-Iturbe B, Rubio L, Garcia R. Attack rate of poststreptococcal glomerulonephritis in families. A prospective study. Lancet. 1981;1:401–5.

69. Tasic V, Polenakovic M. Occurrence of subclinical post-streptococcal glomerulonephritis in family contacts. J Paediatr Child Health. 2003;39:177–9.

70. Yoshizawa N, Suzuki Y, Oshima S, et al. Asymptomatic acute poststreptococcal glomerulonephritis following upper respiratory tract infections caused by Group A streptococci. Clin Nephrol. 1996;46:296–301.

71. Lange K, Azadegan AA, Seligson G, Bovie RC, Majeed H. Asymptomatic poststreptococcal glomerulonephritis in relatives of patients with symptomatic glomerulonephritis. Diagnostic value of endostreptosin antibodies. Child Nephrol Urol. 1988–1989;9:11–5.

72. Goodyer PR, de Chadarevian JP, Kaplan BS. Acute poststreptococcal glomerulonephritis mimicking Henoch-Schonlein purpura. J Pediatr. 1978;93:412–5.

73. Said R, Hussein M, Hassan A. Simultaneous occurrence of acute poststreptococcal glomerulonephritis and acute rheumatic fever. Am J Nephrol. 1986; 6:146–8.

74. Matsell DG, Baldree LA, DiSessa TG, et al. Acute poststreptococcal glomerulonephritis and acute rheumatic fever: occurrence in the same patient. Child Nephrol Urol. 1990;10:112–4.

75. Hiki Y, Tamura K, Shigematsu H, Kobayashi Y. Superimposition of poststreptococcal acute glomerulonephritis on the course of IgA nephropathy. Nephron. 1991;57:358–64.

76. Chadaverian JP, Goodyer PR, Kaplan BS, et al. Acute glomerulonephritis and hemolytic uremic syndrome. CMA J. 1980;123:391–4.

77. Sheridan RJ, Roy S, Stapleton BF. Reflux nephropathy complicated by acute post-streptococcal glomerulonephritis. Int Pediatr Nephrol. 1983;4:119–21.

78. Naito Yoshida Y, Hida M, Maruyama Y, Hori N, Awazu M. Poststreptococcal acute glomerulonephritis superimposed on bilateral renal hypoplasia. Clin Nephrol. 2005;63:477–80.

79. Kaplan BS, Esseltine D. Thrombocytopenia in patients with acute poststreptococcal glomerulonephritis. J Pediatr. 1978;93:974–6.

80. Tasic V, Polenakovic M. Thrombocytopenia during the course of acute poststreptococcal glomerulonephritis. Turk J Pediatr. 2003;45:148–51.

81. Guerrero AP, Musgrave JE, Lee EK. Immune globulin-responsive thrombocytopenia in acute poststreptococcal glomerulonephritis: report of a case in Hawai'i. Hawaii Med J. 2009;68:56–8.

82. Wayatt RJ, Forristal J, West CD, et al. Complement profiles in acute poststreptococcal glomerulonephritis. Pediatr Nephrol. 1988;2:219–23.

83. Kozyro I, Perahud I, Sadallah S, Sukalo A, Titov L, Schifferli J, Trendelenburg M. Clinical value of autoantibodies against C1q in children with glomerulonephritis. Pediatrics. 2006;117:1663–8.

84. Vernon KA, Goicoechea de Jorge E, Hall AE, Fremeaux-Bacchi V, Aitman TJ, Cook HT, Hangartner R, Koziell A, Pickering MC. Acute presentation and persistent glomerulonephritis following streptococcal infection in a patient with heterozygous complement factor H-related protein 5 deficiency. Am J Kidney Dis. 2012;60:121–5.

85. Sethi S, Fervenza FC, Zhang Y, Zand L, Meyer NC, Borsa N, Nasr SH, Smith RJ. Atypical postinfectious glomerulonephritis is associated with abnormalities in the alternative pathway of complement. Kidney Int. 2013;83:293–9.

86. Parra G, Rodriguez-Iturbe B, Colina-Chourio J, Garcia R. Short term treatment with captopril in hypertension due to acute glomerulonephritis. Clin Nephrol. 1988;29:58–62.

87. Yiu V, Orrbine E, Rosychuk RJ, et al. The safety and use of short-acting nifedipine in hospitalized hypertensive children. Pediatr Nephrol. 2004;19:644–50.

88. Roy S, Murphy WM, Arant BS. Poststreptococcal crescentic glomerulonephritis in children: comparison of quintuple therapy versus supportive care. J Pediatr. 1981;98:403–10.

89. Roy S, Wall HP, Etteldorf JN. Second attacks of acute glomerulonephritis. J Pediatr. 1969;75:758–67.

90. Baldwin DS. Poststreptococcal glomerulonephritis. A progressive disease. Am J Med. 1977;62:1–11.

91. Baldwin DS, Gluck MC, Schacht RG, Gallo G. The long-term course of poststreptococcal glomerulonephritis. Ann Intern Med. 1974;80:342–58.

92. Potter E, Lipschultz SA, Abidh S, et al. Twelve to seventeen-year follow-up of patients with poststreptococcal acute glomerulonephritis in Trinidad. N Engl J Med. 1982;307:725–30.

93. Cameron JS. The long-term outcome of glomerular disease. In: Schrier RW, Gottschalk CW, editors. Diseases of the kidney. Boston: Little Brown; 1988. p. 2127–89.

94. Vogl W, Renke M, Mayer-Eichberger D, et al. Long term prognosis for endocapillary glomerulonephritis of poststreptococcal type in children and adults. Nephron. 1986;44:58–65.

95. Clark G, White R, Glasgow EF, et al. Poststreptococcal glomerulonephritis in children: clinicopathological correlations and long term prognosis. Pediatr Nephrol. 1988;2:381–8.

96. Schacht RG, Gluck MC, Gallo GR, et al. Progression to uremia after remission of acute poststreptococcal glomerulonephritis. N Engl J Med. 1976;295:977–81.

97. Gallo GR, Feiner HD, Steele JM, et al. Role of intrarenal vacular sclerosis in progression of poststreptococcal glomerulonephritis. Clin Nephrol. 1980;13:49–57.

98. Rodriguez-Iturbe B, Herrera J, Garcia R. Response to acute protein load in kidney donors and in apparently normal postacute glomerulonephritis patients: evidence for glomerular hyperfiltration. Lancet. 1985;2:461–4.

99. Cleper R, Davidovitz M, Halevi R, Eisenstein B. Renal functional reserve after acute poststreptococcal glomerulonephritis. Pediatr Nephrol. 1997;11:473–6.

100. Rodriguez-Iturbe B, Garcia R, Rubio L, et al. Epidemic glomerulonephritis in Maracaibo. Evidence for progression to chronicity. Clin Nephrol. 1976;5:197–206.

101. Garcia R, Rubio L, Rodriguez-Iturbe B. Long term prognosis of epidemic poststreptococcal glomerulonephritis in Maracaibo: follow-up studies 11–12 years after the acute episode. Clin Nephrol. 1981;15:291–8.

102. Herrera J, Rodríguez-Iturbe B. End-stage renal disease and acute glomerulonephritis in Goajiro Indians. Kidney Int Suppl. 2003;83:S22–6.

103. Dodge WF, Spargo BH, Travis LB, et al. Poststreptococcal glomerulonephritis. A prospective study in children. N Engl J Med. 1971;286:273–8.

104. Travis LB, Dodge WF, Beathard GA, et al. Acute glomerulonephritis in children. A review of the natural history with emphasis on prognosis. Clin Nephrol. 1973;1:169–81.

105. Tasic V, Korneti P, Gucev Z, Korneti B. Stress tolerance test and SDS-PAGE for the analysis of urinary proteins in children and youths. Clin Chem Lab Med. 2001;39:478–3.

106. Perlman LV, Herdman RC, Kleinman H, Vernier RL. Poststreptococcal glomerulo-nephritis. A ten year follow up of an epidemics. JAMA. 1965;194:63–70.

107. Potter EV, Abidh S, Sharrett AR, et al. Clinical healing two to six years after poststreptococcal glomerulonephritis in Trinidad. N Engl J Med. 1978;298:767–72.

108. Nissenson AR, Mayon-White R, Potter EV, et al. Continued absence of clinical renal disease seven to twelve years after poststreptococcal acute glomerulonephritis in Trinidad. Am J Med. 1979;67:255–62.

109. Popovic-Rolovic M, Kostic M, Antic-Peco A, et al. Medium- and long-term prognosis of patients with acute poststreptococcal glomerulonephritis. Nephron. 1991;58:393–9.

110. Tasic V, Polenakovic M, Kuzmanovska D, Sahpazova E, Ristoska N. Prognosis of poststreptococcal glomerulonephritis five to fifteen years after an acute episode. Pediatr Nephrol. 1998;12:C167.

111. Kasahara T, Hayakawa H, Okubo S, et al. Prognosis of acute poststreptococcal glomerulonephritis (APSGN) is excellent in children, when adequately diagnosed. Pediatr Int. 2001;43:364–7.

112. Drukker A, Pomeranz A, Reichenberg J, Mor J, Stankiewicz H. Natriuretic response to i.v. saline

loading after acute poststreptococcal glomerulonephritis. Isr J Med Sci. 1986;22:779–82.

113. Marshall CS, Cheng AC, Markey PG, Towers RJ, Richardson LJ, Fagan PK, Scott L, Krause VL, Currie BJ. Acute post-streptococcal glomerulonephritis in the Northern Territory of Australia: a review of 16 years data and comparison with the literature. Am J Trop Med Hyg. 2011;85:703–10.

114. Wong W, Lennon DR, Crone S, Neutze JM, Reed PW. Prospective population-based study on the burden of disease from post-streptococcal glomerulonephritis of hospitalised children in New Zealand: epidemiology, clinical features and complications. J Paediatr Child Health. 2013;49:850–5.

115. Hoy WE, Kincaid-Smith P, Hughson MD, Fogo AB, Sinniah R, Dowling J, Samuel T, Mott SA, Douglas-Denton RN, Bertram JF. CKD in aboriginal Australians. Am J Kidney Dis. 2010;56:983–93.

116. Hoy WE, White AV, Dowling A, Sharma SK, Bloomfield H, Tipiloura BT, Swanson CE, Mathews JD, McCredie DA. Post-streptococcal glomerulonephritis is a strong risk factor for chronic kidney disease in later life. Kidney Int. 2012;81:1026–32.

117. Tasic V, Polenakovic M, Cakalarovski K, Kuzmanovska D. Progression of crescentic post-streptococcal glomerulonephritis to terminal uremia twelve years after recovery from an acute episode (letter). Nephron. 1988;79:496.

118. Sesso R, Wyton S, Pinto L. Epidemic glomerulonephritis due to Streptococcus zooepidemicus in Nova Serrana, Brazil. Kidney Int Suppl. 2005;97:S132–6.

119. Black JA, Challacombe DN, Ockenden BG. Nephrotic syndrome associated with bacteraemia after shunt operations for hydrocephalus. Lancet. 1965;2(7419):921–4.

120. Haffner D, Schindera F, Aschoff A, Matthias S, Waldherr R, Schärer K. The clinical spectrum of shunt nephritis. Nephrol Dial Transplant. 1997;12:1143–8.

121. Kiryluk K, Preddie D, D'Agati VD, Isom R. A young man with Propionibacterium acnes-induced shunt nephritis. Kidney Int. 2008;73:1434–40.

122. Mantan M, Sethi GR, Batra VV. Post-infectious glomerulonephritis following infective endocarditis: amenable to immunosuppression. Indian J Nephrol. 2013;23:368–70.

123. Bhimma R, Purswani MU, Kala U. Kidney disease in children and adolescents with perinatal HIV-1 infection. J Int AIDS Soc. 2013;16:18596.

124. Ramsuran D, Bhimma R, Ramdial PK, Naicker E, Adhikari M, Deonarain J, Sing Y, Naicker T. The spectrum of HIV-related nephropathy in children. Pediatr Nephrol. 2012;27:821–7.

125. Purswani MU, Chernoff MC, Mitchell CD, Seage 3rd GR, Zilleruelo G, Abitbol C, Andiman WA, Kaiser KA, Spiegel H, Oleske JM, IMPAACT 219/219C Study Team. Chronic kidney disease associated with perinatal HIV infection in children and adolescents. Pediatr Nephrol. 2012;27:981–9.

126. Iduoriyekemwen NJ, Sadoh WE, Sadoh AE. Prevalence of renal disease in Nigerian children infected with the human immunodeficiency virus and on highly active anti-retroviral therapy. Saudi J Kidney Dis Transplant. 2013;24:172–7.

127. Giacomet V, Erba P, Di Nello F, Coletto S, Viganò A, Zuccotti G. Proteinuria in paediatric patients with human immunodeficiency virus infection. World J Clin Cases. 2013;1:13–8.

128. Shah I, Gupta S, Shah DM, Dhabe H, Lala M. Renal manifestations of HIV infected highly active antiretroviral therapy naive children in India. World J Pediatr. 2012;8:252–5.

Rapidly Progressive Glomerulonephritis

22

Arvind Bagga and Shina Menon

Introduction

Rapidly progressive glomerulonephritis (RPGN) is a rare syndrome in children, characterized by clinical features of glomerulonephritis (GN) and rapid loss of renal function. Histology shows crescentic extracapillary proliferation in Bowman space affecting the majority of glomeruli. This course may occur in any form of GN including poststreptococcal GN, renal vasculitis, IgA nephropathy, systemic lupus erythematosus (SLE) and membranoproliferative GN. RPGN is a medical emergency, which if untreated rapidly progresses to irreversible loss of renal function. Prompt evaluation and specific therapy is necessary to ensure satisfactory outcome.

Definition

RPGN is a clinical syndrome characterized by an acute nephritic illness accompanied by rapid loss of renal function (more than 50 % decrease in GFR) over days to weeks [1]. The histological correlate is the presence of crescents (crescentic GN) involving 50 % or more glomeruli. The presence of crescents is a histologic marker of severe glomerular injury, which may occur in a number of conditions including postinfectious GN, IgA nephropathy, SLE, renal vasculitis and membranoproliferative GN [1, 2]. The severity of clinical features correlates with the proportion of glomeruli that show crescents. While patients with circumferential crescents involving more than 80 % of glomeruli present with advanced renal failure, those with crescents in less than 50 % of glomeruli, particularly if these are non-circumferential, have an indolent course.

The terms RPGN and crescentic GN are used interchangeably; similar presentation might occur in conditions without crescents, including hemolytic uremic syndrome (HUS), diffuse proliferative GN and acute interstitial nephritis. Table 22.1 lists common conditions that present with RPGN in childhood.

Pathogenesis of Crescent Formation

Crescents are defined as the presence of two or more layers of cells in Bowman space. The chief components of crescents are coagulation proteins, macrophages, T cells, fibroblasts and parietal and visceral epithelial cells [1, 3]. There is evidence that podocytes also have a role in crescent formation [4]. Perturbations of humoral immunity as well as the Th1 cellular immune

A. Bagga (✉)
Department of Pediatrics,
All India Institute of Medical Sciences,
Ansari Nagar, New Delhi 110029, India
e-mail: arvindbagga@hotmail.com

S. Menon
Assistant Professor, Seattle Children's Hospital,
University of Washington, Seattle, WA 98105, USA
e-mail: shinamenon@gmail.com

© Springer-Verlag Berlin Heidelberg 2016
D.F. Geary, F. Schaefer (eds.), *Pediatric Kidney Disease*, DOI 10.1007/978-3-662-52972-0_22

Table 22.1 Causes of rapidly progressive glomerulonephritis (RPGN)

Immune complex GN
Post infectious GN. Poststreptococcal nephritis, infective endocarditis, shunt nephritis, *Staphylococcus aureus* sepsis, other infections: HIV, hepatitis B and C, syphilis
Systemic disease. Systemic lupus erythematosus, Henoch-Schonlein purpura, cryoglobulinemia, mixed connective tissue disorder, juvenile rheumatoid arthritis
Primary GN. IgA nephropathy, MPGN, membranous nephropathy, C1q nephropathy
Pauci-immune crescentic GN
Microscopic polyangiitis, granulomatosis with polyangiitis (Wegener's granulomatosis), renal limited vasculitis, eosinophilic granulomatosis with polyangiitis (Churg-Strauss disease)
Idiopathic crescentic GN
Medications: penicillamine, hydralazine, hydrocarbons, propylthiouracil
Anti glomerular basement membrane GN
Anti-GBM nephritis, Goodpasture syndrome, post-renal transplantation in Alport syndrome
Post-renal transplantation
Recurrence of IgA nephropathy, Henoch Schonlein purpura, MPGN, systemic lupus
RPGN without crescents
Hemolytic uremic syndrome
Acute interstitial nephritis
Diffuse proliferative GN

GN glomerulonephritis, *MPGN* membranoproliferative GN, *GBM* glomerular basement membrane, *HIV* human immunodeficiency virus

response contribute to the pathogenesis [1, 2]. Various pathways involving T cells, including disturbances in regulatory T cell function and stimulation of toll-like receptor 4 have been described [5, 6].

Initiating Events

The initial event in formation of crescents is the occurrence of a physical gap in the glomerular capillary wall and glomerular basement membrane (GBM), mediated by macrophages and T lymphocytes. Breaks in the integrity of the capillary wall lead to passage of inflammatory mediators and plasma proteins into the Bowman space with fibrin formation, influx of macrophages and

T cells, and release of inflammatory cytokines, e.g., interleukin-1 (IL-1) and tumor necrosis factor-α. Similar breaks in the Bowman capsule allow cells and mediators from the interstitium to enter Bowman space and for contents of the latter to enter the interstitium, resulting in inflammation. It is proposed that podocytes, which are terminally differentiated and stationary cells, change into a migratory phenotype and contribute to crescent formation [7].

Formation

The development of a crescent results from the participation of coagulation factors and different proliferating cells, chiefly macrophages, parietal epithelial cells and interstitial fibroblasts. The presence of coagulation factors in the Bowman space results in formation of a fibrin clot and recruitment of circulating macrophages. Activated neutrophils and mononuclear cells release procoagulant tissue factor, IL-1 and TNF-α, serine proteinases (elastase, PR3) and matrix metalloproteinases. The proteases cause lysis of the GBM proteins and facilitate entry of other mediators in the Bowman space. Release of IL-1 and TNF-α results in expression of adhesion molecules, leading to macrophage recruitment and proliferation. Apart from macrophages, major components of the crescents are proliferating parietal and visceral epithelial cells [8].

Resolution of Crescents

The stage of inflammation is followed by development of fibrocellular and fibrous crescents. The expression of fibroblast growth factors and transforming growth factor-β is important for fibroblast proliferation and production of type I collagen, responsible for transition from cellular to fibrocellular and fibrous crescents. The transition to fibrous crescents, which occurs over days, is important since the latter is not likely to resolve following immunosuppressive therapy. The plasminogen-plasmin system is responsible for fibrinolysis and resolution of crescents.

Causes and Immunopathologic Categories

Based on pathology and immunofluorescence staining patterns, crescentic GN is classified into three categories, which reflect different mechanisms of glomerular injury [1]:

1. Immune-complex GN with granular deposits of immune complexes along capillary wall and mesangium
2. Pauci-immune GN with scant or no immune deposits, and associated with systemic vasculitis
3. Anti-GBM GN with linear deposition of anti-GBM antibodies

Immune Complex Crescentic GN

These patients form a heterogeneous group in which multiple stimuli lead to proliferative GN with crescents. Immunohistology shows granular deposits of immunoglobulin and complement along capillary walls and in the mesangium. The causes include infections, systemic diseases and pre-existing primary GN.

Systemic Infections

Poststreptococcal GN can rarely present with crescentic histology. While most patients recover completely, the presence of nephrotic range proteinuria, sustained hypertension and crescents is associated with an unsatisfactory outcome [9, 10]. Other infectious illnesses associated with crescentic GN include infective endocarditis, infected atrioventricular shunts and visceral abscesses. Crescentic GN may be associated with infection with methicillin resistant *Staphylococcus aureus*, hepatitis B and C virus, leprosy and syphilis.

Systemic Immune Complex Disease

RPGN with glomerular crescents might be seen in patients with class IV and less commonly class III lupus nephritis. Extensive crescent formation is associated with an unsatisfactory outcome in Henoch Schonlein purpura and rheumatoid arthritis.

Primary GN

Patients with IgA nephropathy, membranoproliferative GN and rarely membranous nephropathy may present with rapid loss of renal function and crescentic GN [9–11].

Pauci-Immune Crescentic GN

This form of glomerulonephritis is characterized by few or no immune deposits on immunofluorescence microscopy [2, 12]. This includes renal-limited vasculitis, and the renal manifestations of microscopic polyangiitis, granulomatosis with polyangiitis (formerly Wegener's granulomatosis), or eosinophilic granulomatosis with polyangiitis (formerly Churg-Strauss syndrome). Most (80 %) show antineutrophil cytoplasmic autoantibodies (ANCA) in blood, and are collectively classified as ANCA-associated vasculitides. Some cases of ANCA positive disease might be induced by drugs, including penicillamine, propylthiouracil, minocycline and hydralazine.

In addition, approximately 10–30 % of patients with pauci-immune crescentic GN are ANCA negative [13]. These patients have fewer constitutional and extrarenal symptoms than those who are ANCA-positive. Studies show differences in outcome between these groups suggesting a different pathophysiological basis.

Anti-GBM Crescentic GN

This condition is uncommon in childhood, accounting for less than 10 % cases in children [1, 9, 14–16]. The nephritogenic autoantibody is directed against a 28 kDa monomer located on the $\alpha 3$ chain of type IV collagen (Goodpasture antigen). Pulmonary involvement (Goodpasture syndrome) is uncommon. Approximately 5 % of patients with Alport syndrome who receive a renal allograft show anti-GBM autoantibodies and anti-GBM nephritis within the first year of the transplant [17]. Unlike de novo anti-GBM nephritis, pulmonary hemorrhage is not observed in post-transplant anti-GBM nephritis because the patient's lung tissue does not contain the putative antigen. The risk of post transplantation anti-GBM nephritis is low in subjects with normal hearing, late progression to end stage renal disease, or females with X-linked Alport syndrome.

Idiopathic RPGN

This group includes patients with immune complex crescentic GN who do not fit into any identifiable category, and those with ANCA-negative pauci-immune disease. While both conditions are uncommon, the proportion varies across different regions.

Epidemiology

The incidence of RPGN in children is not known. Crescentic GN comprises about 5 % of unselected renal biopsies in children. While there are no population-based studies in children, a report from Romania suggested an annual incidence of 3.3 per million adult population [18]. The 2010 NAPRTCS Annual Transplant Report shows that idiopathic crescentic GN contributes to 1.7 % of all transplanted patients [19]. This figure is an underestimate since other conditions in the database, including membranoproliferative GN (2.5 %), systemic lupus (1.5 %), systemic immune

disorders (0.3 %), granulomatosis with polyangiitis (0.6 %), chronic GN (3.2 %) and IgA nephropathy and Henoch Schonlein purpura (2.4 %), might present as RPGN.

Table 22.2 outlines the underlying conditions in five series of crescentic GN reported from India [20], United States [14], United Kingdom [16], France [15] and Saudi Arabia [21]. Immune complex GN is the most common pattern of crescentic GN in children accounting for 75–80 % of cases in most reports. Pauci-immune crescentic GN, while common in adults, is less frequent in children, accounting for 15–20 % cases. The decline in the incidence of postinfectious GN has resulted in a change in the profile of crescentic GN. A survey of 73 patients between the ages of 1- and 20-year showed similar frequencies of immune complex (45 %) and pauci-immune crescentic GN (42 %) [1]. The severity of clinical, laboratory and histological features is most with anti-GBM disease, followed by pauci-immune GN and finally immune complex crescentic GN [1, 19].

Clinical Features

The spectrum of presenting features in RPGN is variable, and includes macroscopic hematuria (60–90 % patients), oliguria (60–100 %), hypertension

Table 22.2 Causes of crescentic glomerulonephritis in children (%)

	SPNSG [14] (N=50)	Sinha et al. [20] (N=36)	Niaudet and Levy [12] (N=41)	Jardim et al. [11] (N=30)	Alsaad et al. [21] (N=37)
Immune complex disease					
Unspecified	26	–	4.8	–	13.5
Systemic lupus erythematosus	18	11.1	2.4	3.3	54.1
Poststreptococcal, postinfectious GN	12	8.3	12.1	6.6	16.2
Henoch-Schonlein purpura, IgA nephropathy	14	11.1	34.1	30	
Membranoproliferative GN	4	5.5	21.9	23.3	
Vasculitis, pauci immune GN	6	52.7	7.3	16.6	8.1
Idiopathic crescentic GN	14	11.1	7.3	13.3	
Anti-glomerular basement disease	6		7.3	6.6	
Others	–		2.4	–	8.1

SPNSG Southwest Pediatric Nephrology Study Group, *GN* glomerulonephritis

(60–80%) and edema (60–90%) [9, 12, 14]. The illness is often complicated by occurrence of hypertensive emergencies, pulmonary edema and cardiac failure. Occasionally, RPGN may have an insidious onset with initial symptoms of fatigue or edema. Nephrotic syndrome is rare and seen in patients with less severe renal insufficiency. Systemic complaints, involving the upper respiratory tract (cough, sinusitis), skin (vasculitic rash), musculoskeletal (joint pain, swelling) and nervous system (seizures, altered sensorium) are common in patients with pauci-immune RPGN, with or without ANCA positivity. Relapses of systemic and renal symptoms occur in one-third of patients with vasculitis [2, 12]. Patients with anti-GBM antibody disease present with hemoptysis and, less often, pulmonary hemorrhage. Similar complications are found in granulomatosis with polyangiitis, systemic lupus, Henoch Schonlein purpura and severe GN with pulmonary edema.

Investigations

Hematuria, characterized by dysmorphic red cells and red cell casts is seen in all patients; most also have gross hematuria. A variable degree of non-selective proteinuria (2+ to 4+) is present in more than 65% patients. Urinalysis also shows leukocyte, granular and tubular epithelial cell casts. Renal insufficiency is present at diagnosis, with plasma creatinine concentration often exceeding 3 mg/dL (264 μmol/l). The degree of renal failure is more than that estimated by the serum creatinine. Anemia, if present is mild; peripheral smear shows normocytic normochromic red cells. Non-specific markers of inflammation, including CRP and ESR, are elevated.

Serology

Serological investigations assist in evaluation of the cause and monitoring disease activity (Table 22.3, Fig. 22.1). Low levels of total hemolytic complement (CH50) and complement 3 (C3) are seen in postinfectious GN, systemic lupus and membranoproliferative GN. Patients with lupus and type 1 membranoproliferative GN additionally show reduced levels of C1 and C4 due to activation of the classic complement pathway. Positive antistreptolysin O titers and anti-deoxyribonuclease B suggests streptococcal infection in the past 3 months. Patients with systemic lupus show antinuclear (ANA) and anti-double stranded DNA autoantibodies.

Elevated levels of ANCA suggest an underlying vasculitis, and are present in most patients with pauci-immune crescentic GN. Most ANCA have specificity for myeloperoxidase (MPO) or protein-ase-3 (PR3). ANCA should be screened by indirect immunofluorescence and positive tests confirmed by both PR3-ELISA and MPO-ELISA. In patients with pauci-immune crescentic GN, negative results from immunofluorescence should be tested by ELISA, because 5% serum samples are positive only by the latter. Granulomatosis with polyangiitis is associated with PR3 ANCA, which produces a cytoplasmic staining pattern on immunofluorescence (c-ANCA). Renal limited vasculitis and drug induced pauci-immune crescentic GN are typically associated with MPO ANCA that shows perinuclear staining on immunofluorescence (p-ANCA). Patients with microscopic polyangiitis have equal

Table 22.3 Diagnostic evaluation of patients with rapidly progressive glomerulonephritis

Complete blood counts; peripheral smear for anemia; reticulocyte count; erythrocyte sedimentation rate
Blood levels of urea, creatinine, electrolytes
Urinalysis: proteinuria; microscopy for erythrocytes and leukocytes, casts
Complement levels (C3, C4, CH50)
Antistreptolysin O, antinuclear antibody, anti-double stranded DNA antibodies
Antinuclear cytoplasmic antibodies (ANCA): indirect immunofluorescence, ELISA
Renal biopsy (light microscopy, immunofluorescence, electron microscopy)
Required in specific instances
Anti-GBM IgG antibodies
Blood levels of cryoglobulin, hepatitis B and C serology
Chest: radiograph, CT (patients with Goodpasture syndrome and vasculitides)
Sinuses: radiograph, CT (patients with granulomatosis with polyangiitis)

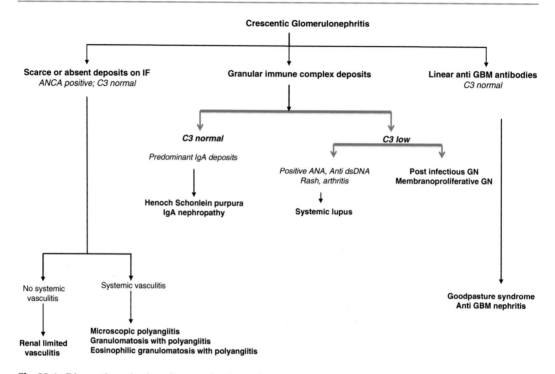

Fig. 22.1 Diagnostic evaluation of crescentic glomerulonephritis, based on renal histology and serological findings

distribution of MPO ANCA/p-ANCA and PR3 ANCA/c-ANCA. Approximately 10% of patients with granulomatosis with polyangiitis or microscopic polyangiitis have negative assays for ANCA. P-ANCA autoantibodies are also found in 20–30% patients with anti-GBM GN, and occasionally in idiopathic immune complex RPGN, inflammatory bowel disease, rheumatoid arthritis and systemic lupus [22].

Apart from diagnosis, ANCA titers have also been used for monitoring activity of systemic vasculitis. Persistent or reappearing ANCA positivity in patients in remission may be associated with disease relapse in ANCA-associated vasculitides. The risk of relapse in patients who show persistently negative ANCA titers is low. An isolated rise in ANCA titers should not be used for modifying treatment in patients with systemic vasculitis [23]. Patients with ANCA-associated crescentic GN in remission, with persistent or reappearing ANCA positivity or rise in its titer, should be closely followed up and diagnostic efforts intensified to detect and treat relapses.

Patients with ANCA-associated vasculitis occasionally show autoantibodies to human lysosome-associated membrane protein-2 (hLAMP-2) [24]. These antibodies were also seen in few patients with pauci-immune focal necrotizing crescentic GN who were negative for ANCA [25]. The hLAMP-2 autoantibodies became undetectable following initiation of immunosuppressive treatment and were detected during clinical relapse.

High titers of anti-GBM IgG antibodies, demonstrated by immunofluorescence or ELISA, are seen in anti-GBM nephritis or Goodpasture syndrome and correlate with disease activity. About 5% of ANCA positive samples are also anti-GBM positive and approximately 20–30% of anti-GBM positive samples are ANCA positive. Serology for ANCA is therefore recommended in all patients with either anti-GBM antibodies in blood or linear IgG deposition along the GBM. The initial clinical outcome for these patients is similar to that of anti-GBM disease, though relapses may occur as in systemic vasculitis [1].

Renal Histology

Light Microscopy

Renal histological findings in various forms of crescentic GN are similar. A glomerular crescent is an accumulation of two or more layers of cells that partially or completely fill the Bowman space. The crescent size varies from circumferential to segmental depending on the plane of the tissue section and the underlying disease. Crescents in anti-GBM nephritis or ANCA associated disease are usually circumferential, while they are often segmental in immune complex GN. Interstitial changes range from acute inflammatory infiltrate to chronic interstitial scarring and tubular atrophy. Once the glomerular capillary loop is compressed by the crescent, tubules that derive their blood flow from that efferent arteriole show ischemic changes.

Crescents may be completely cellular or show variable scarring and fibrosis. Cellular crescents are characterized by proliferation of macrophages, epithelial cells and neutrophils (Fig. 22.2). Fibrocellular crescents show admixture of collagen fibers and membrane proteins amongst the cells (Figs. 22.3 and 22.4). In fibrous crescents, the cells are replaced by collagen. Renal biopsies from patients with vasculitis show crescents in various stages of progression indicating episodic inflammation. Early lesions have segmental fibrinoid necrosis with or without an adjacent small crescent. Severe acute lesions show focal or diffuse necrosis in association with circumferential crescents. Features of small vessel vasculitis, affecting interlobular arteries (Fig. 22.5) and rarely angiitis involving the vasa recta might be seen.

Based on light microscopy findings, a new classification is proposed for ANCA associated GN [26]. Biopsies are categorized as focal, crescentic and sclerotic based on the predominance of normal glomeruli, cellular crescents, and globally sclerotic glomeruli, respectively. A fourth category represents a mixed or heterogeneous phenotype. Although the classification system is believed to have prognostic value for 1- and 5-year renal outcomes, and may guide therapy, it needs to be validated in children.

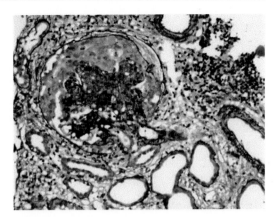

Fig. 22.2 Cellular crescent compressing the glomerular tuft. Silver methanamine stain ×800

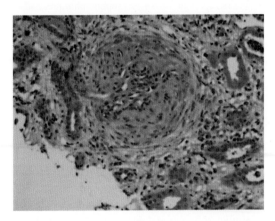

Fig. 22.3 Fibrocellular crescent with compression of glomerular tuft and partial sclerosis. There is chronic interstitial inflammation, tubular atrophy and interstitial fibrosis in surrounding area. H&E ×800

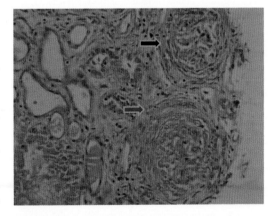

Fig. 22.4 Glomeruli showing cellular (*red arrow*) and fibrocellular crescents (*black arrow*) causing compression of underlying glomerular tuft. Note the disruption of Bowman capsule. H&E ×200

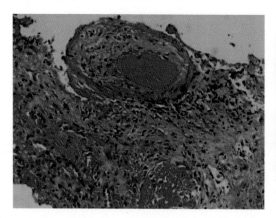

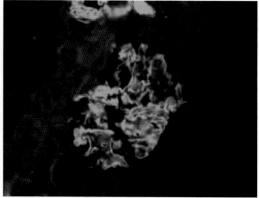

Fig. 22.5 A patient with pauci-immune crescentic glomerulonephritis. A small artery shows features of active vasculitis; its wall shows neutrophil infiltration, fibrin deposition and lumen occluded by a thrombus. Perivascular area shows interstitial hemorrhage and inflammation. H&E ×600

Fig. 22.6 Immunofluorescence microscopy (×1200) in a patient with anti-glomerular basement membrane antibody- mediated crescentic glomerulonephritis showing linear deposition of IgG on the capillary wall

Immunohistology and Electron Microscopy

These investigations assist in determining the cause of crescentic GN, based on presence, location and nature of immune deposits. The crescents stain strongly for fibrin on immunofluorescence [27]. Mesangial deposits of IgA are found in IgA nephropathy and Henoch Schonlein purpura; granular, subepithelial deposits of IgG and C3 in postinfectious GN; mesangial, subendothelial and intramembranous deposits of IgG and C3 in MPGN; and "full house" capillary wall and mesangial deposits of granular IgG, IgA, IgM, C3, C4 and C1q in systemic lupus erythematosus. Glomeruli of patients with vasculitis, both with and without ANCA positivity, have few or no immune deposits. Anti-GBM disease is characterized by linear staining of the GBM with IgG (rarely IgM and IgA) and C3 (Fig. 22.6).

Evaluation and Diagnosis

It is necessary to make an accurate and rapid diagnosis in RPGN as treatment strategies vary and delay in instituting treatment results in risk of irreversible disease. All patients should undergo a kidney biopsy promptly. While the majority shows the presence of crescentic GN, the detection of thrombotic microangiopathy (affecting interlobular arteries and arterioles) or diffuse proliferative GN is not unusual. The diagnosis of the etiology of crescentic GN depends on integration of clinical data and findings on serology and renal histology (Table 22.3, Fig. 22.1). In this way, anti-GBM disease or ANCA-associated RPGN can be distinguished from other conditions.

Treatment

The heterogeneity and unsatisfactory outcome of RPGN has led to institution of multiple treatments. Evidence based data are limited and treatment guidelines for children are based on data from case series and prospective studies in adults [28]. Supportive management includes maintenance of fluid and electrolyte balance, providing adequate nutrition, and control of infections and hypertension.

Specific treatment of RPGN comprises two phases: *induction* of remission and *maintenance* (Table 22.4). The first phase aims at control of inflammation and the associated immune response. Once remission is induced, the maintenance phase attempts to prevent further renal damage and relapses. Combination therapy with high dose steroids and cyclophosphamide is standard *induction* treatment, with additional therapy for those with life or organ threatening disease.

Table 22.4 Treatment of crescentic glomerulonephritis

Induction
Methylprednisolone 15–20 mg/kg (maximum 1 g) IV daily for 3–6 doses
Prednisolone 1.5–2 mg/kg/day PO for 4 weeks; taper to 0.5 mg/kg daily by 3 months; 0.5–1 mg/kg on alternate day for 3 months
[a]Cyclophosphamide 500–750 mg/m² IV every 3–4 weeks for 6 pulses
[b]Plasma exchange (double volume) on alternate days for 2-weeks
[c]Rituximab: 375 mg/m² weekly for 4 weeks
Maintenance
Azathioprine 1.5–2 mg/kg/d for 12–18 months
Alternate day low dose prednisolone
Consider mycophenolate mofetil (1000–1200 mg/m²day) or cyclosporine if disease activity is not controlled with azathioprine or patient does not tolerate azathioprine
Agents for refractory disease
Intravenous immunoglobulin, TNF-α antibody (infliximab), rituximab

[a]The dose of cyclophosphamide may be increased to 750 mg/m² if no leukopenia before next dose. Dose reduction is necessary in patients showing impaired renal function. Alternatively, the medication is given orally at a dose of 2 mg/kg daily for 12 weeks
[b]Plasma exchange should begin early, especially if patient is dialysis dependent at presentation or if biopsy shows severe histological changes (>50 % crescents). Plasma exchange is useful in anti-GBM nephritis and ANCA-associated vasculitis. It should be considered in patients with immune complex crescentic GN if there is unsatisfactory renal recovery after steroid pulses
[c]Rituximab may be used as an alternative initial treatment if cyclophosphamide is contraindicated

Treatment includes IV pulses of methylprednisolone (15–20 mg/kg, maximum 1 g/day) for 3–6 days, followed by high-dose oral prednisone (1.5–2 mg/kg daily) for 4 weeks, with tapering to 0.5 mg/kg daily by 3 months and alternate day prednisone for 6–12 months.

Cyclophosphamide is an important part of the induction regimen, and most centers prefer the use of IV compared to oral therapy. The European Vasculitis Study Group (EUVAS) compared IV pulse cyclophosphamide (15 mg/kg every 2 weeks for three pulses, followed by pulses at 3-week intervals until remission, and then for another 3 months) with daily oral cyclophosphamide (2 mg/kg/day) for induction of remission

[29]. They showed that the time to remission and proportion of patients in remission at 9 months was similar in both groups. The cumulative dose of cyclophosphamide in the daily oral group was twice that in IV group (15.9 g vs. 8.2 g; $P < 0.001$), and the latter had lower rate of leukopenia. A meta-analysis of nonrandomized studies showed that pulse cyclophosphamide was significantly more likely to induce remission and had a lower risk of infection and leukopenia. Pulse cyclophosphamide dosing may, however, be associated with a greater risk of relapses, exposing patients to further immunosuppression [30]. The dose of oral and IV cyclophosphamide is 2 mg/kg/day and 500–750 mg/m² respectively. The dose should be adjusted to maintain a nadir leukocyte count, 2-weeks' post treatment, of 3000–4000/cu mm.

B cell depletion with rituximab is emerging as an important component of induction therapy. It has been used successfully in patients with refractory lupus nephritis and in granulomatosis with polyangiitis [31]. The Rituximab in ANCA-Associated Vasculitis (RAVE) trial compare rituximab with standard therapy for inducing remission in patients with ANCA associated vasculitis [32]. Patients received either rituximab (375 mg/m²/week for 4 weeks) or cyclophosphamide (2 mg/kg/day). Both groups received one to three pulses of methylprednisolone (1000 mg each), followed by tapering dose of prednisone. At 6 months, 64 % in the rituximab group achieved remission without the use of prednisone at 6 months, as compared to 53 % in the control group. Rituximab was efficacious in inducing remission of relapsing disease. The authors concluded that therapy with rituximab was not inferior to treatment with cyclophosphamide for induction of remission, and may be superior in patients with relapsing disease. The RITUXVAS study randomized patients with ANCA associated vasculitis to receive a standard steroid regimen plus either rituximab (375 mg/m²/week for 4 weeks) with two IV cyclophosphamide pulses (n = 33), or IV cyclophosphamide for 3–6 months followed by azathioprine (n = 11) [33]. There was no significant difference in the rate of remission, severe adverse events and death in the two groups.

Therapy with rituximab appears promising in patients with ANCA associated vasculitis.

Mycophenolate mofetil (MMF) has been used in observational studies as part of induction therapy, though it may have a greater role in the maintenance phase. While the rate of remission was high, there was a risk of relapse [34]. Results from the EUVAS MYCYC trial, comparing MMF and cyclophosphamide for induction of remission, are awaited. A number of studies have examined the efficacy of IV immunoglobulin in subjects with ANCA associated vasculitis and RPGN, with benefit lasting for up to 3-months [35]. The exact mechanism of action is unclear with evidence for both non-specific anti-inflammatory and anticytokine effects and specific correction of immunoregulatory defects. In a study on 34 patients with persistent disease activity, 14/17 patients in the IV immunoglobulin group had reduction in disease activity, compared to 6/17 in the placebo group [34]. The precise indications for initial or adjunctive treatment with this agent need to be defined.

The NORAM study compared the effectiveness of orally administered methotrexate and cyclophosphamide in adult patients with early systemic vasculitis and mild renal involvement [36]. Induction of remission was similar at 6 months (90 % versus 94 % respectively), but relapses were more frequent after treatment withdrawal in methotrexate treated patients. Methotrexate is not recommended for patients with moderate to severe renal dysfunction.

The requirement for maintenance therapy in crescentic GN depends on the underlying disease. Most patients with ANCA-associated disease need long-term maintenance immunosuppression due to the risk of relapses. Extended treatment with cyclophosphamide has been used in adults, but carries significant risks and is currently not preferred for children. While azathioprine does not appear to be effective at inducing remission, it is useful for long-term prevention of relapses. The timing of the switch from cyclophosphamide to azathioprine was clarified by the CYCAZAREM trial, which compared switching from cyclophosphamide to maintenance azathioprine at three versus 12 months [37]. Those converted to azathioprine at 3 months had similar remission rates, renal function and patient survival compared to those continuing on cyclophosphamide at 18 months. The duration of maintenance treatment is debatable, with most patients of pauci-immune crescentic GN treated for 2 or more years.

MMF is increasingly being used as an alternative to azathioprine for maintenance therapy in patients with ANCA associated vasculitis. The IMPROVE trial (International Mycophenolate Mofetil Protocol to Reduce Outbreaks of Vasculitides), however, showed that relapses were significantly more common in patients receiving MMF compared to azathioprine (unadjusted hazard ratio 1.69 for MMF), with no difference in severe adverse events [38]. The KDIGO (Kidney Disease: Improving Global Outcomes) Clinical Practice Guideline for Glomerulonephritis recommends using azathioprine as the first choice for maintenance therapy in ANCA vasculitis, and considering MMF as an alternative in patients who are allergic to or intolerant of azathioprine [39].

Plasmapheresis

Plasmapheresis or plasma exchange has been used for the treatment of crescentic GN with variable success. The mechanism of action is not clear, but is believed to involve removal of pathogenic autoantibodies, complement and coagulation factors and cytokines. Plasma exchange has been shown, in controlled trials in adults, to have therapeutic benefit in anti-GBM disease with clearance of antibodies, lower serum creatinine and improved patient and renal survival [40]. However, adults who were anuric with severe azotemia, dialysis dependent or those who had more than 85 % crescents on renal biopsy showed minimal benefit. The role of intensive plasma exchange versus IV methylprednisolone, in addition to oral steroids and cyclophosphamide, was examined by the MEPEX trial in patients with ANCA associated vasculitis and serum creatinine >500 μmol/l (5.65 mg/dl) at presentation [41]. Patients receiving plasma exchange were likely to be off dialysis at 3-months (69 % vs. 49 %) and lower risk of progression to end stage renal failure at 12 months, but with limited benefits on long-term renal function or survival. Another study showed that plasma exchange improved medium-term renal survival, even when initiated in patients with serum creatinine levels >250 μmol/L (2.85 mg/dL) [42].

Retrospective data in children with RPGN show benefits of plasma exchange if commenced within 1 month of onset of the disease [43]. Anecdotal reports confirm the efficacy of plasmapheresis in patients with RPGN due to lupus, Henoch Schonlein purpura and severe proliferative GN, and in life-threatening pulmonary hemorrhage. Prospective studies in patients with pauci-immune crescentic GN suggest that discontinuation of dialysis and renal recovery was better with plasma exchange and immunosuppression *vs.* immunosuppression alone [44]. However, a recent meta-analysis (nine randomized trials; 387 adult patients) on renal vasculitis or idiopathic RPGN, did not show evidence that adjunctive plasma exchange improved renal and patient survival [45]. Despite individual studies showing up to 20 % reduction in risk of progression to ESRD, there were overall too few patients randomized for reliable conclusions.

KDIGO Clinical Practice Guideline for Glomerulonephritis recommends plasma exchange with 60 ml/kg volume replacement [39]. For vasculitis, seven treatments over 14 days are prescribed and for vasculitis with anti-GBM antibodies, daily exchanges are done for 14 days or until anti-GBM antibodies are undetectable.

Immune Complex Crescentic GN

Therapy for these patients depends on the underlying disease. The treatment of IgA nephropathy and lupus nephritis presenting with RPGN is discussed in Chaps. 19 and 28, respectively.

Postinfectious RPGN

Poststreptococcal GN presenting with extensive crescents is rare and the benefits of intensive immunosuppressive therapy are unclear, since most patients recover spontaneously. Nevertheless, immunosuppressive therapy with corticosteroids and alkylating agents has been used in patients with renal failure and extensive glomerular crescents [14, 46]. Despite the lack of evidence-based data, we suggest that patients with postinfectious RPGN and crescents involving 50 % or more glomeruli be treated with three to six IV pulses of methylprednisolone, followed by tapering doses of oral steroids for 6 months. Therapy is combined with cyclophosphamide, administered orally (for 3 months) or IV (monthly for 6 months). Eradication of the infection and/or removal of infected prostheses are necessary for resolution of immune complex GN associated with active infections. Patients with idiopathic immune complex crescentic GN should be treated similarly to those with pauci-immune crescentic GN.

Pauci-Immune Crescentic GN

Induction therapy consists of IV pulses of methylprednisolone (daily for 3–6 days) followed by oral prednisone and cyclophosphamide (orally for 3 months, or IV every 3–4 weeks for 6 months) [2, 28]. Intensive plasma exchanges for 2 weeks have been recommended for children who are dialysis dependent, those with pulmonary hemorrhage or not responding satisfactorily to induction treatment [41]. Therapy during the maintenance phase is comprised of tapering doses of oral prednisolone and azathioprine, usually for 18–24 months. A longer duration of therapy, extended to 3–5 years, is required in patients showing relapses, elevated ANCA titers and those with PR3-ANCA [2]. Approximately one-third patients have one or more relapses, requiring reinstitution of induction therapy with cyclophosphamide. Less intensive treatment with mycophenolate mofetil has been proposed for relapses that are mild and diagnosed early. Since intensive immunosuppression is associated with risk of infection, the use of prophylactic antimicrobials especially against *Pneumocystis carinii* and *Candida* may be required during induction. Patients are also at risk of other complications of therapy with corticosteroids and alkylating agents.

Anti-GBM Crescentic GN

Prompt institution of plasma exchange is necessary in these patients. Double volume exchange is done daily, and subsequently on alternate days until anti-GBM antibodies are no longer detectable (usually 2–3 weeks) [1, 28]. The patients are also treated with IV methylprednisolone (20 mg/kg on alternate days) followed by high-dose oral prednisolone. Co-administration of cyclophosphamide (2 mg/kg daily for 3 months) is effective in suppressing further antibody production. Pulmonary hemorrhage responds to plasma exchange and IV steroids. As anti-GBM disease does not usually have a relapsing course, long-term maintenance therapy is not required and steroids can be tapered over the next 6–9 months. Patients treated early in the course of their illness do satisfactorily. In patients who develop end stage renal disease, transplantation should be deferred until anti-GBM antibodies are undetectable for 12 months, at which point disease recurrence is unlikely.

A proportion of patients with anti-GBM nephritis also show positive ANCA, most often p-ANCA. While the precise significance of the dual positivity is unclear, their outcome is similar to classical anti-GBM disease. In view of a higher risk of relapses, these patients require a longer course of maintenance immunosuppressive therapy (as for ANCA associated GN).

Newer Agents

T lymphocyte depletion with monoclonal anti-CD52 antibody, alemtuzumab or CAMPATH 1-H has been tried with variable success in patients with granulomatosis with polyangiitis and other vasculitides [47]. In a retrospective cohort study 85 % of patients with refractory ANCA associated vasculitis achieved remission after alemtuzumab, but the majority relapsed after a median of 9 months [34]. Patients with refractory granulomatosis with polyangiitis show satisfactory response to therapy with anti-thymocyte globulin and infliximab. Other agents used include gusperimus (15-deoxyspergualin) and newer

monoclonals including humanized anti-CD20 and anti-CD22 antibodies, and an antibody that inhibits B lymphocyte stimulating protein (BLyS).

Outcome

The outcome for patients has improved in the last decades, such that almost 60–70 % of patients show normal renal function on the long term. Patients with poststreptococcal crescentic GN have a better prognosis, with most showing spontaneous improvement. The prognosis is better in patients with poststreptococcal crescentic GN with subepithelial, rather than subendothelial or intramembranous deposits. Outcomes in patients with pauci-immune crescentic GN, MPGN and idiopathic RPGN are less favorable than Henoch Schonlein purpura or systemic lupus. ESRD may occur in the long-term in up to 25 % patients with ANCA associated vasculitis.

The outcome is determined by the severity of renal failure at presentation and promptness of intervention, renal histology and underlying diagnosis [1, 2, 28]. Studies have shown that the use of plasma exchange, high percentage of normal glomeruli, and absence of glomerulosclerosis, tubular atrophy and arteriosclerosis, were associated with better renal recovery [48]. The potential for recovery corresponds with the relative proportion of cellular or fibrous components in the crescents, and the extent of tubulointerstitial scarring and fibrosis.

Post Transplant Recurrence

Based on experience in adult patients, we suggest that patients with ANCA positive vasculitis should have sustained remission for 1-year before considering a transplant [49]. A positive ANCA titer at the time of transplantation does not increase the risk of allograft recurrence. While the use of immunosuppression following transplantation and different antigenic characteristics of the allograft prevent severe recurrences, better graft survival might increase this risk. Conditions associated with a higher risk of histological recurrence include MPGN type II, IgA nephropathy, Henoch Schonlein purpura and lupus. Graft losses are uncommon and occur in <5 % cases.

References

1. Jennette JC. Rapidly progressive crescentic glomerulonephritis. Kidney Int. 2003;63(3):1164–77.
2. Morgan MD, Harper L, Williams J, Savage C. Antineutrophil cytoplasm-associated glomerulonephritis. J Am Soc Nephrol. 2006;17(5):1224–34.
3. Atkins RC, Nikolic-Paterson DJ, Song Q, Lan HY. Modulators of crescentic glomerulonephritis. J Am Soc Nephrol. 1996;7(11):2271–8.
4. Thorner PS, Ho M, Eremina V, Sado Y, Quaggin S. Podocytes contribute to the formation of glomerular crescents. J Am Soc Nephrol. 2008;19(3):495–502.
5. Tipping PG, Holdsworth SR. T cells in crescentic glomerulonephritis. J Am Soc Nephrol. 2006;17(5):1253–63.
6. Paust HJ, Ostmann A, Erhardt A, et al. Regulatory T cells control the Th1 immune response in murine crescentic glomerulonephritis. Kidney Int. 2011;80(2):154–64.
7. Bollée G, Flamant M, Schordan S, et al. Epidermal growth factor receptor promotes glomerular injury and renal failure in rapidly progressive crescentic glomerulonephritis. Nat Med. 2011;17(10):1242–50.
8. Ophascharoensuk V, Pippin JW, Gordon KL, Shankland SJ, Couser WG, Johnson RJ. Role of intrinsic renal cells versus infiltrating cells in glomerular crescent formation. Kidney Int. 1998;54(2):416–25.
9. Srivastava RN, Moudgil A, Bagga A, Vasudev AS, Bhuyan UN, Sundraem KR. Crescentic glomerulonephritis in children: a review of 43 cases. Am J Nephrol. 1992;12(3):155–61.
10. El-Husseini AA, Sheashaa HA, Sabry AA, Moustafa FE, Sobh MA. Acute postinfectious crescentic glomerulonephritis: clinicopathologic presentation and risk factors. Int Urol Nephrol. 2005;37(3):603–9.
11. Hoschek JC, Dreyer P, Dahal S, Walker PD. Rapidly progressive renal failure in childhood. Am J Kidney Dis. 2002;40(6):1342–7.
12. Hattori M, Kurayama H, Koitabashi Y, Nephrology JSfP. Antineutrophil cytoplasmic autoantibody-associated glomerulonephritis in children. J Am Soc Nephrol. 2001;12(7):1493–500.
13. Chen M, Kallenberg CG, Zhao MH. ANCA-negative pauci-immune crescentic glomerulonephritis. Nat Rev Nephrol. 2009;5(6):313–8.
14. A clinico-pathologic study of crescentic glomerulonephritis in 50 children. A report of the Southwest Pediatric Nephrology Study Group. Kidney Int. 1985;27(2):450–8.
15. Niaudet P, Levy M. Glomerulonephritis a croissants diffuse. In: Royer P, Habib R, Mathieu H, Broyer M, editors. Nephrologie Pediatrique. 3rd ed. Paris: Flammarion; 1983. p. 381–94.
16. Jardim HM, Leake J, Risdon RA, Barratt TM, Dillon MJ. Crescentic glomerulonephritis in children. Pediatr Nephrol. 1992;6(3):231–5.
17. Kashtan CE. Renal transplantation in patients with Alport syndrome. Pediatr Transplant. 2006;10(6):651–7.
18. Covic A, Schiller A, Volovat C, et al. Epidemiology of renal disease in Romania: a 10 year review of two regional renal biopsy databases. Nephrol Dial Transplant. 2006;21(2):419–24.
19. Studies NAPRTaC. NAPRTCS 2010 Annual report. 2010. https://web.emmes.com/study/ped/annlrept/annlrept2006.
20. Sinha A, Puri K, Hari P, Dinda AK, Bagga A. Etiology and outcome of crescentic glomerulonephritis. Indian Pediatr. 2013;50(3):283–8.
21. Alsaad K, Oudah N, Al Ameer A, Fakeeh K, Al Jomaih A, Al Sayyari A. Glomerulonephritis with crescents in children: etiology and predictors of renal outcome. ISRN Pediatr. 2011;2011:507298.
22. Bosch X, Guilabert A, Font J. Antineutrophil cytoplasmic antibodies. Lancet. 2006;368(9533):404–18.
23. Schmitt WH, van der Woude FJ. Clinical applications of antineutrophil cytoplasmic antibody testing. Curr Opin Rheumatol. 2004;16(1):9–17.
24. Kain R, Tadema H, McKinney EF, et al. High prevalence of autoantibodies to hLAMP-2 in anti-neutrophil cytoplasmic antibody-associated vasculitis. J Am Soc Nephrol. 2012;23(3):556–66.
25. Peschel A, Basu N, Benharkou A, et al. Autoantibodies to hLAMP-2 in ANCA-negative pauci-immune focal necrotizing GN. J Am Soc Nephrol. 2014;25(3):455–63.
26. Berden AE, Ferrario F, Hagen EC, et al. Histopathologic classification of ANCA-associated glomerulonephritis. J Am Soc Nephrol. 2010;21(10):1628–36.
27. Levy J, Pusey C. Crescentic glomerulonephritis. In: Davison AMA, Cameron JS, Grunfeld J-P, et al., editors. Oxford textbook of clinical nephrology. 3rd ed. Oxford: Oxford University Press; 2005.
28. Jindal KK. Management of idiopathic crescentic and diffuse proliferative glomerulonephritis: evidence-based recommendations. Kidney Int Suppl. 1999;70:S33–40.
29. de Groot K, Harper L, Jayne DR, et al. Pulse versus daily oral cyclophosphamide for induction of remission in antineutrophil cytoplasmic antibody-associated vasculitis: a randomized trial. Ann Intern Med. 2009;150(10):670–80.
30. de Groot K, Adu D, Savage CO, EUVAS (European vasculitis study group). The value of pulse cyclophosphamide in ANCA-associated vasculitis: meta-analysis and critical review. Nephrol Dial Transplant. 2001;16(10):2018–27.
31. Keogh KA, Ytterberg SR, Fervenza FC, Carlson KA, Schroeder DR, Specks U. Rituximab for refractory Wegener's granulomatosis: report of a prospective,

open-label pilot trial. Am J Respir Crit Care Med. 2006;173(2):180–7.

32. Stone JH, Merkel PA, Spiera R, et al. Rituximab versus cyclophosphamide for ANCA-associated vasculitis. N Engl J Med. 2010;363(3):221–32.

33. Jones RB, Tervaert JW, Hauser T, et al. Rituximab versus cyclophosphamide in ANCA-associated renal vasculitis. N Engl J Med. 2010;363(3):211–20.

34. Smith RM, Jones RB, Jayne DR. Progress in treatment of ANCA-associated vasculitis. Arthritis Res Ther. 2012;14(2):210.

35. Ito-Ihara T, Ono T, Nogaki F, et al. Clinical efficacy of intravenous immunoglobulin for patients with MPO-ANCA-associated rapidly progressive glomerulonephritis. Nephron Clin Pract. 2006;102(1):c35–42.

36. De Groot K, Rasmussen N, Bacon PA, et al. Randomized trial of cyclophosphamide versus methotrexate for induction of remission in early systemic antineutrophil cytoplasmic antibody-associated vasculitis. Arthritis Rheum. 2005;52(8):2461–9.

37. Jayne D, Rasmussen N, Andrassy K, et al. A randomized trial of maintenance therapy for vasculitis associated with antineutrophil cytoplasmic autoantibodies. N Engl J Med. 2003;349(1):36–44.

38. Hiemstra TF, Walsh M, Mahr A, et al. Mycophenolate mofetil vs azathioprine for remission maintenance in antineutrophil cytoplasmic antibody-associated vasculitis: a randomized controlled trial. JAMA. 2010;304(21):2381–8.

39. Group KDIGOKGW. KDIGO clinical practice guideline for glomerulonephritis. Kidney Int. 2012;2 (Supplement):139–274.

40. Levy JB, Turner AN, Rees AJ, Pusey CD. Long-term outcome of anti-glomerular basement membrane antibody disease treated with plasma exchange and immunosuppression. Ann Intern Med. 2001;134(11): 1033–42.

41. Jayne DR, Gaskin G, Rasmussen N, et al. Randomized trial of plasma exchange or high-dosage methylprednisolone as adjunctive therapy for severe renal vasculitis. J Am Soc Nephrol. 2007;18(7):2180–8.

42. Szpirt WM, Heaf JG, Petersen J. Plasma exchange for induction and cyclosporine A for maintenance of remission in Wegener's granulomatosis – a clinical randomized controlled trial. Nephrol Dial Transplant. 2011;26(1):206–13.

43. Gianviti A, Trompeter RS, Barratt TM, Lythgoe MF, Dillon MJ. Retrospective study of plasma exchange in patients with idiopathic rapidly progressive glomerulonephritis and vasculitis. Arch Dis Child. 1996;75(3):186–90.

44. Pusey CD, Rees AJ, Evans DJ, Peters DK, Lockwood CM. Plasma exchange in focal necrotizing glomerulonephritis without anti-GBM antibodies. Kidney Int. 1991;40(4):757–63.

45. Walsh M, Catapano F, Szpirt W, et al. Plasma exchange for renal vasculitis and idiopathic rapidly progressive glomerulonephritis: a meta-analysis. Am J Kidney Dis. 2011;57(4):566–74.

46. Raff A, Hebert T, Pullman J, Coco M. Crescentic post-streptococcal glomerulonephritis with nephrotic syndrome in the adult: is aggressive therapy warranted? Clin Nephrol. 2005;63(5):375–80.

47. Jayne D. What place for the new biologics in the treatment of necrotising vasculitides. Clin Exp Rheumatol. 2006;24(2 Suppl 41):S1–5.

48. de Lind van Wijngaarden RA, Hauer HA, Wolterbeek R, et al. Chances of renal recovery for dialysis-dependent ANCA-associated glomerulonephritis. J Am Soc Nephrol. 2007;18(7):2189–97.

49. Little MA, Hassan B, Jacques S, et al. Renal transplantation in systemic vasculitis: when is it safe? Nephrol Dial Transplant. 2009;24(10):3219–25.

Part V

Complement Disorders

The Role of Complement in Disease

23

Christoph Licht and Michael Kirschfink

Abbreviations

aHUS	Atypical hemolytic uremic syndrome
AMR	Antibody-mediated rejection
ANCA	Anti-neutrophil cytoplasmic antibodies
AP	Alternative pathway
C3G	C3 glomerulopathy
C3NeF	C3 nephritic factor
CFB	Complement factor B
CFH	Complement factor H
CFHR	Complement factor H related protein
CFI	Complement factor I
CP	Classical pathway
CR1	Complement receptor 1 (CD35)
CR2	Complement receptor 2 (CD21)
DAF	Decay accelerating factor (CD55)
DDD	Dense deposit disease
DSA	Donor specific antibodies
ESRD	End-stage renal disease
HAE 1/2	Hereditary angioedema type 1/2
IgA-N	IgA nephropathy
LP	Lectin pathway
MAC	Membrane attack complex (C5b-9)
MCP	Membrane cofactor protein (CD46)
MPGN	Membranoproliferative glomerulonephritis
PI	Plasma infusion
PLEX	Plasma exchange
PNH	Paroxysmal nocturnal hemoglobinuria
SCR	Short consensus repeat
STEC HUS	Shiga toxin producing E. coli HUS
THBD	Thrombomodulin (CD141)
TMA	Thrombotic microangiopathy

C. Licht (✉)
Division of Nephrology,
The Hospital for Sick Children,
555 University Avenue, Toronto, ON, M5G 1X8,
Canada
e-mail: christoph.licht@sickkids.ca

M. Kirschfink
Institute of Immunology, University of Heidelberg,
Im Neuenheimer Feld 305, 69120, Heidelberg,
Germany
e-mail: kirschfink@uni-hd.de

The Emerging Concept of Complement-Mediated Diseases

As a key mediator of inflammation complement also significantly contributes to tissue damage in various clinical disorders [1]. Clinical and experimental evidence underlines the prominent role of complement [2–4] in the pathogenesis of numerous inflammatory diseases including immune complex and autoimmune disorders, such as systemic lupus erythematosus and autoimmune arthritis.

© Springer-Verlag Berlin Heidelberg 2016
D.F. Geary, F. Schaefer (eds.), *Pediatric Kidney Disease*, DOI 10.1007/978-3-662-52972-0_23

Complement deficiencies represent approximately 4–5% of all primary immunodeficiencies, in part closely connected with renal disorders.

In clinical practice, overactivation of the complement system is the cause of several inflammatory diseases and life-threatening conditions, such as adult respiratory distress syndrome (ARDS) [5], the systemic inflammatory response syndrome (SIRS), sepsis [6], and multi-organ failure after severe trauma, burns or infections [7]. Complement has also been implicated in neurodegenerative disorders, such as Alzheimer's disease, multiple sclerosis, and Guillain-Barré syndrome. In recent years complement activation has also been recognized as a major effector mechanism of ischemia/reperfusion injury [8, 9].

The inflammatory response induced by artificial surfaces in hemodialysis and other extracorporeal circuits may lead to organ dysfunction. Here, complement activation has been shown to be associated with transient neutropenia, pulmonary vascular leukostasis and even occasionally with anaphylactic shock of variable severity [10, 11].

The Complement System

Complement is a vital part of the body's innate immune system and provides a highly effective means for the destruction of invading microorganisms and immune complex elimination [12, 13]. In addition, complement also modulates the adaptive immune response through modification of T- and B-cell responses employing specific receptors on various immune cells [14]. Moreover, a normally functioning complement system also participates in hematopoiesis, reproduction, lipid metabolism and tissue regeneration [15].

Complement can be activated via three pathways (Fig. 23.1), the classical, the alternative, and the lectin pathway, all of which merge in the activation of complement C3 and subsequently lead to

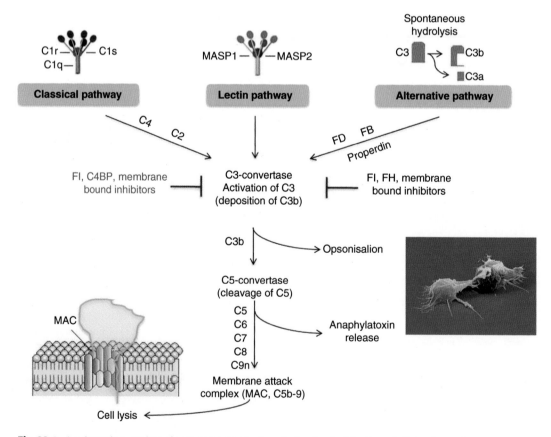

Fig. 23.1 A schematic overview of complement activation via the classical, lectin and alternative pathways

the formation of the cytolytic membrane attack complex (MAC), C5b-9. Following complement activation, the biologically active peptides (anaphylatoxins) C5a and C3a are released and elicit a number of proinflammatory effects, such as chemotaxis of leukocytes, degranulation of phagocytic cells, mast cells and basophils, smooth muscle contraction, and increase of vascular permeabiltiy [16, 17]. Upon cell activation by these complement split products the inflammatory response is further amplified by subsequent generation of toxic oxygen radicals and the induction of synthesis and release of arachidonic acid metabolites and cytokines. Consequently, an over-activated complement system presents a considerable risk of harming the host by directly and indirectly mediating inflammatory tissue destruction [1].

Under physiological conditions, activation of complement is effectively controlled by the coordinated action of soluble as well as membrane-associated regulatory proteins [18]. Soluble complement regulators, such as C1 inhibitor, C4b-binding protein (C4bp), factors H (CFH) and

I (CFI), clusterin and S-protein (vitronectin) restrict the action of complement in body fluids at multiple sites of the cascade (Fig. 23.1). In addition, each individual host cell is protected against the attack of homologous complement by surface proteins, such as the complement receptor 1 (CR1/CD35), the membrane cofactor protein (MCP/CD46) as well as by the glycosylphosphatidylinositol (GPI)-anchored proteins, decay-accelerating factor (DAF/CD55), and protectin (CD59) [18].

Diagnosing Complement-Mediated Diseases

Detecting Complement Activation

In recent years, great progress has been made in complement analysis to better define disease severity, evolution and response to therapy (Tables 23.1 and 23.2) [19]. However, a comprehensive analysis going beyond C3 and C4 is still performed only in specialized laboratories (www.

Table 23.1 Biochemical complement analysis

Functional assays	*Total complement activity (screening for complement deficiency)*	
	CH50 and AH50 hemolytic assays for CP and AP activity	
	Enzyme immunoassays (ELISA) for specific evaluation of CP, LP and AP activity using C5b-9 as readout	
	Functional activity of single components	
	Hemolytic assays for single components (e.g., C3) using corresponding deficient sera as test system	
	ELISA for MBL/MASP functional activity using deposition of C4 as readout	
	C1 inhibitor assay (chromogenic assay or EIA) for diagnosis of HAE	
Proteins	*Concentration of single components by immunoprecipitation (RID, nephelometry, ELISA)*	
	C3 and C4 to detect "hypocomplementemia"	
	Follow-up of a low activity detected in total complement activity screening (any component)	
	C5–C9, properdin, MBL at recurrent neisserial infections	
	C1 inhibitor for diagnosis of HAE type 1 and acquired angioedema	
Activation products	*Concentrations of split products or protein-protein complexes by ELISAs, preferentially based on antibodies to neoepitopes expressed selectively on the activation products*	
	Split products from components after proteolytic cleavage (e.g., C3a, C4a, C5a, Ba, Bb)	
	Complexes between the activated component and its inhibitor (e.g., C1rs-C1 inhibitor)	
	Macromolecular complexes (e.g., the AP convertase C3bBbP and the terminal sC5b-9 complex)	
Autoantibodies	*Assessment of autoantibody concentrations by ELISA or functional assay*	
	Anti-C1q – SLE; anti-C1 inhibitor – angioedema; anti-CFH – aHUS; C3 NeF – C3G/MPGN	
Surface proteins	*Flowcytometric quantification*	
	DAF/CD55 and CD59 for diagnosis of PNH	

Table 23.2 Recommended complement analysis in nephropathies

Disease	Analysis
Systemic lupus erythematosus	CH50, C1q, C4 (C4A/B), C3, C3d or sC5b-9, anti-C1q autoantibodies
Atypical hemolytic uremic syndrome	CH50, AH50, C3, C3a/C3d, sC5b-9, CFH, CFI, CFB
	Anti-CFH autoantibodies
	C3, CFB, CFH, CFHRs, CFI, MCP/CD46, THBD/CD141 (molecular analysis)
C3 glomerulopathy (DDD, C3GN)	CH50, AH50, C3, C3a/C3d, sC5b-9, C3 NeF, CFH
	Anti-CFH autoantibodies
	C3, CFB, CFH, CFHRs, CFI, MCP/CD46, THBD/CD141 (molecular analysis)

IUIS.org). The diagnostic work-up of a patient with a suspected complement-associated disease should start with the assessment of the total activity of the classical (CH50) and alternative (AH50) pathway. For rapid deficiency analysis, an ELISA has been developed that examines all three activation pathways in parallel [20]. These global tests provide information about the integrity of the entire complement cascade. A missing or greatly reduced activity in either test indicates a primary complement deficiency affecting the classical or the alternative or both pathways, but may also be due to a secondary deficiency caused by increased consumption. Analysis of individual components and regulators provide insight, into which portion of the complement cascade either a lack of function or an over-activation occurs.

Analysis of the plasma concentrations of individual complement components, such as C3 and C4 is still performed in many clinical laboratories. These tests, however, detect both native and activated, i.e., already "consumed" complement proteins and are strongly influenced by fluctuations in protein synthesis, in particular during the early acute-phase reaction. Modern complement analyses focus on the quantification of complement-derived split products (e.g., C3a, C3d or Bb) or protein-protein complexes (sC5b-

9) thereby providing a comprehensive insight into the actual activation state of the complement system. By choosing the appropriate parameters, it is possible to determine exactly, which pathway is activated.

Recently, the activation product of the terminal complement cascade, SC5b-9, has received more attention, as unrestricted progression to its final steps has been linked to specific pathology, i.e., aHUS [21], and the efficacy of the recently introduced C5 antibody eculizumab in treating aHUS patients is reflected by sC5b-9 suppression [22]. Thus, like C3a or C3d, sC5b-9 should be utilized as global marker of complement activation and appears to be particularly useful in monitoring patients during (eculizumab) therapy. A recommended algorithm of complement analysis is shown in Fig. 23.2.

Detecting Autoantibodies

Similar to *loss* or *gain of function* mutations in complement regulators or activating components, an overactivation of complement can also be caused by autoantibodies. Autoantibodies to CFH (DEAP HUS) [23], CFB (DDD) [24], C1q (SLE) [25], or to the C1 inhibitor (hereditary angioedema) [26] can be detected by ELISA with the respective purified complement proteins immobilized on a microtiter plate. Results from serial dilutions of patients' sera or plasma should be interpreted in comparison with data from large control panels.

C3 Nephritic Factor (C3NeF), found in all types of MPGN [27], can be measured in a decay assay as C3NeF stabilizes the alternative pathway C3 convertase, C3bBb. In this semi-quantitative screening assay C3NeF stabilizes the C3 convertase on sheep erythrocytes, thereby causing increased complement activation and eventually hemolysis [28]. Fluid-phase conversion of C3 upon mixture of normal serum and C3Nef containing patient's serum can also be visualized as emerging protein bands of C3b and C3c using an immunofixation assay [29].

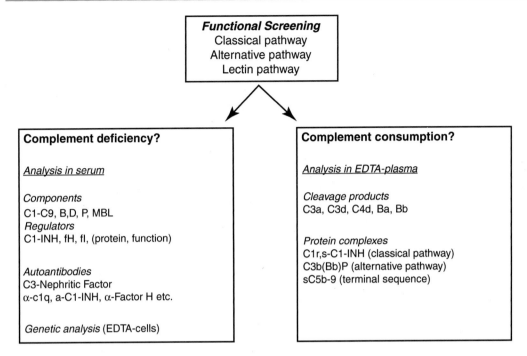

Fig. 23.2   Algorithm of complement analysis

Collecting Blood and Urine Samples

Proper collection of (blood and urine) samples for diagnostic analysis is essential. Sample collection should aim at freezing the complement activation status of the patient at the time of blood draw. Without inhibition, physiological and pathological complement activation would continue, thus obscuring the actual complement activation status and preventing meaningful data interpretation. Therefore, EDTA at ≥10 mM final concentration is used as standard anticoagulant since it blocks the *in vitro* activation of the complement system by way of its Mg^{2+} and Ca^{2+} complexing properties. Heparin and citrate are less useful [30]. Centrifuged plasma should be kept on ice or in a refrigerator if analyzed on the same day; for later processing, the sample should be aliquoted, frozen and stored at −70 °C (−20 °C for short-term [days] storage). Repeated freezing and thawing of aliquots should be avoided because of the risk of

in vitro activation (above). If needed, frozen samples should be shipped on dry ice.

In urine, the measurement of activated complement components or degradation products can be affected by high amounts of urea and urine proteases, so that the addition of protease inhibitors is required. However, as recently shown by van der Pol et al., appearance of complement activation products in proteinuria may also be the consequence of extrarenal (artificial) rather than intrarenal complement activation [31].

Immunohistological Diagnosis

The diagnosis of many autoimmune (or immune complex diseases) is based on the detection of immunoglobulins and complement deposition in various tissues. For immunohistochemical diagnosis, antibodies against C1q, C3b, C4b, C4d, and C5b-9 are suitable and are available for frozen and in part also for paraffin fixed tissue. Positive staining identifies a direct impact of complement in the disease process, indicates disease activity and allows for the differentiation of the complement activation pathways involved . The presence of C3b suggests ongoing inflammation, while C3d deposits in the absence of C3b point to a non-active disease process. While its specificity is debatable, C4d has been accepted as biomarker of humoral renal graft rejection [32, 33].

Complement in Nephropathies

Principles

Complement has been implicated in the pathogenesis of glomerulonephritis and end-stage renal disease (ESRD) [34–36]. The kidney appears particularly vulnerable to complement-mediated injury, and autochthone (i.e., intrarenal) synthesis of complement proteins, often insufficiently counterbalanced by local expression of complement regulatory proteins, contribute to disease progression [37]. Complement associated glomerular inflammation is associated with cell proliferation and influx of inflammatory cells. Complement activation may be the consequence of local – as in aHUS ([21] – or systemic – as in C3GN/DDD [38, 39] – dysregulation of the alternative complement pathway. By contrast, the presence of autoantibodies or immune complexes leads to activation of the classical pathway, as in systemic lupus erythematosis (SLE) [40], anti-glomerular basement membrane (anti-GBM) disease [41], anti-neutrophil cytoplasmic autoantibody (ANCA)-associated vasculitides [42, 43], or in Henoch-Schoenlein purpura (HSP) [36, 39, 44].

Patients suffering from membranoproliferative glomerulonephritis (MPGN), especially the subtype called dense deposit disease (DDD), often show low CH50, AH50 and C3. This results from continuous C3 activation, e.g., due to the C3NeF. High levels of C3 split products in the absence or presence of elevated SC5b-9 may be explained by the presence of nephritic factors (i.e., autoantibodies) with different specificities for C3 and/or C5 convertases. In the absence of

Ig C4d binding may result from lectin pathway activation.

Primary Complement-Mediated Kidney Diseases

Atypical hemolytic uremic syndrome (aHUS) is characterized by microangiopathic hemolytic anemia, thrombocytopenia and acute renal failure. In the majority of cases, loss- or gain-of-function mutations of complement factors (e.g., CFH, CFI, MCP/CD46, THBD/CD141, C3 and CFB), deletions (e.g., CFHRs), or autoantibodies (e.g., against CFH) provide the molecular background for an unrestricted local complement activation at the level of the vascular endothelium [45, 46].

However, also diarrhea-positive HUS, caused by Shiga toxin-producing *Escherichia coli* (STEC HUS) [47, 48]. as well as thrombotic thrombocytopenic purpura (TTP) [49], have been associated with complement alternative pathway activation via mechanisms involving P-selectin and platelet thrombi, respectively.

The diagnostic procedure includes the analysis of total hemolytic activity (CH50, AH50), C3, C3 activation products (C3a or C3d) and SC5b-9, as well as the molecular genetic analysis of *C3, CFB, CFH, CHFR1-5, CFI, MCP/CD46 and THBD/CD141* (Table 23.2) [21].

While in aHUS the regulatory function of factor H in the fluid phase is usually not impaired by the mutations identified, the majority of aHUS related mutations leads to a lack of factor H binding to the endothelial surface or the GBM. This impaired recognition of "self" structures (glycosaminoglycans, anionic phospholipids or sialic acid) by factor H and subsequent targeted attack of the complement alternative pathway against endothelial and blood cells is the underlying cause of aHUS related to CFH mutations. Similarly, defects in the membrane anchored complement regulatory proteins (e.g., MCP/CD46, THBD/CD141) also allow for unrestricted progression of the complement cascade on the vascular endothelium. Finally, gain of function mutations in C3 and CFB result in a decreased decay of the alternative pathway C3 convertase, eventually also fuelling the complement alternative pathway activation.

As recently described, the clinical picture of a TMA can also be mimicked by mutations in diacyl glycerol kinase ε (DGKE), affecing the phosphatidyl-inositol pathway with increased levels of protein kinase C (PKC) [50, 51]. DGKE mutations were so far only identified in infant aHUS patients, typically refractory or poorly responsive to eculizumab treatment. The underlying molecular mechanisms, how these mutations cause disease, are still unclear. It is, however, conceivable, that an increased prothrombotic activity of the target cells may subsequently lead to complement activation. Thus, DGKE mutations should be considered in the panel of genes tested at least in young children.

Dense deposit disease (DDD) – previously called MPGN II – is the first nephropathy, for which excessive activation of the complement alternative pathway was identified [52, 53]. In DDD and less frequently also in other forms of MPGN C3 nephritic factor is found [27]. A severely reduced total complement activity with low C3 plasma levels is typical and warrants testing for C3NeF. Besides C3NeF, additional autoantibodies against C3b and CFB have been detected in DDD. Similar to aHUS, DDD and MPGN I patients can also carry mutations or polymorphisms in the *CFH* [54, 55], *CFHR3-CFHR1* [56], *CFHR5* [57], *CFI* [55, 58], MCP/CD46 [55, 58, 59], and *C3* genes [60]. Different from aHUS, mutations in DDD and MPGN I typically do not impair complement control on endothelial cells but result in complement dysregulation in plasma reflected by significantly decreased C3 levels. This pathogenetic difference is exemplified by the finding of a disease causing CFH mutation (ΔK224 in SCR4) in two siblings with DDD, which abolished CFH cofactor activity while leaving CFH surface binding capacity intact [61, 62]. Similarly, in MPGN patients monoclonal Ig lambda light chain dimers (miniantibodies) binding to SCR3 of CFH were identified, which block one of the CFH C3b binding sites (SCR3) and thus impair CFH cofactor activity [63].

C3 glomerulopathy (C3G) is a recent disease classification comprising several rare types of glomerulonephritis, including dense deposit disease (DDD) and C3 glomerulonephritis (C3GN) [38, 64, 65]. The most common histological feature in these diseases is the glomerular deposition of C3 within the mesangium and along the GBM in the subendothelial area or within the GBM. The key role of the alternative pathway based on the respective acquired or genetic abnormalities has been discussed above [66]. Low serum C3, but normal C4 levels are a common finding. C3NeF activity is found in approximately 80 % of patients with DDD and in 45 % of patients with C3GN [27, 54, 55].

Secondary Complement-Mediated Conditions

Lupus Nephritis

Lupus nephritis develops as a frequent complication of systemic lupus erythematosus (SLE). Impairment of complement-mediated elimination of immune complexes and apoptotic cells, most pronounced in patients with genetic deficiencies of C1q, C2 or C4, are the hallmark of this disease [67–69]. More than 90 % of individuals with hereditary C1q deficiency develop a SLE-like clinical syndrome. Mutations in the C1q gene either lead to the absence of C1q or to the production of a non-functional, low molecular weight C1q [70]. The impaired uptake of apoptotic cells by monocyte-derived macrophages in patients with C1q deficiency could be experimentally corrected by substitution with purified exogenous C1q [71]. Evidence for the protective role of classical pathway components comes from experiments in C4$^{-/-}$ MLR/pr mice (an accepted mouse model for human SLE) where an increase in autoimmunity against self-antigens and subsequent tissue injury was observed [72]. The presence of anti-C1q autoantibodies, found in up to 30–60 % of SLE patients, is strongly associated with hypocomplementaemia, disease activity and the appearance of renal involvement [25, 73].

In the absence of a primary deficiency, active disease in SLE is often accompanied by low levels of C1q and other complement factors of the classical pathway, which indicate consumption of complement by inflammation.

It appears that the complement alternative pathway exacerbates glomerular injury since fB$^{-/-}$ [74] and fD$^{-/-}$ MLR/pr mice [75] are protected from renal disease.

Another susceptibility locus for SLE has been mapped to chromosome 1q31-32 at the position of the genes coding for CFH and the CFHRs [76].

In patients with lupus nephritis complement consumption generally correlates with disease activity. Normalization of CH50, C3 and especially of C4 [77] as well as the reduction of activation products reflect therapeutic efficacy.

IgA Nephropathy

IgA nephropathy (IgA-N) is the most prevalent primary chronic glomerular disease worldwide (for review see: [78]). Since in biopsies C3 and properdin are most often associated with IgA deposits a role for complement was assumed [79]. Low circulating C3 levels correlating with C3 deposition in glomeruli [80] and high urinary levels of MBL [81], sC5b-9, factor H and properdin [82] clearly indicate involvement of complement in the disease process. The presence of C4d in glomeruli, indicative of disease progression [83], derives from the activation of the lectin pathway, as IgA does not initiate the classical complement pathway.

In a study of 128 IgA-N patients, 53 % (68/128) had TMA lesions on biopsy, and 12 % (8/65) showed the typical laboratory findings of TMA [84]. Whereas the pathogenesis of these TMA lesions is unclear, an association with (malignant) hypertension is common. Genetic work-up of the complement alternative pathway has revealed a heterozygous mutation in *CFH*, but others failed to confirm this finding in a cohort of 46 patients [85, 86]. In contrast, a genome-wide association study in IgA nephropathy patients of Chinese ancestry found a highly significant co-segregation of a *CFHR3-CFHR1* deletion and IgA-N. Of note, this *CFHR3-CFHR1* deletion played a protective (i.e., disease averting), rather than a disease promoting role [87].

Renal Transplantation

In the past years a growing understanding of physiology and pathophysiology, a refinement of tissue typing, better surgical techniques and more effective immunosuppressive strategies has favoured prolonged graft survival. However, a significant proportion of grafts still fails because of a progressive and irreversible immune response of the recipient.

The pathogenesis of graft rejection comprises immunological and non-immunological mechanisms, and a complex series of humoral as well as cell-mediated immune reactions have been implicated [88, 89]. Excessive activation of the protein cascade systems has been associated with post-transplant inflammatory disorders. Clinical and experimental data indicate that complement plays a decisive role in humoral kidney rejection. Complement activation, potentially leading to tissue injury, may occur during reperfusion of the organ, and is most pronounced when the donor organ has undergone a significant period of ischaemia [9, 90].

While during recent years T-cell driven allograft rejection has been largely controlled by immunosuppression, antibody-mediated renal injury has become increasingly implicated as a major cause of kidney allograft loss [91] and has been strongly related to complement activation [92]. Sensitized individuals with pre-existing circulating antibodies (e.g., ABO, DAS) are at high risk to develop an immediate complement dependent reaction against the transplant organ. It appears that local synthesis of complement components as well as loss of regulatory mechanisms that limit the activation especially of the pivotal component C3 significantly contributes to renal injury [37]. In acute renal graft rejection increased levels of C3a and C1rsC1-inhibitor complexes indicate complement activation several days before the first clinical signs become obvious, suggesting complement analysis to be of potential diagnostic value in posttransplant immune monitoring [93]. Intragraft detection of complement proteins, such as C3 (and of immunoglobulins) by magnetic resonance imaging may in future substitute for biopsy analysis [94]. Local complement activation with the generation of chemotactic factors C3a and C5a contributes to cell infiltration and activation of the vascular endothelium. As deposition of the membrane attack complex, C5b-9, even at sublytic concentrations induces the expression of adhesion molecules, complement may trigger tissue damage by interference with the anticoagulant and fibrinolytic capacity of the vascular endothelium [95].

Since our knowledge on the mechanisms of tissue injury in acute rejection are well understood, the implication of complement in chronic humoral transplant loss is less clear. Here, donor-specific antibodies (DSA) and C4d in peritubular capillaries, indicating a local complement activation are often associated with interstitial fibrosis and tubular atrophy leading to transplantat glomerulopathy [92]. Microvascular alterations in the early phase after transplantation, potentially induced during reperfusion, may provide the basis for longlasting subclinical inflammation with a high risk for transition to chronic humoral rejection [96].

Targeting Complement in the Treatment of Renal Disease

Unraveling of a key role for complement dysregulation in an increasing spectrum of kidney diseases provides an unprecedented treatment approach to diseases, previously poorly managed and often progressing to ESRD and/or death. Overarching principle is the restitution of proper complement control via replacement of missing or defective complement factors or removal of inhibiting autoantibodies via plasma exchange (PLEX)/plasma infusion (PI). Strategies of interventions include the replacement or supplementation of endogenous soluble complement inhibitors (C1 inhibitor, CFH, recombinant soluble complement receptor 1-rsCR1, TP10), the administration of antibodies to block key proteins of the cascade reaction (e.g., C5) or to neutralize the action of the complement-derived anaphylatoxins (for review see: [97, 98]. The approval of eculizumab, a recombinant humanized monoclonal antibody to C5, for the treatment of paroxysmal nocturnal hemoglobinuria (PNH) and of C1 inhibitor for the treatment of hereditary angioedema have attracted the interest of clinicians to the potential of complement therapeutics for the treatment of severe inflammatory disorders.

Eculizumab prevents the release of the highly potent inflammatory anaphylatoxin C5a and the assembly of the membrane attack complex (MAC; C5b-9) with the advantage of leaving the activation phase of complement up to the generation of the C3 opsonins C3b and iC3b intact. While the treatment of aHUS with eculizumab has been highly successful in most cases [99–101], the use for other complement-mediated renal diseases is still a matter of ongoing clinical research [102, 103].

The successful treatment of DDD and C3G with eculizumab has been reported by several investigators [104–106], but failed to decrease urinary protein excretion.

Recurrence of aHUS after discontinuation of eculizumab administration reflects the uncertainty about duration of treatment with eculizumab. A recently opened aHUS registry (www.clinicaltrials.gov) aims to collect safety and efficacy data specific to the use of eculizumab. Collection of outcome data in patients with aHUS, either receiving eculizumab or other treatment, will certainly help to optimize therapy.

Besides monitoring of eculizumab-treated patients on the basis of traditional parameters such as lactate dehydrogenase (LDH), hemoglobin (Hb), haptoglobin, platelets and serum creatinine, additional analyses of complement activation including CH50 and AH50 (reflect inhibitory efficacy), together with sC5b-9, C3 and C3d (indicating potential ongoing *in vivo* activation) provide valuable information on therapeutic efficacy and may allow – together with drug monitoring – for the re-evaluation of the use and dosage of eculizumab in the heterogeneous group of complement-mediated renal diseases. In sensitized, high risk patients (i.e., DSA; ABO-incompatibility) [107] as well as in aHUS [108] complement inhibition by eculizumab before and during the first stages of transplantation proved to be an important prospect for increasing survival of the kidney transplant.

Novel strategies of treating the donor organ with modified therapeutic regulators that are engineered to be retained by the donor organ after transplantation and prevent an inflammatory injury during the critical early period aim at maintaining the systemic functions of complement, thereby keeping host defence intact. The concept of targeting complement inhibitors to the site of complement activation was first tested with APT070/microcept, where the complement inhibitor sCR1 was bound to the membrane-localizing myristoylated peptide [109]. This provided the first proof that targeting of a complement inhibitor to the site of tissue damage/complement activation is more potent than administration of a non-targeted inhibitor. Improving organ function in a pilot study of renal ransplantation, APT070/microcept is now scheduled for clinical trials [110].

Tissue-bound C3b is cleaved by CFI to C3bi, C3dg and ultimately to C3d, where each of these fragments remains covalently bound to tissue. Complement receptor 2 (CR2, CD21) specifically binds C3bi, C3d and C3dg, allowing complement inhibitors to be targeted to inflamed tissues. The efficacy of CR2-targeted CFH has been demonstrated in various animal models and radiolabelling studies confirmed that CR2 targeted CFH is cleared rapidly from the circulation but binds to and persists in inflamed tissues [111]. Along this line ALXN1102/TT30 has been designed where the ligand binding domain (SCR1-4) of CR2 delivers the complement regulatory domain of CFH (SCR1-5) specifically to tissues, in which complement activation is occurring [103].

This approach may provide a model which combines efficacy with a need for lower dose of drug, thereby potentially decreasing the risk of infections compared to untargeted complement therapy.

References

1. Ricklin D, Lambris JD. Complement in immune and inflammatory disorders: pathophysiological mechanisms. J Immunol. 2013;190:3831–8.
2. Figueroa JE, Densen P. Infectious diseases associated with complement deficiencies. Clin Microbiol Rev. 1991;4:359–95.
3. Abel G, Agnello V. Complement deficiencies: a 2004 update. In: Szebeni J, editor. The complement system novel roles in health and disease. Boston: Kluwer Academic Publishers; 2004. p. 201–28.
4. Botto M, Kirschfink M, Macor P, Pickering MC, Wurzner R, Tedesco F. Complement in human diseases: lessons from complement deficiencies. Mol Immunol. 2009;46:2774–83.
5. Zilow G, Joka T, Obertacke U, Rother U, Kirschfink M. Generation of anaphylatoxin C3a in plasma and bronchoalveolar lavage fluid in trauma patients at risk for the adult respiratory distress syndrome. Crit Care Med. 1992;20:468–73.
6. Ward PA. The dark side of C5a in sepsis. Nat Rev Immunol. 2004;4:133–42.
7. Rittirsch D, Redl H, Huber-Lang M. Role of complement in multiorgan failure. Clin Dev Immunol. 2012;2012, 962927.
8. Farrar CA, Keogh B, McCormack W, O'Shaughnessy A, Parker A, Reilly M, Sacks SH. Inhibition of TLR2 promotes graft function in a murine model of renal transplant ischemia-reperfusion injury. FASEB J. 2012;26:799–807.
9. Farrar CA, Asgari E, Schwaeble WJ, Sacks SH. Which pathways trigger the role of complement in ischaemia/reperfusion injury? Front Immunol. 2012;3:341.
10. Kirschfink M, Kovacs B, Mottaghy K. Extracorporeal circulation: in vivo and in vitro analysis of complement activation by heparin-bonded surfaces. Circ Shock. 1993;40:221–6.
11. Mollnes TE. Biocompatibility: complement as mediator of tissue damage and as indicator of incompatibility. Exp Clin Immunogenet. 1997;14:24–9.
12. Walport MJ. Complement. Second of two parts. N Engl J Med. 2001;344:1140–4.
13. Walport MJ. Complement. First of two parts. N Engl J Med. 2001;344:1058–66.
14. Carol M, Pelegri C, Castellote C, Franch A, Castell M. Immunohistochemical study of lymphoid tissues in adjuvant arthritis (AA) by image analysis; relationship with synovial lesions. Clin Exp Immunol. 2000;120:200–8.
15. Ricklin D, Hajishengallis G, Yang K, Lambris JD. Complement: a key system for immune surveillance and homeostasis. Nat Immunol. 2010;11:785–97.
16. Klos A, Tenner AJ, Johswich KO, Ager RR, Reis ES, Kohl J. The role of the anaphylatoxins in health and disease. Mol Immunol. 2009;46:2753–66.
17. Sacks SH. Complement fragments C3a and C5a: the salt and pepper of the immune response. Eur J Immunol. 2010;40:668–70.
18. Zipfel PF, Skerka C. Complement regulators and inhibitory proteins. Nat Rev Immunol. 2009;9: 729–40.
19. Mollnes TE, Jokiranta TS, Truedsson L, Nilsson B, Rodriguez de Cordoba S, Kirschfink M. Complement analysis in the 21st century. Mol Immunol. 2007; 44:3838–49.
20. Seelen MA, Roos A, Wieslander J, Mollnes TE, Sjoholm AG, Wurzner R, Loos M, Tedesco F, Sim RB, Garred P, Alexopoulos E, Turner MW, Daha MR. Functional analysis of the classical, alternative, and MBL pathways of the complement system: standardization and validation of a simple ELISA. J Immunol Methods. 2005;296:187–98.

21. Noris M, Remuzzi G. Atypical hemolytic-uremic syndrome. N Engl J Med. 2009;361:1676–87.
22. Legendre CM, Licht C, Muus P, Greenbaum LA, Babu S, Bedrosian C, Bingham C, Cohen DJ, Delmas Y, Douglas K, Eitner F, Feldkamp T, Fouque D, Furman RR, Gaber O, Herthelius M, Hourmant M, Karpman D, Lebranchu Y, Mariat C, Menne J, Moulin B, Nurnberger J, Ogawa M, Remuzzi G, Richard T, Sberro-Soussan R, Severino B, Sheerin NS, Trivelli A, Zimmerhackl LB, Goodship T, Loirat C. Terminal complement inhibitor eculizumab in atypical hemolytic-uremic syndrome. N Engl J Med. 2013;368:2169–81.
23. Jozsi M, Licht C, Strobel S, Zipfel SL, Richter H, Heinen S, Zipfel PF, Skerka C. Factor H autoantibodies in atypical hemolytic uremic syndrome correlate with CFHR1/CFHR3 deficiency. Blood. 2008; 111:1512–4.
24. Strobel S, Zimmering M, Papp K, Prechl J, Jozsi M. Anti-factor B autoantibody in dense deposit disease. Mol Immunol. 2010;47:1476–83.
25. Mahler M, van Schaarenburg RA, Trouw LA. Anti-C1q autoantibodies, novel tests, and clinical consequences. Front Immunol. 2013;4:117.
26. Cugno M, Castelli R, Cicardi M. Angioedema due to acquired C1-inhibitor deficiency: a bridging condition between autoimmunity and lymphoproliferation. Autoimmun Rev. 2008;8:156–9.
27. Schwertz R, Rother U, Anders D, Gretz N, Scharer K, Kirschfink M. Complement analysis in children with idiopathic membranoproliferative glomerulonephritis: a long-term follow-up. Pediatr Allergy Immunol. 2001;12:166–72.
28. Rother U. A new screening test for C3 nephritis factor based on a stable cell bound convertase on sheep erythrocytes. J Immunol Methods. 1982;51:101–7.
29. Koch FJ, Jenis EH, Valeski JE. Test for C3 nephritic factor activity by immunofixation electrophoresis. Am J Clin Pathol. 1981;76:63–7.
30. Mollnes TE, Garred P, Bergseth G. Effect of time, temperature and anticoagulants on in vitro complement activation: consequences for collection and preservation of samples to be examined for complement activation. Clin Exp Immunol. 1988;73:484–8.
31. van der Pol P, de Vries DK, van Gijlswijk DJ, van Anken GE, Schlagwein N, Daha MR, Aydin Z, de Fijter JW, Schaapherder AF, van Kooten C. Pitfalls in urinary complement measurements. Transpl Immunol. 2012;27:55–8.
32. Feucht HE, Schneeberger H, Hillebrand G, Burkhardt K, Weiss M, Riethmuller G, Land W, Albert E. Capillary deposition of C4d complement fragment and early renal graft loss. Kidney Int. 1993;43:1333–8.
33. Cohen D, Colvin RB, Daha MR, Drachenberg CB, Haas M, Nickeleit V, Salmon JE, Sis B, Zhao MH, Bruijn JA, Bajema IM. Pros and cons for C4d as a biomarker. Kidney Int. 2012;81:628–39.
34. Cook HT. Complement and kidney disease. Curr Opin Nephrol Hypertens. 2013;22(3):295–301.
35. Koscielska-Kasprzak K, Bartoszek D, Myszka M, Zabinska M, Klinger M. The complement cascade and renal disease. Arch Immunol Ther Exp (Warsz). 2014;62(1):47–57.
36. Brown KM, Sacks SH, Sheerin NS. Mechanisms of disease: the complement system in renal injury – new ways of looking at an old foe. Nat Clin Pract Nephrol. 2007;3:277–86.
37. Zhou W, Marsh JE, Sacks SH. Intrarenal synthesis of complement. Kidney Int. 2001;59:1227–35.
38. Sethi S, Nester CM, Smith RJ. Membranoproliferative glomerulonephritis and C3 glomerulopathy: resolving the confusion. Kidney Int. 2012;81:434–41.
39. Lesher AM, Song WC. Review: complement and its regulatory proteins in kidney diseases. Nephrology (Carlton). 2010;15:663–75.
40. Lech M, Anders HJ. The pathogenesis of lupus nephritis. J Am Soc Nephrol. 2013;24:1357–66.
41. Ma R, Cui Z, Liao YH, Zhao MH. Complement activation contributes to the injury and outcome of kidney in human anti-glomerular basement membrane disease. J Clin Immunol. 2013;33:172–8.
42. Kallenberg CG, Heeringa P. Complement is crucial in the pathogenesis of ANCA-associated vasculitis. Kidney Int. 2013;83:16–8.
43. Gou SJ, Yuan J, Chen M, Yu F, Zhao MH. Circulating complement activation in patients with anti-neutrophil cytoplasmic antibody-associated vasculitis. Kidney Int. 2013;83:129–37.
44. Lin Q, Min Y, Li Y, Zhu Y, Song X, Xu Q, Wang L, Cheng J, Feng Q, Li X. Henoch-Schonlein purpura with hypocomplementemia. Pediatr Nephrol. 2012;27:801–6.
45. Pickering M, Cook HT. Complement and glomerular disease: new insights. Curr Opin Nephrol Hypertens. 2011;20:271–7.
46. Kavanagh D, Goodship TH, Richards A. Atypical hemolytic uremic syndrome. Semin Nephrol. 2013;33:508–30.
47. Orth D, Wurzner R. Complement in typical hemolytic uremic syndrome. Semin Thromb Hemost. 2010;36:620–4.
48. Morigi M, Galbusera M, Gastoldi S, Locatelli M, Buelli S, Pezzotta A, Pagani C, Noris M, Gobbi M, Stravalaci M, Rottoli D, Tedesco F, Remuzzi G, Zoja C. Alternative pathway activation of complement by Shiga toxin promotes exuberant C3a formation that triggers microvascular thrombosis. J Immunol. 2011;187:172–80.
49. Turner NA, Moake J. Assembly and activation of alternative complement components on endothelial cell-anchored ultra-large von Willebrand factor links complement and hemostasis-thrombosis. PLoS One. 2013;8:e59372.
50. Lemaire M, Fremeaux-Bacchi V, Schaefer F, Choi M, Tang WH, Le Quintrec M, Fakhouri F, Taque S, Nobili F, Martinez F, Ji W, Overton JD, Mane SM, Nurnberg G, Altmuller J, Thiele H, Morin D, Deschenes G, Baudouin V, Llanas B, Collard L, Majid MA, Simkova E, Nurnberg P, Rioux-Leclerc

N, Moeckel GW, Gubler MC, Hwa J, Loirat C, Lifton RP. Recessive mutations in DGKE cause atypical hemolytic-uremic syndrome. Nat Genet. 2013;45:531–6.

51. Ozaltin F, Li B, Rauhauser A, An SW, Soylemezoglu O, Gonul II, Taskiran EZ, Ibsirlioglu T, Korkmaz E, Bilginer Y, Duzova A, Ozen S, Topaloglu R, Besbas N, Ashraf S, Du Y, Liang C, Chen P, Lu D, Vadnagara K, Arbuckle S, Lewis D, Wakeland B, Quigg RJ, Ransom RF, Wakeland EK, Topham MK, Bazan NG, Mohan C, Hildebrandt F, Bakkaloglu A, Huang CL, Attanasio M. DGKE variants cause a glomerular microangiopathy that mimics membranoproliferative GN. J Am Soc Nephrol. 2013;24:377–84.

52. Appel GB, Cook HT, Hageman G, Jennette JC, Kashgarian M, Kirschfink M, Lambris JD, Lanning L, Lutz HU, Meri S, Rose NR, Salant DJ, Sethi S, Smith RJ, Smoyer W, Tully HF, Tully SP, Walker P, Welsh M, Wurzner R, Zipfel PF. Membranoproliferative glomerulonephritis type II (dense deposit disease): an update. J Am Soc Nephrol. 2005;16:1392–403.

53. Licht C, Fremeaux-Bacchi V. Hereditary and acquired complement dysregulation in membranoproliferative glomerulonephritis. Thromb Haemost. 2009;101:271–8.

54. Zhang Y, Meyer NC, Wang K, Nishimura C, Frees K, Jones M, Katz LM, Sethi S, Smith RJ. Causes of alternative pathway dysregulation in dense deposit disease. Clin J Am Soc Nephrol. 2012;7:265–74.

55. Servais A, Noel LH, Roumenina LT, Le Quintrec M, Ngo S, Dragon-Durey MA, Macher MA, Zuber J, Karras A, Provot F, Moulin B, Grunfeld JP, Niaudet P, Lesavre P, Fremeaux-Bacchi V. Acquired and genetic complement abnormalities play a critical role in dense deposit disease and other C3 glomerulopathies. Kidney Int. 2012;82:454–64.

56. Malik TH, Lavin PJ, Goicoechea de Jorge E, Vernon KA, Rose KL, Patel MP, de Leeuw M, Neary JJ, Conlon PJ, Winn MP, Pickering MC. A hybrid CFHR3-1 gene causes familial C3 glomerulopathy. J Am Soc Nephrol. 2012;23:1155–60.

57. Gale DP, de Jorge EG, Cook HT, Martinez-Barricarte R, Hadjisavvas A, McLean AG, Pusey CD, Pierides A, Kyriacou K, Athanasiou Y, Voskarides K, Deltas C, Palmer A, Fremeaux-Bacchi V, de Cordoba SR, Maxwell PH, Pickering MC. Identification of a mutation in complement factor H-related protein 5 in patients of Cypriot origin with glomerulonephritis. Lancet. 2010;376:794–801.

58. Servais A, Fremeaux-Bacchi V, Lequintrec M, Salomon R, Blouin J, Knebelmann B, Grunfeld JP, Lesavre P, Noel LH, Fakhouri F. Primary glomerulonephritis with isolated C3 deposits: a new entity which shares common genetic risk factors with haemolytic uraemic syndrome. J Med Genet. 2007;44:193–9.

59. Radhakrishnan S, Lunn A, Kirschfink M, Thorner P, Hebert D, Langlois V, Pluthero F, Licht C. Eculizumab and refractory membranoproliferative glomerulonephritis. N Engl J Med. 2012;366:1165–6.

60. Martinez-Barricarte R, Heurich M, Valdes-Canedo F, Vazquez-Martul E, Torreira E, Montes T, Tortajada A, Pinto S, Lopez-Trascasa M, Morgan BP, Llorca O, Harris CL, Rodriguez de Cordoba S. Human C3 mutation reveals a mechanism of dense deposit disease pathogenesis and provides insights into complement activation and regulation. J Clin Invest. 2010;120:3702–12.

61. Licht C, Heinen S, Jozsi M, Loschmann I, Saunders RE, Perkins SJ, Waldherr R, Skerka C, Kirschfink M, Hoppe B, Zipfel PF. Deletion of Lys224 in regulatory domain 4 of Factor H reveals a novel pathomechanism for dense deposit disease (MPGN II). Kidney Int. 2006;70:42–50.

62. Habbig S, Mihatsch MJ, Heinen S, Beck B, Emmel M, Skerka C, Kirschfink M, Hoppe B, Zipfel PF, Licht C. C3 deposition glomerulopathy due to a functional factor H defect. Kidney Int. 2009;75:1230–4.

63. Jokiranta TS, Solomon A, Pangburn MK, Zipfel PF, Meri S. Nephritogenic lambda light chain dimer: a unique human miniautoantibody against complement factor H. J Immunol. 1999;163:4590–6.

64. Medjeral-Thomas NR, O'Shaughnessy MM, O'Regan JA, Traynor C, Flanagan M, Wong L, Teoh CW, Awan A, Waldron M, Cairns T, O'Kelly P, Dorman AM, Pickering MC, Conlon PJ, Cook HT. C3 glomerulopathy: clinicopathologic features and predictors of outcome. Clin J Am Soc Nephrol. 2014;9(1):46–53.

65. Pickering MC, D'Agati VD, Nester CM, Smith RJ, Haas M, Appel GB, Alpers CE, Bajema IM, Bedrosian C, Braun M, Doyle M, Fakhouri F, Fervenza FC, Fogo AB, Fremeaux-Bacchi V, Gale DP, Goicoechea de Jorge E, Griffin G, Harris CL, Holers VM, Johnson S, Lavin PJ, Medjeral-Thomas N, Paul Morgan B, Nast CC, Noel LH, Peters DK, Rodriguez de Cordoba S, Servais A, Sethi S, Song WC, Tamburini P, Thurman JM, Zavros M, Cook HT. C3 glomerulopathy: consensus report. Kidney Int. 2013;84:1079–89.

66. Sethi S, Fervenza FC, Zhang Y, Zand L, Vrana JA, Nasr SH, Theis JD, Dogan A, Smith RJ. C3 glomerulonephritis: clinicopathological findings, complement abnormalities, glomerular proteomic profile, treatment, and follow-up. Kidney Int. 2012;82:465–73.

67. Pickering MC, Botto M, Taylor PR, Lachmann PJ, Walport MJ. Systemic lupus erythematosus, complement deficiency, and apoptosis. Adv Immunol. 2000;76:227–324.

68. Pickering MC, Walport MJ. Links between complement abnormalities and systemic lupus erythematosus. Rheumatology (Oxford). 2000;39:133–41.

69. Carroll MC. The lupus paradox. Nat Genet. 1998;19:3–4.

70. Petry F, Le DT, Kirschfink M, Loos M. Non-sense and missense mutations in the structural genes of complement component C1q A and C chains are linked with two different types of complete selective C1q deficiencies. J Immunol. 1995;155:4734–8.

71. Taylor PR, Carugati A, Fadok VA, Cook HT, Andrews M, Carroll MC, Savill JS, Henson PM, Botto M, Walport MJ. A hierarchical role for classical pathway complement proteins in the clearance of apoptotic cells in vivo. J Exp Med. 2000;192:359–66.

72. Prodeus AP, Goerg S, Shen LM, Pozdnyakova OO, Chu L, Alicot EM, Goodnow CC, Carroll MC. A critical role for complement in maintenance of self-tolerance. Immunity. 1998;9:721–31.

73. Yin Y, Wu X, Shan G, Zhang X. Diagnostic value of serum anti-C1q antibodies in patients with lupus nephritis: a meta-analysis. Lupus. 2012;21:1088–97.

74. Watanabe H, Garnier G, Circolo A, Wetsel RA, Ruiz P, Holers VM, Boackle SA, Colten HR, Gilkeson GS. Modulation of renal disease in MRL/lpr mice genetically deficient in the alternative complement pathway factor B. J Immunol. 2000;164:786–94.

75. Elliott MK, Jarmi T, Ruiz P, Xu Y, Holers VM, Gilkeson GS. Effects of complement factor D deficiency on the renal disease of MRL/lpr mice. Kidney Int. 2004;65:129–38.

76. Zhao J, Wu H, Khosravi M, Cui H, Qian X, Kelly JA, Kaufman KM, Langefeld CD, Williams AH, Comeau ME, Ziegler JT, Marion MC, Adler A, Glenn SB, Alarcon-Riquelme ME, Pons-Estel BA, Harley JB, Bae SC, Bang SY, Cho SK, Jacob CO, Vyse TJ, Niewold TB, Gaffney PM, Moser KL, Kimberly RP, Edberg JC, Brown EE, Alarcon GS, Petri MA, Ramsey-Goldman R, Vila LM, Reveille JD, James JA, Gilkeson GS, Kamen DL, Freedman BI, Anaya JM, Merrill JT, Criswell LA, Scofield RH, Stevens AM, Guthridge JM, Chang DM, Song YW, Park JA, Lee EY, Boackle SA, Grossman JM, Hahn BH, Goodship TH, Cantor RM, Yu CY, Shen N, Tsao BP. Association of genetic variants in complement factor H and factor H-related genes with systemic lupus erythematosus susceptibility. PLoS Genet. 2011;7:e1002079.

77. Dall'Era M, Stone D, Levesque V, Cisternas M, Wofsy D. Identification of biomarkers that predict response to treatment of lupus nephritis with mycophenolate mofetil or pulse cyclophosphamide. Arthritis Care Res (Hoboken). 2011;63:351–7.

78. Wyatt RJ, Julian BA. IgA nephropathy. N Engl J Med. 2013;368:2402–14.

79. Floege J, Moura IC, Daha MR. New insights into the pathogenesis of IgA nephropathy. Semin Immunopathol. 2014;36(4):431–42.

80. Kim SJ, Koo HM, Lim BJ, Oh HJ, Yoo DE, Shin DH, Lee MJ, Doh FM, Park JT, Yoo TH, Kang SW, Choi KH, Jeong HJ, Han SH. Decreased circulating C3 levels and mesangial C3 deposition predict renal outcome in patients with IgA nephropathy. PLoS One. 2012;7:e40495.

81. Liu LL, Jiang Y, Wang LN, Liu N. Urinary mannose-binding lectin is a biomarker for predicting the progression of immunoglobulin (Ig)A nephropathy. Clin Exp Immunol. 2012;169:148–55.

82. Onda K, Ohsawa I, Ohi H, Tamano M, Mano S, Wakabayashi M, Toki A, Horikoshi S, Fujita T, Tomino Y. Excretion of complement proteins and its activation marker C5b-9 in IgA nephropathy in relation to renal function. BMC Nephrol. 2011;12:64.

83. Espinosa M, Ortega R, Gomez-Carrasco JM, Lopez-Rubio F, Lopez-Andreu M, Lopez-Oliva MO, Aljama P. Mesangial C4d deposition: a new prognostic factor in IgA nephropathy. Nephrol Dial Transplant. 2009;24:886–91.

84. El Karoui K, Hill GS, Karras A, Jacquot C, Moulonguet L, Kourilsky O, Fremeaux-Bacchi V, Delahousse M, Duong Van Huyen JP, Loupy A, Bruneval P, Nochy D. A clinicopathologic study of thrombotic microangiopathy in IgA nephropathy. J Am Soc Nephrol. 2012;23:137–48.

85. Edey M, Strain L, Ward R, Ahmed S, Thomas T, Goodship TH. Is complement factor H a susceptibility factor for IgA nephropathy? Mol Immunol. 2009; 46:1405–8.

86. Schmitt R, Krmar RT, Kristoffersson A, Soderberg M, Karpman D. IgA nephropathy associated with a novel N-terminal mutation in factor H. Eur J Pediatr. 2011;170:107–10.

87. Gharavi AG, Kiryluk K, Choi M, Li Y, Hou P, Xie J, Sanna-Cherchi S, Men CJ, Julian BA, Wyatt RJ, Novak J, He JC, Wang H, Lv J, Zhu L, Wang W, Wang Z, Yasuno K, Gunel M, Mane S, Umlauf S, Tikhonova I, Beerman I, Savoldi S, Magistroni R, Ghiggeri GM, Bodria M, Lugani F, Ravani P, Ponticelli C, Allegri L, Boscutti G, Frasca G, Amore A, Peruzzi L, Coppo R, Izzi C, Viola BF, Prati E, Salvadori M, Mignani R, Gesualdo L, Bertinetto F, Mesiano P, Amoroso A, Scolari F, Chen N, Zhang H, Lifton RP. Genome-wide association study identifies susceptibility loci for IgA nephropathy. Nat Genet. 2011;43:321–7.

88. Ponticelli C. The mechanisms of acute transplant rejection revisited. J Nephrol. 2012;25:150–8.

89. Cornell LD, Smith RN, Colvin RB. Kidney transplantation: mechanisms of rejection and acceptance. Annu Rev Pathol. 2008;3:189–220.

90. Damman J, Seelen MA, Moers C, Daha MR, Rahmel A, Leuvenink HG, Paul A, Pirenne J, Ploeg RJ. Systemic complement activation in deceased donors is associated with acute rejection after renal transplantation in the recipient. Transplantation. 2011;92:163–9.

91. Stegall MD, Gloor JM. Deciphering antibody-mediated rejection: new insights into mechanisms and treatment. Curr Opin Organ Transplant. 2010;15: 8–10.

92. Stegall MD, Chedid MF, Cornell LD. The role of complement in antibody-mediated rejection in kidney transplantation. Nat Rev Nephrol. 2012;8: 670–8.

93. Kirschfink M, Wienert T, Rother K, Pomer S. Complement activation in renal allograft recipients. Transplant Proc. 1992;24:2556–7.

94. Sargsyan SA, Serkova NJ, Renner B, Hasebroock KM, Larsen B, Stoldt C, McFann K, Pickering MC, Thurman JM. Detection of glomerular complement

C3 fragments by magnetic resonance imaging in murine lupus nephritis. Kidney Int. 2012;81:152–9.

95. Tedesco F, Fischetti F, Pausa M, Dobrina A, Sim RB, Daha MR. Complement-endothelial cell interactions: pathophysiological implications. Mol Immunol. 1999;36:261–8.

96. Khan MA, Nicolls MR. Complement-mediated microvascular injury leads to chronic rejection. Adv Exp Med Biol. 2013;735:233–46.

97. Mollnes TE, Kirschfink M. Strategies of therapeutic complement inhibition. Mol Immunol. 2006;43:107–21.

98. Ricklin D, Lambris JD. Progress and trends in complement therapeutics. Adv Exp Med Biol. 2013;734a:1–22.

99. Legendre CM, Licht C, Loirat C. Eculizumab in atypical hemolytic-uremic syndrome. N Engl J Med. 2013;369:1379–80.

100. Nurnberger J, Philipp T, Witzke O, Opazo Saez A, Vester U, Baba HA, Kribben A, Zimmerhackl LB, Janecke AR, Nagel M, Kirschfink M. Eculizumab for atypical hemolytic-uremic syndrome. N Engl J Med. 2009;360:542–4.

101. Gruppo RA, Rother RP. Eculizumab for congenital atypical hemolytic-uremic syndrome. N Engl J Med. 2009;360:544–6.

102. Ricklin D, Lambris JD. Progress and trends in complement therapeutics. Adv Exp Med Biol. 2013;735:1–22.

103. Emlen W, Li W, Kirschfink M. Therapeutic complement inhibition: new developments. Semin Thromb Hemost. 2010;36:660–8.

104. Vivarelli M, Pasini A, Emma F. Eculizumab for the treatment of dense-deposit disease. N Engl J Med. 2012;366:1163–5.

105. Bomback AS, Smith RJ, Barile GR, Zhang Y, Heher EC, Herlitz L, Stokes MB, Markowitz GS, D'Agati VD, Canetta PA, Radhakrishnan J, Appel GB. Eculizumab for dense deposit disease and C3 glomerulonephritis. Clin J Am Soc Nephrol. 2012;7:748–56.

106. Daina E, Noris M, Remuzzi G. Eculizumab in a patient with dense-deposit disease. N Engl J Med. 2012;366:1161–3.

107. Stegall MD, Diwan T, Raghavaiah S, Cornell LD, Burns J, Dean PG, Cosio FG, Gandhi MJ, Kremers W, Gloor JM. Terminal complement inhibition decreases antibody-mediated rejection in sensitized renal transplant recipients. Am J Transplant. 2011;11:2405–13.

108. Zuber J, Fakhouri F, Roumenina LT, Loirat C, Fremeaux-Bacchi V. Use of eculizumab for atypical haemolytic uraemic syndrome and C3 glomerulopathies. Nat Rev Nephrol. 2012;8:643–57.

109. Souza DG, Esser D, Bradford R, Vieira AT, Teixeira MM. APT070 (Mirococept), a membrane-localised complement inhibitor, inhibits inflammatory responses that follow intestinal ischaemia and reperfusion injury. Br J Pharmacol. 2005;145:1027–34.

110. Sacks S, Karegli J, Farrar CA, Asgari E, Schwaeble W, Zhou W, Smith RA. Targeting complement at the time of transplantation. Adv Exp Med Biol. 2013;734a:247–55.

111. Song H, Qiao F, Atkinson C, Holers VM, Tomlinson S. A complement C3 inhibitor specifically targeted to sites of complement activation effectively ameliorates collagen-induced arthritis in DBA/1 J mice. J Immunol. 2007;179:7860–7.

Atypical Hemolytic Uremic Syndrome

24

Chantal Loirat and Véronique Frémeaux-Bacchi

Introduction

The hemolytic uremic syndrome (HUS) is a thrombotic microangiopathy (TMA) characterized by the triad of thrombocytopenia, microangiopathic anemia, and acute renal failure. The most frequent form of HUS in children is secondary to Shiga toxin (Stx) – producing *Escherichia coli* (STEC) and the term atypical HUS (aHUS) was initially used to designate any HUS not caused by STEC. Some forms of non STEC-associated HUS in children are associated with *Streptococcus pneumoniae* infection, cobalamine C (cblC) defect and, rarely, various conditions such as bone marrow transplantation. Atypical HUS without coexisting disease or specific infection was demonstrated during the last decade to be mostly a disease of complement alternative pathway (CAP) overactivation, due to hereditary mutations in complement genes or acquired autoantibodies against complement factor H (FH).

The clinical characteristics of patients, patient outcome and genotype-phenotype correlations were described [1–6]. Therefore the term aHUS is today preferentially used to designate HUS without coexisting disease or specific infection [4, 5, 7–10]. Plasma exchanges (PE) were the mainstay of treatment for aHUS until 2009, with considerable morbidity in children [11, 12]. Since 2009, terminal complement blockade therapy by eculizumab has dramatically changed the dismal outcome of the disease [13, 14]. The aim of this chapter is to review the new knowledge acquired since the early 2000s in the domain of aHUS.

Definition of Atypical HUS

The classification of the various forms of TMA based on etiology and/or physiopathology is recommended since 2006 [15, 16] (Fig. 24.1). Thrombotic thrombocytopenic purpura (TTP) is due to a severe deficiency (<10 %) in ADAMTS13 (A Disintegrin And Metalloproteinase with a ThromboSpondin type 1 motif, member 13) activity, either from a congenital absence of functional protein caused by homozygous or compound heterozygous mutations in the ADAMTS13 gene, or due to anti-ADAMTS13 antibodies. TTP should no longer be classified as a variant of aHUS, but as a diagnosis that has to be ruled out in patients suspected to have

C. Loirat (✉)
Department of Pediatric Nephrology, University Hospital Robert Debre, 48 Boulevard Serurier, Paris 75019, France
e-mail: chantal.loirat@aphp.fr

V. Frémeaux-Bacchi
Laboratoire d'Immunologie, Hopital Europeen Georges Pompidou, 20 Rue Leblanc, 75015 Paris, France
e-mail: veronique.fremeaux-bacchi@aphp.fr

© Springer-Verlag Berlin Heidelberg 2016
D.F. Geary, F. Schaefer (eds.), *Pediatric Kidney Disease*, DOI 10.1007/978-3-662-52972-0_24

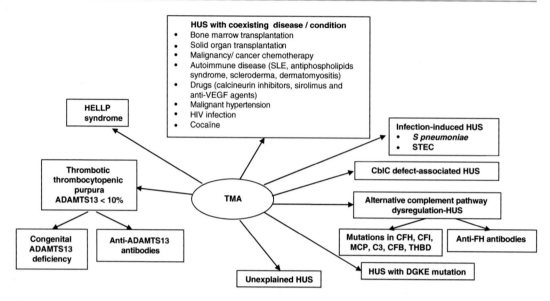

Fig. 24.1 The various forms of thrombotic microangiopathies according to etiology and/or pathophysiology. *ADAMTS 13* A Disintegrin And Metalloproteinase with a ThromboSpondin type 1 motif, member 13, *CblC* cobalamin C, *CFB* complement factor B gene, *CFH* complement factor H gene, *CFI* complement factor I gene, *DGKE* diacylglycerol kinase ε, *HELLP* hemolysis, elevated liver enzymes, and low platelet count ʼsyndrome, *HIV* human immunodeficiency virus, *HUS* hemolytic uremic syndrome, *MCP* membrane cofactor protein (CD46), *SLE* systemic lupus erythematosous, *STEC* Shiga toxin- producing *Escherichia coli*, *THBD* thrombomodulin, *VEGF* vascular endothelium growth factor

aHUS. HUS secondary to coexisting disease/ condition, a frequent situation in adults, is quite exceptional in children except for HUS after bone-marrow transplantation. One must also rule out HUS caused by STEC or other infectious agents in all patients suspected to have aHUS. An agreement has recently emerged that the term aHUS should preferentially be reserved for patients with HUS without a coexisting disease or specific infection [4, 5, 7–10]. This chapter is focused on aHUS according to this definition.

Pathology

The underlying histological lesion of aHUS is TMA involving afferent arterioles and glomerular capillaries. Characteristic features during the acute phase are platelet and fibrin thrombi within glomerular capillaries and the thickening of glomerular capillary walls related to endothelial cell swelling and detachment and the accumulation of flocculent material (proteins and cellular debris) between the endothelial cells and the basement membrane, with double contour appearance. Mesangiolysis (fluffy mesangial expansion) is also common. Bloodless and ischemic glomeruli related to the narrowing or occlusion of the capillary and arteriolar lumen can be observed. Arterial changes range from endothelial swelling to fibrinoid necrosis with occlusive thrombi. Immunofluoresence studies for immunoglobulin G or C3 deposits, though limited, are generally described as negative. However, strong immunostaining for C3 and C9 neoantigen, which reflects C5b-9 formation, were recently reported in kidney biopsies taken during the acute phase in five patients [17]. Late stages are characterized by mesangial sclerosis, thickening of capillary walls with sparce or diffuse double contours, ischemic changes of glomeruli and mucoid intimal hyperplasia and narrowing of the arterial lumen [18, 19]. Due to limited information from sequential biopsies, it is uncertain whether the persistence of diffuse double contours long after the last episode of HUS (e.g., more than 1 year) should be regarded as a marker of ongoing local

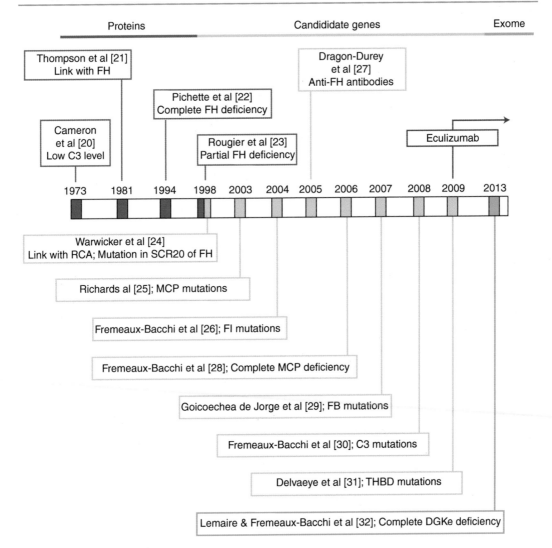

Fig. 24.2 Discoveries that allowed a better understanding of the pathophysiology of aHUS during the last decades. This led to the approval of eculizumab for the treatment of patients with aHUS, to control the overactivation of complement. *FB* complement factor B, *FH* complement factor H, *FI* complement factor I, *DGKE* diacylglycerol kinase ε, *MCP* membrane cofactor protein (CD46), *THBD* thrombomodulin (Data from References [20–32])

TMA process or as a chronic sequel, and sparse or absence of double contours as markers of remission of the TMA process.

Pathophysiology of Atypical HUS

Over the last 40 years, it was demonstrated that the alternative pathway (AP) of the complement system plays a predominant, though not exclusive role in aHUS (Fig. 24.2) [20–32].

The Alternative Pathway of Complement

The complement system is composed of plasma proteins that react with one another to opsonize microbes and induce a series of inflammatory responses that help the immune cells to fight infection. There is mounting evidence that complement participates not only in the defence against pathogens, but also in host homeostasis [33]. The complement cascade can be activated by three different pathways. While the activation of the classical and the lectin pathways occurs after binding to immune complexes or microorganisms respectively, the AP is continuously activated and generates C3b which binds indiscriminately to pathogens and host cells. On a foreign surface, C3b binds factor B (FB), which is then cleaved by Factor D to form the C3 convertase C3bBb. The C3 convertase, which is stabilized by its binding to properdin, induces exponential cleavage of C3b and the generation of C3bBbC3b complexes with C5 convertase activity. The C5 convertase cleaves C5 to generate C5a – the most potent anaphylatoxin – and C5b which initiates the formation of the membrane attack complex (MAC or C5b-9), able to lyse pathogens [34] (Fig. 24.3).

The CAP amplification loop is normally strictly controlled at the surface of the host quiescent endothelium, which is protected from the local formation of the C3 convertase by complement regulatory proteins. These include regulators in serum, such as FH and Factor I (FI), as well as membrane bound CD46 (membrane cofactor protein (MCP)), which cooperate locally to inactivate C3b. FH is the most important protein for the regulation of the CAP. FH consists of 20 short consensus repeats (SCRs) and contain two C3b-binding sites (Fig. 24.4). MCP is a widely expressed transmembrane glycoprotein that binds C3b and inhibits complement activation on host cells. The serine protease FI cleaves C3b in the presence of various cofactors including FH, complement receptor 1 (CR1, CD35) and MCP. Coagulation regulator thrombomodulin (THBD) enhances FI-mediated inactivation of C3b in the presence of FH [31].

Complement Abnormalities in aHUS

A database describing all mutations identified in aHUS is available at http://www.FH.HUS.org and published [35].

CFH Mutations and Anti-FH Antibodies
A role of CFH in aHUS was first suggested more than 40 years ago (Fig. 24.2). A decrease of plasma C3 level was first reported in 1973 in five patients with severe HUS [20] and low FH plasma levels were first reported in 1981 in a 8-month-old boy with HUS [21]. However, it is only in 1998 that Warwicker et al, by linkage analysis, could establish the link between aHUS and the Regulators of Complement Activation (RCA) region in chromosome 1q32, and the presence of mutations in CFH, mainly in the SCR 20, despite normal plasma levels of FH and C3 [24].

During the last 15 years, 163 different mutations of CFH including missense mutations, non sense mutations, short deletions or insertions, located everywhere in the gene, have been identified and referenced in the FH aHUS mutation database. The type I mutations, which induce a quantitative deficiency of the FH protein (low FH plasma levels), are located everywhere in the gene. By contrast, the mutations which induce a decreased ability of FH to bind to endothelial cells-bound C3b while plasma levels of FH are normal (namely type II mutations), are mostly located in SCR 20 (Fig. 24.4). More than 90 % of reported mutations have been heterozygous and plasma C3 levels are decreased in approximately 50 % of patients (Fig. 24.5) [1, 4, 32, 36–42]. Less than 20 children (2–4 % of reported children with aHUS), mostly from consanguineous families, carried a CFH homozygous mutation leading to complete FH deficiency, with permanently very low C3 levels. CFH mutations are the most common among aHUS patients, accounting for 20–30 % of all aHUS cases in registries from the United States and Europe [1–4] (Table 24.1).

The CFH gene is in close proximity to genes encoding for the five CFH Related (CFHR) proteins that are thought to have arisen from several large genomic duplications. All CFHRs share a high degree of homology, which makes the region particularly prone to genomic rearrangement. Mutations (p. Ser1191Leu and p.Val1197Ala) that arose from gene conversion between CFH and CFHR1 or large deletions leading to the formation of hybrid CFH/CFHR1 or CFH/CFHR3 protein have been reported in several unrelated aHUS patients from distinct geographic origins [43–46].

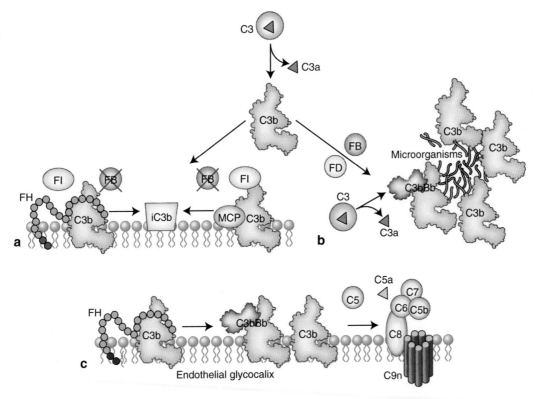

Fig. 24.3 Complement activation and its regulation. aHUS is the prototype of a disease resulting from inefficient protection of endothelial cells against complement activation. (**a**) Protection of cells surface. The AP is permanently active, with a continuous formation of small amounts of the C3 convertase C3bBb at the cell surface. To prevent unopposed complement activation resulting in cell damage, the complement system is tighly regulated. The glycocalyx is a multifunctional thick carbohydrate layer containing glycoaminoglycans (GAG) (heparin sulphate, sialic acid, polyanions) that covers all endothelial cells, in particular the glomerular endothelium in the kidney. FH binds to GAG and C3b. MCP is constitutionally anchored to endothelial membrane. Under normal conditions, the C3 convertase formation is stopped by the interaction of FH or MCP with C3b, which makes further binding of FB to C3b impossible. C3b is then cleaved by FI to iC3b, which cannot bind FB. (**b**) Activation of complement and covalent attachment of C3b to the microbial surfaces. The major function of complement is to act as a defence mechanism against microbes. Very small amounts of C3b are normally present in plasma due to low levels of spontaneous C3 cleavage but C3b can bind to bacteria. Once C3b is covalently bound to the surface of microorganisms, FB binds to it and becomes susceptible to cleavage by Factor D (FD). The resulting C3bBb complex is a C3 convertase that will continue to generate more C3b, thus amplifying C3b production. C3b attaches to bacterial surfaces for opsonization by phagocytes and simultaneous activation of the cytolytic terminal complement cascade. (**c**) In the case of aHUS, AP activation is uncontrolled and C3 convertase C3bBb and C5 convertase C3bC3bBb are formed. During complement activation, C5 is split into C5a and C5b. C5b together with complement proteins C6, C7, C8 and C9 form the C5b9 complex in sublytic quantities that activate endothelial cells to produce prothrombotic factors. *AP* alternative pathway, *C3bBb* C3 convertase, *C3bC3bBb* C5 convertase, *FB* complement factor B, *FD* complement factor D, *FH* complement factor H, *FI* complement factor I, *MCP* membrane cofactor protein (CD46)

An acquired dysfunction of FH due to anti-FH autoantibodies has been described in 6–25 % of patients in European cohorts [4, 38, 39, 42], up to 50 % in India [40], mostly in children. The antibodies bind mostly to SCR 19 and 20 of FH but also to other epitopes of FH and thus inhibit the majority of regulatory functions of FH at cell surfaces [47]. Plasma C3 level is decreased in 40–60 % of patients with anti-FH antibodies during the acute phase (Fig. 24.5), while FH levels are decreased in only approximately 20 % of patients [38]. C3 levels are significantly lower in patients with very high anti-FH titer, while no correlation has

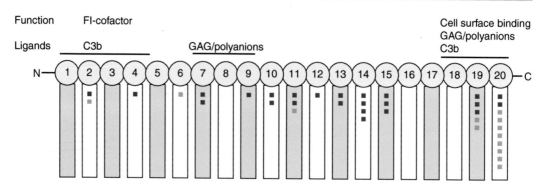

Fig. 24.4 Complement factor H. FH is a plasma protein consisting in 20 domains called short consensus repeats (SCRs) (*numbered circles*). FH has two C3b binding sites: one is localized within the N-terminal SCR 1–4, implicated in the clivage of C3b by FI and the other in the C-terminal SCR 19, implicated in cell surface binding. FH also contains two polyanion-binding sites in SCR 7 and SCR 20 implicated in GAG binding. FH regulates the formation, stability and decay of the C3 convertase C3bBb.

CFH mutations identified in the French aHUS cohort [4] are shown within columns. Blue squares indicate mutations associated with decreased FH plasma level, orange squares indicate mutations associated with normal FH level. Mutations in the C-terminus SCR 20 are mostly associated with normal FH plasma level. *FH* complement factor H, *FI* complement factor I, *GAG* glycoaminoglycans, *SCR* short consensus repeat

been found between FH plasma levels and the anti-FH antibody titer [38, 40].

Ninety percent of patients with anti-FH antibodies have a complete deficiency of CFHR1 and CFHR3 due to a homozygous deletion of *CFHR1-R3*, a polymorphism carried by 2–9 % of European, 16 % of African and ≤2 % of Chinese healthy controls [48]. The reason why individuals with *CFHR1-R3* deletion develop anti-FH antibodies is uncertain.

CFI Mutations and Anti-FI Antibodies

To date 57 *CFI* mutations have been published, located everywhere in the gene. All but one mutation are heterozygous [4]. *CFI* mutations induce either a default of secretion of the mutant protein or disrupt its cofactor activity, with altered degradation of C3b in the fluid phase and on surfaces. However, 40 % of *CFI* mutations have no identified functional consequences and their link with the disease remains unclear. Plasma C3 levels are below the normal range in approximately 50 % of patients with *CFI* mutation (Fig. 24.5) and FI levels are slightly decreased in 30 %. *CFI* mutations account for 4–8 % of aHUS cases (Table 24.1). Two cases of anti-FI antibody-associated HUS have been reported [49].

MCP Mutations

Forty nine mutations have been identified in *MCP* gene. Fifty percent of mutations identified in MCP gene are splice site mutations. One third of *MCP* mutations are homozygous and two-thirds are heterozygous. Over 80 % of the reported mutations induce a reduction in MCP expression. Plasma C3 level is normal in patients with isolated *MCP* mutations (Fig. 24.5). *MCP* mutations are more frequent in children with aHUS than in adults (10–15 % versus 4–6 %) (Table 24.1).

C3 Mutations

Forty seven mutations have been identified in C3 gene, but few functional studies have been reported. Mutations demonstrated to have a functional consequence were all shown to be gain of function mutations that induce either a defect in the ability of C3 to bind to regulatory proteins MCP and FH (indirect gain of function mutation) or an increase in the capacity of C3 to bind FB (direct gain of function mutation). In both cases, the mutation induces enhanced C3bBb convertase formation and complement activation on cell surfaces [50]. From 5 % to 8 % of aHUS patients carry a C3 mutation (Table 24.1) and the majority (approximately 80 %) has persistently low plasma C3 levels (Fig. 24.5).

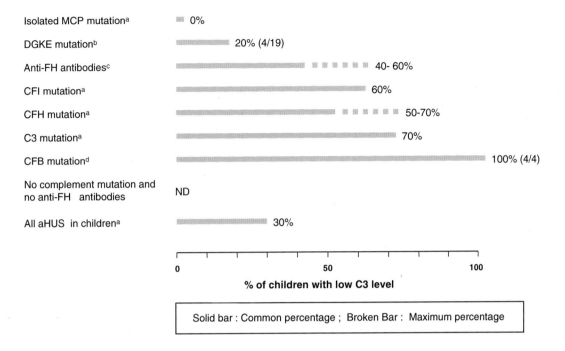

Fig. 24.5 Percentage of children with low C3 levels according to the mutation identified or the presence of anti-FH antibodies. Persistently very low C3 levels (<100 mg/ml) are observed only in patients with homozygous *CFH* mutations. The percentage of CFH-mutated patients who have low C3 is approximately 50 % in children and adults with heterozygous *CFH* mutation and may reach 70 % in pediatric cohorts including children with homozygous *CFH* mutation [1, 4]. C3 level is inversely correlated with anti-FH antibody titer in patients with anti-FH antibody-associated HUS. *CFB* complement factor B gene, *CFH* complement factor H gene, *CFI* complement factor I gene, *DGKE* diacylglycerol kinase ε gene, *MCP* membrane cofactor protein (CD46). [a]Reference [4], including 89 children with aHUS (19 with *CFH* mutation, 12 with isolated *MCP* mutation, 6 with *CFI* mutation, 7 with *C3* mutation and 2 with *CFB* mutation). [b]References [32, 36, 37], including 13, 2 and 4 patients with *DGKE* mutation, respectively. [c]References [38–40], including 45, 19 and 138 patients with anti-FH antibodies, respectively. [d]Reference [41], including 4 children with *CFB* gain of function mutation (Data from References [1, 4, 32, 36–42])

Mutations with Low Frequency

Few mutations in *THBD* affecting the functions of the protein have been identified, with a frequency varying from 0 % to 5 % of all aHUS cases [1, 2, 31] (Table 24.1).

Only four mutations of *CFB* with functional consequences have been identified. Therefore *CFB* mutations account for only 1–2 % of aHUS patients (Table 24.1). Functional analyses demonstrated that aHUS-associated *CFB* mutations are exclusively gain of function mutations that result in enhanced formation of the C3bBb convertase [41, 51]. CFB-mutated patients exhibit a permanent activation of the alternative pathway with very low C3 (Fig. 24.5).

Combined Mutations

Interestingly, combined mutations (mutations in two genes) were identified in 3.4 % of 795 patients with aHUS from a large European cohort. Only 8–10 % of patients with mutations in *CFH*, *C3*, or *CFB* had combined mutations, whereas approximately 25 % of patients with mutations in *MCP* or *CFI* had combined mutations [52].

Mode of Inheritance and Penetrance of Complement: Mediated HUS

Twenty to 30 % of patients have a familial history of aHUS. More frequently the disease is sporadic with only one case per family. However, de novo mutations are exceptional [51]. Among pedigrees

Table 24.1 Frequency of complement and DGKE abnormalities in children and adults with atypical hemolytic uremic syndrome in four cohorts from Europe and the USA

	[1]			[4][a]			[3]	[2]
	Total	Children	Adults	Total	Children	Adults	Children	Children + adults
Number of patients	256	152	104	214	89	125	45	144
CFH mutation, %	25.3	25.6	25	27.5	21.3	32	11	27
Homozygous	4.2	–	–	1.8	4.4	0	–	
Heterozygous	21.1	–	–	25.7	16.8	32	–	
MCP mutation, %	7	9.2	3.8	9.3	13.5	6.4	9	5
Homozygous	–	–	–	2.8	5.6	0.8	–	–
Heterozygous	–	–	–	6.5	7.8	5.6	–	–
CFI mutation, %	3.9	2.6	5.7	8.4	6.7	9.6	7	8
C3 mutation, %	4.6	3.9	5.7	8.4	7.8	8.8	9	2
CFB mutation, %	0.4	–	–	1.4	1	2.4	4	4
Anti-CFH antibodies, %	3.1	3.9	1.9	6.5	11	3.2	13	–
THBD mutation, %	5	7.8	0.9	0	0	0	0	3
Combined mutations, %	3	–	–	4.2	3.4	4.8	4	5.5
Complement-mediated HUS, %	52.3	53	43	65.7	64.7	67.2	55	46
DGKE mutation, %	–	–	–	3.2	7.9	0	–	–
No identified abnormality, %	47.7	47	57	31.1	27.4	32.8	45	54

CFB complement factor B, CFH complement factor H, CFI complement factor I, DGKE diacylglycerol kinase ε, MCP membrane cofactor protein (CD46), THBD thrombomodulin
% percentage of patients, –: not documented
[a]DGKE mutations were identified in seven children who were previously within the group with no complement mutation identified [4]

with familial aHUS, transmission of the disease is autosomal recessive in cases with homozygous or compound heterozygous mutations in *CFH* or *MCP*. Transmission is autosomal dominant in cases with a heterozygous mutation. Disease penetrance in family members who carry the heterozygous mutation has been evaluated to be approximately 50 %, as only half of these subjects develop the disease. The identified mutation therefore appears to be a risk factor for the disease rather than its direct and unique cause and aHUS has to be regarded as a complex polygenic disease which results from a combination of genetic risk factors. Homozygous haplotypes (defined by five frequent genetic variants transmitted in block) in CFH (CFH tgtgt), MCP (MCP ggaac) [53] and CFHR1*B allele [54] have been demonstrated to be more frequent in patients with aHUS than in controls. Some variants of plasminogen and ADAMTS 13 may also have a predisposing role [55, 56]. In addition, precipitating events or triggers appear required for the disease to manifest in patients genetically at risk.

Complement Alternative Pathway Dysregulation Causes TMA Lesions

Mutations in the genes *CFH*, *MCP* and *CFI* impair the mechanisms that regulate CAP activation and gain of function mutations increase CAP activation. Whatever the mutations identified, endothelial cells are no longer protected from complement activation [57, 58]. The increased production of MAC at the endothelial cell surface induces alterations of these cells, which become procoagulant by producing high molecular weight multimers of von Willebrand Factor, thus triggering the formation of thrombi [59–61]. In addition, complement activation at the surface of platelets triggers platelet activation and aggregation and this contributes to the formation of thrombi within the microcirculation [62]. This physiopathological model is corroborated by transgenic animal models. Mice which express FH variant lacking the C-terminal 16–20 domain responsible for the interaction of FH with C3b and the endothelium develop HUS similar to the human disease [63].

DGKE Mutations

Using exome sequencing, deficiency in diacylglycerol kinase ε (DGKε) was established as a novel cause of pediatric-onset aHUS in 2013 [32]. Following this first publication of 13 aHUS children from 9 kindreds, who carried mutations in *DGKE* gene, 6 new cases from 4 kindreds have been identified [36, 37]. Transmission of *DGKE* mutations is autosomic recessive. The 19 patients reported to date carry homozygous or compound heterozygous nonsense, splice sites or frameshift mutations. The penetrance of *DGKE* mutation-associated HUS is complete. Interestingly, 3 of the 19 reported children had a heterozygous mutation of *THBD* (2 siblings) or a *C3* variant (1 case) in addition to compound heterozygous *DGKE* mutation [37].

DGKε protein is an intracellular lipid kinase highly expressed in glomerular capillaries, podocytes and platelets of healthy mice and humans. DGKs are enzymes that phosphorylate diacylglycerol molecules to phosphatidic acid. A likely explanation is that the loss of DGKε enhances protein kinase C activation in endothelial cells, platelets and podocytes, which may result in upregulation of prothrombic factors and platelet activation and altered podocyte function [32, 64]. Whether complement activation is indirectly involved in this form of HUS – as suggested by decreased C3 levels not only in one patient with combined C3 variant and *DGKE* mutation [37], but also in three patients with isolated *DGKE* mutation [32, 36]- remains to be confirmed.

Incidence of Atypical HUS

aHUS defined as indicated above is an ultra-rare disease. In the United States, aHUS is considered to have an annual incidence rate of two new pediatric cases per million total population [65]. This incidence was estimated from the number of children screened between 1997 and 2001 for enrollment in a multicenter trial of SYNSORB-Pk in post-diarrheal HUS, but who were not eligible because of lack of diarrhea prodrome (27/247). Thirty eight per cent of them (9/24 documented) had *S pneumoniae*-HUS, and one patient had post-bone marrow transplantation HUS. Assays for STEC infection, ADAMTS13 deficiency or cblC defect were not available at that time. More recent data from the French aHUS Registry (including only patients without ADAMTS 13 deficiency, coexisting disease or specific infection) suggested a lower incidence of 0.23 new cases (adult or pediatric onset) per million total population per year between 2000 and 2008 (mean number of new cases: 15 (8–21) per year, for a total population of 65 millions). As 42 % of new patients were children at onset of the disease (<16 years), the incidence in children could be estimated to be at least 0.10 new cases per million total population per year [4]. An incidence of approximately 0.11 new pediatric cases per million total population per year was also observed between July 2009 and December 2010 in an exhaustive cohort of children with aHUS from France, the United Kingdom, Spain, Netherlands and Canada [12]. Even though incidence may be underestimated in the latter two series, it probably is not more than 0.20 per million total population in children. Notice that the assumption that aHUS is a predominantly pediatric disease is not valid. Onset during adulthood was only slightly less frequent than during childhood in one series (44 % versus 56 %, respectively) [1], and was more frequent in another one (58 % versus 42 %) [4].

Clinical Characteristics at Onset

Age and Gender

Atypical HUS in children is a disease of early childhood: mean age at onset was 1.5 years (0 to <15) and 56% (50/89) of children had onset between birth and 2 years of age (28% between birth and 6 months, 28% between 6 months and 2 years) in one series [4], similar to the proportion of 22% (10/45) of children having onset between 1 month and 1 year in another series [3]. aHUS in children is as frequent in females as in males (female-to-male ratio 0.9), in contrast with the female preponderance when the disease starts at the adult age (female-to-male ration 3) [3, 4].

Age at onset in children varies according to the underlying complement abnormality. Onset between birth and 1 year of age has been reported in all aHUS patients (19/19) reported to date with *DGKE* mutation [32, 36, 37] and all children with homozygous *CFH* mutation. It is also frequent in children with heterozygous *CFH* or *CFI* mutation-associated HUS. Conversely, *MCP* mutation -associated HUS in children exceptionally starts before the age of 1 year but most often between age 2 and 12 years. HUS with anti-FH antibodies is also mostly a disease of late childhood and adolescence (onset between 5 and 12 years, mean age 7.9–9 years in three series including a total of 202 patients with this form of aHUS [38–40, 42]. *C3* or *CFB* mutation-associated HUS and aHUS with no complement mutation and no anti-FH antibodies appear to start at any age (Fig. 24.6) [1, 4, 32, 36–40, 42, 66, 67].

Familial History

As indicated above, despite aHUS being a genetic disease, a familial history of HUS is present in only 20–30% of patients [1, 3, 4]. The disease may touch siblings, one parent and his/her child, or show incomplete penetrance, touching cousins, aunt/uncle and nephew/niece, grandparent and grandchild. The diagnosis of HUS may be unknown in the family and questioning should ask about cases of uremia, anemia, hypertension, dialysis and graft failure in the pedigree as well as about consanguinity. Consanguinity explains all homozygous mutations identified in aHUS (*CFH*, *MCP* and *DGKE*). No familial case of anti-FH antibody-associated HUS has been reported.

Triggering Events

aHUS episodes in children are frequently triggered by intercurrent infections, whatever the genetic background. Diarrhoea triggers onset of aHUS in at least one third of children and upper respiratory tract infections in at least 10% [3, 4] (Fig. 24.6). This frequency of diarrhea at onset of aHUS explains why the former post-diarrheal or non post-diarrheal criterion to differentiate STEC-HUS from aHUS was frequently misleading. It is, however, often unclear whether gastrointestinal symptoms in aHUS are linked to an infectious trigger or whether they are manifestations of intestinal TMA. Bloody diarrhea preceding HUS is probably much more frequent in STEC-HUS than in aHUS; however, this is not precisely documented in series of pediatric aHUS. Rare patients (approximately 1%) have been reported in whom the first episode of aHUS was caused by STEC gastroenteritis, with the diagnosis of aHUS being retained because the patient (one patient with *MCP* mutation) had subsequent relapses and a familial history of aHUS [4], a severe course possibly favoured by the genetic complement abnormality (one patient with *CFH* mutation) [68] or recurrence after kidney transplantation (two patients with *CFI* or *MCP* mutation – the latter also in the mother who donated the kidney) [69]. Further studies might help to clarify the role of rare variants in complement genes in patients with STEC-HUS, especially in case of a fulminant outcome [70]. STEC has also been the trigger of HUS in a couple of patients with anti-FH antibody-associated HUS [38, 42]. Interestingly, the association of homozygous *MCP* mutation with common variable immunodeficiency has been reported [28].

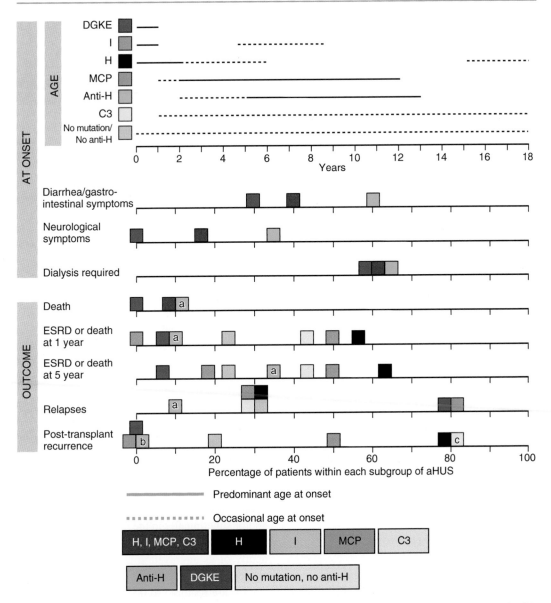

Fig. 24.6 Clinical characteristics at onset and outcome (pre-complement blockade therapy era) in children with aHUS and complement or DGKE mutation, anti-FH antibodies or no mutation and no anti-FH antibody identified. *aHUS* atypical hemolytic uremic syndrome, *anti-H* anti-factor H antibody, *H* complement factor H, *I* complement factor I, *DGKE* diacylglycerol kinase ε, *MCP* membrane cofactor protein (CD46). References: aHUS in children with or without complement mutation: [4]; aHUS with *DGKE* mutation: [32, 36, 37]; aHUS with anti-FH antibodies: [38–40, 42]; post- kidney transplant recurrence of aHUS: [42, 66, 67]. (*a*) Anti-FH antibody-associated HUS treated with PE + immunosuppressants + corticosteroids. (*b*) Anti-FH antibody-associated HUS transplanted with negativated or low titer of anti-FH antibodies. (*c*) *C3/CFB* gain of function mutation-associated HUS

Therefore patients with homozygous *MCP* mutation should be investigated for immunodeficiency that may require immunoglobulin therapy to prevent infections –and thus decrease the frequency of HUS relapses triggered by infections.

Lastly, pregnancy is the trigger of aHUS in 20 % of adult women [4] and 86 % of women with pregnancy-HUS (mostly in the post-partum) have a complement mutation [71]. For this reason, pregnancy-HUS is now classified as aHUS.

Clinical Presentation

The majority of children with aHUS present with the complete triad of HUS (mechanical hemolytic anemia with haemoglobin <10 g/dl, presence of schizocytes, high lacticodeshydrogenase (LDH), decreased haptoglobin levels, plus platelet count <150 Giga (G)/L plus serum creatinine above the upper limit of normal (ULN)); approximately 60 % of them require dialysis at the first episode (Fig. 24.6). Severe hypertension is common. However, the complete triad may be missing at admission and a gradual onset is possible. Particularly, platelet count may be >150 G/L (approximately 15 % of patients) and hemoglobin may be >10 g/dL (approximately 5 % of patients) [4]. Children (approximately 15 %) may also have normal serum creatinine at presentation [72] and/or present with proteinuria/nephrotic syndrome/hematuria/hypertension as the only renal manifestations. Thus any association of 2 components of the triad with the third one missing can be a manifestation of HUS. While kidney biopsy is not required to establish the diagnosis when full-blown HUS is present, it is useful when hematologic criteria are missing or incomplete and any time the diagnosis of HUS is uncertain, to document that the underlying histological lesion is TMA.

Extra-renal Manifestations

Although the TMA process predominates in the renal vasculature, other organs may be involved. The most frequent extra-renal manifestation during acute episodes of aHUS is brain involvement, reported in 15–20 % of children with aHUS (Fig. 24.6) [4, 73, 74]. Symptoms can be seizures, altered mental status, altered consciousness, visual problems (diplopia, sudden visual loss), paresis and coma. Computed tomography scan is useful to rule out cerebral bleeding. Magnetic resonance imaging (MRI) shows hyperdensities of variable severity and extension. Focal cerebral infarction is possible. The prognostic significance of MRI abnormalities is generally uncertain. The frequency of cardiac involvement is poorly documented, but life threatening ischemic myocardiopathy may occur, which makes sequential troponine level assay, electrocardiography and echocardiography mandatory during acute episodes [74–77]. Peripheral acute ischemia leading to gangrene of fingers/hands and toes/feet [78], skin necrosis [79–81] or retinal ischemia with sudden visual loss [82] have been reported in a few patients. Extrarenal manifestations may also include pancreatitis (increase in pancreatic enzymes with or without clinical/radiologic signs) and/or hepatitis (increase of hepatic enzymes) (5–10 % of patients) and, exceptionally, intra-alveolar hemorrhage, severe gastro-intestinal manifestations including intestinal perforation or life-threatening multiorgan failure (2–3 % of patients [4, 79]. Severe gastrointestinal symptoms (abdominal pain, vomiting, diarrhea, biological pancreatitis and hepatitis), myocardial and neurological manifestations appear to be particularly frequent in patients with anti-FH antibodies [38–40, 42, 76, 78] (Fig. 24.6).

Four children have been reported who developed cerebral ischemic events due to stenoses of cerebral arteries after several years on dialysis [83–86]. One of them also had stenoses of coronary, pulmonary and digestive arteries [83]. These observations have suggested that local complement activation during acute episodes and/or subclinically in the long term, may lead to such macrovascular complications, independently or as aggravating factors of the vascular consequences of long term dialysis. Prospective studies are required to document whether aHUS patients have an increased risk of cardio-or cerebro vascular events and of arterial disease due to the local complement activation [87].

Diagnosis of Atypical Hemolytic Uremic Syndrome

In children, the medical history and physical examination usually eliminate HUS secondary to a coexisting condition – mostly bone marrow transplantation- and generally suffice for the diagnosis of *Streptococcus pneumoniae*-HUS, that occurs mostly in children less than 2 years of age presenting with symptoms of invasive infection (pneumonia, meningitis, bacteremia) (see Part VI, Chap. 26). The clinical context and baseline laboratory assays also generally are sufficient to allow the diagnosis of STEC-HUS (see Chap. 26), TTP, cblC defect or aHUS with a good degree of certainty. However, age at onset and the clinical presentation of these various forms of pediatric TMA may overlap, while outcome and first line treatment are different (Fig. 24.7) [66, 88–101]. Therefore confirmatory investigations are necessary to rule out all the other causes of TMA in any patient suspected to have aHUS (Fig. 24.8) [102].

Biological Assays to Confirm the Clinical Diagnosis of aHUS

STEC infection should be ruled out as soon as possible when aHUS is suspected. Stools should be collected at admission or rectal swab performed if no stools are available, allowing stool culture and faecal polymerase chain reaction (PCR) or immunologic assay for Stx (see Chap. 26). Negative results, mostly due to delayed stool collection, are observed in at least 30 % of cases classified clinically as STEC-HUS [89]: in such cases, the clinical diagnosis should prevail. Congenital TTP requires urgent plasma infusion (PI) and acquired TTP urgent PE plus corticosteroids ± rituximab. Blood samples collected before PE/PI are required for ADAMTS13 activity assays, which most commonly rely on the cleavage by plasma ADAMTS13 of the von Willebrand Factor (VWF) peptide containing the cleaving site of VWF (Fret-VWF 73). Results can be available within a few hours [103]. A limitation is the interference of hyperbilirubinemia [104]. Results of commercial kits show reasonable though not full agreement (80–90 % concordance) with Fret-VWF73 [105, 106]. Lastly, assays to detect cblC defect should be part of the initial biological sampling in any child suspected to have aHUS. CblC defect – associated HUS, which can be rescued by hydroxocobalamine treatment, may occur in

neonatal forms presenting with neurological, cardiac or multivisceral involvement, but at least as frequently in late-onset forms presenting with predominant or isolated HUS during childhood or early adulthood [99–101] (Figs. 24.7 and 24.8).

Complement Investigations in Patients Suspected to Have aHUS

All patients suspected of having aHUS should have blood sampling before PE/PI for measurement of C3, C4, FH, FI and FB plasma levels and screening for anti-FH antibodies. A recent publication from seven European laboratories reports the standardization of the enzyme linked immunosorbent assay technique for anti-FH antibodies [107], which could be developed in other countries. MCP surface expression on polynuclear or mononuclear leucocytes is also required.

As indicated above, decreased C3 levels are observed in only 30 % of children with aHUS [1, 3–5] (Fig. 24.5). Therefore, a normal C3 level does not rule out the diagnosis of aHUS. Normal C4 concentration associated with decreased C3 level confirms activation of the CAP as would a decreased FB concentration. As the C3 level is normal in patients with isolated MCP mutation and decreased in patients with high titer anti-FH antibodies, aHUS in a pre-adolescent or adolescent child – the age of onset in these two subgroups of complement-dependent HUS – is most likely MCP mutation-associated-HUS if C3 level is normal or anti-FH antibody-associated HUS if C3 level is low.

As indicated above, decreased FH or FI plasma levels are observed in approximately 50 % and 30 % of patients with mutation in *CFH* or *CFI* genes, respectively [4, 5, 108]. Therefore, a normal FH or FI plasma level does not exclude a mutation in the corresponding gene.

Recent data suggest that levels of C5a and soluble C5b-9 (sC5b-9) are elevated during acute episodes of aHUS and may be biological markers to differentiate aHUS from TTP [109]. Increased C5a and sC5b-9 plasma levels have been confirmed in approximately half of aHUS patients

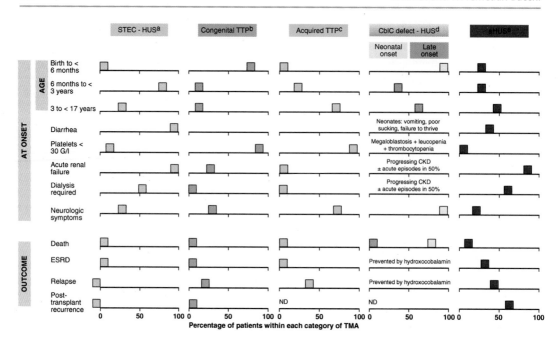

Fig. 24.7 Clinical characteristics at onset in children with STEC-HUS, congenital or acquired TTP, cblC defect-HUS or atypical HUS. [a]STEC-HUS: Incidence: 23/10[6] children <2 years, 8/10[6]children <15 years [89]. Bloody diarrhea in ≥60% of cases, preceeding onset of HUS. At 5 years follow-up, ESRD rate is 2–3%, but 30–40% of patients have proteinuria, hypertension or GFR <90 ml/min/1.73 m[2] [90, 91]. Treatment relies on supportive care. [b]Congenital TTP (Upshaw-Schulman syndrome): Low incidence, though not precisely documented. Neonatal jaundice+hemolytic anemia+thrombocytopenia in 50–75% of cases. Transient hematuria, hemoglobinuria, proteinuria with normal or slightly elevated serum creatinine are frequent during acute episodes, but acute renal failure requiring dialysis is rare. First line treatment is plasma infusion (PI) (10–15 ml/kg). Outcome indicated here is in children receiving PI. Relapses were common (≥80% of patients) in patients with neonatal onset not receiving prophylactic PI, but are unfrequent under prophylactic PI (generally given twice monthly). Infections require additional PI. Death and ESRD rates are ~ zero with prophylactic PI. Some mild cases (late onset or mild thrombocytopenia as the only manifestation) require only on demand PI. Recurrence after transplantation is prevented by PI. Recombinant ADAMTS13 therapy will reduce treatment burden [92–94]. [c]Acquired TTP: Incidence: 0.09/10[6] children <18 years (30-fold lower than in adults) [95]. More common in females and older children. Severe renal failure requiring dialysis is rare (<10%). Additional diagnosis of SLE in 19% of children. First line treatment: PE. Outcome indicated here is in children receiving PE (+ corticosteroids ± rituximab). Patients with persistant severe ADAMTS13 deficiency in remission are at high risk of relapse. Rituximab decreases relapse rate [92, 93, 95, 96]. [d]CblC defect-HUS: a rare disease, with 22 patients reported, including 11 with neonatal (<28 days) onset, 10 with onset during childhood (1.5–14 years) and 1 in a 20 year-old adult [97–100]. In addition, HUS occurred, generally at onset, in 9 of 88 (10%) patients with cblC defect (5% of cases with neonatal onset, 12% of cases with onset between 1 month and <1 year and 25% of cases with onset after 1 year) [101]. In neonatal forms, hypotonia, lethargy, feeding difficulties, developmental delay ± micro or hydrocephalus preceedes onset of HUS and mortality rate is high (from multivisceral failure, cardiomyopathy and neurologic involvement). Early treatment with intramuscular hydroxocobalamin+betaine+folic acid may allow survival, but neurologic and visual impairment (pigmentary retinopathy, optic atrophy) generally persist. Late onset cases may present as isolated HUS and early treatment may allow full recovery. A frequent complication in late forms is pulmonary hypertension (two thirds of patients) [99–101]. [e]aHUS in children: outcome indicated here is in children not receiving complement-blockade therapy. *aHUS* atypical hemolytic uremic syndrome, *Cbl-C* cobalamin C, *ESRD* end stage renal disease, *HUS* hemolytic uremic syndrome, *PE* plasma exchange, *PI* plasma infusion, *STEC* Shiga toxin- producing *Escherichia coli*, *TTP* Thrombotic thrombocytopenic purpura

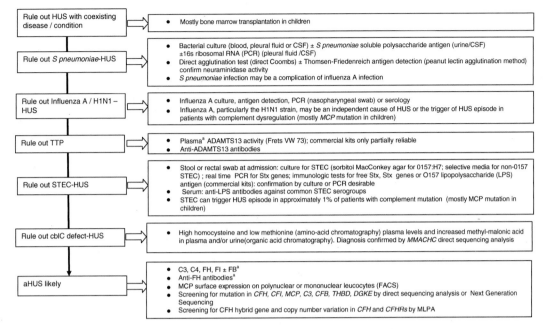

Fig. 24.8 Diagnosis algorithm for atypical HUS in children. *ADAMTS13* A Disintegrin And Metalloproteinase with a ThromboSpondin type 1 motif, member 13, *aHUS* atypical hemolytic uremic syndrome, *Cbl-C* cobalamin C, *CFB* complement factor B gene, *CFH* complement factor H gene, *CFHRs* complement factor H related proteins, *CFI* complement factor I gene, *CSF* cerebrospinal fluid, *DGKE* diacylglycerol kinase ε, *FACS* Fluorescence Activated Cell Sorting, *HUS* hemolytic uremic syndrome, *MCP* membrane cofactor protein (CD46), *MLPA* multiplex ligation dependent probe amplification, *PCR* polymerase chain reaction, *STEC* Shiga toxin- producing *Escherichia coli, Stx* shigatoxin. [a]Blood sampling to be collected before plasma exchange/plasma infusion (Used with permission of Springer Science + Business Media from Loirat et al. [102])

during acute phases of the disease and also during remission [17]. However, a normalization of complement activation products levels after remission, including sC5b-9, has been reported by another group [110]. Thus the usefulness of these markers for routine clinical care remains to be determined.

Genetic Screening in Patients Confirmed to Have aHUS

Genetic screening results are not required for urgent therapeutic decisions but are necessary to establish whether the disease is complement-dependent or not, prognosis, risk of relapses and of progression to end stage renal disease (ESRD), genetic councelling, decisions for complement blockade treatment duration and for kidney transplantation. The six complement genes identified as susceptibility factors for aHUS (*CFH, CFI, MCP, C3, CFB* and *THBD*) should be analysed by direct sequencing or next generation sequencing analysis. Multiplex ligation dependent probe amplification (MLPA) is required to detect hybrid *CFH* genes (5 % of patients) and copy number variations in *CFH* and *CFHRs* genes. Because of the frequency of combined mutations indicated above, all six genes should be screened for mutation in all patients. Screening for *DGKE* mutation should be performed in children with onset of aHUS before the age of 1–2 years and maybe in older children if further reports indicate *DGKE* mutation-associated HUS may occur later in life. Sequence variants in complement genes have been identified in 5 of 13 patients with anti-FH antibody –associated HUS in one series [111], but none of 26 patients in another series [38]. Genetic analyses even when anti-FH antibodies are present may be justified. If the patient has anti-FH antibodies and a mutation, treatment should be decided according to the antibody titer and the functional consequences of the mutation [102].

Next-generation sequencing analysis allows the simultaneous study of all potentially relevant genes and will probably decrease the delay for results and the cost of genetic analysis. Exome sequencing, which was successfully used to identify *DGKE* mutations [32], is still limited to research laboratories.

Outcome of Atypical HUS in the Pre-complement Blockade Therapy Era

Mortality and Renal Outcome

The death rate in children with aHUS was 8 % [4], 9 % [3] and 14 % [1] in three recent pediatric series, at follow-up 45 months (median), 7.5 years (mean) and 3 years (median), respectively. Most deaths occurred in children less than 1 year of age and at first episode or during the first year after onset. This shows that despite medical progress, the disease is still life-threatening, especially in very young children. Approximately 20 % of children progressed to ESRD or died at first episode or within <1 month after onset, 30 % within 1 year and 40 % at 5 years follow-up. The most severe outcome was in children with *CFH* mutation, of whom one third progressed to ESRD or died at first episode, half at 1 year and two thirds at 5 years follow-up. The prognosis of *CFI* and *C3* mutation-associated HUS was hardly less severe than that of *CFH* mutation-associated HUS. *MCP* mutation-associated HUS in children had the best prognosis, with a risk of ESRD of 25 % at median follow-up 17.8 years. HUS in children with no complement mutation identified also had a relatively favourable outcome [4] (Fig. 24.6). Among patients with *CFH* or *CFI* mutations, the presence of mutations in other genes did not modify prognosis. In contrast, 50 % of patients with combined *MCP* mutations developed ESRD within 3 years from onset compared with 19 % of patients with an isolated *MCP* mutation [52].

Less than 10 % of children with *DGKE* mutation-associated HUS progress to ESRD in the first year after onset, but patients with this form of aHUS develop proteinuria and nephrotic syndrome, severe hypertension and progress to chronic kidney disease (CKD) stages 4–5 (estimated glomerular filtration rate 15–29 ml/min/1.73 m^2 or ESRD) between the age of 20 and 25 years [32]. Lastly, outcome of anti-FH antibody–associated HUS was poor when treatment was limited to PE, including death in 10 % of patients, CKD in 40 % and ESRD in one third at mean follow-up 39 months [38]. In recent years, early treatment with a combination of PE, corticosteroids and immunosuppressants has allowed a more favourable outcome, similar to that of *MCP* mutation – associated HUS [4, 40] (Fig. 24.6).

Relapses

Recent series suggest that approximately half of children with aHUS have relapses [3, 4]. Among children who had not died or reached ESRD at first episode or at 1 year follow-up, 25 % had relapses during the first year and 47 % after the first year. However, a high relapse rate after the first year was mostly in patients with *DGKE* mutation (83 % during the first year, 50 % up to 5 years) or *MCP* mutation (25 % during the first year, 92 % after the first year), while relapse rate after the first year was 20–30 % in other genetic subgroups [4, 32]. Despite this risk of relapses in the long term, *MCP* mutation-associated HUS has the best prognosis in children, as indicated above. Last, aHUS with anti-FH antibodies had a relapsing course in two third of patients when untreated or treated only with PE/PI [38, 42], which has been reduced to approximately 10 % by early treatment combining PE + immunosuppressants + corticosteroids [4, 40] (Fig. 24.6).

Treatment of Atypical HUS in the Pre-complement Blockade Therapy Era

Plasma Exchange/Plasma Infusion

PE (or PI when PE was not possible) has been first line treatment for aHUS until recent years. The aim was to infuse a large amount of non-mutated complement factors by using frozen plasma for volume substitution (60 ml/kg /PE session) and to withdraw mutated factors and other potential thrombogenic factors. A guideline for early (within 24 h) and intensive PE (or PI, 10–15 ml/kg, if PE was not possible) during the first month of the disease was published in 2009 by the European Pediatric Study Group for HUS [11]. A recent audit of this guideline showed that among 71 patients treated for aHUS in European and North American university hospitals between 1 July 2009 and 31 December 2010, 51 received plasmatherapy through a central venous catheter. Sixteen of them (31 %) had 17 catheter-related complications (infection in 8, thrombosis in 3, ischemic limb in 1, hemorrhage in 2, chylothorax in 1). In addition, eight children developed plasma hypersensitivity leading to treatment cessation in 1 case. This confirms that PE continues to be a source of severe complications in children [12]. Approximately 15 case reports, mostly in children with *CFH* mutation, showed that early plasmatherapy, generally consisting of daily PE until platelet count, hemolysis and LDH level normalized and renal function improved, followed by maintenance PE/PI, could prevent relapses and preserve renal function at follow-up up to 6 years [7, 8, 108]. However, although plasmatherapy was associated with complete or partial remission (hematologic remission with renal sequelae) in approximately 80 % of aHUS episodes in children, half of them had died or reached ESRD at 3 years follow-up [1]. The rate of progression to ESRD at first episode was not significantly different in children with CFH mutation who received high-intensity plasmatherapy compared to those who did not [4]. The benefit of PE/PI is also uncertain in *DGKE* mutation-associated HUS, as proteinuria, the main marker of a progressing course in *DGKE* mutation–associated HUS, persisted in 9 of the 12 patients who received plasmatherapy [32, 36, 37].

Kidney Transplantation

The risk of post-transplant recurrence of aHUS was 60 % in the pre-complement blockade era [1, 66]. Forty percent of recurrences occurred during the first month after transplantation and 70 % during the first year. Graft survival was 30 % at 5 years follow-up in patients with recurrence, compared to 68 % in those without recurrence [66]. Eighty percent of patients who had lost a prior graft from recurrence had recurrence after retransplantation. The main independent risk factor for recurrence was the presence of a complement mutation (Fig. 24.6). The highest risk (approximately 80 %) was in patients with *CFH* and *C3* or *CFB* gain of function mutation, the risk in patients with *CFI* mutation was approximately 50 % and patients with no complement mutation identified had the lowest risk (approximately 20 %) [66]. The risk of post-transplant recurrence in patients with *MCP* mutation has been shown to be low (<10 %) if the mutation is isolated (the graft brings the non-mutated MCP protein), while it is approximately 30 % if the *MCP* mutation is associated with a mutation in *CFH*, *CFI* or *C3* [52]. No post-transplant recurrence was observed in three patients with *DGKE* mutation [32]. The risk is low in anti-FH antibody-associated HUS if the antibody titer is low at the time of transplantation, while substantial if elevated [38, 42, 67, 111, 112] (Fig. 24.6). One patient with *THBD* mutation has been reported to have post-transplant recurrence [113].

This shows that genetic screening is necessary before listing a patient for kidney transplantation, to predict the risk of post-transplant recurrence and guide decisions for the choice of the donor and the prevention of recurrence.

PE/PI for post-transplant recurrence generally failed to avoid graft loss [1, 66]. Therefore prophylactic PE/PI was recommended [114]. The efficacy of this strategy is poorly documented. However, graft survival rate free of recurrence was significantly higher in 9 patients who received prophylactic PE/PI than in 62 patients without prophylactic PE/PI [66]. Interestingly, calcineurin inhibitors (CNI) regimen did not increase significantly the risk of recurrence in a recent series, while mTOR inhibitors use was an independent significant risk factor for recurrence, possibly related to the anti-VEGF (vascular endothelium growth factor) action of these drugs [66]. The current consensus is that aHUS is not per se a contraindication to CNI; however, strict monitoring of blood levels and overdosage avoidance is recommended, while CNI-free mTOR based immunosuppressive regimens should be avoided [115].

Terminal Complement Blockade Therapy

Eculizumab, a monoclonal humanized anti-C5 antibody, prevents C5 cleavage and the formation of C5a and C5b-9, thus blocking the C5a pro-inflammatory and the C5b-9 pro-thrombotic consequences of complement activation. It is the accepted treatment of paroxysmal nocturnal hemoglobinuria (PNH), another complement dependent disease, with more than 1000 patients treated in the world, a number of them for more than 10 years [116]. The first two aHUS patients treated with eculizumab were published in 2009 [117, 118]. As of June 2014, approximately 180 aHUS patients treated with eculizumab have been reported, including 100 patients treated within 4 prospective single-arm, non-randomized trials conducted by Alexion Pharmaceuticals. Eculizumab is approved for the treatment of aHUS in a number of countries worldwide, including the European Union and the USA [119, 120]. Recommended treatment schedule in patients with aHUS [119, 120] is indicated in Table 24.2.

Prospective Trials of Eculizumab in Patients with aHUS

The trials design, definitions of primary endpoints and baseline patients' characteristics are summarized in Table 24.3 and results of the trials in Table 24.4. All patients received the recommended treatment schedule [119, 120] (Table 24.2).

In trial 1 comprising patients with progressive TMA resistant to PE/PI, platelet count normalized after 7 days (median; range 1–218 days) and LDH activity after 14 days (range 0–56 days) after the first dose of eculizumab. Eighty eight

Table 24.2 Body weight-based dosing recommendations for intravenous eculizumab in patients with atypical HUS

Patient body weight	Induction regimen	Maintenance regimen
40 kg and over	900 mg weekly × 4 doses	1200 mg at week 5; then 1200 mg every 2 weeks
30 kg to less than 40 kg	600 mg weekly × 2 doses	900 mg at week 3; then 900 mg every 2 weeks
20 kg to less than 30 kg	600 mg weekly × 2 doses	600 mg at week 3; then 600 mg every 2 weeks
10 kg to less than 20 kg	600 mg weekly × 1 dose	300 mg at week 2; then 300 mg every 2 weeks
5 kg to less than 10 kg	300 mg weekly × 1 dose	300 mg at week 2; then 300 mg every 3 weeks

Eculizumab (Soliris®) should be administered at the recommended dosage regimen time points, or within 2 days of these time points

Data from Soliris:summary of product characteristics http://www.medicines.org.uk/emc/medicine/19966; and from Soliris.net.U.S. prescribing information http://soliris.net/sites/default/files/assets/soliris_pi.pdf

per cent of patients maintained normal platelet count and hematologic remission over a median of 2 years treatment duration. Eighty per cent (4/5) of patients on dialysis at baseline became free of dialysis. Mean gain (95 % CI) in estimated glomerular filtration rate (eGFR) was 32 (14–49) ml/min/1.73 m^2 at 26 weeks (p=0.001 versus baseline eGFR). The gain in eGFR was subsequently maintained and only 12 % of patients (2/17) were on chronic dialysis after 2 years treatment duration (Table 24.4). Earlier initiation of eculizumab was associated with a significantly greater improvement in eGFR (p<0.01) [14, 121]. Improvement in eGFR was less in transplanted than in non-transplanted patients (14.8±18.7 ml/min/1.73 m^2 versus 48.3±38.4) and a shorter duration between onset of HUS episode and treatment initiation correlated with greater gain in eGFR in both groups (p=0.008) [122].

In trial 2 comprising patients with CKD under long-term PE/PI, who were switched to eculi-

Table 24.3 Trial design and baseline patients' characteristics in four prospective, single-arm, non-randomized, multi-national phase 2 trials of the efficacy of eculizumab in atypical HUS

	Trial 1	Trial 2	Trial 3	Trial 4
	Adults/adolescents with progressing TMA despite PE/PI (n=17) [14, 121]	Adults/adolescents with long disease duration and CKD under long-term PE/PI (n=20) [14, 121]	Children (n=22) [124]	Adults (n=41) [123]
Baseline patients characteristics				
Median age, year (range)	28 (17–68)	28 (13–63)	Mean 6.5 (0.5–17.0)	Mean 40.3 (18–80)
Identified complement mutation or anti-FH antibodies (%)	76	70	45	49
History of kidney transplant (%)	41	40	9	22
Median time from diagnosis of aHUS to screening, months (range)	9.7 (0.3–236)	48.3 (0.7–286)	0.6 (0.03–191)	0.79 (0.03–311)
Median time from onset of current aHUS manifestation to screening, months (range)	0.75 (0.2–3.7)	8.6 (1.2–45)	0.2 (0.03–4.3)	0.5 (0.0–19.2)
Median (range) or mean (SD) platelet count, G/L	Median 118 (62–161)	Median 218 (105–421)	Mean 87.5 (42.3)	Mean 119.1 (66.1)
Mean eGFR, ml/min/1.73 m^2 (SD)	23 (14.5)	31 (19)	32.7 (30.3)	17.3 (12.1)
Dialysis within 8 weeks prior to first eculizumab dose or at baseline prior to first eculizumab dose (%)	35 (within 8 weeks)	10 (within 8 weeks)	55 (at baseline)	59 (at baseline)
Median number of PE/PI prior to first eculizumab dose (range)	6 (0–7) during the week prior to first eculizumab dose	1.3 (1–3) during the week prior to first eculizumab dose	None in 55% of patients during current manifestation of HUS prior to first eculizumab dose	None in 15% of patients during current manifestation of HUS prior to first eculizumab dose
Study design[a]	Screening period ≤3 days, then PE/PI stopped and eculizumab initiated, 26-week treatment period followed by a long-term extension	Screening period ≤2 weeks, then 8- week observation period, then PE/PI stopped and eculizumab initiated, 26-week treatment period followed by a long-term extension	Screening period 0–7 days, then PE/PI (if any) stopped and eculizumab initiated, 26-week treatment period followed by a long-term extension	
	No requirement for identified complement mutation or antibody	No requirement for identified complement mutation or antibody	No requirement for identified complement mutation or antibody	

(continued)

Table 24.3 (continued)

	Trial 1	Trial 2	Trial 3	Trial 4
	Adults/adolescents with progressing TMA despite PE/PI (n = 17) [14, 121]	Adults/adolescents with long disease duration and CKD under long-term PE/PI (n = 20) [14, 121]	Children (n = 22) [124]	Adults (n = 41) [123]
Key inclusion criteria	Age ≥12 years; Progressing TMA measured by low platelet count (<150G/L) and a decrease of >25 % lower than the average of 3 platelet counts before the most recent HUS manifestation, despite ≥4 PE/PI in the week before screening; Evidence of hemolysis: LDH ≥ ULN, haptoglobin < LLN or schizocytes and impaired renal function (Screatinine ≥ ULN)	Age ≥12 years; No platelet decrease >25 % during the 8-week observation period under ≥1 PE/PI every 2 weeks but ≤3 times per week for ≥8 weeks; Evidence of hemolysis: LDH ≥ ULN, haptoglobin < LLN or schizocytes and impaired renal function (Screatinine ≥ ULN)	Age ≥1 month to <18 years; Body weight ≥5 kg; Platelet count <150 G/L; Hemoglobin < LLN; LDH ≥1.5×ULN; Screatinine ≥ ULN; No PE/PI for >5 weeks prior to enrollment	Age ≥18 years; Platelet count <150 G/L; Hemoglobin < LLN; LDH ≥1.5×ULN; Screatinine ≥ ULN; No specification for PE/PI prior to enrollment
Key exclusion criteria	ADAMTS13 activity ≤5 %; STEC-HUS; prior eculizumab exposure			
Primary efficacy endpoints	Change in platelet count	TMA event-free status defined as: absence for ≥12 consecutive weeks of a decrease of platelet count of >25 %, no PE/PI while receiving eculizumab and no initiation of new dialysis	Complete TMA response with improvement of renal function, defined as: Platelet count normalization (≥150G/L)+ LDH normalization (≤ULN)+ Improved renal function (≥25 % decrease of Screatinine from baseline), sustained for ≥2 consecutive measurements obtained ≥4 weeks apart	Complete TMA response with preservation of renal function, defined as: Platelet count normalization (≥150G/L)+ LDH normalization (≤ULN)+ Preserved renal function (<25 % increase of Screatinine from baseline), sustained for ≥2 consecutive measurements obtained ≥4 weeks apart
	Proportion of patients with platelet count normalization (≥150G/L) sustained for ≥2 consecutive measurements for ≥4 weeks	Proportion of patients with hematologic normalization defined as: Platelet count ≥150 G/L and LDH ≤ ULN sustained for ≥2 consecutive measurements obtained ≥4 weeks apart		
	Proportion of patients with hematologic normalization defined as: Platelet count ≥150 G/L and LDH ≤ ULN sustained for ≥2 consecutive measurements obtained ≥4 weeks apart			

Used with permission of Springer Science + Business Media from Loirat et al. [102]

Eculizumab was administered at the recommended dosage regimen time points [119, 120] (See Table 24.2) during the total trial duration

Table 24.4 Efficacy of eculizumab in patients with atypical HUS. Results of four prospective, single-arm, non-randomized, multinational trials at week 26 and after continued treatment in the extension phase

	Trial 1 [14, 121]		Trial 2 [14, 121]		Trial 3 [124]	Trial 4 [123]
Median treatment duration[a]	26 weeks	2 years	26 weeks	2 years	26 weeks	26 weeks
Mean change in platelet count from baseline (G/L)	73[c]	75[c]	/	/	164	135
Normalization of platelet count[b] (% patients)	82[c]	88[c]	90	90	95	98
Median time to endpoint, days (range)	7 (1–218)				7 (1–80)	8 (0–84)
Hematologic normalization[b] (% patients)	76[c]	88[c]	90[c]	90[c]	82	88
Median time to endpoint, days (range)					55 (1–153)	55 (2–146)
TMA event-free status[b] (% patients)	88	88	85[c]	95[c]	/	90
Complete TMA response with preserved renal function[b] (% patients)	/	/	/	/	/	73[c]
Complete TMA response with improved renal function[b] (% patients)	65	76	25	55	64[c]	56
Mean increase in eGFR from baseline, ml/min/1.73 m^2 (95 % CI)	32 (14–49)	35 (17–53)	6 (3–9)	7 (0.8–14)	64 (50–79)	29 (SD24)
Patients on dialysis at data cutoff (%)		12		10	9	15

Used with permission of Springer Science + Business Media from Loirat et al. [102]
[a]Eculizumab was administered at the recommended dosage regimen time points [119, 120] (See Table 24.2) during the total trial duration
[b]See Table 24.3 for definition
[c]Primary efficacy endpoint

zumab long after onset of the current aHUS episode, 85 % of patients maintained TMA event-free status (see definition in Table 24.3) at 26 weeks and 95 % at 2 years and 90 % maintained hematologic remission over a median of 2 years treatment duration. Mean (95 % CI) gain in eGFR was only 6 (3–9) ml/min/1.73 m^2 at 26 weeks (p=0.0001 versus baseline eGFR). However, eGFR gain was maintained after 2 years of continued treatment (Table 24.4) and also correlated with shorter time from onset of HUS episode to treatment (p=0.001) [14, 121].

The two subsequent trials (trials 3 and 4) allowed rapid treatment initiation (no obligation for the patient to receive prior plasmatherapy and brief screening period for enrollment). The efficacy of eculizumab to induce hematologic normalization was confirmed. Complete TMA response with improved renal function (see definition in Table 24.3) was maintained at 26 weeks in 64 % of children (trial 3), while improved or preserved renal function was maintained in 56 % and 73 % adult patients, respectively (trial 4). While mean eGFR at baseline was 33 ± 30 ml/min/1.73 m^2 in children and 17 ± 12 ml/min/1.73 m^2 in adults, a greater gain in eGFR was observed in children than in adults (64 ml/min/1.73 m^2 versus 29.3 ml/min/1.73 m^2 at week 26, respectively). After 26 weeks of continued eculizumab treatment, only 9 % (2/22) of children and 15 % (6/41) of adults were on chronic dialysis [121, 123, 124] (Table 24.4).

Taken together, the four trials demonstrated the efficacy of eculizumab to stop the TMA process, allowing sustained remission of aHUS with improved or preserved renal function in the majority of patients. Data from the trials also suggest that an early switch from PE/PI to eculizumab or the use of eculizumab as first line therapy may be warranted to offer patients the best chance of full recovery of renal function. Treatment was well tolerated, with no increase of adverse events over time. However, 2 of the 100 patients who entered these trials developed meningococcal meningitis [123].

Case Reports of Eculizumab to Treat aHUS in Native Kidneys or to Treat or Prevent Post-kidney Transplant Recurrence of aHUS

Case reports have brought data consistant with those of the prospective trials just discussed. Among approximately 35 case reports of patients who received eculizumab to treat HUS in native kidneys (cases with anti-FH antibodies not included), 19 described children, including 9 aged ≤1 year at treatment initiation (Table 24.5) [13, 73–75, 77–79, 125–130]. After a median follow-up of 13 months on eculizumab therapy, all children were free of HUS relapse, only one child (5 %) was on dialysis and median serum creatinine was 43 μmol/l in the 18 other children. In a recently published series, the outcome of 19 adults treated with eculizumab was compared with that of paired historical controls treated only with PE (63 % of cases). Among eculizumab-treated patients, 17 % had progressed to ESRD at 3 months and 25 % at

Table 24.5 Eculizumab for atypical HUS on native kidneys. Pooled analysis of 19 case reports of pediatric patients treated outside of prospective trials

Patients characteristics at baseline N = 19	
Median age at eculizumab initiation, years (range)	1.5 (11 days–11 years)
	(≤1 year in 9 cases)
Complement mutation identified, n (%)	15 /18 (83); *CFH*, n = 10; *CFI*, n = 2 *MCP*, n = 1; *C3*, n = 1; *CFB*, n = 1
Prior PE/PI or first line eculizumab, n	PE/PI resistant, n = 12
	PE/PI dependent, n = 2
	1st line eculizumab, n = 5
Median duration from current HUS onset to eculizumab initiation, days (range)	19 (<1–225)
Dialysis required, n (%)	13 (68)
Median serum creatinine (6 non-dialysed patients), μmol/l (range)	99 (20–264)
Outcome under eculizumab	
Hematological remission, n (%)	19 (100)
Dialysis required, n (%)	1 (5)
Median serum creatinine (18 non-dialysed patients), μmol/l (range)	43 (20–90)
Serum creatinine <50 μmol/l, n (%) (18 non-dialysed patients)	13 (72)
Median follow-up, months (range)	13 (2.5–42)

Data from References [13, 73–75, 77–79, 125–130]
Conversion factor for serum creatinine in μmol/l to mg/dl, × 0.011
CFH complement factor H, *CFI* complement factor I, *MCP* membrane cofactor protein (CD46), *PE* plasma exchange, *PI* plasma infusion

1 year follow-up, compared to 46 % (p = 0.02) and 63 % (p = 0.04) of historical controls, respectively. Patients treated with eculizumab within 6 days of onset tended to have lower final serum creatinine levels than those treated later [131]. Lastly, no clear benefit from eculizumab treatment was observed in seven patients with isolated *DGKE* mutation [32], while the benefit was uncertain – clinical improvement but persistant proteinuria – in one patient with associated C3 variant [37]. Eculizumab efficacy

needs to be studied in a larger number of patients with DGKE mutation before reaching a conclusion about its benefits.

Experience of eculizumab to treat extra-renal manifestations of aHUS is limited. However, eculizumab was impressively effective in two children with acute distal ischemia [78] or skin necrosis and intestinal perforation [79], respectively. Eculizumab may rescue central nervous system manifestations, as suggested by nine case reports, including four in children [73, 74, 76, 132–136]. Eculizumab also appeared life-saving in four children with myocardial involvement [74–77]. Lastly, two children who had developed cerebral arteries stenosis stopped having ischemic events under eculizumab therapy, with non-progression of arterial stenosis documented in one [84, 85].

Most of the 19 patients who received eculizumab to treat post-transplant recurrence were adults who carried high risk mutations and/or had lost prior grafts from recurrence (Table 24.6) [112, 113, 137–139]. Remission of HUS was obtained in all and earlier initiation of treatment was correlated with greater gain of graft function [112]. However, similar to transplanted patients included in prospective trials, many patients did not achieve full rescue of graft function. This may be due to the variety of factors, particularly ischemia-reperfusion injury, that induce endothelial damage to the graft and local complement activation, perhaps with more severe consequences in patients with pre-existing complement dysregulation [115].

These observations suggested prophylactic eculizumab treatment might be an appropriate option for patients at very high risk of post-transplant recurrence of HUS. Fifteen patients (nine children) (median age 11 years (3–41)) at high risk of post-transplant recurrence (*CFH* mutation (all in C terminus) or hybrid *CFH* (n = 13), *C3* gain of function mutation (n = 1) or *CFB + CFI* (n = 1) mutation; 8/8 prior grafts in five patients lost from recurrence) have been reported who received deceased donor (n = 11) or living related (n = 1) or non-related (n = 3) donor kidney transplantation. Patients generally received a first dose a few hours before surgery

Table 24.6 Eculizumab for post-transplant recurrence of atypical HUS. Pooled analysis of 19 case reports of patients treated outside of prospective trials

Patients characteristics at baseline N = 19	
Median age, years (range)	32 (6–57) (3 children, 16 adults)
Previous grafts (22 in 13 patients)	18/22 (82 %) lost for recurrence
Complement abnormalities (14/18 patients)	Mutation of *CFH*, n = 8; *C3*, n = 2; *CFI*, n = 1; *MCP*, n = 1; *THBD*, n = 1; anti-FH antibodies, n = 1; No mutation identified, n = 4
Median duration from onset of recurrence to eculizumab initiation, days (range) (17 patients)	21 (1 day–14 months)
Median serum creatinine before eculizumab initiation, μmol/l (range) (17 patients)	237 (89–752)
Graft outcome under eculizumab	
Patients on dialysis, n (%)	2 (10.5)
Median serum creatinine at last-follow-up, μmol/l (range) (16 patients not on dialysis)	117 (48–238)
Median follow-up, months (range) (19 patients)	17 (4.5–120)

Conversion factor for serum creatinine in μmol/l to mg/dl, × 0.011
Data from References [112, 113, 137–139]
CFH complement factor H, *CFI* complement factor I, *MCP* membrane cofactor protein (CD46), *PE* plasma exchange

and second dose within the next 24 h, to guarantee full complement blockade during the per and post-operative period, when maximum complement activation is likely to occur, followed by the recommended treatment schedule (Table 24.2). Three patients received one PE before the pre-operative eculizumab dose(s). In four patients (three scheduled for living donor-transplantation and one on urgent list), eculizumab treatment was initiated 1–3 weeks before surgery. Two other children were receiving eculizumab since 7 and 9 months while on chronic dialysis. Except for one patient who had graft artery thrombosis related to technical difficulties and was ultimately successfully re-transplanted under prophylactic eculizumab (communication of M. Hourmant, Nantes, France, with permission), all patients had a recurrence-free post-transplant course, with median serum creatinine level 65 ± 37 µmol/l at median follow-up 17.5 (range 2–39) months [85, 112, 139–143].

The Risk of Meningococcal Infection Under Eculizumab

Defense against *Neisseria meningitis* depends on the lytic terminal complement complex C5b-9. The incidence of meningococcal infections in patients with congenital complete deficiency in terminal complement factors is 0.5 % per year, a relative risk of 5000 compared to the normal population [34]. Patients under eculizumab treatment have the same risk as these patients. Therefore prevention of meningococcal infection is crucial, relying on vaccination and antibiotic prophylaxis. Tetravalent conjugated vaccines protect against serogroups A, C, W135 and Y, but not against serogroup B which predominates in Europe, North America, Australia and New Zealand. A vaccine against *N meningitis* B is now available in some countries, but its clinical efficacy and duration of protection under complement blockade is not yet documented. The frequency of invasive meningococcal infection has been approximately 0.5/100 patients year in patients with PNH treated with eculizumab, despite meningococcal vaccination (not anti-B) [116]. Two of the 100 aHUS patients treated within protocols [123] and one among approximately 80 case reports [144] developed invasive meningococcal infection despite being vaccinated. The later patient had received a polysaccharide vaccine and no patient received the anti-B vaccine. However, the efficacy of anti-meningococcal (vaccine) antibodies is uncertain in patients with complement deficiency, complement blockade or immunosuppressive therapy. Therefore antibiotic prophylaxis is recom-

mended, allowing prompt initiation of eculizumab. Continuous antibiotic prophylaxis -with methyl-penicillin- is obligatory in some countries and strongly recommended for children [102]. Neither vaccines nor antibiotic prophylaxis guarantee full protection, hence the importance of patient and family education on signs of meningococcal infection and of the information card to be carried by the patient or his care giver.

New Clinical Practice for Treatment of Children with aHUS

A consensus approach was recently proposed for the management of aHUS in children, which can serve as a basis for individual decisions [102].

First Line Treatment for Children with a Clinical Diagnosis of aHUS

Eculizumab should be proposed as first line treatment for children with a clinical diagnosis of aHUS, to avoid PE and the complications of central catheters. Confirmation of a complement mutation is not required for the decision of treatment initiation in such cases. As treatment delay may affect GFR recovery, eculizumab treatment should be initiated within 24–48 h of onset or admission. If eculizumab treatment is not available, PE (or PI if PE is not possible) should be started as recommended in the 2009 guideline [11]. The only urgently needed complement investigation is anti-FH antibody assay, as a positive result opens specific treatment options.

Treatment of Anti-FH Antibody-Associated HUS

As discussed above, outcome was poor in the first large series of patients with anti-FH antibody-associated HUS treated mostly with PE without immunosuppressants [38] and a much more favourable outcome, similar to that of

MCP mutation-associated HUS, has been recently reported in children with this form of HUS treated early with PE, immunosuppressants and corticosteroids [4]. A recent report of 138 Indian children showed that combined PE and immunosuppression (oral prednisone with cyclophosphamide or rituximab) reduced antibody titer to ≤1000 arbitrary units (AU)/ml (positive threshold 100–150 AU/ml [38, 40]) within a median of 32 (interquartile range 11–84) days. This was associated with hematological remission and a significant decrease of adverse outcomes (defined as eGFR <30 ml/min/1.73 m^2 or death) from 71 % to 33 % after a mean follow-up of 14.5 (range 3–95) months. Maintenance treatment with corticosteroids and mycophenolate mofetyl (MMF) or azathioprine significantly decreased the risk of relapses, from 87 % to 46 % at last follow-up [40]. Interestingly, four patients have been reported who went into remission after a short course of cyclophosphamide pulse therapy (two pulses of 0.5 g/1.73 m^2 in three patients, five pulses of 1 g/1.73 m^2 in one patient resistant to PE+rituximab) combined with PE and corticosteroids, and maintained full renal recovery up to 6 years, 4 years, 4 years and 4 months without additional maintenance therapy [145]. This shows that the best immunosuppressive regimen and its duration remain to be defined for anti-FH antibody-associated HUS. In addition, although experience is limited, eculizumab is also efficient in anti-FH antibody-associated HUS [76, 131, 146, 147]. However, eculizumab is not expected to inhibit anti-FH antibodies production and a spontaneous decrease of antibodies is rare [38, 42]. Therefore immunosuppressive therapy should be included in an attempt to reduce antibody titer, thus allowing cessation of eculizumab. Lastly, eculizumab has to be considered in patients with anti-FH antibody- associated HUS and acute, severe injury of vital organs such as brain or heart [76]. Further studies are required to establish the respective place of eculizumab, PE, cyclophosphamide pulses and MMF to control anti-FH antibodies titer and offer the best chance of favourable outcome in anti-FH antibody associated-HUS.

Reasons to Consider a Switch from PE/PI to Eculizumab in Children Who Received PE or PI as First Therapy

Children who received PE or PI as first line therapy because the clinical diagnosis of aHUS was uncertain should be switched to eculizumab when the diagnosis of aHUS is established. An exception to this recommendation could be patients with anti-FH antibodies.

Patients showing resistance to PE/PI should be switched to eculizumab: the patient who, after approximately 5 daily PE/PI, has no consistent trend upwards of platelet count (especially if the platelet count remains <150 G/L) or no consistent trend downwards of LDH level (especially if LDH remains > ULN) or no decrease of serum creatinine (at least a decrease of ≥25 %) should be prescribed eculizumab [10, 13, 102]. This recommendation is based on the data reviewed above suggesting that this offers the patient the best chance of optimal recovery of renal function.

For patients on long term PE/PI, there is no reason to change therapy in those who show full remission and normal renal function (eGFR >90 ml/min/1.73 m^2, no proteinuria, no hematuria, no hypertension requiring a combination of drugs) under a schedule of PE/PI compatible with their daily activity, without catheter–related complications or plasma intolerance. Conversely, the switch to eculizumab should be considered if any sign of subclinical hematological (LDH > ULN, haptoglobin < lower limit of normal) or renal TMA (isolated proteinuria or slowly increasing serum creatinine level with active TMA confirmed at renal biopsy [148]) appears. Eculizumab should also be prescribed to patients with normalized hematologic markers but residual CKD despite PE/PI [14] and in case of extra-renal manifestations of TMA (neurologic, cardiac, vascular, etc.) [102].

Complement Blockade Assessment in Patients Treated with Eculizumab

Data from the prospective studies show that complete complement blockade is obtained within one hour after the first dose and is maintained long term in patients receiving the recommended treatment schedule (doses and intervals adjusted according to weight as indicated in Table 24.2 [119, 120]) [14, 121]. At the acute phase of HUS, it may be useful to check complement blockade at day 7 after the first dose (just before the second dose). Incomplete blockade may be due to insufficient dose (especially in children with a weight just below a weight threshold requiring a higher dose) or heavy proteinuria with nephrotic syndrome (leakage of the drug in the urine). A genetic cause might also have to be considered in aHUS patients of Japanese or Asian origin with poor response to eculizumab and/or complement non-blockade, such as the C5 variant which impairs the binding of eculizumab to C5, as recently described [149]. For the long term, complement blockade assessment is mostly required in cases of apparent resistance to eculizumab, including relapse of HUS but also isolated abnormalities in platelet count, LDH and/or haptoglobin levels, appearance or increase of proteinuria or serum creatinine, especially if renal biopsy suggests ongoing TMA.

Currently available assays of complement blockade under eculizumab are a CH50 or other haemolytic-based assays or the Wieslab Complement System [150]. Due to the site of action of eculizumab, low C3 levels as observed in some mutations are not expected to normalize under eculizumab, and this has been confirmed recently [17]. Soluble C5b-9 remains detectable or increased in aHUS patients under eculizumab and therefore cannot be recommended to monitor the efficacy of eculizumab [17, 128]. Most aHUS patients treated within the prospective trials who received the protocol schedule had suppression of CH50 activity and eculizumab trough levels ≥ 150 µg/ml [14]. However, the correlation between drug levels and complement activity in aHUS patients is not fully established and the availability of eculizumab levels determination is currently limited.

In current clinical practice, increasing the interval between doses should be considered only in patients who maintain CH50 activity <10 % despite the longer intervals or lower doses, as recently reported [150].

Duration of Complement Blockade Therapy in Children with aHUS in Their Native Kidneys

Life long treatment has been the accepted paradigm until recently. This recommendation is being reconsidered for patients treated for aHUS in their native kidneys, for the following reasons: the risk of relapse after treatment discontinuation is unknown in patients who have preserved renal function under eculizumab, while the risk of meningococcal infection under complement blockade therapy is high and the cost of eculizumab treatment enormous. Experience with eculizumab discontinuation is currently limited, but the risk of early relapse seems to be high in patients with *CFH* mutation, while it seems lower in patients with no mutation identified [73, 125, 131, 134–136, 151–153] (Table 24.7). Prospective studies are required to establish whether eculizumab treatment discontinuation is feasible, in whom and when.

Kidney Transplantation for aHUS Patients Today

Complement blockade therapy has deeply modified the approach to kidney transplantation for aHUS patients:

1. Deceased donor or non-related living donor can now be considered provided that eculizumab will be available to prevent or treat HUS post-transplant recurrence
2. Former contra-indication to related living donor transplantation has to be reconsidered, with the decision relying on a carefull assessment of the risk of aHUS in the donor after kidney donation. This requires full genetic screening of the recipient and the donor, leading to three possible issues: i. If the mutation found in the recipient is undeniably responsible for the occurrence of HUS (e.g., *CFH* mutation in C terminus SCR 19 or 20) and is not found in the recipient, the risk of HUS is low for the donor and living-related donor transplantation can be done. ii. If the donor has the same mutation as the recipient, the risk

Table 24.7 Outcome after eculizumab discontinuation, in 20 case reports of patients with atypical HUS in their native kidneys

Author [Reference]	Age (years)	Complement anomaly	Eculizumab treatment duration before withdrawal (months)	Relapse of HUS after eculizumab withdrawal	Delay between eculizumab withdrawal and relapse (months)	Change in Screatinine at relapse (μmol/l)	Screatinine at last follow-up (μmol/l)	Follow-up after eculizumab withdrawal or re-initiation[d] (months)
Carr et al. [151]	20 (PP)	CFH mutation	9 months	Yes	6	Normal→451 (3 weeks dialysis)	ND (free of dialysis)	ND
Fakhouri et al. (Patient 1) [131]	26 (PP)	CFH + CFI mutation	18 months	No	NA	NA	70	18
Ardissino et al. [152] Patient 1	4.3	CFH mutation	5.5 months	Yes	1.5	71→248	71	25
Ardissino et al. [152] Patient 2	37.7	CFH mutation	14 months	Yes	0.9	124→203	115	10
Cayci et al. [125][a]	11	CFI mutation	2 weeks	No	NA	NA	48	11
Ardissino et al. [152] Patient 3	52.7	CFI mutation	1.5 month	No	NA	NA	88.5	22
Ardissino et al. [152] Patient 4	34.8	CFI mutation	11.5 months	No	NA	NA	221	10
Ardissino et al. [152] Patient 5	2.6	CFI mutation	5.5 months	No	NA	NA	35	15.5
Guleroglu et al. [73] Patient 2	6	MCP mutation	5 weeks	No	NA	NA	Normal	9
Fakhouri et al. [131] Patient 2	22	MCP mutation	8 weeks	No	NA	NA	84	11
Ardissino et al. [152] Patient 8	5.4	MCP mutation	0.5 month	No	NA	NA	44	13.5
Fakhouri et al. [131] Patient 4	49	Anti-FH Ab[b]	8 weeks	No	NA	NA	88.5	10
Ardissino et al. [152] Patient 7	19.1	Anti-FH Ab[b]	5.5 months	No	NA	NA	106	14.5
Ardissino et al. [152] Patient 9	13.3	Anti-FH Ab[c]	2.5 months	No	NA	NA	53	8.5

(continued)

Table 24.3 (continued)

Author [Reference]	Age (years)	Complement anomaly	Eculizumab treatment duration before withdrawal (months)	Relapse of HUS after eculizumab withdrawal	Delay between eculizumab withdrawal and relapse (months)	Change in Screatinine at relapse (µmol/l)	Screatinine at last follow-up (µmol/l)	Follow-up after eculizumab withdrawal or re-initiation[d] (months)
Ardissino et al. [152] Patient 10	10.9	Anti-FH Ab[c]	0.4 months	Yes	1	62 →301	53	5
Pu et al. [135]	85	None identified	3 months	No	NA	NA	Normal	12
Beye et al. [134]	64	ND	13 weeks	No	NA	NA	60	6
Canigral et al. [153]	32 (PP)	None identified	6 months	No	NA	NA	88.5	12
Chaudhary et al. [136]	20	None identified	9 months	No	NA	NA	70.8	≈9
Ardissino et al. [152] Patient 6	1.3	None identified	13.5 months	No	NA	NA	26	6.5

Data from References [73, 125, 131, 134–136, 151–153]

Used with permission of Springer Science + Business Media from Loirat et al. [102]

Conversion factor for serum creatinine in µmol/l to mg/dl, × 0.011

Ab antibody, *CFH* complement factor H, *CFI* complement factor I, *MCP* membrane cofactor protein (CD46), *NA* non applicable

[a]Follow-up information provided by FS Altugan-Cayci, Ankara, Turkey

[b]Negative or low anti-FH antibody titer (Communication of G. Ardissino, Milan, Italy)

[c]High anti-FH antibody titer (Communication of G. Ardissino, Milan, Italy)

[d]Eculizumab was reinitiated in the four patients who relapsed after eculizumab withdrawal

of HUS is high for the donor and living-related donor transplantation should not be done. iii. If the role of the variant found in the recipient is uncertain (not reported in databases, unknown functional consequences) or no mutation is identified in the recipient and the donor, the risk of HUS is intermediate for the donor, who may share with the recipient an unknown risk factor, and living-related donor transplantation should not be done.

3. Prophylactic eculizumab treatment should be considered for patients at high risk of recurrence, i.e., patients with *CFH* or *C3/CFB* gain of function mutation and patients with prior graft lost from recurrence. Prophylatic treatment (eculizumab or PE) should also be considered for patients at intermediate risk of recurrence, i.e., patients with *CFI* or combined *MCP* mutation.

4. No prophylaxis is required for patients at low risk of recurrence, i.e., patients with *DGKE* or isolated *MCP* mutation, no mutation identified or low anti-FH antibody titer.

5. Avoidance of additional endothelial damaging factors is recommended, such as delayed graft function (prolonged ischemia time, non-heartbeating donor), cytomegalovirus (CMV) infection (CMV prophylactic treatment when required), overdosage of CNI and the association of CNI + mTOR inhibitors, hypertension/atherosclerosis (angiotensin-converting enzyme inhibitors/angiotensin receptor antagonist/statins).

6. For patients treated for post-transplant recurrence or who received prophylactic treatment because they were at high risk of recurrence, the current recommendation is that complement blockade therapy should not be discontinued.

7. Liver or combined liver-kidney transplantation (CLKT) for aHUS patients in 2014

Liver or CLKT is the only option to cure the disease in patients with severe HUS and mutations in factors synthetized in the liver (FH, C3 and FB). Pre-operative PE (+ per-operative PI) to provide large amounts of the deficient complement factor, or pre-operative eculizumab, is required to prevent extensive microvascular thrombosis due to the massive complement activation associated with hepatic reperfusion. We are aware of 22 patients with *CFH* (n=20), *CFB* (n=1) or *C3* (n=1) mutations who received CLKT (n=20) or liver transplantation (n=2) under PE/PI (n=19) or eculizumab (n=3, 2 of them with 1 PE just before eculizumab). Four of the 20 patients (20%) who received CLKT died, mostly (n=3) from post-operative complications [102, 154, 155]. Even though kidney transplantation under eculizumab would be favoured by most groups, the CKLT – or isolated liver transplantation in patients with a severe course of the disease but preserved renal function – options should be discussed with patients and families. The decision can only be taken on a case by case basis, determined by local experience, benefits/risks assessment and for some patients the country's ability to cover the cost of long-term eculizumab treatment in patients with their native kidneys or after isolated kidney transplantation [115].

Some Secondary Forms of HUS Are Emerging as Potential Indications of Complement-Blockade Treatment

Although secondary forms of HUS are out of the scope of this chapter, pediatricians should be aware that some of them might benefit from complement blockade therapy. In particular, eculizumab therapy has been efficient and life-saving in six of eight patients (one adult, seven children) with severe hematopoietic stem cell transplantation (HSCT)-associated TMA, all during severe acute graft versus host disease [156–158]. Although a possible role of anti-FH antibodies in HSCT-associated TMA has been suggested [159], none of the eight patients treated with eculizumab had anti-FH antibodies. Increased eculizumab doses/reduced intervals between doses were necessary to reach therapeutic levels and complete complement blockade in four out of six children. Two critically ill children failed to reach therapeutic levels and subsequently died. Although the benefit from complement-blockade in this form of TMA has to be confirmed in a larger number of patients, eculizumab therapy should be considered as a first-line therapy for patients with severe HSCT-associated TMA [157].

Conversely, although complement activation has been demonstrated in TTP [160–162], treatment of congenital TTP is PI and treatment of acquired TTP is PE + corticosteroids ± rituximab. The single adult patient with TTP resistant to current therapy who went into remission under eculizumab [163] was subsequently found to have anti-FH antibodies associated with anti-ADAMTS13 antibodies, but without severe ADAMTS13 deficiency [164]. Interestingly, this association of anti-FH and anti-ADAMTS13 antibodies has also been reported in one child [12].

Conclusion

Atypical HUS is a striking demonstration that understanding the pathophysiology of a disease opens the way to new therapies. The demonstration that aHUS was mostly a disease of complement dysregulation paralleled the development of the anti-C5 monoclonal antibody eculizumab. Prospective trials as well as off-label clinical experience confirmed the efficacy of complement blockade to prevent progression to ESRD in aHUS patients and allow successful kidney transplantation in those on dialysis. This new era in the field of aHUS emphasizes the need for an etiology/pathophysiology-based classification of the various forms of TMAs. Hopefully, new discoveries will identify the etiology of the 30 % of aHUS cases that remain unexplained today, and the aHUS denomination will then disappear. An important question today is that of eculizumab treatment duration and prospective studies are needed to define whether discontinuation can be considered, in which patients and when. Should withdrawal be shown as feasible in some patients, this would decrease the burden and risks of continuous treatment for patients, but also the cost for health care systems.

References

1. Noris M, Caprioli J, Bresin E, Mossali C, Pianetti G, Gamba S, et al. Relative role of genetic complement abnormalities in sporadic and familial aHUS and their impact on clinical phenotype. Clin J Am Soc Nephrol. 2010;5(10):1844–59.
2. Maga TK, Nishimura CJ, Weaver AE, Frees KL, Smith RJ. Mutations in alternative pathway complement proteins in American patients with atypical hemolytic uremic syndrome. Hum Mutat. 2010;31(6):E1445–60.
3. Geerdink LM, Westra D, van Wijk JA, Dorresteijn EM, Lilien MR, Davin JC, et al. Atypical hemolytic uremic syndrome in children: complement mutations and clinical characteristics. Pediatr Nephrol. 2012;27(8):1283–91.
4. Fremeaux-Bacchi V, Fakhouri F, Garnier A, Bienaime F, Dragon-Durey MA, Ngo S, et al. Genetics and outcome of atypical hemolytic uremic syndrome: a nationwide French series comparing children and adults. Clin J Am Soc Nephrol. 2013;8(4):554–62.
5. Kavanagh D, Goodship TH, Richards A. Atypical hemolytic uremic syndrome. Semin Nephrol. 2013;33(6):508–30.
6. Rodríguez de Córdoba S, Hidalgo MS, Pinto S, Tortajada A. Genetics of atypical hemolytic uremic syndrome (aHUS). Semin Thromb Hemost. 2014;40(4):422–30.
7. Nester CM, Thomas CP. Atypical hemolytic uremic syndrome: what is it, how is it diagnosed, and how is it treated? Hematol Educ Prog Am Soc Hematol. 2012;2012:617–25.
8. Campistol JM, Arias M, Ariceta G, Blasco M, Espinosa M, Grinyo JM, et al. An update for atypical haemolytic uraemic syndrome: diagnosis and treatment. A consensus document. Nefrologia. 2013;33(1):27–45.
9. Scully M, Goodship T. How I treat thrombotic thrombocytopenic purpura and atypical haemolytic uraemic syndrome. Br J Haematol. 2014;164(6):759–66.
10. Cataland SR, Wu HM. How I treat: the clinical differentiation and initial treatment of adult patients with atypical hemolytic uremic syndrome. Blood. 2014;123(16):2478–84.
11. Ariceta G, Besbas N, Johnson S, Karpman D, Landau D, Licht C, European Paediatric Study Group for HUS, et al. Guideline for the investigation and initial therapy of diarrhea-negative hemolytic uremic syndrome. Pediatr Nephrol. 2009;24(4):687–96.
12. Johnson S, Stojanovic J, Ariceta G, Bitzan M, Besbas N, Frieling M, et al. An audit analysis of a guideline for the investigation and initial therapy of diarrhea negative (atypical) hemolytic uremic syndrome. Pediatr Nephrol. 2014;29(10):1967–78.

13. Zuber J, Fakhouri F, Roumenina LT, Loirat C, Frémeaux-Bacchi V, French Study Group for aHUS/C3G. Use of eculizumab for atypical haemolytic uraemic syndrome and C3 glomerulopathies. Nat Rev Nephrol. 2012;8(11):643–57.

14. Legendre CM, Licht C, Muus P, Greenbaum LA, Babu S, Bedrosian C, et al. Terminal complement inhibitor eculizumab in atypical hemolytic-uremic syndrome. N Engl J Med. 2013;368(23): 2169–81.

15. Besbas N, Karpman D, Landau D, Loirat C, Proesmans W, Remuzzi G, et al. A classification of hemolytic uremic syndrome and thrombotic thrombocytopenic purpura and related disorders. Kidney Int. 2006;70(3):423–31.

16. George JN, Nester CM. Syndromes of thrombotic microangiopathy. N Engl J Med. 2014;371(7):654–66.

17. Noris M, Galbusera M, Gastoldi S, Macor P, Banterla F, Bresin E, et al. Dynamics of complement activation in aHUS and how to monitor eculizumab therapy. Blood. 2014;124(11):1715–26.

18. Benz K, Amann K. Pathological aspects of membranoproliferative glomerulonephritis (MPGN) and haemolytic uraemic syndrome (HUS)/thrombocytic thrombopenic purpura (TTP). Thromb Haemost. 2009;101(2):265–70.

19. Sethi S, Fervenza FC. Pathology of renal diseases associated with dysfunction of the alternative pathway of complement: C3 glomerulopathy and atypical hemolytic uremic syndrome (aHUS). Semin Thromb Hemost. 2014;40(4):416–21.

20. Cameron JS, Vick R. Letter: plasma-C3 in haemolytic-uraemic syndrome and thrombotic thrombocytopenic purpura. Lancet. 1973;2(7835):975.

21. Thompson RA, Winterborn MH. Hypocomplementaemia due to a genetic deficiency of beta 1H globulin. Clin Exp Immunol. 1981;46(1):110–9.

22. Pichette V, Quérin S, Schürch W, Brun G, Lehner-Netsch G, Delâge JM. Familial hemolytic-uremic syndrome and homozygous factor H deficiency. Am J Kidney Dis. 1994;24(6):936–41.

23. Rougier N, Kazatchkine MD, Rougier JP, Frémeaux-Bacchi V, Blouin J, Deschenes G, et al. Human complement factor H deficiency associated with hemolytic uremic syndrome. J Am Soc Nephrol. 1998;9(12):2318–26.

24. Warwicker P, Goodship TH, Donne RL, Pirson Y, Nicholls A, Ward RM, et al. Genetic studies into inherited and sporadic hemolytic uremic syndrome. Kidney Int. 1998;53(4):836–44.

25. Richards A, Kemp EJ, Liszewski MK, Goodship JA, Lampe AK, Decorte R, et al. Mutations in human complement regulator, membrane cofactor protein (CD46), predispose to development of familial hemolytic uremic syndrome. Proc Natl Acad Sci U S A. 2003;100(22):12966–71.

26. Fremeaux-Bacchi V, Dragon-Durey MA, Blouin J, Vigneau C, Kuypers D, Boudailliez B, et al. Complement factor I: a susceptibility gene for atypical haemolytic uraemic syndrome. J Med Genet. 2004;41(6):e84.

27. Dragon-Durey MA, Loirat C, Cloarec S, Macher MA, Blouin J, Nivet H, et al. Anti-Factor H autoantibodies associated with atypical hemolytic uremic syndrome. J Am Soc Nephrol. 2005;16(2):555–63.

28. Fremeaux-Bacchi V, Moulton EA, Kavanagh D, Dragon-Durey MA, Blouin J, Caudy A, et al. Genetic and functional analyses of membrane cofactor protein (CD46) mutations in atypical hemolytic uremic syndrome. J Am Soc Nephrol. 2006;17(7):2017–25.

29. Goicoechea de Jorge E, Harris CL, Esparza-Gordillo J, Carreras L, Arranz EA, Garrido CA, et al. Gain-of-function mutations in complement factor B are associated with atypical hemolytic uremic syndrome. Proc Natl Acad Sci U S A. 2007;104(1):240–5.

30. Frémeaux-Bacchi V, Miller EC, Liszewski MK, Strain L, Blouin J, Brown AL, et al. Mutations in complement C3 predispose to development of atypical hemolytic uremic syndrome. Blood. 2008;112(13):4948–52.

31. Delvaeye M, Noris M, De Vriese A, Esmon CT, Esmon NL, Ferrell G, et al. Thrombomodulin mutations in atypical hemolytic-uremic syndrome. N Engl J Med. 2009;361(4):345–57.

32. Lemaire M, Frémeaux-Bacchi V, Schaefer F, Choi M, Tang WH, Le Quintrec M, et al. Recessive mutations in DGKE cause atypical hemolytic-uremic syndrome. Nat Genet. 2013;45(5):531–6.

33. Ricklin D, Hajishengallis G, Yang K, Lambris JD. Complement: a key system for immune surveillance and homeostasis. Nat Immunol. 2010;11(9):785–97.

34. Walport MJ. Complement. First of two parts. N Engl J Med. 2001;344(14):1058–66.

35. Rodriguez E, Rallapalli PM, Osborne A, Perkins SJ. New functional and structural insights from updated mutational databases for complement factor H, factor I, membrane cofactor protein and C3. Biosci Rep. 2014;22:34(5).

36. Westland R, Bodria M, Carrea A, Lata S, Scolari F, Fremeaux-Bacchi V, et al. Phenotypic expansion of DGKE-associated diseases. J Am Soc Nephrol. 2014;25(7):1408–14.

37. Sánchez Chinchilla D, Pinto S, Hoppe B, Adragna M, Lopez L, Justa Roldan ML, et al. Complement mutations in diacylglycerol kinase-ε-associated atypical hemolytic uremic syndrome. Clin J Am Soc Nephrol. 2014;9(9):1611–9.

38. Dragon-Durey MA, Sethi SK, Bagga A, Blanc C, Blouin J, Ranchin B, et al. Clinical features of anti-factor H autoantibody-associated hemolytic uremic syndrome. J Am Soc Nephrol. 2010;21(12):2180–7.

39. Hofer J, Janecke AR, Zimmerhackl LB, Riedl M, Rosales A, Giner T, et al. Complement factor H-related protein 1 deficiency and factor H antibodies in pediatric patients with atypical hemolytic uremic syndrome. Clin J Am Soc Nephrol. 2013;8(3):407–15.

40. Sinha A, Gulati A, Saini S, Blanc C, Gupta A, Gurjar BS, et al. Prompt plasma exchanges and immunosuppressive treatment improves the outcomes of anti-factor H autoantibody-associated hemolytic uremic syndrome in children. Kidney Int. 2014;85(5):1151–60.

41. Marinozzi MC, Vergoz L, Rybkine T, Ngo S, Bettoni S, Pashov A, et al. Complement factor B mutations in atypical hemolytic uremic syndrome-disease-relevant or benign? J Am Soc Nephrol. 2014;25(9):2053–65.

42. Hofer J, Giner T, Józsi M. Complement factor h-antibody-associated hemolytic uremic syndrome: pathogenesis, clinical presentation, and treatment. Semin Thromb Hemost. 2014;40(4):431–43.

43. Venables JP, Strain L, Routledge D, Bourn D, Powell HM, Warwicker P, et al. Atypical haemolytic uraemic syndrome associated with a hybrid complement gene. PLoS Med. 2006;3(10):e431.

44. Maga TK, Meyer NC, Belsha C, Nishimura CJ, Zhang Y, Smith RJ. A novel deletion in the RCA gene cluster causes atypical hemolytic uremic syndrome. Nephrol Dial Transplant. 2011;26(2):739–41.

45. Francis NJ, McNicholas B, Awan A, Waldron M, Reddan D, Sadlier D, et al. A novel hybrid CFH/CFHR3 gene generated by a microhomology-mediated deletion in familial atypical hemolytic uremic syndrome. Blood. 2012;119(2):591–601.

46. Eyler SJ, Meyer NC, Zhang Y, Xiao X, Nester CM, Smith RJ. A novel hybrid CFHR1/CFH gene causes atypical hemolytic uremic syndrome. Pediatr Nephrol. 2013;28(11):2221–5.

47. Blanc C, Roumenina LT, Ashraf Y, Hyvärinen S, Sethi SK, Ranchin B, et al. Overall neutralization of complement factor H by autoantibodies in the acute phase of the autoimmune form of atypical hemolytic uremic syndrome. J Immunol. 2012;189(7):3528–37.

48. Holmes LV, Strain L, Staniforth SJ, Moore I, Marchbank K, Kavanagh D, et al. Determining the population frequency of the CFHR3/CFHR1 deletion at 1q32. PLoS One. 2013;8(4):e60352.

49. Kavanagh D, Pappworth IY, Anderson H, Hayes CM, Moore I, Hunze EM, et al. Factor I autoantibodies in patients with atypical hemolytic uremic syndrome: disease-associated or an epiphenomenon? Clin J Am Soc Nephrol. 2012;7(3):417–26.

50. Roumenina LT, Frimat M, Miller EC, Provot F, Dragon-Durey MA, Bordereau P, et al. A prevalent C3 mutation in aHUS patients causes a direct C3 convertase gain of function. Blood. 2012;119(18):4182–91.

51. Roumenina LT, Jablonski M, Hue C, Blouin J, Dimitrov JD, Dragon-Durey MA, et al. Hyperfunctional C3 convertase leads to complement deposition on endothelial cells and contributes to atypical hemolytic uremic syndrome. Blood. 2009;114(13):2837–45.

52. Bresin E, Rurali E, Caprioli J, Sanchez-Corral P, Fremeaux-Bacchi V, Rodriguez de Cordoba S, et al. Combined complement gene mutations in atypical hemolytic uremic syndrome influence clinical phenotype. J Am Soc Nephrol. 2013;24(3): 475–86.

53. Fremeaux-Bacchi V, Kemp EJ, Goodship JA, Dragon-Durey MA, Strain L, Loirat C, et al. The development of atypical haemolytic-uraemic syndrome is influenced by susceptibility factors in factor H and membrane cofactor protein: evidence from two independent cohorts. J Med Genet. 2005;42(11):852–6.

54. Abarrategui-Garrido C, Martínez-Barricarte R, López-Trascasa M, de Córdoba SR, Sánchez-Corral P. Characterization of complement factor H-related (CFHR) proteins in plasma reveals novel genetic variations of CFHR1 associated with atypical hemolytic uremic syndrome. Blood. 2009;114(19):4261–71.

55. Bu F, Maga T, Meyer NC, Wang K, Thomas CP, Nester CM, et al. Comprehensive genetic analysis of complement and coagulation genes in atypical hemolytic uremic syndrome. J Am Soc Nephrol. 2014;25(1):55–64.

56. Feng S, Eyler SJ, Zhang Y, Maga T, Nester CM, Kroll MH, et al. Partial ADAMTS13 deficiency in atypical hemolytic uremic syndrome. Blood. 2013;122(8):1487–93.

57. Meri S. Complement activation in diseases presenting with thrombotic microangiopathy. Eur J Intern Med. 2013;24(6):496–502.

58. Riedl M, Fakhouri F, Le Quintrec M, Noone DG, Jungraithmayr TC, Fremeaux-Bacchi V, et al. Spectrum of complement-mediated thrombotic microangiopathies: pathogenetic insights identifying novel treatment approaches. Semin Thromb Hemost. 2014;40(4):444–64.

59. Turner NA, Moake J. Assembly and activation of alternative complement components on endothelial cell-anchored ultra-large von Willebrand factor links complement and hemostasis-thrombosis. PLoS One. 2013;8(3):e59372.

60. Rayes J, Roumenina LT, Dimitrov JD, Repessé Y, Ing M, Christophe O, et al. The interaction between factor H and VWF increases factor H cofactor activity and regulates VWF prothrombotic status. Blood. 2014;123(1):121–5.

61. Feng S, Liang X, Cruz MA, Vu H, Zhou Z, Pemmaraju N, et al. The interaction between factor H and Von Willebrand factor. PLoS One. 2013;8(8):e73715.

62. Ståhl AL, Vaziri-Sani F, Heinen S, Kristoffersson AC, Gydell KH, Raafat R, et al. Factor H dysfunction in patients with atypical hemolytic uremic syndrome contributes to complement deposition on platelets and their activation. Blood. 2008;111(11): 5307–15.

63. Pickering MC, de Jorge EG, Martinez-Barricarte R, Recalde S, Garcia-Layana A, Rose KL, et al. Spontaneous hemolytic uremic syndrome triggered by complement factor H lacking surface recognition domains. J Exp Med. 2007;204(6):1249–56.

64. Quaggin SE. DGKE and atypical HUS. Nat Genet. 2013;45(5):475–6.
65. Constantinescu AR, Bitzan M, Weiss LS, Christen E, Kaplan BS, Cnaan A, et al. Non-enteropathic hemolytic uremic syndrome: causes and short-term course. Am J Kidney Dis. 2004;43(6):976–82.
66. Le Quintrec M, Zuber J, Moulin B, Kamar N, Jablonski M, Lionet A, et al. Complement genes strongly predict recurrence and graft outcome in adult renal transplant recipients with atypical hemolytic and uremic syndrome. Am J Transplant. 2013;13(3):663–75.
67. Khandelwal P, Sinha A, Hari P, Bansal VK, Dinda AK, Bagga A. Outcomes of renal transplant in patients with anti-complement factor H antibody-associated hemolytic uremic syndrome. Pediatr Transplant. 2014;18(5):E134–9.
68. Edey MM, Mead PA, Saunders RE, Strain L, Perkins SJ, Goodship TH, et al. Association of a factor H mutation with hemolytic uremic syndrome following a diarrheal illness. Am J Kidney Dis. 2008;51(3):487–90.
69. Alberti M, Valoti E, Piras R, Bresin E, Galbusera M, Tripodo C, et al. Two patients with history of STEC-HUS, posttransplant recurrence and complement gene mutations. Am J Transplant. 2013;13(8): 2201–6.
70. Fang CJ, Fremeaux-Bacchi V, Liszewski MK, Pianetti G, Noris M, Goodship TH, et al. Membrane cofactor protein mutations in atypical hemolytic uremic syndrome (aHUS), fatal Stx-HUS, C3 glomerulonephritis, and the HELLP syndrome. Blood. 2008;111(2):624–32.
71. Fakhouri F, Roumenina L, Provot F, Sallée M, Caillard S, Couzi L, et al. Pregnancy-associated hemolytic uremic syndrome revisited in the era of complement gene mutations. J Am Soc Nephrol. 2010;21(5):859–67.
72. Sellier-Leclerc AL, Fremeaux-Bacchi V, Dragon-Durey MA, Macher MA, Niaudet P, Guest G, et al. Differential impact of complement mutations on clinical characteristics in atypical hemolytic uremic syndrome. J Am Soc Nephrol. 2007;18(8):2392–400.
73. Gulleroglu K, Fidan K, Hançer VS, Bayrakci U, Baskin E, Soylemezoglu O. Neurologic involvement in atypical hemolytic uremic syndrome and successful treatment with eculizumab. Pediatr Nephrol. 2013;28(5):827–30.
74. Hu H, Nagra A, Haq MR, Gilbert RD. Eculizumab in atypical haemolytic uraemic syndrome with severe cardiac and neurological involvement. Pediatr Nephrol. 2014;29(6):1103–6.
75. Vilalta R, Lara E, Madrid A, Chocron S, Muñoz M, Casquero A, et al. Long-term eculizumab improves clinical outcomes in atypical hemolytic uremic syndrome. Pediatr Nephrol. 2012;27(12):2323–6.
76. Diamante Chiodini B, Davin JC, Corazza F, Khaldi K, Dahan K, Ismaili K, Adams B. Eculizumab in anti-factor h antibodies associated with atypical hemolytic uremic syndrome. Pediatrics. 2014;133(6):e1764–8.
77. Michaux K, Bacchetta J, Javouhey E, Cochat P, Frémaux-Bacchi V, Sellier-Leclerc AL. Eculizumab in neonatal hemolytic uremic syndrome with homozygous factor H deficiency. Pediatr Nephrol. 2014;29(12):2415–9.
78. Malina M, Gulati A, Bagga A, Majid MA, Simkova E, Schaefer F. Peripheral gangrene in children with atypical hemolytic uremic syndrome. Pediatrics. 2013;131(1):e331–5.
79. Ariceta G, Arrizabalaga B, Aguirre M, Morteruel E, Lopez-Trascasa M. Eculizumab in the treatment of atypical hemolytic uremic syndrome in infants. Am J Kidney Dis. 2012;59(5):707–10.
80. Ardissino G, Tel F, Testa S, Marzano AV, Lazzari R, Salardi S, et al. Skin involvement in atypical hemolytic uremic syndrome. Am J Kidney Dis. 2014;63(4):652–5.
81. Santos C, Lopes D, Gomes A, Venturaa A, Tente D, Seabra J. Cutaneous involvement in haemolytic uraemic syndrome. Clin Kidney J. 2013;0:1–2.
82. Larakeb A, Leroy S, Frémeaux-Bacchi V, Montchilova M, Pelosse B, Dunand O, et al. Ocular involvement in hemolytic uremic syndrome due to factor H deficiency – are there therapeutic consequences? Pediatr Nephrol. 2007;22(11): 1967–70.
83. Loirat C, Macher MA, Elmaleh-Berges M, Kwon T, Deschênes G, Goodship TH, et al. Non-atheromatous arterial stenoses in atypical haemolytic uraemic syndrome associated with complement dysregulation. Nephrol Dial Transplant. 2010;25(10):3421–5.
84. Davin JC, Majoie C, Groothoff J, Gracchi V, Bouts A, Goodship TH, et al. Prevention of large-vessel stenoses in atypical hemolytic uremic syndrome associated with complement dysregulation. Pediatr Nephrol. 2011;26(1):155–7.
85. Békássy ZD, Kristoffersson AC, Cronqvist M, Roumenina LT, Rybkine T, Vergoz L, et al. Eculizumab in an anephric patient with atypical haemolytic uraemic syndrome and advanced vascular lesions. Nephrol Dial Transplant. 2013;28(11): 2899–907.
86. Ažukaitis K, Loirat C, Malina M, Adomaitienė I, Jankauskienė A. Macrovascular involvement in a child with atypical hemolytic uremic syndrome. Pediatr Nephrol. 2014;29(7):1273–7.
87. Noris M, Remuzzi G. Cardiovascular complications in atypical haemolytic uraemic syndrome. Nat Rev Nephrol. 2014;10(3):174–80.
88. Mele C, Remuzzi G, Noris M. Hemolytic uremic syndrome. Semin Immunopathol. 2014;36(4): 399–420.
89. Espié E, Grimont F, Mariani-Kurkdjian P, Bouvet P, Haeghebaert S, Filliol I, et al. Surveillance of hemolytic uremic syndrome in children less than 15 years of age, a system to monitor O157 and non-O157 Shiga toxin-producing Escherichia coli infections in

France, 1996–2006. Pediatr Infect Dis J. 2008;27(7): 595–601.

90. Rosales A, Hofer J, Zimmerhackl LB, Jungraithmayr TC, Riedl M, Giner T, et al. Need for long-term follow-up in enterohemorrhagic Escherichia coli-associated hemolytic uremic syndrome due to late-emerging sequelae. Clin Infect Dis. 2012;54(10): 1413–21.

91. Spinale JM, Ruebner RL, Copelovitch L, Kaplan BS. Long-term outcomes of Shiga toxin hemolytic uremic syndrome. Pediatr Nephrol. 2013;28(11): 2097–105.

92. Yagi H, Matsumoto M, Fujimura Y. Paradigm shift of childhood thrombotic thrombocytopenic purpura with severe ADAMTS13 deficiency. Presse Med. 2012;41(3 Pt 2):e137–55.

93. Loirat C, Coppo P, Veyradier A. Thrombotic thrombocytopenic purpura in children. Curr Opin Pediatr. 2013;25(2):216–24.

94. Hassenpflug WA, Budde U, Schneppenheim S, Schneppenheim R. Inherited thrombotic thrombocytopenic purpura in children. Semin Thromb Hemost. 2014;40(4):487–92.

95. Reese JA, Muthurajah DS, Kremer Hovinga JA, Vesely SK, Terrell DR, George JN. Children and adults with thrombotic thrombocytopenic purpura associated with severe, acquired Adamts13 deficiency: comparison of incidence, demographic and clinical features. Pediatr Blood Cancer. 2013;60(10):1676–82.

96. Hie M, Gay J, Galicier L, Provôt F, Presne C, Poullin P, et al. Preemptive rituximab infusions after remission efficiently prevent relapses in acquired thrombotic thrombocytopenic purpura. Blood. 2014;124(2):204–10.

97. Sharma AP, Greenberg CR, Prasad AN, Prasad C. Hemolytic uremic syndrome (HUS) secondary to cobalamin C (cblC) disorder. Pediatr Nephrol. 2007;22(12):2097–103.

98. Menni F, Testa S, Guez S, Chiarelli G, Alberti L, Esposito S. Neonatal atypical hemolytic uremic syndrome due to methylmalonic aciduria and homocystinuria. Pediatr Nephrol. 2012;27(8):1401–5.

99. Cornec-Le Gall E, Delmas Y, De Parscau L, Doucet L, Ogier H, Benoist JF, et al. Adult-onset eculizumab-resistant hemolytic uremic syndrome associated with cobalamin C deficiency. Am J Kidney Dis. 2014;63(1):119–23.

100. Kömhoff M, Roofthooft MT, Westra D, Teertstra TK, Losito A, van de Kar NC, et al. Combined pulmonary hypertension and renal thrombotic microangiopathy in cobalamin C deficiency. Pediatrics. 2013;132(2):e540–4.

101. Fischer S, Huemer M, Baumgartner M, Deodato F, Ballhausen D, Boneh A, et al. Clinical presentation and outcome in a series of 88 patients with the cblC defect. J Inherit Metab Dis. 2014;37(5):831–40.

102. Loirat C, Fakhouri F, Ariceta G, Besbas N, Bitzan M, Bjerre A, et al. An international consensus approach to the management of atypical hemolytic uremic syndrome in children. Pediatr Nephrol. 2016;31(1):15–39.

103. Kokame K, Nobe Y, Kokubo Y, Okayama A, Miyata T. FRETS-VWF73, a first fluorogenic substrate for ADAMTS13 assay. Br J Haematol. 2005;129(1): 93–100.

104. Meyer SC, Sulzer I, Lämmle B, Kremer Hovinga JA. Hyperbilirubinemia interferes with ADAMTS-13 activity measurement by FRETS-VWF73 assay: diagnostic relevance in patients suffering from acute thrombotic microangiopathies. J Thromb Haemost. 2007;5(4):866–7.

105. Mackie I, Langley K, Chitolie A, Liesner R, Scully M, Machin S, et al. Discrepancies between ADAMTS13 activity assays in patients with thrombotic microangiopathies. Thromb Haemost. 2013;109(3):488–96.

106. Thouzeau S, Capdenat S, Stépanian A, Coppo P, Veyradier A. Evaluation of a commercial assay for ADAMTS13 activity measurement. Thromb Haemost. 2013;110(4):852–3.

107. Watson R, Lindner S, Bordereau P, Hunze EM, Tak F, Ngo S, et al. Standardisation of the factor H autoantibody assay. Immunobiology. 2014;219(1):9–16.

108. Loirat C, Frémeaux-Bacchi V. Atypical hemolytic uremic syndrome. Orphanet J Rare Dis. 2011;6:60.

109. Cataland SR, Holers VM, Geyer S, Yang S, Wu HM. Biomarkers of terminal complement activation confirm the diagnosis of aHUS and differentiate aHUS from TTP. Blood. 2014;123(24):3733–8.

110. Volokhina EB, Westra D, van der Velden TJ, van de Kar NC, Mollnes TE, van den Heuvel LP. Complement activation patterns in atypical hemolytic uremic syndrome during acute phase and in remission. Clin Exp Immunol. 2015;181(2):306–13.

111. Moore I, Strain L, Pappworth I, Kavanagh D, Barlow PN, Herbert AP, et al. Association of factor H autoantibodies with deletions of CFHR1, CFHR3, CFHR4, and with mutations in CFH, CFI, CD46, and C3 in patients with atypical hemolytic uremic syndrome. Blood. 2010;115(2):379–87.

112. Zuber J, Le Quintrec M, Krid S, Bertoye C, Gueutin V, Lahoche A, et al. Eculizumab for atypical hemolytic uremic syndrome recurrence in renal transplantation. Am J Transplant. 2012;12(12):3337–54.

113. Sinibaldi S, Guzzo I, Piras R, Bresin E, Emma F, Dello Strologo L. Post-transplant recurrence of atypical hemolytic uremic syndrome in a patient with thrombomodulin mutation. Pediatr Transplant. 2013;17(8):E177–81.

114. Saland JM, Ruggenenti P, Remuzzi G, Consensus Study Group. Liver-kidney transplantation to cure atypical hemolytic uremic syndrome. J Am Soc Nephrol. 2009;20(5):940–9.

115. Zuber J, Le Quintrec M, Morris H, Frémeaux-Bacchi V, Loirat C, Legendre C. Targeted strategies in the prevention and management of atypical HUS recurrence after kidney transplantation. Transplant Rev (Orlando). 2013;27(4):117–25.

116. Hillmen P, Muus P, Röth A, Elebute MO, Risitano AM, Schrezenmeier H, et al. Long-term safety and efficacy of sustained eculizumab treatment in patients with paroxysmal nocturnal haemoglobinuria. Br J Haematol. 2013;162(1):62–73.

117. Gruppo RA, Rother RP. Eculizumab for congenital atypical hemolytic-uremic syndrome. N Engl J Med. 2009;360(5):544–6.

118. Nürnberger J, Philipp T, Witzke O, Opazo Saez A, Vester U, Baba HA, et al. Eculizumab for atypical hemolytic-uremic syndrome. N Engl J Med. 2009;360(5):542–4.

119. Soliris: summary of product characteristics. http://www.medicines.org.uk/emc/medicine/19966.

120. Soliris.net.U.S. prescribing information. http://soliris.net/sites/default/files/assets/soliris_pi.pdf.

121. Licht C, Greenbaum LA, Muus P, Babu S, Bedrosian CL, Cohen D, et al. Efficacy and safety of eculizumab in atypical hemolytic uremic syndrome: 2-year results from extensions of phase 2 studies. Kidney Int. 2015;87(5):1061–73.

122. Legendre C, Greenbaum L, Sheerin N, Cohen D, Gaber O, Eitner F, et al. Eculizumab efficacy in aHUS patients with progressing TMA, with or without prior renal transplant. American Transplant Congress, Poster A822, 18–22 May 2013, Seattle, WA.

123. Fakhouri F, Hourmant M, Campistol JM, Cataland SR, Espinosa M, Gaber AO, et al. Eculizumab inhibits TMA and improves hematologic parameters and renal function in adult patients with aHUS. American Society of Nephrology, Abstract 5593 and Presentation FR-OR057, 5–9 Nov 2013, Atlanta.

124. Greenbaum L, Fila M, Tsimaratos M, Ardissino G, Al-Akash SI, Evans J, et al. eculizumab inhibits TMA and improves renal function in pediatric aHUS patients. American Society of Nephrology, Abstract 5579 and Poster SA-PO849, 5–9 Nov 2013, Atlanta.

125. Cayci FS, Cakar N, Hancer VS, Uncu N, Acar B, Gur G. Eculizumab therapy in a child with hemolytic uremic syndrome and CFI mutation. Pediatr Nephrol. 2012;27(12):2327–31.

126. Giordano M, Castellano G, Messina G, Divella C, Bellantuono R, Puteo F, et al. Preservation of renal function in atypical hemolytic uremic syndrome by eculizumab: a case report. Pediatrics. 2012;130(5):e1385–8.

127. Besbas N, Gulhan B, Karpman D, Topaloglu R, Duzova A, Korkmaz E, et al. Neonatal onset atypical hemolytic uremic syndrome successfully treated with eculizumab. Pediatr Nephrol. 2013;28(1):155–8.

128. Gilbert RD, Fowler DJ, Angus E, Hardy SA, Stanley L, Goodship TH. Eculizumab therapy for atypical haemolytic uraemic syndrome due to a gain-of-function mutation of complement factor B. Pediatr Nephrol. 2013;28(8):1315–8.

129. Vaisbich MH, Henriques Ldos S, Watanabe A, Pereira LM, Metran CC, Malheiros DA, et al. Eculizumab for the treatment of atypical hemolytic uremic syndrome: case report and revision of the literature. J Bras Neurol. 2013;35(3):237–41.

130. Christmann M, Hansen M, Bergmann C, Schwabe D, Brand J, Schneider W. Eculizumab as first-line therapy for atypical hemolytic uremic syndrome. Pediatrics. 2014;133(6):e1759–63.

131. Fakhouri F, Delmas Y, Provot F, Barbet C, Karras A, Makdassi R, et al. Insights from the use in clinical practice of eculizumab in adult patients with atypical hemolytic uremic syndrome affecting the native kidneys: an analysis of 19 cases. Am J Kidney Dis. 2014;63(1):40–8.

132. Ohanian M, Cable C, Halka K. Eculizumab safely reverses neurologic impairment and eliminates need for dialysis in severe atypical hemolytic uremic syndrome. Clin Pharmacol. 2011;3:5–12.

133. Salem G, Flynn JM, Cataland SR. Profound neurological injury in a patient with atypical hemolytic uremic syndrome. Ann Hematol. 2013;92(4):557–8.

134. Beye F, Malbranche C, Tramecon D, Pernot C, Zanetta G, Mousson C. Eculizumab: effectiveness of a shortened dosing schedule in the treatment of atypical haemolytic uremic syndrome of unknown origin. Therapie. 2013;68(2):119–22.

135. Pu JJ, Sido A. Successful discontinuation of eculizumab therapy in a patient with aHUS. Ann Hematol. 2014;93(8):1423–5.

136. Chaudhary P, Hepgur M, Sarkissian S, Smith RJ, Weitz IC. Atypical haemolytic-uraemic syndrome due to heterozygous mutations of CFH/CFHR1-3 and complement factor H 479. Blood Transfus. 2014;12(1):111–3.

137. Hodgkins KS, Bobrowski AE, Lane JC, Langman CB. Clinical grand rounds: atypical hemolytic uremic syndrome. Am J Nephrol. 2012;35(5):394–400.

138. Reuter S, Heitplatz B, Pavenstädt H, Suwelack B. Successful long-term treatment of TMA with eculizumab in a transplanted patient with atypical hemolytic uremic syndrome due to MCP mutation. Transplantation. 2013;96(10):e74–6.

139. Matar D, Naqvi F, Racusen LC, Carter-Monroe N, Montgomery RA, Alachkar N. Atypical hemolytic uremic syndrome recurrence after kidney transplantation. Transplantation. 2014;98(11):1205–12.

140. Xie L, Nester CM, Reed AI, Zhang Y, Smith RJ, Thomas CP. Tailored eculizumab therapy in the management of complement factor H-mediated atypical hemolytic uremic syndrome in an adult kidney transplant recipient: a case report. Transplant Proc. 2012;44(10):3037–40.

141. Pelicano MB, de Córdoba SR, Diekmann F, Saiz M, Herrero S, Oppenheimer F, et al. Anti-C5 as prophylactic therapy in atypical hemolytic uremic syndrome in living-related kidneytransplantation. Transplantation. 2013;96(4):e26–9.

142. Román-Ortiz E, Mendizabal Oteiza S, Pinto S, López-Trascasa M, Sánchez-Corral P, Rodríguez de Cordoba S. Eculizumab long-term therapy for pediatric renal transplant in aHUS with CFH/CFHR1 hybrid gene. Pediatr Nephrol. 2014;29(1):149–53.

143. Ranch D, Crowther B, Arar M, Assanasen C. Prophylactic eculizumab for kidney transplantation in a child with atypical hemolytic uremic syndrome due to complement factor H mutation. Pediatr Transplant. 2014;18(6):E185–9.

144. Struijk GH, Bouts AH, Rijkers GT, Kuin EA, ten Berge IJ, Bemelman FJ. Meningococcal sepsis complicating eculizumab treatment despite prior vaccination. Am J Transplant. 2013;13(3):819–20.

145. Sana G, Dragon-Durey MA, Charbit M, Bouchireb K, Rousset-Rouvière C, Bérard E, et al. Long-term remission of atypical HUS with anti-factor H antibodies after cyclophosphamide pulses. Pediatr Nephrol. 2014;29(1):75–83.

146. Noone D, Waters A, Pluthero FG, Geary DF, Kirschfink M, Zipfel PF, et al. Successful treatment of DEAP-HUS with eculizumab. Pediatr Nephrol. 2014;29(5):841–51.

147. Green H, Harari E, Davidovits M, Blickstein D, Grossman A, Gafter U, et al. Atypical HUS due to factor H antibodies in an adult patient successfully treated with eculizumab. Ren Fail. 2014;36(7):1119–21.

148. Belingheri M, Possenti I, Tel F, Paglialonga F, Testa S, Salardi S, et al. Cryptic activity of atypical hemolytic uremic syndrome and eculizumab treatment. Pediatrics. 2014;133(6):e1769–71.

149. Nishimura J, Yamamoto M, Hayashi S, Ohyashiki K, Ando K, Brodsky AL, et al. Genetic variants in C5 and poor response to eculizumab. N Engl J Med. 2014;370(7):632–9.

150. Cugno M, Gualtierotti R, Possenti I, Testa S, Tel F, Griffini S, et al. Complement functional tests for monitoring eculizumab treatment in patients with atypical hemolytic uremic syndrome. J Thromb Haemost. 2014;12(9):1440–8.

151. Carr R, Cataland SR. Relapse of aHUS after discontinuation of therapy with eculizumab in a patient with aHUS and factor H mutation. Ann Hematol. 2013;92(6):845–6.

152. Ardissino G, Testa S, Possenti I, Tel F, Paglialonga F, Salardi S, et al. Discontinuation of eculizumab maintenance treatment for atypical hemolytic uremic syndrome: a report of 10 cases. Am J Kidney Dis. 2014;64(4):633–7.

153. Cañigral C, Moscardó F, Castro C, Pajares A, Lancharro A, Solves P, et al. Eculizumab for the treatment of pregnancy-related atypical hemolytic uremic syndrome. Ann Hematol. 2014;93(8):1421–2.

154. Saland J. Liver-kidney transplantation to cure atypical HUS: still an option post-eculizumab? Pediatr Nephrol. 2014;29(3):329–32.

155. Park SH, Kim GS. Anesthetic management of living donor liver transplantation for complement factor H deficiency hemolytic uremic syndrome: a case report. Korean J Anesthesiol. 2014;66(6):481–5.

156. Peffault de Latour R, Xhaard A, Fremeaux-Bacchi V, Coppo P, Fischer AM, Helley D, et al. Successful use of eculizumab in a patient with post-transplant thrombotic microangiopathy. Br J Haematol. 2013;161(2):279–80.

157. Jodele S, Fukuda T, Vinks A, Mizuno K, Laskin BL, Goebel J, et al. Eculizumab therapy in children with severe hematopoietic stem cell transplantation-associated thrombotic microangiopathy. Biol Blood Marrow Transplant. 2014;20(4):518–25.

158. Okano M, Sakata N, Ueda S, Takemura T. Recovery from life-threatening transplantation-associated thrombotic microangiopathy using eculizumab in a patient with very severe aplastic anemia. Bone Marrow Transplant. 2014;49(8):1116–8.

159. Jodele S, Licht C, Goebel J, Dixon BP, Zhang K, Sivakumaran TA, et al. Abnormalities in the alternative pathway of complement in children with hematopoietic stem cell transplant-associated thrombotic microangiopathy. Blood. 2013;122(12):2003–7.

160. Réti M, Farkas P, Csuka D, Rázsó K, Schlammadinger Á, Udvardy ML, et al. Complement activation in thrombotic thrombocytopenic purpura. J Thromb Haemost. 2012;10(5):791–8.

161. Wu TC, Yang S, Haven S, Holers VM, Lundberg AS, Wu H, et al. Complement activation and mortality during an acute episode of thrombotic thrombocytopenic purpura. J Thromb Haemost. 2013;11(10):1925–7.

162. Tati R, Kristoffersson AC, Ståhl AL, Rebetz J, Wang L, Licht C, et al. Complement activation associated with ADAMTS13 deficiency in human and murine thrombotic microangiopathy. J Immunol. 2013;191(5):2184–93.

163. Chapin J, Weksler B, Magro C, Laurence J. Eculizumab in the treatment of refractory idiopathic thrombotic thrombocytopenic purpura. Br J Haematol. 2012;157(6):772–4.

164. Tsai E, Chapin J, Laurence JC, Tsai HM. Use of eculizumab in the treatment of a case of refractory, ADAMTS13-deficient thrombotic thrombocytopenic purpura: additional data and clinical follow-up. Br J Haematol. 2013;162(4):558–9.

C3 Glomerulopathies

25

Christoph Licht, Marina Vivarelli,
and Sanjeev Sethi

Pathology of C3 Glomerulopathies

Membranoproliferative Glomerulonephritis

Membranoproliferative glomerulonephritis
(MPGN) refers to a pattern of injury occurring as
response to deposition of immunoglobulins (Ig)/
immune-complexes (IC) and/or complement factors in the mesangium and/or along the glomerular capillary walls [1]. The deposition of Ig/IC and
complement factors results in an inflammatory
response due to: (1) proliferation of indigenous
glomerular cells such as mesangial cells, endothelial cells, and infiltration and proliferation of leukocytes, and (2) synthesis of matrix material such
as mesangial matrix material, basement membrane material and fibrin. The MPGN pattern is
thus characterized by (1) increased cellularity
in the mesangium (mesangial proliferation) and
within the capillary lumen (endocapillary proliferation), and (2) mesangial expansion by matrix
material and capillary wall remodelling with formation of double contours. The MPGN pattern is
distinguished from a diffuse (endocapillary) proliferative pattern by the finding that in MPGN at
the time of diagnosis the injury is often chronic,
resulting in a healing or remodeling phase in the
mesangium (mesangial expansion, often with
nodule formation) and along the glomerular capillaries (double contour formation) [2].

Glomerular deposition of Ig/IC originates
from three basic pathogenic mechanisms (see
later in this chapter Fig. 25.3a–d): (1) deposition
of monoclonal Ig as a result of a monoclonal
gammopathy due to a plasma cell or B cell disorder [3–6]; (2) deposition of antigen-antibody or
IC as a result of an infection [7]; and (3) IC
deposition as a result of an autoimmune disease
[8, 9]. Immunofluorescence studies can often
confirm the underlying pathogenic mechanism
of Ig/IC deposition based on the type of Ig
detected. Complement factors are also noted
along with the Ig/IC, due to activation of the
complement system via the *classical pathway* by
the Ig/IC. On the other hand, glomerular deposition of complement factors alone or in the presence of scant Ig results from dysregulation of the
complement alternative pathway (CAP). The
term C3 glomerulopathy (C3G) is used to define
this entity [10].

C. Licht (✉)
Department of Nephrology,
The Hospital for Sick Children,
555 University Avenue, Toronto M5G 1X8, Canada
e-mail: christoph.licht@sickkids.ca

M. Vivarelli
Department of Nephrology and Dialysis,
Ospedale Pediatrico Bambino Gesu,
Pizza S.Onofrio 4, Rome 00165, Italy
e-mail: marina.vivarelli@opbg.net

S. Sethi
Laboratory Medicine and Pathology Department,
Mayo Clinic, 200 1st Street SW,
Rochester, MN 55902, USA
e-mail: sethi.sanjeev@mayo.edu

© Springer-Verlag Berlin Heidelberg 2016
D.F. Geary, F. Schaefer (eds.), *Pediatric Kidney Disease*, DOI 10.1007/978-3-662-52972-0_25

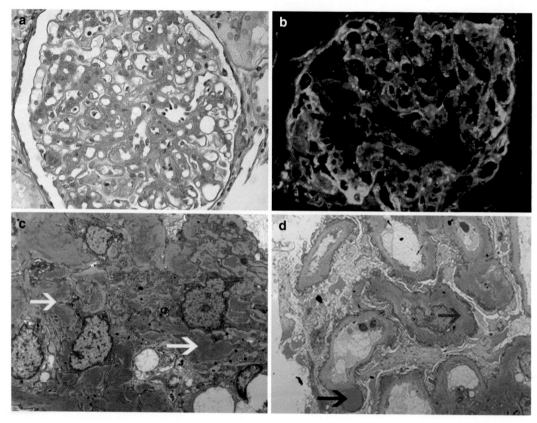

Fig. 25.1 C3 glomerulonephritis. (**a**) Light microscopy showing a MPGN pattern of injury (periodic acid Schiff 60×). (**b**) Immunofluorescence microscopy showing mesangial and capillary wall staining for C3. Immunofluorescence studies were negative for Igs. (**c, d**) EM showing (**c**) Numerous mesangial electron dense deposits (*white arrows*) and (**d**) Capillary wall deposits (*red arrow*-intramembranous and subendothelial deposits, *black arrow*-subepithelial deposit/hump) (**c** 4,200×, **d** 2,500)

Based on these findings MPGN has recently been classified into- Ig/IC-mediated glomerulonephritis and complement-mediated glomerulonephritis (C3 glomerulopathy, C3G) [11]. Thus, immunofluorescence studies of the kidney biopsy are the key to the classification of MPGN into Ig/IC-mediated or complement-mediated MPGN.

C3 Glomerulopathy

While the pathogenesis of MPGN includes a variety of causes, the pathogenesis of C3G is now thought to be predominantly linked to defects in the control of the complement system, in particular its alternative pathway (CAP). Deposition of complement factors in the mesangium and/or along the glomerular capillary walls results in a proliferative glomerulonephritis. The term "C3 glomerulopathy" (C3G) is now used to define the entity of a glomerulonephritis characterized by C3 accumulation, with absent or scanty Ig deposition [10, 12, 13]. C3G encompasses the entities of C3 glomerulonephritis (C3GN) and dense deposit disease (DDD) [10, 12, 14]. On kidney biopsy, C3GN (Fig. 25.1a–d) and DDD (Fig. 25.2a–c) present as a proliferative glomerulonephritis [1]. The most common pattern on light microscopy for both C3GN and DDD is that of MPGN. Other patterns of injury include mesangial proliferative glomerulonephritis, diffuse proliferative glomerulonephritis or even a necrotizing and crescentic glomerulonephritis [15]. Two or more patterns of injury may be seen on the same biopsy. On immu-

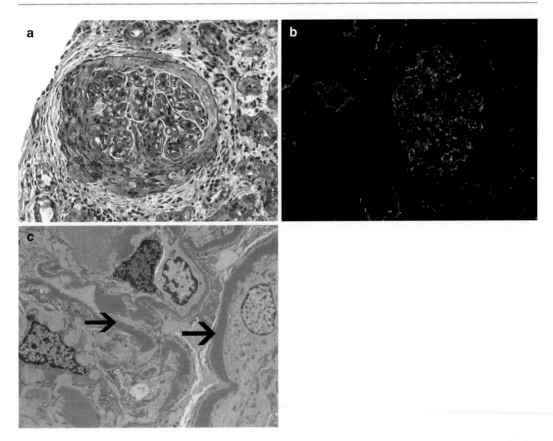

Fig. 25.2 Dense deposit disease. (**a**) Light microscopy showing an MPGN pattern of injury (periodic acid Schiff 40×). Note cellular crescent. (**b**) Immunofluorescence microscopy showing mesangial and capillary wall stain-ing for C3. Immunofluorescence studies were negative for Ig's. (**c**) EM showing dense osmiophilic deposits along the glomerular basement membranes and in the mesan-gium (11,100×). *Arrows* point to the deposits

nofluorescence studies, both C3GN and DDD are characterized by bright mesangial and capillary wall staining for C3. In DDD, C3 staining may also be seen along the tubular basement membrane. Tubular basement membrane staining for C3 is uncommon in C3GN. The main differentiating factor between C3GN and DDD lies in the EM findings. In C3GN, the complement deposits are discrete and are located in the mesangium and along the capillary wall in the subendothelial region of the GBM. Subepithelial (humps) and few intramembranous deposits are also often present. The deposits often assume a lobular shape and have a waxy appearance with ill-defined margins. On the other hand, in DDD the deposits are intensely osmiophilic and are located in the mesangium and within the GBM (intra-membranous deposits) often forming large dense ribbon/sausage shaped bands that can completely transform the GBM.

Lessons Learned from Proteomics in C3GN and DDD Patients

Both C3GN and DDD are diseases resulting from CAP dysregulation. Recent studies using the technique of laser microdissection of glomeruli followed by mass spectrometry showed accumulation of complement factors of the CAP including the terminal pathway and regulating proteins such as CFHR1 and CFHR5 as well as vitronectin and clusterin in both conditions [16, 17]. There was little or no significant accumulation of complement factors of the classical complement pathway, such as C1, C2 or C4. In addition, there was little or no Ig present. Of note, there was no CFB present either, indicating absence of C3 and C5 convertase in the glomeruli, findings suggesting that CAP activation in C3G occurs in fluid phase rather than locally (as on the glomerular endothelial cells in aHUS).

Post-infectious Glomerulonephritis and C3GN

Post-infectious glomerulonephritis (PIGN) is characterized by a proliferative glomerulonephritis on light microscopy, staining for granular IgG and C3 on IF microscopy, and mesangial, subendothelial and subepithelial "hump" like deposits on EM. However, in some cases IF studies show dominant C3 with scant or no Ig staining while EM shows the characteristic "hump" like subepithelial deposits. Thus, in this setting the IF findings are similar to C3GN.

In the past, many of these cases with the "hump" like subepithelial deposits and bright C3 staining were deemed PIGN. Terms such as "resolving," "persistent" or "chronic" PIGN were used when decreased serum C3 levels, hematuria and proteinuria persisted or when there was deterioration of kidney function, as PIGN typically resolves within weeks. Recently, it was shown that cases with "hump" like subepithelial deposits, bright C3 staining and scant/no Ig and persistent decreased serum C3 levels and hematuria/proteinuria, were associated with CAP abnormalities. The term "atypical" PIGN – in analogy to aHUS – was introduced to highlight the underlying CAP abnormalities in these patients [18]. The key differentiating feature between PIGN and "atypical" PIGN is the presence of both Ig and C3 in PIGN while there is only C3 with scant or no Ig in "atypical" PIGN, even though subepithelial humps are common to both entities. It is postulated that infections activate the CAP in atypical PIGN. However, due to an underlying defect in the regulatory mechanisms, there is persistent CAP activation with resultant deposition of complement factors and ensuing inflammation in the glomeruli. Of note, subepithelial humps are also seen in DDD [19]. Thus, it is conceivable that DDD and C3GN may be triggered by an infection. However, it is the underlying regulatory CAP defect which then drives the glomerular inflammation even after the infection is controlled.

C3G Recurrence After Transplantation

DDD and C3GN have a high recurrence rate in kidney transplant recipients. For DDD, there is a 60–85 % recurrence risk, resulting in allograft failure in 45–50 % within 5 years of transplantation [20–22]. Information on C3GN recurrence is scarce. In a recent study, there was recurrence of C3GN in 66.7 % of patients, with graft loss in 33 % within 5 years [6]. Kidney biopsy of early recurrent C3GN, detected mainly on routine/protocol biopsies, shows a mesangial proliferative glomerulonephritis on light microscopy, mesangial C3 deposition on IF and mesangial electron dense deposits on EM. MPGN is more common at later stages or when the biopsy is done for clinical indications. This is similar to the findings of recurrent MPGN in general [23].

Immune (Ig/IC)-Mediated MPGN

The three main causes of glomerular Ig/IC deposition are monoclonal Ig deposition as a result of paraproteinemia, immune-complexes (IC) as result of infection, or autoimmune diseases. Monoclonal Ig is rare in the pediatric population. On the other hand, MPGN may result from chronic infections or autoimmune diseases (Table 25.1).

On LM (Fig. 25.3a–d), the glomeruli appear enlarged and show mesangial expansion with increase in cellularity. The capillary walls are thickened and show double contour formation. The capillary tufts have a distinctly lobular appearance and present with increased endocapillary cellularity. IF studies are the key to define the underlying etiology: granular polyclonal IgM, with smaller amounts of IgG along the capillary walls, with or without C3, is typical of chronic viral infections such as hepatitis C;

Table 25.1   Secondary MPGN – synopsis

Conditions underlying secondary MPGN	Type of MPGN[a]
Infectious diseases: bacterial/viral/protozoal	
Hepatitis B, C, EBV, HIV	I, III
Endocarditis/visceral abcesses	I
Infected ventriculoatrial/ventriculoperitoneal shunts/empyema	I
Malaria, schistosomiasis, mycoplasma	I
Tuberculosis, leprosy	I, II
EBV infection	I
Brucellosis	MPGN-like pattern
Systemic immune diseases	
Cryoglobulinemia	I, III
Systemic lupus erythematosus	I, III, II
Sjögren's syndrome	III, I
Rheumatoid arthritis	I
Heriditary deficiencies of complement components	I, II
X-linked agammaglobulinemia	MPGN-like pattern
Neoplasms/dysproteinemias	
Plasma cell dyscrasia	MPGN-like pattern
Fibrillary and immunotactoid glomerulonephritis	MPGN-like pattern
Light chain deposition disease	MPGN-like pattern
Heavy chain deposition disease	MPGN-like pattern
Light and heavy chain deposition disease	MPGN-like pattern
Leukemias and lymphomas (with cryoglobulinemia)	I, III
Waldenstrom macroglobulinemia	I, III
Carcinomas, Wilms' tumor, malignant melanoma	II
Chronic liver disease	
Chronic active hepatitis (B, C)	I, III
Cirrhosis	I, III
Alpha-1-antitrypsin deficiency	I
Miscellaneous	
All conditions leading to thrombotic microangiopathy	MPGN-like pattern
Sickle cell disease	I
Partial lipodystrophy (mainly dense deposit disease)	II, I, III
Transplant glomerulopathy	MPGN-like pattern
Niemann-Pick disease (type C)	II

[a]Listed according to frequency – nomenclature based on original references

multiple immunoglobulins, such as IgM, IgG, and sometimes IgA, along with C3 and C4, are noted in autoimmune diseases, such as Sjogren Syndrome, rheumatoid arthritis, etc. Lupus nephritis, with polyclonal Ig of all classes, along with C3 and C1q, may also present with an MPGN picture. EM shows glomerular capillary wall thickening with subendothelial deposits, cellular elements, and new basement membrane material resulting in double contours. Foot process effacement may be extensive. Tubulo-reticular inclusions in endothelial cells point to an autoimmune etiology. The mesangium is expanded and often contains electron dense deposits which are often more sharp and discrete compared to the waxy and lobular appearance of such deposits in C3G. Deposits in small arteries and along the tubular basement membranes may be present in IC-mediated MPGN due to autoimmune diseases.

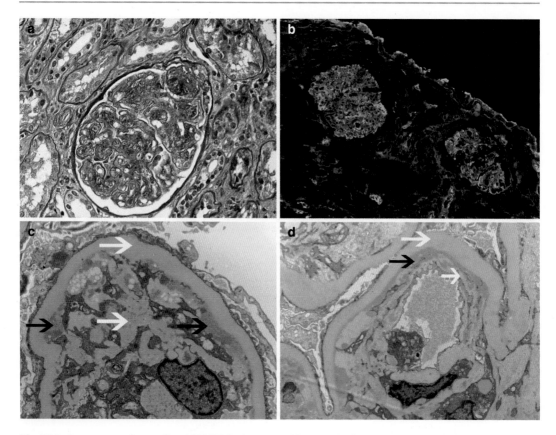

Fig. 25.3 Immune complex-mediated MPGN, in the setting of rheumatoid arthritis. (**a**) Light microscopy showing an MPGN pattern of injury (periodic acid Schiff 40×). Note lobular accentuation of glomerular tufts and thickened capillary walls. (**b**) Immunofluorescence microscopy showing mesangial and capillary wall staining for IgM (20×). (**c**, **d**) EM showing subendothelial deposits and capillary wall thickening with double conotur formation. *Black arrows* point to subendothelial deposits, and *white arrows* point at original and new basement membrane formation (double contour) (**c**-11,100×, **d**-7,830×)

Classification Summary

The classification of C3G is based on the pattern and intensity of immunofluorescence seen on renal biopsy (Figs. 25.1, 25.2, and 25.3). Prevalent Ig staining prompts the diagnosis of a *secondary* MPGN (above), and work-up including a panel of auto-antibodies, viral serologies and, exceptionally in pediatric patients, searching for cryoglobulins and monoclonal gammopathies is warranted (Table 25.1). However, predominant C3 staining prompts the diagnosis of a primary disease, referred to as C3G. Within this category, EM assessment allows for the differentiation of patients with dense deposit disease (DDD; previously known as MPGN II), in whom dense, sausage-like very intensely osmiophilic deposits are present along the glomerular basement membrane, from patients with predominant mesangial C3 staining and possible presence of subepithelial humps as described in post-infectious mesangial glomerulonephritis. The latter group is diagnosed with MPGN I or C3GN, with MPGN I traditionally being favored in patients with membranoproliferative lesions. Of note, C3G may be familial or sporadic.

Clinical Presentation

While the clinical presentation of C3G is very heterogenous reflecting the variety of the underlying causes for CAP dysregulation, the initial manifestation of C3G is typically characterized by (possibly nephrotic range) proteinuria, hematuria and hypertension coupled with low circulating C3 levels [24, 25]. Age of disease onset is very variable, with the earliest reported case being at age 1 [26]. In the most comprehensive clinical overview of cases [27] disease onset was below the age of 16 years in about 40 % of cases with the youngest reported age at onset of 5 years and a slight prevalence of males (60 %). Family history of glomerulonephritis was present in 11 % of cases. At onset, 41 % of patients had nephrotic-range proteinuria (>3 g/day), 61 % had microhematuria. The frequency of macrohematuria in this cohort was not reported, but was around 16 % in other reports [19]. High blood pressure was present in 30.5 % of patients. Renal function was impaired at disease onset in 45.5 % of cases, with a mean eGFR of 69.3 ml/min per 1.73 m². Evaluation of circulating C3 and C4 levels showed low C3 plasma levels in 46 % of all patients, more frequently in patients with DDD (60 %), in whom C3 levels were on average also lower. Low C4 was rare (only about 2 % of cases).

Disease precipitation is often associated with an infection as described in a report of children with DDD, in whom the appearance of renal symptoms was preceded by a respiratory infection in 57 % of cases [19].

Variable age at presentation is probably linked to the fact that C3G can have an indolent and remitting course, so that microhematuria and low-grade proteinuria can remain undetected for years, leading to a delayed diagnosis when proteinuria becomes nephrotic or when renal failure develops. However, early onset with nephrotic proteinuria and renal failure, though less common, has been reported [28]. Recurrent macrohematuria during banal infections is not uncommon [29, 30].

C3G can present as *nephritic syndrome*: a child with macrohematuria, glomerular microhematuria (dysmorphic red blood cells) and proteinuria of variable intensity appearing within 2–3 weeks of an infectious episode (such as upper or lower respiratory tract or gastroenteritis). Laboratory exams usually reveal low circulating C3 with normal C4 and a variable degree of renal impairment. Hypertension may be present. This picture is (clinically) compatible with post-infectious glomerulonephritis (PIGN), IgA nephropathy (if C3

is normal), or (especially in adolescent females with decreased C4) lupus nephritis.

C3G can also present as *nephrotic syndrome*: patients present with peripheral edema (and weight gain), abdominal pain, and in some cases reduced urine output and usually marked hypertension. Laboratory exams show nephrotic-range proteinuria (>40 mg/h/m² or urinary protein/creatinine >2 mg/mg, respectively) with microhematuria, typically some degree of (acute) renal failure, hypoalbuminemia, elevated cholesterol, triglycerides and platelets, and low immunoglobulins. C3 levels are typically low. This presentation can lead to treatment with steroids, and only subsequently, in the absence of response to this treatment, be deemed an indication for a renal biopsy.

In other cases, C3G presents with *microhematuria and low-grade proteinuria* only. In this case examination of the patient will be unremarkable, and laboratory evaluations may be normal except for low circulating C3 (with normal C4) levels.

In general, a family history of glomerulonephritis must be investigated, as familial forms of C3G are described and genetic investigations may be channeled more effectively in these cases. In addition, establishing the diagnosis of C3G not only warrants a renal biopsy (histopathological findings described in detail above) but also detailed work-up of the complement system including (Table 25.2) [10, 14]:

1. Complement factors (CFH; CFB)
2. CAP activation markers (C3; C4; APH50; CH50; C3d; C5a; SC5b9)
3. Circulating autoantibodies (C3 Nephritic Factor (C3NeF), anti-CFH autoantibodies [31] and anti-CFB autoantibodies [32])
4. Mutations in factors involved in CAP regulation (Factor H [CFH]; Factor I [CFI]; membrane cofactor protein [MCP/CD46]; C3 and Factor B [CFB])
5. Copy number variations and hybrid gene formation within the complement CFH related (CFHR) gene locus, in particular internal duplications within *CFHR5* [33, 34], *CFHR3-1* [35], or other rearrangements (reviewed in [10]).

Servais et al. identified mutations in complement genes in 18 % of patients, while the presence

Table 25.2 Diagnostic evaluation of a patient with suspected diagnosis of C3G: *complement system*

Complement factors	Complement activation markers	Antibodies	Mutations	Copy number variations and hybrid genes
CFH	C3	C3NeF	CFH	CFHR3-1
CFI	C3d	Anti-CFH	Cfi	CFHR5
	C4	Anti-CFB	MCP/CD46	
	C5a		C3	
	C5b-9		CFB	
	APH50			
	CH50			

of circulating C3Nef was detected in 59 % of cases [13]. C3Nef is an autoantibody capable of binding the CAP C3 convertase, C3BbB, thus conferring resistance to its inactivation by regulatory factors such as CFH.

Of note, more than half of the patients carrying complement gene mutations were also C3NeF positive. C3Nef was more frequent in patients with DDD (86 %) and was associated with significantly lower levels of circulating C3. A report of three patients with DDD showed a correlation of moderate increases in C3Nef and slight reduction on C3 with disease recurrence post-transplant [36]. In other reports, lower circulating levels of C3 were found in patients with a membranoproliferative pattern of disease [28], while others have reported that children have significantly lower C3 levels and more frequent C3Nef positivity compared to adults [19]. C3NeF can be detected in different ways [37, 38]. Some assays use patient purified immunoglobulins to screen for autoantibodies that stabilize C3bBb [38], others infer the presence of C3bBb-stabilizing autoantibodies by detection of C3 breakdown products [38]. It is possible that patients may be positive in some but not all of these assays, and C3Nef levels have been found occasionally also in healthy individuals [39]. Therefore, the significance of C3Nef in the pathophysiology of C3G and its correlation with disease course and treatment response is still debated and warrants further investigation [10, 40].

Symptoms

C3G is a complement-mediated disease, secondary to CAP dysregulation. Given that this dysregulation occurs in the fluid phase of blood, extra-renal features of disease are to be expected. In DDD, patients may develop acquired partial lipodystrophy (APL) [39, 41, 42] and ocular lesions similar to soft drusen seen in age-related macular degeneration (AMD) [43]. Moreover, the presence of C3 deposits has also been described in the spleen of patients with DDD [44].

Acquired partial lipodystrophy – like DDD and C3GN – is associated with dysregulation of CAP on adipocytes and becomes manifest in the loss of subcutaneous fat tissue, which typically occurs in the upper half of the body (starting from the face and extending to involve the neck, shoulders, arms and thorax) and precedes the onset of renal disease by several years. Median interval between the onset of APL and DDD is about 8 years [45]. The majority of APL patients presents with low C3 levels and are C3NeF positive. Patients with combined disease are more likely to present with decreased C3 levels and develop APL earlier in life (about 7.7 years of age) [45]. A common cause – unrestricted CAP activation – for both APL and DDD is suggested, and complement mediated destruction of adipocytes has been shown [39, 42].

Patients with DDD can also develop ocular lesions in the form of drusen. Drusen are retinal changes seen as crystalline yellow or white dots, which lie between the retinal pigment epithelium and Bruch's membrane [46]. Drusen can develop in the second decade of life and are responsible for visual disturbances in up to 10 % of DDD patients [43]. The drusen seen in DDD patients are similar to those in age-related macular degeneration (AMD), which represents the major cause of blindness in the Western aging population. In the early phase of AMD, drusen can develop without any visual problems (i.e., soft drusen), but can progress to visual loss after 65 years of age [47, 48]. Genome scan studies have linked AMD to the "regulators of complement" (RCA) gene cluster on chromosome 1q32 [49]. Moreover, recently a single-nucleotide *CFH* polymorphism (Y402H) was found to be crucial in the development of AMD [49–52]. Studies of the composition of drusen support this link by confirming the presence of CFH in drusen of AMD patients [46, 49].

Outcome and Risk of Relapse Post-transplantation

The natural history of C3G is still quite obscure, but available data do not indicate a favorable outcome. Fifty percent of DDD patients with disease for 10 years or more progress to end-stage renal disease (ESRD), with young girls having the greatest risk for renal failure [22]. Forty-five percent of renal allografts are lost within 5 years of transplant [22]. Concerning risk of relapse following renal transplantation for DDD, in one study the degree of proteinuria was strongly associated with disease recurrence, and the presence of glomerular crescents in biopsies of renal allografts had a significant negative correlation with graft survival [21]. However, a correlation with the severity of hypocomplementemia either at initial presentation or at the time of disease recurrence in the renal allograft was not found [21].

In reports evaluating C3G [27, 28], at last follow-up about 37 % of patients were on dialysis. Median time from first observation to ESRD was about 10 years, and in the patients that underwent renal transplantation, disease recurrence was observed in >50 % of cases, with an additional 17 % experiencing thrombotic microangiopathy (TMA). In the familial form of C3G secondary to CFHR5 mutations described in individuals of Cypriot descent [33] there was a significant difference in prognosis between sexes: among mutation carriers, men were by far more likely to progress to chronic kidney disease (CKD) and ESRD than women (78 % vs 22 %).

Currently, the available data on C3G are too limited to correlate findings on genetic, autoantibody, and complement function screening with prognosis or progression of disease [53]. As the number of identified cases increases, it is likely that some of these pathogenetic parameters will be found to be biomarkers of disease progression. In small case series, however, the best available predictors for disease outcome remain the standard clinical parameters, such as degree of renal dysfunction, measured by serum creatinine or estimated glomerular filtration rate (eGFR), proteinuria and blood pressure at the time of diagnosis [43]. In one series of patients with DDD, older age at diagnosis also emerged as an independent predictor of ESRD in a multivariate analysis [19]. Others have suggested that patients with C3GN may have a more benign course than patients with DDD, indicating differences in the degree or nature of CAP activation that correlate with the differences in histology [1, 12, 27]. Thus, the formal assessment of a newly diagnosed C3G must consider traditional predictors of renal outcomes, particularly when trying to gauge prognosis and evaluate the need for therapy [53].

Differential Diagnosis

The presentation of a nephritic/nephrotic clinical picture is compatible with a variety of diagnoses at disease onset (Table 25.3). The clinical picture can be indistinguishable from IgA nephropathy (IgAN), particularly if the circulating C3 is normal and macrohematuria is observed [29]. The presence of familial disease does not exclude the diagnosis of C3G, particularly but not exclusively in patients of Cypriot descent [33, 35]. Renal biopsy, in particular the immunofluorescence, allows clear discrimination between C3G and IgAN.

In the presence of reduced C3 levels, particularly in context of a recent infection, the diagnosis of acute post-infectious glomerulonephritis (PIGN) needs to be considered. In this case, a renal biopsy may not be definitive as the presence of "humps" in the EM is common to both, C3G and PIGN [54]. The latter presents with reduced circulating C3 levels, which typically normalize within 1–3 months from disease onset. As C3 levels may be normal also in C3G and given the heterogeneity of the clinical picture of this disease

Table 25.3 Diagnostic evaluation of a patient with suspected diagnosis of C3G: *non-complement aspects*

History	Family history of hematuria, proteinuria, renal failure
	Macrohematuria (if yes, concomitant to infection?)
	Infection (especially URTI) in the preceding weeks
	Reduction in urine output, frothy urine
	Symptoms of systemic disease (e.g., weight loss, fever, arthralgia, rash, petechiae)
Clinical examination	Signs of nephrotic syndrome (peripheral edema; bloodwork)
	Blood pressure
	Urine dipstick
	Ocular examination (drusen)
	Partial lipodystrophy
Laboratory work-up	Urinalysis, spot urine or 24-h PCR and ACR
	Complete blood count, urea, creatinine, protein, IgG, IgA, IgM
	Serum C3, C4
	Auto-antibodies (ANA, anti-dsDNA, ANCA)
	ASOT
	Renal ultrasound

entity, we suggest that in the case of a clinical picture common to C3G and PIGN, even with normalizing C3 levels and absent proteinuria, patients be advised to perform urinalysis e.g., every 3–6 months for 2 years following resolution of the acute clinical picture and to seek medical attention if macrohematuria or significant proteinuria (>20 mg/dl) re-appear.

Management

At present, there is no treatment standard or therapeutic agent of proven effectiveness in C3G available. The rarity of this disease, coupled with its protracted and variable natural history, make clinical trials logistically challenging. Moreover, performing a literature review has to consider the fact that with advanced pathogenetic insights the nomenclature in the field has changed, and literature specifically referring to C3G is consequently very scarce. However, considering that about

50 % of patients proceed to ESRD and may face a high risk of disease recurrence post-renal transplant, concerted efforts to define effective treatment strategies are necessary.

Searches performed on the existing literature using the terms "dense deposit disease" and "idiopathic membranoproliferative glomerulonephritis" show that randomized clinical trials are very few, and the use of different end-points make uniform interpretation of results difficult [55]. Several therapeutic regimens have been employed, utilizing immunosuppressive agents (glucocorticoids, mycophenolate mofetil, calcineurin inhibitors), anti-platelet agents, plasma exchange or infusion and, much more recently, complement blockers [56, 57]. Renoprotective agents (such as angiotensin-converting-enzyme inhibitors, ACEI, or angiotensin II receptor antagonists, ARB) are associated with these treatments almost invariably. As our understanding of the pathophysiology of C3G is rapidly expanding and changing, while reviewing published cases is reasonable, its usefulness in guiding future therapeutic strategies may be limited [10].

The therapeutic strategy should be driven by clinical parameters, such as the degree of proteinuria and impairment in renal function, and also by diagnostic test results. In the near future, the availability of new therapeutic agents may drastically alter this strategy. Clinicians need to be aware that clinical practices in this field may evolve rapidly.

In the following paragraphs regarding treatment, for all options except eculizumab the literature cited is about different forms of idiopathic or primary MPGN, including DDD.

Immunosuppressive Agents

Prednisone

There are no published trials on the use of prednisone in C3G. Existing literature pertains to primary MPGN of all subtypes. In children with primary MPGN, prednisone – specifically, long-term low-dose use of prednisone – was found to have a beneficial effect with respect to the degree of proteinuria and renal survival [58–61]. This observation was confirmed by subsequent studies, in which therapy with prolonged alternate day prednisone delayed deterioration of renal function [60, 62].

However, response of MPGN patients to corticosteroids is not homogenous. A MPGN subtype specific analysis of the effect of corticosteroid treatment revealed a lack of efficacy in patients with MPGN II/DDD, despite a beneficial effect on all MPGN patients irrespective of the MPGN subtype [60].

Altogether, in forms of C3G other than DDD, glucocorticoids may be effective, but their non-specific nature and adverse effects mean that a high price is paid for any beneficial effect on the renal lesion [63]. A reasonable approach based on current knowledge may be that of utilizing 40 mg/m^2 alternate-day prednisone for 6–12 months in patients with a C3G that presents with nephrotic-range proteinuria, with or without renal failure. If no significant reduction of proteinuria is observed, steroids should be tapered and discontinued [64]. It is important to recognize that a number of patients with C3G will not respond to this therapeutic approach [10].

Other Immunosuppressive Agents

In idiopathic MPGN patients, MMF was administered alone or in combination with corticosteroids, and generated encouraging results [65]. Another report of 13 adult patients with idiopathic MPGN resistant to glucocorticoid treatment (8 weeks at 1 mg/kg/day) showed that adding MMF led to significant reduction of proteinuria and increase of eGFR [66]. MMF in addition to pulse and long-term steroid treatment was also found effective in a pediatric patient [67]. No published reports on the effectiveness of MMF in DDD are available. In a recently published metaanalysis of 60 patients with C3GN with a median follow-up of 47 months, 22 patients were treated with a combination of corticosteroids and MMF. Compared to patients with no treatment or other immunosuppressive regimens, patients treated with corticosteroids and MMF showed the best outcome with respect to disease progression (i.e. decline in kidney function) and renal survival.

Calcineurin inhibitors (i.e., cyclosporine and tacrolimus) are also used in the treatment of MPGN. The efficacy of cyclosporine was recently tested with encouraging results in a trial involving 18 patients with refractory MPGN who also received small doses of prednisolone (0.15 mg/kg/day). Long-term reductions in proteinuria with preservation of renal function was observed in 17 of the patients [68]. In two children with idiopathic MPGN with suboptimal response to a prolonged course of steroids, rapid and complete remission of the nephrotic syndrome was achieved after initiation of tacrolimus [69].

Contradictory results are published about the efficacy of cyclosporine A in the treatment of patients with MPGN II/DDD. While Kiyomasu et al. report recovery from nephrotic syndrome using a combination of alternate-day low-dose prednisone and cyclosporine [70], a beneficial effect of calcineurin inhibitors was not seen in other patients [43].

The use of rituximab has been suggested in the presence of circulating C3NeF. However, to the best of our knowledge, while there are no published results showing this treatment to be effective, there are a few single case reports of its inefficacy [71, 72].

Altogether, limited uncontrolled data suggest that MMF or CNI may be of use in patients with C3G and high-grade proteinuria resistant to glucocorticoids and at present there is insufficient evidence to support the use of cyclophosphamide or rituximab in children with this disease [64].

Plasma Infusion or Plasma Exchange

As reviewed by Smith et al. [40] in CFH-deficient mice with C3G, renal C3 deposition and its depletion in plasma are rapidly reversed when (either mouse or human) CFH is administered [73, 74]. These data are in keeping with observations made in the first naturally occurring animal model of DDD in Norwegian pigs, in which a truncating *Cfh* mutation in SCR15 resulted in the absence of CFH from plasma [75–77]. Treatment with purified porcine or human CFH delayed onset of the DDD phenotype and progression to ESRD significantly [76, 77]. These outcomes suggest that in some C3G patients with CFH mutations, CFH replacement therapy could restore the underlying defect and correct the disease. This has been shown in two siblings with DDD secondary to a functional CFH defect in whom chronic plasma infusion prevented disease progression and development of ESRD [30, 78] as well as in a MPGN I patient with a MCP/CD46 mutation refractory to conventional treatments who also responded favorably to chronic plasma infusion [79].

Purified CFH preparations may be available for therapeutic use in the future [80, 81]. Whether administration of exogenous CFH to patients without *CFH* mutations would be therapeutically successful is unclear; however, patients with C3 mutations rendering the C3 convertase resistant to regulation by CFH, are expected to be refractory to treatment with CFH [82].

In all scenarios characterized by deficiency or functional defect of one or more complement components, replacement of this factor/these factors by either plasma infusion or plasma exchange could theoretically be effective [83]. For plasma infusion, volumes of 10–20 ml/kg/treatment (fresh frozen, solvent-detergent or cryosupernatant plasma), and treatment intervals of 14 days based on the measured CFH half life of about 6 days [84], seemed to be adequate [30, 78].

Plasma exchange allows removal of either dysfunctional endogenous complement factors, which – in addition to their functional impairment – might also compete for potential binding partners/receptors, thus possibly weakening the efficacy of plasma replacement therapy. Furthermore, plasma exchange removes antibodies like the IgG autoantibody C3NeF and CFH/CFB autoantibodies. Plasmapheresis/plasma exchange has been reported to be beneficial in MPGN I [85], and MPGN II/DDD [21, 86]. Conversely, McCaughan et al. reported an inability to establish remission in DDD despite the documented removal of C3Nef via plasmapheresis [72].

Because of discordant reports in the literature and the absence of definitive therapy, it is likely that plasma therapy will continue to be used on a case-by-case basis in C3G [10]. However, this therapy may be attempted, in the absence of response to immunosuppression, in rapidly progressive forms, particularly if defective CFH or anti-CFH autoantibodies are found.

Complement Inhibitors

Our advanced understanding of C3G pathogenesis suggests therapeutic targeting of CAP dysregulation by complement inhibition. Based on the pathophysiology of disease, anticomplement therapy warrants consideration. This could include (1) C3 convertase inhibition, which may have its greatest utility in limiting C3 breakdown product deposition on (glomerular) basement membranes; (2) C5 or terminal complement pathway inhibition [10].

While somewhat conflicting with *in vivo* observations, in *cfh,cfi* double knock out mice, which identified a critical role for uncontrolled C3 conversion in MPGN (vs. uncontrolled C5 conversion in aHUS) [87], effectiveness of anti-C5 therapy in a mouse model of DDD (*Cfh* deficient mice) [88] provided the rationale and led to the use of a humanized anti-C5 monoclonal antibody (eculizumab) in patients with different forms of C3G [71, 72, 79, 89–91].

Eculizumab is a humanized monoclonal antibody directed against C5, which blocks C5 cleavage, thus preventing the release of C5a, a potent anaphylatoxin, and C5b, the initial protein of the cytotoxic membrane attack complex (MAC; C5b-9). Its use has been recently approved for aHUS, the classic model of renal disease mediated by the CAP. Up to now its use has been reported in 11 C3G patients, including six cases of C3G affecting the native kidneys [71, 79, 89, 91] and five cases of C3G recurring in the renal graft [72, 90, 91]. The results from these studies are encouraging in 8/11 patients, in whom treatment with eculizumab led to some improvement in renal parameters (proteinuria and/or renal function and/or histology). Nonetheless, response in most cases appears to be less transformative than what has been reported so far concerning the use of eculizumab in patients with aHUS. Interestingly, an increased level of circulating SC5b-9 tended to correlate with a beneficial effect of eculizumab on the course of C3G. The other most relevant factor in predicting response to eculizumab appears to be disease duration, which was longer in non-responders. The limited available pathological data indicate that eculizumab decreased endocapillary proliferation and inflammatory cell infiltration in four out of six patients who underwent repeat kidney biopsy [89, 92]. Taken together, while encouraging, the limited data available does not allow for proposing eculizumab as standard therapy for C3G yet, and a prospective treatment trial will be needed to answer this question.

Recently, a report was published on the effectiveness of Tripterygium wilfordii (TW or triptolide), a herbal extract shown to have in vitro immunomodulatory effects and the ability to reduce renal complement expression [93], in reducing proteinuria in different degrees in eight out of ten patients with DDD [94]. The broader therapeutic use of this option, that has been employed for rheumatoid arthritis, is limited by reports of severe side effects in about half of treated patients [43].

A potential benefit of complement inhibition in the treatment of complement-mediated diseases needs to be balanced against the detrimental effect of complement inhibition in situations when complement activation is required as part of the physiological immune defense of the host, and clinical trials are required before the use of these novel substances in children can be recommended.

Renoprotective Agents

About 80 % of C3G patients are placed on ACEIs or ARBs as first line agents used to improve renal dynamics, decrease proteinuria, control blood pressure and limit glomerular leukocyte infiltration [40]. This approach is recommended as exclusive treatment in two cases:

1. Non-nephrotic proteinuria with or without microhematuria and normal renal function/absence of acute renal failure. Close follow-up is needed to assess progression of disease based on renal function, proteinuria, and urine microscopy.

2. Histological evidence of advanced chronicity of the renal lesions on the biopsy.
   Patients with advanced CKD, severe tubulointerstitial fibrosis (TIF), or other findings consistent with chronic disease sequel should – in the absence of systemic disease manifestations – not be treated with immunosuppression [64].

Treatment of Recurrence Post-renal Transplantation

There is no proven beneficial therapy for recurrent C3G in the renal allograft following transplantation. Therapeutic approaches are similar to those used in primary disease manifestation and are therefore not discussed in detail here.

Reported treatment of *recurrent idiopathic MPGN*, besides conservative medications, include antiplatelet/anticoagulant agents [95], corticosteroids [96], cyclosporine [97], cyclophosphamide [98], and plasmapheresis [96, 99]. Reported treatments of *recurrent DDD* include dose reduction, discontinuation or switch (cyclosporine to tacrolimus) of the CNI used as part of the posttransplant immunosuppression regimen, modification of the prednisone dose (increase; switch from daily to alternate-day), pulse methylprednisolone, or plasmapheresis/plasma exchange [21, 86].

In summary, the therapeutic options in C3G depend on the level of proteinuria and kidney failure and on the results of the diagnostic tests performed. In the vast majority of patients, the empiric use of ACEI or ARB as drugs of first choice to treat hypertension and decrease proteinuria is a common practice, which may delay the progression of renal disease [63]. Plasma therapy or, in the future, purified CFH may be useful in some cases in which there is clear evidence of a CFH deficiency or of the presence of anti-CFH autoantibodies. There is little evidence of the effectiveness of immunosuppression, which should therefore be employed only in cases where disease is very active and proliferative with intense inflammation in the renal biopsy and nephrotic-range proteinuria. Preliminary results on the use of complement blockers such as eculizumab are encouraging in some but not in all patients.

References

1. Sethi S, Fervenza FC. Membranoproliferative glomerulonephritis: a new look at an old entity. N Engl J Med. 2012;366:1119–31.
2. Sethi S. Etiology-based diagnostic approach to proliferative glomerulonephritis. Am J Kidney Dis. 2014;63:561–6.
3. Nasr SH, Satoskar A, Markowitz GS, Valeri AM, Appel GB, Stokes MB, Nadasdy T, D'Agati VD. Proliferative glomerulonephritis with monoclonal IgG deposits. J Am Soc Nephrol. 2009;20: 2055–64.
4. Sethi S, Zand L, Leung N, Smith RJH, Jevremonic D, Herrmann SS, Fervenza FC. Membranoproliferative glomerulonephritis secondary to monoclonal gammopathy. Clin J Am Soc Nephrol. 2010;5:770–82.
5. Sethi S, Rajkumar SV. Monoclonal gammopathy – associated proliferative glomerulonephritis. Mayo Clin Proc. 2013;88:1284–93.
6. Zand L, Lorenz EC, Cosio FG, Fervenza FC, Nasr SH, Gandhi MJ, Smith RJ, Sethi S. Clinical findings, pathology, and outcomes of C3GN after kidney transplantation. J Am Soc Nephrol. 2014;25(5):1110–7.
7. Rennke HG. Secondary membranoproliferative glomerulonephritis. Kidney Int. 1995;47:643–56.
8. Weening JJ, D'Agati VD, Schwartz MM, Seshan SV, Alpers CE, Appel GB, Balow JE, Bruijn JA, Cook T, Ferrario F, Fogo AB, Ginzler EM, Hebert L, Hill G, Hill P, Jennette JC, Kong NC, Lesavre P, Lockshin M, Looi L-M, Makino H, Moura LA, Nagata M. The classification of glomerulonephritis in systemic lupus erythematosus revisited. J Am Soc Nephrol. 2004;15:241–50.
9. Zand L, Fervenza FC, Nasr SH, Sethi S. Membranoproliferative glomerulonephritis associated with autoimmune diseases. J Nephrol. 2014;27(2):165–71.
10. Pickering MC, D'Agati VD, Nester CM, Smith RJ, Haas M, Appel GB, Alpers CE, Bajema IM, Bedrosian C, Braun M, Doyle M, Fakhouri F, Fervenza FC, Fogo AB, Fremeaux-Bacchi V, Gale DP, Goicoechea de Jorge E, Griffin G, Harris CL, Holers VM, Johnson S, Lavin PJ, Medjeral-Thomas N, Paul Morgan B, Nast CC, Noel L-H, Peters DK, Rodriguez de Cordoba S, Servais A, Sethi S, Song W-C, Tamburini P, Thurman JM, Zavros M, Cook HT. C3 glomerulopathy: consensus report. Kidney Int. 2013;84(6):1079–89.
11. Sethi S, Fervenza FC. Membranoproliferative glomerulonephritis: pathogenetic heterogeneity and proposal for a new classification. Semin Nephrol. 2011;31:341–8.
12. Sethi S, Nester CM, Smith RJH. Membranoproliferative glomerulonephritis and C3 glomerulopathy: resolving the confusion. Kidney Int. 2012;81:434–41.
13. Servais A, Noel L, Fremeaux-Bacch IV, Lesavre P. C3 glomerulopathy. Contrib Nephrol. 2013;181:185–93.
14. Fakhouri F, Fremeaux-Bacchi V, Noel L-H, Cook HT, Pickering MC. C3 glomerulopathy: a new classification. Nat Rev Nephrol. 2010;6:494–9.
15. Fervenza FC, Smith RJH, Sethi S. Association of a novel complement factor H mutation with severe crescentic and necrotizing glomerulonephritis. Am J Kidney Dis. 2012;60:126–32.
16. Sethi S, Vrana JA, Theis JD, Dogan A. Mass spectrometry based proteomics in the diagnosis of kidney disease. Curr Opin Nephrol Hypertens. 2013;22:273–80.
17. Sethi S, Gamez JD, Vrana JA, Theis JD, Bergen III HR, Zipfel PF, Dogan A, Smith RJH. Glomeruli of dense deposit disease contain components of the alternative and terminal complement pathway. Kidney Int. 2009;75:952–60.
18. Sethi S, Fervenza FC, Zhang Y, Zand L, Meyer NC, Borsa N, Nasr SH, Smith RJH. Atypical postinfectious glomerulonephritis is associated with abnormalities in the alternative pathway of complement. Kidney Int. 2013;83:293–9.
19. Nasr SH, Valeri AM, Appel GB, Sherwinter J, Stokes MB, Said SM, Markowitz GS, D'Agati VD. Dense deposit disease: clinicopathologic study of 32 pediatric and adult patients. Clin J Am Soc Nephrol. 2009;4:22–32.
20. Andresdottir MB, Assmann KJ, Hoitsma AJ, Koene RA, Wetzels JF. Renal transplantation in patients with dense deposit disease: morphological characteristics of recurrent disease and clinical outcome. Nephrol Dial Transplant. 1999;14:1723–31.
21. Braun MC, Stablein DM, Hamiwka LA, Bell L, Bartosh SM, Strife CF. Recurrence of membranoproliferative glomerulonephritis type II in renal allografts: the North American Pediatric Renal Transplant Cooperative Study experience. J Am Soc Nephrol. 2005;16:2225–33.
22. Lu D-F, Moon M, Lanning L, McCarthy A, Smith RH. Clinical features and outcomes of 98 children and adults with dense deposit disease. Pediatr Nephrol. 2012;27:773–81.
23. Lorenz EC, Sethi S, Leung N, Dispenzieri A, Fervenza FC, Cosio FG. Recurrent membranoproliferative glomerulonephritis after kidney transplantation. Kidney Int. 2010;77:721–8.
24. Schwertz R, Rother U, Anders D, Gretz N, Scharer K, Kirschfink M. Complement analysis in children with idiopathic membranoproliferative glomerulonephritis: a long-term follow-up. Pediatr Allergy Immunol. 2001;12:166–72.
25. Schwertz R, de Jong R, Gretz N, Kirschfink M, Anders D, Scharer K. Outcome of idiopathic membranoproliferative glomerulonephritis in children. Arbeitsgemeinschaft Padiatrische Nephrologie. Acta Paediatr. 1996;85:308–12.
26. Servais A, Noel LH, Dragon-Durey MA, Gubler MC, Remy P, Buob D, Cordonnier C, Makdassi R, Jaber W, Boulanger E, Lesavre P, Fremeaux-Bacchi V. Heterogeneous pattern of renal disease associated

with homozygous factor H deficiency. Hum Pathol. 2001;42:1305–11.

27. Servais A, Noel LH, Roumenina LT, Le Quintrec M, Ngo S, Dragon-Durey MA, Macher MA, Zuber J, Karras A, Provot F, Moulin B, Grunfeld JP, Niaudet P, Lesavre P, Fremeaux-Bacchi V. Acquired and genetic complement abnormalities play a critical role in dense deposit disease and other C3 glomerulopathies. Kidney Int. 2012;82:454–64.

28. Servais A, Fremeaux-Bacchi V, Lequintrec M, Salomon R, Blouin J, Knebelmann B, Grunfeld JP, Lesavre P, Noel LH, Fakhouri F. Primary glomerulonephritis with isolated C3 deposits: a new entity which shares common genetic risk factors with haemolytic uraemic syndrome. J Med Genet. 2007;44:193–9.

29. Karumanchi SA, Thadhani R. A complement to kidney disease: CFHR5 nephropathy. Lancet. 2010;376:748–50.

30. Habbig S, Mihatsch MJ, Heinen S, Beck B, Emmel M, Skerka C, Kirschfink M, Hoppe B, Zipfel PF, Licht C. C3 deposition glomerulopathy due to a functional factor H defect. Kidney Int. 2009;75:1230–4.

31. Jokiranta TS, Solomon A, Pangburn MK, Zipfel PF, Meri S. Nephritogenic lambda light chain dimer: a unique human miniautoantibody against complement factor H. J Immunol. 1999;163:4590–6.

32. Strobel S, Zimmering M, Papp K, Prechl J, Jozsi M. Anti-factor B autoantibody in dense deposit disease. Mol Immunol. 2010;47:1476–83.

33. Gale DP, de Jorge EG, Cook HT, Martinez-Barricarte R, Hadjisavvas A, McLean AG, Pusey CD, Pierides A, Kyriacou K, Athanasiou Y, Voskarides K, Deltas C, Palmer A, Fremeaux-Bacchi V, de Cordoba SR, Maxwell PH, Pickering MC. Identification of a mutation in complement factor H-related protein 5 in patients of Cypriot origin with glomerulonephritis. Lancet. 2010;376:794–801.

34. Medjeral-Thomas N, Malik TH, Patel MP, Toth T, Cook HT, Tomson C, Pickering MC. A novel CFHR5 fusion protein causes C3 glomerulopathy in a family without Cypriot ancestry. Kidney Int. 2014;85:933–7.

35. Malik TH, Lavin PJ, Goicoechea de Jorge E, Vernon KA, Rose KL, Patel MP, de Leeuw M, Neary JJ, Conlon PJ, Winn MP, Pickering MC. A hybrid CFHR3-1 gene causes familial C3 glomerulopathy. J Am Soc Nephrol. 2012;23:1155–60.

36. West CD, Bissler JJ. Nephritic factor and recurrence in the renal transplant of membranoproliferative glomerulonephritis type II. Pediatr Nephrol. 2008;23:1867–76.

37. Paixao-Cavalcante D, Lopez-Trascasa M, Skattum L, Giclas PC, Goodship TH, de Cordoba SR, Truedsson L, Morgan BP, Harris CL. Sensitive and specific assays for C3 nephritic factors clarify mechanisms underlying complement dysregulation. Kidney Int. 2012;82:1084–92.

38. Zhang Y, Meyer NC, Wang K, Nishimura C, Frees K, Jones M, Katz LM, Sethi S, Smith RJ. Causes of alternative pathway dysregulation in dense deposit disease. Clin J Am Soc Nephrol. 2012;7:265–74.

39. Mathieson PW, Wurzner R, Oliveria DB, Lachmann PJ, Peters DK. Complement-mediated adipocyte lysis by nephritic factor sera. J Exp Med. 1993;177:1827–31.

40. Smith RJ, Harris CL, Pickering MC. Dense deposit disease. Mol Immunol. 2011;48:1604–10.

41. Meri S. Loss of self-control in the complement system and innate autoreactivity. Ann N Y Acad Sci. 2007;1109:93–105.

42. Mathieson PW, Peters DK. Lipodystrophy in MCGN type II: the clue to links between the adipocyte and the complement system. Nephrol Dial Transplant. 1997;12:1804–6.

43. Appel GB, Cook HT, Hageman G, Jennette JC, Kashgarian M, Kirschfink M, Lambris JD, Lanning L, Lutz HU, Meri S, Rose NR, Salant DJ, Sethi S, Smith RJ, Smoyer W, Tully HF, Tully SP, Walker P, Welsh M, Wurzner R, Zipfel PF. Membranoproliferative glomerulonephritis type II (dense deposit disease): an update. J Am Soc Nephrol. 2005;6:1392–403.

44. Thorner P, Baumal R. Extraglomerular dense deposits in dense deposit disease. Arch Pathol Lab Med. 1982;106:628–31.

45. Misra A, Peethambaram A, Garg A. Clinical features and metabolic and autoimmune derangements in acquired partial lipodystrophy: report of 35 cases and review of the literature. Medicine (Baltimore). 2004;83:18–34.

46. de Jong PT. Age-related macular degeneration. N Engl J Med. 2006;355:1474–85.

47. Hogg RE, Chakravarthy U. Visual function and dysfunction in early and late age-related maculopathy. Prog Retin Eye Res. 2006;25:249–76.

48. Magnusson KP, Duan S, Sigurdsson H, Petursson H, Yang Z, Zhao Y, Bernstein PS, Ge J, Jonasson F, Stefansson E, Helgadottir G, Zabriskie NA, Jonsson T, Bjornsson A, Thorlacius T, Jonsson PV, Thorleifsson G, Kong A, Stefansson H, Zhang K, Stefansson K, Gulcher JR. CFH Y402H confers similar risk of soft drusen and both forms of advanced AMD. PLoS Med. 2006;3:e5.

49. Hageman GS, Anderson DH, Johnson LV, Hancox LS, Taiber AJ, Hardisty LI, Hageman JL, Stockman HA, Borchardt JD, Gehrs KM, Smith RJ, Silvestri G, Russell SR, Klaver CC, Barbazetto I, Chang S, Yannuzzi LA, Barile GR, Merriam JC, Smith RT, Olsh AK, Bergeron J, Zernant J, Merriam JE, Gold B, Dean M, Allikmets R. A common haplotype in the complement regulatory gene factor H (HF1/CFH) predisposes individuals to age-related macular degeneration. Proc Natl Acad Sci U S A. 2005;102:7227–32.

50. Edwards AO, Ritter 3rd R, Abel KJ, Manning A, Panhuysen C, Farrer LA. Complement factor H polymorphism and age-related macular degeneration. Science. 2005;308:421–4.

51. Haines JL, Hauser MA, Schmidt S, Scott WK, Olson LM, Gallins P, Spencer KL, Kwan SY, Noureddine M, Gilbert JR, Schnetz-Boutaud N, Agarwal A, Postel

EA, Pericak-Vance MA. Complement factor H variant increases the risk of age-related macular degeneration. Science. 2005;308:419–21.

52. Klein RJ, Zeiss C, Chew EY, Tsai JY, Sackler RS, Haynes C, Henning AK, SanGiovanni JP, Mane SM, Mayne ST, Bracken MB, Ferris FL, Ott J, Barnstable C, Hoh J. Complement factor H polymorphism in age-related macular degeneration. Science. 2005;308:385–9.

53. Bomback AS, Appel GB. Pathogenesis of the C3 glomerulopathies and reclassification of MPGN. Nat Rev Nephrol. 2012;8:634–42.

54. Sethi S, Fervenza FC, Zhang Y, Zand L, Vrana JA, Nasr SH, Theis JD, Dogan A, Smith RJ. C3 glomerulonephritis: clinicopathological findings, complement abnormalities, glomerular proteomic profile, treatment, and follow-up. Kidney Int. 2012;82:465–73.

55. Noris M, Remuzzi G. Translational mini-review series on complement factor H: therapies of renal diseases associated with complement factor H abnormalities: atypical haemolytic uraemic syndrome and membranoproliferative glomerulonephritis. Clin Exp Immunol. 2008;151:199–209.

56. Nester CM, Smith RJ. Diagnosis and treatment of C3 glomerulopathy. Clin Nephrol. 2013;80:395–403.

57. Nester CM, Smith RJ. Treatment options for C3 glomerulopathy. Curr Opin Nephrol Hypertens. 2013;22: 231–7.

58. McEnery PT. Membranoproliferative glomerulonephritis: the Cincinnati experience – cumulative renal survival from 1957 to 1989. J Pediatr. 1990;116:S109–14.

59. West CD. Childhood membranoproliferative glomerulonephritis: an approach to management. Kidney Int. 1986;29:1077–93.

60. Tarshish P, Bernstein J, Tobin JN, Edelmann Jr CM. Treatment of mesangiocapillary glomerulonephritis with alternate-day prednisone – a report of the International Study of Kidney Disease in Children. Pediatr Nephrol. 1992;6:123–30.

61. Ford DM, Briscoe DM, Shanley PF, Lum GM. Childhood membranoproliferative glomerulonephritis type I: limited steroid therapy. Kidney Int. 1992;41:1606–12.

62. Yanagihara T, Hayakawa M, Yoshida J, Tsuchiya M, Morita T, Murakami M, Fukunaga Y. Long-term follow-up of diffuse membranoproliferative glomerulonephritis type I. Pediatr Nephrol. 2005;20:585–90.

63. Alchi B, Jayne D. Membranoproliferative glomerulonephritis. Pediatr Nephrol. 2010;25:1409–18.

64. Beck L, Bomback AS, Choi MJ, Holzman LB, Langford C, Mariani LH, Somers MJ, Trachtman H, Waldman M. KDOQI US commentary on the 2012 KDIGO clinical practice guideline for glomerulonephritis. Am J Kidney Dis. 2013;62:403–41.

65. Jones G, Juszczak M, Kingdon E, Harber M, Sweny P, Burns A. Treatment of idiopathic membranoproliferative glomerulonephritis with mycophenolate mofetil and steroids. Nephrol Dial Transplant. 2004;19:3160–4.

66. Yuan M, Zou J, Zhang X, Liu H, Teng J, Zhong Y, Ding X. Combination therapy with mycophenolate mofetil and prednisone in steroid-resistant idiopathic membranoproliferative glomerulonephritis. Clin Nephrol. 2010;73:354–9.

67. De S, Al-Nabhani D, Thorner P, Cattran D, Piscione TD, Licht C. Remission of resistant MPGN type I with mycophenolate mofetil and steroids. Pediatr Nephrol. 2009;24:597–600.

68. Bagheri N, Nemati E, Rahbar K, Nobakht A, Einollahi B, Taheri S. Cyclosporine in the treatment of membranoproliferative glomerulonephritis. Arch Iran Med. 2008;11:26–9.

69. Haddad M, Lau K, Butani L. Remission of membranoproliferative glomerulonephritis type I with the use of tacrolimus. Pediatr Nephrol. 2007;22:1787–91.

70. Kiyomasu T, Shibata M, Kurosu H, Shiraishi K, Hashimoto H, Hayashidera T, Akiyama Y, Takeda N. Cyclosporin A treatment for membranoproliferative glomerulonephritis type II. Nephron. 2002;91:509–11.

71. Daina E, Noris M, Remuzzi G. Eculizumab in a patient with dense-deposit disease. N Engl J Med. 2012;366:1161–3.

72. McCaughan JA, O'Rourke DM, Courtney AE. Recurrent dense deposit disease after renal transplantation: an emerging role for complementary therapies. Am J Transplant. 2012;12:1046–51.

73. Fakhouri F, de Jorge EG, Brune F, Azam P, Cook HT, Pickering MC. Treatment with human complement factor H rapidly reverses renal complement deposition in factor H-deficient mice. Kidney Int. 2010;78: 279–86.

74. Paixao-Cavalcante D, Hanson S, Botto M, Cook HT, Pickering MC. Factor H facilitates the clearance of GBM bound iC3b by controlling C3 activation in fluid phase. Mol Immunol. 2009;46:1942–50.

75. Hegasy GA, Manuelian T, Hogasen K, Jansen JH, Zipfel PF. The molecular basis for hereditary porcine membranoproliferative glomerulonephritis type II: point mutations in the factor H coding sequence block protein secretion. Am J Pathol. 2002;161:2027–34.

76. Jansen JH, Hogasen K, Grondahl AM. Porcine membranoproliferative glomerulonephritis type II: an autosomal recessive deficiency of factor H. Vet Rec. 1995;137:240–4.

77. Hogasen K, Jansen JH, Mollnes TE, Hovdenes J, Harboe M. Hereditary porcine membranoproliferative glomerulonephritis type II is caused by factor H deficiency. J Clin Invest. 1995;95:1054–61.

78. Licht C, Heinen S, Jozsi M, Loschmann I, Saunders RE, Perkins SJ, Waldherr R, Skerka C, Kirschfink M, Hoppe B, Zipfel PF. Deletion of Lys224 in regulatory domain 4 of Factor H reveals a novel pathomechanism for dense deposit disease (MPGN II). Kidney Int. 2006;70:42–50.

79. Radhakrishnan S, Lunn A, Kirschfink M, Thorner P, Hebert D, Langlois V, Pluthero F, Licht C. Eculizumab and refractory membranoproliferative glomerulonephritis. N Engl J Med. 2012;366:1165–6.

80. Buttner-Mainik A, Parsons J, Jerome H, Hartmann A, Lamer S, Schaaf A, Schlosser A, Zipfel PF, Reski R, Decker EL. Production of biologically active recom-

binant human factor H in Physcomitrella. Plant Biotechnol J. 2011;9:373–83.

81. Schmidt CQ, Slingsby FC, Richards A, Barlow PN. Production of biologically active complement factor H in therapeutically useful quantities. Protein Expr Purif. 2011;76:254–63.

82. Martinez-Barricarte R, Heurich M, Valdes-Canedo F, Vazquez-Martul E, Torreira E, Montes T, Tortajada A, Pinto S, Lopez-Trascasa M, Morgan BP, Llorca O, Harris CL, Rodriguez de Cordoba S. Human C3 mutation reveals a mechanism of dense deposit disease pathogenesis and provides insights into complement activation and regulation. J Clin Invest. 2010;120:3702–12.

83. Licht C, Schlotzer-Schrehardt U, Kirschfink M, Zipfel PF, Hoppe B. MPGN II – genetically determined by defective complement regulation? Pediatr Nephrol. 2007;22:2–9.

84. Licht C, Weyersberg A, Heinen S, Stapenhorst L, Devenge J, Beck B, Waldherr R, Kirschfink M, Zipfel PF, Hoppe B. Successful plasma therapy for atypical hemolytic uremic syndrome caused by factor H deficiency owing to a novel mutation in the complement cofactor protein domain 15. Am J Kidney Dis. 2005; 45:415–21.

85. McGinley E, Watkins R, McLay A, Boulton-Jones JM. Plasma exchange in the treatment of mesangiocapillary glomerulonephritis. Nephron. 1985;40:385–90.

86. Oberkircher OR, Enama M, West JC, Campbell P, Moran J. Regression of recurrent membranoproliferative glomerulonephritis type II in a transplanted kidney after plasmapheresis therapy. Transplant Proc. 1988;20:418–23.

87. Rose KL, Paixao-Cavalcante D, Fish J, Manderson AP, Malik TH, Bygrave AE, Lin T, Sacks SH, Walport MJ, Cook HT, Botto M, Pickering MC. Factor I is required for the development of membranoproliferative glomerulonephritis in factor H-deficient mice. J Clin Invest. 2008;118:608–18.

88. Pickering MC, Warren J, Rose KL, Carlucci F, Wang Y, Walport MJ, Cook HT, Botto M. Prevention of C5 activation ameliorates spontaneous and experimental glomerulonephritis in factor H-deficient mice. Proc Natl Acad Sci U S A. 2006;103: 9649–54.

89. Vivarelli M, Pasini A, Emma F. Eculizumab for the treatment of dense-deposit disease. N Engl J Med. 2012;366:1163–5.

90. Gurkan S, Fyfe B, Weiss L, Xiao X, Zhang Y, Smith RJ. Eculizumab and recurrent C3 glomerulonephritis. Pediatr Nephrol. 2013;28:1975–81.

91. Bomback AS, Smith RJ, Barile GR, Zhang Y, Heher EC, Herlitz L, Stokes MB, Markowitz GS, D'Agati VD, Canetta PA, Radhakrishnan J, Appel GB. Eculizumab for dense deposit disease and C3 glomerulonephritis. Clin J Am Soc Nephrol. 2012;7: 748–56.

92. Herlitz LC, Bomback AS, Markowitz GS, Stokes MB, Smith RN, Colvin RB, Appel GB, D'Agati VD. Pathology after eculizumab in dense deposit disease and C3 GN. J Am Soc Nephrol. 2012;23:1229–37.

93. Hong Y, Zhou W, Li K, Sacks SH. Triptolide is a potent suppressant of C3, CD40 and B7h expression in activated human proximal tubular epithelial cells. Kidney Int. 2002;62:1291–300.

94. Wang J, Tang Z, Luo C, Hu Y, Zeng C, Chen H, Liu Z. Clinical and pathological features of dense deposit disease in Chinese patients. Clin Nephrol. 2012;78: 207–15.

95. Glicklich D, Matas AJ, Sablay LB, Senitzer D, Tellis VA, Soberman R, Veith FJ. Recurrent membranoproliferative glomerulonephritis type 1 in successive renal transplants. Am J Nephrol. 1987;7:143–9.

96. Saxena R, Frankel WL, Sedmak DD, Falkenhain ME, Cosio FG. Recurrent type I membranoproliferative glomerulonephritis in a renal allograft: successful treatment with plasmapheresis. Am J Kidney Dis. 2000;35:749–52.

97. Tomlanovich S, Vincenti F, Amend W, Biava C, Melzer J, Feduska N, Salvatierra O. Is cyclosporine effective in preventing recurrence of immune-mediated glomerular disease after renal transplantation? Transplant Proc. 1988;20:285–8.

98. Lien YH, Scott K. Long-term cyclophosphamide treatment for recurrent type I membranoproliferative glomerulonephritis after transplantation. Am J Kidney Dis. 2000;35:539–43.

99. Muczynski KA. Plasmapheresis maintained renal function in an allograft with recurrent membranoproliferative glomerulonephritis type I. Am J Nephrol. 1995;15:446–9.

Part VI

The Kidney and Systemic Disease

Postinfectious Hemolytic Uremic Syndrome

26

Martin Bitzan and Anne-Laure Lapeyraque

Abbreviations

A/E	Attaching and effacing
ACE(i)	Angiotensin converting enzyme (inhibitor)
ADAMTS13	A disintegrin and metalloprotease with a thrombospondin type 1 motif, member 13
ADC	Apparent diffusion coefficient
aHUS	Atypical hemolytic uremic syndrome
AIDS	Acquired immunodeficiency syndrome
AKI	Acute kidney injury
ALT	Alanine amino transferase
AP	Alternative pathway (of complement)
ARDS	Acute respiratory distress syndrome
Bcl-2	B-cell lymphoma protein-2
BP	Blood pressure
C1q	Complement factor 1q
C3	Complement factor 3
C4	Complement factor 4
C5	Complement factor 5
CBC	Complete blood cell (count)
CDC	Centers for Disease Control and Prevention
CFB	Complement factor B
CFH	Complement Factor H
CFHL-1	Complement factor H-like 1
CFHR-1	Complement factor H-related protein 1
CI	Confidence interval
CKD	Chronic kidney disease
CNS	Central nervous system
CPKDRC	Canadian Pediatric Kidney Disease Research Centre
CrI	Credible interval
CRP	C-reactive protein
CRRT	Continuous renal replacement therapy
DAF	Decay-accelerating factor
DGKE	Diacylglycerol kinase-epsilon
DIC	Disseminated intravascular coagulation
DNA	Deoxyribonucleic acid
DWI	Diffusion-weighted images
EAEC	Enteroaggregative *E. coli*
eGFR	Estimated glomerular filtration rate

M. Bitzan (✉)
Division of Nehprology, Montreal Children's Hospital, 1001, Boulevard Decarie, Room B RC.6651, Montreal H4A 3JI, Canada
e-mail: martin.bitzan@mcgill.ca

A.-L. Lapeyraque
Division of Nephrology, Hopital Sainte Justine, 3175 Cote Sainte Catherine, Montreal H4A 3M7, Canada
e-mail: anne.laure.lapeyraque@umontreal.ca

© Springer-Verlag Berlin Heidelberg 2016
D.F. Geary, F. Schaefer (eds.), *Pediatric Kidney Disease*, DOI 10.1007/978-3-662-52972-0_26

EHEC	Enterohemorrhagic *Escherichia coli*	NA	Neuraminidase
eHUS	Enteropathogen (or *Escherichia coli*) induced hemolytic uremic syndrome	NanA	Neuraminidase A
		NM	Non-motile
		NSAID(s)	Non-steroidal anti-inflammatory drug(s)
EhxA	Enterohemolysin	NYED	Not yet etiologically defined
ELISA	Enzyme-linked immunosorbent assay	OR	Odds ratio
		PAI-1	Plasminogen activator inhibitor type 1
EPEC	Enteropathogenic *Escherichia coli*	PCR	Polymerase chain reaction
ER	Endoplasmic reticulum	PD	Peritoneal dialysis
ESA	Erythropoiesis-stimulating agent	PE	Plasma exchange
Esp	Extracellular serine proteases	PEITC	Phenethyl isothiocyanate
ESRD	End stage renal disease	PI	Plasma infusion
FDA	Federal Drug Agency	pnHUS	Pneumococcal (*Streptococcus pneumoniae*) hemolytic uremic syndrome
FLAIR	Fluid-attenuated inversion recovery		
Gb3	Globotriaosylceramide	PO	Per oral
Gb4	Globotetraosylceramide	PRBC	Packed red blood cell(s)
GI	Gastrointestinal	PRES	Posterior reversible leukoencephalopathy syndrome
Hb	Hemoglobin		
HC	Hemorrhagic colitis	PSGL-1	P-selectin soluble ligand 1
HD	Hemodialysis	PT	Prothrombin time
HLA	Human leukocyte antigen	PTT	Partial thromboplastin time
HUS	Hemolytic uremic syndrome	RAS	Renin-angiotensin system
IA	Immunoabsorption	RBC	Red blood cell(s)
Iha	Iron-regulated gene A (IrgA) homolog adhesin	RNA	Ribonucleic acid
		RRT	Renal replacement therapy
iHUS	Influenza-induced hemolytic uremic syndrome	rTM	Recombinant thrombomodulin
		Saa	STEC autoagglutinating adhesin
IPD	Invasive pneumococcal disease	SC5b-9	Serum (soluble complement factor) C5b to 9 complex (see TCC)
IQR	Interquartile range		
IrgA	Iron-regulated gene A	SCR	Short consensus repeat(s)
IV	Intravenous	sCR1	Soluble complement receptor 1
JNK	c-Jun N-terminal kinase	SD1	*Shigella dysenteriae* type 1
KatP	Catalase/peroxidase	SLT	Shiga-like toxin
LDH	Lactate dehydrogenase	SMAC	Sorbitol MacConkey (agar)
LEE	Locus of enterocyte effacement	SMX/TMP	Sulfamethoxazole/trimethoprim
LPS	Lipopolysaccharide	STEC	Shiga toxin producing *Escherichia coli*
MAHA	Microangiopathic hemolytic anemia		
		STPB	Shiga toxin producing bacteria
MAP(K)	Mitogen-activated protein (kinase)	Stx	Shiga toxin
MCP	Membrane cofactor protein	SubA	Subtilase A
MIC	Minimal inhibitory concentration	T3SS	Type III secretion system
MMACHC	Methylmalonic aciduria and homocystinuria, cblC type (gene)	TCC	Terminal complement complex
		TF	Thomsen-Friedenreich (antigen)
MRI	Magnetic resonance imaging	*THBD*	Thrombomodulin (gene)
mRNA	Messenger ribonucleic acid	Tir	Translocated intimin receptor

TM	Thrombomodulin
TMA	Thrombotic microangiopathy
TNF-α	Tumor necrosis factor alpha
TTP	Thrombotic thrombocytopenic purpura
UK	United Kingdom
US	United States (of America)
USS	Upshaw Shulman syndrome
UTI	Urinary tract infection
VEGF	Vascular endothelial growth factor
VT	Vero(cyto)toxin
VTEC	Vero(cyto)toxin producing *Escherichia coli*
WBC	White blood cell

Introduction

For the purpose of this section, we define postinfectious hemolytic uremic syndrome as HUS [1] caused by specific infectious organisms in patients with no identifiable HUS-associated genetic mutation or autoantibody. Major triggers of postinfectious HUS are Shiga toxin (Stx) producing bacteria (STPB, mainly *Escherichia coli* and *Shigella dysenteriae* type 1) [2, 3] and neuraminidase (NA) producing organisms (mainly *Streptococcus pneumoniae*) [4, 5]. Stx and NA are thought to injure vascular endothelial and perhaps circulating red blood cells and platelets leading to thrombotic microangiopathy with intravascular hemolysis (TMA). In children, more than 80 % of cases of HUS are due to STEC infection. This contrasts with HUS causally linked to the deficiency of proteins that regulate the alternative pathway of complement, either due to genetic mutations or the presence of autoantibodies (mainly to complement factor H), or to other genetic and metabolic causes (Box 26.1). However, HUS can arise following infection by a "specific" agent in a patient with a complement defect; the "atypical" nature of such HUS is usually uncovered by its atypical presentation (relapsing course, recurrence after transplantation or family history).

Box 26.1 Classification of HUS/TMA and TTP

1. Infection-induced HUS (caused by endothelial injury due to specific infectious agents)

   (a) Shiga toxin-producing bacteria (STPB)

      (i) Shiga toxin-producing / enterohemorrhagic *Escherichia coli* (STEC/EHEC)

      (ii) *Shigella dysenteriae* type 1

      (iii) *Citrobacter freundii* and others

   (b) Neuraminidase-producing bacteria

      (i) *Streptococcus pneumoniae*

      (ii) *Clostridium perfringens* and others

   (c) Influenza A virus (A/H3N2, A/H1N1)[a]

   (d) Human immunodeficiency virus (HIV)[b]

2. Hereditary/genetic forms of HUS

   (a) HUS associated with mutations of regulatory proteins and components of the complement and coagulation pathways[c]

      (i) Soluble regulator deficiencies (examples: CFH, CFI etc.)

      (ii) Membrane-bound regulator deficiencies (examples: MCP)

      (iii) Thrombomodulin, plasminogen[d]

   (b) Genetic abnormalities without known complement dysregulation, usually autosomal recessive (examples: defective cobalamin metabolism due to mutations in *MMACHC* [methylmalonic aciduria and homocystinuria, cblC type]; mutation of *DGKE* [diacylglycerol kinase-epsilon])[e]

3. Autoimmune HUS

   (a) Autoantibodies against complement regulatory proteins (example: anti-CFH antibody)

4. Thrombotic thrombocytopenic purpura (TTP)

   (a) Hereditary TTP (Upshaw Shulman Syndrome [USS], autosomal recessive mutation of *ADAMS13*)

   (b) Autoimmune TTP (due to anti-ADAMS13 antibody)

5. NYED (not yet etiologically defined)

   (a) Spontaneous forms without known co-morbidities

   (b) "Secondary forms" (examples: HUS associated with bone marrow transplantation,[f] anti-phospholipid syndrome, malignant hypertension etc.

(c) HUS caused by endotheliotoxic therapeutics (examples: cancer drugs, endotheliotropic antibodies, such as anti-VEGF)

[a]While influenza virus expresses neuraminidase (NA), its causal role in HUS has yet to be proven
[b]The mechanism underlying HIV HUS is not clear; the majority of patients appear to present HUS-like features [6–8]
[c]Forms involving unregulated alternative pathway of complement activation are differentiated from others for therapeutic purposes; combinations of various factor mutations and/or autoantibodies exist
[d]For details, see [9]
[e]A recent publication implicates cases with DGKE mutation that demonstrate complement consumption [10]
[f]Combination with genetic complement regulator mutations have been described [11]

The historical terms diarrhea-positive (D[+]) and diarrhea-negative (D[−]) HUS, introduced to distinguish STEC-induced HUS from "atypical" forms, should be abandoned since at least one third of patients with complement-mediated "atypical" HUS present with diarrhea or even colitis [12]. The D[+]/D[−] dichotomy fails to differentiate postinfectious forms, such as *S. pneumonia* HUS, from "atypical" HUS, and could delay the necessary workup and potentially deprive patients of effective treatment. An etiology-based classification is preferred.

Finally, there is emerging evidence of (transient) complement activation in post-infectious forms of HUS in the absence of a demonstrable genetic defect or anti-CFH autoantibodies. The precise mechanism of complement activation and its pathological significance are presently under investigation. With the evolving understanding of the complement system and of the pathogenesis of different forms of HUS, some of the descriptions and assumptions in this chapter will have to be revised in the future [12–15].

Shigatoxin Producing *Escherichia coli*-HUS

History of HUS and Definitions

The term "hemolytic uremic syndromes" was first used in 1955 by the Swiss hematologist Dr. C. Gasser, who described five children presenting with the triad of acute hemolytic anemia, thrombocytopenia and renal failure [1]. The largest early series of patients with HUS originated from Argentina, the country with the highest incidence of HUS [16].

It was not until 1983 when two major discoveries led to the recognition of a specific microbial etiology as the predominant cause of HUS in children: Dr. Karmali and his group from the Hospital for Sick Children in Toronto, Canada reported the isolation of *Escherichia coli* strains from children with "idiopathic" (typical) HUS that produced a filterable agent that was toxic to cultured Vero (African Green Monkey kidney) cells (verocytotoxin or VT) [2, 17]. VT detected in the stools of children with HUS (free fecal VT) and lysates from VT producing *E. coli* (VTEC) [18] were neutralized by convalescent patient and rabbit immune sera [2, 17]. In the same year, Dr. Allison O'Brien from the Armed Services, Bethesda, recognized that a toxin, elaborated by a newly described *E. coli* strain (*E. coli* O157:H7), bore close similarity with the toxin produced by *Shigella dysenteriae* type 1 (Shiga toxin) which she termed Shiga-like toxin (SLT) [19]. The prototypic disease caused by *E. coli* O157:H7 became known as hemorrhagic colitis [20–23] and the organism was termed "enterohemorrhagic *E. coli*" or EHEC. Subsequent work by Karmali, O'Brien, Karch and others showed that verotoxin, SLT and the classic Shiga toxin belonged to a family of closely-related bacterial protein exotoxins with the major subdivisions of SLT-I or VT1, now termed Stx1, and SLT-II or VT2, now termed Stx2 (and variants) [24] as outlined in Table 26.1. We will use the terms STEC-HUS, Stx-HUS or enteropathogenic HUS (eHUS) to describe patients with the "typical" or "classical" form of HUS.

Table 26.1 Shiga toxins: nomenclature, reservoir and clinical relevance

Stx family	Current nomenclature[a]	Type strain	Stx synonyms	Sequence homology[b]		Clinical association	References
Stx types	*Stx subtypes*			*A subunit*	*B subunit*		
Stx 1	Stx1	*S. dysenteriae* type 1 (SD1)	Stx	100%	100%	Dysentery, HUS	[25, 26]
	Stx1a	*E. coli* O157:H7	STL1, VT1	99%	100%	Hemorrhagic colitis (HC), HUS	[27–29]
	Stx1c	*E. coli* O128:H2	SLT1c, VT1c	97%	97%	Uncomplicated diarrhea/ asymptomatic humans, ovine, deer	[30, 31]
Stx 2	Stx2a	*E. coli* O157:H7	SLTII, VT2, Stx2	100% (homology to Stx 55%)	100% (homology to Stx 57%)	HC, diarrhea, HUS	[25, 32, 33]
	Stx2b	*E. coli* O118:H12	SLTIIb, VT2b, [VT2d]	94%	89%	Low pathogenicity in humans	[34]
	Stx2c	*E. coli* O157:H7	SLTIIc, VT2c	100%	97%	HC, HUS; often expressed jointly with Stx2a	[35, 36]
	Stx2d (Stx2d$_{activatable}$)	*E. coli* O91:H21	SLTIId, VT2d	99%	97%	HC, HUS	[34, 37]
	Stx2e	*E. coli* O139	SLTIIe, VT2e	94%	87%	Porcine edema disease; rare human diarrhea or HUS; binds to Gb3 and Gb4	[38, 39]

Nomenclature base on References [24, 40]

[b]Additional Shiga toxins variants, produced primarily by non-human *E. coli* strains are Stx1d (ONT:H19, a bovine isolate), recognized by commercial ELISA, but not by prototypic anti-Stx1 mAb 13C4 [41], Stx2f (*E. coli* 128:H2, isolated from pigeon droppings) [42], and Stx2g (*E. coli* O2:H25, bovine isolate) [43]

[b]DNA sequence homology to prototypic Shiga toxin (Stx from *S. dysenteriae* 1) and Stx2a (STEC O157:H7 EDL)

There is some confusion about the designation of *E. coli* strains associated with hemorrhagic colitis (HC) and HUS. More than 200 serotypes have been described carrying Stx phage(s) and producing Stx, but only a limited number has been associated with human diseases [44]. The term STEC (Stx producing *E. coli*) describes *E. coli* strains harboring one or more Stx phages and producing Stx *in vivo*. EHEC (enterohemorrhagic *E. coli*) are defined by the disease they induce in humans, bloody (hemorrhagic) colitis [45]. STPB (Shiga toxin producing bacteria) encompass STEC and *S. dysenteriae* type 1 (SD1), and the occasional *Citrobacter freundii* [46–49], *Salmonella* or *Shigella* (enterobacteriaceae) isolates capable of Stx production [50].

While *E. coli* O157:H7 is worldwide the most important STPB and responsible for the majority of sporadic HC and HUS cases and outbreaks, non-O157:H7 STEC serotypes, including *E. coli* O111:H11/NM and O26H11/NM have been likewise implicated in (severe) human disease [49–61]. The large-scale *E. coli* O104:H4 outbreak in Germany in 2011 [62, 63] with >850 mostly adult victims of HUS and 50 deaths [64] represents a unique scenario where an enteroaggregative *E. coli* (EAEC) incorporated an *stx2* phage; this novel strain was propagated in a bean-sprouting facility and contaminated a product (sprouts), that is usually eaten raw [63, 65].

Epidemiology of STEC Infections and STEC HUS

Global estimates of the disease burden by human STEC infections and deaths did not exist until recently. Majowicz et al. recently published a study assessing the annual number of illnesses worldwide due to pathogenic STEC and the resulting cases of HUS, end-stage renal disease (ESRD) and death [66] using various online resources, including databases from 21 countries and WHO regions. According to the authors' (conservative) accounts, STEC causes about 2.8 million acute illnesses annually (95 % credible interval [CrI$_{95\%}$]: 1.7; 5.2 million), and leads to 3890 cases of HUS (CrI$_{95\%}$ 2400; 6700), 270 cases of ESRD (CrI$_{95\%}$ 20; 800), and 230 deaths (CrI$_{95\%}$ 130; 420).

One of the earliest and most comprehensive epidemiological studies of STEC infection and HUS was launched by the Canadian Pediatric Kidney Disease Research Centre (CPKDRC) in Ottawa following the discovery by Karmali and his group in Toronto, with the collaborative efforts of many Canadian centers [67]. The study revealed an annual incidence of sporadic (STEC) HUS in children younger than 15 years of 1.44 per 100,000. The vast majority of patients was diagnosed between the months April and September (82 % of cases); 72 % of patients were <5 years of age (median age 2.7 years). Diarrhea was present in 95 %; it was bloody in 74 % of patients. STEC O157:H7 was isolated in 51 % of those screened for this organism. Dialysis was performed in 48 %, and the mortality rate of this cohort was 2.7 % [67, 68].

During a 3-year, prospective CPKDRC study aimed at determining the risk of developing HUS after sporadic *E. coli* O157:H7 infection among 19 pediatric centers between 1991 and 1994, 582 children were identified with uncomplicated STEC gastroenteritis, 18 with isolated hemolytic anemia/partial HUS, and 205 with HUS (77 % with evidence of STEC infection) [69]. A complete cohort was available for Alberta, the Canadian province with the highest incidence of STEC infections. The risk of HUS after *E. coli* O157:H7 infection in Alberta was 8.1 % (95 % confidence interval, 5.3–11.6). The highest age-specific risk of HUS or hemolytic anemia was 12.9 % in young children <5 years of age [69]. This contrasted with a reported HUS risk of 31.4 % in participating tertiary care centers outside Alberta most likely reflecting referral bias; it highlights the need to critically read epidemiological studies in this field. In another CPKDRC study, 34 consecutive children with HUS were enrolled at 8 hospitals over a 4-month period; 16 patients were treated with dialysis (47 %), and 1 patient died (2.9 %). STEC O157:H7 was isolated from 26 patients, non-O157 from 4 patients, and 4 patients had no growth of STEC [68].

Additional case series, cohort studies and prospective, matched case-control, registry and comparative studies have uncovered important epidemiological aspects of STEC infections and HUS. Detailed microbiological and molecular analyses of isolates obtained during outbreaks have identified the genetic signatures of pathogenic clones, ecological features and modes of transmission, and clinical phenotypes caused by the organism, mainly diarrhea, HC and HUS [52, 57, 58, 70–94].

STEC infections and STEC-HUS show a marked seasonal variation with a peak during the summer and early fall and only few cases during the winter of the Northern and Southern hemispheres. STEC infections and HUS are endemic in moderate climate zones and in areas of high-density cattle raising, such as Argentina, the pacific Northwest of the United States or Alberta in Canada, and Scotland, among others [95, 96]. Studies from Ontario, Canada showed that the prevalence of anti-Stx antibodies was greater in children from rural compared to urban areas suggesting earlier or more frequent exposure to STPB in the rural population. These and other surveys further suggest that the development of immunity to the toxin and/or the organism confers protection against Stx-mediated complications [97].

The majority of STEC-HUS cases appear to occur spontaneously. However, family members or close contacts often report a history of recent diarrhea. These endemic or "spontaneous" cases of HUS are epidemiological markers for the prevalence and (epidemic) transmission of STEC in the community or region. Its primary reservoir is cattle and cattle manure that contaminate produce and drinking water. STEC O157:H7 can survive for months or years and multiply at low rates even under adverse conditions [98].

The first etiologically defined epidemics of STEC infections and (fatal cases) of HUS in the early 1990s were linked to the consumption of contaminated ground beef [70, 72]. The outbreaks led to widespread media attention and expensive lawsuits, and eventually resulted in improved hygiene in slaughterhouses and warnings against the consumption of undercooked meat. A comprehensive review of 350 outbreaks of STEC O157:H7 infections in the United States between 1982 and 2002 [99] identified 8598 cases; 17 % of the patients were hospitalized, 4 % developed HUS, and 0.5 % died. The transmission was foodborne in 52 %, person-to-person in 14 %, waterborne in 9 %, and direct animal contact in 3 %. No vehicle was identified in 21 %. Of the foodborne outbreaks, 41 % were due to ground beef, and 21 % due to produce [99]. The role of processed meat as the predominant outbreak vehicle is diminishing, and more recent, large epidemics were due to contaminated well water [100] or agricultural produce, such as bean sprout (Sakai outbreak) [101, 102], lettuce [103] and fenugreek [63, 104, 105].

Non-O157:H7 STEC

While *E. coli* O157:H7 has been associated with the majority of outbreaks and of sporadic cases of STEC infections in many countries in North and South America, Central and Northern Europe, and China, non-O157:H7 STEC serotypes are increasingly recognized as a cause of sporadic as well as epidemic colitis and HUS. They belong to more than 50 *E. coli* serogroups [106–109].

Isolation frequencies of non-O157:H7 STEC strains approach or exceed those of O157:H7 strains in North America, Europe and elsewhere [55, 110, 111]. A study from the Centers for Disease Control and Prevention (CDC) in Atlanta, published in 2014, summarized outbreaks by non-O157 STEC infections in the US [109]. The authors defined "outbreak" as ≥2 epidemiologically linked, culture-confirmed non-O157 STEC infections. They reported 46 outbreaks with 1727 illnesses and 144 hospitalizations. Of 38 single-etiology outbreaks, two-third were caused by STEC O111:NM or O111:H8 (n=14), and O26:NM or O26:H8 (n=11); 84 % were transmitted in about equal proportions through food and person-to-person spread. Food vehicles included dairy products, produce (mainly fruits and vegetables) and meats, while the most common setting for person-to-person spread was childcare centers. About one-third of all STEC isolates were recovered in multiple-etiology outbreaks [108].

Severe hemorrhagic colitis is typically seen in infections by (enterohemorrhagic) *E. coli*

O157:H7 and O26:NM/H11 and less often with other STEC serotypes [65, 112, 113]. Per definition, all STEC strains have the potential to produce Stx. However, STEC serotypes and clones variably express additional pathogenic factors that mediate bacterial adherence in the gut and *in vivo* toxin production and delivery [114]. Deadly outbreaks by other non-O157 STEC strains have been reported, and the large *E. coli* O104:H4 epidemic in Northern Germany in 2011 was a powerful reminder that non-O157:H7 Stx producing *E. coli*, when introduced into widely distributed food items, can have devastating consequences.

HUS Risk

The HUS risk related to STEC infection varies substantially between STEC serotypes: in pediatric populations, it is between 8 % and 15 % for O157:H7 [69, 115]; it is generally lower, albeit less well defined, for most non-O157:H7 serotypes [109, 116]. A study from Germany estimated that *E. coli* O157:H7 imparts overall an approximately tenfold greater HUS risk compared with non-O157 STEC strains (<1 % versus 8–15 %) [116]. Nevertheless, there is substantial variation in the HUS risk according to the infecting (non-O157) STEC clone. In the cited US-based, CDC analysis [109] a greater percentage of persons infected by Stx2-positive non-O157:H7 STEC developed HUS compared with persons infected by Stx1-only producing strains (7 % vs. 0.8 %; $P<0.001$) [109]. Infections by the emerging, highly pathogenic, Stx2-producing *E. coli* O26:NM/H11 [93, 117, 118] and, in particular, by the sorbitol-fermenting (SF) non-motile *E. coli* O157 clone [119], carry high case fatality rates between 11 % and 50 % [88, 120]. No animal reservoir has been identified for the "German" *E. coli* SF O157:NM strain, which has also been isolated from HUS patients in the Czech Republic and Finland [88, 121, 122].

Table 26.2 summarizes large or clinically significant outbreaks of STEC infections highlighting the spectrum of involved STEC serotypes and toxins, the vehicle of transmission and the calculated HUS risks.

Public Health Initiatives and Tools for Monitoring STEC Infections and Outbreaks

Since the recognition of the public health importance of STEC, national and international surveillance networks have been created with the goal to capture incipient outbreaks by comparing isolates from different laboratories. These networks are often linked to specialized, national or international reference laboratories using the full spectrum of serological, biochemical and advanced molecular typing technologies. Examples of surveillance networks are the CDC-sponsored FoodNet (http://www.cdc.gov/foodnet/) consisting of a network of pediatric nephrologists and hospital infection control personnel that catches 15 % of the US population with sites in ten states [142, 143], the Food- and Waterborne Diseases and Zoonoses Network (FSW-Net), FoodNet Canada [144], Eurosurveillance of the European Center for Disease Prevention and Control (ECDC) in Stockholm, Sweden (www.ecdc.europa.eu/), the "Institut de veille sanitaire" in France [145], and the OzFoodNet network in Australia (www.ozfoodnet.gov.au/) and others worldwide. These networks and their on-line and print publications are valuable sources of up-to-date trends and outbreak information.

Pathogenesis of STEC Disease and HUS

STEC are among the most dreaded enteric pathogens in moderate climates of the Northern and Southern hemispheres due to their potential to cause severe colitis and HUS. They display a sophisticated machinery involving bacterial and host proteins, high contagiosity and resistance to environmental factors. The central pathogenic factor leading to HC and HUS is the ability to produce Stx and to deliver the toxin into the circulation.

STEC are not tissue invasive, and bacteremia is not a feature of STEC diarrhea or HUS. The vascular (endothelial) injury and clinical and pathological changes are believed to result from

Table 26.2 STEC-HUS outbreaks and epidemics

Location (year)	Vehicle	Outbreak strain (Stx type)	# of cases (hospitalization)	# of HUS	HUS risk ratio	# deaths/HUS mortality	Ref
Upper Bavaria, (Germany) [Sept–Nov 1988]	?	E. coli O157:NM[b] (stx2)	6	6 (4–17 months; dialysis 6)	100%	0/6	[123]
Lombardia, Italy [Apr–May 1992]	?	E. coli O111:NM (stx1 and stx2)	?	9	?	1/9 (11.1%)	[124]
State of Washington/West Coast (USA) [Jan–Feb 1993]	Beef patties (Hamburger; errors in meat processing and cooking)	E. coli O157:H7 (stx1 and stx2)	501 (151; 31%) Children 278	45 (37 children)	9.0% (Children 13.3%)	3/45 (6.7%) 3/501 (0.60%)	[72] See also [125–128]
South Australia [Jan–Feb 1995]	Dry fermented sausage (Mettwurst)	E. coli O111:NM (stx1 and stx2)	?	21	?	1/21 (4.8%)	[75, 76]
Sakai, Osaka Prefecture (Japan) [July 1996]	Bean sprout	E. coli O157:H7 (stx1 and stx2)	12,680 (425; 3.4%)	12	0.09%	0/12	[101, 102, 129–131]
Scotland[a] (UK) [Nov–Dec 1996]	Cold cooked meat from single butcher	E. coli O157:H7 (stx2, phage type 2)	512 (120; 23.4%)	HUS/TMA 36 (children 6)	7.0%	17/36 (47.2%) 17/512 (3.32%; all deaths >65 years)	[132–134]
Walkerton, Ontario (Canada) [May 2000]	Contaminated municipal drinking water [135]	E. coli O157:H7, Campylobacter jejuni	Symptomatic Self-reported 2300 (65; 2.8%)	HUS 30 (Children 22)	1.3% (total)	6/30 (20%) 6/2300 (0.26%)	[136–138]
Germany [2002]	Unknown	SF (sorbitol-fermenting) EHEC O157:NM	Unknown	38	Unknown	4/38 (10.5%)	[88]
Oklahoma (USA) [August 2008]	Food (diseased food workers in restaurant)	E. coli O111:NM (stx1 and stx2)	344 (70; 20.3%)	25	7.3%	1/25 (4.0%) 1/344 (0.29%)	[139]
Northern Germany [May–June 2011]	Fenugreek	E. coli O104:H4 (stx2; STEC/EAEC hybrid strain)	3842	855 (children 90)	22.2%	54/855 (6.3%) 54/3842 (1.41%) Pediatric HUS 1/90 (1.11%)	[63, 105, 140, 141]

[a]There are some discrepancies in the reported numbers between publications
[b]NM (non-motile or H−)

the effects of the circulating toxin, both locally (HC) and systemically (HUS). Shiga toxinemia appears to occur early during the illness. It is short-lived with an estimated serum half-life of <5 min [146, 147] and has largely ceased when the patient presents with HUS [115]. Of note, coagulopathy, measured as thrombin generation, plasminogen activator inhibitor type 1 (PAI-1) activity, intravascular fibrin deposition and other events can be demonstrated well before – or even in the absence of – the clinical manifestation of HUS [148, 149].

STEC counts and free fecal toxin excretion often diminish or become undetectable during early, acute stages of HUS [115, 150, 151]. The amount of measurable, circulating toxin is extremely low. The difficulty of measuring active toxin in the circulation is likely due to its avid binding to the (microvascular) endothelium, and to plasma proteins or glycolipids. Shiga toxinemia has been demonstrated 24 h after the experimental (oral) inoculation of streptomycin-treated, starved mice with a large dose of the highly virulent Stx2d-producing E. coli O91:H21 strain B2F1 [152]. Intravascular binding of circulating toxin by neutralizing antibodies or receptor analogues decreased Stx-induced mortality in these mice when the Stx neutralizing agent was injected during the first 72 h after inoculation [152–155].

STEC: Host Interaction in the Gut

Ingested STEC bind to epithelial cells in terminal ileum and Payer's patches. Bacterial/host cell interaction elicits signals that enhance bacterial colonization and release of bacterium-derived pathogenic factors including lipopolysaccharide (LPS) and Stx. STPB express and excrete various enzymes, additional toxins, such as subtilase, extracellular serine proteases (Esp) and hemolysins [156–168]. Their contribution to hemorrhagic colitis and HUS is subject to ongoing research.

Bacterial Adherence

The first important step in the pathologic process leading to HC and HUS is the adherence of STPB to the intestinal epithelium. Various factors have been identified that facilitate initial attachment.

The key set of proteins is described as Type III secretion system (T3SS) [169]. The T3SS is encoded by the locus of enterocyte effacement (LEE); LEE comprises the genes for "intimin," a 94 kDa outer membrane protein involved in intimate enterocyte adherence (eae, "enterocyte attachment and effacement"), "translocated intimin receptor" (Tir), a protein injected by attaching bacteria into the gut epithelial cell, and the type III secretion apparatus (Esp B and D). The bacterial proteins work in tandem to form characteristic attaching and effacing (A/E) lesions (actin "pedestals") upon intestinal adhesion (Fig. 26.1a–c). LEE-related genes are shared with related enterobacteriacea, such as enteropathogenic E. coli (EPEC) and Citrobacter freundii [114, 169–172].

LEE-negative STEC strains [173] use alternative adhesion strategies to host enterocytes, including an iron-regulated gene A (IrgA) homolog adhesin (Iha) [174] and STEC autoagglutinating adhesin (Saa) [175].

Human pathogenic STEC elaborate additional toxins, such as an enterohemolysin (EhxA) [176–179] and subtilase (SubA) [168, 180–182] EhxA, are encoded by a gene located in the pO157 megaplasmid, present in a large proportion of STEC strains [179, 183–185], along with the putative virulence factors EspP that cleaves human coagulation factor V [156], a catalase/peroxidase (KatP) [186], and a metalloprotease that contributes to intimate adherence of EHEC O157:H7 to host cells (StcE) [187].

Shiga Toxin Delivery

The tight adherence of STPB to the epithelium of the gut facilitates toxin translocation into local microvasculature and systemic circulation. Stx binds to Gb3 on Paneth cells and transverses the intestinal barrier without killing the epithelial cell [188, 189]. The microaerobic conditions in the gut reduce bacterial Stx production and release, but enhance Stx translocation across the epithelial monolayer [190]. Inflammatory host response of the gut and resulting diarrhea can be viewed as an attempt of the host to clear out pathogenic bacteria. Interestingly, STEC appear to counteract their removal from the gut by dampening the cytokine response [191].

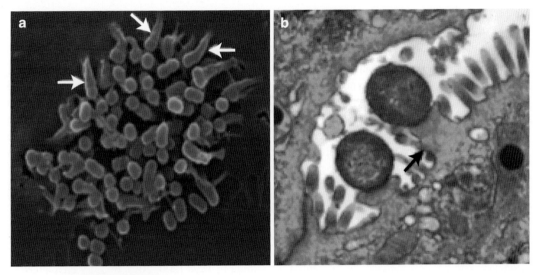

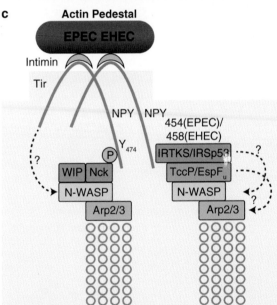

Fig. 26.1 STEC and related attaching and effacing (A/E) pathogens, such as enteropathogenic E. coli (EPEC), induce distinct histopathological lesions using the (bacterial) type III secretion system (T3SS) encoded by the "locus of enterocyte effacement" (LEE). (**a**) Scanning electron micrograph of pedestals induced by adherent bacteria (*arrows*). (**b**) Transmission electron micrograph showing intestinal A/E lesions (*arrow*). (**c**) Diagram depicting the actions of a subset of T3SS effectors of A/E pathogens on host cytoskeletal pathways and structures. *Green circles* represent actin filaments (Used with permission of Jonn Wiley and Sons from Wong et al. [170])

Classification of Pathogenic STEC

Several authors have attempted to classify STEC according to their pathogenic potential in humans [192]. Karmali et al. [193] proposed to group STEC isolates into "seropathotypes" A through E. Seropathotype A is composed of *E. coli* O157:H7 and O157:NM, that are the most common causes of severe STEC disease and outbreaks. Strains assigned to seropathotype B, including O26:H11, O103:H2, O111:NM, O121:H19, and O145:NM, are associated with outbreaks and severe disease but at a lower incidence compared with seropathotype A strains, while seropathotype E isolates are not associated with human disease [193, 194].

STEC virulence factors are encoded by genes located in mobile genetic elements (prophages, genomic islands, plasmids) that can dramatically alter the virulence of *E. coli* [195]. A revised classification by Kobayashi et al. [194] differentiates STEC strains according to "clusters" 1 through 8 that are defined by virulence gene profiles. In addition to genes located in LEE, the authors identified both *katP* and *stcE* as key attributes of the top pathogenic STEC genotypes. Despite up to 80 % overlap with the seropathotype classification, the proposed "clusters" may more accurately reflect the virulence potential of a given isolate [194].

Stx-Negative STEC

An interesting finding is the loss of *stx2*-containing phages during human disease, originally reported by Dr. Karch's group: Initially *stx*-positive STEC O26:H11/NM and (sorbitol-fermenting) O157:NM patient isolates became *stx* negative during the course of the disease [84, 196]. Similar observations have been reported for STEC O103:H2/NM and O145:H28/NM strains. Thus, *stx* gene content (and Stx production) can fluctuate, with evolutionary, diagnostic, and clinical implications [197].

Shiga Toxin and Its Glycolipid Receptor

Shiga Toxin

Shiga toxins are AB_5 protein toxins consisting of an enzymatically active 32.2 kDa "A" subunit and a (receptor-binding) "B" subunit, which consists of five identical 7.7 kDa proteins. The pentameric B-subunit forms a central pore that anchors the C-terminus of the A subunit (Fig. 26.2a–c). B monomers expose three distinct binding sites that recognize and interact in a lectin-like fashion with the terminal sugars of the glycolipid receptor, globotriaosylceramide (Gb3) [198, 199].

Stx was first discovered in the lysates of cultured *Shigella dysenteriae* named after Kiyoshi Shiga in 1898 [200, 201]. Initially characterized as a neurotoxin, its propensity for endothelial cells was recognized >50 years after the initial publication [202, 203], followed by its description as an enterotoxin in 1972 [204]. Antiserum against Stx from *S. dysenteriae* 1 neutralizes Stx and all Stx1 variants, but not Stx2 or Stx2 variants. In contrast, antibodies raised against Stx2 neutralize most Stx2 variants but not Shiga toxin or Stx1 [24, 35, 205].

Subsequently, numerous *E. coli* strains were characterized that express Stxs with varied amino acid sequences, some of which confer unique biological properties. Because serious outcomes of infection have been attributed to certain Stx

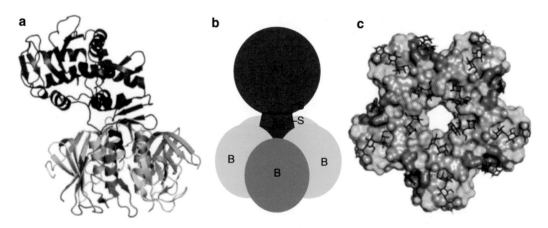

Fig. 26.2 (a) The structure of Shiga holotoxin as determined by X-ray crystallography. The A moiety is shown in *red*, the five B subunits in *green*, and the disulfide bridge linking the A1 and A2 fragments in *blue*. (b) Schematic representation of the Shiga toxin structure. (c) The surface of the B5 pentamer indicating the location of the 15 potential receptor binding sites, based on the structure of Shiga toxin 1 (Used with permission of Elsevier from Bergan et al. [198])

subtypes, an international working group defined the toxin subtypes by comparing the level of relatedness of a large collection of sequence variants comprising three Stx/Stx1 and seven Stx2 subtypes and developed a practical PCR subtyping method [40]. Table 26.1 provides an updated list of members of the Stx "family" associated with human disease.

Shiga Toxin Globotriaosyl Ceramide Receptor

Principles of mammalian cell membrane binding, translocation and downstream effects are identical across all Stxs. The toxins' lectin-like recognition and binding to Gb3 (Galα1-4Galβ1-4Glc ceramide) induces the formation of lipid rafts with clathrin-coated pits that mediate the internalization of membrane-bound toxin into the target cell. Gb3 is identical with CD77 or the P^k blood group antigen [206–209] (Fig. 26.3a, b). There are subtle differences between Stx1 and Stx2 and its variants in their affinity to Gb3 and related glycolipids that influence binding to susceptible tissues and intracellular cell sorting [210–215]. However, these differences do not easily explain why severe disease and HUS are more often associated with STPB producing Stx2 (or Stx1 and Stx2) [216]. Not all Stx subtypes have been isolated from humans with colitis or HUS (Table 26.1).

Gb3 is the only functional receptor for Stx1 and most Stx2 variants in mammals, including humans. Knockout mice for Gb3 synthase, the enzyme that ligates galactose to lactosylceramide (Fig. 26.3a, b), are resistant to the toxic actions of Stx [217, 218]. Expression of Gb3 is

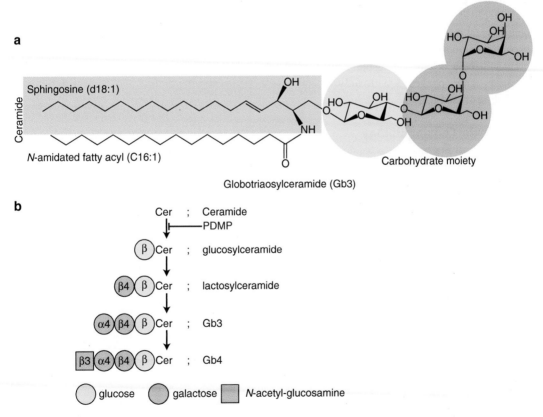

Fig. 26.3 (a) Structure of the Shiga toxin receptor Gb3. Glucose and galactose of the carbohydrate moiety are shown in *blue* and *yellow*, respectively. The ceramide moiety consists of a sphingosine backbone (in *pink*) and a variable fatty acid chain. (b) The steps in the synthesis of the globo-series of glycosphingolipids from ceramide, showing the sequential addition of carbohydrates represented by the glycan symbol system (Used with permission of Elsevier from Bergan et al. [198])

cell-restricted. It is found on microvascular endothelial cells (including glomerular and peritubular capillary endothelium), glomerular epithelial cells (podocytes), platelets and germinal center B-lymphocytes [219], and peripheral and central neurons [220, 221]. Only the efficient transport to the endoplasmic reticulum and subsequent rRNA depurination result in cell toxicity. Platelets, and possibly red blood cells (RBCs), can bind Stx (and LPS) [208, 209, 222, 223]. Newer ex vivo studies suggest a link between platelet Stx binding, complement activation and microparticle-induced endothelial injury and microvascular thrombosis in patients with eHUS [223–225].

Stx2e, the toxin responsible for porcine edema disease of weanling piglets [226] binds to globotetraosylceramide (GalNAcβ1-3Galα1,4 Galβ1-4Glc Ceramide; Gb4) in addition to Gb3. Gb4 is abundantly expressed in various porcine issues and involved in cerebral vascular injury and neurological disturbance [227]. Although Gb4 is present in human tissues, involvement of Stx2e in human disease is rare and usually mild, likely because *stx2e* phages are mainly found in porcine-restricted pathogens [228–231].

Shiga Toxin: Cellular Biology

The process of Stx binding to the cell membrane and internalization has been described in the 1980s [232–234]. Ongoing research is concerned with details of Gb3 expression and presentation in the lipid bilayer, and intracellular effects [235–240].

Intracellular Toxin Trafficking and Action

Upon its transport across the cell membrane, the toxin subunits disassemble. The "binding" B subunit is marked for ubiquitin-mediated degradation. The A subunit is nicked by the intracellular protease furin [241] and is chaperoned to the endoplasmic reticulum (ER), where the disulfide bond linking the A1 and A2 fragments is reduced. Stx endocytosis and transport to the Golgi apparatus are facilitated by various second messenger (phosphorylation) events that include Stx-induced tyrosine kinases as well as remodeling of cytoskeleton components

[198, 242]. The processed A1 fragment then cleaves a specific adenine residue from the 3′ region of the 28S rRNA of the mammalian 60S ribosomal subunit of actively translating ribosomes. Loss of the adenine residue causes a conformational change of the ribosomal RNA resulting in the effective inhibition of protein biosynthesis in toxin-sensitive cells [243] (Fig. 26.4). Very few molecules are needed to paralyze the cell making it one of the most potent known toxins.

The action of Stx on the ribosome not only leads to protein synthesis inhibition, but induces a separable cascade of cell biological effects known as ribotoxic stress response; it is characterized by the activation of the MAP kinase pathway, specifically c-Jun N-terminal kinase (JNK) and p38 [245–252], similar to ricin [253]. The observed biological effects are tissue dependent. For example, bovine intestinal epithelial cells express Gb3 but are insensitive to Shiga cytotox-

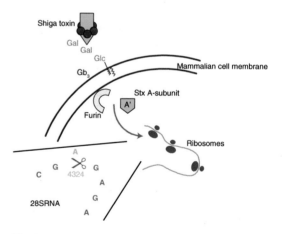

Fig. 26.4 Schematic diagram of the biological action of Stx in susceptible mammalian cells. The holotoxin binds to lipid raft-associated membrane globotriasosyl ceramide (Gb3) and enters the cell via clathrin-mediated endocytosis. A and B subunits become disengaged and the A submit is cleaved and activated by intracellular furin. Upon "retrograde" passage through the Golgi apparatus, the A′ subunit selectively removes a specific adenine residue from the 28S RNA of the large ribosomal subunit (N-glycosidase activity). This results in (1) blockade of active (translating) ribosomes (translational inhibition), and (2) a ribotoxic cellular stress response with activation of c-jun and p38 (MAP) kinases and/or apoptotic cell death (Used with permission of author and Elsevier from Loirat et al. [244]. Copyrighted by Martin Bitzan)

icity, possibly due to their sorting of the toxin to lysosomes instead of the endoplasmic reticulum [254]. Other tissues that are relatively resistant to the cytotoxic effect of Stx may still respond with an "activated" phenotype [255–258]. These effects are in part mediated by an Stx-induced increase in mRNA stability and enhanced protein expression of select (inducible) mRNA transcripts [255, 257–259].

Apoptosis

As outlined above, Stx activates a stress response in sensitive mammalian cells. Intracellular signaling occurs at the plasma cell membrane following Stx binding to Gb3 via the pentameric B-subunit resulting in lipid raft formation, during the course of retrotranslocation of the Stx A subunit, and/or as a result of the purine residue cleavage at the alpha-sarcin/ricin loop of the 28S rRNA [198]. It has become evident that Stx-mediated protein synthesis inhibition is dissociated from cell death signaling and cytotoxicity and that the ribotoxic stress response induced by ribosomal depurination or by the presence of unfolded proteins within the ER (ER stress) induces apoptosis (programmed cell death) [260, 261].

Initiation of apoptosis entails multiple changes to cell morphology, such as cell shrinkage, cytoplasmic vacuolization, chromatin condensation (pyknosis), nuclear fragmentation (karyorrhexis), phosphatidylserine exposure at the plasma membrane, cell blebbing and extrusion of apoptotic bodies [261]. Stx-induced apoptotic signaling is believed to occur mainly via the intrinsic, mitochondrial pathway. It is regulated by B-cell lymphoma protein-2 (Bcl-2) family proteins and results in the downstream activation of cysteine-dependent aspartate-directed proteases (caspases) and the deactivation of anti-apoptotic proteins [198, 248, 261–264]. Pharmacological blockade of MAP kinase and its upstream kinases weakens the Stx-induced cytotoxic (apoptotic) effect *in vitro* [245, 248, 250, 265].

Evidence of apoptosis in renal and other tissues has been demonstrated ex vivo in kidney biopsies from patients with STEC-HUS and in animal models of STEC infection [266–268].

Endothelial Injury in STEC-HUS

Microvascular endothelial cell injury is believed to be the major pathological pathway leading to eHUS. Experimental results from cell culture experiments, animal models of HUS and observations in humans suggest that the endothelium becomes prothrombotic due to injury and apoptotic events. Cultured microvascular endothelial cells, including glomerular and renal tubular endothelial cells, are exquisitely sensitive to nM concentrations of both Stx1 and 2 [269, 270], even in the absence of LPS or TNF-α [271].

The mechanism leading to intravascular hemolysis through the sudden intravascular destruction of RBCs and acute thrombocytopenia is less well understood. Stx (and LPS) interact with platelets, monocytes and neutrophils, and possibly RBCs and plasma proteins (serum amyloid proteins) or glycolipids [205, 223, 225, 272–279]. There is little evidence that Stx modulates neutrophil or monocyte function under *in vivo* conditions [280–284]. The previously postulated "transfer" of toxin from low affinity receptors on circulating leukocytes to high affinity receptors on small vessel endothelial cells [274, 285, 286] may be (too) simplistic [279, 287]. However, investigators have demonstrated more recently that Stx (and LPS) induce the formation of platelet and monocyte microparticles loaded with tissue factor and complement [223, 288]. Biologically active microparticles and (direct) Stx-induced apoptosis of endothelial cells, including the externalization of plasma membrane phosphatidylserine [289], may provide a mechanism how localized (colon) or systemic microvascular thrombosis is initiated in the gut and kidney [290]. Endothelial cell injury or activation may induce or modulate vasoactive mediators, including chemokines and their receptors [255, 258, 259, 290–294] which would then result in a prothrombotic and vasoconstrictive endothelial phenotype known as thrombotic microangiopathy.

The *in vitro* susceptibility of podocytes and of proximal renal tubular cells is similar to that of microvascular endothelial cells [295, 296]. There is a long-standing debate, if tubular injury is a primary feature of eHUS, i.e., directly

Stx-mediated, or secondary to the renovascular (thrombotic) events. Animal experiments suggest that Stx exerts direct effects on renal tubular epithelium [297–299]. Data from the German *E. coli* O104:H4 HUS outbreak support this view [300].

Stx and Cytokines

Stx can lead to enhanced cytokine expression *in vitro* and in experimental mouse models [301, 302]. Conversely, exposure to cytokines, specifically TNF-α, may increase Gb3 in endothelial cells of various vascular beds and enhance Stx sensitivity [303–306]. The release of LPS and (other) exogenous or endogenous inflammatory agents during STEC infection is thought to contribute to or facilitate Stx toxicity and, potentially, the development of HUS [307]. Indirect support for the concept of generalized inflammation is gleaned from the association between HUS risk and margination of peripheral neutrophils (neutrophil count) and acute phase reactants during STEC colitis [129, 308–313] and from *in vitro* and animal experimental data linking the generation of cyto- and chemokines to tissue toxicity.

Data to support the importance of LPS or cytokines in animal models of HUS or Stx-induced renal failure are conflicting [299, 314]. While there is good evidence for direct and indirect cytokine-aided renal parenchymal injury in various forms of glomerulonephritis [315, 316], attempts to detect (increased) circulating LPS, TNF-α or other cytokines in patients with HUS were generally unsuccessful [280, 317–320]. The role of proinflammatory cytokines in the pathogenesis of acute kidney injury (AKI) of human HUS remains inconclusive [300, 306, 321].

Stx Genetics and Stx Phages

Shiga toxins are encoded by bacteriophages (Stx phages) that are closely related to phage lambda (lambdoid) with similar promoters, repressors, terminators, antiterminators, lysis genes, and structural proteins [322, 323]. Lambdoid bacteriophages constitute a heterogeneous group of mobile genetic elements that integrate into specific sites of the bacterial (host) chromosome, with the exception of *stx2e* [228]. The *stx* genes

are always located in the same region of these lambdoid phages as part of a late expressed module under the control of anti-terminator Q [324].

Stx phages are lytic and can propagate in receptive *E. coli* and other enterobacteriaceae present in the gut, such as *C. freundii* or *Shigella sonnei* [325–327]. *E. coli* can carry multiple Stx phages leading to the simultaneous production of two or more different Stxs. These conditions are conducive to the creation of novel phages and genome diversification [198, 328]. The genes encoding Stx and enzymes needed for its release are controlled by phage promoters that also regulate the replication cycle of the phage. Phage-mediated bacteriolysis releases the toxin [329, 330]. Stx2 (but not Stx1) can be released from viable *E. coli* using a specific bacterial secretion system [331].

Antibiotics and STEC

Certain antimicrobial and chemotherapeutic drugs induce Stx phage replication and toxin release. This phenomenon has been exploited in the laboratory to increase the yield of Stx for experimental purposes [332, 333], as well as for diagnostic testing of stool isolates [334, 335]. Rare cases of HUS during chemotherapy with mitomycin have been linked to this phenomenon [336–338].

Stx genes are expressed together with bacteriophage SOS response genes [330, 339–341]. Some antibiotics, such as (fluoro)quinolones, sulfamethoxazole/trimethoprim (SMX/TMP) and others lead to prophage induction and Stx production by several orders of magnitude within 2–4 h [342–345]. The SOS response is initiated when damaged bacterial DNA binds and activates the (bacterial) RecA protein. Activated RecA induces the degradation (cleavage) of key repressor molecules, LexA and CI, leading to the temporary arrest of DNA synthesis, cell division and error-prone DNA repair. Cleavage of the CI phage repressor/activator protein results in the coordinately regulated induction and expression of previously silent phage encoded genes (including Stx A and B subunit genes), the production of phage particles, and bacterial cell lysis [330, 340, 345]. Experiments in mice infected with RecA mutated STEC strains [341] have demonstrated the importance of the bacterial SOS system under *in vivo* conditions.

Antibiotics have been noted to induce an SOS response and phage/Stx expression at levels below minimal inhibitory as well as suprainhibitory concentrations [345]. One study employing subinhibitory norfloxacin concentrations revealed profound effects on the ensemble of the bacterial gene transcripts (transcriptome) of the model *E. coli* O157:H7 strain EDL 933: the vast majority of the upregulated genes was *stx* phage-borne, with up to 158-fold induction of *stxA₂*; conversely, the expression of bacterial genes responsible for bacterial metabolism, cell division and amino acid biosynthesis was down-regulated [346].

Concerns have been raised that the use of antimicrobials that induce an *stx* phage SOS response in patients with (bloody) diarrhea may increase the risk of HUS [347]. Some authors speculated the presence of (putative) triggers of Stx (bacterio)phage in the intestinal lumen may add to the variability of the risk of developing severe hemorrhagic colitis or HUS [344]. The use of antibiotics in this patient population is discussed in detail below.

Laboratory Diagnosis of STEC Infections

STEC infections warrant fast diagnosis; tests must be sensitive, specific and easily accessible. An etiological diagnosis is important for early treatment decisions, particularly by separating STEC-HUS from other HUS forms, and impacts on the long-term clinical follow-up [12, 244, 348]. STEC detection affects close contacts, particularly family and daycare, healthcare institutions, and occasionally schools, restaurants/kitchens and the food industry. STEC infections are notifiable and require isolation measures [349, 350]; results also inform the search for the source of infection and preventive measures to curb further transmission during an epidemic. In the bigger picture, bacterial isolation allows monitoring of epidemiological changes, such as the emergence of new strains and virulence traits.

Identification and management of STEC infection depends on the availability of laboratories testing for STEC and physicians ordering and correctly interpreting results of Stx tests [351, 352]. Current recommendations stipulate that stools are plated simultaneously on an *E. coli* O157:H7 selective agar and tested for the presence of Stx using a fresh stool suspension or overnight broth culture [56, 353]. An Stx immunoassay is not an adequate stand-alone test for detection of STEC in clinical samples [354]. Where available, real-time PCR for the detection of *stx* and other virulence factor encoding genes (if available) in stool or overnight culture should be added. Vero cell or other cell toxicity assays, although highly sensitive and specific, when combined with a neutralization step, are not routinely performed. Stx detection and PCR are important tools for the identification of non-O157:H7 STEC infections.

E. coli O157:H7 are most efficiently isolated by plating fresh stool on Sorbitol MacConkey [SMAC] agar, with or without added cefixime-tellurite [355]. Prior to the use of Shiga toxin assays and PCR, the isolation of non-O157:H7 STEC strains among commensal gut flora by traditional microbiological techniques was laborious, which contributed to the delayed appreciation of non-O157:H7 STEC clones as a cause of enterocolitis and HUS. Another potential barrier to the efficient isolation of non-O157:H7 STEC strains are variable toxin production and instability or loss of toxin producing phages. The latter phenomenon was first noted in subcultures of STEC isolates, but was subsequently shown to occur *in vivo* as well [84, 326]. In fact, the gut appears to be a veritable hot bed for the exchange of phage material and other mobile genetic elements [325, 356].

In addition to STPB identification from stool, testing for (free) fecal Stx is recommended. The classical cytotoxicity assay using Vero or other cell cultures, is time-consuming, labor intensive, and requires cell culture facilities; it has therefore been replaced in most diagnostic labs by ELISA based and other (rapid) diagnostic tests with variable sensitivity and specificity [357–362].

The probability of successfully identifying STPB in children with HUS rises when the first stool samples is tested less than 4 days after diarrhea onset, the patient is 12 months or older, the infection is part of an outbreak, bloody diarrhea is present and onset is during June through September [142]. STEC isolation and free fecal toxin detection rates diminish soon after the onset of HUS [115, 150, 151]. If stool culture or toxin assay(s) are delayed or negative, serological assays can be employed to search for elevated (or rising) IgM class antibodies to one of the more common STEC O-groups (LPS antigens) by ELISA, hemagglutination assay or Western blot [150, 222, 363–366]. Saliva IgA (and IgM) provide a suitable alternative to serum antibodies [366–368]. Testing for serum antibodies to Stx has been used as an epidemiological tool [97, 369], but its diagnostic utility in the clinical setting is limited [142]. Additional STEC-expressed or secreted proteins may elicit an antibody response [370], but are rarely used diagnostically. Serological tests are generally offered in reference laboratories (Table 26.3).

Rapid diagnosis of STEC diarrhea is essential. When sending stools for culture, the clinician should inform the laboratory with clear written and verbal information [372], including the presence of painful or bloody diarrhea, or signs of HUS. "Routine" stool cultures from patients with diarrhea should always include at least a SMAC agar. If the stool culture of an index patient is STEC negative, the pathogen may be identified in other, including asymptomatic, family members. Stools, or broth culture, and serum should be preserved and sent to a reference laboratory in case of negative results, particularly if additional (or suspected) cases of HC or HUS have been identified in the community.

Urinalysis contributes little to the diagnosis of HUS. However, occasionally, a urinary tract infection (UTI) must be ruled out. A patient with moderate to severe hemolysis will present proteinuria and hematuria (hemoglobinuria and erythrocyturia). A documented UTI or the presence of an abnormal urinalysis should not delay the stool-based, etiological diagnosis or the diagnosis of HUS. Macroscopic hematuria is rare in Stx-HUS. Anecdotal reports have described the occurrence of HUS following an STEC UTI without documented diarrhea [373–376].

In conclusion, early stool collection for the culture of *E coli* O157:H7 and, if negative, other STEC serotypes, and testing for the presence of (fecal) Stx should be attempted in all patients with HUS and diarrhea, and in siblings or contacts of index the patient(s). Relying on a clinical diagnosis ("D+ HUS") and omission of microbiological testing is inadequate. A prerequisite for the correct microbiological diagnosis is the dialogue with the microbiologist. The diagnostic workup should not be limited to free Stx [377]. Where available, stool samples should be screened (by PCR) for Stx genes and/or specific STEC "virulence"-associated genes. In the absence of microbiological evidence of STEC, serological testing for serum or saliva IgM or IgA antibodies against defined O-group (LPS) antigens or other virulence proteins may aid in the diagnosis. Although new and more sensitive diagnostic techniques continue to be developed, a combination of methods will still be necessary for optimal yield [353, 378, 379].

From Colitis to HUS

Clinical Presentation and Evolution

The spectrum of STEC disease ranges from mild diarrhea and hemorrhagic colitis to severe HUS, and death. Fatal outcomes have also been reported in patients with STEC infection without HUS [380, 381].

Most clinical descriptions and risk estimates are based on *E. coli* O157:H7 infections. Severity and incidence of diarrhea or colitis and of HUS by non-O157:H7 serotypes vary due to the heterogeneity of this group of pathogens [65, 81]. The HUS risk is 8–15 % for EHEC O157:H7 colitis [69, 72, 115, 382], but substantially lower for non-O157 STEC infections [111, 113, 383]. The sorbitol-fermenting, Stx2 producing non-motile EHEC O157:NM clone, almost exclusively found in central Europe, appears to be exceptionally dangerous with a HUS risk that exceeds 30 % [88, 120].

The interval between EHEC O157:H7 ingestion and diarrhea is 3–8 days [102, 115, 384]. The diarrhea is typically painful and frequent, with

Table 26.3 Laboratory diagnostic of STEC infections and HUS

STEC disease	Material	Test	Details	Comments
Diarrhea/colitis	Stool	*E. coli* O157:H7	Sorbitol/tellurite MacConkey agar or similar selective medium)	*E. coli* O157:H7 colonies are distinct due to lack of sorbitol metabolism; tellurite suppresses growth of irrelevant flora
		Free fecal Stx	ELISA, Vero cell tissue culture assay	Fresh stool preferred to prevent decay of toxin protein and activity
		Non-O157:H7 STEC	PCR (for *stx*, structural or phage genes) [40]	Most non-O157:H7 STEC strains ferment sorbitol and cannot be visually or metabolically differentiated on sorbitol containing media
			Colony blot hybridization or blotting	Keep stool sample, colony sweep or broth at -80 °C for reference laboratory
			O-group agglutination	
			Toxin testing of lysates/supernatant	
	Blood	CBC, smear	Baseline hemoglobin and platelets; presence of schistocytes	
		Creatinine	Baseline renal function	
	Urine	Urinalysis	Baseline/early changes	
Acute HUS	Stool		See above	Stool culture may become negative early during HUS
				STPB may loose *stx* phage during course of infection [326, 371]
	Blood	Hematology	CBC, differential, smear, reticulocyte count	
			Consider coagulation screen and d-dimers	
		Biochemistry	Creatinine, electrolytes, albumin, LDH, haptoglobin	Elevated plasma AST and (indirect) bilirubin indicate vigorous hemolysis, not hepatopathy
			Liver enzymes	Detailed complement analysis and/or metabolic or genetic work-up if presentation is "atypical"
			Amylase or lipase	
			Troponin	
			Blood glucose	
			CRP (or other acute phase reactant)	
		Blood bank	Cross and type	
	Urine		Urinalysis	During recovery and follow-up: protein/creatinine
				Acute proteinuria indicates hemoglobinuria with or without glomerular and tubular injury
"Atypical" presentation			Detailed complement analysis and/or metabolic or genetic workup	Relapse (native) or recurrence of HUS (graft kidney)
				Prolonged or waxing and waning course of thrombocytopenia/hemolysis
				Family history of "asynchronous" HUS

>15 discharges of small amounts of mucous or liquid stools daily; the stools turn bloody by day 2 or 3 in >80 % of children. The amount of (visible) blood varies from a few specks to frank hemorrhage. About 50 % of patients develop nausea and vomiting; fever is present in one third [65, 115, 148, 372, 384]. The evolution of infections by non-O157:H7 STEC serotypes is generally milder compared with *E. coli* O157:H7 [65]. Exceptions are infections by EHEC clones belonging to serogroups O26, O55, O91, O111, among others, that can be clinically indiscernible from infections by classical EHEC O157:H7 [78, 81, 88, 91, 93, 111, 197, 385, 386].

The HUS risk is greatest at the extremes of age, in children <3–5 years and the elderly [115, 132, 380]; it decreases during childhood and adolescence, and is <0.1 % in young and middle aged adults. Conversely, STEC colitis can lead to acute kidney injury (AKI) and death without the picture of HUS, particularly in the elderly [380, 381]. Other variables impacting on the HUS risk are the STEC serotype or clone (as outlined above), the toxin type(s) produced, and preexisting immunity [97, 387]. Experimental animal data indicate that a high Stx "load" exceeding binding to natural protectants and acquired antibodies, is the major precipitant of HUS [152].

Biomarkers and Predictors of Severe STEC Disease

Predictive clinical and biological markers of HUS are the degree of systemic inflammation during the preceding colitis, particularly neutrophilia with a high-percentage shift to band forms, and a sharp rise of acute phase reactants, such as C-reactive protein or calcitonin [102, 129, 309, 310, 312, 313, 388]. Patients who progress to HUS demonstrate significantly more often a peripheral neutrophil count in excess of 20×10^9/L than patients with colitis only [125, 129, 389, 390]. Human and experimental animal data suggest that STEC infection as well as parenteral Stx administration induce a cytokine response that mediates some of the observed pathological effects [293, 301, 391–393]. Some, but not all inbred mouse strains [299] require the combination of Stx and added LPS or TNF-α to produce an HUS-like disease [394–399], while no such dependency on added cytokines was noted in primate models of HUS [392, 393, 400, 401].

Clinical features associated with an increased HUS risk are vomiting, diminished extracellular fluid volume [402, 403] and ingestion of antimotility agents or antibiotics during the first 3–4 days of the diarrheal illness [347, 404]. Female gender, although noted by some authors [68, 405], does not seem to predispose to HUS. The German *E. coli* O104:H4 epidemic represents an exception due to specific features of transmission (vehicle) and consumer habits of many of the victims of this outbreak [140].

HUS mediated by Stx starts abruptly, about 3–10 days (median 6 days) after the onset of diarrhea [115, 129] (Fig. 26.5). Patients present from 1 day to the other with fatigue and pallor; they become listless and may develop petechiae, often after transient clinical improvement of the colitis.

Fig. 26.5 Schematic diagram of the development of diarrhea and HUS due to Shiga toxin-producing E. coli (STEC) (Used with permission of Elsevier from Loirat et al. [244])

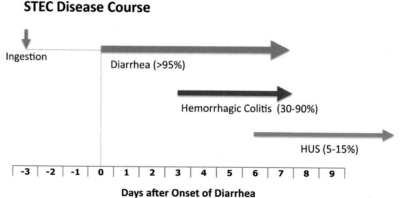

Absent bowel movements during the acute phase of HUS should raise the suspicion of intussusception or ileus.

The clinical diagnosis of HUS is generally straightforward, once the HUS-defining triad of (intravascular) hemolysis, thrombocytopenia and acute kidney injury is recognized. Hemolytic anemia of HUS – characterized by RBC fragmentation with schistocytes (burr or helmet cells) in the peripheral blood smear – with or without thrombocytopenia – is known as microangiopathic hemolytic anemia (MAHA). With disease progression, the serum creatinine concentration rises and oligoanuria, hypertension and edema may become apparent, usually within 1–2 days after onset of symptoms. Some patients may recover before the full picture of HUS develops. They may only demonstrate hemolytic anemia without apparent AKI, while platelets may briefly dip within and slightly below the reference range ("partial HUS") [69, 406].

The etiological diagnosis of HUS is important, particularly in patients with atypical presentation, because of the differential prognosis and management of different forms of HUS [12, 348]. Diarrhea has been noted in one third of patients with atypical HUS, occasionally with features of ischemic colitis [407–409]. Conversely, viral or bacterial diarrhea, including STEC infection, can trigger HUS in persons with a genetic defect in the alternative pathway of complement. Such patients should be treated as aHUS [12].

Hematologic Manifestations of STEC HUS

Commonly, the hemoglobin level drops precipitously to <80 g/L with a nadir of <60 g/L. Hemolysis is accompanied by a rapid fall of platelet numbers, usually <50, at times $<30 \times 10^9$/L. Direct and indirect Coombs (antiglobulin) tests are negative. Rising indirect bilirubin, free plasma hemoglobin and serum lactate dehydrogenase (LDH) (the latter often more than five times the upper normal), and haptoglobin depletion are consistent with a rapid hemolytic process. The peripheral white blood cell (neutrophil) count, already increased during the colitis phase, may continue to rise and, if associated

with a leukemoid reaction, can herald a severe course with poor intestinal or renal outcome [68, 308, 410]. The severity of anemia and thrombocytopenia does not correlate with the degree of acute or chronic kidney injury. Some authors noted an inverse relationship between hematocrit (Hb level) and disease severity [410, 411]. A plausible explanation for the latter observation is the hemoconcentration seen in patients with intravascular volume depletion during the first 4 days of STEC colitis [402, 410]. A retrospective study of 137 children with STEC-HUS from Argentina, performed to determine whether dehydration at admission is associated with an increased need for dialysis, indeed showed that "dehydrated" children had a higher rate of vomiting and an increased risk of being dialysed than normovolemic children (70.6 versus 40.7 %, $P = 0.0007$) [412].

Thrombocytopenia and active hemolysis usually resolve within 2 weeks. Indeed, a rising platelet count heralds the cessation of active HUS; platelets may transiently rebound to $>500 \times 10^9$/L. Anemia can persist for weeks after disease recovery without signs of active hemolysis.

AKI in HUS

Renal injury in HUS ranges from microscopic hematuria and proteinuria to severe renal failure and oligoanuria. Up to 50 % of children with STEC-HUS will need acute dialysis [67, 68, 413]. Arterial hypertension is common in the acute phase of HUS and may not be volume-dependent. Blood pressure instability and hypotension with ongoing fever is not a typical feature of STEC-HUS and should raise the suspicion of primary sepsis, complicated by thrombocytopenia and hemolysis, or sepsis from gangrenous (perforating) colitis and peritonitis. Time to recovery of kidney function ranges from a few days to weeks or even months. The risk of long-term renal impairment (CKD, chronic hypertension) increases with the duration of oliguria (dialysis). A commonly cited threshold for the risk of diminished renal recovery is 2–3 weeks [414, 415]. Primary endstage renal disease (ESRD) is rare and should prompt investigations into a genetic or atypical form of HUS. The results will inform the planning of future kidney transplantation [244, 416].

Extrarenal Manifestations

There is hardly an organ system that has not been affected in STEC infection or HUS. Clinically rare, but important extrarenal and extraintestinal manifestations include myocarditis and (congestive) heart failure, cardiac tamponade, pulmonary hemorrhage, pancreatitis and hepatic involvement, and CNS complications [417–428]. Patients with multiple organ involvement generally also have severe renal injury and often a poor outcome [389, 418, 426]. Postulated mechanisms underlying organ injury in HUS are Stx load and direct tissue toxicity and/or microvascular thrombosis and ischemic injury [418]. Histological and morphological evidence is largely based on autopsy findings (see below).

Rectal prolapse and intussusception may result in transmural bowel necrosis with perforation and peritonitis [429, 430]. In a large study from Argentina, 35 of 987 children with post-diarrheal HUS underwent abdominal surgery requiring bowel resection in 17. Transverse and ascending colon were most frequently affected. Bowel necrosis was noted in 18 and perforation in 12 patients by macroscopic evaluation; histologically, transmural necrosis was present in 21 patients [431].

Serum amylase and lipase activities, considered evidence of exocrine pancreatopathy, are elevated in up to 20 % of patients [429]. Islet injury with transient glucose intolerance or, albeit rare, chronic insulin-dependent diabetes mellitus has been reported [424, 430, 432, 433]. Hepatomegaly and/or rising serum alanine amino transferase (ALT) are noted in up to 40 % of cases; high serum LDH activities may originate not only from RBC lysis, but also from solid tissue ischemia, specifically of liver and skeletal muscle [434]. Acute myocardial insufficiency occurs in less than 1 % of cases [418, 421, 422, 435]. Elevated troponin levels may reflect the degree of myocardial ischemia [436, 437]. Skeletal muscle involvement is exceedingly rare and may manifest as rhabdomyolysis.

The reported incidence of central nervous system (CNS) manifestations varies widely, between 3 % and >41 % [313, 438]. Most case series are retrospective, with variable definitions of CNS injury, frequency and timing of imaging or EEG, or neurological and psychological testing [423, 438–442]. Signs and symptoms can be vague and nonspecific, and are probably underappreciated. Patients may present with irritability, lethargy or decreased level of consciousness; short seizures are relatively common and may reflect fluid and electrolyte imbalances related to AKI and inadequate volume replacement. Abnormal electroencephalograms have been reported in up to 50 % of patients with HUS. Prolonged seizure activity, usually associated with acute respiratory deterioration or palsy, is an ominous sign and may indicate a cerebral stroke or hemorrhage. Acute, transient or persistent (isolated) palsy, dysphasia, diplopia, retinal injury or cortical blindness has been noted [426, 438]. Evident neurological complications or "catastrophic" events are associated with a poor prognosis [426, 439]. Identification of clinical parameters predicting severe neurological events is desirable. A proposed composite score including WBC count, and serum sodium, total protein and CRP concentrations during "early" HUS [441] needs independent validation in a better defined, prospective cohort.

Magnetic resonance imaging (MRI) of the brain is helpful in the differentiation of structural from ischemic or transient injury. However, the predictive value of MRI findings in STEC-HUS remains to be confirmed [427, 443]. In the acute phase, basal ganglia and white matter abnormalities with apparent diffusion coefficient (ADC) restriction are a common and reversible MRI finding. They consist characteristically of bilateral hyperintensities on diffusion-weighted imaging and T2-weighted sequences located in the basal ganglia and thalami, and can extend to the white matter [443]; they can be associated with decreased signal intensity on T1-weighted images of basal ganglia, thalami, and brainstem [427, 428, 443–446] (Fig. 26.6a–f). However, the described changes do not appear to be specific for

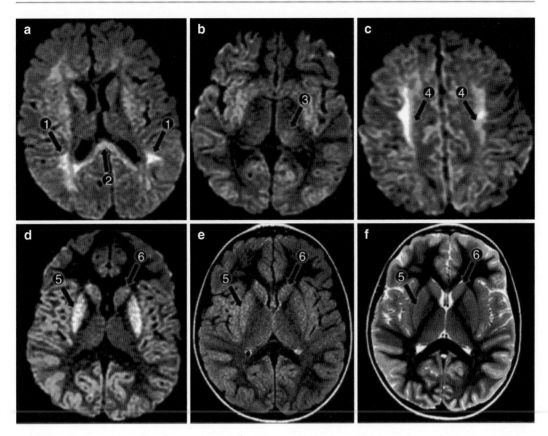

Fig. 26.6 Brain magnetic resonance imaging (MRI) of patients with STEC-HUS acquired within the first 24 h after the onset of neurological symptoms. (**a–d**) Diffusion-weighted images (DWI) which demonstrate (*1*) hypersignal involving deep white matter; (*2*) corpus callosum; (*3*) thalamus, (*4*) centrum semiovale; (*5*) putamen; and (*6*) caudate nucleus. (**d–f**) Brain MRI of one of the two patients who died. (**d**) The images of this patient demonstrate deep hypersignal on DWI in putamen (*5*) and caudate nucleus (*6*), that can be detected in T2- (**e**) and fluid-attenuated inversion recovery (FLAIR) (**f**) weighted classical imaging. T2- and FLAIR-weighted images of all the surviving patients were normal (not shown) (Used with permission of John Wiley and Sons from Gitiaux et al. [443])

STEC-HUS and often revert over a period of weeks or months [443]. Images can be variable, with or without ADC decrease due to the presence of posterior reversible encephalopathy syndrome or hemodialysis in addition to primary, Stx or STEC-HUS induced lesions [443].

The *E. coli* O104:H4 HUS outbreak in Europe also highlighted the occurrence of psychiatric symptoms [447, 448]. Described manifestations include cognitive impairment [449] and, in a few cases, hallucinations, and affective disorders, such as severe panic attacks. Psychiatric symptoms were associated with higher age ($P < 0.0001$),

higher degree of inflammation (level of CRP) ($P < 0.05$), and positive family history of heart disease ($P < 0.05$) [447].

Renal Pathology

Few pathological descriptions are available from renal biopsies of patients with acute STEC HUS [130, 268, 300, 450–452]. Patients with a clinical diagnosis of HUS are not routinely biopsied, except in cases of progressive or chronic renal injury. Most pathological reports have been published prior to 1990, and they do not distinguish between colitis (Stx-) associated and other forms of HUS.

Macroscopically, the kidneys may appear swollen, with numerous petechial hemorrhages on the external surface; on section, the cortex will show areas of hemorrhage and infarction. Focal hemorrhage has also been noted in the collecting system and ureters (Chantal Bernard, unpublished communication).

Prominent *light microscopic* features are the presence of fragmented RBC in *glomerular* capillary loops. Glomerular capillary and renal arteriolar (microvascular) thrombosis may demonstrate prominent fibrin staining, but their extent varies considerably. Endothelial and mesangial cell changes are also evident by *electron microscopy* (Fig. 26.7a–c).

Immunofluorescence is variably positive for fibrin. Immune deposits containing immunoglobulins and/or C1q, C3 or C4 are not a feature of STEC-HUS.

While glomerular histological changes dominate, the *tubulo-interstitial compartment* can also be affected. In fact, all biopsies from a series of patients during the 2011 German HUS outbreak, including those without evidence of TMA, showed severe acute tubular injury [300]. Apoptosis of renal tubular cells has been noted in a few reported cases [266, 452]. Renal cortical "necrosis" and tubular destruction has been shown in cases of clinically severe kidney injury. While the tubulo-interstitial changes are reminiscent of a mouse model of Stx-induced renal injury [297, 299],

the mechanism underlying these changes has not been determined in human HUS.

Extrarenal Histopathological Aspects

Few histopathological descriptions are available of Stx-mediated changes in extrarenal tissue, mostly post-mortem (autopsy) studies that variably include colon, CNS, pancreas, skeletal and myocardium [450, 451, 453]. These findings demonstrate that STEC-HUS is a systemic disease (microangiopathy) characterized by endothelial cell swelling and injury.

The most consistent changes are demonstrated in the gut: the colon (and rectum) shows diffuse hemorrhagic colitis with mucoal ulcerations and hemorrhagic infiltration of the bowel wall as well as congestion of the serosa and extensive vascular thrombosis. Changes of the small bowel consist of submucosal edema with congested mucosa, with or without intussusception, but may also show the presence of TMA [450]. The pancreas may appear enlarged and swollen, with areas of necrosis and haemorrhage (Chantal Bernard, unpublished observations). Changes in lung and heart may not be specific and may reflect complications prior to death. Descriptions of central nervous system changes in STEC-HUS are scarce. Reported findings consist of brain swelling and bilateral, symmetrical necrotic lesions mainly of the corpus striatum (putamen, globus pallidus) and scattered necrotic lesions in the cortex and other cerebral structures [454].

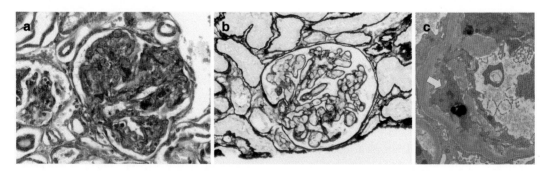

Fig. 26.7 Kidney biopsy, culture-proven STEC-HUS. (**a**) Trichrome stain of glomerulus showing fibrin and RBCs (*orange* and *red*, respectively). (**b**) Silver stain, emphasizing glomerular and tubulular basement membrane structures. (**c**) Electron microscopy; a glomerular capillary is shown. *Arrow* indicates fibrin and proteinaceous material pushing toward the capillary lumen and creating the impression of double contours of the glomerular basement membrane (Courtesy of Dr. Natacha Patey CHU Ste-Justine)

Prevention and Treatment of STEC Disease

There is currently no specific therapy for STEC colitis or STEC-HUS. Nevertheless, best supportive treatment [455] mitigates – if not the development of HUS – at least the severity of the illness and its complications. STEC colitis is a medical emergency [372]. Prompt diagnosis of STEC infection allows initiation of supportive treatment, monitor for signs of HUS, and limit the spread of the organism. In a broader context, the definitive etiological diagnosis, i.e., the isolation and characterization of the infecting organism, is essential for the recognition and control of outbreaks.

Prevention of STEC Infection

Exposure Prophylaxis

Treatment of Stx-HUS starts with the prevention of STEC (STPB) infections. Preventive strategies focus on the implementation of hygienic measures. This applies to cattle farming, the management of drinking water and agricultural produce, and safe practices of food preparation and consumption to containment of the spread of the organism in case of recognized infections [349, 456–459]. The UK Health Protection Agency has established guidelines aimed at the reduction of person-to-person transmission for healthcare providers [460, 461]. The risk of transmission is reduced by adherence to essential hygiene (frequent hand washing and avoiding of touching the face) [458]. Children with proven STEC infection should only return to childcare or school 48 h after the cessation of diarrhea. A thorough review of preventive measures and advice for patients and caregivers can be found in various publications [457, 458, 462, 463].

Vaccines

Active immunization of humans, targeting the O157 LPS antigen [464, 465] and/or Stx and other bacterial antigens [466, 467] remains an elusive goal [468, 469]. Progress has been reported, however, in the vaccination of cattle, e.g., targeting type III secreted proteins, siderophore receptor, porin and intimin [470–472]. Mice and goats, immunized with a promising novel fusion protein, termed Stx2B–Tir–Stx1B–Zot, that carries the immunogenic Stx1 and Stx2 B-subunits, the intimin receptor Tir, and the *Vibrio cholerae* bacteriophage-derived zonula occludens toxin (Zot) which reversibly increases mucosal permeability and acts as mucosal adjuvant, showed substantially reduced colonization and shedding of *E. coli* O157:H7 [473, 474].

Therapeutic Interventions During STEC Colitis

Considerable work has been invested to better understand factors that facilitate the progression from colitis to HUS and to intervene at a stage where the process can be reversed and HUS prevented or at least, ameliorated. Potential strategies are the elimination of STPB from the gut, the binding of free Stx prior to its translocation into the circulation and/or neutralization in the blood stream, thus minimizing the amount of toxin injuring the vascular endothelium. Additional strategies have targeted the coagulation system to prevent microvascular thrombosis and ischemia. Although some of the earlier trials were underpowered, none of these strategies have shown convincing results or promising clinical signals [244, 475, 476]. The conduction of definitive, randomized controlled HUS prevention trials of any intervention in a conventional format is extremely challenging due to the low prevalence of STEC infections and the overall low risk of progression to HUS [153, 403, 477, 478].

Volume Therapy

Volume expansion with isotonic saline administered intravenously during early STEC colitis may ameliorate the severity of HUS. In a retrospective cohort study of 29 unselected children with *E. coli* O157:H7 HUS, Tarr and his group [402] showed that patients who became oligoanuric and needed dialysis had received significantly less intravenous fluid during the first 4 days of diarrhea than children who had preserved urine output and who were not dialyzed. The authors concluded that early parenteral volume expansion before the onset of HUS attenuates

AKI and reduces the need for dialysis. The original findings were reproduced in a prospective multicenter cohort of 50 children with STEC O157:H7 colitis. The treated group received a median volume of 1.7 (0–7.5) vs. 0 (0–4.9) L/m^2 ($P=0.02$) and 189 (0–483) vs. 0 (0–755) mmol sodium/m^2 surface area ($P=0.05$). None of the enrolled patients required ventilatory assistance because of acute pulmonary edema or other volume-related complications [403]. The authors postulated that the oligoanuria of HUS results from renal parenchymal hypoperfusion and ischemia using the analogy of myocardial infarction; and that intravenous volume expansion is an underused intervention that has the potential to decrease the frequency of oligoanuric renal failure in patients at risk of HUS [403]. Support for the "volume hypothesis" comes from an independent study from Argentina [479] and observations linking higher Hb concentrations at presentation with severe HUS, including neurological complications [405, 411].

The administration of isotonic solutions is not expected to affect bacterial toxin production, delivery into the circulation and target tissue binding; however, the intended alleviation of incipient AKI is plausible in view of similar strategies commonly used to prevent or ameliorate acute tubular necrosis and AKI in other scenarios involving potentially nephrotoxic agents [480, 481]. In addition, there are hints that saline infusion may also mitigate the abdominal cramps caused by STEC induced ischemic colitis [482].

Figure 26.8 shows an abbreviated, practical algorithm to estimate the individual child's risk of HUS, initial (minimal) investigations (stool

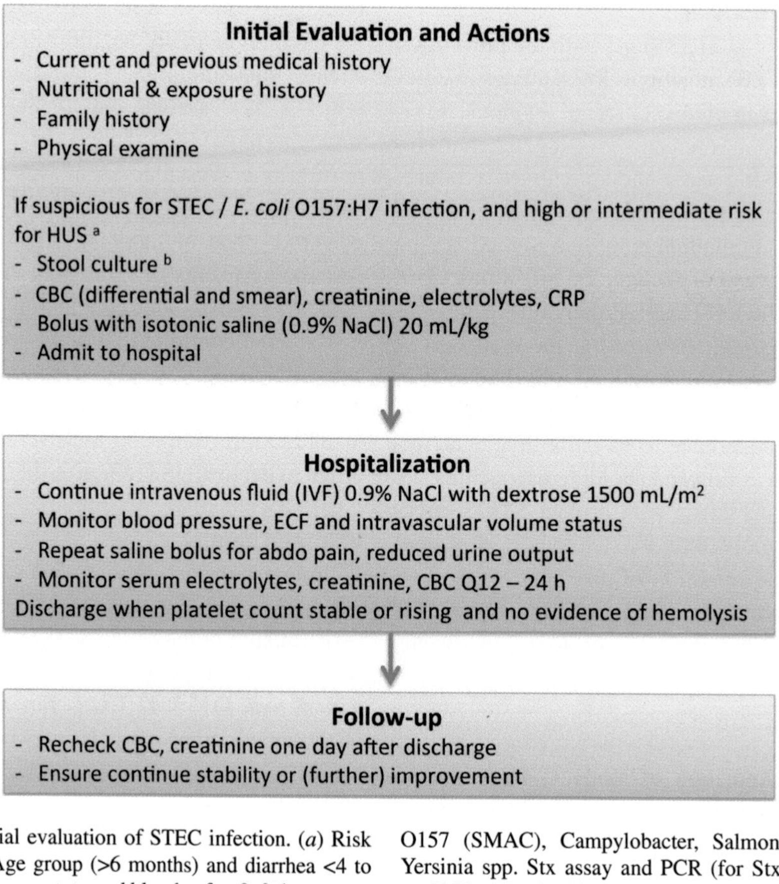

Fig. 26.8 Initial evaluation of STEC infection. (*a*) Risk of Stx HUS: Age group (>6 months) and diarrhea <4 to 7 days that is frequent, turned bloody after 2–3 days, associated with abdominal cramps, or recent HC/HUS in family of community. (*b*) Culture stool for (at least): E. coli O157 (SMAC), Campylobacter, Salmonella, Shigella, Yersinia spp. Stx assay and PCR (for Stx sequences) if available (Used with permission of AGA Institute from Holtz et al. [372])

culture, CBC, renal function, and electrolytes) and the size of the isotonic saline bolus (20 mL/kg body weight) as soon as STEC colitis is diagnosed or suspected [65, 372]. The risk of fluid overload and cardiopulmonary complications due to saline infusion is minimal, provided the patient is hospitalized and supervised diligently by an experienced team [403]. Hospital admission does not only simplify patient monitoring, it may also alleviate parental anxiety and reduce the spreading of the potentially dangerous organisms from the family and community (see above) [349, 350].

Analgesia

Abdominal, typically cramping pain can be severe. Where volume expansion with isotonic saline fails to alleviate the ischemic colitis pain, pharmacological therapy may be warranted. Acetaminophen can be tried, unless there is evidence of hepatopathy. Morphine, found to be effective in children with severe abdominal pain due other etiologies [483], may be administered sparingly, although it tends to worsen post-colitis constipation or ileus. Although there are no separate studies about the effect of morphine in STEC colitis, antimotility drugs in general have been associated with adverse outcome (see below).

Anti-motility Drugs and NSAIDs

Cimolai et al. reported, in a retrospective review of 91 children with HUS from British Columbia, that the prolonged use (>24 h) of a variety of antimotility drugs collectively increased the risk of central nervous system complications, including seizures, encephalopathy or death (multivariate analysis; OR 8.5, 95 % $CI_{95\%}$ 1.7–42.8) [405]. A subsequent study of 118 children with STEC colitis (28 with HUS) from the same center revealed that the prolonged use of antidiarrheal agents was associated with development of HUS (multivariate analysis; relative risk 44.1; $CI_{95\%}$ 8.5–229.4) [484]. An independent analysis of 278 children with HUS from the US confirmed the association between antimotility drug use and HUS (OR 2.9; $CI_{95\%}$ 1.2–7.5) [125].

Antimotility drugs do not shorten the duration of diarrhea; their use may prolong bloody diarrhea and increase the risk of systemic complications and should therefore be avoided [125, 485].

Non-steroidal anti-inflammatory analgesic drugs (NSAIDs) have no place in the treatment of patients with STEC colitis or HUS who are often intravascularly volume depleted and at risk of ischemic injury of the gastrointestinal (GI) tract and the kidneys [115, 125, 486–490]. NSAIDs impair renal perfusion and glomerular filtration, and increase the risk of intestinal bleeding.

Antibiotic Therapy of STEC Infection

It is widely accepted that patients with STEC colitis should not be treated with antibiotics. This recommendation is based on clinical observations linking antimicrobial therapy to an increased HUS risk and fatal outcomes [65, 347, 380, 491] and supported by experimental studies demonstrating that certain antibiotics stimulate Stx phage induction and toxin production. Stx induction can occur at levels below or above the minimal inhibitory concentrations of these antibiotics [345, 492, 493].

There is only one published randomized and placebo-controlled trial assessing the efficacy of antibiotics to prevent HUS, by Proulx et al. [494]: 47 children with E. coli O157:H7 colitis (mean age 5.3 years, range 3 months to 17.8 years) received TMP/SMX 4/20 mg/kg/dose twice daily (n=22) or placebo (n=25) for 5 days. The relative HUS risk in the treatment group was 0.57 (CI 0.09–3.46, p=0.67). The study was underpowered and treatment allocation was not concealed. Importantly, the mean time to treatment initiation was 7 days from the onset of diarrhea, which may have been too late to influence the evolution of the disease (Fig. 26.5) [115, 129].

A multicenter, prospective registry study of 259 children with E. coli O157:H7 infection, with laboratory signs of TMA and the occurrence of oligoanuric HUS as primary and secondary endpoints, respectively, showed that children treated with antibiotics during the first week of diarrhea progressed more often to HUS than those who did not receive antibiotics (multivariable analysis; adjusted Odd's ratio 3.62; $CI_{95\%}$ 1.23–10.6). Antibiotic use was further associated with the development of oligoanuric HUS

[347, 404]. When authors compared different antibiotic classes, the association with HUS remained significant for cotrimoxazole and metronidazole, but not for betalactams or azithromycin. Antibiotic therapy also failed to shorten the duration of gastrointestinal symptoms [404]. The latter analysis replicated the results of a retrospective case-control study of an institutional outbreak of STEC O157:H7 HUS, where eight residents developed HUS; five of these eight patients had received TMP/SMX compared to none of the seven residents with diarrhea, whose colitis was not complicated by HUS ($p = 0.026$). As the authors point out, antimicrobial treatment may have been given to patients with more severe illness [70].

Two systematic reviews [495, 496] contend that antibiotics confer neither benefit nor a risk of complications. An instructive, prospective cohort study [390] originated from the 1996 outbreak of *E. coli* O157:H7 infection among school children via contaminated bean sprout in Sakai City, Japan, where antibiotics were used extensively during the diarrhea phase [102]. Children infected with the outbreak strain, who were given fosfomycin within the first 2 days of illness (diarrhea), developed HUS significantly less often than those who did not receive antibiotics (adjusted OR 0.15; $CI_{95\%}$ 0.03–0.78). In contrast, fosfomycin started on and after the third day of illness was not associated with HUS prevention [390]. Others suggested a beneficial effect of oral fluoroquinolones compared with IV or PO fosfomycin during the same outbreak [497]. While the latter (retrospective) study has important limitations, it draws attention to the difficulties predicting minimal inhibitory (MIC) and sub-inhibitory concentrations in the (anaerobic) milieu of the gut.

During the enteroaggregative/Stx producing *E. coli* O104:H4 epidemic in Germany, one center chose a deliberately aggressive approach combining intravenous meropenem and ciprofloxacin (and additional oral rifaximin for those admitted to the intensive care unit) [141]. The duration of STEC excretion appears to have been shortened from 22.6 to 14.8 days in patients treated with antibiotics after the diagnosis of HUS [141, 498]. The authors emphasized the

presence of less morbidity, including fewer neurological complications (seizures), and a reduced mortality rate [141]. Another cohort study from the same epidemic comprised 65 patients, 22 receiving oral azithromycin and 43 no antibiotics. STEC shedding >28 days was observed in 1 of the 22 treated patients (4.5 %; $CI_{95\%}$, 0–13.3 %) compared with 35 untreated patients (81.4 %; $CI_{95\%}$ 69.8–93.0 %) ($P < 0.001$) [498].

It should be emphasized that fluoroquinolones represent the one class of antibiotics consistently found to stimulate toxin production (mainly Stx2) *in vitro* and in experimental animal models, and that little is known about the interaction of co-administered antibiotics. Furthermore, the outbreak strain represents a unique hybrid pathogen (enteroaggregative Stx producing *E. coli*), and most patients described in the above studies were treated after the diagnosis of HUS.

Rifaximin, a semisynthetic derivative of rifamycin with minimal oral bioavailability and proven efficacy in the prevention and treatment of enterotoxic *E. coli* (traveler's diarrhea) [499–501] that interferes with (bacterial) transcription by binding to the β-subunit of bacterial RNA polymerase is an interesting agent for further studies in patients with STEC infection, as is chloramphenicol – although fallen out of favor in Western countries for its rare, but severe hematological adverse effects – due to its suppression of Stx phage induction, *stx2* transcription, and Stx2 production in a number of STPB strains [324].

The potential importance of the interactions of antibiotics and other phage-activating agents *in vivo* has been demonstrated in mouse models of STEC disease. While fluoroquinolones and fosfomycin, given to mice infected with *E. coli* O157:H7, resulted in reduced excretion of the colonizing STEC strain, ciprofloxacin – but not fosfomycin – markedly increased both the presence of free fecal Stx and lethality in the treated animals. Ciprofloxacin treatment also enhanced the transfer of *Stx2* prophage to other *E. coli* the gut [502].

In a mouse model of STEC encephalopathy, oral administration of a single azithromycin dose 2 h after the oral instillation of a 100 % lethal infective dose of the Stx2c-producing STEC strain E325211/HSC protected all animals. Using the same model, fosfomycin, ofloxacin and ciprofloxacin failed to protect STEC infected mice, while kanamycin and norfloxacin improved survival, albeit less effectively than azithromycin [503]. Similar results were shown in the gnotobiotic piglet model of oral Stx2 (but not Stx1) producing STEC O157:H7 infection [504].

Novel, non-antibiotic agents are on the horizon and may offer an alternative strategy. One such experimental compound is phenethyl isothiocyanate (PEITC), a dietary anticancer compound derived from common vegetables [505, 506]. It has been shown *in vitro* to suppress STEC growth, phage induction and Stx production by effecting a stringent bacterial response mediated by massive production of a global regulator, guanosine tetraphosphate (ppGpp) [507].

Consensus on the use of antimicrobial therapy in children with hemorrhagic colitis is lacking and the hypothetical benefit of antibiotics in the prevention of STEC HUS remains controversial. Controlled, prospective studies with select antimicrobial agents are necessary to resolve this important caveat [508, 509]. Rifaximin and few other agents, such as azithromycin or fosfomycin may be suitable to limit the spread of the organism and, potentially, to reduce the rate of complications during STEC epidemics. Based on the experience during the Sakai outbreak in Japan, the antibiotic should be given immediately, i.e., within 48 h after the onset of diarrhea to be effective [390]. Only agents that do not induce a bacterial SOS response or augment Stx production at any concentration should be used [141, 324, 510]. All other antimicrobial agents should be discontinued after STEC identification if already started [115, 509, 511]. Until additional data become available, caution is advised in prescribing antibiotics empirically to children with bloody diarrhea, except in *Shigella dysentereriae* endemic regions.

STEC-HUS: Therapy and Management

The presence of diarrhea ("D+ HUS") is not synonymous with STEC (Stx, enteropathogenic)

HUS; a rigorous search for the etiology of any HUS is important for therapeutic decision-making and the prognosis. Any patient with a second episode of HUS or with an "asynchronous" family history of HUS and (thorough) exclusion of STEC infection (Table 26.3) should be screened for genetic mutations of complement regulatory and related proteins as well as for ADAMTS13 activity, and presumptively diagnosed and treated as "atypical HUS" [12]. As the recent discovery of a (homozygous) mutation in the gene encoding the protein triacylglycerol kinase epsilon (*DGKE*) among patients with infantile aHUS showed, additional causes of (a)HUS will be identified with time.

Current Therapeutic Approach and Best Supportive Care

Symptomatic treatment of manifest HUS follows general principles established for patients with AKI, however with some specific recommendations related to the often rapid hemolytic process and thrombocytopenia. All patients need careful monitoring of vital signs, fluid intake and excretion, and signs of cardiac, respiratory and neurological deterioration. Treatment focuses on the stabilization of vital functions, intravascular volume status, acid-base, serum electrolytes (potassium, sodium, calcium and phosphate) and uric acid. Patients may develop pleural or pericardial effusion, or cardiac insufficiency, in addition to potentially serious complications of the colitis, requiring careful monitoring and intervention. As with other critically ill children, nutrition – already compromised during the diarrhea phase – is part of the treatment.

In the wake of the German 2011 HUS outbreak, "best supportive care" for patients with HUS was defined as "volume replacement, parenteral nutrition and dialysis" [455, 508]. This care is best provided in a center with experienced (pediatric) nephrologists where extracorporeal purification techniques and a Critical Care environment can be provided around the clock. Referral to such a center early in the disease course is strongly recommended.

Management of Hematological Manifestations

The large majority of patients with HUS receive packed red blood cells [413]. The threshold for PRBC infusions is clinically defined: symptoms (tachycardia and tachypnea) and/or the velocity of intravascular RBC destruction as gauged by frequent Hb determinations, rising LDH and free plasma Hb levels. A practical cut-off is a Hb of 60 g/L (hematocrit <18%). Twelve to 15 mL of PRBC per kg body weight can be transfused over 2–4 h; a loop diuretic can be given in case of fluid overload or hyperkalemia (such as furosemide 0.5 mg/kg IV). If necessary, PRBC transfusions can be timed to coincide with hemodialysis sessions, particularly if hyperkalemia or volume overload are a concern, or when a blood prime is needed for (small) children undergoing HD. PRBCs should be deplete of leucocytes and platelets, as practiced in most pediatric hospitals. Transfusion of PRBC and platelets has to be weighed against the HLA alloimmunization risk, particularly in children with severe AKI who may not recover kidney function.

Erythropoiesis-stimulating agents (ESA) may provide a benefit beyond the reduction of PRBC transfusions [512]. However, a more recent study from South America failed to demonstrate a difference in the number and frequency of blood transfusions following the use of ESA [513].

Platelet transfusions during the acute HUS phase should be limited to (rare) active bleeding and to (some) surgical procedures. A reptrospective, single-center cohort analysis of children with acute HUS requiring dialysis access, revealed no difference with respect to bleeding complications or catheter survival in patients who did (30%) or did not receive platelets (70%) prior to the procedure [514]; the authors concluded that peritoneal and central venous catheter placement can be accomplished safely in most children with HUS, without a need for platelet transfusion, despite the associated thrombocytopenia. Previously expressed concerns that transfused platelets accelerate microvascular thrombus formation and promote tissue ischemia as reported in adulthood TTP [515, 516] have not

born out in practice [479]. Platelets may be concentrated (volume-reduced) to avoid fluid overload; however, most oliguric patients will need dialysis, making this a lesser concern.

AKI Management in HUS

AKI treatment pertains to the management of fluids and electrolytes, hypertension and nutrition. About 50% of children with eHUS will need some form of renal replacement therapy.

Fluid and Electrolyte Management

Assessment of intravascular volume status helps guide initial treatment toward fluid replacement or restriction, and administration of diuretics or dialysis. Patients are monitored for fluid intake and changes in urine output, along with frequent measurements of BP and heart rate. Weight changes correlate poorly with effective circulatory volume. Intravascular volume may be decreased secondary to intestinal losses and reduced oral intake during the early phase of the disease and may result in hypoperfusion of the kidneys. Third spacing, especially in the gut, and generalized edema – due to endothelial injury and capillary leak – may mask intravascular depletion and, if not corrected, aggravate ischemic injury. Patients warrant diligent intravascular volume expansion to improve organ perfusion, particularly of the gut, kidneys and brain. Systemic hypotension is rare and should raise suspicion of an alternative diagnosis or secondary sepsis, e.g., from gangrenous colitis or line infection.

Fluid restriction may be necessary in patients with fluid overload secondary to oliguric renal failure. If intravascular volume is replete, a trial with furosemide at a dose of 1–2 mg/kg may be attempted to induce diuresis and delay dialysis, particularly in patients with pulmonary or cardiac compromise, or to bridge the time to catheter placement.

Aggressive challenge with high-dose loop diuretics has been advocated in the past to prevent progression to oligoanuric failure and avoid dialysis [517]. However, clinical trials and meta-analyses of studies in patients with AKI due to a variety etiologies, primarily in intensive care settings, have failed to document a beneficial effect of furosemide on short or long-term renal outcome [518–520].

It seems best to follow a pragmatic path and use a loop diuretic to bridge the time to safe hemo- or peritoneal dialysis catheter placement while avoiding harm (toxicity, intravascular volume depletion). General indications to initiate RRT are electrolyte disturbances including hyperkalemia, hyperphosphatemia and metabolic acidosis; fluid overload unresponsive to medical treatment; and symptomatic azotemia. Some investigators believe that hyperuricemia contributes to renal function deterioration and discuss the benefit of removing uric acid [521, 522].

Antihypertensive Therapy

Arterial hypertension occurs commonly in acute (STEC) HUS. It may be caused by renal microvascular thrombosis, Stx-mediated, direct vascular endothelial cell injury or activation, or intravascular fluid overload. Cerebral complications may contribute to hypertension. Conversely, systemic hypertension can lead to CNS complications, such as posterior reversible leukoencephalopathy syndrome (PRES) [523–526] or facial palsy [527]. PRES and co-existing cerebral vasoconstriction syndrome may also represent manifestations of similar underlying pathophysiologic mechanisms [528].

Although activation of the renin-angiotensin system (RAS) has been invoked [529–531], several clinical and genetic studies have failed to demonstrate a relationship between plasma renin activity and the course of HUS. Specifically, activation of the RAS in HUS was noted to occur irrespective of hypertension [532]. While the interpretation of renin measurements is complicated by physiological, age-related differences [533], hypertension in HUS does not appear to be directly linked to RAS activation. Furthermore, earlier studies also noted that the BP did not correlate well with the estimated degree of hydration in children with HUS [529].

Where antihypertensive therapy is needed during the acute phase of HUS, it is reasonable to use dihydropyridine calcium channel blockers (nifedipine, amlodipine or PO/IV nicardipine). While acute treatment with ACE inhibitors has to be balanced against concerns over the impairment of renal perfusion and hyperkalemia, RAS blockers are a rationale choice for patients with HUS-induced chronic hypertension with or without residual CKD or proteinuria [534–536].

Renal Replacement Therapy

Up to 50 % of children with STEC-HUS will need dialysis treatment [102, 413, 537, 538], but higher rates, up to 70 %, have been reported in registries and select HUS outbreaks [81, 91, 105]. The North American Synsorb Pk® (Synsorb Biotech, Calgary, Canada) trial (Synsorb Biotech, Calgary, Canada) protocol mandated that dialysis be delayed until 72 h post diagnosis of HUS, if clinically acceptable to the responsible physician. Under these restrictive conditions, 39 % of the 49 placebo-treated patients were dialyzed for a mean of 3.6 days [413].

There is no evidence that early dialysis changes the evolution of acute eHUS or long-term outcome. However, delaying dialysis unduly increases the risk of complications of kidney injury. Indications for dialysis initiation in HUS are similar to those for other causes of AKI and may evolve rapidly: severe electrolyte imbalance (hyperkalemia, hyperphosphatemia), acidosis or fluid overload refractory to medical/diuretic therapy, symptomatic uremia and, possibly, hyperuricemia. The presence of profound thrombocytopenia, anemia and (rare) gangrenous colitis will influence the choice of dialysis modality and anticoagulation.

Dialysis Modality

The choice of the dialysis technique depends on patient-related, clinical and practical aspects, such as availability of HD and adequately trained personnel, patient size for (central) access creation, local preference and experience, particularly when dialyzing young children and infants. Factors favoring PD are young age (infants), lack of pediatric-trained HD facilities, and avoidance of anticoagulation. Diarrhea or colitis is not considered a contraindication for PD [153, 413].

Continuous Renal Replacement Therapy (CRRT)

CRRT is rarely needed, but may offer an alternative approach to conventional dialysis in children who present contraindications to PD or where PD has failed. HUS patients with severe fluid overload, cardiovascular instability, with or without sepsis, and multiorgan failure may benefit from CRRT. "Slow" hemodialysis offers an alternative where CRRT is not possible. Both are typically performed in a critical care setting. During the acute stage, when patients are thrombocytopenic, HD and CRRT can be tried with minimal heparin, provided there is sufficient blood flow. Regional, citrate-based anticoagulation offers an alternative to heparin, specifically in patients with cerebral stroke or hemorrhage, or after surgery.

Apheresis Modalities

Plasma Exchange (PE) Therapy

Some pediatric centers consider severe, life-threatening STEC-HUS an indication for PE as "rescue" therapy, especially in patients with CNS complications [153, 539]; this approach may have been influenced by the success of PE in patients with TTP (see below). However, the benefit of PE in eHUS remains unproven [476, 540–542], unless aHUS is suspected [348]. The European Paediatric Study Group for HUS excluded other forms, specifically STEC-HUS, from this form of invasive therapy [348]. In young children, PE necessitates the insertion of a large-bore central venous access (hemodialysis line), which confers additional morbidity to children not already undergoing HD [409].

Although PE has no proven benefit in children with STEC-HUS, it is commonly used in the treatment of adult patients. Reports of its efficacy in (adult) patients with STEC-HUS are limited to uncontrolled observations, including data published after the Scotland outbreak [133, 543–546], and none of the more recent (adult) recommendations to initiate PE [543, 544, 546] is based on controlled trials [508]. Nevertheless, large-scale PE administration occurred during the E. coli O104:H4 epidemic.

One reason for this variation in practice between pediatric and adult nephrologists is the traditional view of HUS as part of the TTP spectrum ("HUS/TTP") [547–549]. The previously dismal prognosis of (classical) TTP [550], now known to be caused by anti-ADAMTS13 (auto) antibodies [551–553], has improved dramatically with the introduction of intensive PE therapy (and immunosuppression) [554, 555].

A careful, comprehensive analysis of the treatment strategies during the E. coli O104:H4 HUS outbreak concluded that PE failed to improve the outcome of adult HUS patients [141], Furthermore (and in keeping with the pediatric experience [409]), prolonged PE was found to be potentially harmful [104, 476]. Consequently, the latest, 2013 guidelines on the use of apheresis by the American Society for Apheresis (ASFA) categorized STEC-HUS as a disorder where apheresis treatment is ineffective or harmful (category IV) with 1C evidence [556].

Hypothetically, PE would remove inflammatory mediators, bacterial toxins and plasma microparticles, and – if performed against frozen plasma – replenish coagulation and complement factors [557]. However, the concentration of Stx in the circulation amenable to apheresis is minute due to rapid toxin binding and uptake by endothelial cells. Some authors noted that PE removes platelet- and leukocyte-derived plasma microparticles [288], while others associated the procedure with increased microparticle generation [558, 559]. Although the concept of microparticle removal may be appealing for specific diseases, the pathological importance of (prothrombotic) particles and the benefit of their removal for the outcome of HUS is currently far from clear.

Extracorporeal Immunoabsorption

Immunoabsorption (IA) is a specialized apheresis technique aimed at the removal of IgG from plasma by specific binding to a column loaded with (purified or recombinant) staphylococcal protein A; it has been advocated by some centers for the treatment of HUS associated with severe CNS disease. In a recent, uncontrolled series, the authors speculated that pathogenic (autoimmune

?) antibodies may be responsible for the neurological symptoms in STEC-HUS [560]. While this hypothesis remains to be tested, the usually rapid clinical resolution of acute neurological signs unrelated to detectable infarction or hemorrhage with and without IA (or PE) argues against this speculation.

Antithrombotic and Antiplatelet Agents

Treatment with anticoagulation/antithrombotic agents (heparin, urokinase, or antiplatelet drugs such as aspirin or dipyridamole) has failed to ameliorate the course of HUS or to decrease the mortality rate, neurological events or long-term sequelae [476, 561]. These (negative) findings correspond to experimental Stx-HUS in primates [562, 563]. On the contrary, heparin and antithrombotic agents have been associated with an increased risk of bleeding in at least two trials (RR, 25.9; $CI_{95\%}$ 3.7–183) [476]. However, these earlier studies were underpowered, and interventions started late during the course of the disease. Without a beneficial "signal," none of the latter agents can be currently recommended in the treatment of STEC-HUS [153, 469, 476].

Non-medical Supportive Therapies

Nutritional Support

Appetite and nutritional intake are already limited when infants or children present with HUS due to the preceding colitis, with or without vomiting. Patients usually continue to experience abdominal pain, likely due to ischemia, often with constipation, partial ileus or persistent colitis. Nausea and inability to eat can be accentuated by uremia, surgical intervention and opiates given for pain relief, or by PD. Nutritional support with nasogastric feeding or total parenteral nutrition should be initiated early in the course of the disease. Insulin therapy may be required in case of endocrine pancreatic involvement.

Psychosocial Support

Patient and familial anxiety and (valid) concerns about the disease process, prolonged hospitalization, repeated invasive procedures and the prognosis of the HUS – paired with information in the lay press and the internet, specifically during outbreaks – warrant the support by a social worker or psychologist.

Experimental Therapies and Novel Mechanisms of STEC-HUS

Shiga Toxin Neutralizing Agents

The concept of binding Stx in the blood stream or, preferably, prior to its translocation from the gut into the circulation, is not new. Receptor analogues, e.g., for TNF-α (etanercept), or toxin neutralizing antibodies (e.g., *Clostridium botulinum* or *C. tetani* toxin antibodies) are well established treatment modalities. Animal studies support the feasibility of this approach in STEC disease, at least in an experimental setting [153].

Stx Receptor Analogues

Predicated on its effective toxin binding *in vitro* and a reduction of the fecal toxin load in experimentally infected mice [564, 565] synthetic Gb3 linked to an inert, non-resorbable carrier (Synsorb-Pk®) has been studied in a randomized controlled North American (US/Canada) trial [413]. The investigators hypothesized that the agent, administered orally soon after the diagnosis of HUS, would diminish continued toxin absorption and result in disease amelioration. Primary endpoints were decreased rates of death, serious extrarenal events and dialysis frequency. The trial was stopped when the interim analysis revealed no difference between treatment and placebo groups. Several consideration may explain the negative trial outcome: (a) the binder may not reach the site of toxin production and delivery by STEC that adhere tightly to the mucosa via "attaching and effacing" lesions [566], (b) the binding affinity and capacity may have been insufficient and/or the chosen dose too small, and (c) the timing after HUS onset may have been too late. New, multi-branched (clustered trisaccharide), high-capacity oral and systemic Gb3 analogs (e.g., "Starfish," "Daisy," "Super Twigs") [567–570], peptides that prevent intracellular Stx targeting when bound to the circulating toxin [571–573], and genetically modified, Gb3-expressing *E. coli* and (other) probiotics are being developed [574–576], but no new clinical trial initiatives have been announced or published [154, 155].

Shiga Toxin Antibodies

In murine and newborn piglet models of STEC-HUS, infusion of toxin-neutralizing monoclonal antibodies up to 3 days after orogastric infection protects against hematological and renal disease, but efficacy decreases rapidly with delayed antibody administration [152, 577]. No important adverse effects were noted when the anti-Stx2 antibody TMA-15 (Urtoxazumab) was infused in children with documented STEC colitis [578]. Another phase II trial (NCT01252199, "Shigatec") with a monoclonal antibody combination against Stx1 and 2 (Shigamabs®, Thallion Pharmaceuticals Inc.) [579–581] showed likewise good tolerance [478]. Further development and clinical testing of each antibody product was stalled due to corporate decisions. Newest developments include the generation of highly effective single domain antibodies that recognize and neutralize Stx1 and 2 [582].

The theoretical window for meaningful intervention is narrow. It is still debated if relevant toxin absorption from the gut continues, once HUS has become manifest, and whether toxin neutralization at that stage has any ameliorating effect on the disease course and outcome.

Considering the low incidence of STEC-HUS and the multicentric logistic infrastructure needed to conduct a traditional randomized controlled trial as demanded by the FDA (in 2006) and other regulatory agencies (http://www.fda.gov/ohrms/dockets/ac/07/minutes/2007-4286m1.pdf), despite its orphan drug status (http://www.medscape.com/viewarticle/521133), makes it unlikely that anti-toxin antibodies will become available anytime soon for patients with STEC infection at risk of HUS.

Anticomplement Therapy in STEC-HUS

Complement and STEC-HUS

The potential role of the complement system in the pathogenesis of STEC-HUS gained traction over the past few years. Several events stimulated scientific inquiry and clinical interest: progress in the understanding of atypical HUS caused by genetic or acquired dysregulation of the alternative pathway; availability of a potent, well tolerated anti-complement (anti-C5) antibody (eculizumab); and the eruption of the *E. coli* O104:H4 epidemic in Northern Germany which coincided with a report in the New England Journal describing three children with STEC-HUS and severe CNS involvement who recovered after the infusion of eculizumab [583].

Clinical Observations

Reports of decreased plasma C3 concentrations in children with presumed STEC-HUS appeared since the 1970s [584–586]. The first reports predated the recognition of the central role of STEC infection in children with (typical) HUS. Several authors described glomerular deposition of C3 in (kidney) biopsies obtained during the acute phase of HUS [587]. Nonetheless, the majority of eHUS patients demonstrate C3 serum levels within the reference range. The employment of more sensitive assays confirmed the activation of complement in eHUS. For example, Monnens et al. detected elevated levels of breakdown products of the two components of the alternative pathway C3-convertase, C3 (C3b, C3c, C3d) and CFB (Ba) in the serum of children with "post-diarrhea" HUS [585]. More recently, increased plasma levels of the CFB activation product Bb and the soluble form of the terminal complement complex sC5b-9 were demonstrated in 17 children with acute STEC-HUS that normalized by day 28 of the disease [588]. Comparable results were obtained in a Swedish cohort of 10 children, all of whom displayed elevated C3a and sC5b-9 (terminal complement complex) concentrations in plasma as well as C3 and C9 bearing, mainly platelet-derived microparticles (measured as mean fluorescent intensities) during acute STEC-HUS that normalized with disease recovery [223]. A detailed case study of one patient with acute eHUS by the same authors revealed the presence of C3, Stx2 and LPSO157 on a larger number of platelet-neutrophil and platelet-monocyte complexes (by flow cytometry) compared with healthy controls [223]. The cited findings suggest the recruitment of complement components, together with Stx and bacterial LPS, on the surface of platelets [589] and, to a lesser degree, neutrophils and monocytes, and alternative pathway activation in acute STEC-HUS [223]. Stahl et al. speculated that while complement activation is not the primary event occurring during EHEC infection, it may contribute to blood cell activation and renal injury, through the release of microparticles, free radicals and cytokines. Deposition of the terminal complement complex (TCC or sC5b-9), demonstrated in post-mortem tissue from a child with STEC-HUS (Fig. 26.9a–f) further suggests that complement is activated in this disease.

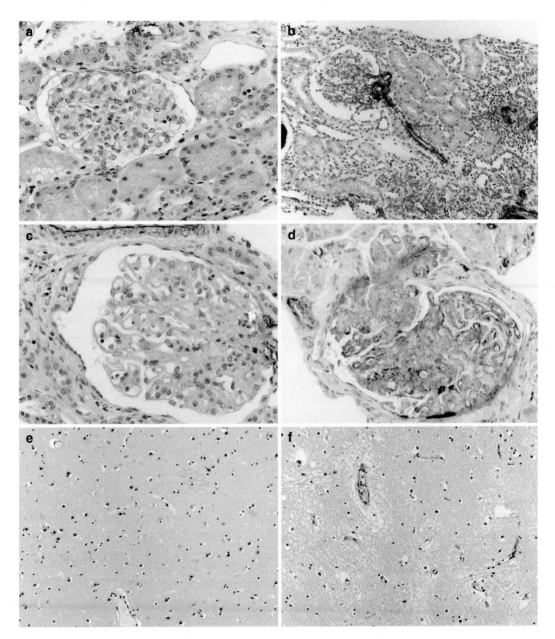

Fig. 26.9 C5b-9 (membrane attack complex, MAC) deposition in kidney and CNS sections of a child who died of STEC O157:H7 HUS. (**a**) Control (kidney). (**b**) Strong staining of renal arteriole and glomerular capillaries with anti-MAC antibody (1:200). (**c**) Staining of afferent and efferent arterioles, minor staining within the glomerulus. (**d**) Ubiquitous glomerular capillary staining with anti-MAC antibody. (**e**) control (brain). (**f**) Staining of cerebral capillaries with anti-MAC antibody (Courtesy of Dr. Natacha Patey CHU Ste-Justine)

Interestingly, no correlation was found between the levels of activated complement products in plasma or on platelet derived microparticles and the presence or absence of renal or extrarenal complications [223, 588].

Experimental Studies

The hypothesis that complement is activated in STEC-HUS has been addressed by several laboratories. Morigi et al. reported that Stx1 induced cultured microvascular endothelial cells to express the membrane adhesion molecule P-selectin which bound and activated C3 (via the alternative pathway). The resultant C3 cleavage generated C3a, a potent chemokine, which conversely upregulated P-selectin expression and thrombus formation under flow conditions, along with a reduction of endothelial cell thrombomodulin (TM) expression [399]. This study confirmed results previously published by others using glomerular endothelial cells [590].

In this animal model, Stx may directly contribute to complement activation: C3 was found to be deposited when Stx1-treated microvascular endothelial cells were exposed to normal human serum [399]. Perfusion of Stx-treated endothelial cells with whole blood led to increased surface thrombus formation compared to monolayers not exposed to toxin; thrombus formation was prevented by the complement inhibitor sCR1. Endothelial complement deposition and loss of thromboresistance was dependent on Stx-induced P-selectin expression and high-affinity C3 binding and alternative pathway activation [399, 591], and was blocked by a P-selectin antibody and the P-selectin soluble ligand PSGL-1. The findings were reproduced in the authors' mouse model of HUS induced by the combined injection of Stx2 and LPS [399]. The absence of CFB (injection of genetically modified mice deficient of CFB with Stx2 and LPS) mitigated the degree of thrombocytopenia and protected against glomerular microangiopathy and renal function impairment, further supporting the involvement of alternative pathway of complement activation in this HUS model [399].

Another mechanism underlying activation in patients with STEC-HUS is the interaction of Stx and LPS with platelets and leucocytes as outlined above [223]. *In vitro* experiments by the same group showed that soon after incubation of human whole blood with purified Stx1 or Stx2 or O157 LPS, platelet-leucocyte complexes and platelet-leucocyte-derived microparticles bearing complement C3 and C9 on their surfaces became detectable, along with the generation of C3a and soluble C5b-9 complex. This effect was enhanced in the presence of LPS compared with Stx alone [223].

Based on experimental studies showing that Stx2 binds CFH, specifically the short consensus repeats (SCRs) 6-8 and SCRs18-20, domains required for CFH surface recognition [592], Würzner and Orth promoted the idea that interference with this functionally and quantitatively most important inhibitor of unregulated AP activation causes – or contributes to – complement activation in STEC-HUS [593]. The same laboratory subsequently demonstrated that CFHR-1 and CFHL-1, complement proteins with partial homology to CFH, also bind Stx2, and compete with Stx2 binding to CFH [593, 594].

The above experimental and human data are at variance with the results reported by Kurosawa and Stearns-Kurosawa's group in Boston, who employed a non-human primate (baboon) model of Stx-TMA that closely resembles human HUS. Importantly, in this model HUS is induced by the infusion of purified Stx without the addition of LPS or TNF-α [400]. To their surprise, the authors failed to discover significant increases in soluble terminal complement complex levels (TCC or SC5b-9) after lethal challenges with Stx1 or Stx2 [595]. Complement activation and disseminated intravascular coagulation (DIC) were, however, evident in baboons with sublethal *E. coli* bacteremia. Complement inhibition with compstatin, a peptide that prevents C3 cleavage and activation, reduced consumptive coagulopathy, inflammation and microvascular thrombosis in the bacteremia model, and improved cardiac and renal function [596, 597]. It should be remembered, however, that bacteremia is not a feature of (typical) childhood STEC-HUS.

The complement system is a fundamental bacterial defense mechanism [595]. Human HUS is characterized by STEC-induced colitis with intestinal injury, hemorrhage and leucocytosis that may contribute to complement activation [595], likely involving C3a and C5a [597, 598]. Further research is warranted to identify complement activation pathways and effectors in human HUS and the therapeutic benefit of various anti-complement agents [595, 599]. Currently available evidence does not support the general use of complement blockers in the treatment of STEC-HUS [141, 600–602].

Thrombomodulin (THBD) and Complement Activation

THBD (CD141) is a multidomain, constitutively expressed endothelial integral membrane type-1 glycoprotein. It acts as receptor for the serine protease thrombin and mediates anticoagulant and antifibrinolytic properties of the endothelium. In addition, it dampens the inflammatory response through its anti-inflammatory properties [603, 604]. TM can also negatively regulate the complement system by accelerating factor I-mediated inactivation of C3b [604, 605].

Inactivating mutations of TM, although exceedingly rare, have been identified in patients with aHUS [606], both in isolation or combined with mutations of cognate complement proteins. Apart from its role in aHUS, evidence is emerging for an involvement of TM in STEC-HUS. Experimental data indicate that TM expression is decreased in Stx2 exposed human glomerular microvascular endothelial cells that had been sensitized with pro-inflammatory mediators [590]. In the Bergamo mouse model of HUS, induced by the combined injection of Stx2 and LPS, reduced glomerular TM expression was observed in association with fibrin and platelets deposition [399]. Zoja et al. further demonstrated that mutation of the lectin-like TM domain worsened murine Stx-HUS [607]. Mice lacking the lectin-like domain exhibited excess glomerular C3 deposition indicating impaired complement regulation and local generation of complement-derived, pro-inflammatory peptides, such as the chemokines C3a and C5a. Binding of C3a to endothelial cells leads to impaired endothelial thromboresistance and may contribute to the TMA in the authors' model [399].

Soluble, recombinant TM (rTM) has been administered successfully to septic patients with DIC [608]. Honda et al. reported the use of rTM-α in a small, uncontrolled series of pediatric patients with severe STEC-HUS [609]. While the authors observed clinical resolution and favorable disease outcome in all three cases, efficacy and benefit of this novel therapeutic agents remain to be established.

Membrane-Bound Regulators of Complement Alternative Pathway

Experiments using cultured glomerular endothelial and immortalized human proximal tubular cells, revealed that Stx "down regulated" the expression of CD59 (protectin), but not of the decay-accelerating factor (DAF, CD55) or membrane cofactor protein (MCP/CD46) [610]. Studies in survivors of E. coli O104:H4 HUS, examined after recovery, showed increased CD59 expression on granulocytes and monocytes. The same group noted, however, abundant CD59 on the patients' RBCs that were studied during the acute HUS [611].

Therapeutic Complement Blockade in STEC-HUS

Eculizumab has been tried as "rescue" therapy in a few patients with severe neurological manifestations of HUS due to E. coli O157:H7 infection. The authors of the first publication detailing this approach reported rapid neurological improvement, which was unexpected considering the natural history of this complication, along with the cessation of hemolysis and normalization of the platelet count [583]. All three patients recovered without neurological or renal sequelae. The generalizability of these encouraging finding remains unclear. Several pediatric and many adult patients with HUS received eculizumab during the E. coli O104:H4 epidemic, mainly on compassionate grounds. Careful analysis of a large cohort from this HUS outbreak comparing the clinical findings and outcomes of patients receiving eculizumab versus "best supportive care", with or without plasma exchange failed to demonstrate that complement blockade with the anti-C5 antibody (or plasma exchange therapy) changed the course of the disease [141].

In the absence of a controlled trial with pre-defined endpoints, it is currently premature to recommend anti-complement therapy for the treatment of (typical) STEC-HUS. Exceptions are patients with a severe, fluctuating or pro-longed course of "diarrhea-associated" HUS with or without proven STEC infection: some of these patients may indeed experience an exaggerated or uncontrolled activation of the alternative path-way of complement induced by Stx or other STEC-derived proteins [223], or by an underly-ing (or unrecognized) genetic defect of the com-plement or coagulation cascade, including thrombomodulin [612, 613],

In conclusion, experimental and ex-vivo studies suggest that Stx may interact directly with CFH and CFH-related proteins, or induce alternative pathway of complement activation, secondary to endothelial cell injury, and inter-fere with endothelial thromboresistance. The putative roles of TM and complement-derived chemokines require additional studies both to better understand the pathogenesis of this form of HUS and to design effective therapeutic inter-ventions. However, there is no doubt that Stx itself can injure the microvascular endothelium and trigger the activation of various cellular and plasmatic cascades, including the platelet/coagulation and complement systems. With a few documented exceptions [612–614], STEC-HUS patients do not have underlying comple-ment regulator deficiencies or autoantibodies, nor does the generally acute and self-limited course justify treatment with anticomplement agents [141].

Outlook and Future Research

Currently, there is no specific therapy to pre-vent or treat STEC-HUS. The testing of new therapeutics for the prevention or mitigation of (severe) HUS poses important challenges due to the relatively rare occurrence and the acuity of the disease. Such studies require an innova-tive trial design and international collaborative efforts. Candidate therapeutic agents that may be tested in the future include, among others, fluid therapy, (intravenous) toxin binders (Gb3 receptor analogues, Stx-neutralizing antibodies), recombinant thrombomodulin and complement inhibitors (anti-C5 antibody, recombinant com-plement receptors), and select, non-phage induc-ing antibiotics during the early diarrhea phase.

Complications and Long-Term Outcome

Acute Prognosis

STEC-HUS represents an important cause of AKI in young children. Its course is generally self-limited. Hematological improvement (decreasing LDH activity, rising numbers of platelets in the circulation) may herald the begin-ning of renal recovery, but normalization of kid-ney function typically lags a few days to weeks behind the resolution of thrombocytopenia and hemolysis.

Overall, the outcome of STEC-HUS has improved substantially since its first description [1, 615, 616]. Reported mortality rates vary between <1 % and 5 % (and up to 12 %; median 1–4 %) [617], mostly secondary to CNS or car-diac involvement, or catastrophic colitis. About 70 % of patients recover completely from the acute episode; the remainder suffers varying degrees of sequelae [389, 410, 422, 423, 426, 430, 435, 617, 618].

While early diagnosis and supportive inter-vention, such as fluid management during the colitis phase and better dialysis techniques may have improved outcome, shifts in endemic STEC clones and the occurrence of epidemics may con-found comparisons between periods. Sustained oligoanuria, a WBC $>20 \times 10^9$/L and hematocrit >23 % were found significantly more often in patients who died during acute *E. coli* O157:H7 HUS (or later, due to severe complications) than in survivors [132, 410]. A large registry study from central Europe identified seven deaths among 490 enrolled, EHEC-positive patients (1.4 %; $CI_{95\%}$ 0.01–0.04) during the acute phase (2–30 days after diagnosis; median age 3.6 years [IQR, 2.7–4.7 years]). All seven patients had been dialyzed; five presented neurological mani-festations, including three who died of cerebral edema [91]. The authors of another series of children with STEC-HUS from France reported a lethality of 17 % among patients with CNS complications [426].

Complications and mortality rates appear to be greater in adult patients than in children with HUS. Lethality of STEC-HUS in the elderly population may be as high as 50 % [132, 140, 619, 620].

Long-Term Outcome

Despite its importance, the long-term renal prognosis of patients with HUS is controversial [621]. There is consensus that children who have recovered from the acute phase of HUS are at risk of long-term complications including CKD, arterial hypertension, neurological impairment or diabetes mellitus [410, 622, 623]. Long-term renal complications have been reported in 5–25 % of patients ranging from persistent microalbuminuria or proteinuria and hypertension to CKD and ESRD secondary to nephron loss. Fifteen to 30 % of patients demonstrate (usually mild) proteinuria and 5–15 % arterial hypertension; chronic (CKD) or endstage renal disease has been noted in approximately 10 % of surviving patients [91, 389], and ESRD in 3 % [617].

A carefully conducted, prospective long-term follow-up study of the drinking water *E. coli* O157:H7 epidemic from 2000 by the Nephrology group at the University of Western Ontario (Walkerton Health Study), found that 5 years after the event, 20 % of pediatric HUS survivors had microalbuminuria; the HUS cohort had an average 10-mL/min/1.73 m^2 decrease in GFR compared with age-matched controls from the same community [621]. The observed prognosis was better than reported in other studies; none of the children with HUS had overt proteinuria or GFR less than 80 mL/min/1.73 m^2 (1.33 mL/s/1.73 m^2) or blood pressures higher than expected for community norms.

Possible reasons contributing to the discrepancies found in the literature are sampling bias and loss of follow-up, differences in the infecting STPB strains (single outbreak scenarios, i.e., homogenous exposure, versus variable strain exposure in spontaneous cases). Comparison between reported outcomes is also hampered by the lack of clear definitions [617]. The cited European registry study [91] defined "poor" outcome as the presence of arterial hypertension (systolic or diastolic blood pressure >95th percentile according to age, sex, and height), neurological abnormalities (seizures, coma, stroke, or delayed motor development), impaired renal function (estimated glomerular filtration rate [eGFR] <80 mL/min/1.73 m^2), or presence of proteinuria (positive dipstick analysis or protein-to-creatinine ratio >0.15 g/g). Based on these criteria, 30 % of 274 prospectively followed patients were found to have sequelae 5 years after the initial diagnosis: 9 % of the study population had persistent hypertension, 4 % neurological symptoms, 18 % proteinuria without or with (7 %) decreased eGFR. Of importance, hypertension and proteinuria was noted in 18 % of patients who had been free of renal sequelae at the end of the first year following HUS (CI$_{95\%}$ 0.12–0.26) [91].

Predictors of Long-Term Renal Outcome

The risk of long-term renal complications is commonly thought to be related to the duration of anuria (or dialysis) during the acute phase of HUS. Frequently cited cut-offs are 10 or 14 days of oligoanuria [415, 617]. However, substantial overlap exists, and individual predictions are prone to errors [415]. For example, Rosales et al. noted that the duration of dialysis correlated with the risk of presenting with sequelae at the 1-year, 2-year, and 3-year follow-up ($P=0.0004$; Odds ratio [OR] for each 1-day increase in dialysis period, 1.04–1.08). Patients presenting with long-term complications were dialyzed for a median period of 15 days (IQR, 7–22 days) compared with 9 days for those with favorable (uncomplicated) outcome (IQR, 6–14 days; $P=0.01$) [91].

Registry studies from Utah [414, 415] and from the UK [624] noted that up to one-third of children with severe HUS (defined as anuria >8 days and oliguria >15 days) developed long-term sequelae. Oakes et al. analyzed a cohort of 159 children with HUS from 1970 to 2003 and at least 1 year of follow-up (mean 8.75 years) [415].

The authors of the latter study defined oliguria as urine output <240 mL/m²/day, and anuria as urine output <15 mL/day. In this cohort, 90 children (57%) had at least 1 day of oliguria and 69 (43%) at least 1 day of anuria. The occurrence of chronic sequelae (proteinuria, low GFR [estimated GFR <90 mL/min/1.73 m²], hypertension [BP >95th percentile for height and age]) increased stepwise with the duration of anuria, markedly with >5 days of anuria or >10 days of oliguria with anuria performing better as a predictor of sequelae than oliguria. Hypertension was present in 55.6% of patients with >10 days of anuria versus 8.9% in those without anuria (OR 12.8; CI$_{95\%}$ 2.9–57.5). Anuria >10 days was associated with combined GFR loss and proteinuria in 44% versus 2.2% of patients without anuria (OR 35.2; CI$_{95\%}$ 5.1–240.5). On the other hand, 36% of children with no recorded oliguria or anuria were left with sequelae, and 10% of those with no recorded oliguria or anuria were found to have proteinuria [415].

Histological studies of kidney biopsies from patients with HUS suggest a correlation between the extent of glomerular microangiopathy and long-term renal prognosis: the prognosis was noted to be poor when >50% of glomeruli were affected and in the presence of arterial microangiopathy and/or cortical necrosis [451]. However, a biopsy is rarely performed during the acute stage.

Outcome of Extrarenal Manifestations

Up to 30% of children with CNS manifestations during the acute phase of HUS develop long-term neurological sequelae [423]. Subtle neurological problems attributable to HUS are probably underdiagnosed, such as learning and behavioral difficulties, reduced fine motor coordination, or attention deficit and hyperactivity disorder [625].

Long-term gastrointestinal complications after STEC-HUS are colonic strictures and bilirubin gallstones, insulin-dependent diabetes mellitus, exocrine pancreatopathy [429, 430, 432, 433].

Myocardial insufficiency, attributed to previous eHUS, has been described [421, 422, 626].

Post-HUS Monitoring and Long-Term Interventions

Delayed renal function deterioration >1 year after the HUS has been reported in patients who appeared to have completely recovered [91, 415, 627]. Furthermore, a normal GFR does not exclude nephron loss with compensatory hyperfiltration in the surviving nephrons. Rosales et al. found late-onset hypertension and (chronic) proteinuria in 18% of their cohort [91]. Although not formally studied, angiotensin converting enzyme (ACE) inhibition is a rationale therapeutic strategy in patients with hypertension and/or proteinuria, with the aim to reduce glomerular pressure [621]. Yearly evaluation of kidney function, blood pressure and urinalysis (with quantitative urine protein or albumin measurements) has been recommended for at least 5 years, and indefinitely for patients with renal sequelae and/or hypertension [91, 424, 617].

STEC-HUS and Kidney Transplantation

Consistent with the observation that most patients with STEC-HUS recover kidney function after the acute episode, the number of patients with kidney transplantation following this form of HUS is limited. Of 274 STEC-HUS patients followed longitudinally through the German-Austrian HUS registry [91], seven patients (1.4%) required chronic dialysis and received a kidney allograft (one patient had developed ESRD within 2 months, five within the first year, and one 2 years after disease onset).

Renal transplantation in patients with STEC-HUS is safe without specific precautions, as demonstrated in several case series and registry reports [91, 628]. In a series from Argentina, no difference was observed between pediatric transplant recipients with and without a history of HUS with respect to graft survival and function, number of rejections and patient survival over up to 20 years; none had evidence of HUS recurrence [628, 629].

However, there is a caveat to the general principle. A few cases have now been described where STEC-induced HUS led to ESRD and subsequent recurrence of HUS in the graft [416, 613, 630]. Detailed genetic screening of two of these cases demonstrated the presence of disease-associated mutations of complement regulator genes [613]. As emphasized elsewhere, a second episode of HUS, even with microbiologically proven STEC infection, and HUS recurrence in the graft, indicate another (primary) etiology. These patients cannot be classified as "typical HUS" or (typical) "STEC-HUS", and genetic complement regulator abnormalities should be suspected and searched for [416].

Shigella dysenteriae HUS

Clinical Presentation and Epidemiology

HUS is a rare, but recognized complication of *Shigella dysenteriae* type 1 (SD1) infection. The first traceable descriptions of HUS following shigellosis appeared in the 1970s [631–634]. While some of its features resemble those of STEC-HUS, the reported disease course is generally more severe. The account of 81 cases of HUS during the 1994–1996 SD1 epidemic in

South Africa shows acute oliguric renal failure in 90.1% and dialysis in 42 (51.6%). Disseminated intravascular coagulation (DIC) was recorded in 21% [635]. Additional complications are listed in Table 26.4.

The age range at presentation is wide (median 3 years). HUS is diagnosed more than a week (range 4–17 days) after the onset of bloody diarrhea (colitis), and occasionally after diarrhea has improved. Reported incidences of HUS related to all dysentery cases range from 6% to 45% (median 13%) [636]. However, much lower figures emerge from prospective cohort studies [637] (Table 26.5).

Pathogenesis of *Shigella dysenteriae* HUS

Unlike STEC, *S. dysenteriae* is an invasive organism that penetrates the bowel wall, enters the blood stream and spreads hematogenously. Patients with SD1 infection should be treated with appropriate antibiotics. Shiga toxin (Stx) is likely involved in

Table 26.4 Organ involvement in *Shigella dysenteriae* (SD1) HUS

Organ involvement	Details	Percentage (of SD1 HUS cases)[a]
Generalized	Septicemia	18.5
	Disseminated intravascular coagulation (DIC)	21.0
	Hyponatremia	69.1
	Hypoalbuminemia	82.7
Gastrointestinal	Toxic megacolon	4.9
	Gastrointestinal perforation	9.9
	Protein-loosing enteropathy	32.1
	Rectal prolapse	6.2
	Hepatitis	13.6
Renal	Oliguric AKI	90.1
	Dialysis	51.6
Central nervous system	Encephalopathy	37.0
	Convulsions	14.8
	Hemiplegia	2.3
Heart	Myocarditis	6.2
	Congestive cardiac failure	3.7
	Cardiomyopathy	3.7
	Infective endocarditis	1.2
Hematological	Leukemoid reaction	91.3

[a]Extracted from Bhimma et al. [635]. Percentages are from 81 of 107 cases of HUS, admitted between July 1994 and February 1996, following an outbreak of *S. dysenteriae* type 1 dysentery in Kwazulu/Natal

Table 26.5 Pediatric *Shigella dysenteriae* type 1 (SD1) HUS

Country	# of reported cases	Age in years (mean or median)	Interval between onset of diarrhea and diagnosis of HUS (days)	Case fatality rate (%)	References
South Africa	151	4.6	7	17	[635, 638–640]
Zimbabwe	110	1.5	11	41	[641, 642]
India	74	2.3	8	59	[643, 644]
Nepal	55	2.1	17	23	[645, 646]
Saudi Arabia	33	3.0	8	26	[647, 648]
Bangla Desh	30	3.3	6	37	[649]
Kenya	21	1.6	4	52	[650]

Used with permission of Oxford University Press from Butler [636]

the pathogenesis of *S. dysenteriae* colitis and HUS. The release of lipopolysaccharide (LPS) during the invasive infection is thought to potentiate the ribotoxic effect of Stx and disease severity [651, 652]. Children with SD1-HUS can demonstrate impressive neutrophilia and left shift [635, 641]. As with STEC-HUS, a high peripheral neutrophil count has been associated with the development and severity of HUS [649, 653]. Some patients manifest the full DIC picture [3, 654]. Although STEC can induce subtle coagulation activation [148], full-blown DIC is not seen in STEC-HUS in the absence of gangrenous or perforating colitis and secondary sepsis or peritonitis.

Morbidity and mortality of SD1-HUS appear to be substantially higher than of HUS due to STEC infection [636]. The estimated case fatality rate is 36 % and by far exceeds that of shigellosis without HUS [635–637, 641, 655]. According to some authors, HUS has emerged as the principal cause of death in epidemics of SD1 dysentery [636]. However, *S. dysenteriae* is endemic in areas with limited resources and access to health care, and affected children may be malnourished and suffer from additional morbidities [656]. Severe fluid volume loss, hypernatremia and lack of dialysis may contribute to the previously reported poor outcome, described particularly in Sub-Saharan epidemics.

Antibiotic Therapy and HUS Risk in *S. dysenteriae* colitis

Antimicrobial therapy is the standard of care for patients with shigellosis. SD1 Stx is encoded in a defective lambdoid prophage unable to become lysogenic, which leads to constitutive Stx production [25, 637, 657, 658]. Thus, exposure of *S. dysenteriae* type 1 to antibiotics is not expected to increase Stx expression via phage induction. However, bacterial killing by antibiotics and subsequent lysis could augment stool toxin concentrations. In an attempt to estimate the risk of HUS attributable to antibiotic use, investigators at the International Centre for Diarrhoeal Disease Research in Dhaka, Bangladesh analyzed a well-defined group of children with SD1 infection who were treated early in the course of illness. Free fecal Stx levels decreased after the administration of antibiotics in 85 % of enrolled children, and none of the studied patients developed HUS [637].

The same authors reviewed the results of seven shigellosis drug trials, most of them performed in Bangladesh, during 1988–2000. Antimicrobials were administered within 96 h of the onset of dysentery. A total of 378 patients had proven SD1 infection (66 % children) [637]. The list of antibiotics used in these studies comprises nalidixic acid, ciprofloxacin, cefixime, ampicillin and other betalactams, and azithromycin. A single child, treated with ciprofloxacin, developed HUS, corresponding to a calculated risk of 0.004 (95 % $CI_{95\%}$ 0.001–0.022) in children and of 0.0026 (95 % $CI_{95\%}$ <0.001–0.015) in all participants. For persons with *S. dysenteriae* type 1 colitis, early administration of effective antimicrobial agents, including fluoroquinolones, is associated with decreasing Stx concentrations in stool and a low risk of HUS [637, 659].

Non-SD1 Shigellosis and HUS

Severe intestinal disease and extra-intestinal manifestations occur with infections by any of the four Shigella species, but most commonly with *S. dysenteriae* type 1. In a study of hospitalized pediatric patients <15 years old in Dhaka, Bangla Desh, *S. flexneri*, *S. boydii* and *S. sonnei* were significantly less likely ($P < 0.05$) to cause grossly bloody stools (33 versus 78 %), frequent stools in the 24 h before admission (median 11 vs. 25), rectal prolapse (15 versus 52 %), or extra-intestinal manifestations, including leukemoid reactions (2 versus 22 %), severe hypernatremia (26 versus 58 %) and neurologic manifestations (16 versus 24 %) [656]. The same authors calculated an incidence of HUS of 1 % by non-SD1 *Shigellae* versus 8 % by *S. dysenteriae* type 1. Death rates due to infections by any of the four *Shigella spp.* were similar (10 %). Factors significantly associated with death were younger age, lower stool frequency before admission, poor nutrition, hyponatremia, documented seizure and unconsciousness [656].

Streptococcus pneumoniae HUS

Epidemiology

Invasive pneumococcal disease (IPD) may lead to HUS, variably referred to as pneumococcal (pnHUS, pHUS) or *Streptococcus pneumoniae* HUS (SpHUS). It occurs in <0.6 % of IPD episodes [660] and affects mostly infants and young children with a median age at presentation of 13 months (range 5–39 months) [661]. Authors from New Zealand reported a 10-year cumulative incidence rate of 1.2 per 100,000 children under 15 years ($CI_{95\%}$ 0.5–2.0) [662]. The majority of patients (three fourths) present during the cold season (October to March in the Northern hemisphere) [661, 663].

pnHUS accounts for approximately 5 % of all pediatric HUS, and 40 % of all non-STEC HUS cases in children [663, 664]. Relative incidence estimates from the Canada, the UK and New Zealand range from 3 % to 11 % of all HUS cases [661, 662, 665]. Indigenous populations, such as Maori and Pacific Islanders may have a higher disease burden than other groups [662].

While increased vaccine coverage may have led to a decline in the incidence of pnHUS, *S. pneumoniae* serotype 19A has emerged as the predominant isolate during the last decade [661, 666–668]. Serotype 19A is missing in the first generation pneumococcal 7-valent conjugate vaccine (PCV7 [Prevnar®, Pfizer Inc., New York, NY]; serotypes 4, 6B, 9V, 14, 18C, 19F, and 23F) [669], but has been incorporated into the current 13-valent vaccine (PCV13; pneumococcal polysaccharide serotypes 1, 3, 4, 5, 6A, 6B, 7F, 9V, 14, 18C, 19A, 19F and 23F) [670] and the 23-valent pneumococcal polysaccharide vaccine (PPV23; Pneumovax®, Kenilworth, New Jersey, USA).

Pathogenesis

More than 85 years after the discovery of the T agglutination phenomenon [671], and more than 40 years after the report linking microangiopathic (intravascular) hemolytic anemia and HUS with *S. pneumoniae* infection and *in vivo* neuraminidase production [4], the pathogenesis of pnHUS is only partially understood, and the approach to treatment remains controversial [244, 672, 673].

pnHUS typically develops in a patient with pneumonia, often with pleural empyema (70 %), or meningitis (up to 30 %) [661, 668, 673, 674]. HUS has been linked to abundant in situ production of bacterial neuraminidase [4, 675], in particular neuraminidase A (NanA) [676]. Neuraminidase cleaves terminal sialyl (*N*-acetyl neuraminic acid, Neu5Ac) residues from membrane glycoproteins and glycolipids of red and white blood cells, endothelial cells, and other tissues [676–678]. The exposed O-glycan core 1 (Gal β1-3 GalNAc α-O-) is known as (asialo)glycophorin A [660, 679] or Thomsen-Friedenreich disaccharide (T or TF antigen) [671] (Fig. 26.10). The TF antigen is recognized by the lectin *Arachis hypogaea* which has been used to detect the *in vivo* effect of neuraminidase on RBCs and tissues in patients with pnHUS [4, 5, 676] and to

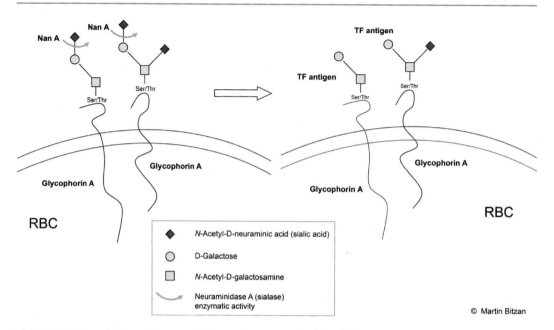

Fig. 26.10 Neuraminidase action on RBC membrane. Nan A (pneumococcal neuraminidase A) removes the terminal sialic acid. The Arachis hypogea lectin specifically recognizes the residual disaccharide β-D-galactose (1-3)-N-acetyl-D-galactosamine (Thomsen-Friedenreich antigen) that is O-glycosidically linked to the serine/threonine residue of glycophorin A (Used with permission of author and Elsevier from Loirat et al. [244]; Copyrighted by Martin Bitzan)

titrate circulating neuraminidase activity by exposing control RBCs to serially diluted plasma from patients with pnHUS [680].

Klein et al. postulated that the interaction of preformed anti-TF antibodies with the exposed neoantigen induces hemolysis, platelet agglutination, microvascular thrombosis, and tissue injury [5]. However, anti-TF antibodies are generally of the IgM class and of low affinity at body temperature [672, 681, 682]. Furthermore, desialylation of RBCs is not specific for HUS: it can be found in patients with IPD without progression to HUS [680, 683, 684], and pnHUS can develop in the absence of TF antibodies [678].

Classification of pnHUS

A practical classification of pnHUS is shown in Table 26.6. It is based on previous publications [665, 668] and refers to coagulation test results at the time of diagnosis, in addition to Coombs test and TF antigen detection. Since other pathogens capable of neuraminidase production, such

as *Clostridium perfringens* and influenza A virus, have been identified as causes of HUS [679, 685–689], we suggest the term "pnHUS" for "pneumococcal/neuraminidase (associated) HUS" and distinguish it from "atypical" and other "non-enteropathic" forms of HUS [348, 663, 690].

Presentation of pnHUS and Clinical Course

Patients with pnHUS typically (70–80%) present with fever and respiratory distress due to lobar pneumonia (70–80%) that is complicated in two thirds of patients by pleural effusion or empyema [661, 691]. The remaining 20–30% evolve during bacterial (pneumococcal) meningitis, acute otitis media [660] or pneumococcal sepsis. In one series, 12% of patients presented with pneumonia and proven or suspected meningitis [661]. The majority (80%) is bacteremic at the time of diagnosis [692]. The interval between onset of illness attributable to *S. pneumoniae* and the manifestation of HUS is 1–2 weeks; oliguria develops within 2 weeks of IPD onset [683].

The disease course can be severe or even fatal. A large proportion of patients is admitted to the intensive care unit, of whom >50% require mechanical ventilation and chest tube placement. About 70–85% of patients become oliguric or anuric, often with rapid clinical deterioration, and need acute dialysis [661, 691, 692]. Median time of dialysis in the largest reported series was 10 days (range 2–240 days) [661].

In addition to evidence of microangiopathic hemolytic anemia with profound thrombocytopenia, the laboratory profile is characterized by a rapid rise of acute phase reactants in plasma (CRP, procalcitonin) and an elevated white blood cell count with neutrophilia; however, leucocytopenia may be found in a third of patients [683]. Elevated liver and pancreatic enzymes (amylase/lipase) indicate additional organ involvement. The direct Coombs is positive in 58–90% of patients during the early phase of pnHUS [673, 693–695].

Critically ill patients may present features of HUS and of disseminated intravascular coagulation (DIC) [673, 694, 696, 697]. *S. pneumoniae* sepsis with (mild) anemia, thrombocytopenia, DIC, hypotension and acute kidney injury can masquerade as HUS. Furthermore, Coombs-test positive hemolytic anemia may occur without thrombocytopenia and apparent kidney injury [679, 680]. Investigators therefore felt a need for the definition and classification pnHUS [665, 668, 673] (Table 26.6).

Laboratory Studies and Biomarkers

The defining criterion and most important diagnostic result is the detection of *S. pneumoniae* in physiologically sterile fluids (blood, pleural effusion, CSF, middle ear aspirate, etc.). In case of preceding antibiotic therapy, PCR for pneumococcal-specific nucleic acid sequences or pneumococcal antigen detection should be attempted using pleural fluid, CSF and/or urine.

Laboratory workup of patients with suspected or proven HUS due to neuraminidase-producing organisms should include demonstration of TF exposure and direct Coombs test, in addition to

Table 26.6 Diagnostic criteria for pnHUS

pnHUS	Criteria		Details
Definite	1	Evidence of HUS	Intravascular hemolytic anemia, thrombocytopenia and acute kidney injury (AKI)
	2	Evidence of invasive *S. pneumoniae* infection	Pneumococcal growth/antigen detection or positive PCR from physiologically sterile biological fluid
	3	No evidence of disseminated intravascular coagulation (DIC)	Fibrinogen consumption, prolonged prothrombin (PT) or partial thromboplastin time (PTT), and/or d-dimers *at the time of diagnosis*
Probable	1	Evidence of HUS	See above
	2	Evidence of invasive *S. pneumoniae* infection	See above
	3	(a) Evidence of DIC *and*	Usually cold agglutinins; TF (Thomsen-Friedenreich) antigen detection by *Arachis hypogaea* or specific lectin/monoclonal antibody binding [679]
		(b) Positive Coombs test and/or evidence of TF antigen exposure	
Possible	1	Evidence of HUS	See above
	2	Suspected (unproven) invasive *S. pneumoniae* infection	Negative culture/antigen detection or PCR from sterile fluid
	3	(a) No evidence of DIC, *or*	
		(b) Positive Coombs test and/or TF antigen exposure	With or without evidence of DIC (see above)

Data in Copelovitch and Kaplan [668]; and in Spinale et al. [673]

routine coagulation tests, fibrinogen, and d-dimers. Recommended are also C3, C4, CH50, and serum immunoglobulins to exclude congenital or acquired immune deficiencies. Serial CRP measurements, if available, are useful to monitor effective antimicrobial therapy.

No other form of HUS presents with positive Coombs test or TF antigen exposure. However, the frequency of Coombs test positivity in IPD (without evidence of HUS) is not known [673]. Sensitivity and specificity of TF antigen detection was reported as 86 % and 57 %, respectively, for pnHUS or isolated hemolytic anemia. The positive predictive value was 76 %. Conversely, in children with IPD, positive and negative predictive values of TF antigen detection for pnHUS were 52 and 100 % [684].

Complement and pnHUS

Informative studies of the complement system in pnHUS patients are scarce. In one series, two of five previously healthy children with pnHUS were found to carry known, heterozygous mutations in *CFI* and *CFH* and one had a possibly damaging variant in the gene coding for thrombomodulin (*THBD*); three patients had a CFH related protein one third (*CFHR1/3*) deletion (two in combination with a *CFH* or *CFI* mutation), but none had detectable anti-CFH antibodies. All five patients were Coombs positive and demonstrated mild to moderate depression of serum C3 and C4. ADAMTS13 (a disintegrin and metalloprotease with a thrombospondin type 1 motif, member 13) activity was preserved [698]. Another group reported two patients with pnHUS, both with transiently depressed serum C3, but normal C4 concentrations, normal ADAMTS13 activity and no detectable mutations in the studied alternative pathway of complement regulator genes [699].

Complement consumption, primarily due to activation of the alternative pathway, appears to be a frequent, but not obligatory event in patients with pnHUS. However, *S. pneumoniae* infection can trigger HUS in children with damaging mutations of complement regulator genes, similar

to non-specific agents in patients with "atypical" HUS. Interestingly, disease relapses due to *S. pneumoniae* have not been described. The emergence of specific immunity is surmised, not only to the pneumococcal serotype but common virulence factors.

Treatment of pnHUS

Treatment of patients with pnHUS includes appropriate antibiotics and best supportive care [244]. As with eHUS, symptomatic anemia, significant bleeding or surgery are indications for PRBC and platelet transfusions, respectively. Dialysis (hemodialysis or peritoneal dialysis, depending on local expertise and preference) is required in up to 80 % of patients. Some patients with *S. pneumoniae* sepsis or sepsis due to a secondary organisms and hemodynamic instability may benefit from CRRT.

Previous recommendations to only transfuse "washed" RBCs and to avoid administration of plasma (which contains anti-TF antibodies) – or to select plasma with low anti-TF titers [700, 701] – are not based on evidence [14, 244, 662, 673]. Indeed, plasma therapy (plasma infusion or plasma exchange) has been described in pnHUS patients without apparent worsening of hemolysis or renal function [661, 702, 703].

Although reported, currently available data do not suggest that patients with pnHUS should be subjected to therapeutic complement blockade, unless there is a proven or suspected complement regulator defect [699].

Outcome

Unfavorable outcome is expected in about 20 % of patients in the largest case series comprising 43 patients from the UK in 2007 [661]. From a recent North American series, 10 % of patients with ≥6 months follow-up had undergone kidney transplantation, 13 % had neurologic sequelae, and 3 % had died [692]. Important CNS complications are intracranial hemorrhage and infarction, leading to obstructive hydrocephalus in some patients and sensorineural hearing loss [661, 662]. Waters et al. reported that only 2 of 13 patients with pnHUS and meningitis demonstrated a normal neurodevelopmental outcome [661]. Pulmonary complications in addition to empyema include pneumatoceles and necrotic pneumonic changes [662].

Investigators from France, the UK and New Zealand noted mortality rates of 27 %, 11 % and 9 %, respectively [661, 662, 704]. In contrast, no fatalities were recorded in patients with *S. pneumoniae*-related HUS during the SYNSORB Pk^R clinical trial [663]. There is substantial variability of the reported mortality rates (0–13 %), which is best explained by the small number of cases even in the largest reported series [673, 690]. Most deaths are not caused directly by HUS or renal injury, but are related to complicating pneumococcal meningitis and sepsis/shock.

Although the clinical course tends to be more severe in HUS following *S. pneumoniae* than STEC infection, as indicated by frequency of PRBC transfusions and dialysis [661, 691, 704], the long-term renal outcome in surviving patients does not appear to be worse than in patients with STEC-HUS [663, 690]. Residual renal dysfunction, reflected by decreased GFR and the presence of proteinuria, has been variably reported in 20–25 % [661, 690]. Kidney transplantation following pnHUS is very rare, and experience is limited [705, 706].

Influenza HUS

Epidemiology and Importance

Few proven cases of HUS triggered by influenza virus infection (iHUS) have been published. In all instances with appropriate viral diagnostic, HUS was associated with influenza A strains, mainly A(H3N2) and A(H1N1) (Table 26.7). The first retrievable description is from a 20 year-old kidney transplant recipient, from 1971 [707]. The patient was diagnosed with microangiopathic hemolytic anemia and graft failure 1–2 weeks

Table 26.7 Demographic and clinical data of influenza HUS

Demographic and clinical features	Details	Median (range), frequencies[a]
Age (years)		14.5 (3–34) years, n = 12
Influenza strains	A(H3N2)	2
	A(H1N1)	7
	A (serology only)	3
Renal status	Native kidneys	9/12 (75 %)
	Kidney allografts [707–709]	3/12 (25 %)
Hematology	Hemoglobin (nadir)	78 (50–111) g/L (n = 11)[a]
	Platelets (nadir)	29 (8–80) × 10⁹/L (n = 12)
	LDH (peak)	2888 (300–13,188) U/L (n = 7)
	Positive Coombs test	None (n = 8)
AKI	Serum creatinine (peak)	309 (230–701) μmol/L (n = 10)
Complement	Low C3	3/8 (27 %)[a,b]
	Low C4	None (n = 5)[a,b]
	Complement regulator deficiency or relapsing HUS[b]	2
Treatment	Dialysis	7/12 (58 %)
	Plasma infusion	4/12 (33 %)
	Plasma exchange	3/12 (25 %)
	Eculizumab	1/12 (8 %)
Outcome	Complete recovery	10/12 (83 %)
	CKD	1/11 (9 %)[c]
	Death	1/12 (8 %)
	Graft loss	1/3 (33 %)

Data from References [688, 689, 707–715]
[a]Number of patients with reported results. Three additional cases, not included in this table, have been reported as TTP (see text) [716–718]
[b]Mutation of C3 (Transplant recipient); iHUS in third graft [709]; relapsing HUS (native kidney) without identified complement mutation; fourth episode triggered by influenza A/H1N1 infection [715]; decreased C3 (complement mutation studies not reported) [713]
[c]Graft loss (transplant recipient); deceased patient excluded

after the onset of influenza, almost 2 years after transplantation; additional laboratory features included cold agglutinins (with negative direct Coombs test) and transiently reduced plasma C3 concentration. A graft biopsy 5 weeks after HUS onset revealed thrombosis of small renal arteries and glomerular capillaries. The graft was removed 8 weeks after HUS onset, followed by swift normalization of the hematological parameters. A subsequent graft from a deceased donor (DD) was tolerated well without recurrence of HUS.

Several cases of iHUS were noted during the pandemic influenza A(H1N1). A typical scenario is that of a previously healthy, 7-year-old boy with febrile pneumonitis and transient respiratory failure who developed severe AKI, profound microangiopathic hemolytic anemia and thrombocytopenia associated with hypertensive encephalopathy 5 days after the onset of respiratory symptoms. Coagulation profile, plasma fibrinogen, Coombs test and C3 concentration were normal as was the screening for MCP expression, plasma ADAMTS13 activity and CFB, CFH and CFI concentrations. He recovered completely after 2 weeks of peritoneal dialysis [710]. Additional patients with influenza A-associated HUS demonstrated elevated d-dimers [688, 711, 712]. None of the tested patients had a positive Coombs test [689, 707, 708, 710, 713, 714], but cold agglutinins were reported once [707]. It is currently unclear if A(H1N1) has a greater propensity to induce HUS than other influenza strains.

Pathogenesis

There is an established link between influenza virus infection and HUS, but the mechanism that triggers iHUS remains speculative [13]. Influenza virus shares with *S. pneumoniae* the ability to express neuraminidase (NA). Hemagglutinin (HA) and NA are defining and important (viral) pathogenicity factors in human (and animal) infections. NA shedding in influenza infection is minimal compared to *S. pneumoniae*, and it remains to be shown if it contributes to the pathogenesis HUS.

Influenza A virus attachment to sialic acid residues on host (target) cells is mediated by viral surface-exposed HA. Once endocytosed, virus redirects the host cell machinery to serve its replication and turns host cell RNA transcription and translation off. NA is responsible for virion release and propagation of the infection through the cleavage of sialic acid residues on host cells [719]. Autopsy studies during the 2009 A(H1N1) pandemic showed viral antigen in endothelial cells [720, 721]. *In vitro* infection of endothelial cell by influenza virus [722] can trigger apoptosis [723], a process known to stimulate platelet adhesion directly and via the exposure of extracellular matrix [289, 724].

In addition to injuring or activating vascular endothelial cells, influenza virus may directly affect platelets. A(H3N2) virus induces clumping of human and rabbit platelets *in vitro* and a rapid drop of platelet counts *in vivo* after injection of the virus into rabbits [725]. More recent studies confirmed the potential of influenza virus to activate platelets and generate thrombin, among others [726, 727]. In a prospective study comparing patients with ARDS due to severe influenza A(H1N1) and bacterial pneumonia with healthy controls, influenza showed the greatest degree of platelet activation measured as formation of platelet-monocyte aggregates and activation of $\alpha IIb\beta 3$ integrin on platelets [726].

Influenza-Associated HUS and Complement Dysregulation

Plasma C3 levels have been reported in eight patients, based on a review of the accessible literature; they were reduced in three of eight cases. Three patients were found (or suspected) to have genetic complement regulator defects: a 15 year-old boy with a gain-of-function mutation in the C3 locus, who had lost two previous kidney allografts due to HUS recurrences (treated with eculizumab) [709], a 17 year-old boy with reduced plasma C3 and heterozygous CD46 deficiency (second episode of HUS) [714] and a 15 year-old girl with incomplete genetic workup (normal C3 and C4, factor H, and factor I levels, undetectable CFH autoantibody, and lack of *CHF* mutation), who had four preceding spontaneously resolving episodes of HUS (Table 26.7) [715]. In these instances, HUS should be viewed as "atypical," triggered by influenza A infection. The remaining nine patients, including a transplant recipient with HUS, had no preceding episodes of HUS. Thus, the majority of the reported cases iHUS appear to occur spontaneously, without known complement regulator defect. However, only two of the reported patients have been screened for alternative pathway regulator abnormalities. The question, whether genetic (host) factors confer susceptibility and whether complement plays a role in iHUS warrants further studies.

Influenza and Streptococcus Pneumoniae Infection

Influenza virus infections are known to increase the susceptibility of the host to the propagation of *S. pneumonia* [728]. Co-infection can pose a challenge determining which of the pathogens is responsible for pulmonary complications and HUS [13].

Influenza and TTP

Influenza A virus infections, including A(H1N1) have been invoked as a cause of TTP in at least three published cases [716–718]. TTP is defined by nearly absent (<10%) ADAMTS13 activity [729]. Kosugi [716] reported a 68 year-old patient with influenza A infection–associated TTP with <0.5% ADAMTS13 activity and increased inhibitor concentration. The TTP diagnosis of the remaining two cases was based on the presence of neurological manifestations, such as headache and mental confusion [718] or hemiplegia [717]. However, neither ADAMTS13 activities or anti-ADAMTS13 antibody measurements nor complement genetic studies were reported in the latter cases. It therefore remains to be shown if influenza virus can induce TTP, based on current definitions (lack of active ADAMTS13) or

whether these were cases of HUS with CNS manifestations.

Laboratory Diagnosis

All patients with HUS due to infections by seasonal or epidemic influenza strains should undergo rapid testing for plasma C3 and, if available, SC5b-9 concentrations, and ADAMTS13 activity and autoantibodies. TTP is suspected in patients with minimal or no renal injury [553, 729]. The presence of concomitant or complicating pneumococcal pneumonia or sepsis must be ruled out in any case of (suspected) iHUS (see above).

Therapeutic Management

Best supportive care includes judicious transfusion of RBCs and platelets, dialysis and other supportive measures. It is unknown if the NA inhibitor oseltamivir prevents or ameliorates iHUS. Where its administration has been reported, it has been given at or after the onset of HUS [713, 714]. The role of plasma therapy (PI, PLEX) or of eculizumab in iHUS is unproven. However, recommendations for the treatment of "atypical" HUS should be followed if the patient presents evidence of complement dysregulation, i.e., known complement gene mutation or CFH antibody, preceding HUS episode(s) or positive family history of (a) HUS, or recurrence of HUS after kidney transplantation [12, 244, 348].

HIV HUS

Epidemiology and Clinical Presentation

TMA in the context of AIDS has been variably described as HUS or TTP. In fact, TTP has been listed as an AIDS defining condition [730, 731]. However, AIDS-related infections or complications can present clinical features that resemble TMA [732].

One of the first reports of TTP in a patient with AIDS appeared in 1984 [733]. In a large series by Moore et al. [732], 350 consecutive, hospitalized adult patients with AIDS in the mid-1990s were evaluated for the presence of a TTP-like syndrome, i.e., anemia, thrombocytopenia, fragmented erythrocytes, renal and neurologic dysfunction, and fever [732]. Schistocytosis was present in 24%, and the full clinical picture of TTP in 7% of the patients. Patients with TMA were more likely to have a low CD4 lymphocyte count, CDC stage C disease, and bacterial sepsis [732].

Based on the number of published reports, the incidence of HIV TMA has decreased since the advent of ART and HAART therapies [6]. A study from the Oklahoma TTP-HUS Registry covering an 18-year period, from 1989 to 2007 [7], found evidence of HIV infection in 6 of 326 patients with a diagnosis of TTP (1.84%; $CI_{95\%}$ 0.68%–4.01%). The authors calculated a period prevalence for 1989–2007 of HIV infection among all adults in the Oklahoma TTP-HUS Registry region of 0.30%. One patient had multiple relapses. However, there was a large overlap between TTP-like conditions and other AIDS-related complications [7].

Pathogenesis

Measurements of ADAMTS13 activity or antibodies, of complement activation, anti-CFH antibodies, or the presence of neuraminidase/NA-mediated desialylation (TF antigen) have not been studied. The direct Coombs test appears to be negative [733]. None of the described children presented with bloody diarrhea or evidence of STEC O157:H7 infection. The evolution of the HUS and its severity are variable.

Clinical observation and animal experimentation suggest that HIV can directly cause HUS [734]. The mechanism(s) leading to HUS remain unclear. HIV infects glomerular endothelial and mesangial but not epithelial cells *in vitro* [735]. Intriguingly, a viral surface glycoprotein, pg120, binds to Gb3, the Stx receptor; this interaction has been linked with the occurrence of HIV HUS [215, 734, 736]. Conversely, Gb3 has been described as natural resistance factor for the prevention of HIV infection, e.g., when given as soluble agent [737, 738].

ADAMTS13 deficiency, characteristic for TTP [739], has rarely been reported in patients with HIV TMA. Some authors noted difficulties in the interpretation of ADAMTS13 activity levels which may develop after repeat episodes or independent of clinical signs of TMA, leading to the conclusion that measurement of ADAMTS13 activity cannot distinguish patients with "typical TTP" from those where TMA is subsequently attributed to another etiology [7, 740].

Clinical Presentation and Outcome

Clinical information of HIV HUS or HUS-like conditions is limited to a few anecdotal reports and summary statistics. An instructive case is that of a 12-year-old boy with transfusion-associated HIV infection [8]. He presented with fever, abdominal pain, and cough, 8 months after the detection of HIV infection. The absolute CD4 count was 10 cells/mm^3. HUS was diagnosed based on the presence of (severe) intravascular hemolysis, moderate thrombocytopenia, and gradually rising serum creatinine with mild oliguria. There was no infectious focus. Stool cultures failed to grow common enteropathogens, and *E. coli* O157 LPS serology was non-diagnostic. Blood and urine cultures were negative. Both kidneys appeared echogenic by ultrasound.

Treatment consisted of daily infusions of frozen plasma, 10 ml/kg per dose over 10 days. Hemolysis and the need for PRBC infusions diminished 2 weeks after the first plasma infusion. The platelet count increased a week after discontinuation of plasma infusions. However, he became dialysis-dependent and subsequently died after treatment withdrawal [8].

The second case was that of a 6-month old infant. She too experienced gradual loss of renal function despite plasma infusions for 10 days. She succumbed to unstoppable gastrointestinal bleeding 17 days after diagnosis [8].

A third report describes a previously undiagnosed adult male with HIV infection presenting with fever, nausea, diarrhea and reduced urinary output [6]. HUS was diagnosed and treatment with plasmapheresis and hemodialysis started. Hb, platelets, LDH and renal function normalized after four daily treatment sessions.

Renal Pathology

The kidney biopsy of the first case of pediatric HIV described above [8], revealed marked thickening of the walls of glomerular capillaries, arterioles and small arteries, vacuolar endothelial changes, luminal thrombosis and presence of intravascular red cell fragments. There was focal tubular atrophy, interstitial fibrosis, and a mild focal mononuclear interstitial infiltrate composed, predominantly, of lymphocytes and a few plasma cells. Immunofluorescent staining for IgG and IgM was negative, but there was 1+ focal staining of the capillary walls for fibrinogen and C3. Electron microscopy showed no electron-dense deposits.

Therapeutic Management of HIV TMA

Some authors found HIV TTP to be highly responsive to PLEX therapy [741]. Given the overall limited evidence, others suggested cautious consideration of plasma exchange for HUS or TTP in AIDS patients [6–8]. There are no guidelines for children with TMA-like disorders associated with HIV infection. Effective treatment of the HIV infection is expected to help recovery from HIV-associated TMA. Careful evaluation is recommended to exclude alternative diagnoses, such as malignant hypertension or disseminated Kaposi sarcoma [7].

References

1. Gasser C, Gautier E, Steck A, Siebenmann RE, Oechslin R. Hemolytic-uremic syndrome: bilateral necrosis of the renal cortex in acute acquired hemolytic anemia. Schweiz Med Wochenschr. 1955; 85(38–39):905–9.

2. Karmali MA, Petric M, Lim C, Fleming PC, Arbus GS, Lior H. The association between idiopathic hemolytic uremic syndrome and infection by verotoxin-producing Escherichia coli. J Infect Dis. 1985;151(5):775–82.

3. Koster F, Levin J, Walker L, Tung KS, Gilman RH, Rahaman MM, et al. Hemolytic-uremic syndrome after shigellosis. Relation to endotoxemia and circulating immune complexes. N Engl J Med. 1978;298(17):927–33.

4. Fischer K, Poschmann A, Oster H. Severe pneumonia with hemolysis caused by neuraminidase. Detection of cryptantigens by indirect immunofluorescent technic. Monatsschr Kinderheilkd. 1971;119(1):2–8.

5. Klein PJ, Bulla M, Newman RA, Muller P, Uhlenbruck G, Schaefer HE, et al. Thomsen-Friedenreich antigen in haemolytic-uraemic syndrome. Lancet. 1977;2(8046):1024–5.

6. Gomes AM, Ventura A, Almeida C, Correia M, Tavares V, Mota M, et al. Hemolytic uremic syndrome as a primary manifestation of acute human immunodeficiency virus infection. Clin Nephrol. 2009;71(5):563–6.

7. Benjamin M, Terrell DR, Vesely SK, Voskuhl GW, Dezube BJ, Kremer Hovinga JA, et al. Frequency and significance of HIV infection among patients diagnosed with thrombotic thrombocytopenic purpura. Clin Infect Dis. 2009;48(8):1129–37.

8. Turner ME, Kher K, Rakusan T, D'Angelo L, Kapur S, Selby D, et al. A typical hemolytic uremic syndrome in human immunodeficiency virus-1-infected children. Pediatr Nephrol. 1997;11(2):161–3.

9. Bu F, Maga T, Meyer NC, Wang K, Thomas CP, Nester CM, et al. Comprehensive genetic analysis of complement and coagulation genes in atypical hemolytic uremic syndrome. J Am Soc Nephrol. 2014;25(1):55–64.

10. Westland R, Bodria M, Carrea A, Lata S, Scolari F, Fremeaux-Bacchi V, et al. Phenotypic expansion of DGKE-associated diseases. J Am Soc Nephrol. 2014;25(7):1408–14.

11. Jodele S, Licht C, Goebel J, Dixon BP, Zhang K, Sivakumaran TA, et al. Abnormalities in the alternative pathway of complement in children with hematopoietic stem cell transplant-associated thrombotic microangiopathy. Blood. 2013;122(12):2003–7.

12. Loirat C, Fakhouri F, Ariceta G, Besbas N, Bitzan M, Bjerre A, et al. An international consensus approach to the management of atypical hemolytic uremic syndrome in children. Pediatr Nephrol. 2016;31(1):15–39.

13. Allen U, Licht C. Pandemic H1N1 influenza A infection and (atypical) HUS – more than just another trigger? Pediatr Nephrol. 2011;26(1):3–5.

14. Johnson S, Waters A. Is complement a culprit in infection-induced forms of haemolytic uraemic syndrome? Immunobiology. 2012;217(2):235–43.

15. Mele C, Remuzzi G, Noris M. Hemolytic uremic syndrome. Semin Immunopathol. 2014;36(4): 399–420.

16. Gianantonio CA, Vitacco M, Mendilaharzu F, Gallo GE, Sojo ET. The hemolytic-uremic syndrome. Nephron. 1973;11(2):174–92.

17. Karmali MA, Steele BT, Petric M, Lim C. Sporadic cases of haemolytic-uraemic syndrome associated with faecal cytotoxin and cytotoxin-producing Escherichia coli in stools. Lancet. 1983;1(8325): 619–20.

18. Konowalchuk J, Speirs JI, Stavric S. Vero response to a cytotoxin of Escherichia coli. Infect Immun. 1977;18(3):775–9.

19. O'Brien AD, Lively TA, Chang TW, Gorbach SL. Purification of Shigella dysenteriae 1 (Shiga)-like toxin from Escherichia coli O157:H7 strain associated with haemorrhagic colitis. Lancet. 1983;2(8349):573.

20. Riley LW, Remis RS, Helgerson SD, McGee HB, Wells JG, Davis BR, et al. Hemorrhagic colitis associated with a rare Escherichia coli serotype. N Engl J Med. 1983;308(12):681–5.

21. Karmali MA, Petric M, Lim C, Fleming PC, Steele BT. Escherichia coli cytotoxin, haemolytic-uraemic syndrome, and haemorrhagic colitis. Lancet. 1983;2(8362):1299–300.

22. Johnson WM, Lior H, Bezanson GS. Cytotoxic Escherichia coli O157:H7 associated with haemorrhagic colitis in Canada. Lancet. 1983; 1(8314–5):76.

23. Griffin PM, Olmstead LC, Petras RE. Escherichia coli O157:H7-associated colitis. A clinical and histological study of 11 cases. Gastroenterology. 1990;99(1):142–9.

24. Scheutz F, Beutin L, Piérard D, Karch H, Tozzoli R, Caprioli A, et al., editors. Nomenclature of verocytotoxins: a review, a proposal, and a protocol for typing Vtx genes. 4th Annu Workshop Commun Ref Lab E coli VTEC, Rome; 2009.

25. Strockbine NA, Jackson MP, Sung LM, Holmes RK, O'Brien AD. Cloning and sequencing of the genes for Shiga toxin from Shigella dysenteriae type 1. J Bacteriol. 1988;170(3):1116–22.

26. Newland JW, Strockbine NA, Miller SF, O'Brien AD, Holmes RK. Cloning of Shiga-like toxin structural genes from a toxin converting phage of Escherichia coli. Science. 1985;230(4722):179–81.

27. Jackson MP, Newland JW, Holmes RK, O'Brien AD. Nucleotide sequence analysis of the structural genes for Shiga-like toxin I encoded by bacteriophage 933 J from Escherichia coli. Microb Pathog. 1987;2(2):147–53.

28. Calderwood SB, Auclair F, Donohue-Rolfe A, Keusch GT, Mekalanos JJ. Nucleotide sequence of the Shiga-like toxin genes of Escherichia coli. Proc Natl Acad Sci U S A. 1987;84(13):4364–8.

29. Takao T, Tanabe T, Hong YM, Shimonishi Y, Kurazono H, Yutsudo T, et al. Identity of molecular structure of Shiga-like toxin I (VT1) from Escherichia coli O157:H7 with that of Shiga toxin. Microb Pathog. 1988;5(5):57–69.

30. Zhang W, Bielaszewska M, Kuczius T, Karch H. Identification, characterization, and distribution of a Shiga toxin 1 gene variant (stx(1c)) in Escherichia coli strains isolated from humans. J Clin Microbiol. 2002;40(4):1441–6.

31. Brett KN, Ramachandran V, Hornitzky MA, Bettelheim KA, Walker MJ, Djordjevic SP. stx1c Is the most common Shiga toxin 1 subtype among Shiga toxin-producing Escherichia coli isolates from sheep but not among isolates from cattle. J Clin Microbiol. 2003;41(3):926–36.

32. Newland JW, Strockbine NA, Neill RJ. Cloning of genes for production of Escherichia coli Shiga-like toxin type II. Infect Immun. 1987;55(11):2675–80.

33. Downes FP, Barrett TJ, Green JH, Aloisio CH, Spika JS, Strockbine NA, et al. Affinity purification and characterization of Shiga-like toxin II and production of toxin-specific monoclonal antibodies. Infect Immun. 1988;56(8):1926–33.

34. Pierard D, Muyldermans G, Moriau L, Stevens D, Lauwers S. Identification of new verocytotoxin type 2 variant B-subunit genes in human and animal Escherichia coli isolates. J Clin Microbiol. 1998;36(11):3317–22.

35. Head SC, Karmali MA, Roscoe ME, Petric M, Strockbine NA, Wachsmuth IK. Serological differences between verocytotoxin 2 and shiga-like toxin II. Lancet. 1988;2(8613):751.

36. Schmitt CK, McKee ML, O'Brien AD. Two copies of Shiga-like toxin II-related genes common in enterohemorrhagic Escherichia coli strains are responsible for the antigenic heterogeneity of the O157:H- strain E32511. Infect Immun. 1991;59(3): 1065–73.

37. Teel LD, Melton-Celsa AR, Schmitt CK, O'Brien AD. One of two copies of the gene for the activatable shiga toxin type 2d in Escherichia coli O91:H21 strain B2F1 is associated with an inducible bacteriophage. Infect Immun. 2002;70(8):4282–91.

38. Gyles CL, De Grandis SA, MacKenzie C, Brunton JL. Cloning and nucleotide sequence analysis of the genes determining verocytotoxin production in a porcine edema disease isolate of Escherichia coli. Microb Pathog. 1988;5(6):419–26.

39. Weinstein DL, Jackson MP, Samuel JE, Holmes RK, O'Brien AD. Cloning and sequencing of a Shiga-like toxin type II variant from Escherichia coli strain responsible for edema disease of swine. J Bacteriol. 1988;170(9):4223–30.

40. Scheutz F, Teel LD, Beutin L, Pierard D, Buvens G, Karch H, et al. Multicenter evaluation of a sequence-based protocol for subtyping Shiga toxins and standardizing Stx nomenclature. J Clin Microbiol. 2012;50(9):2951–63.

41. Burk C, Dietrich R, Acar G, Moravek M, Bulte M, Martlbauer E. Identification and characterization of a new variant of Shiga toxin 1 in Escherichia coli ONT:H19 of bovine origin. J Clin Microbiol. 2003;41(5):2106–12.

42. Schmidt H, Scheef J, Morabito S, Caprioli A, Wieler LH, Karch H. A new Shiga toxin 2 variant (Stx2f) from Escherichia coli isolated from pigeons. Appl Environ Microbiol. 2000;66(3):1205–8.

43. Leung PH, Peiris JS, Ng WW, Robins-Browne RM, Bettelheim KA, Yam WC. A newly discovered verotoxin variant, VT2g, produced by bovine verocytotoxigenic Escherichia coli. Appl Environ Microbiol. 2003;69(12):7549–53.

44. Prager R, Fruth A, Busch U, Tietze E. Comparative analysis of virulence genes, genetic diversity, and phylogeny of Shiga toxin 2 g and heat-stable enterotoxin STIa encoding Escherichia coli isolates from humans, animals, and environmental sources. Int J Med Microbiol. 2011;301(3):181–91.

45. Karch H, Tarr PI, Bielaszewska M. Enterohaemorrhagic Escherichia coli in human medicine. Int J Med Microbiol. 2005;295(6–7): 405–18.

46. Schmidt H, Montag M, Bockemuhl J, Heesemann J, Karch H. Shiga-like toxin II-related cytotoxins in Citrobacter freundii strains from humans and beef samples. Infect Immun. 1993;61(2):534–43.

47. Tschape H, Prager R, Streckel W, Fruth A, Tietze E, Bohme G. Verotoxinogenic Citrobacter freundii associated with severe gastroenteritis and cases of haemolytic uraemic syndrome in a nursery school: green butter as the infection source. Epidemiol Infect. 1995;114(3):441–50.

48. Paton AW, Paton JC. Enterobacter cloacae producing a Shiga-like toxin II-related cytotoxin associated with a case of hemolytic-uremic syndrome. J Clin Microbiol. 1996;34(2):463–5.

49. Wickham ME, Lupp C, Mascarenhas M, Vazquez A, Coombes BK, Brown NF, et al. Bacterial genetic determinants of non-O157 STEC outbreaks and hemolytic-uremic syndrome after infection. J Infect Dis. 2006;194(6):819–27.

50. Albaqali A, Ghuloom A, Al Arrayed A, Al Ajami A, Shome DK, Jamsheer A, et al. Hemolytic uremic syndrome in association with typhoid fever. Am J Kidney Dis. 2003;41(3):709–13.

51. Miceli S, Jure MA, de Saab OA, de Castillo MC, Rojas S, de Holgado AP, et al. A clinical and bacteriological study of children suffering from haemolytic uraemic syndrome in Tucuman, Argentina. Jpn J Infect Dis. 1999;52(2):33–7.

52. Elliott EJ, Robins-Browne RM, O'Loughlin EV, Bennett-Wood V, Bourke J, Henning P, et al. Nationwide study of haemolytic uraemic syndrome: clinical, microbiological, and epidemiological features. Arch Dis Child. 2001;85(2):125–31.

53. McCarthy TA, Barrett NL, Hadler JL, Salsbury B, Howard RT, Dingman DW, et al. Hemolytic-uremic syndrome and Escherichia coli O121 at a Lake in Connecticut, 1999. Pediatrics. 2001;108(4):E59.

54. Misselwitz J, Karch H, Bielazewska M, John U, Ringelmann F, Ronnefarth G, et al. Cluster of hemolytic-uremic syndrome caused by Shiga toxin-producing Escherichia coli O26:H11. Pediatr Infect Dis J. 2003;22(4):349–54.

55. Brooks JT, Sowers EG, Wells JG, Greene KD, Griffin PM, Hoekstra RM, et al. Non-O157 Shiga toxin-producing Escherichia coli infections in the United States, 1983–2002. J Infect Dis. 2005;192(8):1422–9.

56. (CDC) CfDCaP. Laboratory-confirmed non-O157 Shiga toxin-producing Escherichia coli – Connecticut, 2000–2005. MMWR Morb Mortal Wkly Rep. 2007;56(2):29–31.

57. Rivas M, Miliwebsky E, Chinen I, Roldan CD, Balbi L, Garcia B, et al. Characterization and epidemiologic subtyping of Shiga toxin-producing Escherichia coli strains isolated from hemolytic uremic syndrome and diarrhea cases in Argentina. Foodborne Pathog Dis. 2006;3(1):88–96.

58. Espie E, Grimont F, Vaillant V, Montet MP, Carle I, Bavai C, et al. O148 Shiga toxin-producing Escherichia coli outbreak: microbiological investigation as a useful complement to epidemiological investigation. Clin Microbiol Infect. 2006;12(10): 992–8.

59. Orth D, Grif K, Zimmerhackl LB, Wurzner R. Sorbitol-fermenting Shiga toxin-producing Escherichia coli O157 in Austria. Wien Klin Wochenschr. 2009;121(3–4):108–12.

60. Wahl E, Vold L, Lindstedt BA, Bruheim T, Afset JE. Investigation of an Escherichia coli O145 outbreak in a child day-care centre – extensive sampling and characterization of eae- and stx1-positive E. coli yields epidemiological and socioeconomic insight. BMC Infect Dis. 2011;11:238.

61. Taylor EV, Nguyen TA, Machesky KD, Koch E, Sotir MJ, Bohm SR, et al. Multistate outbreak of Escherichia coli O145 infections associated with romaine lettuce consumption, 2010. J Food Prot. 2013;76(6):939–44.

62. Bielaszewska M, Mellmann A, Zhang W, Kock R, Fruth A, Bauwens A, et al. Characterisation of the Escherichia coli strain associated with an outbreak of haemolytic uraemic syndrome in Germany, 2011: a microbiological study. Lancet Infect Dis. 2011;11(9):671–6.

63. Buchholz U, Bernard H, Werber D, Bohmer MM, Remschmidt C, Wilking H, et al. German outbreak of Escherichia coli O104:H4 associated with sprouts. N Engl J Med. 2011;365(19):1763–70.

64. Koch-Institut R. EHEC/HUS O104:H4 – Der Ausbruch wird als beendet betrachtet 2011 [updated 2011-07-26]. Available from: http://www.rki.de/DE/Content/Service/Presse/Pressemitteilungen/2011/|11_2011.html.

65. Davis TK, McKee R, Schnadower D, Tarr PI. Treatment of Shiga toxin-producing Escherichia coli infections. Infect Dis Clin North Am. 2013;27(3):577–97.

66. Majowicz SE, Scallan E, Jones-Bitton A, Sargeant JM, Stapleton J, Angulo FJ, et al. Global incidence

of human Shiga toxin-producing Escherichia coli infections and deaths: a systematic review and knowledge synthesis. Foodborne Pathog Dis. 2014; 11(6):447–55.

67. McLaine PN, Rowe PC, Orrbine E. Experiences with HUS in Canada: what have we learned about childhood HUS in Canada? Kidney Int Suppl. 2009;112:S25–8.

68. Rowe PC, Orrbine E, Wells GA, McLaine PN. Epidemiology of hemolytic-uremic syndrome in Canadian children from 1986 to 1988. The Canadian Pediatric Kidney Disease Reference Centre. J Pediatr. 1991;119(2):218–24.

69. Rowe PC, Orrbine E, Lior H, Wells GA, Yetisir E, Clulow M, et al. Risk of hemolytic uremic syndrome after sporadic Escherichia coli O157:H7 infection: results of a Canadian collaborative study. Investigators of the Canadian Pediatric Kidney Disease Research Center. J Pediatr. 1998;132(5): 777–82.

70. Pavia AT, Nichols CR, Green DP, Tauxe RV, Mottice S, Greene KD, et al. Hemolytic-uremic syndrome during an outbreak of Escherichia coli O157:H7 infections in institutions for mentally retarded persons: clinical and epidemiologic observations. J Pediatr. 1990;116(4):544–51.

71. Rowe PC, Orrbine E, Lior H, Wells GA, McLaine PN. A prospective study of exposure to verotoxin-producing Escherichia coli among Canadian children with haemolytic uraemic syndrome. The CPKDRC co-investigators. Epidemiol Infect. 1993;110(1):1–7.

72. Bell BP, Goldoft M, Griffin PM, Davis MA, Gordon DC, Tarr PI, et al. A multistate outbreak of Escherichia coli O157:H7-associated bloody diarrhea and hemolytic uremic syndrome from hamburgers. The Washington experience. JAMA. 1994;272(17):1349–53.

73. Gianviti A, Rosmini F, Caprioli A, Corona R, Matteucci MC, Principato F, et al. Haemolytic-uraemic syndrome in childhood: surveillance and case-control studies in Italy. Italian HUS Study Group. Pediatr Nephrol. 1994;8(6):705–9.

74. Tozzi AE, Niccolini A, Caprioli A, Luzzi I, Montini G, Zacchello G, et al. A community outbreak of haemolytic-uraemic syndrome in children occurring in a large area of northern Italy over a period of several months. Epidemiol Infect. 1994;113(2): 209–19.

75. (CDC) CfDCaP. Community outbreak of hemolytic uremic syndrome attributable to Escherichia coli O111:NM – South Australia 1995. MMWR Morb Mortal Wkly Rep. 1995;44(29):550–1. 7-8.

76. Paton AW, Ratcliff RM, Doyle RM, Seymour-Murray J, Davos D, Lanser JA, et al. Molecular microbiological investigation of an outbreak of hemolytic-uremic syndrome caused by dry fermented sausage contaminated with Shiga-like toxin-producing Escherichia coli. J Clin Microbiol. 1996;34(7):1622–7.

77. Boudailliez B, Berquin P, Mariani-Kurkdjian P, Ilef D, Cuvelier B, Capek I, et al. Possible person-to-person transmission of Escherichia coli O111 – associated hemolytic uremic syndrome. Pediatr Nephrol. 1997;11(1):36–9.

78. Verweyen HM, Karch H, Allerberger F, Zimmerhackl LB. Enterohemorrhagic Escherichia coli (EHEC) in pediatric hemolytic-uremic syndrome: a prospective study in Germany and Austria. Infection. 1999;27(6):341–7.

79. Decludt B, Bouvet P, Mariani-Kurkdjian P, Grimont F, Grimont PA, Hubert B, et al. Haemolytic uraemic syndrome and Shiga toxin-producing Escherichia coli infection in children in France. The Societe de Nephrologie Pediatrique. Epidemiol Infect. 2000;124(2):215–20.

80. Verweyen HM, Karch H, Brandis M, Zimmerhackl LB. Enterohemorrhagic Escherichia coli infections: following transmission routes. Pediatr Nephrol. 2000;14(1):73–83.

81. Gerber A, Karch H, Allerberger F, Verweyen HM, Zimmerhackl LB. Clinical course and the role of shiga toxin-producing Escherichia coli infection in the hemolytic-uremic syndrome in pediatric patients, 1997–2000, in Germany and Austria: a prospective study. J Infect Dis. 2002;186(4):493–500.

82. (CDC) CfDCaP. Outbreaks of Escherichia coli O157:H7 associated with petting zoos – North Carolina, Florida, and Arizona, 2004 and 2005. MMWR Morb Mortal Wkly Rep. 2005;54(50): 1277–80.

83. Besbas N, Karpman D, Landau D, Loirat C, Proesmans W, Remuzzi G, et al. A classification of hemolytic uremic syndrome and thrombotic thrombocytopenic purpura and related disorders. Kidney Int. 2006;70(3):423–31.

84. Friedrich AW, Zhang W, Bielaszewska M, Mellmann A, Kock R, Fruth A, et al. Prevalence, virulence profiles, and clinical significance of Shiga toxin-negative variants of enterohemorrhagic Escherichia coli O157 infection in humans. Clin Infect Dis. 2007;45(1):39–45.

85. Espie E, Vaillant V, Mariani-Kurkdjian P, Grimont F, Martin-Schaller R, De Valk H, et al. Escherichia coli O157 outbreak associated with fresh unpasteurized goats' cheese. Epidemiol Infect. 2006;134(1): 143–6.

86. Leotta GA, Miliwebsky ES, Chinen I, Espinosa EM, Azzopardi K, Tennant SM, et al. Characterisation of Shiga toxin-producing Escherichia coli O157 strains isolated from humans in Argentina, Australia and New Zealand. BMC Microbiol. 2008;8:46.

87. Rivas M, Sosa-Estani S, Rangel J, Caletti MG, Valles P, Roldan CD, et al. Risk factors for sporadic Shiga toxin-producing Escherichia coli infections in children, Argentina. Emerg Infect Dis. 2008;14(5): 763–71.

88. Alpers K, Werber D, Frank C, Koch J, Friedrich AW, Karch H, et al. Sorbitol-fermenting enterohaemorrhagic Escherichia coli O157:H- causes another

outbreak of haemolytic uraemic syndrome in children. Epidemiol Infect. 2009;137(3):389–95.

89. Goode B, O'Reilly C, Dunn J, Fullerton K, Smith S, Ghneim G, et al. Outbreak of escherichia coli O157: H7 infections after Petting Zoo visits, North Carolina State Fair, October–November 2004. Arch Pediatr Adolesc Med. 2009;163(1):42–8.

90. King LA, Mailles A, Mariani-Kurkdjian P, Vernozy-Rozand C, Montet MP, Grimont F, et al. Community-wide outbreak of Escherichia coli O157:H7 associated with consumption of frozen beef burgers. Epidemiol Infect. 2009;137(6):889–96.

91. Rosales A, Hofer J, Zimmerhackl LB, Jungraithmayr TC, Riedl M, Giner T, et al. Need for long-term follow-up in enterohemorrhagic Escherichia coli-associated hemolytic uremic syndrome due to late-emerging sequelae. Clin Infect Dis. 2012;54(10): 1413–21.

92. Vally H, Hall G, Dyda A, Raupach J, Knope K, Combs B, et al. Epidemiology of Shiga toxin producing Escherichia coli in Australia, 2000–2010. BMC Public Health. 2012;12:63.

93. Bielaszewska M, Mellmann A, Bletz S, Zhang W, Kock R, Kossow A, et al. Enterohemorrhagic Escherichia coli O26:H11/H-: a new virulent clone emerges in Europe. Clin Infect Dis. 2013;56(10): 1373–81.

94. Rivero M, Passucci J, Lucchesi P, Signorini M, Alconcher L, Rodriguez E, et al. Epidemiology of hemolytic uremic syndrome in two regions of Buenos Aires Province. Medicina. 2013;73(2):127–35.

95. Frank C, Kapfhammer S, Werber D, Stark K, Held L. Cattle density and Shiga toxin-producing Escherichia coli infection in Germany: increased risk for most but not all serogroups. Vector Borne Zoonotic Dis. 2008;8(5):635–43.

96. Haus-Cheymol R, Espie E, Che D, Vaillant V, De Valk H, Desenclos JC. Association between indicators of cattle density and incidence of paediatric haemolytic-uraemic syndrome (HUS) in children under 15 years of age in France between 1996 and 2001: an ecological study. Epidemiol Infect. 2006;134(4):712–8.

97. Karmali MA, Mascarenhas M, Petric M, Dutil L, Rahn K, Ludwig K, et al. Age-specific frequencies of antibodies to Escherichia coli verocytotoxins (Shiga toxins) 1 and 2 among urban and rural populations in southern Ontario. J Infect Dis. 2003;188(11):1724–9.

98. Williams AP, Avery LM, Killham K, Jones DL. Persistence, dissipation, and activity of Escherichia coli O157:H7 within sand and seawater environments. FEMS Microbiol Ecol. 2007;60(1):24–32.

99. Rangel JM, Sparling PH, Crowe C, Griffin PM, Swerdlow DL. Epidemiology of Escherichia coli O157:H7 outbreaks, United States, 1982–2002. Emerg Infect Dis. 2005;11(4):603–9.

100. Salvadori MI, Sontrop JM, Garg AX, Moist LM, Suri RS, Clark WF. Factors that led to the Walkerton tragedy. Kidney Int Suppl. 2009;112:S33–4.

101. Yukioka H, Kurita S. Escherichia coli O157 infection disaster in Japan, 1996. Eur J Emerg Med: Off J Eur Soc Emerg Med. 1997;4(3):165.

102. Fukushima H, Hashizume T, Morita Y, Tanaka J, Azuma K, Mizumoto Y, et al. Clinical experiences in Sakai City Hospital during the massive outbreak of enterohemorrhagic Escherichia coli O157 infections in Sakai City, 1996. Pediatr Int: Off J Jpn Pediatr Soc. 1999;41(2):213–7.

103. Ackers ML, Mahon BE, Leahy E, Goode B, Damrow T, Hayes PS, et al. An outbreak of Escherichia coli O157:H7 infections associated with leaf lettuce consumption. J Infect Dis. 1998;177(6):1588–93.

104. Kemper MJ. Outbreak of hemolytic uremic syndrome caused by E. coli O104:H4 in Germany: a pediatric perspective. Pediatr Nephrol. 2012; 27(2):161–4.

105. Loos S, Ahlenstiel T, Kranz B, Staude H, Pape L, Hartel C, et al. An outbreak of Shiga toxin-producing Escherichia coli O104:H4 hemolytic uremic syndrome in Germany: presentation and short-term outcome in children. Clin Infect Dis. 2012;55(6): 753–9.

106. Mingle LA, Garcia DL, Root TP, Halse TA, Quinlan TM, Armstrong LR, et al. Enhanced identification and characterization of non-O157 Shiga toxin-producing Escherichia coli: a six-year study. Foodborne Pathog Dis. 2012;9(11):1028–36.

107. Byrne L, Vanstone GL, Perry NT, Launders N, Adak GK, Godbole G, et al. Epidemiology and microbiology of Shiga toxin-producing Escherichia coli other than serogroup O157 in England, 2009–2013. J Med Microbiol. 2014;63(Pt 9):1181–8.

108. Luna-Gierke RE, Wymore K, Sadlowski J, Clogher P, Gierke RW, Tobin-D'Angelo M, et al. Multiple-aetiology enteric infections involving non-O157 Shiga toxin-producing Escherichia coli – FoodNet, 2001–2010. Zoonoses Public Health. 2014;61(7): 492–8.

109. Luna-Gierke RE, Griffin PM, Gould LH, Herman K, Bopp CA, Strockbine N, et al. Outbreaks of non-O157 Shiga toxin-producing Escherichia coli infection: USA. Epidemiol Infect. 2014:1–11.

110. Scallan E, Hoekstra RM, Angulo FJ, Tauxe RV, Widdowson MA, Roy SL, et al. Foodborne illness acquired in the United States – major pathogens. Emerg Infect Dis. 2011;17(1):7–15.

111. Gould LH, Mody RK, Ong KL, Clogher P, Cronquist AB, Garman KN, et al. Increased recognition of non-O157 Shiga toxin-producing Escherichia coli infections in the United States during 2000–2010: epidemiologic features and comparison with E. coli O157 infections. Foodborne Pathog Dis. 2013;10(5):453–60.

112. Werber D, Fruth A, Liesegang A, Littmann M, Buchholz U, Prager R, et al. A multistate outbreak of Shiga toxin-producing Escherichia coli O26:H11 infections in Germany, detected by molecular subtyping surveillance. J Infect Dis. 2002;186(3): 419–22.

113. Werber D, Fruth A, Heissenhuber A, Wildner M, Prager R, Tschape H, et al. Shiga toxin-producing Escherichia coli O157 more frequently cause bloody diarrhea than do non-O157 strains. J Infect Dis. 2004;189(7):1335–6. author reply 6-7.

114. Croxen MA, Law RJ, Scholz R, Keeney KM, Wlodarska M, Finlay BB. Recent advances in understanding enteric pathogenic Escherichia coli. Clin Microbiol Rev. 2013;26(4):822–80.

115. Tarr PI, Gordon CA, Chandler WL. Shiga-toxin-producing Escherichia coli and haemolytic uraemic syndrome. Lancet. 2005;365(9464):1073–86.

116. Preussel K, Hohle M, Stark K, Werber D. Shiga toxin-producing Escherichia coli O157 is more likely to lead to hospitalization and death than non-O157 serogroups – except O104. PLoS One. 2013;8(11):e78180.

117. Bielaszewska M, Zhang W, Mellmann A, Karch H. Enterohaemorrhagic Escherichia coli O26:H11/H-: a human pathogen in emergence. Berl Munch Tierarztl Wochenschr. 2007;120(7–8): 279–87.

118. Chase-Topping ME, Rosser T, Allison LJ, Courcier E, Evans J, McKendrick IJ, et al. Pathogenic potential to humans of bovine Escherichia coli O26, Scotland. Emerg Infect Dis. 2012;18(3):439–48.

119. Feng PC, Monday SR, Lacher DW, Allison L, Siitonen A, Keys C, et al. Genetic diversity among clonal lineages within Escherichia coli O157:H7 stepwise evolutionary model. Emerg Infect Dis. 2007;13(11):1701–6.

120. Werber D, Bielaszewska M, Frank C, Stark K, Karch H. Watch out for the even eviler cousin-sorbitol-fermenting E coli O157. Lancet. 2011; 377(9762):298–9.

121. Eklund M, Bielaszewska M, Nakari UM, Karch H, Siitonen A. Molecular and phenotypic profiling of sorbitol-fermenting Escherichia coli O157:H- human isolates from Finland. Clin Microbiol Infect. 2006;12(7):634–41.

122. Nielsen S, Frank C, Fruth A, Spode A, Prager R, Graff A, et al. Desperately seeking diarrhoea: outbreak of haemolytic uraemic syndrome caused by emerging sorbitol-fermenting shiga toxin-producing Escherichia coli O157:H-, Germany, 2009. Zoonoses Public Health. 2011;58(8):567–72.

123. Karch H, Wiß R, Gloning H, Emmrich P, Aleksic S, Bockemuhl J. Hemolytic-uremic syndrome in infants due to verotoxin-producing Escherichia coli. Dtsch Med Wochenschr. 1990;115(13):489–95.

124. Caprioli A, Luzzi I, Rosmini F, Resti C, Edefonti A, Perfumo F, et al. Community-wide outbreak of hemolytic-uremic syndrome associated with non-O157 verocytotoxin-producing Escherichia coli. J Infect Dis. 1994;169(1):208–11.

125. Bell BP, Griffin PM, Lozano P, Christie DL, Kobayashi JM, Tarr PI. Predictors of hemolytic uremic syndrome in children during a large outbreak of Escherichia coli O157:H7 infections. Pediatrics. 1997;100(1):E12.

126. Shefer AM, Koo D, Werner SB, Mintz ED, Baron R, Wells JG, et al. A cluster of Escherichia coli O157:H7 infections with the hemolytic-uremic syndrome and death in California. A mandate for improved surveillance. West J Med. 1996; 165(1–2):15–9.

127. Slutsker L, Ries AA, Maloney K, Wells JG, Greene KD, Griffin PM. A nationwide case-control study of Escherichia coli O157:H7 infection in the United States. J Infect Dis. 1998;177(4):962–6.

128. Tuttle J, Gomez T, Doyle MP, Wells JG, Zhao T, Tauxe RV, et al. Lessons from a large outbreak of Escherichia coli O157:H7 infections: insights into the infectious dose and method of widespread contamination of hamburger patties. Epidemiol Infect. 1999;122(2):185–92.

129. Ikeda K, Ida O, Kimoto K, Takatorige T, Nakanishi N, Tatara K. Predictors for the development of haemolytic uraemic syndrome with Escherichia coli O157:H7 infections: with focus on the day of illness. Epidemiol Infect. 2000;124(3):343–9.

130. Yoshioka K, Yagi K, Moriguchi N. Clinical features and treatment of children with hemolytic uremic syndrome caused by enterohemorrhagic Escherichia coli O157:H7 infection: experience of an outbreak in Sakai City, 1996. Pediatr Int: Off J Jpn Pediatr Soc. 1999;41(2):223–7.

131. Higami S, Nishimoto K, Kawamura T, Tsuruhara T, Isshiki G, Ookita A. Retrospective analysis of the relationship between HUS incidence and antibiotics among patients with Escherichia coli O157 enterocolitis in the Sakai outbreak. Kansenshogaku zasshi J Jpn Assoc Infect Dis. 1998;72(3):266–72.

132. Dundas S, Todd WT, Stewart AI, Murdoch PS, Chaudhuri AK, Hutchinson SJ. The central Scotland Escherichia coli O157:H7 outbreak: risk factors for the hemolytic uremic syndrome and death among hospitalized patients. Clin Infect Dis. 2001;33(7):923–31.

133. Dundas S, Murphy J, Soutar RL, Jones GA, Hutchinson SJ, Todd WT. Effectiveness of therapeutic plasma exchange in the 1996 Lanarkshire Escherichia coli O157:H7 outbreak. Lancet. 1999; 354(9187):1327–30.

134. Cowden JM, Ahmed S, Donaghy M, Riley A. Epidemiological investigation of the central Scotland outbreak of Escherichia coli O157 infection, November to December 1996. Epidemiol Infect. 2001;126(3):335–41.

135. Auld H, MacIver D, Klaassen J. Heavy rainfall and waterborne disease outbreaks: the Walkerton example. J Toxicol Environ Health A. 2004;67(20–22): 1879–87.

136. Ali SH. A socio-ecological autopsy of the E. coli O157:H7 outbreak in Walkerton, Ontario, Canada. Soc Sci Med. 2004;58(12):2601–12.

137. Garg AX, Macnab J, Clark W, Ray JG, Marshall JK, Suri RS, et al. Long-term health sequelae following E. coli and campylobacter contamination of municipal water. Population sampling and assessing

non-participation biases. Can J Public Health. 2005;96(2):125–30.

138. Richards A. The Walkerton Health Study. Can Nurse. 2005;101(5):16–21.

139. Bradley KK, Williams JM, Burnsed LJ, Lytle MB, McDermott MD, Mody RK, et al. Epidemiology of a large restaurant-associated outbreak of Shiga toxin-producing Escherichia coli O111:NM. Epidemiol Infect. 2012;140(9):1644–54.

140. Frank C, Werber D, Cramer JP, Askar M, Faber M, an der Heiden M, et al. Epidemic profile of Shiga-toxin-producing Escherichia coli O104:H4 outbreak in Germany. N Engl J Med. 2011;365(19):1771–80.

141. Menne J, Nitschke M, Stingele R, Abu-Tair M, Beneke J, Bramstedt J, et al. Validation of treatment strategies for enterohaemorrhagic Escherichia coli O104:H4 induced haemolytic uraemic syndrome: case-control study. BMJ. 2012;345:e4565.

142. Mody RK, Luna-Gierke RE, Jones TF, Comstock N, Hurd S, Scheftel J, et al. Infections in pediatric post-diarrheal hemolytic uremic syndrome: factors associated with identifying shiga toxin-producing Escherichia coli. Arch Pediatr Adolesc Med. 2012;166(10):902–9.

143. (CDC) CfDCaP. National Shiga toxin-producing Escherichia coli (STEC) surveillance overview. Atlanta: US Department of Health and Human Services, CDC; 2012. Available from: http://www.cdc.gov/ncezid/dfwed/pdfs/national-stec-surveillance-overiew-508c.pdf.

144. Canada PHAo. FoodNet Canada 2013 [updated 2013-11-15]. Available from: http://www.phac-aspc.gc.ca/foodnetcanada/index-eng.php.

145. sanitaire Idv. SYNDROME HÉMOLYTIQUE ET URÉMIQUE 2006 [updated 2014-07-31]. Available from: http://www.invs.sante.fr/Dossiers-thematiques/Maladies-infectieuses/Risques-infectieux-d-origine-alimentaire/Syndrome-hemolytique-et-uremique.

146. Richardson SE, Rotman TA, Jay V, Smith CR, Becker LE, Petric M, et al. Experimental verocyto-toxemia in rabbits. Infect Immun. 1992;60(10):4154–67.

147. Lopez EL, Contrini MM, Glatstein E, Ayala SG, Santoro R, Ezcurra G, et al. An epidemiologic surveillance of Shiga-like toxin-producing Escherichia coli infection in Argentinean children: risk factors and serum Shiga-like toxin 2 values. Pediatr Infect Dis J. 2012;31(1):20–4.

148. Chandler WL, Jelacic S, Boster DR, Ciol MA, Williams GD, Watkins SL, et al. Prothrombotic coagulation abnormalities preceding the hemolytic-uremic syndrome. N Engl J Med. 2002;346(1):23–32.

149. Tsai HM, Chandler WL, Sarode R, Hoffman R, Jelacic S, Habeeb RL, et al. von Willebrand factor and von Willebrand factor-cleaving metalloprotease activity in Escherichia coli O157:H7-associated hemolytic uremic syndrome. Pediatr Res. 2001;49(5):653–9.

150. Bitzan M, Ludwig K, Klemt M, Konig H, Buren J, Muller-Wiefel DE. The role of Escherichia coli O

151. infections in the classical (enteropathic) haemolytic uraemic syndrome: results of a Central European, multicentre study. Epidemiol Infect. 1993;110(2):183–96.

151. Cornick NA, Jelacic S, Ciol MA, Tarr PI. Escherichia coli O157:H7 infections: discordance between filterable fecal shiga toxin and disease outcome. J Infect Dis. 2002;186(1):57–63.

152. Yamagami S, Motoki M, Kimura T, Izumi H, Takeda T, Katsuura Y, et al. Efficacy of postinfection treatment with anti-Shiga toxin (Stx) 2 humanized monoclonal antibody TMA-15 in mice lethally challenged with Stx-producing Escherichia coli. J Infect Dis. 2001;184(6):738–42.

153. Bitzan M, Schaefer F, Reymond D. Treatment of typical (enteropathic) hemolytic uremic syndrome. Semin Thromb Hemost. 2010;36(6):594–610.

154. Nishikawa K. Recent progress of Shiga toxin neutralizer for treatment of infections by Shiga toxin-producing Escherichia coli. Arch Immunol Ther Exp (Warsz). 2011;59(4):239–47.

155. Stearns-Kurosawa DJ, Collins V, Freeman S, Debord D, Nishikawa K, Oh SY, et al. Rescue from lethal Shiga toxin 2-induced renal failure with a cell-permeable peptide. Pediatr Nephrol. 2011; 26(11):2031–9.

156. Brunder W, Schmidt H, Karch H. EspP, a novel extracellular serine protease of enterohaemorrhagic Escherichia coli O157:H7 cleaves human coagulation factor V. Mol Microbiol. 1997;24(4):767–78.

157. Harama D, Koyama K, Mukai M, Shimokawa N, Miyata M, Nakamura Y, et al. A subcytotoxic dose of subtilase cytotoxin prevents lipopolysaccharide-induced inflammatory responses, depending on its capacity to induce the unfolded protein response. J Immunol. 2009;183(2):1368–74.

158. Brockmeyer J, Spelten S, Kuczius T, Bielaszewska M, Karch H. Structure and function relationship of the autotransport and proteolytic activity of EspP from Shiga toxin-producing Escherichia coli. PLoS One. 2009;4(7):e6100.

159. Orth D, Ehrlenbach S, Brockmeyer J, Khan AB, Huber G, Karch H, et al. EspP, a serine protease of enterohemorrhagic Escherichia coli, impairs complement activation by cleaving complement factors C3/C3b and C5. Infect Immun. 2010;78(10):4294–301.

160. May KL, Paton JC, Paton AW. Escherichia coli subtilase cytotoxin induces apoptosis regulated by host Bcl-2 family proteins Bax/Bak. Infect Immun. 2010;78(11):4691–6.

161. Brockmeyer J, Aldick T, Soltwisch J, Zhang W, Tarr PI, Weiss A, et al. Enterohaemorrhagic Escherichia coli haemolysin is cleaved and inactivated by serine protease EspPalpha. Environ Microbiol. 2011;13(5):1327–41.

162. Shames SR, Croxen MA, Deng W, Finlay BB. The type III system-secreted effector EspZ localizes to host mitochondria and interacts with the translocase of inner mitochondrial membrane 17b. Infect Immun. 2011;79(12):4784–90.

163. Zhao Y, Tian T, Huang T, Nakajima S, Saito Y, Takahashi S, et al. Subtilase cytotoxin activates MAP kinases through PERK and IRE1 branches of the unfolded protein response. Toxicol Sci: Off J Soc Toxicol. 2011;120(1):79–86.

164. Wong AR, Raymond B, Collins JW, Crepin VF, Frankel G. The enteropathogenic E. coli effector EspH promotes actin pedestal formation and elongation via WASP-interacting protein (WIP). Cell Microbiol. 2012;14(7):1051–70.

165. Amaral MM, Sacerdoti F, Jancic C, Repetto HA, Paton AW, Paton JC, et al. Action of shiga toxin type-2 and subtilase cytotoxin on human microvascular endothelial cells. PLoS One. 2013;8(7):e70431.

166. In J, Lukyanenko V, Foulke-Abel J, Hubbard AL, Delannoy M, Hansen AM, et al. Serine protease EspP from enterohemorrhagic Escherichia coli is sufficient to induce shiga toxin macropinocytosis in intestinal epithelium. PLoS One. 2013;8(7):e69196.

167. Wang H, Rogers TJ, Paton JC, Paton AW. Differential effects of Escherichia coli subtilase cytotoxin and Shiga toxin 2 on chemokine and proinflammatory cytokine expression in human macrophage, colonic epithelial, and brain microvascular endothelial cell lines. Infect Immun. 2014;82(9):3567–79.

168. Marquez LB, Velazquez N, Repetto HA, Paton AW, Paton JC, Ibarra C, et al. Effects of Escherichia coli subtilase cytotoxin and Shiga toxin 2 on primary cultures of human renal tubular epithelial cells. PLoS One. 2014;9(1):e87022.

169. Battle SE, Brady MJ, Vanaja SK, Leong JM, Hecht GA. Actin pedestal formation by enterohemorrhagic Escherichia coli enhances bacterial host cell attachment and concomitant type III translocation. Infect Immun. 2014;82(9):3713–22.

170. Wong AR, Pearson JS, Bright MD, Munera D, Robinson KS, Lee SF, et al. Enteropathogenic and enterohaemorrhagic Escherichia coli: even more subversive elements. Mol Microbiol. 2011; 80(6):1420–38.

171. Newton HJ, Pearson JS, Badea L, Kelly M, Lucas M, Holloway G, et al. The type III effectors NleE and NleB from enteropathogenic E. coli and OspZ from Shigella block nuclear translocation of NF-kappaB p65. PLoS Pathog. 2010;6(5):e1000898.

172. Wong AR, Clements A, Raymond B, Crepin VF, Frankel G. The interplay between the Escherichia coli Rho guanine nucleotide exchange factor effectors and the mammalian RhoGEF inhibitor EspH. MBio. 2012;3(1).

173. Schmidt H, Zhang WL, Hemmrich U, Jelacic S, Brunder W, Tarr PI, et al. Identification and characterization of a novel genomic island integrated at selC in locus of enterocyte effacement-negative, Shiga toxin-producing Escherichia coli. Infect Immun. 2001;69(11):6863–73.

174. Tarr PI, Bilge SS, Vary Jr JC, Jelacic S, Habeeb RL, Ward TR, et al. Iha: a novel Escherichia coli O157:H7 adherence-conferring molecule encoded

on a recently acquired chromosomal island of conserved structure. Infect Immun. 2000;68(3):1400–7.

175. Paton AW, Srimanote P, Woodrow MC, Paton JC. Characterization of Saa, a novel autoagglutinating adhesin produced by locus of enterocyte effacement-negative Shiga-toxigenic Escherichia coli strains that are virulent for humans. Infect Immun. 2001;69(11):6999–7009.

176. Eklund M, Leino K, Siitonen A. Clinical Escherichia coli strains carrying stx genes: stx variants and stx-positive virulence profiles. J Clin Microbiol. 2002;40(12):4585–93.

177. Taneike I, Zhang HM, Wakisaka-Saito N, Yamamoto T. Enterohemolysin operon of Shiga toxin-producing Escherichia coli: a virulence function of inflammatory cytokine production from human monocytes. FEBS Lett. 2002;524(1–3):219–24.

178. Aldick T, Bielaszewska M, Zhang W, Brockmeyer J, Schmidt H, Friedrich AW, et al. Hemolysin from Shiga toxin-negative Escherichia coli O26 strains injures microvascular endothelium. Microbes Infect. 2007;9(3):282–90.

179. Bielaszewska M, Aldick T, Bauwens A, Karch H. Hemolysin of enterohemorrhagic Escherichia coli: structure, transport, biological activity and putative role in virulence. Int J Med Microbiol. 2014;304(5–6):521–9.

180. Paton AW, Srimanote P, Talbot UM, Wang H, Paton JC. A new family of potent AB(5) cytotoxins produced by Shiga toxigenic Escherichia coli. J Exp Med. 2004;200(1):35–46.

181. Paton AW, Beddoe T, Thorpe CM, Whisstock JC, Wilce MC, Rossjohn J, et al. AB5 subtilase cytotoxin inactivates the endoplasmic reticulum chaperone BiP. Nature. 2006;443(7111):548–52.

182. Funk J, Stoeber H, Hauser E, Schmidt H. Molecular analysis of subtilase cytotoxin genes of food-borne Shiga toxin-producing Escherichia coli reveals a new allelic subAB variant. BMC Microbiol. 2013;13:230.

183. Burland V, Shao Y, Perna NT, Plunkett G, Sofia HJ, Blattner FR. The complete DNA sequence and analysis of the large virulence plasmid of Escherichia coli O157:H7. Nucleic Acids Res. 1998;26(18): 4196–204.

184. Brunder W, Schmidt H, Frosch M, Karch H. The large plasmids of Shiga-toxin-producing Escherichia coli (STEC) are highly variable genetic elements. Microbiology. 1999;145(Pt 5):1005–14.

185. Perna NT, Plunkett 3rd G, Burland V, Mau B, Glasner JD, Rose DJ, et al. Genome sequence of enterohaemorrhagic Escherichia coli O157:H7. Nature. 2001;409(6819):529–33.

186. Brunder W, Schmidt H, Karch H. KatP, a novel catalase-peroxidase encoded by the large plasmid of enterohaemorrhagic Escherichia coli O157:H7. Microbiology. 1996;142(Pt 11):3305–15.

187. Grys TE, Siegel MB, Lathem WW, Welch RA. The StcE protease contributes to intimate adherence of

enterohemorrhagic Escherichia coli O157:H7 to host cells. Infect Immun. 2005;73(3):1295–303.

188. Schuller S, Heuschkel R, Torrente F, Kaper JB, Phillips AD. Shiga toxin binding in normal and inflamed human intestinal mucosa. Microbes Infect. 2007;9(1):35–9.

189. Bekassy ZD, Calderon Toledo C, Leoj G, Kristoffersson A, Leopold SR, Perez MT, et al. Intestinal damage in enterohemorrhagic Escherichia coli infection. Pediatr Nephrol. 2011;26(11): 2059–71.

190. Schuller S, Phillips AD. Microaerobic conditions enhance type III secretion and adherence of entero-haemorrhagic Escherichia coli to polarized human intestinal epithelial cells. Environ Microbiol. 2010;12(9):2426–35.

191. Bellmeyer A, Cotton C, Kanteti R, Koutsouris A, Viswanathan VK, Hecht G. Enterohemorrhagic Escherichia coli suppresses inflammatory response to cytokines and its own toxin. Am J Physiol Gastrointest Liver Physiol. 2009;297(3):G576–81.

192. Mellmann A, Bielaszewska M, Kock R, Friedrich AW, Fruth A, Middendorf B, et al. Analysis of collection of hemolytic uremic syndrome-associated enterohemorrhagic Escherichia coli. Emerg Infect Dis. 2008;14(8):1287–90.

193. Karmali MA, Mascarenhas M, Shen S, Ziebell K, Johnson S, Reid-Smith R, et al. Association of genomic O island 122 of Escherichia coli EDL 933 with verocytotoxin-producing Escherichia coli seropathotypes that are linked to epidemic and/or serious disease. J Clin Microbiol. 2003;41(11):4930–40.

194. Kobayashi N, Lee K, Yamazaki A, Saito S, Furukawa I, Kono T, et al. Virulence gene profiles and population genetic analysis for exploration of pathogenic serogroups of Shiga toxin-producing Escherichia coli. J Clin Microbiol. 2013;51(12):4022–8.

195. Grad YH, Godfrey P, Cerquiera GC, Mariani-Kurkdjian P, Gouali M, Bingen E, et al. Comparative genomics of recent Shiga toxin-producing Escherichia coli O104:H4: short-term evolution of an emerging pathogen. MBio. 2013;4(1): e00452–12.

196. Mellmann A, Bielaszewska M, Zimmerhackl LB, Prager R, Harmsen D, Tschape H, et al. Enterohemorrhagic Escherichia coli in human infection: in vivo evolution of a bacterial pathogen. Clin Infect Dis. 2005;41(6):785–92.

197. Bielaszewska M, Kock R, Friedrich AW, von Eiff C, Zimmerhackl LB, Karch H, et al. Shiga toxin-mediated hemolytic uremic syndrome: time to change the diagnostic paradigm? PLoS One. 2007;2(10):e1024.

198. Bergan J, Dyve Lingelem AB, Simm R, Skotland T, Sandvig K. Shiga toxins. Toxicon: Off J Int Soc Toxinology. 2012;60(6):1085–107.

199. Bast DJ, Banerjee L, Clark C, Read RJ, Brunton JL. The identification of three biologically relevant globotriaosyl ceramide receptor binding sites on the Verotoxin 1 B subunit. Mol Microbiol. 1999;32(5):953–60.

200. Shiga K. Über den Dysenterie-bacillus (Bacillus dysenteriae). Centralblatt Bakteriologie Parasitenkunde Infektionskr Erste Abt Med-Hygienische Bakter-iologie Tierische Parasitenkunde. 1898;24:913–8.

201. Neisser M, Shiga K. Über freie Rezeptoren von Typhus- und Dysenterie-Bazillen und über das Dysenterie-Toxin. Dtsch Med Wochenschr. 1903;29:61–2.

202. Bridgwater FA, Morgan RS, Rowson KE, Wright GP. The neurotoxin of Shigella shigae: morphological and functional lesions produced in the central nervous system of rabbits. Br J Exp Pathol. 1955;36(5):447–53.

203. Howard JG. Observations on the intoxication produced in mice and rabbits by the neurotoxin of Shigella shigae. Br J Exp Pathol. 1955;36(5):439–46.

204. Keusch GT, Grady GF, Mata LJ, McIver J. The pathogenesis of Shigella diarrhea. I. Enterotoxin production by Shigella dysenteriae I. J Clin Invest. 1972;51(5):1212–8.

205. Bitzan M, Klemt M, Steffens R, Muller-Wiefel DE. Differences in verotoxin neutralizing activity of therapeutic immunoglobulins and sera from healthy controls. Infection. 1993;21(3):140–5.

206. Taylor CM, Milford DV, Rose PE, Roy TC, Rowe B. The expression of blood group P1 in post-enteropathic haemolytic uraemic syndrome. Pediatr Nephrol. 1990;4(1):59–61.

207. Armstrong GD, Fodor E, Vanmaele R. Investigation of Shiga-like toxin binding to chemically synthesized oligosaccharide sequences. J Infect Dis. 1991;164(6):1160–7.

208. Bitzan M, Richardson S, Huang C, Boyd B, Petric M, Karmali MA. Evidence that verotoxins (Shiga-like toxins) from Escherichia coli bind to P blood group antigens of human erythrocytes in vitro. Infect Immun. 1994;62(8):3337–47.

209. Cooling LL, Walker KE, Gille T, Koerner TA. Shiga toxin binds human platelets via globotriaosylceramide (Pk antigen) and a novel platelet glycosphingolipid. Infect Immun. 1998;66(9):4355–66.

210. Kiarash A, Boyd B, Lingwood CA. Glycosphingolipid receptor function is modified by fatty acid content. Verotoxin 1 and verotoxin 2c preferentially recognize different globotriaosyl ceramide fatty acid homologues. J Biol Chem. 1994;269(15):11138–46.

211. Rutjes NW, Binnington BA, Smith CR, Maloney MD, Lingwood CA. Differential tissue targeting and pathogenesis of verotoxins 1 and 2 in the mouse animal model. Kidney Int. 2002;62(3):832–45.

212. Schweppe CH, Bielaszewska M, Pohlentz G, Friedrich AW, Buntemeyer H, Schmidt MA, et al. Glycosphingolipids in vascular endothelial cells: relationship of heterogeneity in Gb3Cer/CD77 receptor expression with differential Shiga toxin 1 cytotoxicity. Glycoconj J. 2008;25(4):291–304.

213. Tam P, Mahfoud R, Nutikka A, Khine AA, Binnington B, Paroutis P, et al. Differential intracellular transport and binding of verotoxin 1 and verotoxin 2 to globotriaosylceramide-containing lipid assemblies. J Cell Physiol. 2008;216(3):750–63.

214. Khan F, Proulx F, Lingwood CA. Detergent-resistant globotriaosyl ceramide may define verotoxin/glomeruli-restricted hemolytic uremic syndrome pathology. Kidney Int. 2009;75(11):1209–16.

215. Lingwood CA, Binnington B, Manis A, Branch DR. Globotriaosyl ceramide receptor function – where membrane structure and pathology intersect. FEBS Lett. 2010;584(9):1879–86.

216. Boerlin P, McEwen SA, Boerlin-Petzold F, Wilson JB, Johnson RP, Gyles CL. Associations between virulence factors of Shiga toxin-producing Escherichia coli and disease in humans. J Clin Microbiol. 1999;37(3):497–503.

217. Okuda T, Nakayama K. Identification and characterization of the human Gb3/CD77 synthase gene promoter. Glycobiology. 2008;18(12):1028–35.

218. Okuda T, Tokuda N, Numata S, Ito M, Ohta M, Kawamura K, et al. Targeted disruption of Gb3/CD77 synthase gene resulted in the complete deletion of globo-series glycosphingolipids and loss of sensitivity to verotoxins. J Biol Chem. 2006;281(15):10230–5.

219. Engedal N, Skotland T, Torgersen ML, Sandvig K. Shiga toxin and its use in targeted cancer therapy and imaging. Microb Biotechnol. 2011;4(1):32–46.

220. Arab S, Murakami M, Dirks P, Boyd B, Hubbard SL, Lingwood CA, et al. Verotoxins inhibit the growth of and induce apoptosis in human astrocytoma cells. J Neurooncol. 1998;40(2):137–50.

221. Obata F, Tohyama K, Bonev AD, Kolling GL, Keepers TR, Gross LK, et al. Shiga toxin 2 affects the central nervous system through receptor globotriaosylceramide localized to neurons. J Infect Dis. 2008;198(9):1398–406.

222. Bitzan M, Moebius E, Ludwig K, Muller-Wiefel DE, Heesemann J, Karch H. High incidence of serum antibodies to Escherichia coli O157 lipopolysaccharide in children with hemolytic-uremic syndrome. J Pediatr. 1991;119(3):380–5.

223. Stahl AL, Sartz L, Karpman D. Complement activation on platelet-leukocyte complexes and microparticles in enterohemorrhagic Escherichia coli-induced hemolytic uremic syndrome. Blood. 2011;117(20):5503–13.

224. Karpman D, Papadopoulou D, Nilsson K, Sjogren AC, Mikaelsson C, Lethagen S. Platelet activation by Shiga toxin and circulatory factors as a pathogenetic mechanism in the hemolytic uremic syndrome. Blood. 2001;97(10):3100–8.

225. Stahl AL, Sartz L, Nelsson A, Bekassy ZD, Karpman D. Shiga toxin and lipopolysaccharide induce platelet-leukocyte aggregates and tissue factor release, a thrombotic mechanism in hemolytic uremic syndrome. PLoS One. 2009;4(9):e6990.

226. DeGrandis S, Law H, Brunton J, Gyles C, Lingwood CA. Globotetraosylceramide is recognized by the pig edema disease toxin. J Biol Chem. 1989;264(21):12520–5.

227. Meisen I, Rosenbruck R, Galla HJ, Huwel S, Kouzel IU, Mormann M, et al. Expression of Shiga toxin 2e glycosphingolipid receptors of primary porcine brain endothelial cells and toxin-mediated breakdown of the blood-brain barrier. Glycobiology. 2013;23(6):745–59.

228. Muniesa M, Recktenwald J, Bielaszewska M, Karch H, Schmidt H. Characterization of a shiga toxin 2e-converting bacteriophage from an Escherichia coli strain of human origin. Infect Immun. 2000;68(9):4850–5.

229. Friedrich AW, Bielaszewska M, Zhang WL, Pulz M, Kuczius T, Ammon A, et al. Escherichia coli harboring Shiga toxin 2 gene variants: frequency and association with clinical symptoms. J Infect Dis. 2002;185(1):74–84.

230. Sonntag AK, Bielaszewska M, Mellmann A, Dierksen N, Schierack P, Wieler LH, et al. Shiga toxin 2e-producing Escherichia coli isolates from humans and pigs differ in their virulence profiles and interactions with intestinal epithelial cells. Appl Environ Microbiol. 2005;71(12):8855–63.

231. Muthing J, Meisen I, Zhang W, Bielaszewska M, Mormann M, Bauerfeind R, et al. Promiscuous Shiga toxin 2e and its intimate relationship to Forssman. Glycobiology. 2012;22(6):849–62.

232. Jacewicz M, Clausen H, Nudelman E, Donohue-Rolfe A, Keusch GT. Pathogenesis of shigella diarrhea. XI. Isolation of a shigella toxin-binding glycolipid from rabbit jejunum and HeLa cells and its identification as globotriaosylceramide. J Exp Med. 1986;163(6):1391–404.

233. Lindberg AA, Brown JE, Stromberg N, Westling-Ryd M, Schultz JE, Karlsson KA. Identification of the carbohydrate receptor for Shiga toxin produced by Shigella dysenteriae type 1. J Biol Chem. 1987;262(4):1779–85.

234. Lingwood CA, Law H, Richardson S, Petric M, Brunton JL, De Grandis S, et al. Glycolipid binding of purified and recombinant Escherichia coli produced verotoxin in vitro. J Biol Chem. 1987;262(18):8834–9.

235. Muthing J, Schweppe CH, Karch H, Friedrich AW. Shiga toxins, glycosphingolipid diversity, and endothelial cell injury. Thromb Haemost. 2009;101(2):252–64.

236. Johannes L, Romer W. Shiga toxins – from cell biology to biomedical applications. Nat Rev Microbiol. 2010;8(2):105–16.

237. Betz J, Bauwens A, Kunsmann L, Bielaszewska M, Mormann M, Humpf HU, et al. Uncommon membrane distribution of Shiga toxin glycosphingolipid receptors in toxin-sensitive human glomerular microvascular endothelial cells. Biol Chem. 2012;393(3):133–47.

238. Karve SS, Weiss AA. Glycolipid binding preferences of Shiga toxin variants. PLoS One. 2014;9(7):e101173.

239. Sandvig K, Bergan J, Kavaliauskiene S, Skotland T. Lipid requirements for entry of protein toxins into cells. Prog Lipid Res. 2014;54:1–13.

240. Watkins EB, Gao H, Dennison AJ, Chopin N, Struth B, Arnold T, et al. Carbohydrate conformation and lipid condensation in monolayers containing glycosphingolipid gb3: influence of acyl chain structure. Biophys J. 2014;107(5):1146–55.

241. Becker GL, Lu Y, Hardes K, Strehlow B, Levesque C, Lindberg I, et al. Highly potent inhibitors of proprotein convertase furin as potential drugs for treatment of infectious diseases. J Biol Chem. 2012;287(26):21992–2003.

242. Sandvig K, Skotland T, van Deurs B, Klokk TI. Retrograde transport of protein toxins through the Golgi apparatus. Histochem Cell Biol. 2013;140(3):317–26.

243. Endo Y, Tsurugi K, Yutsudo T, Takeda Y, Ogasawara T, Igarashi K. Site of action of a Vero toxin (VT2) from Escherichia coli O157:H7 and of Shiga toxin on eukaryotic ribosomes. RNA N-glycosidase activity of the toxins. Eur J Biochem. 1988; 171(1–2):45–50.

244. Loirat C, Saland J, Bitzan M. Management of hemolytic uremic syndrome. Presse Med. 2012;41(3 Pt 2):e115–35.

245. Cherla RP, Lee SY, Mees PL, Tesh VL. Shiga toxin 1-induced cytokine production is mediated by MAP kinase pathways and translation initiation factor eIF4E in the macrophage-like THP-1 cell line. J Leukoc Biol. 2006;79(2):397–407.

246. Foster GH, Tesh VL. Shiga toxin 1-induced activation of c-Jun NH(2)-terminal kinase and p38 in the human monocytic cell line THP-1: possible involvement in the production of TNF-alpha. J Leukoc Biol. 2002;71(1):107–14.

247. Smith WE, Kane AV, Campbell ST, Acheson DW, Cochran BH, Thorpe CM. Shiga toxin 1 triggers a ribotoxic stress response leading to p38 and JNK activation and induction of apoptosis in intestinal epithelial cells. Infect Immun. 2003;71(3):1497–504.

248. Bitzan M, Foster G. Shiga toxin causes Bcl-2 phosphorylation and apoptosis of renal epithelial cells via c-Jun kinase. J Am Soc Nephrol. 2005;16:160A.

249. Brigotti M, Carnicelli D, Ravanelli E, Vara AG, Martinelli C, Alfieri RR, et al. Molecular damage and induction of proinflammatory cytokines in human endothelial cells exposed to Shiga toxin 1, Shiga toxin 2, and alpha-sarcin. Infect Immun. 2007;75(5):2201–7.

250. Jandhyala DM, Ahluwalia A, Obrig T, Thorpe CM. ZAK: a MAP3Kinase that transduces Shiga toxin- and ricin-induced proinflammatory cytokine expression. Cell Microbiol. 2008;10(7):1468–77.

251. Leyva-Illades D, Cherla RP, Lee MS, Tesh VL. Regulation of cytokine and chemokine expression by the ribotoxic stress response elicited by Shiga toxin type 1 in human macrophage-like THP-1 cells. Infect Immun. 2012;80(6):2109–20.

252. Tesh VL. Activation of cell stress response pathways by Shiga toxins. Cell Microbiol. 2012;14(1):1–9.

253. Iordanov MS, Pribnow D, Magun JL, Dinh TH, Pearson JA, Chen SL, et al. Ribotoxic stress response: activation of the stress-activated protein kinase JNK1 by inhibitors of the peptidyl transferase reaction and by sequence-specific RNA damage to the alpha-sarcin/ricin loop in the 28S rRNA. Mol Cell Biol. 1997;17(6):3373–81.

254. Hoey DE, Sharp L, Currie C, Lingwood CA, Gally DL, Smith DG. Verotoxin 1 binding to intestinal crypt epithelial cells results in localization to lysosomes and abrogation of toxicity. Cell Microbiol. 2003;5(2):85–97.

255. Bitzan MM, Wang Y, Lin J, Marsden PA. Verotoxin and ricin have novel effects on preproendothelin-1 expression but fail to modify nitric oxide synthase (ecNOS) expression and NO production in vascular endothelium. J Clin Invest. 1998;101(2):372–82.

256. Thorpe CM, Hurley BP, Lincicome LL, Jacewicz MS, Keusch GT, Acheson DW. Shiga toxins stimulate secretion of interleukin-8 from intestinal epithelial cells. Infect Immun. 1999;67(11):5985–93.

257. Thorpe CM, Smith WE, Hurley BP, Acheson DW. Shiga toxins induce, superinduce, and stabilize a variety of C-X-C chemokine mRNAs in intestinal epithelial cells, resulting in increased chemokine expression. Infect Immun. 2001;69(10):6140–7.

258. Petruzziello TN, Mawji IA, Khan M, Marsden PA. Verotoxin biology: molecular events in vascular endothelial injury. Kidney Int Suppl. 2009;112: S17–9.

259. Petruzziello-Pellegrini TN, Moslemi-Naeini M, Marsden PA. New insights into Shiga toxin-mediated endothelial dysfunction in hemolytic uremic syndrome. Virulence. 2013;4(6):556–63.

260. Lee SY, Lee MS, Cherla RP, Tesh VL. Shiga toxin 1 induces apoptosis through the endoplasmic reticulum stress response in human monocytic cells. Cell Microbiol. 2008;10(3):770–80.

261. Tesh VL. The induction of apoptosis by Shiga toxins and ricin. Curr Top Microbiol Immunol. 2012;357:137–78.

262. Cherla RP, Lee SY, Tesh VL. Shiga toxins and apoptosis. FEMS Microbiol Lett. 2003;228(2):159–66.

263. Wilson C, Foster GH, Bitzan M. Silencing of Bak ameliorates apoptosis of human proximal tubular epithelial cells by Escherichia coli-derived Shiga toxin 2. Infection. 2005;33(5–6):362–7.

264. Lee MS, Cherla RP, Leyva-Illades D, Tesh VL. Bcl-2 regulates the onset of shiga toxin 1-induced apoptosis in THP-1 cells. Infect Immun. 2009;77(12): 5233–44.

265. Stricklett PK, Hughes AK, Kohan DE. Inhibition of p38 mitogen-activated protein kinase ameliorates cytokine up-regulated shigatoxin-1 toxicity in

human brain microvascular endothelial cells. J Infect Dis. 2005;191(3):461–71.

266. Karpman D, Hakansson A, Perez MT, Isaksson C, Carlemalm E, Caprioli A, et al. Apoptosis of renal cortical cells in the hemolytic-uremic syndrome: in vivo and in vitro studies. Infect Immun. 1998;66(2):636–44.

267. Kaneko K, Kiyokawa N, Ohtomo Y, Nagaoka R, Yamashiro Y, Taguchi T, et al. Apoptosis of renal tubular cells in Shiga-toxin-mediated hemolytic uremic syndrome. Nephron. 2001;87(2):182–5.

268. Te Loo DM, Monnens LA, van den Heuvel LP, Gubler MC, Kockx MM. Detection of apoptosis in kidney biopsies of patients with D+ hemolytic uremic syndrome. Pediatr Res. 2001;49(3):413–6.

269. Yoshida T, Fukada M, Koide N, Ikeda H, Sugiyama T, Kato Y, et al. Primary cultures of human endothelial cells are susceptible to low doses of Shiga toxins and undergo apoptosis. J Infect Dis. 1999;180(6): 2048–52.

270. Pijpers AH, van Setten PA, van den Heuvel LP, Assmann KJ, Dijkman HB, Pennings AH, et al. Verocytotoxin-induced apoptosis of human microvascular endothelial cells. J Am Soc Nephrol. 2001;12(4):767–78.

271. van Setten PA, van Hinsbergh VW, van der Velden TJ, van de Kar NC, Vermeer M, Mahan JD, et al. Effects of TNF alpha on verocytotoxin cytotoxicity in purified human glomerular microvascular endothelial cells. Kidney Int. 1997;51(4):1245–56.

272. van Setten PA, Monnens LA, Verstraten RG, van den Heuvel LP, van Hinsbergh VW. Effects of verocytotoxin-1 on nonadherent human monocytes: binding characteristics, protein synthesis, and induction of cytokine release. Blood. 1996;88(1):174–83.

273. te Loo DM, Monnens LA, van Der Velden TJ, Vermeer MA, Preyers F, Demacker PN, et al. Binding and transfer of verocytotoxin by polymorphonuclear leukocytes in hemolytic uremic syndrome. Blood. 2000;95(11):3396–402.

274. Te Loo DM, van Hinsbergh VW, van den Heuvel LP, Monnens LA. Detection of verocytotoxin bound to circulating polymorphonuclear leukocytes of patients with hemolytic uremic syndrome. J Am Soc Nephrol. 2001;12(4):800–6.

275. Kimura T, Tani S, Matsumoto Yi Y, Takeda T. Serum amyloid P component is the Shiga toxin 2-neutralizing factor in human blood. J Biol Chem. 2001;276(45):41576–9.

276. Marcato P, Vander Helm K, Mulvey GL, Armstrong GD. Serum amyloid P component binding to Shiga toxin 2 requires both a subunit and B pentamer. Infect Immun. 2003;71(10):6075–8.

277. Armstrong GD, Mulvey GL, Marcato P, Griener TP, Kahan MC, Tennent GA, et al. Human serum amyloid P component protects against Escherichia coli O157:H7 Shiga toxin 2 in vivo: therapeutic implications for hemolytic-uremic syndrome. J Infect Dis. 2006;193(8):1120–4.

278. Griener TP, Mulvey GL, Marcato P, Armstrong GD. Differential binding of Shiga toxin 2 to human and murine neutrophils. J Med Microbiol. 2007;56(Pt 11):1423–30.

279. Geelen JM, van der Velden TJ, Te Loo DM, Boerman OC, van den Heuvel LP, Monnens LA. Lack of specific binding of Shiga-like toxin (verocytotoxin) and non-specific interaction of Shiga-like toxin 2 antibody with human polymorphonuclear leucocytes. Nephrol Dial Transplant. 2007;22(3):749–55.

280. Fitzpatrick MM, Shah V, Trompeter RS, Dillon MJ, Barratt TM. Interleukin-8 and polymorphoneutrophil leucocyte activation in hemolytic uremic syndrome of childhood. Kidney Int. 1992;42(4):951–6.

281. Fitzpatrick MM, Shah V, Filler G, Dillon MJ, Barratt TM. Neutrophil activation in the haemolytic uraemic syndrome: free and complexed elastase in plasma. Pediatr Nephrol. 1992;6(1):50–3.

282. Hughes DA, Smith GC, Davidson JE, Murphy AV, Beattie TJ. The neutrophil oxidative burst in diarrhoea-associated haemolytic uraemic syndrome. Pediatr Nephrol. 1996;10(4):445–7.

283. Holle JU, Williams JM, Harper L, Savage CO, Taylor CM. Effect of verocytotoxins (Shiga-like toxins) on human neutrophils in vitro. Pediatr Nephrol. 2005;20(9):1237–44.

284. Geelen J, Valsecchi F, van der Velden T, van den Heuvel L, Monnens L, Morigi M. Shiga-toxin-induced firm adhesion of human leukocytes to endothelium is in part mediated by heparan sulfate. Nephrol Dial Transplant. 2008;23(10):3091–5.

285. te Loo DM, Levtchenko E, Furlan M, Roosendaal GP, van den Heuvel LP. Autosomal recessive inheritance of von Willebrand factor-cleaving protease deficiency. Pediatr Nephrol. 2000;14(8–9):762–5.

286. Brigotti M, Caprioli A, Tozzi AE, Tazzari PL, Ricci F, Conte R, et al. Shiga toxins present in the gut and in the polymorphonuclear leukocytes circulating in the blood of children with hemolytic-uremic syndrome. J Clin Microbiol. 2006;44(2):313–7.

287. Geelen JM, van der Velden TJ, van den Heuvel LP, Monnens LA. Interactions of Shiga-like toxin with human peripheral blood monocytes. Pediatr Nephrol. 2007;22(8):1181–7.

288. Ge S, Hertel B, Emden SH, Beneke J, Menne J, Haller H, et al. Microparticle generation and leucocyte death in Shiga toxin-mediated HUS. Nephrol Dial Transplant. 2012;27(7):2768–75.

289. Bombeli T, Schwartz BR, Harlan JM. Endothelial cells undergoing apoptosis become proadhesive for nonactivated platelets. Blood. 1999;93(11): 3831–8.

290. Zoja C, Buelli S, Morigi M. Shiga toxin-associated hemolytic uremic syndrome: pathophysiology of endothelial dysfunction. Pediatr Nephrol. 2010;25(11):2231–40.

291. Matussek A, Lauber J, Bergau A, Hansen W, Rohde M, Dittmar KE, et al. Molecular and functional analysis of Shiga toxin-induced response patterns in

human vascular endothelial cells. Blood. 2003;102(4):1323–32.

292. Petruzziello-Pellegrini TN, Yuen DA, Page AV, Patel S, Soltyk AM, Matouk CC, et al. The CXCR4/CXCR7/SDF-1 pathway contributes to the pathogenesis of Shiga toxin-associated hemolytic uremic syndrome in humans and mice. J Clin Invest. 2012;122(2):759–76.

293. Ramos MV, Auvynet C, Poupel L, Rodero M, Mejias MP, Panek CA, et al. Chemokine receptor CCR1 disruption limits renal damage in a murine model of hemolytic uremic syndrome. Am J Pathol. 2012;180(3):1040–8.

294. Page AV, Tarr PI, Watkins SL, Rajwans N, Petruzziello-Pellegrini TN, Marsden PA, et al. Dysregulation of angiopoietin 1 and 2 in Escherichia coli O157:H7 infection and the hemolytic-uremic syndrome. J Infect Dis. 2013;208(6):929–33.

295. Sood A, Mathew R, Trachtman H. Cytoprotective effect of curcumin in human proximal tubule epithelial cells exposed to shiga toxin. Biochem Biophys Res Commun. 2001;283(1):36–41.

296. Bitzan M, Bickford BB, Foster GH. Verotoxin (shiga toxin) sensitizes renal epithelial cells to increased heme toxicity: possible implications for the hemolytic uremic syndrome. J Am Soc Nephrol. 2004;15(9):2334–43.

297. Wadolkowski EA, Sung LM, Burris JA, Samuel JE, O'Brien AD. Acute renal tubular necrosis and death of mice orally infected with Escherichia coli strains that produce Shiga-like toxin type II. Infect Immun. 1990;58(12):3959–65.

298. Wolski VM, Soltyk AM, Brunton JL. Mouse toxicity and cytokine release by verotoxin 1 B subunit mutants. Infect Immun. 2001;69(1):579–83.

299. Wolski VM, Soltyk AM, Brunton JL. Tumour necrosis factor alpha is not an essential component of verotoxin 1-induced toxicity in mice. Microb Pathog. 2002;32(6):263–71.

300. Porubsky S, Federico G, Muthing J, Jennemann R, Gretz N, Buttner S, et al. Direct acute tubular damage contributes to Shigatoxin-mediated kidney failure. J Pathol. 2014;234(1):120–33.

301. Harel Y, Silva M, Giroir B, Weinberg A, Cleary TB, Beutler B. A reporter transgene indicates renal-specific induction of tumor necrosis factor (TNF) by shiga-like toxin. Possible involvement of TNF in hemolytic uremic syndrome. J Clin Invest. 1993; 92(5):2110–6.

302. Bielaszewska M, Karch H. Consequences of enterohaemorrhagic Escherichia coli infection for the vascular endothelium. Thromb Haemost. 2005;94(2):312–8.

303. van de Kar NC, Monnens LA, Karmali MA, van Hinsbergh VW. Tumor necrosis factor and interleukin-1 induce expression of the verocytotoxin receptor globotriaosylceramide on human endothelial cells: implications for the pathogenesis of the hemolytic uremic syndrome. Blood. 1992;80(11):2755–64.

304. van de Kar NC, Kooistra T, Vermeer M, Lesslauer W, Monnens LA, van Hinsbergh VW. Tumor necrosis factor alpha induces endothelial galactosyl transferase activity and verocytotoxin receptors. Role of specific tumor necrosis factor receptors and protein kinase C. Blood. 1995;85(3):734–43.

305. Eisenhauer PB, Chaturvedi P, Fine RE, Ritchie AJ, Pober JS, Cleary TG, et al. Tumor necrosis factor alpha increases human cerebral endothelial cell Gb3 and sensitivity to Shiga toxin. Infect Immun. 2001;69(3):1889–94.

306. Clayton F, Pysher TJ, Lou R, Kohan DE, Denkers ND, Tesh VL, et al. Lipopolysaccharide upregulates renal shiga toxin receptors in a primate model of hemolytic uremic syndrome. Am J Nephrol. 2005;25(6):536–40.

307. Karpman D, Connell H, Svensson M, Scheutz F, Alm P, Svanborg C. The role of lipopolysaccharide and Shiga-like toxin in a mouse model of Escherichia coli O157:H7 infection. J Infect Dis. 1997; 175(3):611–20.

308. Walters MD, Matthei IU, Kay R, Dillon MJ, Barratt TM. The polymorphonuclear leucocyte count in childhood haemolytic uraemic syndrome. Pediatr Nephrol. 1989;3(2):130–4.

309. Proulx F, Turgeon JP, Litalien C, Mariscalco MM, Robitaille P, Seidman E. Inflammatory mediators in Escherichia coli O157:H7 hemorrhagic colitis and hemolytic-uremic syndrome. Pediatr Infect Dis J. 1998;17(10):899–904.

310. Buteau C, Proulx F, Chaibou M, Raymond D, Clermont MJ, Mariscalco MM, et al. Leukocytosis in children with Escherichia coli O157:H7 enteritis developing the hemolytic-uremic syndrome. Pediatr Infect Dis J. 2000;19(7):642–7.

311. Westerholt S, Hartung T, Tollens M, Gustrau A, Oberhoffer M, Karch H, et al. Inflammatory and immunological parameters in children with haemolytic uremic syndrome (HUS) and gastroenteritis-pathophysiological and diagnostic clues. Cytokine. 2000;12(6):822–7.

312. Decaluwe H, Harrison LM, Mariscalco MM, Gendrel D, Bohuon C, Tesh VL, et al. Procalcitonin in children with Escherichia coli O157:H7 associated hemolytic uremic syndrome. Pediatr Res. 2006;59(4 Pt 1):579–83.

313. Yamamoto T, Satomura K, Okada S, Ozono K. Risk factors for neurological complications in complete hemolytic uremic syndrome caused by Escherichia coli O157. Pediatr Int: Off J Jpn Pediatr Soc. 2009;51(2):216–9.

314. Yamamoto ET, Mizuno M, Nishikawa K, Miyazawa S, Zhang L, Matsuo S, et al. Shiga toxin 1 causes direct renal injury in rats. Infect Immun. 2005;73(11):7099–106.

315. Vielhauer V, Anders HJ, Schlondorff D. Chemokines and chemokine receptors as therapeutic targets in lupus nephritis. Semin Nephrol. 2007;27(1): 81–97.

316. Heller F, Lindenmeyer MT, Cohen CD, Brandt U, Draganovici D, Fischereder M, et al. The contribution of B cells to renal interstitial inflammation. Am J Pathol. 2007;170(2):457–68.

317. van Wieringen PM, Monnens LA, Bakkeren JA. Hemolytic-uremic syndrome: absence of circulating endotoxin. Pediatrics. 1976;58(4):561–3.

318. van de Kar NC, Sauerwein RW, Demacker PN, Grau GE, van Hinsbergh VW, Monnens LA. Plasma cytokine levels in hemolytic uremic syndrome. Nephron. 1995;71(3):309–13.

319. van Setten PA, van Hinsbergh VW, van den Heuvel LP, Preyers F, Dijkman HB, Assmann KJ, et al. Monocyte chemoattractant protein-1 and interleukin-8 levels in urine and serum of patents with hemolytic uremic syndrome. Pediatr Res. 1998;43(6):759–67.

320. Westerholt S, Pieper AK, Griebel M, Volk HD, Hartung T, Oberhoffer R. Characterization of the cytokine immune response in children who have experienced an episode of typical hemolytic-uremic syndrome. Clin Diagn Lab Immunol. 2003;10(6):1090–5.

321. Fernandez GC, Ramos MV, Landoni VI, Bentancor LV, Fernandez-Brando RJ, Exeni R, et al. Cytokine production is altered in monocytes from children with hemolytic uremic syndrome. J Clin Immunol. 2012;32(3):622–31.

322. Recktenwald J, Schmidt H. The nucleotide sequence of Shiga toxin (Stx) 2e-encoding phage phiP27 is not related to other Stx phage genomes, but the modular genetic structure is conserved. Infect Immun. 2002;70(4):1896–908.

323. Schmidt H. Shiga-toxin-converting bacteriophages. Res Microbiol. 2001;152(8):687–95.

324. Ochoa TJ, Chen J, Walker CM, Gonzales E, Cleary TG. Rifaximin does not induce toxin production or phage-mediated lysis of Shiga toxin-producing Escherichia coli. Antimicrob Agents Chemother. 2007;51(8):2837–41.

325. Herold S, Karch H, Schmidt H. Shiga toxin-encoding bacteriophages – genomes in motion. Int J Med Microbiol. 2004;294(2–3):115–21.

326. Bielaszewska M, Prager R, Kock R, Mellmann A, Zhang W, Tschape H, et al. Shiga toxin gene loss and transfer in vitro and in vivo during enterohemorrhagic Escherichia coli O26 infection in humans. Appl Environ Microbiol. 2007;73(10):3144–50.

327. Beutin L, Hammerl JA, Strauch E, Reetz J, Dieckmann R, Kelner-Burgos Y, et al. Spread of a distinct Stx2-encoding phage prototype among Escherichia coli O104:H4 strains from outbreaks in Germany, Norway, and Georgia. J Virol. 2012;86(19):10444–55.

328. Johansen BK, Wasteson Y, Granum PE, Brynestad S. Mosaic structure of Shiga-toxin-2-encoding phages isolated from Escherichia coli O157:H7 indicates frequent gene exchange between lambdoid phage genomes. Microbiology. 2001;147(Pt 7):1929–36.

329. Neely MN, Friedman DI. Arrangement and functional identification of genes in the regulatory region of lambdoid phage H-19B, a carrier of a Shiga-like toxin. Gene. 1998;223(1–2):105–13.

330. Neely MN, Friedman DI. Functional and genetic analysis of regulatory regions of coliphage H-19B: location of shiga-like toxin and lysis genes suggest a role for phage functions in toxin release. Mol Microbiol. 1998;28(6):1255–67.

331. Shimizu T, Ohta Y, Noda M. Shiga toxin 2 is specifically released from bacterial cells by two different mechanisms. Infect Immun. 2009;77(7):2813–23.

332. Yee AJ, De Grandis S, Gyles CL. Mitomycin-induced synthesis of a Shiga-like toxin from enteropathogenic Escherichia coli H.I.8. Infect Immun. 1993;61(10):4510–3.

333. Al-Jumaili I, Burke DA, Scotland SM, Al-Mardini H, Record CO. A method of enhancing verocytotoxin production by Escherichia coli. FEMS Microbiol Lett. 1992;72(2):121–5.

334. Karch H, Strockbine NA, O'Brien AD. Growth of Escherichia coli in the presence of trimethoprim-sulfamethoxazole facilitates detection of Shiga-like toxin-producing strains by colony blot assay. FEMS Microbiol Lett. 1986;35:141–5.

335. Karmali MA, Petric M, Lim C, Cheung R, Arbus GS. Sensitive method for detecting low numbers of verotoxin-producing Escherichia coli in mixed cultures by use of colony sweeps and polymyxin extraction of verotoxin. J Clin Microbiol. 1985;22(4):614–9.

336. Verweij J, van der Burg ME, Pinedo HM. Mitomycin C-induced hemolytic uremic syndrome. Six case reports and review of the literature on renal, pulmonary and cardiac side effects of the drug. Radiother Oncol. 1987;8(1):33–41.

337. Acheson DW, Donohue-Rolfe A. Cancer-associated hemolytic uremic syndrome: a possible role of mitomycin in relation to Shiga-like toxins. J Clin Oncol: Off J Am Soc Clin Oncol. 1989;7(12):1943.

338. Lesesne JB, Rothschild N, Erickson B, Korec S, Sisk R, Keller J, et al. Cancer-associated hemolytic-uremic syndrome: analysis of 85 cases from a national registry. J Clin Oncol: Off J Am Soc Clin Oncol. 1989;7(6):781–9.

339. Muhldorfer I, Hacker J, Keusch GT, Acheson DW, Tschape H, Kane AV, et al. Regulation of the Shiga-like toxin II operon in Escherichia coli. Infect Immun. 1996;64(2):495–502.

340. Plunkett 3rd G, Rose DJ, Durfee TJ, Blattner FR. Sequence of Shiga toxin 2 phage 933 W from Escherichia coli O157:H7: Shiga toxin as a phage late-gene product. J Bacteriol. 1999;181(6):1767–78.

341. Fuchs S, Muhldorfer I, Donohue-Rolfe A, Kerenyi M, Emody L, Alexiev R, et al. Influence of RecA on in vivo virulence and Shiga toxin 2 production in Escherichia coli pathogens. Microb Pathog. 1999;27(1):13–23.

342. Lewin CS, Amyes SG. The role of the SOS response in bacteria exposed to zidovudine or trimethoprim. J Med Microbiol. 1991;34(6):329–32.

343. Quillardet P, Hofnung M. The SOS chromotest: a review. Mutat Res. 1993;297(3):235–79.

344. Matsushiro A, Sato K, Miyamoto H, Yamamura T, Honda T. Induction of prophages of enterohemorrhagic Escherichia coli O157:H7 with norfloxacin. J Bacteriol. 1999;181(7):2257–60.

345. Kimmitt PT, Harwood CR, Barer MR. Toxin gene expression by shiga toxin-producing Escherichia coli: the role of antibiotics and the bacterial SOS response. Emerg Infect Dis. 2000;6(5):458–65.

346. Herold S, Siebert J, Huber A, Schmidt H. Global expression of prophage genes in Escherichia coli O157:H7 strain EDL933 in response to norfloxacin. Antimicrob Agents Chemother. 2005;49(3):931–44.

347. Wong CS, Jelacic S, Habeeb RL, Watkins SL, Tarr PI. The risk of the hemolytic-uremic syndrome after antibiotic treatment of Escherichia coli O157:H7 infections. N Engl J Med. 2000;342(26):1930–6.

348. Ariceta G, Besbas N, Johnson S, Karpman D, Landau D, Licht C, et al. Guideline for the investigation and initial therapy of diarrhea-negative hemolytic uremic syndrome. Pediatr Nephrol. 2009;24(4):687–96.

349. Werber D, Mason BW, Evans MR, Salmon RL. Preventing household transmission of Shiga toxin-producing Escherichia coli O157 infection: promptly separating siblings might be the key. Clin Infect Dis. 2008;46(8):1189–96.

350. Ahn CK, Klein E, Tarr PI. Isolation of patients acutely infected with Escherichia coli O157:H7: low-tech, highly effective prevention of hemolytic uremic syndrome. Clin Infect Dis. 2008;46(8): 1197–9.

351. Pollock KG, Stewart A, Beattie TJ, Todd WT, Ahn CK, Tarr PI, et al. From diarrhoea to haemolytic uraemic syndrome – when to seek advice. J Med Microbiol. 2009;58(Pt 4):397–8.

352. Clogher P, Hurd S, Hoefer D, Hadler JL, Pasutti L, Cosgrove S, et al. Assessment of physician knowledge and practices concerning Shiga toxin-producing Escherichia coli infection and enteric illness, 2009, Foodborne Diseases Active Surveillance Network (FoodNet). Clin Infect Dis. 2012;54 Suppl 5: S446–52.

353. Gould LH, Bopp C, Strockbine N, Atkinson R, Baselski V, Body B, et al. Recommendations for diagnosis of shiga toxin – producing Escherichia coli infections by clinical laboratories. MMWR Recomm Rep. 2009;58(RR-12):1–14.

354. Schindler EI, Sellenriek P, Storch GA, Tarr PI, Burnham CA. Shiga toxin-producing Escherichia coli: a single-center, 11-year pediatric experience. J Clin Microbiol. 2014;52(10):3647–53.

355. Chapman PA, Siddons CA. A comparison of immunomagnetic separation and direct culture for the isolation of verocytotoxin-producing Escherichia coli O157 from cases of bloody diarrhoea, non-bloody diarrhoea and asymptomatic contacts. J Med Microbiol. 1996;44(4):267–71.

356. Brunder W, Karch H. Genome plasticity in Enterobacteriaceae. Int J Med Microbiol. 2000;290(2):153–65.

357. Mackenzie AM, Lebel P, Orrbine E, Rowe PC, Hyde L, Chan F, et al. Sensitivities and specificities of premier E. coli O157 and premier EHEC enzyme immunoassays for diagnosis of infection with verotxin (Shiga-like toxin)-producing Escherichia coli. The SYNSORB Pk Study investigators. J Clin Microbiol. 1998;36(6):1608–11.

358. Teel LD, Daly JA, Jerris RC, Maul D, Svanas G, O'Brien AD, et al. Rapid detection of Shiga toxin-producing Escherichia coli by optical immunoassay. J Clin Microbiol. 2007;45(10):3377–80.

359. Chui L, Lee MC, Malejczyk K, Lim L, Fok D, Kwong P. Prevalence of shiga toxin-producing Escherichia coli as detected by enzyme-linked immunoassays and real-time PCR during the summer months in northern Alberta, Canada. J Clin Microbiol. 2011;49(12):4307–10.

360. Staples M, Jennison AV, Graham RM, Smith HV. Evaluation of the meridian premier EHEC assay as an indicator of Shiga toxin presence in direct faecal specimens. Diagn Microbiol Infect Dis. 2012;73(4):322–5.

361. Chui L, Lee MC, Allen R, Bryks A, Haines L, Boras V. Comparison between ImmunoCard STAT!((R)) and real-time PCR as screening tools for both O157:H7 and non-O157 Shiga toxin-producing Escherichia coli in Southern Alberta, Canada. Diagn Microbiol Infect Dis. 2013;77(1):8–13.

362. He X, Patfield S, Hnasko R, Rasooly R, Mandrell RE. A polyclonal antibody based immunoassay detects seven subtypes of Shiga toxin 2 produced by Escherichia coli in human and environmental samples. PLoS One. 2013;8(10):e76368.

363. Chart H, Smith HR, Scotland SM, Rowe B, Milford DV, Taylor CM. Serological identification of Escherichia coli O157:H7 infection in haemolytic uraemic syndrome. Lancet. 1991;337(8734): 138–40.

364. Chart H, van der Kar NC, Tolboom JJ, Monnens LM, Rowe B. Serological detection of verocytotoxin-producing Escherichia coli in patients with haemolytic uraemic syndrome in western Europe. Eur J Clin Microbiol Infect Dis. 1993;12(9):707–9.

365. Ludwig K, Bitzan M, Zimmermann S, Kloth M, Ruder H, Muller-Wiefel DE. Immune response to non-O157 Vero toxin-producing Escherichia coli in patients with hemolytic uremic syndrome. J Infect Dis. 1996;174(5):1028–39.

366. Chart H, Cheasty T. Human infections with verocytotoxin-producing Escherichia coli O157–10 years of E. coli O157 serodiagnosis. J Med Microbiol. 2008;57(Pt 11):1389–93.

367. Ludwig K, Grabhorn E, Bitzan M, Bobrowski C, Kemper MJ, Sobottka I, et al. Saliva IgM and IgA are a sensitive indicator of the humoral immune response to Escherichia coli O157 lipopolysaccharide

in children with enteropathic hemolytic uremic syndrome. Pediatr Res. 2002;52(2):307–13.

368. Chart H, Perry NT, Willshaw GA, Cheasty T. Analysis of saliva for antibodies to the LPS of Escherichia coli O157 in patients with serum antibodies to E. coli O157 LPS. J Med Microbiol. 2003;52(Pt 7):569–72.

369. Karmali MA, Petric M, Winkler M, Bielaszewska M, Brunton J, van de Kar N, et al. Enzyme-linked immunosorbent assay for detection of immunoglobulin G antibodies to Escherichia coli Vero cytotoxin 1. J Clin Microbiol. 1994;32(6):1457–63.

370. Karpman D, Bekassy ZD, Sjogren AC, Dubois MS, Karmali MA, Mascarenhas M, et al. Antibodies to intimin and Escherichia coli secreted proteins A and B in patients with enterohemorrhagic Escherichia coli infections. Pediatr Nephrol. 2002;17(3):201–11.

371. Mellmann A, Lu S, Karch H, Xu JG, Harmsen D, Schmidt MA, et al. Recycling of Shiga toxin 2 genes in sorbitol-fermenting enterohemorrhagic Escherichia coli O157:NM. Appl Environ Microbiol. 2008;74(1):67–72.

372. Holtz LR, Neill MA, Tarr PI. Acute bloody diarrhea: a medical emergency for patients of all ages. Gastroenterology. 2009;136(6):1887–98.

373. Tarr PI, Fouser LS, Stapleton AE, Wilson RA, Kim HH, Vary Jr JC, et al. Hemolytic-uremic syndrome in a six-year-old girl after a urinary tract infection with Shiga-toxin-producing Escherichia coli O103:H2. N Engl J Med. 1996;335(9):635–8.

374. Starr M, Bennett-Wood V, Bigham AK, de Koning-Ward TF, Bordun AM, Lightfoot D, et al. Hemolytic-uremic syndrome following urinary tract infection with enterohemorrhagic Escherichia coli: case report and review. Clin Infect Dis. 1998;27(2):310–5.

375. Scheutz F, Olesen B, Norgaard A. Two cases of human urinary tract infection complicated by hemolytic uremic syndrome caused by verotoxin-producing Escherichia coli. Clin Infect Dis. 2000;31(3):815–6.

376. Toval F, Schiller R, Meisen I, Putze J, Kouzel IU, Zhang W, et al. Characterization of urinary tract infection-associated Shiga toxin-producing Escherichia coli. Infect Immun. 2014;82(11):4631–42.

377. Klein EJ, Stapp JR, Neill MA, Besser JM, Osterholm MT, Tarr PI. Shiga toxin antigen detection should not replace sorbitol MacConkey agar screening of stool specimens. J Clin Microbiol. 2004;42(9):4416. author reply -7.

378. Lindsay B, Pop M, Antonio M, Walker AW, Mai V, Ahmed D, et al. Survey of culture, goldengate assay, universal biosensor assay, and 16S rRNA Gene sequencing as alternative methods of bacterial pathogen detection. J Clin Microbiol. 2013;51(10):3263–9.

379. Bitzan M. Glomerular diseases. In: Phadke KD, Goodyer PR, Bitzan M, editors. Manual of pediatric nephrology. Heidelberg: Springer; 2014. p. 141–229.

380. Carter AO, Borczyk AA, Carlson JA, Harvey B, Hockin JC, Karmali MA, et al. A severe outbreak of Escherichia coli O157:H7 – associated hemorrhagic colitis in a nursing home. N Engl J Med. 1987;317(24):1496–500.

381. Blanco JE, Blanco M, Alonso MP, Mora A, Dahbi G, Coira MA, et al. Serotypes, virulence genes, and intimin types of Shiga toxin (verotoxin)-producing Escherichia coli isolates from human patients: prevalence in Lugo, Spain, from 1992 through 1999. J Clin Microbiol. 2004;42(1):311–9.

382. Boyce TG, Swerdlow DL, Griffin PM. Escherichia coli O157:H7 and the hemolytic-uremic syndrome. N Engl J Med. 1995;333(6):364–8.

383. Werber D, Fruth A, Buchholz U, Prager R, Kramer MH, Ammon A, et al. Strong association between shiga toxin-producing Escherichia coli O157 and virulence genes stx2 and eae as possible explanation for predominance of serogroup O157 in patients with haemolytic uraemic syndrome. Eur J Clin Microbiol Infect Dis. 2003;22(12):726–30.

384. Scheiring J, Andreoli SP, Zimmerhackl LB. Treatment and outcome of Shiga-toxin-associated hemolytic uremic syndrome (HUS). Pediatr Nephrol. 2008;23(10):1749–60.

385. Jelacic JK, Damrow T, Chen GS, Jelacic S, Bielaszewska M, Ciol M, et al. Shiga toxin-producing Escherichia coli in Montana: bacterial genotypes and clinical profiles. J Infect Dis. 2003;188(5):719–29.

386. Bielaszewska M, Friedrich AW, Aldick T, Schurk-Bulgrin R, Karch H. Shiga toxin activatable by intestinal mucus in Escherichia coli isolated from humans: predictor for a severe clinical outcome. Clin Infect Dis. 2006;43(9):1160–7.

387. Karmali MA, Arbus GS, Ish-Shalom N, Fleming PC, Malkin D, Petric M, et al. A family outbreak of hemolytic-uremic syndrome associated with verotoxin-producing Escherichia coli serotype O157:H7. Pediatr Nephrol. 1988;2(4):409–14.

388. Kawamura N, Yamazaki T, Tamai H. Risk factors for the development of Escherichia coli O157:H7 associated with hemolytic uremic syndrome. Pediatr Int: Off J Jpn Pediatr Soc. 1999;41(2):218–22.

389. Siegler RL. The hemolytic uremic syndrome. Pediatr Clin North Am. 1995;42(6):1505–29.

390. Ikeda K, Ida O, Kimoto K, Takatorige T, Nakanishi N, Tatara K. Effect of early fosfomycin treatment on prevention of hemolytic uremic syndrome accompanying Escherichia coli O157:H7 infection. Clin Nephrol. 1999;52(6):357–62.

391. Barrett TJ, Potter ME, Strockbine NA. Evidence for participation of the macrophage in Shiga-like toxin II-induced lethality in mice. Microb Pathog. 1990;9(2):95–103.

392. Siegler RL, Pysher TJ, Lou R, Tesh VL, Taylor Jr FB. Response to Shiga toxin-1, with and without lipopolysaccharide, in a primate model of hemolytic uremic syndrome. Am J Nephrol. 2001;21(5):420–5.

393. Siegler RL, Obrig TG, Pysher TJ, Tesh VL, Denkers ND, Taylor FB. Response to Shiga toxin 1 and 2 in a baboon model of hemolytic uremic syndrome. Pediatr Nephrol. 2003;18(2):92–6.

394. Palermo M, Alves-Rosa F, Rubel C, Fernandez GC, Fernandez-Alonso G, Alberto F, et al. Pretreatment of mice with lipopolysaccharide (LPS) or IL-1beta exerts dose-dependent opposite effects on Shiga toxin-2 lethality. Clin Exp Immunol. 2000;119(1):77–83.

395. Kita E, Yunou Y, Kurioka T, Harada H, Yoshikawa S, Mikasa K, et al. Pathogenic mechanism of mouse brain damage caused by oral infection with Shiga toxin-producing Escherichia coli O157:H7. Infect Immun. 2000;68(3):1207–14.

396. Alves-Rosa F, Beigier-Bompadre M, Fernandez G, Barrionuevo P, Mari L, Palermo M, et al. Tolerance to lipopolysaccharide (LPS) regulates the endotoxin effects on Shiga toxin-2 lethality. Immunol Lett. 2001;76(2):125–31.

397. Isogai E, Isogai H, Hirose K, Kubota T, Kimura K, Fujii N, et al. Therapeutic effect of anti-TNF-alpha antibody and levofloxacin (LVFX) in a mouse model of enterohemorrhagic Escherichia coli O157 infection. Comp Immunol Microbiol Infect Dis. 2001;24(4):217–31.

398. Keepers TR, Psotka MA, Gross LK, Obrig TG. A murine model of HUS: Shiga toxin with lipopolysaccharide mimics the renal damage and physiologic response of human disease. J Am Soc Nephrol. 2006;17(12):3404–14.

399. Morigi M, Galbusera M, Gastoldi S, Locatelli M, Buelli S, Pezzotta A, et al. Alternative pathway activation of complement by Shiga toxin promotes exuberant C3a formation that triggers microvascular thrombosis. J Immunol. 2011;187(1):172–80.

400. Stearns-Kurosawa DJ, Collins V, Freeman S, Tesh VL, Kurosawa S. Distinct physiologic and inflammatory responses elicited in baboons after challenge with Shiga toxin type 1 or 2 from enterohemorrhagic Escherichia coli. Infect Immun. 2010;78(6):2497–504.

401. Stearns-Kurosawa DJ, Oh SY, Cherla RP, Lee MS, Tesh VL, Papin J, et al. Distinct renal pathology and a chemotactic phenotype after enterohemorrhagic Escherichia coli shiga toxins in non-human primate models of hemolytic uremic syndrome. Am J Pathol. 2013;182(4):1227–38.

402. Ake JA, Jelacic S, Ciol MA, Watkins SL, Murray KF, Christie DL, et al. Relative nephroprotection during Escherichia coli O157:H7 infections: association with intravenous volume expansion. Pediatrics. 2005;115(6):e673–80.

403. Hickey CA, Beattie TJ, Cowieson J, Miyashita Y, Strife CF, Frem JC, et al. Early volume expansion during diarrhea and relative nephroprotection during subsequent hemolytic uremic syndrome. Arch Pediatr Adolesc Med. 2011;165(10):884–9.

404. Wong CS, Mooney JC, Brandt JR, Staples AO, Jelacic S, Boster DR, et al. Risk factors for the hemolytic uremic syndrome in children infected with Escherichia coli O157:H7: a multivariable analysis. Clin Infect Dis. 2012;55(1):33–41.

405. Cimolai N, Morrison BJ, Carter JE. Risk factors for the central nervous system manifestations of gastroenteritis-associated hemolytic-uremic syndrome. Pediatrics. 1992;90(4):616–21.

406. Lopez EL, Contrini MM, Devoto S, de Rosa MF, Grana MG, Aversa L, et al. Incomplete hemolytic-uremic syndrome in Argentinean children with bloody diarrhea. J Pediatr. 1995;127(3):364–7.

407. Edey MM, Mead PA, Saunders RE, Strain L, Perkins SJ, Goodship TH, et al. Association of a factor H mutation with hemolytic uremic syndrome following a diarrheal illness. Am J Kidney Dis. 2008;51(3): 487–90.

408. Gupta A, Khaira A, Rathi OP, Mahajan S, Bhowmik D, Agarwal SK, et al. Diarrhea-related hemolytic uremic syndrome: unmasking antifactor H antibodies. Saudi J Kidney Dis Transpl. 2011;22(5): 1017–8.

409. Johnson S, Stojanovic J, Ariceta G, Bitzan M, Besbas N, Frieling M, et al. An audit analysis of a guideline for the investigation and initial therapy of diarrhea negative (atypical) hemolytic uremic syndrome. Pediatr Nephrol. 2014;29(10):1967–78.

410. Oakes RS, Siegler RL, McReynolds MA, Pysher T, Pavia AT. Predictors of fatality in postdiarrheal hemolytic uremic syndrome. Pediatrics. 2006;117(5): 1656–62.

411. Ardissino G, Dacco V, Testa S, Civitillo CF, Tel F, Possenti I, et al. Hemoconcentration: a major risk factor for neurological involvement in hemolytic uremic syndrome. Pediatr Nephrol. 2015;30(2): 345–52.

412. Balestracci A, Martin SM, Toledo I, Alvarado C, Wainsztein RE. Dehydration at admission increased the need for dialysis in hemolytic uremic syndrome children. Pediatr Nephrol. 2012;27(8):1407–10.

413. Trachtman H, Cnaan A, Christen E, Gibbs K, Zhao S, Acheson DW, et al. Effect of an oral Shiga toxin-binding agent on diarrhea-associated hemolytic uremic syndrome in children: a randomized controlled trial. JAMA. 2003;290(10):1337–44.

414. Siegler RL, Milligan MK, Burningham TH, Christofferson RD, Chang SY, Jorde LB. Long-term outcome and prognostic indicators in the hemolytic-uremic syndrome. J Pediatr. 1991;118(2):195–200.

415. Oakes RS, Kirkham JK, Nelson RD, Siegler RL. Duration of oliguria and anuria as predictors of chronic renal-related sequelae in post-diarrheal hemolytic uremic syndrome. Pediatr Nephrol. 2008;23(8):1303–8.

416. Loirat C, Niaudet P. The risk of recurrence of hemolytic uremic syndrome after renal transplantation in children. Pediatr Nephrol. 2003;18(11):1095–101.

417. Siegler RL, Brewer ED, Swartz M. Ocular involvement in hemolytic-uremic syndrome. J Pediatr. 1988;112(4):594–7.

418. Siegler RL. Spectrum of extrarenal involvement in postdiarrheal hemolytic-uremic syndrome. J Pediatr. 1994;125(4):511–8.

419. Siegler RL, Loghman-Adham M, Timmons OD. Acute respiratory failure in the hemolytic uremic syndrome. Clin Pediatr (Phila). 1995;34(12): 660–2.

420. Abu-Arafeh I, Gray E, Youngson G, Auchterlonie I, Russell G. Myocarditis and haemolytic uraemic syndrome. Arch Dis Child. 1995;72(1):46–7.

421. Walker AM, Benson LN, Wilson GJ, Arbus GS. Cardiomyopathy: a late complication of hemolytic uremic syndrome. Pediatr Nephrol. 1997;11(2):221–2.

422. Eckart P, Guillot M, Jokic M, Maragnes P, Boudailliez B, Palcoux JB, et al. Cardiac involvement during classic hemolytic uremic syndrome. Arch Pediatr. 1999;6(4):430–3.

423. Eriksson KJ, Boyd SG, Tasker RC. Acute neurology and neurophysiology of haemolytic-uraemic syndrome. Arch Dis Child. 2001;84(5):434–5.

424. Repetto HA. Long-term course and mechanisms of progression of renal disease in hemolytic uremic syndrome. Kidney Int Suppl. 2005;97:S102–6.

425. Mohammed J, Filler G, Price A, Sharma AP. Cardiac tamponade in diarrhoea-positive haemolytic uraemic syndrome. Nephrol Dial Transplant. 2009;24(2): 679–81.

426. Nathanson S, Kwon T, Elmaleh M, Charbit M, Launay EA, Harambat J, et al. Acute neurological involvement in diarrhea-associated hemolytic uremic syndrome. Clin J Am Soc Nephrol. 2010;5(7):1218–28.

427. Donnerstag F, Ding X, Pape L, Bultmann E, Lucke T, Zajaczek J, et al. Patterns in early diffusion-weighted MRI in children with haemolytic uraemic syndrome and CNS involvement. Eur Radiol. 2012;22(3):506–13.

428. Meuth SG, Gobel K, Kanyshkova T, Ehling P, Ritter MA, Schwindt W, et al. Thalamic involvement in patients with neurologic impairment due to Shiga toxin 2. Ann Neurol. 2013;73(3):419–29.

429. de Buys Roessingh AS, de Lagausie P, Baudoin V, Loirat C, Aigrain Y. Gastrointestinal complications of post-diarrheal hemolytic uremic syndrome. Eur J Pediatr Surg: Off J Austrian Assoc Pediatr Surg [et al] = Z Kinderchir. 2007;17(5):328–34.

430. Krogvold L, Henrichsen T, Bjerre A, Brackman D, Dollner H, Gudmundsdottir H, et al. Clinical aspects of a nationwide epidemic of severe haemolytic uremic syndrome (HUS) in children. Scand J Trauma Resusc Emerg Med. 2011;19:44.

431. Rahman RC, Cobenas CJ, Drut R, Amoreo OR, Ruscasso JD, Spizzirri AP, et al. Hemorrhagic colitis in postdiarrheal hemolytic uremic syndrome: retrospective analysis of 54 children. Pediatr Nephrol. 2012;27(2):229–33.

432. Suri RS, Clark WF, Barrowman N, Mahon JL, Thiessen-Philbrook HR, Rosas-Arellano MP, et al. Diabetes during diarrhea-associated hemolytic uremic syndrome: a systematic review and meta-analysis. Diabetes Care. 2005;28(10):2556–62.

433. Suri RS, Mahon JL, Clark WF, Moist LM, Salvadori M, Garg AX. Relationship between Escherichia coli O157:H7 and diabetes mellitus. Kidney Int Suppl. 2009;112:S44–6.

434. Cohen JA, Brecher ME, Bandarenko N. Cellular source of serum lactate dehydrogenase elevation in patients with thrombotic thrombocytopenic purpura. J Clin Apher. 1998;13(1):16–9.

435. Thayu M, Chandler WL, Jelacic S, Gordon CA, Rosenthal GL, Tarr PI. Cardiac ischemia during hemolytic uremic syndrome. Pediatr Nephrol. 2003;18(3):286–9.

436. Askiti V, Hendrickson K, Fish AJ, Braunlin E, Sinaiko AR. Troponin I levels in a hemolytic uremic syndrome patient with severe cardiac failure. Pediatr Nephrol. 2004;19(3):345–8.

437. Patschan D, Witzke O, Dührsen U, Erbel R, Philipp T, Herget-Rosenthal S. Acute myocardial infarction in thrombotic microangiopathies–clinical characteristics, risk factors and outcome. Nephrol Dial Transplant. 2006;21(6):1549–54.

438. Weissenborn K, Donnerstag F, Kielstein JT, Heeren M, Worthmann H, Hecker H, et al. Neurologic manifestations of E coli infection-induced hemolytic-uremic syndrome in adults. Neurology. 2012;79(14):1466–73.

439. Gianviti A, Tozzi AE, De Petris L, Caprioli A, Rava L, Edefonti A, et al. Risk factors for poor renal prognosis in children with hemolytic uremic syndrome. Pediatr Nephrol. 2003;18(12):1229–35.

440. Kamioka I, Yoshiya K, Satomura K, Kaito H, Fujita T, Iijima K, et al. Risk factors for developing severe clinical course in HUS patients: a national survey in Japan. Pediatr Int: Off J Jpn Pediatr Soc. 2008;50(4):441–6.

441. Teramoto T, Fukao T, Hirayama K, Asano T, Aoki Y, Kondo N. Escherichia coli O-157-induced hemolytic uremic syndrome: Usefulness of SCWP score for the prediction of neurological complication. Pediatr Int: Off J Jpn Pediatr Soc. 2009;51(1):107–9.

442. Trachtman H, Austin C, Lewinski M, Stahl RA. Renal and neurological involvement in typical Shiga toxin-associated HUS. Nat Rev Nephrol. 2012;8(11):658–69.

443. Gitiaux C, Krug P, Grevent D, Kossorotoff M, Poncet S, Eisermann M, et al. Brain magnetic resonance imaging pattern and outcome in children with haemolytic-uraemic syndrome and neurological impairment treated with eculizumab. Dev Med Child Neurol. 2013;55(8):758–65.

444. Toldo I, Manara R, Cogo P, Sartori S, Murer L, Battistella PA, et al. Diffusion-weighted imaging findings in hemolytic uremic syndrome with central nervous system involvement. J Child Neurol. 2009;24(2):247–50.

445. Weissenborn K, Bultmann E, Donnerstag F, Giesemann AM, Gotz F, Worthmann H, et al. Quantitative MRI shows cerebral microstructural damage in hemolytic-uremic syndrome patients with severe neurological symptoms but no changes in conventional MRI. Neuroradiology. 2013;55(7): 819–25.

446. Wengenroth M, Hoeltje J, Repenthin J, Meyer TN, Bonk F, Becker H, et al. Central nervous system involvement in adults with epidemic hemolytic uremic syndrome. AJNR Am J Neuroradiol. 2013;34(5):1016–21. S1.

447. Kleimann A, Toto S, Eberlein CK, Kielstein JT, Bleich S, Frieling H, et al. Psychiatric symptoms in patients with Shiga toxin-producing E. coli O104:H4 induced haemolytic-uraemic syndrome. PLoS One. 2014;9(7):e101839.

448. Simova O, Weineck G, Schuetze T, Wegscheider K, Panzer U, Stahl RA, et al. Neuropsychological outcome after complicated Shiga toxin-producing Escherichia coli infection. PLoS One. 2014;9(7): e103029.

449. Bauer A, Loos S, Wehrmann C, Horstmann D, Donnerstag F, Lemke J, et al. Neurological involvement in children with E. coli O104:H4-induced hemolytic uremic syndrome. Pediatr Nephrol. 2014;29(9):1607–15.

450. Richardson SE, Karmali MA, Becker LE, Smith CR. The histopathology of the hemolytic uremic syndrome associated with verocytotoxin-producing Escherichia coli infections. Hum Pathol. 1988;19(9):1102–8.

451. Gagnadoux MF, Habib R, Gubler MC, Bacri JL, Broyer M. Long-term (15–25 years) outcome of childhood hemolytic-uremic syndrome. Clin Nephrol. 1996;46(1):39–41.

452. Inward CD, Howie AJ, Fitzpatrick MM, Rafaat F, Milford DV, Taylor CM. Renal histopathology in fatal cases of diarrhoea-associated haemolytic uraemic syndrome. Br Assoc Paediatr Nephrol Pediatr Nephrol. 1997;11(5):556–9.

453. Burns JC, Berman ER. Pancreatic islet HUS. J Pediatr J Pediatr. 1982;100:582–4.

454. Hrynchak M, ANg LC, Munoz DG. Bilateral striatal necrosis in hemolytic-uremic syndrome. Clin Neuropathol. 1992;11(1):45–8.

455. Kielstein JT, Beutel G, Fleig S, Steinhoff J, Meyer TN, Hafer C, et al. Best supportive care and therapeutic plasma exchange with or without eculizumab in Shiga-toxin-producing E. coli O104:H4 induced haemolytic-uraemic syndrome: an analysis of the German STEC-HUS registry. Nephrol Dial Transplant. 2012;27(10):3807–15.

456. Health Q. Shiga toxin-producing Escherichia coli (STEC) infection 2013 [updated Full revision of guideline, June 2013; September 14, 2014]. Available from: http://www.health.qld.gov.au/cdcg/index/stec.asp.

457. Centers for Disease Control and Prevention. Shiga toxin-producing E. coli and Food Safety. www.cdc.gov/features/ecoliinfection/index.html.

458. Thomas DE, Elliott EJ. Interventions for preventing diarrhea-associated hemolytic uremic syndrome: systematic review. BMC Public Health. 2013;13:799.

459. Perrin F, Tenenhaus-Aziza F, Michel V, Miszczycha S, Bel N, Sanaa M. Quantitative risk assessment of haemolytic and uremic syndrome linked to O157:H7 and non-O157:H7 Shiga-toxin producing Escherichia coli strains in raw milk soft cheeses. Risk Anal: Off Publ Soc Risk Anal. 2015;35(1): 109–28.

460. Infections PACoG. Preventing person-to-person spread following gastrointestinal infections: guidelines for public health physicians and environmental health officers. Commun Dis Pub Health/PHLS. 2004;7(4):362–84.

461. Infections WGotfPACoG. Preventing person-to-person spread following gastrointestinal infections: guidelines for public health physicians and environmental health officers 2004. Available from: http://webarchive.nationalarchives.gov.uk/20140714084352/http://www.hpa.org.uk/cdph/issues/CDPHvol7/No4/guidelines2_4_04.pdf.

462. Agency HP. The management of potential VTEC infection: Health Protection Agency; 2011 [updated July 2011]. Available from: https://www.gov.uk/government/uploads/system/uploads/attachment_data/file/342344/management_of_acute_bloody_diarrhoea.pdf.

463. (HPSC) HPSC. Infectious intestinal disease: public health & clinical guidance: Health Protection Surveillance Centre (HPSC) 25-27 Middle Gardiner Street Dublin 1, Ireland; 2012. Available from: http://www.hpsc.ie/A-Z/Gastroenteric/GastroenteritisorIID/GuidanceIIDPublicHealthandClinicalGuidanceappendices/File,13509,en.pdf.

464. Konadu EY, Parke Jr JC, Tran HT, Bryla DA, Robbins JB, Szu SC. Investigational vaccine for Escherichia coli O157: phase 1 study of O157 O-specific polysaccharide-Pseudomonas aeruginosa recombinant exoprotein A conjugates in adults. J Infect Dis. 1998;177(2):383–7.

465. Ahmed A, Li J, Shiloach Y, Robbins JB, Szu SC. Safety and immunogenicity of Escherichia coli O157 O-specific polysaccharide conjugate vaccine in 2-5-year-old children. J Infect Dis. 2006; 193(4):515–21.

466. Smith MJ, Teel LD, Carvalho HM, Melton-Celsa AR, O'Brien AD. Development of a hybrid Shiga holotoxoid vaccine to elicit heterologous protection against Shiga toxins types 1 and 2. Vaccine. 2006;24(19):4122–9.

467. Wen SX, Teel LD, Judge NA, O'Brien AD. A plant-based oral vaccine to protect against systemic intoxication by Shiga toxin type 2. Proc Natl Acad Sci U S A. 2006;103(18):7082–7.

468. Goldwater PN. Treatment and prevention of entero-hemorrhagic Escherichia coli infection and hemolytic uremic syndrome. Expert Rev Anti Infect Ther. 2007;5(4):653–63.

469. Bitzan M. Treatment options for HUS secondary to Escherichia coli O157:H7. Kidney Int Suppl. 2009;112:S62–6.

470. Judge NA, Mason HS, O'Brien AD. Plant cell-based intimin vaccine given orally to mice primed with intimin reduces time of Escherichia coli O157:H7 shedding in feces. Infect Immun. 2004;72(1):168–75.

471. Snedeker KG, Campbell M, Sargeant JM. A systematic review of vaccinations to reduce the shedding of Escherichia coli O157 in the faeces of domestic ruminants. Zoonoses Public Health. 2012;59(2):126–38.

472. Varela NP, Dick P, Wilson J. Assessing the existing information on the efficacy of bovine vaccination against Escherichia coli O157:H7 – a systematic review and meta-analysis. Zoonoses Public Health. 2013;60(4):253–68.

473. Zhang XH, He KW, Zhang SX, Lu WC, Zhao PD, Luan XT, et al. Subcutaneous and intranasal immunization with Stx2B-Tir-Stx1B-Zot reduces colonization and shedding of Escherichia coli O157:H7 in mice. Vaccine. 2011;29(22):3923–9.

474. Zhang XH, He KW, Zhao PD, Ye Q, Luan XT, Yu ZY, et al. Intranasal immunisation with Stx2B-Tir-Stx1B-Zot protein leads to decreased shedding in goats after challenge with Escherichia coli O157:H7. Vet Rec. 2012;170(7):178.

475. Michael M, Elliott EJ, Craig JC, Ridley G, Hodson EM. Interventions for hemolytic uremic syndrome and thrombotic thrombocytopenic purpura: a systematic review of randomized controlled trials. Am J Kidney Dis. 2009;53(2):259–72.

476. Michael M, Elliott EJ, Ridley GF, Hodson EM, Craig JC. Interventions for haemolytic uraemic syndrome and thrombotic thrombocytopenic purpura. Cochrane Database Syst Rev. 2009;1:CD003595.

477. Lopez EL, Contrini MM, Glatstein E, Gonzalez Ayala S, Santoro R, Allende D, et al. Safety and pharmacokinetics of urtoxazumab, a humanized monoclonal antibody, against Shiga-like toxin 2 in healthy adults and in pediatric patients infected with Shiga-like toxin-producing Escherichia coli. Antimicrob Agents Chemother. 2010;54(1):239–43.

478. Bitzan M, Mellmann A, Karch H, Reymond D. SHIGATEC: a phase II study evaluating Shigamabs in STEC-infected children. Zoonoses Public Health. 2012;59 Suppl 1:18.

479. Balestracci A, Martin SM, Toledo I, Alvarado C, Wainsztein RE. Impact of platelet transfusions in children with post-diarrheal hemolytic uremic syndrome. Pediatr Nephrol. 2013;28(6):919–25.

480. Goldstein SL, Chawla LS. Renal angina. Clin J Am Soc Nephrol. 2010;5(5):943–9.

481. Basu RK, Zappitelli M, Brunner L, Wang Y, Wong HR, Chawla LS, et al. Derivation and validation of the renal angina index to improve the prediction of acute kidney injury in critically ill children. Kidney Int. 2014;85(3):659–67.

482. Washington C, Carmichael JC. Management of ischemic colitis. Clin Colon Rectal Surg. 2012;25(4):228–35.

483. Green R, Bulloch B, Kabani A, Hancock BJ, Tenenbein M. Early analgesia for children with acute abdominal pain. Pediatrics. 2005;116(4):978–83.

484. Cimolai N, Basalyga S, Mah DG, Morrison BJ, Carter JE. A continuing assessment of risk factors for the development of Escherichia coli O157:H7-associated hemolytic uremic syndrome. Clin Nephrol. 1994;42(2):85–9.

485. Cimolai N, Carter JE. Antimotility agents for paediatric use. Lancet. 1990;336(8719):874.

486. Brown JW. Toxic megacolon associated with loperamide therapy. JAMA. 1979;241(5):501–2.

487. Tarr PI, Neill MA. Escherichia coli O157:H7. Gastroenterol Clin North Am. 2001;30(3):735–51.

488. Eronen M, Putkonen H, Hallikainen T, Vartiainen H. Lethal gastroenteritis associated with clozapine and loperamide. Am J Psychiatry. 2003;160(12):2242–3.

489. Thorpe CM. Shiga toxin-producing Escherichia coli infection. Clin Infect Dis. 2004;38(9):1298–303.

490. Nelson JM, Griffin PM, Jones TF, Smith KE, Scallan E. Antimicrobial and antimotility agent use in persons with shiga toxin-producing Escherichia coli O157 infection in FoodNet Sites. Clin Infect Dis. 2011;52(9):1130–2.

491. Wong CS, Brandt JR. Risk of hemolytic uremic syndrome from antibiotic treatment of Escherichia coli O157:H7 colitis. JAMA. 2002;288(24):3111. author reply 2.

492. Walterspiel JN, Ashkenazi S, Morrow AL, Cleary TG. Effect of subinhibitory concentrations of antibiotics on extracellular Shiga-like toxin I. Infection. 1992;20(1):25–9.

493. Yoh M, Frimpong EK, Voravuthikunchai SP, Honda T. Effect of subinhibitory concentrations of antimicrobial agents (quinolones and macrolide) on the production of verotoxin by enterohemorrhagic Escherichia coli O157:H7. Can J Microbiol. 1999;45(9):732–9.

494. Proulx F, Turgeon JP, Delage G, Lafleur L, Chicoine L. Randomized, controlled trial of antibiotic therapy for Escherichia coli O157:H7 enteritis. J Pediatr. 1992;121(2):299–303.

495. Safdar N, Said A, Gangnon RE, Maki DG. Risk of hemolytic uremic syndrome after antibiotic treatment of Escherichia coli O157:H7 enteritis: a meta-analysis. JAMA. 2002;288(8):996–1001.

496. Panos GZ, Betsi GI, Falagas ME. Systematic review: are antibiotics detrimental or beneficial for the treatment of patients with Escherichia coli O157:H7 infection? Aliment Pharmacol Ther. 2006;24(5):731–42.

497. Shiomi M, Togawa M, Fujita K, Murata R. Effect of early oral fluoroquinolones in hemorrhagic colitis due to Escherichia coli O157:H7. Pediatr Int: Off J Jpn Pediatr Soc. 1999;41(2):228–32.

498. Nitschke M, Sayk F, Hartel C, Roseland RT, Hauswaldt S, Steinhoff J, et al. Association between azithromycin therapy and duration of bacterial shedding among patients with Shiga toxin-producing enteroaggregative Escherichia coli O104:H4. JAMA. 2012;307(10):1046–52.

499. Gerard L, Garey KW, DuPont HL. Rifaximin: a nonabsorbable rifamycin antibiotic for use in nonsystemic gastrointestinal infections. Expert Rev Anti Infect Ther. 2005;3(2):201–11.

500. Ruiz J, Mensa L, Pons MJ, Vila J, Gascon J. Development of Escherichia coli rifaximin-resistant mutants: frequency of selection and stability. J Antimicrob Chemother. 2008;61(5):1016–9.

501. Hong KS, Kim JS. Rifaximin for the treatment of acute infectious diarrhea. Ther Adv Gastroenterol. 2011;4(4):227–35.

502. Zhang X, McDaniel AD, Wolf LE, Keusch GT, Waldor MK, Acheson DW. Quinolone antibiotics induce Shiga toxin-encoding bacteriophages, toxin production, and death in mice. J Infect Dis. 2000;181(2):664–70.

503. Amran MY, Fujii J, Kolling GL, Villanueva SY, Kainuma M, Kobayashi H, et al. Proposal for effective treatment of Shiga toxin-producing Escherichia coli infection in mice. Microb Pathog. 2013;65: 57–62.

504. Zhang Q, Donohue-Rolfe A, Krautz-Peterson G, Sevo M, Parry N, Abeijon C, et al. Gnotobiotic piglet infection model for evaluating the safe use of antibiotics against Escherichia coli O157:H7 infection. J Infect Dis. 2009;199(4):486–93.

505. Fenwick GR, Heaney RK, Mullin WJ. Glucosinolates and their breakdown products in food and food plants. Crit Rev Food Sci Nutr. 1983;18(2): 123–201.

506. Wang D, Upadhyaya B, Liu Y, Knudsen D, Dey M. Phenethyl isothiocyanate upregulates death receptors 4 and 5 and inhibits proliferation in human cancer stem-like cells. BMC Cancer. 2014;14:591.

507. Nowicki D, Maciag-Dorszynska M, Kobiela W, Herman-Antosiewicz A, Wegrzyn A, Szalewska-Palasz A, et al. Phenethyl isothiocyanate inhibits shiga toxin production in enterohemorrhagic Escherichia coli by stringent response induction. Antimicrob Agents Chemother. 2014;58(4):2304–15.

508. Tarr PI, Karpman D. Editorial commentary: Escherichia coli O104:H4 and hemolytic uremic syndrome: the analysis begins. Clin Infect Dis. 2012;55(6):760–3.

509. DuPont HL. Approach to the patient with infectious colitis. Curr Opin Gastroenterol. 2012;28(1):39–46.

510. Bielaszewska M, Idelevich EA, Zhang W, Bauwens A, Schaumburg F, Mellmann A, et al. Effects of antibiotics on Shiga toxin 2 production and bacterio-phage induction by epidemic Escherichia coli O104:H4 strain. Antimicrob Agents Chemother. 2012;56(6):3277–82.

511. Tarr PI, Sadler JE, Chandler WL, George JN, Tsai HM. Should all adult patients with diarrhoea-associated HUS receive plasma exchange? Lancet. 2012;379(9815):516. author reply -7.

512. Pape L, Ahlenstiel T, Kreuzer M, Drube J, Froede K, Franke D, et al. Early erythropoietin reduced the need for red blood cell transfusion in childhood hemolytic uremic syndrome: a randomized prospective pilot trial. Pediatr Nephrol. 2009;24(5):1061–4.

513. Balestracci A, Martin SM, Toledo I, Alvarado C, Wainsztein RE. Early erythropoietin in post-diarrheal hemolytic uremic syndrome: a case-control study. Pediatr Nephrol. 2015;30(2):339–44.

514. Weil BR, Andreoli SP, Billmire DF. Bleeding risk for surgical dialysis procedures in children with hemolytic uremic syndrome. Pediatr Nephrol. 2010;25(9):1693–8.

515. Harkness DR, Byrnes JJ, Lian EC, Williams WD, Hensley GT. Hazard of platelet transfusion in thrombotic thrombocytopenic purpura. JAMA. 1981; 246(17):1931–3.

516. Lind SE. Thrombocytopenic purpura and platelet transfusion. Ann Intern Med. 1987;106(3):478.

517. Rousseau E, Blais N, O'Regan S. Decreased necessity for dialysis with loop diuretic therapy in hemolytic uremic syndrome. Clin Nephrol. 1990;34(1):22–5.

518. Ho KM, Sheridan DJ. Meta-analysis of frusemide to prevent or treat acute renal failure. BMJ. 2006; 333(7565):420.

519. Bagshaw SM, Bellomo R, Kellum JA. Oliguria, volume overload, and loop diuretics. Crit Care Med. 2008;36(4 Suppl):S172–8.

520. Karajala V, Mansour W, Kellum JA. Diuretics in acute kidney injury. Minerva Anestesiol. 2009;75(5): 251–7.

521. O'Regan S, Rousseau E. Hemolytic uremic syndrome: urate nephropathy superimposed on an acute glomerulopathy? An hypothesis. Clin Nephrol. 1988;30(4):207–10.

522. Acosta AA, Hogg RJ. Rasburicase for hyperuricemia in hemolytic uremic syndrome. Pediatr Nephrol. 2012;27(2):325–9.

523. Taylor MB, Jackson A, Weller JM. Dynamic susceptibility contrast enhanced MRI in reversible posterior leukoencephalopathy syndrome associated with haemolytic uraemic syndrome. Br J Radiol. 2000;73(868):438–42.

524. Gomez-Lado C, Martinon-Torres F, Alvarez-Moreno A, Eiris-Punal J, Carreira-Sande N, Rodriguez-Nunez A, et al. Reversible posterior leukoencephalopathy syndrome: an infrequent complication in the course of haemolytic-uremic syndrome. Rev Neurol. 2007;44(8):475–8.

525. Fujii K, Matsuo K, Takatani T, Uchikawa H, Kohno Y. Multiple cavitations in posterior reversible leukoencephalopathy syndrome associated with

hemolytic-uremic syndrome. Brain Dev. 2012;34(4): 318–21.

526. Gera DN, Patil SB, Iyer A, Kute VB, Gandhi S, Kumar D, et al. Posterior reversible encephalopathy syndrome in children with kidney disease. Indian J Nephrol. 2014;24(1):28–34.

527. Siegler RL, Brewer ED, Corneli HM, Thompson JA. Hypertension first seen as facial paralysis: case reports and review of the literature. Pediatrics. 1991;87(3):387–9.

528. Agarwal R, Davis C, Altinok D, Serajee FJ. Posterior reversible encephalopathy and cerebral vasoconstriction in a patient with hemolytic uremic syndrome. Pediatr Neurol. 2014;50(5):518–21.

529. Grunfeld B, Gimenez M, Liapchuc S, Mendilaharzu J, Gianantonio C. Systemic hypertension and plasma renin activity in children with the hemolytic-uremic syndrome. Int J Pediatr Nephrol. 1982;3(3):211–4.

530. Nestoridi E, Kushak RI, Tsukurov O, Grabowski EF, Ingelfinger JR. Role of the renin angiotensin system in TNF-alpha and Shiga-toxin-induced tissue factor expression. Pediatr Nephrol. 2008;23(2):221–31.

531. Taranta A, Gianviti A, Palma A, De Luca V, Mannucci L, Procaccino MA, et al. Genetic risk factors in typical haemolytic uraemic syndrome. Nephrol Dial Transplant. 2009;24(6):1851–7.

532. Grunfeld B, Gimenez M, Simsolo R, Mendilaharzu F, Becu L. Urinary kallikrein in hypertension secondary to hemolytic uremic syndrome: response to diuretic stimulus. Int J Pediatr Nephrol. 1984;5(4): 205–8.

533. Proesmans W, VanCauter A, Thijs L, Lijnen P. Plasma renin activity in haemolytic uraemic syndrome. Pediatr Nephrol. 1994;8(4):444–6.

534. Molinaro G, Adam A, Lepage Y, Hammerschmidt D, Koenigbauer U, Eastlund T. Hypotensive reaction during staphylococcal protein A column therapy in a patient with anomalous degradation of bradykinin and Des-Arg9-bradykinin after contact activation. Transfusion. 2002;42(11):1458–65.

535. Caletti MG, Lejarraga H, Kelmansky D, Missoni M. Two different therapeutic regimes in patients with sequelae of hemolytic-uremic syndrome. Pediatr Nephrol. 2004;19(10):1148–52.

536. Caletti MG, Balestracci A, Missoni M, Vezzani C. Additive antiproteinuric effect of enalapril and losartan in children with hemolytic uremic syndrome. Pediatr Nephrol. 2013;28(5):745–50.

537. Cobenas CJ, Alconcher LF, Spizzirri AP, Rahman RC. Long-term follow-up of Argentinean patients with hemolytic uremic syndrome who had not undergone dialysis. Pediatr Nephrol. 2007;22(9): 1343–7.

538. Bertholet-Thomas A, Ranchin B, King LA, Bacchetta J, Belot A, Gillet Y, et al. Post-diarrheal haemolytic uremic syndrome: when shall we consider it? Which follow-up? Arch Pediatr. 2011;18(7):823–30.

539. Nakatani T, Tsuchida K, Yoshimura R, Sugimura K, Takemoto Y. Plasma exchange therapy for the treat-

540. Loirat C, Sonsino E, Hinglais N, Jais JP, Landais P, Fermanian J. Treatment of the childhood haemolytic uraemic syndrome with plasma. A multicentre randomized controlled trial. The French Society of Paediatric Nephrology. Pediatr Nephrol. 1988;2(3):279–85.

541. Rizzoni G, Claris-Appiani A, Edefonti A, Facchin P, Franchini F, Gusmano R, et al. Plasma infusion for hemolytic-uremic syndrome in children: results of a multicenter controlled trial. J Pediatr. 1988; 112(2):284–90.

542. Loirat C. Hemolytic uremic syndrome caused by Shiga-toxin-producing Escherichia coli. Rev Prat. 2013;63(1):11–6.

543. Colic E, Dieperink H, Titlestad K, Tepel M. Management of an acute outbreak of diarrhoea-associated haemolytic uraemic syndrome with early plasma exchange in adults from southern Denmark: an observational study. Lancet. 2011;378(9796): 1089–93.

544. Ruggenenti P, Remuzzi G. A German outbreak of haemolytic uraemic syndrome. Lancet. 2011; 378(9796):1057–8.

545. Bambauer R, Latza R, Schiel R. Therapeutic apheresis in the treatment of hemolytic uremic syndrome in view of pathophysiological aspects. Ther Apher Dial: Off Peer-Rev J Int Soc Apher Jpn Soc Apher Jpn Soc Dial Ther. 2011;15(1):10–9.

546. (DGfN) GSoN. Therapeutische Apheresebehandlung bei EHEC assoziiertem HUS. [Therapeutic plasma exchange in EHEC-HUS] 2011. Available from: http://www.dgfn.eu/aktuell/ehec-informationen/fuer-das-fachpublikum/therapeutische-apheresebehandlung-bei-ehec-assoziiertem-hus.html.

547. Remuzzi G. HUS and TTP: variable expression of a single entity. Kidney Int. 1987;32(2):292–308.

548. Fakhouri F, Fremeaux-Bacchi V. Does hemolytic uremic syndrome differ from thrombotic thrombocytopenic purpura? Nat Clin Pract Nephrol. 2007;3(12):679–87.

549. Forzley BR, Clark WF. TTP/HUS and prognosis: the syndrome and the disease(s). Kidney Int Suppl. 2009;112:S59–61.

550. Moschcowitz E. An acute febrile pleiochromic anemia with hyaline thrombosis of the terminal arterioles and capillaries: an undescribed disease. 1925. Mt Sinai J Med NY. 2003;70(5):352–5.

551. Tsai HM. Physiologic cleavage of von Willebrand factor by a plasma protease is dependent on its conformation and requires calcium ion. Blood. 1996;87(10):4235–44.

552. Furlan M, Robles R, Lammle B. Partial purification and characterization of a protease from human plasma cleaving von Willebrand factor to fragments produced by in vivo proteolysis. Blood. 1996;87(10): 4223–34.

553. Tsai HM. Untying the knot of thrombotic thrombocytopenic purpura and atypical hemolytic uremic syndrome. Am J Med. 2013;126(3):200–9.

ment of Escherichia coli O-157 associated hemolytic uremic syndrome. Int J Mol Med. 2002;10(5):585–8.

554. Rock G, Shumak K, Nair R. A study of plasma exchange in TTP. The Canadian Apheresis Study Group. Prog Clin Biol Res. 1990;337:125–7.

555. Knobl P. Inherited and acquired thrombotic thrombocytopenic purpura (TTP) in adults. Semin Thromb Hemost. 2014;40(4):493–502.

556. Schwartz J, Winters JL, Padmanabhan A, Balogun RA, Delaney M, Linenberger ML, et al. Guidelines on the use of therapeutic apheresis in clinical practice-evidence-based approach from the Writing Committee of the American Society for Apheresis: the sixth special issue. J Clin Apher. 2013;28(3):145–284.

557. Karpman D. Management of Shiga toxin-associated Escherichia coli-induced haemolytic uraemic syndrome: randomized clinical trials are needed. Nephrol Dial Transplant. 2012;27(10):3669–74.

558. Wun T, Paglieroni T, Holland P. Prolonged circulation of activated platelets following plasmapheresis. J Clin Apher. 1994;9(1):10–6.

559. Hanafusa N, Satonaka H, Doi K, Yatomi Y, Noiri E, Fujita T. Platelet-derived microparticles are removed by a membrane plasma separator. ASAIO J. 2010;56(4):323–5.

560. Greinacher A, Friesecke S, Abel P, Dressel A, Stracke S, Fiene M, et al. Treatment of severe neurological deficits with IgG depletion through immunoadsorption in patients with Escherichia coli O104:H4-associated haemolytic uraemic syndrome: a prospective trial. Lancet. 2011;378(9797): 1166–73.

561. Monnens L, van Collenburg J, de Jong M, Zoethout H, van Wieringen P. Treatment of the hemolytic-uremic syndrome. Comparison of the results of heparin treatment with the results of streptokinase treatment. Helv Paediatr Acta. 1978;33(4–5):321–8.

562. Siegler RL, Pysher TJ, Tesh VL, Taylor FB. Renal prostacyclin biosynthesis in a baboon model of Shiga toxin mediated hemolytic uremic syndrome. Nephron. 2002;92(2):363–8.

563. Siegler RL, Pysher TJ, Tesh VL, Denkers ND, Taylor FB. Prophylactic heparinization is ineffective in a primate model of hemolytic uremic syndrome. Pediatr Nephrol. 2002;17(12):1053–8.

564. Heerze LD, Kelm MA, Talbot JA, Armstrong GD. Oligosaccharide sequences attached to an inert support (SYNSORB) as potential therapy for antibiotic-associated diarrhea and pseudomembranous colitis. J Infect Dis. 1994;169(6):1291–6.

565. Armstrong GD, Rowe PC, Goodyer P, Orrbine E, Klassen TP, Wells G, et al. A phase I study of chemically synthesized verotoxin (Shiga-like toxin) Pk-trisaccharide receptors attached to chromosorb for preventing hemolytic-uremic syndrome. J Infect Dis. 1995;171(4):1042–5.

566. Abu-Ali GS, Ouellette LM, Henderson ST, Lacher DW, Riordan JT, Whittam TS, et al. Increased adherence and expression of virulence genes in a lineage of Escherichia coli O157:H7 commonly associated with human infections. PLoS One. 2010;5(4):e10167.

567. Kitov PI, Sadowska JM, Mulvey G, Armstrong GD, Ling H, Pannu NS, et al. Shiga-like toxins are neutralized by tailored multivalent carbohydrate ligands. Nature. 2000;403(6770):669–72.

568. Nishikawa K, Matsuoka K, Kita E, Okabe N, Mizuguchi M, Hino K, et al. A therapeutic agent with oriented carbohydrates for treatment of infections by Shiga toxin-producing Escherichia coli O157:H7. Proc Natl Acad Sci U S A. 2002;99(11): 7669–74.

569. Mulvey GL, Marcato P, Kitov PI, Sadowska J, Bundle DR, Armstrong GD. Assessment in mice of the therapeutic potential of tailored, multivalent Shiga toxin carbohydrate ligands. J Infect Dis. 2003;187(4):640–9.

570. Nishikawa K, Matsuoka K, Watanabe M, Igai K, Hino K, Hatano K, et al. Identification of the optimal structure required for a Shiga toxin neutralizer with oriented carbohydrates to function in the circulation. J Infect Dis. 2005;191(12):2097–105.

571. Nishikawa K, Watanabe M, Kita E, Igai K, Omata K, Yaffe MB, et al. A multivalent peptide library approach identifies a novel Shiga toxin inhibitor that induces aberrant cellular transport of the toxin. Faseb J. 2006;20(14):2597–9.

572. Watanabe-Takahashi M, Sato T, Dohi T, Noguchi N, Kano F, Murata M, et al. An orally applicable Shiga toxin neutralizer functions in the intestine to inhibit the intracellular transport of the toxin. Infect Immun. 2010;78(1):177–83.

573. Tsutsuki K, Watanabe-Takahashi M, Takenaka Y, Kita E, Nishikawa K. Identification of a peptide-based neutralizer that potently inhibits both Shiga toxins 1 and 2 by targeting specific receptor-binding regions. Infect Immun. 2013;81(6):2133–8.

574. Paton AW, Morona R, Paton JC. Neutralization of Shiga toxins Stx1, Stx2c, and Stx2e by recombinant bacteria expressing mimics of globotriose and globotetraose. Infect Immun. 2001;69(3):1967–70.

575. Paton AW, Morona R, Paton JC. Bioengineered bugs expressing oligosaccharide receptor mimics: toxin-binding probiotics for treatment and prevention of enteric infections. Bioeng Bugs. 2010;1(3):172–7.

576. Hostetter SJ, Helgerson AF, Paton JC, Paton AW, Cornick NA. Therapeutic use of a receptor mimic probiotic reduces intestinal Shiga toxin levels in a piglet model of hemolytic uremic syndrome. BMC Res Notes. 2014;7:331.

577. Sauter KA, Melton-Celsa AR, Larkin K, Troxell ML, O'Brien AD, Magun BE. Mouse model of hemolytic-uremic syndrome caused by endotoxin-free Shiga toxin 2 (Stx2) and protection from lethal outcome by anti-Stx2 antibody. Infect Immun. 2008;76(10):4469–78.

578. López EL, Contrini MM, Glatstein E, González Ayala S, Santoro R, Allende D, et al. Safety and pharmacokinetics of urtoxazumab, a humanized monoclonal antibody against Shiga-like toxin 2 in healthy adults and pediatric STEC- infected patients. Antimicrob Agents Chemother. 2010;54(1):239–43.

579. Dowling TC, Chavaillaz PA, Young DG, Melton-Celsa A, O'Brien A, Thuning-Roberson C, et al. Phase 1 safety and pharmacokinetic study of chimeric murine-human monoclonal antibody c alpha Stx2 administered intravenously to healthy adult volunteers. Antimicrob Agents Chemother. 2005;49(5):1808–12.

580. Bitzan M, Poole R, Mehran M, Sicard E, Brockus C, Thuning-Roberson C, et al. Safety and pharmacokinetics of chimeric anti-Shiga toxin 1 and anti-Shiga toxin 2 monoclonal antibodies in healthy volunteers. Antimicrob Agents Chemother. 2009;53(7):3081–7.

581. Taylor C, Bitzan M, Reymond D. Shigatec: a Phase II study assessing monoclonal antibodies against Shiga toxin 1 and 2 in Shiga toxin- producing *E. coli*-infected children. Pediatr Nephrol. 2011;26:1595–6.

582. Tremblay JM, Mukherjee J, Leysath CE, Debatis M, Ofori K, Baldwin K, et al. A single VHH-based toxin-neutralizing agent and an effector antibody protect mice against challenge with Shiga toxins 1 and 2. Infect Immun. 2013;81(12):4592–603.

583. Lapeyraque AL, Malina M, Fremeaux-Bacchi V, Boppel T, Kirschfink M, Oualha M, et al. Complement blockade in severe Shiga-toxin-associated HUS. N Engl J Med. 2011. Letter published May 25, 2011. Published at NEJM.org.

584. Kim Y, Miller K, Michael AF. Breakdown products of C3 and factor B in hemolytic-uremic syndrome. J Lab Clin Med. 1977;89(4):845–50.

585. Monnens L, Molenaar J, Lambert PH, Proesmans W, van Munster P. The complement system in hemolytic-uremic syndrome in childhood. Clin Nephrol. 1980;13(4):168–71.

586. Robson WL, Leung AK, Fick GH, McKenna AI. Hypocomplementemia and leukocytosis in diarrhea-associated hemolytic uremic syndrome. Nephron. 1992;62(3):296–9.

587. McCoy RC, Abramowsky CR, Krueger R. The hemolytic uremic syndrome, with positive immunofluorescence studies. J Pediatr. 1974;85(2):170–4.

588. Thurman JM, Marians R, Emlen W, Wood S, Smith C, Akana H, et al. Alternative pathway of complement in children with diarrhea-associated hemolytic uremic syndrome. Clin J Am Soc Nephrol. 2009;4(12):1920–4.

589. Ghosh SA, Polanowska-Grabowska RK, Fujii J, Obrig T, Gear AR. Shiga toxin binds to activated platelets. J Thromb Haemost: JTH. 2004;2(3):499–506.

590. Fernandez GC, Te Loo MW, van der Velden TJ, van der Heuvel LP, Palermo MS, Monnens LL. Decrease of thrombomodulin contributes to the procoagulant state of endothelium in hemolytic uremic syndrome. Pediatr Nephrol. 2003;18(10):1066–8.

591. Del Conde I, Cruz MA, Zhang H, Lopez JA, Afshar-Kharghan V. Platelet activation leads to activation and propagation of the complement system. J Exp Med. 2005;201(6):871–9.

592. Orth D, Khan AB, Naim A, Grif K, Brockmeyer J, Karch H, et al. Shiga toxin activates complement and binds factor H: evidence for an active role of complement in hemolytic uremic syndrome. J Immunol. 2009;182(10):6394–400.

593. Orth-Holler D, Wurzner R. Role of complement in enterohemorrhagic Escherichia coli-Induced hemolytic uremic syndrome. Semin Thromb Hemost. 2014;40(4):503–7.

594. Poolpol K, Orth-Holler D, Speth C, Zipfel PF, Skerka C, de Cordoba SR, et al. Interaction of Shiga toxin 2 with complement regulators of the factor H protein family. Mol Immunol. 2014;58(1):77–84.

595. Lee BC, Mayer CL, Leibowitz CS, Stearns-Kurosawa DJ, Kurosawa S. Quiescent complement in nonhuman primates during E coli Shiga toxin-induced hemolytic uremic syndrome and thrombotic microangiopathy. Blood. 2013;122(5):803–6.

596. Silasi-Mansat R, Zhu H, Popescu NI, Peer G, Sfyroera G, Magotti P, et al. Complement inhibition decreases the procoagulant response and confers organ protection in a baboon model of Escherichia coli sepsis. Blood. 2010;116(6):1002–10.

597. Lupu F, Keshari RS, Lambris JD, Coggeshall KM. Crosstalk between the coagulation and complement systems in sepsis. Thromb Res. 2014;133 Suppl 1:S28–31.

598. Ward PA, Guo RF, Riedemann NC. Manipulation of the complement system for benefit in sepsis. Crit Care Res Pract. 2012;2012:427607.

599. Thurman JM. New anti-complement drugs: not so far away. Blood. 2014;123(13):1975–6.

600. Keir LS, Saleem MA. Current evidence for the role of complement in the pathogenesis of Shiga toxin haemolytic uraemic syndrome. Pediatr Nephrol. 2014;29(10):1895–902.

601. Delmas Y, Vendrely B, Clouzeau B, Bachir H, Bui HN, Lacraz A, et al. Outbreak of Escherichia coli O104:H4 haemolytic uraemic syndrome in France: outcome with eculizumab. Nephrol Dial Transplant. 2014;29(3):565–72.

602. Igarashi T, Ito S, Sako M, Saitoh A, Hataya H, Mizuguchi M, et al. Guidelines for the management and investigation of hemolytic uremic syndrome. Clin Exp Nephrol. 2014;18(4):525–57.

603. Conway EM. Thrombomodulin and its role in inflammation. Semin Immunopathol. 2012;34(1):107–25.

604. Martin FA, Murphy RP, Cummins PM. Thrombomodulin and the vascular endothelium: insights into functional, regulatory, and therapeutic aspects. Am J Physiol Heart Circ Physiol. 2013;304(12):H1585–97.

605. Wang H, Vinnikov I, Shahzad K, Bock F, Ranjan S, Wolter J, et al. The lectin-like domain of thrombomodulin ameliorates diabetic glomerulopathy via complement inhibition. Thromb Haemost. 2012;108(6):1141–53.

606. Delvaeye M, Noris M, De Vriese A, Esmon CT, Esmon NL, Ferrell G, et al. Thrombomodulin muta-

tions in atypical hemolytic-uremic syndrome. N Engl J Med. 2009;361(4):345–57.

607. Zoja C, Locatelli M, Pagani C, Corna D, Zanchi C, Isermann B, et al. Lack of the lectin-like domain of thrombomodulin worsens Shiga toxin-associated hemolytic uremic syndrome in mice. J Immunol. 2012;189(7):3661–8.

608. Vincent JL, Ramesh MK, Ernest D, LaRosa SP, Pachl J, Aikawa N, et al. A randomized, double-blind, placebo-controlled, Phase 2b study to evaluate the safety and efficacy of recombinant human soluble thrombomodulin, ART-123, in patients with sepsis and suspected disseminated intravascular coagulation. Crit Care Med. 2013;41(9):2069–79.

609. Honda T, Ogata S, Mineo E, Nagamori Y, Nakamura S, Bando Y, et al. A novel strategy for hemolytic uremic syndrome: successful treatment with thrombomodulin alpha. Pediatrics. 2013;131(3):e928–33.

610. Ehrlenbach S, Rosales A, Posch W, Wilflingseder D, Hermann M, Brockmeyer J, et al. Shiga toxin 2 reduces complement inhibitor CD59 expression on human renal tubular epithelial and glomerular endothelial cells. Infect Immun. 2013;81(8):2678–85.

611. Dammermann W, Schipper P, Ullrich S, Fraedrich K, Schulze Zur Wiesch J, Frundt T, et al. Increased expression of complement regulators CD55 and CD59 on peripheral blood cells in patients with EAHEC O104:H4 infection. PLoS One. 2013;8(9):e74880.

612. Fang CJ, Fremeaux-Bacchi V, Liszewski MK, Pianetti G, Noris M, Goodship TH, et al. Membrane cofactor protein mutations in atypical hemolytic uremic syndrome (aHUS), fatal Stx-HUS, C3 glomerulonephritis, and the HELLP syndrome. Blood. 2008;111(2):624–32.

613. Alberti M, Valoti E, Piras R, Bresin E, Galbusera M, Tripodo C, et al. Two patients with history of STEC-HUS, posttransplant recurrence and complement gene mutations. Am J Transplant. 2013;13(8): 2201–6.

614. Brockleband V, Wong EKS, RFielding R, Goodship THJ, Kavanagh D. Atypical haemolytic uraemic syndrome associated with a CD46 mutation triggered by Shigella flexneri. Clin Kidney J. 2014;7: 286–8.

615. Gianantonio CA, Vitacco M, Mendilaharzu F, Gallo G. The hemolytic-uremic syndrome. Renal status of 76 patients at long-term follow-up. J Pediatr. 1968;72(6):757–65.

616. Kaplan BS, Katz J, Krawitz S, Lurie A. An analysis of the results of therapy in 67 cases of the hemolytic-uremic syndrome. J Pediatr. 1971;78(3):420–5.

617. Spinale JM, Ruebner RL, Copelovitch L, Kaplan BS. Long-term outcomes of Shiga toxin hemolytic uremic syndrome. Pediatr Nephrol. 2013;28(11): 2097–105.

618. Garg AX, Suri RS, Barrowman N, Rehman F, Matsell D, Rosas-Arellano MP, et al. Long-term renal prognosis of diarrhea-associated hemolytic uremic syndrome: a systematic review, meta-analysis, and meta-regression. Jama. 2003;290(10):1360–70.

619. Schieppati A, Ruggenenti P, Cornejo RP, Ferrario F, Gregorini G, Zucchelli P, et al. Renal function at hospital admission as a prognostic factor in adult hemolytic uremic syndrome. The Italian Registry of Haemolytic Uremic Syndrome. J Am Soc Nephrol. 1992;2(11):1640–4.

620. Havelaar AH, Van Duynhoven YT, Nauta MJ, Bouwknegt M, Heuvelink AE, De Wit GA, et al. Disease burden in The Netherlands due to infections with Shiga toxin-producing Escherichia coli O157. Epidemiol Infect. 2004;132(3):467–84.

621. Garg AX, Salvadori M, Okell JM, Thiessen-Philbrook HR, Suri RS, Filler G, et al. Albuminuria and estimated GFR 5 years after Escherichia coli O157 hemolytic uremic syndrome: an update. Am J Kidney Dis. 2008;51(3):435–44.

622. Siegler R, Oakes R. Hemolytic uremic syndrome; pathogenesis, treatment, and outcome. Curr Opin Pediatr. 2005;17(2):200–4.

623. Sharma AP, Filler G, Dwight P, Clark WF. Chronic renal disease is more prevalent in patients with hemolytic uremic syndrome who had a positive history of diarrhea. Kidney Int. 2010;78(6):598–604.

624. Fitzpatrick MM, Shah V, Trompeter RS, Dillon MJ, Barratt TM. Long term renal outcome of childhood haemolytic uraemic syndrome. BMJ. 1991;303(6801):489–92.

625. Buder K, Latal B, Nef S, Neuhaus TJ, Laube GF, Spartà G. Neurodevelopmental long-term outcome in children after hemolytic uremic syndrome. Pediatr Nephrol. 2015;30(3):503–13. Doi:10.1007/s00467-014-2950-0. Epub 2014 Sep 19.

626. Clark WF, Sontrop JM, Macnab JJ, Salvadori M, Moist L, Suri R, et al. Long term risk for hypertension, renal impairment, and cardiovascular disease after gastroenteritis from drinking water contaminated with Escherichia coli O157:H7: a prospective cohort study. BMJ. 2010;341:c6020.

627. Small G, Watson AR, Evans JH, Gallagher J. Hemolytic uremic syndrome: defining the need for long-term follow-up. Clin Nephrol. 1999;52(6): 352–6.

628. Bassani CE, Ferraris J, Gianantonio CA, Ruiz S, Ramirez J. Renal transplantation in patients with classical haemolytic-uraemic syndrome. Pediatr Nephrol. 1991;5(5):607–11.

629. Ferraris JR, Ramirez JA, Ruiz S, Caletti MG, Vallejo G, Piantanida JJ, et al. Shiga toxin-associated hemolytic uremic syndrome: absence of recurrence after renal transplantation. Pediatr Nephrol. 2002;17(10):809–14.

630. Siegler RL, Griffin PM, Barrett TJ, Strockbine NA. Recurrent hemolytic uremic syndrome secondary to Escherichia coli O157:H7 infection. Pediatrics. 1993;91(3):666–8.

631. Ullis KC, Rosenblatt RM. Shiga bacillus dysentery complicated by bacteremia and disseminated intravascular coagulation. J Pediatr. 1973;83(1):90–3.

632. Chesney R. Letter: hemolytic-uremic syndrome with shigellosis. J Pediatr. 1974;84(2):312–3.

633. Wimmer LE. Hemolytic-uremic syndrome with shigella antecedent. J Am Osteopath Assoc. 1974;74(2):139–43.

634. Raghupathy P, Date A, Shastry JC, Sudarsanam A, Jadhav M. Haemolytic-uraemic syndrome complicating shigella dystentery in south Indian children. Br Med J. 1978;1(6126):1518–21.

635. Bhimma R, Rollins NC, Coovadia HM, Adhikari M. Post-dysenteric hemolytic uremic syndrome in children during an epidemic of Shigella dysentery in Kwazulu/Natal. Pediatr Nephrol. 1997;11(5):560–4.

636. Butler T. Haemolytic uraemic syndrome during shigellosis. Trans R Soc Trop Med Hyg. 2012;106(7):395–9.

637. Bennish ML, Khan WA, Begum M, Bridges EA, Ahmed S, Saha D, et al. Low risk of hemolytic uremic syndrome after early effective antimicrobial therapy for Shigella dysenteriae type 1 infection in Bangladesh. Clin Infect Dis. 2006;42(3):356–62.

638. Bloom PD, MacPhail AP, Klugman K, Louw M, Raubenheimer C, Fischer C. Haemolytic-uraemic syndrome in adults with resistant Shigella dysenteriae type I. Lancet. 1994;344(8916):206.

639. Rollins NC, Wittenberg DF, Coovadia HM, Pillay DG, Karas AJ, Sturm AW. Epidemic Shigella dysenteriae type 1 in Natal. J Trop Pediatr. 1995;41(5):281–4.

640. Zimbabwe BSADSG. Multicenter, randomized, double blind clinical trial of short course versus standard course oral ciprofloxacin for Shigella dysenteriae type 1 dysentery in children. Pediatr Infect Dis J. 2002;21(12):1136–41.

641. Nathoo KJ, Sanders JA, Siziya S, Mucheche C. Haemolytic uraemic syndrome following Shigella dysenteriae type 1 outbreak in Zimbabwe: a clinical experience. Cent Afr J Med. 1995;41(9):267–74.

642. Oneko M, Nyathi MN, Doehring E. Post-dysenteric hemolytic uremic syndrome in Bulawayo, Zimbabwe. Pediatr Nephrol. 2001;16(12):1142–5.

643. Srivastava RN, Moudgil A, Bagga A, Vasudev AS. Hemolytic uremic syndrome in children in northern India. Pediatr Nephrol. 1991;5(3):284–8.

644. Taneja N, Lyngdoh VW, Sharma M. Haemolytic uraemic syndrome due to ciprofloxacin-resistant Shigella dysenteriae serotype 1. J Med Microbiol. 2005;54(Pt 10):997–8.

645. Jha DK, Singh R, Raja S, Kumari N, Das BK. Clinico-laboratory profile of haemolytic uremic syndrome. Kathmandu Univ Med J (KUMJ). 2007;5(4):468–74.

646. Baranwal AK, Ravi R, Singh R. Diarrhea associated hemolytic uremic syndrome: a 3-year PICU experience from Nepal. Indian J Pediatr. 2009;76(11):1180–2.

647. Bin Saeed AA, El Bushra HE, Al-Hamdan NA. Does treatment of bloody diarrhea due to Shigella dysenteriae type 1 with ampicillin precipitate hemolytic uremic syndrome? Emerg Infect Dis. 1995;1(4):134–7.

648. Al-Qarawi S, Fontaine RE, Al-Qahtani MS. An outbreak of hemolytic uremic syndrome associated with antibiotic treatment of hospital inpatients for dysentery. Emerg Infect Dis. 1995;1(4):138–40.

649. Butler T, Islam MR, Azad MA, Jones PK. Risk factors for development of hemolytic uremic syndrome during shigellosis. J Pediatr. 1987;110(6):894–7.

650. Olotu AI, Mithwani S, Newton CR. Haemolytic uraemic syndrome in children admitted to a rural district hospital in Kenya. Trop Doct. 2008;38(3):165–7.

651. Yuhas Y, Weizman A, Dinari G, Ashkenazi S. An animal model for the study of neurotoxicity of bacterial products and application of the model to demonstrate that Shiga toxin and lipopolysaccharide cooperate in inducing neurologic disorders. J Infect Dis. 1995;171(5):1244–9.

652. Butler T, Rahman H, Al-Mahmud KA, Islam M, Bardhan P, Kabir I, et al. An animal model of haemolytic – uraemic syndrome in shigellosis: lipopolysaccharides of Shigella dysenteriae I and S. flexneri produce leucocyte-mediated renal cortical necrosis in rabbits. Br J Exp Pathol. 1985;66(1):7–15.

653. Azim T, Islam LN, Halder RC, Hamadani J, Khanum N, Sarker MS, et al. Peripheral blood neutrophil responses in children with shigellosis. Clin Diagn Lab Immunol. 1995;2(5):616–22.

654. Badami KG, Srivastava RN, Kumar R, Saraya AK. Disseminated intravascular coagulation in post-dysenteric haemolytic uraemic syndrome. Acta Paediatr Scand. 1987;76(6):919–22.

655. Bennish ML, Harris JR, Wojtyniak BJ, Struelens M. Death in shigellosis: incidence and risk factors in hospitalized patients. J Infect Dis. 1990;161(3):500–6.

656. Khan WA, Griffiths JK, Bennish ML. Gastrointestinal and extra-intestinal manifestations of childhood shigellosis in a region where all four species of Shigella are endemic. PLoS One. 2013;8(5):e64097.

657. Mizutani S, Nakazono N, Sugino Y. The so-called chromosomal verotoxin genes are actually carried by defective prophages. DNA Res: Int J Rapid Publ Rep Genes Genomes. 1999;6(2):141–3.

658. Greco KM, McDonough MA, Butterton JR. Variation in the Shiga toxin region of 20th-century epidemic and endemic Shigella dysenteriae 1 strains. J Infect Dis. 2004;190(2):330–4.

659. Taylor CM. Enterohaemorrhagic Escherichia coli and Shigella dysenteriae type 1-induced haemolytic uraemic syndrome. Pediatr Nephrol. 2008;23(9):1425–31.

660. Cabrera GR, Fortenberry JD, Warshaw BL, Chambliss CR, Butler JC, Cooperstone BG. Hemolytic uremic syndrome associated with invasive Streptococcus pneumoniae infection. Pediatrics. 1998;101(4 Pt 1):699–703.

661. Waters AM, Kerecuk L, Luk D, Haq MR, Fitzpatrick MM, Gilbert RD, et al. Hemolytic uremic syndrome associated with invasive pneumococcal disease: the

United kingdom experience. J Pediatr. 2007;151(2): 140–4.

662. Prestidge C, Wong W. Ten years of pneumococcal-associated haemolytic uraemic syndrome in New Zealand children. J Paediatr Child Health. 2009;45(12): 731–5.

663. Constantinescu AR, Bitzan M, Weiss LS, Christen E, Kaplan BS, Cnaan A, et al. Non-enteropathic hemolytic uremic syndrome: causes and short-term course. Am J Kidney Dis. 2004;43(6):976–82.

664. Mizusawa Y, Pitcher LA, Burke JR, Falk MC, Mizushima W. Survey of haemolytic-uraemic syndrome in Queensland 1979–1995. Med J Aust. 1996;165(4):188–91.

665. Proulx F, Sockett P. Prospective surveillance of Canadian children with the haemolytic uraemic syndrome. Pediatr Nephrol. 2005;20(6):786–90.

666. Brueggemann AB, Pai R, Crook DW, Beall B. Vaccine escape recombinants emerge after pneumococcal vaccination in the United States. PLoS Pathog. 2007;3(11):e168.

667. Van Effelterre T, Moore MR, Fierens F, Whitney CG, White L, Pelton SI, et al. A dynamic model of pneumococcal infection in the United States: implications for prevention through vaccination. Vaccine. 2010;28(21):3650–60.

668. Copelovitch L, Kaplan BS. Streptococcus pneumoniae-associated hemolytic uremic syndrome: classification and the emergence of serotype 19A. Pediatrics. 2010;125(1):e174–82.

669. Cohen R, Levy C, Bonnet E, Thollot F, Boucherat M, Fritzell B, et al. Risk factors for serotype 19A carriage after introduction of 7-valent pneumococcal vaccination. BMC Infect Dis. 2011;11:95.

670. Hanquet G, Kissling E, Fenoll A, George R, Lepoutre A, Lernout T, et al. Pneumococcal serotypes in children in 4 European countries. Emerg Infect Dis. 2010;16(9):1428–39.

671. Vaith P, Uhlenbruck G. The Thomsen agglutination phenomenon: a discovery revisited 50 years later. Z Immunitatsforsch Immunobiol. 1978;154(1):1–15.

672. Eder AF, Manno CS. Does red-cell T activation matter? Br J Haematol. 2001;114(1):25–30.

673. Spinale JM, Ruebner RL, Kaplan BS, Copelovitch L. Update on Streptococcus pneumoniae associated hemolytic uremic syndrome. Curr Opin Pediatr. 2013;25(2):203–8.

674. Bender JM, Ampofo K, Byington CL, Grinsell M, Korgenski K, Daly JA, et al. Epidemiology of Streptococcus pneumoniae-induced hemolytic uremic syndrome in Utah children. Pediatr Infect Dis J. 2010;29(8):712–6.

675. O'Toole RD, Goode L, Howe C. Neuraminidase activity in bacterial meningitis. J Clin Invest. 1971;50(5):979–85.

676. Coats MT, Murphy T, Paton JC, Gray B, Briles DE. Exposure of Thomsen-Friedenreich antigen in Streptococcus pneumoniae infection is dependent on pneumococcal neuraminidase A. Microb Pathog. 2011;50(6):343–9.

677. Klein PJ, Newman RA, Muller P, Uhlenbruck G, Schaefer HE, Lennartz KJ, et al. Histochemical methods for the demonstration of Thomsen-Friedenreich antigen in cell suspensions and tissue sections. Klin Wochenschr. 1978;56(15):761–5.

678. Eber SW, Polster H, Quentin SH, Rumpf KW, Lynen R. Hemolytic-uremic syndrome in pneumococcal meningitis and infection. Importance of T-transformation. Monatsschr Kinderheilkd. 1993; 141(3):219–22.

679. Seitz RC, Poschmann A, Hellwege HH. Monoclonal antibodies for the detection of desialylation of erythrocyte membranes during haemolytic disease and haemolytic uraemic syndrome caused by the in vivo action of microbial neuraminidase. Glycoconj J. 1997;14(6):699–706.

680. Poschmann A, Fischer K, Grundmann A, Vongjirad A. Neuraminidase induced hemolytic anemia. Experimental and clinical observations (author's transl). Monatsschr Kinderheilkd. 1976;124(1):15–24.

681. Crookston KP, Reiner AP, Cooper LJ, Sacher RA, Blajchman MA, Heddle NM. RBC T activation and hemolysis: implications for pediatric transfusion management. Transfusion. 2000;40(7):801–12.

682. Bitzan M, AlKandari O, Whittemore B. Variable complement consumption and Coombs test positivity in pneumococcal hemolytic uremic syndrome. 47th Annual Scientific Meeting of the European Society of Pediatric Nephrology (ESPN), Porto (Portugal). 2014;18–20, (Poster # 1057).

683. Huang YH, Lin TY, Wong KS, Huang YC, Chiu CH, Lai SH, et al. Hemolytic uremic syndrome associated with pneumococcal pneumonia in Taiwan. Eur J Pediatr. 2006;165(5):332–5.

684. Huang DT, Chi H, Lee HC, Chiu NC, Huang FY. T-antigen activation for prediction of pneumococcus-induced hemolytic uremic syndrome and hemolytic anemia. Pediatr Infect Dis J. 2006;25(7):608–10.

685. Seger R, Joller P, Bird GW, Wingham J, Wuest J, Kenny A, et al. Necrotising enterocolitis and neuraminidase-producing bacteria. Helv Paediatr Acta. 1980;35(2):121–8.

686. Eversole M, Nonemaker B, Zurek K, South S, Simon T. Uneventful administration of plasma products in a recipient with T-activated red cells. Transfusion. 1986;26(2):182–5.

687. Poschmann A, Fischer K. Exchange transfusion with heparinised fresh blood in necrotising enterocolitis. Lancet. 1979;1(8120):824–5.

688. Trachtman H, Sethna C, Epstein R, D'Souza M, Rubin LG, Ginocchio CC. Atypical hemolytic uremic syndrome associated with H1N1 influenza A virus infection. Pediatr Nephrol. 2011;26(1):145–6.

689. Watanabe T. Hemolytic uremic syndrome associated with influenza A virus infection. Nephron. 2001;89(3):359–60.

690. Geary DF. Hemolytic uremic syndrome and streptococcus pneumoniae: improving our understanding. J Pediatr. 2007;151(2):113–4.

691. Brandt J, Wong C, Mihm S, Roberts J, Smith J, Brewer E, et al. Invasive pneumococcal disease and hemolytic uremic syndrome. Pediatrics. 2002;110(2 Pt 1):371–6.

692. Banerjee R, Hersh AL, Newland J, Beekmann SE, Polgreen PM, Bender J, et al. Streptococcus pneumoniae-associated hemolytic uremic syndrome among children in North America. Pediatr Infect Dis J. 2011;30(9):736–9.

693. von Vigier RO, Seibel K, Bianchetti MG. Positive Coombs test in pneumococcus-associated hemolytic uremic syndrome. A review of the literature. Nephron. 1999;82(2):183–4.

694. Lee CS, Chen MJ, Chiou YH, Shen CF, Wu CY, Chiou YY. Invasive pneumococcal pneumonia is the major cause of paediatric haemolytic-uraemic syndrome in Taiwan. Nephrology (Carlton). 2012;17(1): 48–52.

695. Loupiac A, Elayan A, Cailliez M, Adra AL, Decramer S, Thouret MC, et al. Diagnosis of Streptococcus pneumoniae-associated hemolytic uremic syndrome. Pediatr Infect Dis J. 2013; 32(10):1045–9.

696. Moorthy B, Makker SP. Hemolytic-uremic syndrome associated with pneumococcal sepsis. J Pediatr. 1979;95(4):558–9.

697. Beattie KM, Lewis PE, Briski JE, Strauch BM. Detection of circulating T-activating enzyme in the serum of a patient having hemolytic-uremic syndrome and disseminated intravascular coagulation. Am J Clin Pathol. 1985;84(2):244–8.

698. Szilagyi A, Kiss N, Bereczki C, Talosi G, Racz K, Turi S, et al. The role of complement in Streptococcus pneumoniae-associated haemolytic uraemic syndrome. Nephrol Dial Transplant. 2013;28(9):2237–45.

699. Gilbert RD, Nagra A, Haq MR. Does dysregulated complement activation contribute to haemolytic uraemic syndrome secondary to Streptococcus pneumoniae? Med Hypotheses. 2013;81(3):400–3.

700. Cochran JB, Panzarino VM, Maes LY, Tecklenburg FW. Pneumococcus-induced T-antigen activation in hemolytic uremic syndrome and anemia. Pediatr Nephrol. 2004;19(3):317–21.

701. Oliver JW, Akins RS, Bibens MK, Dunn DM. Pneumococcal Induced T-activation with Resultant Thrombotic Microangiopathy. Clin Med Insights Pathol. 2010;3:13–7.

702. Herrero-Morin JD, Fernandez N, Santos F, Rey C, Malaga S. Hemolytic uremic syndrome by Streptococcus pneumoniae. Nefrologia. 2007;27(4): 505–8.

703. Petras ML, Dunbar NM, Filiano JJ, Braga MS, Chobanian MC, Szczepiorkowski ZM. Therapeutic plasma exchange in Streptococcus pneumoniae-associated hemolytic uremic syndrome: a case report. J Clin Apher. 2012;27(4):212–4.

704. Nathanson S, Deschenes G. Prognosis of Streptococcus pneumoniae-induced hemolytic uremic syndrome. Pediatr Nephrol. 2001;16(4):362–5.

705. Krysan DJ, Flynn JT. Renal transplantation after Streptococcus pneumoniae-associated hemolytic uremic syndrome. Am J Kidney Dis. 2001;37(2):E15.

706. Fabregas Martori A, Moraga-Llop F, Nieto Rey J, Figueras Nadal C, Soler Palacin P, Roqueta Mas J. Invasive pneumococcal disease and hemolytic uremic syndrome. An Pediatr (Barc). 2008;68(3): 269–72.

707. Petersen VP, Olsen TS. Late renal trnsplant failure due to the hemolytic-uremic syndrome. Acta Med Scand. 1971;189(5):377–80.

708. Asaka M, Ishikawa I, Nakazawa T, Tomosugi N, Yuri T, Suzuki K. Hemolytic uremic syndrome associated with influenza A virus infection in an adult renal allograft recipient: case report and review of the literature. Nephron. 2000;84(3):258–66.

709. Al-Akash SI, Almond PS, Savell Jr VH, Gharaybeh SI, Hogue C. Eculizumab induces long-term remission in recurrent post-transplant HUS associated with C3 gene mutation. Pediatr Nephrol. 2011;26(4):613–9.

710. Printza N, Roilides E, Kotsiou M, Zafeiriou D, Hatzidimitriou V, Papachristou F. Pandemic influenza A (H1N1) 2009-associated hemolytic uremic syndrome. Pediatr Nephrol. 2011;26(1):143–4.

711. Davison AM, Thomson D, Robson JS. Intravascular coagulation complicating influenza A virus infection. Br Med J. 1973;1(5854):654–5.

712. Golubovic E, Miljkovic P, Zivic S, Jovancic D, Kostic G. Hemolytic uremic syndrome associated with novel influenza A H1N1 infection. Pediatr Nephrol. 2011;26(1):149–50.

713. Rhee H, Song SH, Lee YJ, Choi HJ, Ahn JH, Seong EY, et al. Pandemic H1N1 influenza A viral infection complicated by atypical hemolytic uremic syndrome and diffuse alveolar hemorrhage. Clin Exp Nephrol. 2011;15(6):948–52.

714. Bento D, Mapril J, Rocha C, Marchbank KJ, Kavanagh D, Barge D, et al. Triggering of atypical hemolytic uremic syndrome by influenza A (H1N1). Ren Fail. 2010;32(6):753–6.

715. Caltik A, Akyuz SG, Erdogan O, Demircin G. Hemolytic uremic syndrome triggered with a new pandemic virus: influenza A (H1N1). Pediatr Nephrol. 2011;26(1):147–8.

716. Kosugi N, Tsurutani Y, Isonishi A, Hori Y, Matsumoto M, Fujimura Y. Influenza A infection triggers thrombotic thrombocytopenic purpura by producing the anti-ADAMTS13 IgG inhibitor. Intern Med. 2010;49(7):689–93.

717. Mammas IN, Koutsaftiki C, Papantzimas K, Symeonoglou Z, Koussouri M, Theodoridou M, et al. Thrombocytic thrombocytopenic purpura in a child with A/H1N1 influenza infection. J Clin Virol. 2011;51(2):146–7.

718. Koh YR, Hwang SH, Chang CL, Lee EY, Son HC, Kim HH. Thrombotic thrombocytopenic purpura triggered by influenza A virus subtype H1N1 infection. Transfus Apher Sci. 2012;46(1):25–8.

719. Kamali A, Holodniy M. Influenza treatment and pro-phylaxis with neuraminidase inhibitors: a review. Infect Drug Resist. 2013;6:187–98.

720. Shieh WJ, Blau DM, Denison AM, Deleon-Carnes M, Adem P, Bhatnagar J, et al. 2009 pandemic influenza A (H1N1): pathology and pathogenesis of 100 fatal cases in the United States. Am J Pathol. 2010;177(1):166–75.

721. Nicholls JM. The battle between influenza and the innate immune response in the human respiratory tract. Infect Chemother. 2013;45(1):11–21.

722. Chan MC, Chan RW, Yu WC, Ho CC, Chui WH, Lo CK, et al. Influenza H5N1 virus infection of polarized human alveolar epithelial cells and lung microvascular endothelial cells. Respir Res. 2009;10:102.

723. Armstrong SM, Wang C, Tigdi J, Si X, Dumpit C, Charles S, et al. Influenza infects lung microvascular endothelium leading to microvascular leak: role of apoptosis and claudin-5. PLoS One. 2012;7(10): e47323.

724. Armstrong SM, Darwish I, Lee WL. Endothelial activation and dysfunction in the pathogenesis of influenza A virus infection. Virulence. 2013;4(6): 537–42.

725. Terada H, Baldini M, Ebbe S, Madoff MA. Interaction of influenza virus with blood platelets. Blood. 1966;28(2):213–28.

726. Rondina MT, Brewster B, Grissom CK, Zimmerman GA, Kastendieck DH, Harris ES, et al. In vivo platelet activation in critically ill patients with primary 2009 influenza A(H1N1). Chest. 2012;141(6):1490–5.

727. Boilard E, Pare G, Rousseau M, Cloutier N, Dubuc I, Levesque T, et al. Influenza virus H1N1 activates platelets through FcgammaRIIA signaling and thrombin generation. Blood. 2014;123(18):2854–63.

728. Lei TH, Hsia SH, Wu CT, Lin JJ. Streptococcus pneumoniae-associated haemolytic uremic syndrome following influenza A virus infection. Eur J Pediatr. 2010;169(2):237–9.

729. Tsai HM. Thrombotic thrombocytopenic purpura and the atypical hemolytic uremic syndrome: an update. Hematol Oncol Clin North Am. 2013;27(3): 565–84.

730. Leaf AN, Laubenstein LJ, Raphael B, Hochster H, Baez L, Karpatkin S. Thrombotic thrombocytopenic purpura associated with human immunodeficiency virus type 1 (HIV-1) infection. Ann Intern Med. 1988;109(3):194–7.

731. Tamkus D, Jajeh A, Osafo D, Hadad L, Bhanot B, Yogore MG. Thrombotic microangiopathy syndrome as an AIDS-defining illness: the experience of J. Stroger Hospital of Cook County. Clin Adv Hematol Oncol. 2006; 145–149.

732. Moore RD. Schistocytosis and a thrombotic microangiopathy-like syndrome in hospitalized HIV-infected patients. Am J Hematol. 1999;60(2): 116–20.

733. Boccia RV, Gelmann EP, Baker CC, Marti G, Longo DL. A hemolytic-uremic syndrome with the acquired immunodeficiency syndrome. Ann Intern Med. 1984;101(5):716–7.

734. Ray PE. Shiga-like toxins and HIV-1 'go through' glycosphingolipids and lipid rafts in renal cells. Kidney Int. 2009;75(11):1135–7.

735. Green DF, Resnick L, Bourgoignie JJ. HIV infects glomerular endothelial and mesangial but not epithelial cells in vitro. Kidney Int. 1992;41(4):956–60.

736. Liu XH, Lingwood CA, Ray PE. Recruitment of renal tubular epithelial cells expressing verotoxin-1 (Stx1) receptors in HIV-1 transgenic mice with renal disease. Kidney Int. 1999;55(2):554–61.

737. Lund N, Branch DR, Mylvaganam M, Chark D, Ma XZ, Sakac D, et al. A novel soluble mimic of the glycolipid, globotriaosyl ceramide inhibits HIV infection. Aids. 2006;20(3):333–43.

738. Lingwood CA, Branch DR. The role of glycosphingolipids in HIV/AIDS. Discov Med. 2011; 11(59):303–13.

739. Lammle B, Kremer Hovinga JA, Alberio L. Thrombotic thrombocytopenic purpura. J Thromb Haemost: JTH. 2005;3(8):1663–75.

740. Gunther K, Garizio D, Nesara P. ADAMTS13 activity and the presence of acquired inhibitors in human immunodeficiency virus-related throm-botic thrombocytopenic purpura. Transfusion. 2007;47:1710–6.

741. Novitzky N, Thomson J, Abrahams L, du Toit C, McDonald A. Thrombotic thrombocytopenic purpura in patients with retroviral infection is highly responsive to plasma infusion. Br J Haematol. 2005;128:373–9.

Shori Takahashi, Michio Nagata, and Hiroshi Saito

Abbreviations

AAGN	ANCA-associated glomerulonephritis
AAV	ANCA-associated vasculitis
ANCA	Antineutrophil cytoplasmic antibody
CPA	Oral cyclophosphamide
EGP	Eosinophilic granuloma with polyangiitis (Churg-Strauss syndrome)
ENT	Ear nose, and throat
GBM	Glomerular basement membrane
GN	Glomerulonephritis
GPA	Granulomatous polyangiitis (WG)
HSPN	Henoch-Schönlein purpura nephritis
LAMP-2	Lysosome-associated membrane protein-2
MHC	Major histocompatibility complex
MMI	Methimazole
MPA	Microscopic polyangiitis
MPO	Myeloperoxidase
NCGN	Necrotizing crescentic glomerulonephritis
NETs	Neutrophil extracellular traps
PAN	Polyarteritis nodosa
PE	Plasma exchange
PR3	Proteinase-3
PTU	Propylthiouracil
RLV	Renal-limited vasculitis
RPGN	Rapidly progressive glomerulonephritis
SNP	Single nucleotide polymorphism
SOV	Single-organ vasculitis
VVV	Variable vessel vasculitis
WG	Wegener's granulomatosis (GPA)

S. Takahashi (✉)
Department of Pediatrics, Nihon University Itabashi Hospital, 30-1, Kamichou, Oyaguchi, Itabashi-ku, Tokyo 173-8610, Japan
e-mail: shori@med.nihon-u.ac.jp

M. Nagata
Department of Kidney and Vascular Pathology, University of Tsukuba,
Tennodai 1-1-1, Tsukuba-City,
Ibaraki 305-8575, Japan
e-mail: nagatam@md.tsukuba.ac.jp

H. Saito
Department of Pediatrics, Nihon University School of Medicine, 30-1, Kamichou, Oyaguchi, Itabashi-ku, Tokyo 173-8610, Japan
e-mail: saito.hiroshi54@nihon-u.ac.jp

Historical Changes in the Entity of Renal Vasculitis

Glomerulonephritis is a manifestation of vasculitis occurring in glomeruli.

© Springer-Verlag Berlin Heidelberg 2016
D.F. Geary, F. Schaefer (eds.), *Pediatric Kidney Disease*, DOI 10.1007/978-3-662-52972-0_27

The Era of Subacute Glomerulonephritis to Rapidly Progressive Glomerulonephritis

In 1914, Volhard and Fahr described a combination of severe renal disease and glomerular crescents; they gave this the clinical expression "subacute glomerulonephritis" [1]. Renal vasculitis seems to have been included in the category of subacute glomerulonephritis during the 1930s [2] to the 1960s because of its progressive nature toward renal failure. In 1942, Ellis referred to this aggressive category of glomerulonephritis with pathological epithelial crescent formation, as "rapidly progressive glomerulonephritis" [3].

In the 1960s, the term "rapidly progressive glomerulonephritis" was widely used for patients with acute glomerulonephritis, Henoch-Shönlein purpura nephritis, IgA nephritis, lupus nephritis, Goodpasture disease, and pulmonary renal syndrome if those nephritides exhibited a rapidly progressive disease course. In 1965, Duncan et al. [4] and Sturgill and Westervelt [5] described the pathogenesis of Goodpasture syndrome (glomerulonephritis and hemorrhagic pneumonitis) as an anti-glomerular and pulmonary basement membrane disease. Most of the kidney pathology from patients with this condition showed crescents, characteristic of "subacute" glomerulonephritis [5].

Diagnosis and Definition of Crescentic Glomerulonephritis in the 1960s and 1970s

The term "crescentic glomerulonephritis" appeared in the 1960s, prompted by the pathology of kidney biopsies taken from patients who had been clinically diagnosed as having RPGN. Therefore, "crescentic glomerulonephritis" was thought to be a synonym of RPGN and included all of the above glomerulonephritides, if over 50% of the glomeruli in a biopsied specimen showed crescent formation.

In 1968, Bacani et al. illustrated the characteristic lesion of non-streptococcal rapidly progressive glomerulonephritis as a marked extracapillary cell proliferation with pronounced crescent formation [6]. Thus, extensive extracapillary proliferation came to be regarded as synonymous with RPGN.

In 1971, Martinez et al. published a case series with the title "Variant Goodpasture's syndrome?" [7]. In this report, Martinez et al. discussed a patient who showed no anti-glomerular basement membrane (GBM) antibody deposition, despite immune complex pathogenesis suggested by the presence of mixed cryoglobulinemia. However, the patient showed intermittent purpura, Raynaud's phenomenon, and evidence of vasculitis involving the small renal arteries. The combination of hemorrhagic pneumonitis and mixed cryoglobulinemia with glomerulonephritis as well as vasculitis was first reported in this paper.

In 1976, Whitworth et al. reported their review of 60 cases of crescentic glomerulonephritis excluding polyarteritis nodosa (PAN), lupus, and Henoch-Shönlein purpura nephritis (HSPN), in which crescentic nephritis was defined as the presence of ≥50% crescent formation in the glomeruli. They showed that the outcome was significantly related to the percentage of crescentic involvement, and that the clinical course was not always the same as that of RPGN in crescentic glomerulonephritis [8].

In 1979, Stilmant et al. reported an RPGN case series, in which they observed that 16 out of 46 RPGN patients displayed no immune deposits in the glomeruli [9]. Those patients were similar to the reported cases of anti-GBM nephritis. In addition, Stilmant et al. showed that idiopathic acute crescentic glomerulonephritis without immune deposits was more common than immune complex or anti-GBM nephritis. A pediatric case series of 13 RPGN patients of variable etiology – post streptococcal acute glomerulonephritis (seven patients), membranoproliferative glomerulonephritis (two patients) and idiopathic glomerulonephritis (four patients) was subsequently published by Cunningham et al. in 1980 [10]. All of those patients showed crescent formation. Cunningham et al. concluded that "the severity of crescent formation, not the presumed etiology, appeared to be a reliable prognosticator," which was the same conclusion reached by Whitworth et al. in 1976 [8].

Discovery of Antineutrophil Cytoplasmic Antibody (ANCA) and the Development of ANCA-Related Vasculitis/Glomerulonephritis During the 1980s and 1990s

In 1982, Davies et al. first reported the diagnostic role of ANCA in eight patients who presented with generalized illness and segmental necrotizing glomerulonephritis of unknown etiology [11].

In 1987, Croker et al. used the term "primary crescentic and necrotizing glomerulonephritis" for a kidney-limited form of polyarteritis nodosa [12]. Almost at the same time, Chen et al. also suggested that there was a "renal-limited variant of polyarteritis nodosa; primary crescentic and necrotizing glomerulonephritis" [13]. However, those disease entities were later reclassified into microscopic polyangiitis (MPA) at the Chapel Hill Consensus Conference (CHCC) in 1994 [14]. Also in 1987, a case of microscopic polyarteritis associated with antineutrophil cytoplasmic antibodies (ANCA) was reported by Feehally et al. [15]. A pediatric case series of "three children with crescentic glomerulonephritis in whom ANCA concentrations were raised at presentation" was reported by Walters et al. in the next year [16].

In 1988, Falk and Jennette identified two types of anti-neutrophil autoantibodies (anti-myeloperoxidase antibodies that show perigranular immunostaining of alcohol-fixed neutrophils [P-ANCA], and another type [C-ANCA] with no reactivity with myeloperoxidase on enzyme-linked immunosorbent assay (ELISA)-produced diffuse cytoplasmic immunostaining) [17]. In 1989, Goldschmeding et al. reported the antigen of C-ANCA to be proteinase 3 (PR3) [18]. In this way, the difference in the indirect immunostaining pattern between C-ANCA and P-ANCA was clarified.

The term "pauci-immune necrotizing and crescentic glomerulonephritis" was used by the Jennette group in 1989 [19]. However, in the early 1990s, there was still no universally accepted nomenclature for systemic vasculitides, and this became a major communication problem [14].

Actually, in the early 1990s, pauci-immune glomerulonephritis, necrotizing glomerulonephritis, rapidly progressive glomerulonephritis, and crescentic glomerulonephritis were used concurrently. These diagnostic names sometimes indicated the same disease entity and at other times indicated different entities, varying among MPA, Wegener's granulomatosis (WG), renal limited vasculitis (RLV), HSPN, lupus nephritis, Goodpasture syndrome, and more.

Another reason for this confusion was that the vasculitis that affects the medium-sized vessels often affects the small-sized vessels; i.e., the arterioles, venules, and capillaries, whereas the medium-sized vessels of many patients with small-sized vessel vasculitis showing ANCA-associated glomerulonephritis are not affected [20]. A final reason for the confusing terminology was that there seemed to be three points of view: first from the field of nephrology, second from rheumatology, and third from pathology, all of which have different scientific backgrounds and points of view.

Ultimately, when laboratory examination of ANCA became popular and accurate, the use of such clinicopathologic names as ANCA-positive pauci-immune (crescentic) glomerulonephritis or ANCA-associated glomerulonephritis became popular in the literature.

Renal Vasculitis in the Twenty-First Century

In 2002, investigation of the differences between the diagnostic subgroups of ANCA-associated vasculitis was reported by the European Vasculitis Study Group (EUVAS) [21]. From an analysis of 173 patients (histopathological diagnosis of the patients is shown in Fig. 27.1) with renal disease in MPA or Wegener granulomatosis (WG), the EUVAS investigators showed that both active and chronic lesions are more abundantly present in MPO-ANCA-positive patients than in patients with PR3-ANCA positivity, and described the differences in the pathogenesis of these two ANCA subsets. The EUVAS investigators also suggested that ANCA test results could be useful in classifying ANCA-associated vasculitis.

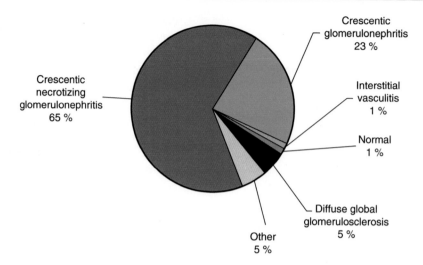

Fig. 27.1 Histopathological diagnosis of renal biopsy findings of ANCA-associated vasculitis from 173 patients (Used with permission of American Society of Nephrology from Hauer et al. [21])

Clinical and histological relationships among ANCA subsets were also reported by Vizjak et al. in 2003 [22]. These authors studied 135 ANCA-positive subjects who presented with renal histological changes; the results revealed the differences in renal histology between the ANCA subsets. The Vizjak study indicated that PR3-ANCA-positive patients tend to show focal crescentic glomerulonephritis and glomerular necrosis, whereas MPO-ANCA-positive patients tend to show diffuse crescentic glomerulonephritis, glomerular sclerosis, and tubulo-interstitial fibrosis. Vizjak et al. concluded that the differences in histopathology were related to the timing of biopsy, because PR3-ANCA-positive patients underwent their renal biopsies earlier and showed mainly focal active lesions, while the MPO-ANCA-positive patients had predominantly diffuse chronic sclerotic lesions.

The rarity of pauci-immune glomerulonephritis became an issue for discussion in 2004, because Haas et al. found that over half of patients with ANCA (PR3 or MPO) -positive crescentic/necrotizing glomerulonephritis showed immune complex deposition by electron microscopy and immunofluorescence [23]. This topic was discussed later at the 2012 CHCC. Although Conference participants could not precisely establish the break point, it was concluded that the presence of fewer versus more immune deposits distinguishes between ANCA-associated vasculitis (AAV, with fewer immune deposits in vessel walls) and immune complex small vessel vasculitis (SVV, with more immune deposits in vessel walls) [24].

In 2010, Berden et al. (an international working group of renal pathologists) described a histological classification of ANCA-associated glomerulonephritis (AAGN) in relation to patient prognosis [25]. This research group investigated 100 biopsies from patients with clinically and histologically confirmed AAGN. The resulting classification proposed four general categories of AAGN: focal, crescentic, mixed, and sclerotic (Table 27.1). The results of this investigation clearly showed that the classification was of predictive value for 1- and 5-year renal outcome. The renal survival data were obtained from 82 of 100 patients. A total of 25 patients with AAGN developed end-stage renal disease (ESRD) during 5 years of observation; one of 14 patients with focal AAGN, 11 of 45 with crescentic AAGN, 6 of 13 with mixed AAGN, and 7 of 10 with sclerotic AAGN (Fig. 27.2). Berden et al. also illustrated that patients with sclerotic ANCA-associated glomerulonephritis not only had a decreased chance of renal survival but also were at a higher risk of death.

Table 27.1 Classification schema for ANCA-associated glomerulonephritis

Class	Inclusion criteria[a]
Focal	≥50% normal glomeruli
Crescentic	≥50% glomeruli with crescents
Mixed	<50% normal, <50% crescentic, <50% globally sclerotic glomeruli
Sclerotic	≥50% globally sclerotic glomeruli

Used with permission of American Society of Nephrology from Berden et al. [25]

[a]Pauci-immune staining pattern on immunofluorescence micrography and ≥1 glomerulus with necrotizing or crescentic glomerulonephritis on light microscopy are required for inclusion in all four classes

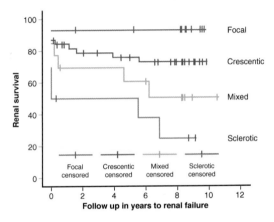

Fig. 27.2 Renal survival is depicted according to the four histological categories (Used with permission of American Society of Nephrology from Berden et al. [25])

The accumulation of knowledge concerning vasculitis led to the requirement for standardized nomenclature. Accordingly, the 2012 Revised International Chapel Hill Consensus Conference, Nomenclature of Vasculitides was produced by the CHCC, to improve the CHCC 1994 Nomenclature, change names and definitions as appropriate, and add important categories of vasculitis that were not included in CHCC 1994. The 2012 revised nomenclature provided a more precise categorization, definition and nomenclature of vasculitides [24].

According to the CHCC 2012, ANCA-associated vasculitis (AAV) is defined as necrotizing vasculitis, with few or no immune deposits, predominantly affecting small vessels (i.e., capillaries, venules, arterioles, and small arteries), associated with MPO-ANCA or PR3-ANCA. Because not all patients have ANCA, a prefix was added in the nomenclature to indicate ANCA reactivity, e.g., PR3 (proteinase 3)-ANCA, MPO (myeloperoxidase)-ANCA, and ANCA-negative.

At CHCC 2012, the size of vessels was defined as shown in Figs. 27.3, 27.4a, and 27.5 (CHCC 1994), which indicate the relationships between vascular size and the disease nomenclature.

In addition, the following four categories of vasculitides were defined in CHCC 2012 (Fig. 27.6):

1. Variable vessel vasculitis (VVV): vasculitis without any predominance of vessel size (large, medium, or small) and type (arteries, veins, or capillaries).
2. Single-organ vasculitis (SOV): vasculitis in arteries or veins of any size in a single organ, with no features that indicate it is a limited expression of a systemic vasculitis.
3. Vasculitis associated with systemic diseases: Vasculitis can be associated with and may be caused by a systemic disease.
4. Vasculitis associated with probable etiology: vasculitis can be associated with probable underlying condition.

Thus, the nomenclature system of vasculitides has been updated on the basis of the latest knowledge.

The first categorization level is based on the predominant vessels involved. In addition, CHCC 2012 determined that a key concept of the categorization was that vasculitis in all three major categories (based on vascular size) can affect any size of artery (i.e., large-vessel vasculitis affects large arteries more often than medium- or small-vessel vasculitis). However, there is some inconsistency with the above description in CHCC 2012, because the definition of polyarteritis nodosa (PAN) in CHCC 2012 excluded glomerulonephritis or vasculitis in arterioles, capillaries, or venules [24]. Eleftheriou et al. reported on systemic polyarteritis nodosa in the young, in which they showed that 8 of 69 patients with PAN had glomerular lesions such as focal segmental glomerulonephritis,

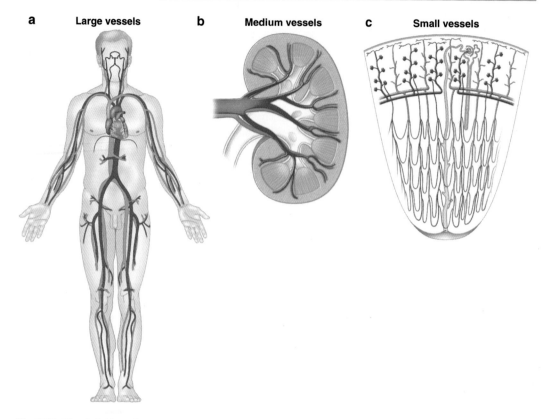

Fig. 27.3 The definition of vessel size (Used with permission of John Wiley and Sons from Jennette et al. [24])

crescent formation, and membranoproliferative glomerulonephritis, in the same journal and the same year [26]. Thus, the nomenclature of vasculitides still needs improvement.

Disease Spectrum and Classification of Vasculitides

As described above, vasculitis has been classified into three groups according to the size of the affected vasculature: large, medium, or small (Fig. 27.3):

(a) Large-vessel vasculitis comprises Takayasu arteritis and giant cell vasculitis.
(b) Medium-sized vasculitis includes polyarteritis nodosa, Kawasaki disease, and primary central nervous system arteritis.
(c) Small-vessel vasculitis comprises eosinophilic granulomatosis with polyangiitis (Churg-Strauss syndrome), granulomatosis with polyangiitis (Wegener's granulomatosis), microscopic polyangiitis (microscopic polyangiitis and renal-limited vasculitis; pauci-immune glomerulonephritis), Henoch-Shönlein purpura (IgA vasculitis), and cryogobulinemia.

Jennette and Falk clearly illustrated this classification with simple graphics (Fig. 27.4a) [24]. Figure 27.4b [14] shows their previous classification, illustrated in 1994.

On the other hand, there are many disease names that have been used in the past to describe progressive renal diseases, including ANCA-associated glomerulonephritis (ANCA-associated GN), subacute glomerulonephritis (subacute GN), rapidly progressive glomerulonephritis (RPGN), necrotizing and crescentic glomerulonephritis (necrotizing and crescentic GN), crescentic glomerulonephritis (crescentic GN), renal-limited vasculitis (RLV), and pauci-immune glomerulonephritis (pauci-immune GN); all but

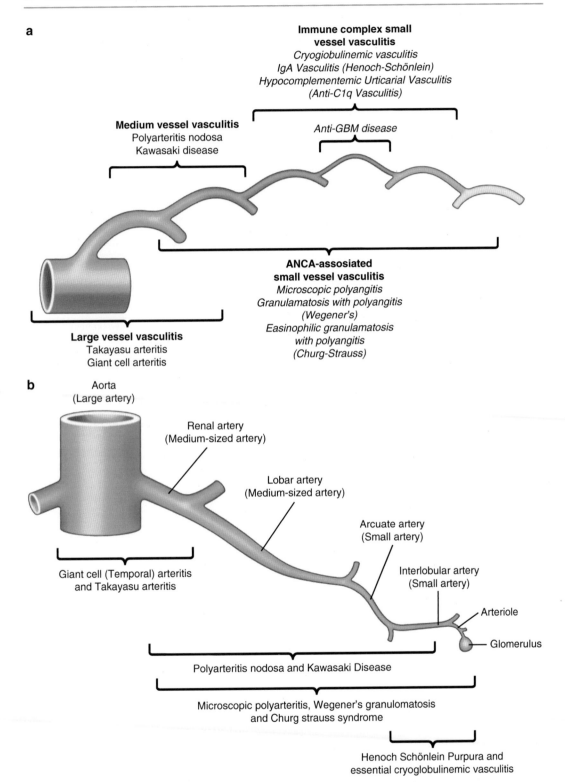

Fig. 27.4 (**a**, **b**) Vasculitis and vascular size (CHCC 2012) (Used with permission of John Wiley and Sons from Jennette et al. [24]); (**b**) Vascular size and vasculitides (CHCC 1994) (Used with permission of Elsevier from Jennette and Falk [14])

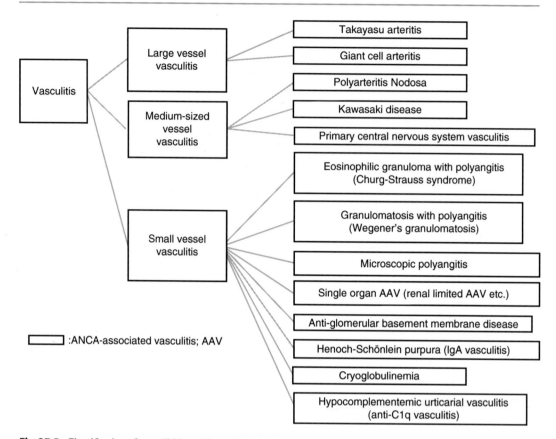

Fig. 27.5 Classification of vasculitides with vascular size (Used with permission of John Wiley and Sons from Jennette et al. [24])

subacute GN continue to be widely used in the field of nephrology (Fig. 27.7). These diagnostic names were derived from clinical practice (subacute GN, RPGN, and ANCA-associated GN), and from the field of pathology (crescentic GN, necrotizing and crescentic GN, RLV, and pauci-immune GN). From the rheumatology perspective, ANCA-associated GN (AAGN) is considered to be a renal manifestation of ANCA-associated vasculitis (AAV).

The Definition of Pauci-Immune

Falk and Jennette have defined "pauci-immune" as 2+ or less staining of any immunoglobulins (on a scale of 0–4+) and absence of immune complex type electron-dense deposits by electron microscopy [27]. However, Haas et al. studied the electron micrographs of 124 cases of ANCA-associated crescentic GN and revealed that 68

(54 %) of the biopsies showed glomerular immune complex deposition [23], although the immuno-fluorescence staining was relatively weak (≤2+).

Difference in Perspective of the Fields of Nephrology, Rheumatology and Pathology on Vasculitides

Patients with vasculitides had been treated by internists until the early twentieth century. However, with the sub-specialist development of nephrology and rheumatology, such patients have been treated by nephrologists and rheumatologists over the past half century. It is likely that the patients with predominantly renal symptoms, such as glomerulonephritis or impaired renal function, would have been referred to nephrologists, and patients with vasculitis symptoms and fewer renal

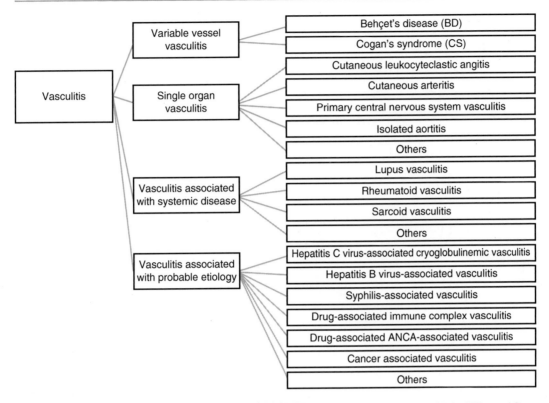

Fig. 27.6 Four categories (other than vascular size) and vasculitides (Used with permission of John Wiley and Sons from Jennette et al. [24])

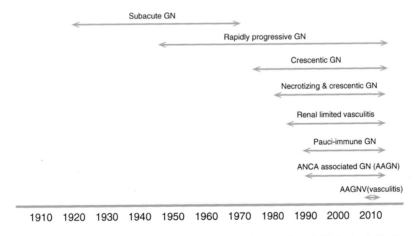

Fig. 27.7 The disease names that were used for ANCA-associated Glomerulonephritis in the field of nephrology. *GN* glomerulonephritis

symptoms would have been referred to rheumatologists. On the other hand, pathologists may have been able to integrate the pathology of these vasculitides objectively. Therefore, the perspectives on vasculitides are thought to be different among nephrologists, rheumatologists, and pathologists (Fig. 27.8). These different perspectives may have played an important role in the longstanding confusion of the nomenclature system for vasculitides.

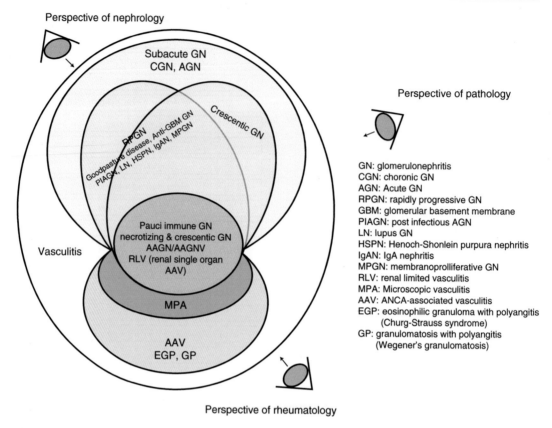

Fig. 27.8 Three different perspectives (nephrologists, rheumatologists and pathologists) for the same pathophysiology

As shown in Figs. 27.3 and 27.7 and mentioned above, there are now many diagnostic names, such as pauci-immune GN, necrotizing and crescentic GN, crescentic GN, AAGN, AAGNV (AAGN and vasculitis), RLV (renal single organ AAV), and RPGN for a common renal manifestation, regardless of the causes of the disease. However, based upon recent accumulating knowledge of clinical features, it seems better for nephrologists to use the unifying term of AAGN on behalf of these diagnostic names, at least with respect to glomerular lesions.

Classification of Childhood Vasculitis

CHCC 2012 currently provides a basic classification of vasculitis. However, there is another general classification of vasculitis specifically for

children [28], based on modification of the CHCC 1994 criteria. This classification is listed below:

I. Predominantly large-vessel vasculitis
   • Takayasu arteritis
II. Predominantly medium-vessel vasculitis
   • Childhood polyarteritis nodosa
   • Cutaneous polyarteritis
   • Kawasaki disease
III. Predominantly small-vessel arteritis
   (A) Granulomatous
      • Wegener's granulomatosis
      • Churg-Strauss syndrome
   (B) Non-granulomatous
      • Microscopic polyangiitis
      • Henoch-Schönlein purpura
      • Isolated cutaneous leukocytoclastic vasculitis
      • Hypocomplementemic urticarial vasculitis

IV. Other vasculitides
- Beçhet's disease
- Vasculitis secondary to infection (including hepatitis B-associated polyarteritis nodosa), malignancies, and drugs, including hypersensitivity vasculitis
- Vasculitis associated with connective tissue disease
- Isolated vasculitis of the central nervous system
- Cogan's syndrome
- Unclassified

The above classification was based on the CHCC 1994, which was fully revised and published as CHCC 2012. In our opinion pediatric nephrologists should use CHCC 2012 nomenclature in order to be consistent with adult vasculitis.

Pathogenesis of Vasculitis

Toxicity of ANCA

Since the discovery of ANCA, ANCA itself has been a target of research using both in vitro and animal models, because it was not known whether the presence of ANCA was an epiphenomenon or if it played a pathogenic role. In 1990, Falk et al. reported that cytoplasmic-pattern ANCA and myeloperoxidase-specific ANCA induce neutrophil activation [29]. The activation of neutrophils by ANCA results in the generation of reactive oxygen intermediators such as superoxide anions, lysosomal enzymes, and ANCA antigens themselves [30]. MPO-ANCA was also proven to stimulate neutrophils, leading to damage of human umbilical vein endothelial cells (HUVEC) [31]. Endothelial cells upregulate the expression of adhesion molecules (Mac-1) via stimulation of the IgG fraction of MPO-ANCA [32]. The sera of patients with ANCA-positive vasculitis has also been seen to induce upregulation of intercellular adhesion molecule-1 (ICAM-1) in HUVEC by stimulating neutrophils via Fcγ receptors [32].

ANCA also affects cytokine production of neutrophils, such as interleukin (IL)-1β, which stimulates local inflammatory processes [33].

A recent study revealed that the development of anti-MPO antibody-induced necrotizing crescentic glomerulonephritis (NCGN) requires neutrophil serine protease (NPS)-dependent IL-1β generation [34].

Thus, ANCA itself has been shown to play a significant role in the pathogenesis of idiopathic pauci-immune glomerulonephritis and vasculitis via neutrophil activation, and stimulating and damaging endothelial cells.

There is an important case report of neonatal ANCA-associated pulmonary-renal syndrome caused by maternal-neonatal transmission of MPO-ANCA IgG [35]. This case report is direct proof of the toxicity of MPO-ANCA to humans.

It is also suggested that ANCA-associated GN is an immune complex-mediated glomerulonephritis, despite half of patients lacking IgG immune deposition [23]. In an animal model of necrotizing crescentic glomerulonephritis using Brown-Norway rats immunized by human MPO, immune complex deposits were observed in the kidneys shortly after perfusion, but the deposits were dissolved at the peak of renal damage [36]. Thus, the immune-complex mediated mechanism possibly works on ANCA-associated GN.

The Role of LAMP-2

In 1995, Kain et al. found antibodies direct to lysosomal membrane protein-2 (LAMP-2) from necrotizing crescent GN patients' sera in a systematic search for autoantibodies to neutrophil or glomerular basement membrane proteins [37]. LAMP-2 is integrated into the membranes of myeloperoxidase- and proteinase-3-containing intracellular vesicles; therefore, autoantibodies to human LAMP-2 (hLAMP-2) give positive results in the immunofluorescence ANCA assay. The antibodies to LAMP-2 had been proven to cause pauci-immune focal and necrotizing glomerulonephritis when injected into rats. Additionally, monoclonal antibodies to human LAMP-2 induce apoptosis of human microvascular endothelium in vitro [38]. Recently, a high prevalence of hLAMP-2 autoantibodies in AAV patients was shown by Kain et al. [39].

NETs and ANCA-Associated Vasculitis (AAV)

In 2004, Brinkmann et al. discovered a unique type of neutrophil cell death in order to kill bacteria, and named it neutrophil extracellular traps (NETs) [40]. These investigators suggested that NETs appeared to be a form of innate response that binds microorganisms, prevents them from spreading, and ensures a high local concentration of antimicrobial agents to degrade virulence factors and kill bacteria.

The major structural component of NETs is DNA (DNA web). NETs contain proteins from azurophilic granules such as neutrophil elastase, cathepsin G, and myeloperoxidase, as well as proteins from specific granules and tertiary granules such as lactoferrin and gelatinase. This DNA web can stick to the endothelium and cause tissue damage. As NETs contain proteinase 3 and myeloperoxidase, the autoantigens of AAV, it seems likely that NETs are easily targeted by MPO- and PR3-ANCA, provoking local inflammation. This interaction was subsequently proven by Kessenbrock et al. in 2009 [41]. Kessenbrock et al. also demonstrated the deposition of NETs in inflamed kidneys and circulating MPO-DNA complexes in patients with small-vessel vasculitis (SVV; AAV). This evidence suggested that the formation of NETs triggers vasculitis and promotes the autoimmune response against neutrophil components in patients with SVV (AAV).

Genetics of ANCA-Associated Vasculitis (AAV)

The genetic contribution to the pathogenesis of ANCA vasculitis has been a target of research in recent years. A familial association with Wegener's granulomatosis (GPA) was shown by Knight et al. in 2008 [42]. These authors found a relative risk of 1.56 for first degree relatives of patients. The major histocompatibility complex (MHC) of AAV has also been studied extensively with respect to the genetic background of the disease [43]. Among many studies of MHC and AAV, a single nucleotide polymorphism (SNP) of the HLA-DPB1 locus has been found to have a significant association with GPA [44]. Alpha-1 antitrypsin is the major inhibitor of PR3. Once generated from neutrophils, PR3 directly damages the endothelial cells. Therefore, the association of the S and Z alleles of ATT (the gene encoding α1-antitrypsin) with GPA, those which are known to reduce the function of α1-antitrypsin, and AAV was also investigated. As a result, neither anti-PR3 antibodies nor the clinical features of WG were detected in 191 α1-antitrypsin Z homozygotes. Therefore, the association of the S and Z alleles of gene encoding α1-antitrypsin (SERPINA1) with GPA, those which are known to reduce the function of α1-antitrypsin, and AAV was also investigated. Neither anti-PR3 antibodies nor the clinical features of WG were detected in 191α1-antitrypsin Z homozygotes. This finding suggests that the deficiency contributes to, but is not the sole genetic determinant of, the risk for AAV [45].

In 2012, an English group generated conclusive data using genome-wide association analysis [46]. This study by Lyons et al. showed that PR3-ANCA was associated with HLA-DP and the genes encoding α-antitrypsin (SERPINA1) and proteinase 3 (PRTN3), and that MPO-ANCA was associated with HLA-DQ. From the above evidence, Lyons et al. proposed the concept that MPO-AAV and PR3-AAV are genetically distinct autoimmune syndromes. There are many clinically overlapping symptoms between MPO-AAV and PR3-AAV; however, Lyons et al. speculated that either type of ANCA drives a similar pathologic process that is largely independent of precise antigen specificity but is due to antigen similarity.

Propylthiouracil-Induced ANCA-Associated Glomerulonephritis

Propylthiouracil (PTU) is a commonly used drug for the treatment of hyperthyroidism. However, this drug has variable adverse effects. A case of propylthiouracil-related fatal periarteritis was first reported by McCormick R.V in 1950 [47]. The patient had nephrosclerosis with hyaline necrosis of the arterioles. After the discovery of

ANCA, vasculitis, and antineutrophil cytoplasmic autoantibodies associated with PTU, therapy for this condition was reported by Dolman et al. in 1993 [48]. A pediatric case report of PTU-related ANCA-positive crescentic glomerulonephritis (GN) was subsequently published by Vogt et al. in 1994 [49].

The clinical characteristics of PTU-related ANCA-positive GN in comparison with PTU-unrelated primary ANCA-positive GN are as follows:

1. Female predominance (However, this seems to be a result of the female predominance of Graves' disease).
2. Fewer patients with rapidly progressive GN (fewer glomeruli with crescents)
3. MPO-ANCA-positive (MPO-directed antibodies induced by PTU)
4. eGFR is usually higher (lower serum creatinine)
5. Renal pathology is less severe

A pediatric case series from Japan showed that the clinical disease spectrum of PTU-related ANCA-positive disease is similar in pediatric and adult patients, and that the overall prognosis may be better than that in primary ANCA-positive disease [50]. The clinical findings of this case series are shown in Table 27.2. All seven patients showed renal involvement. Three of them showed systemic symptoms such as flu-like fever and malaise within 2 months before the onset of overt vasculitis or GN. Three had pulmonary hemorrhage, two had a purpuric rash, and two had arthralgia and arthritis. One had ocular involvement (Table 27.3).

The reason why PTU-induced AAV is less severe than primary AAV has been investigated. A recent study by Wang et al. indicated that this variation could result from the difference of the target epitope of the MPO molecule between these two types of AAV [51].

The treatment of PTU-related AAV or AAGN is the discontinuation of PTU, oral prednisolone, pulse methylprednisolone, and cyclophosphamide. This strategy has resulted in favorable prognosis [52].

Other Environmental Factors of AAV (Silica, Cocaine, FimH)

Air pollutants, drugs, and infections are thought to be causative factors of AAV. Silica is a well-known air pollutant that causes MPA with MPO-ANCA positivity [53]. Cocaine is a known causative drug of AAV other than PTU. The influence of infection on AAV has also been investigated because nearly two thirds of patients presenting with WG are nasal carriers of Staphylococcus aureus, of which nasal colonization increases the risk for disease relapse [54]. On the other hand, Escherichia coli (E. coli) has been found to be a causal candidate bacteria of AAV, as found through a systematic search for autoantibodies to neutrophil or glomerular basement membrane proteins [37]. Antibodies to lysosome-associated membrane protein-2 (LAMP-2) were discovered from this research, and LAMP-2 (epitope P41–49) had been shown to possess 100 % homology to FimH (amino acid 72–80 of mature FimH) expressed on the fimbriae of Gram-negative bacteria such as E. coli, Klebsiella pneumonia and Proteus mirabilis. LAMP-2 is a heavily glycosylated type I membrane protein and is expressed on human neutrophils as well as on endothelial cells [38]. Kain et al. reported that there were 9 (69 %) out of 13 pauci-immune focal necrotizing glomerulonephritis (FNGN) patients of their cohort who had microbiologically confirmed diagnosis of FimH-expressing bacterial infection during the 12 weeks before presentation with pauci-immune FNGN [38].

Clinical Features and Diagnosis of ANCA-Associated GN (AAGN) in Pediatric Patients

AAGN is a generic name for glomerulonephritis associated with AAV such as MPA (including RLV), granulomatosis with polyangiitis (GPA), and eosinophilic granulomatosis with polyantiitis (EGP). EGP is very rare in childhood, and the ANCA titer is often negative [55]. Although EGP

Table 27.2 Clinical findings of seven ANCA-positive patients with NCGN or NCGN with extra renal organ system vasculitis associated with PTU treatment

Patient	Age/gender (year)	Clinical manifestation at onset[a]	Organ system involvement	Duration of PTU therapy (month)	Antithyroid drug	Therapy	Response to therapy
1	16/F	None	R	48	PTU reduced	PE+PSL	Remission (46 months)[b]
2	11/M	None	R	24	PTU discontinued	PE+mPSL+PSL	Remission on therapy
3	15/F	Erythema	R	42	PTU discontinued	mPSL+PSL	Remission (10 months)
4	14/F	Macrohematuria edema hypertension	R, S, P, C	3	PTU discontinued→MMI	mPSL+PSL	Remission (62 months)
5	16/F	Conjunctivitis arthralgia	R, S, P, M, O	21	PTU discontinued→MMI	mPSL+PSL	Remission (1 month)
6	13/F	Hemoptysis	R, S, P	43	PTU discontinued→MMI	mPSL+PSL+CPA	Remission (28 months)
7	13/F	Purpura arthralgia	R, C, M	60	PTU discontinued	PSL+CPA	Remission (33 months)

Used with permission of American Society of Nephrology Fujieda et al. [50]

ANCA antineutrophil cytoplasmic autoantibody, PTU propulthyouracil, R renal involvement, S systemic involvement, P pulmonary involvement, C cutaneous involvement, M musculoskeletal involvement, O ocular involvement, NCGN necrotizing crescentic glomerulonephritis, MMI methimazole, PE plasma exchange, PSL oral prednisolone, mPSL pulse methylprednisolone, CPA oral cyclophosphamide

[a]None, two patients were asymptomatically detected by a national urine screening program

[b]Duration of remission after stopping immunosuppressive treatment

Table 27.3 Organ involvement of patients with PTU-associated ANCA-positive and primary ANCA-associated vasculitis

Organ involvement	PTU-associated	Primary ANCA associated	P
Kidney	15/15 (100%)	59/59 (100%)	1
Systemic involvement	13/15 (87%)	52/59 (88%)	0.88
Skin	9/15 (60%)	25/59 (42%)	0.22
Eye	2/15 (13%)	19/59 (32%)	0.15
Ear	3/15 (20%)	14/59 (24%)	0.76
Nose	1/15 (7%)	15/59 (25%)	0.11
Lung	8/15 (53%)	39/59 (66%)	0.36
Digestive system	2/15 (13%)	22/59 (37%)	0.08
Nervous system	1/17 (7%)	8/59 (14%)	0.47

Used with permission of Elsevier from Yu et al. [52]

is very rare in childhood, the diagnosis of EGP may not be very difficult because of the characteristic eosinophilia and eosinophilic granuloma. Therefore, EGP will not be discussed in detail.

Vanoni et al. summarized the clinical features of pediatric AAV, as shown in Table 27.4 [56].

Clinical Features of GPA

The triad of clinical features of GPA is upper and lower respiratory tract inflammation, systemic or focal necrotizing vasculitis, and renal disease. GPA is diagnosed when three of the following six conditions are satisfied: (1) Abnormal urinalysis (hematuria and/or significant proteinuria); (2) Granulomatous inflammation on biopsy (necrotizing pauci-immune GN on renal biopsy); (3) Nasal sinus inflammation; (4) Subglottic, tracheal, or endobronchial stenosis; (5) Abnormal chest x-ray or computed tomography (CT) scan; and (6) PR3-ANCA or C-ANCA staining [28].

Clinical Features of Childhood MPA and NCGN (AAGN)

According to a nationwide retrospective study conducted by the Japanese Society of Pediatric Nephrology from 1990 to 1997 in Japan [57], 34 ANCA-positive pauci-immune necrotizing and crescentic glomerulonephritis patients were identified. Among the 34 patients, 21 had MPA, 9 had necrotizing and crescentic GN alone, and 3 had GPA (Wegener's granulomatosis). In this case series, the positivity of MPO-ANCA was 90% in patients excluding GPA. A diagnosis of AAGN was based on pathology of pauci-immune necrotizing and crescentic glomerulonephritis with or without ANCA positivity. AAGN can also be diagnosed as glomerulonephritis accompanied by AAV.

Most patients with MPA and NCGN (AAGN) experience prodromal symptoms (malaise, fever, anorexia, and weight loss) days to weeks before the onset of overt vasculitic or nephritic disease. Predominant symptoms are hemoptysis and pulmonary hemorrhage. Purpuric rash, arthralgia, arthritis, and abdominal pain with or without intestinal bleeding frequently occur in patients with MPA. The distribution of organ involvement in pediatric patients with NCGN (AAGN) and MPA is shown in Table 27.5 [57]. All ten patients with NCGN (AAGN) in the study by Hattori et al. have not yet shown any extra renal organ involvement.

There are many clinical features in common between MPA and GPA such as nephritis, respiratory symptoms, skin lesions, eye, nose, and throat symptoms, abdominal symptoms, and more. Therefore, it is difficult to distinguish between MPA and GPA by clinical features except in extreme cases. In cases of this difficulty, it seems better to use the diagnostic name of (MPO-/PR3-) AAGN or pauci-immune GN in patients with ANCA negativity.

Typical Pathology of AAGN and Small-Vessel Vasculitis

The renal vasculature has a characteristic structural arrangement that directly affects renal function. Vasculitis is a general term for

Table 27.4 Features in pediatric patients with GPA, MPA, and EGP

Feature	GPA	MPA	EGP
IgG/ANCA positivity	90%	70%	$\leq$0–50%
Antigen	Proteinase 3	Myeloperoxidase	?
Peripheral eosinophilia	Rather rare (and mild)	–	Very often (and severe)
Histology	Necrotizing vasculitis, granulomatous inflammation	Necrotizing vasculitis, no granulomatous inflammation	Necrotizing vasculitis, granulomatous inflammation, tissue eosinophilia
Fever, weight loss	Very often	Very often	Very often
Ear, nose, throat	Sinusitis, saddle nose, epistaxis, oral or nasal ulcer, otitis, conductive hearing loss, subglottic stenosis	Absent or mild	Nasal polyp, allergic rhinitis, conductive hearing loss
Lung	Nodules, infiltrates, cavitary lesions, rarely alveolar hemorrhage	Alveolar hemorrhage	Asthma, nonfixed infiltrates, rarely alveolar hemorrhage
Kidney	Segmental necrotizing glomerulonephritis (granulomatous inflammation rarely seen in biopsy specimen)	Segmental necrotizing glomerulonephritis	Segmental necrotizing glomerulonephritis
Eye	Conjunctivitis, (epi)scleritis, orbital inflammatory disease	Occasionally (epi)scleritis, uveitis	Occasionally (epi)scleritis, uveitis
Peripheral nerve	Occasionally vasculitic neuropathy	Often vasculitic neuropathy	Often vasculitic neuropathy
Heart	Occasionally valvular lesions	Rare	Often cardiomyopathy, pericardial effusion or valvular lesions

Used with permission of Springer Science + Business Media from Vanoni et al. [56]
GPA granulomatous polyangiitis (Wegener's syndrome), MPA microscopic polyangiitis, EGP eosinophilic granuloma with polyangiitis (Churg-Strauss syndrome)

Table 27.5 Distribution of organ system involvement in 31 pediatric patients with [a]NCGN and [b]MPA

Organ system involvement	NCGN (n=10)	MPA (n=21)
Systemic	3	18
Renal	10	20
Pulmonary	0	13
Cutaneous	0	8
Musculoskeletal	0	7
Gastrointestinal	0	7
Upper respiratory	0	2
Ocular	0	2
Neurologic	0	1

Used with permission of American Society of Nephrology from Hattori et al. [57]
[a]NCGN necrotizing and crescentic glomerulonephritis
[b]MPA microscopic polyangiitis

vessel wall inflammation. It can occur in any of the vascular segments, including the arterioles, veins, and capillaries, and is associated secondarily with a variety of systemic diseases.

There are various systemic diseases that potentially cause renal vasculitis in children; the major diseases are IgA vasculitis, AAV, vasculitis with autoimmune diseases, and infections.

The pathology of renal vasculitis is characterized by its grade of morphology (severity) in relation to the anatomical location. Although there may be several stimuli that trigger vasculitis, endothelial cells are the basic target in the cause of vasculitis. The early or incipient pathology appears as endotheliitis, which is frequently seen with any endothelial injury. The more severe

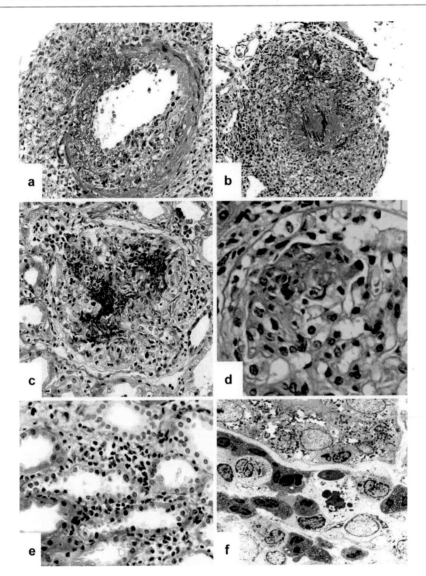

Fig. 27.9 Necrotizing angiitis and glomerulonephritis in patients with ANCA-associated vasculitis/glomerulonephritis. (**a**) Necrotizing vasculitis. Interlobular artery is affected by intimal inflammatory infiltrates particularly neutrophils. Note rupture of vascular wall with substantial fibrin deposition (Masson Trichrome Stain, ×400). (**b**) Severe vasculitis involves entire glomerulus with granulomatous changes (Periodic Acid Methenamine-Silver Stain, ×400). (**c**) Necrotizing capillaritis in the glomerulus. Note numerous neutrophils accumulation at the site of fibrinoid necrosis (Masson Trichrome Stain, ×400). (**d**) Segmental fibrinoid necrosis with nuclear fragmentation in the neutrophils (Periodic Acid Schiff Stain, ×550). (**e**) Peritubular capillaritis and interstitial inflammatory infiltrates (Masson Trichrome Stain, ×400). (**f**) Interstitial inflammatory infiltrates by electron microscopy. Note neutrophils predominant infiltration (×2,000)

phenotypes are fibrinoid necrosis and occasional rupture of the corresponding vasculature, resulting in interstitial hemorrhage (Fig. 27.9a). In some cases, vasculitis is recognized by severe inflammatory infiltrates in the vascular wall; other cases show fewer inflammatory infiltrates with necrosis, such as PAN (very rare) or Kawasaki disease. Giant cell arteritis is very rare in the kidney. IgG4-related kidney disease, as well as cryoglobulinemia, reveal a kind of vasculitis that fits the usual definition; this only rarely occurs in children.

Endoarteritis

Histology shows endothelial cell swelling/
proliferation and inflammatory cell infiltration
in the subendothelial space. Intimal edema
and occasional luminal stenosis are seen. In
this lesion, the profiles of the inflammatory
cells depend on the systemic condition and the
phase of inflammation. Neutrophils are typically seen in AAV, while mononuclear cells
are dominant in transplant rejection. The
lesion can be seen in any of the types of renal
vasculitis.

Microscopic Polyangiitis (AAV)

Various morphological features are seen in
AAV. The pathology is not determined by the
type of ANCA (PR3 or MPO). There are three
typical sites of vasculitis in this disease: arterioles, glomeruli, and peritubular capillaries. In
the arteriolar changes, a wide range of morphology can be seen. Very incipient changes show
endothelial cell swelling without apparent
inflammatory infiltrates. More severe changes
include intimal thickening due to accumulation
of inflammatory cells, deposition of active coagulation product (fibrinoid necrosis and thrombotic formations; Fig. 27.9b), and defect or
rupture of the vascular wall. The most severe
form of AAV affecting the glomeruli is angiitis
that targets the glomerular hilum, resulting in
the destruction of the entire glomerular structure, which is replaced by granulomatous
inflammation (Fig. 27.9b). In the glomeruli,
capillaritis causes NCGN, which frequently
develops into glomerulosclerosis (Fig. 27.9c, d).
Peritubular capillaritis (Fig. 27.9e) has been
recently recognized as an important lesion relating to renal function. The morphology is characterized by dilatation and adherence of
inflammatory cells on the endothelium; this is
limited to the cortex. Occasional rupture leads
to interstitial hemorrhage. Electron micrography shows neutrophil infiltration into the interstitium (Fig. 27.9f).

IgA Vasculitis

IgA vasculitis, formerly called Henoch-Shönlein
purpura, is an important disease in children since it
occurs frequently and in some cases causes kidney
failure. Although vasculitis is possibly seen in the
vasculature, most of the lesions are seen in the
glomeruli as capillaritis. Endocapillary proliferation
and occasional tuft necrosis with crescents are
changes that occur in the acute phase. Mesangial
proliferation is seen either in patients with mild disease, with mild changes, or in the subacute to
chronic phase. Although polymorphonuclear cells
are seen in endocapillary proliferation, macrophages seem to be predominant. Immunofluorescence
reveals IgA and C3 deposition in the glomerular
mesangium, but in active glomerular changes, such
deposition tends to shift to capillaries in a granular
pattern. Although many pediatric cases of acute IgA
vasculitis are self-limiting, renal biopsy should be
obtained in the acute phase, and pathology-based
therapy should be considered. Renal outcome can
be predicted by the appearance of crescents and
progressive interstitial changes.

Lupus Vasculitis

Lupus is a typical autoimmune disease attacking
the renal vasculature. Lupus vasculitis is triggered by immune-complex deposition and complement activation. Serum ANCA elevation is
occasionally associated with lupus, along with
renal vasculitis and NCGN. In such cases, glomerular immune deposition is basically absent if
ANCA is contributing to GN. Vascular changes
often occur in patients with lupus, including in
patients with thrombotic microangiopathy as
well as lupus vasculopathy. These conditions
should be categorized as types of vasculitis, even
though the endothelial alterations are similar.

Infectious Vasculitis

Infectious vasculitis is caused by the direct
involvement of microbes in the kidney, but not

immune complex deposition triggered by infection. Although systemic infection is very rare, it may cause renal vascular endothelial cell injury that initiates vasculitis. Another possible cause of renal vasculitis may be urinary tract infection, including fungal pyelonephritis seen in neonates, which is often accompanied by renal parenchymal damage.

Treatment and Outcome

As described above, the ANCA-associated vasculitides (AAV) include Churg-Strauss syndrome, Wegener's syndrome, microscopic vasculitis, and renal-limited microscopic vasculitis, also known as pauci-immune or idiopathic crescentic glomerulonephritis (GN). Pauci-immune GN is a rare and fulminant relapsing disease in children [58, 59], and is frequently associated with rapidly progressive glomerulonephritis (RPGN), characterized by clinical features of glomerulonephritis and rapid decline of renal function, with pathology exhibiting crescent formation affecting the majority of glomeruli. Pauci-immune GN accounts for 42% of patients in the category of RPGN who are less than 20 years of age. The outcome of pediatric patients with pauci-immune GN and positive ANCA has been reported by Hattori et al. [57], who suggested that these patients have a poor renal prognosis despite treatment. In the Hattori report, 6 of 31 patients (19.4%) had reduced renal function, 9 (29%) progressed to end-stage renal disease (ESRD), and 15 (48.4%) had normal renal function at the last observation. The evidence-based data are limited, and specific treatment for pauci-immune GN in children is mainly based on the data in adults. The treatment of pauci-immune GN broadly comprises two phases: induction of remission and maintenance of remission. Early progressive treatment for induction of remission is recommended to control the inflammation of vasculitides. The current initial therapeutic regimen for pediatric pauci-immune GN consists of cyclophosphamide, corticosteroids, and plasmapheresis.

Cyclophosphamide and corticosteroids are well-established as induction agents (level of evidence 1A) [60]. The Kidney Disease: Improving Global Outcomes (KDIGO) guidelines recommend that rituximab and corticosteroids be used as initial treatment in patients without severe disease or in whom cyclophosphamide is contraindicated (1B). The guidelines also recommend the addition of plasmapheresis for patients requiring dialysis or with rapidly increasing serum creatinine (1C), patients with diffuse pulmonary hemorrhage (2C), and patients with overlap syndrome of ANCA vasculitis and anti-GBM GN, according to proposed criteria and regimen for anti-GBM GN (2D) [60].

Induction Treatment (Table 27.6)

Cyclophosphamide and Corticosteroids (Pulse Methylprednisolone)

Cyclophosphamide and corticosteroids are well-established as induction treatments. Combination therapy with cyclophosphamide and prednisolone for 3–6 months was found to lead to clinical remission in 93% of adult patients with AAV [61]. It has also been reported that this combination therapy improved the remission rate from 56 to 84.7%, and decreased the relapse rate by approximately half [62]. Although the efficacy of pulse methylprednisolone for induction therapy has not been evaluated sufficiently, in view of the fulminant nature of pauci-immune GN, induction therapy for pediatric pauci-immune GN should be started with high-dose corticosteroids and cyclophosphamide. It has been reported that combination therapy with cyclophosphamide and pulse methylprednisolone resulted in a significant remission rate and low mortality in pediatric ANCA-associated GN [57, 63, 64]. The only randomized study of pulse methylprednisolone was reported in the MEPEX trial [65]. This study investigated whether the addition of plasma exchange to oral corticosteroids and cyclophosphamide was more effective than pulse methylprednisolone (1 g×3) for renal recovery in patients who presented with renal failure. In this study, there was no difference in mortality and

Table 27.6 Induction treatment

Agent	Route	Administration dosage and duration
Induction treatment		
Pulse	i.v.	400–600 mg/m^2/day (max 1,000 mg/day) for 3–5 consecutive days
Methylprednisolone[a]		
Prednisone[a]	Oral	1.5–2.0 mg/kg/day (max 60 mg/day) for 4 weeks
Prednisolone[a]		Gradually taper down over 6–12 months
Cyclophosphamide[b]	i.v.	Start at 500 mg/m^2/day
		Increase monthly by 125 mg/m^2/day to 750–1,000 mg/m^2/day (max 1,000 mg/day) for 6–10 times
Cyclophosphamide	Oral	2 mg/kg/day for 2–3 months
Rituximab[c]	i.v.	375 mg/mg/m^2/day weekly for four times
Plasmapheresis		Double volume on alternate day for 2 weeks
Maintenance treatment		
Azathioprine	Oral	2.0 mg/kg/day for 9 months
		Switch from cyclophosphamide at 3 months

i.v. intravenous
[a]Methylprednisolone pulses followed by oral prednisone or prednisolone 1.5–2.0 mg/kg/day for 4 weeks, with gradually tapering until discontinuation over 6–12 months
[b]Cyclophosphamide followed by azathioprine switching from cyclophosphamide at 3–6 months
[c]Given with pulse and oral corticosteroids

safety, but plasma exchange was more effective than pulse methylprednisolone in preserving kidney function.

Induction therapy regimens include methylprednisolone pulses and cyclophosphamide. Methylprednisolone pulses consist of intravenous methylprednisolone 400–600 mg/m^2/day (maximum dose 1,000 mg/day) for 3–5 consecutive days, followed by oral prednisone or prednisolone 1.5–2.0 mg/ideal body weight daily (maximum dose 60 mg/day) for 4 weeks, with gradually tapering until discontinuation over 6–12 months. Cyclophosphamide is administered in oral or intravenous pulse regimens. A regimen of daily oral cyclophosphamide should start at a dose of 2 mg/kg/day and continue for 2–3 months while adjusting the dose to keep the nadir leukocyte count above 3,000/mm^3. When a regimen of intravenous pulsed cyclophosphamide is used, the initial dose should be approximately 500 mg/m^2 and increased monthly by 125 to 750–1,000 mg/m^2 (maximum dose 1,000 mg/day) every 4 weeks for six to ten times. The subsequent

doses should be adjusted depending on the 2-week post-treatment nadir leukocyte count. A randomized controlled trial of intravenous pulse cyclophosphamide versus daily oral cyclophosphamide regimens for induction of remission against AAV with renal involvement has been conducted [66]. This trial demonstrated that pulse and daily oral regimens for cyclophosphamide had similar remission rates and times to remission. Patients receiving the pulse regimen were administered approximately one-half the cumulative dose of cyclophosphamide of the oral regimen and experienced a significantly lower rate of leukopenia for the same duration of therapy [66]. In a meta-analysis of randomized controlled trials (RCTs), the pulse regimen was associated with fewer infections, increased risk of relapse, less leukopenia, and a trend toward a higher rate of requiring renal replacement therapy [67]. Because of a lower cumulative dose and a lower risk of side effects, the pulse regimen is recommended as the first line of induction therapy for pediatric pauci-immune GN.

Rituximab

Rituximab is a chimeric monoclonal antibody that targets the CD20 antigen on the surface of B cells. Several case series and small studies have reported the efficacy of rituximab in refractory AAV. Recently, two randomized trials examined rituximab as induction therapy for AAV. In the RITUXVAS trial, 44 patients with newly diagnosed AAV were randomized to either rituximab or cyclophosphamide groups. The rituximab group regimen consisted of rituximab at a dose of 375 mg/m^2 infusion once weekly for a total of four times, in addition to intravenous cyclophosphamide at a dose of 15 mg/kg, 2 weeks apart for a total of two doses. The cyclophosphamide group regimen consisted of intravenous cyclophosphamide at a dose of 15 mg/kg every 2 weeks for a total of three times, then every 3 weeks for a maximum total of ten doses. Both groups received the same regimen of intravenous methylprednisolone 1,000 mg, followed by oral corticosteroids. There were no significant differences in the rates of remission and serious adverse events [68]. In the RAVE trial, 197 ANCA-positive patients with either Wegener's granulomatosis or microscopic polyangiitis were randomized to treatment with either rituximab or conventional cyclophosphamide–azathioprine groups. The rituximab group regimen consisted of rituximab at a dose of 375 mg/m^2, with infusions once weekly for a total of four times. The cyclophosphamide group regimen included oral cyclophosphamide at a dose of 2 mg/kg/day for 3 months, followed by oral azathioprine at a dose of 2 mg/kg/day for 3 months. The two treatment groups received the same glucocorticoid regimens: one to three pulses of methylprednisolone (1,000 mg each), followed by prednisone at a dose of 1 mg/kg/day, tapered by 5 months. A total of 64 % of the patients in the rituximab group, compared with 53 % of the patients in the cyclophosphamide–azathioprine group, experienced complete remission by 6 months without prednisone. There were no significant differences between the two treatment groups in the rates of complete remission, adverse events, or relapse rates at 6 months [69]. At 12 and 18 months, 48 % and 39 %, respectively, of the patients in the rituximab group had maintained complete remission, compared with 39 % and 33 %, respectively, in the cyclophosphamide–azathioprine group. There were no significant differences between the two groups in the duration of complete remission, the frequency or severity of relapses, and adverse events. Rituximab shows equivalent efficacy to cyclophosphamide for the induction and maintenance of remission over 18 months [70].

Plasmapheresis

The KDIGO guidelines recommend the addition of plasmapheresis for patients requiring dialysis or with rapidly increasing serum creatinine (SCr >5.66 mg/dl [>500 µmol/l]), patients with diffuse pulmonary hemorrhage, and patients with overlap syndrome of ANCA vasculitis and anti-GBM GN, according to the proposed criteria and regimen for anti-GBM GN [58].

In an RTC comparing a group of patients who received immunosuppressive treatment (corticosteroids, cyclophosphamide, and azathioprine) to a group of patients with histologically confirmed rapidly progressive crescentic glomerulonephritis who received immunosuppressive treatment plus plasma exchange, no statistically significant differences were found between the two groups [71]. In another RTC comparing intravenous methylprednisolone, prednisone, and azathioprine with and without plasma exchange, plasma exchange produced no additional therapeutic benefit to patients with idiopathic RPGN who were not dialysis-dependent at presentation [72]. These studies of plasmapheresis as adjunctive therapy in patients with mild to moderate renal dysfunction have not shown more benefit with plasmapheresis as adjunctive therapy than immunosuppressive treatment alone, but the studies were underpowered to provide definitive evidence. However, a meta-analysis of trials of plasma exchange for renal vasculitis and idiopathic rapidly progressive glomerulonephritis suggested a beneficial effect on the risk for ESRD, but no effect on mortality [73]. In the EUVAS MEPEX trial, which compared plasma exchange to pulse methylprednisolone in addition to oral prednisolone and oral cyclophosphamide, in patients with a new diagnosis of ANCA vasculitis and serum creatinine >500 μmol/L (5.8 mg/dl), plasmapheresis was associated with a significantly higher rate of kidney recovery at 3 months (69 % of patients with plasmapheresis vs. 49 % with pulse methylprednisolone), and was also associated with dialysis-free survival at 12 months. Plasma exchange was associated with a reduction in risk for progression to ESRD of 24 % (from 43 to 19 %) at 12 months. On the other hand, patient survival and the rate of severe adverse events were similar in both groups [65].

Maintenance Treatment

Cyclophosphamide

Maintenance therapy to prevent relapse is required after induction of remission, but exposure to an excessive amount of cyclophosphamide causes hemorrhagic cystitis and infertility, and increases the risk for bladder cancer and lymphoproliferative disorders. Combination therapy with oral cyclophosphamide (2 mg/kg/day) and prednisolone (initially 1 mg/kg/day, with the dose tapered to 0.25 mg/kg/day by 12 weeks) was found to lead to clinical remission in 77 % of study patients by 3 months, and 93 % by 6 months [61]. Thus, the duration of continuous oral cyclophosphamide should usually be limited to 3 months, with a maximum of 6 months, but whether the same duration can be applied to intravenous pulsed cyclophosphamide is unclear [60].

Azathioprine

While azathioprine does not appear to be effective for induction therapy, it is less toxic than cyclophosphamide and has been used for the maintenance of remission in patients with AAV [74]. Based on a RCT of maintenance treatment, which compared switching from cyclophosphamide to azathioprine at 3–6 versus 12 months, the withdrawal of cyclophosphamide and the substitution of azathioprine after remission did not increase the rate of relapse. Both study groups received the same induction therapy consisting of oral cyclophosphamide and prednisolone. Those patients in whom remission had been achieved by

3 months, or between 3 and 6 months, were randomly assigned to treatment with azathioprine as a substitute for cyclophosphamide (azathioprine group) or to continued cyclophosphamide therapy (cyclophosphamide group). After randomization, patients received either continued cyclophosphamide (1.5 mg/kg/day) or azathioprine (2 mg/kg/day), with the same dose of prednisolone (10 mg/day). Both groups received azathioprine (1.5 mg/kg/day) and prednisolone (7.5 mg/kg/day) after 12 months. The azathioprine group had similar remission rates, renal function, and patient survival compared with the cyclophosphamide group at 18 months [61].

Mycophenolate Mofetil

Mycophenolate mofetil (MMF) has been found to be less effective than azathioprine for maintaining disease remission. In the IMPROVE trial comparing MMF and azathioprine for maintenance treatment of 156 patients with AAV who attained remission with cyclophosphamide and prednisolone, the patients were randomized to either MMF at a dose of 2,000 mg/day or azathioprine at a dose of 2 mg/kg/day after induction of remission. Relapse was more common in the MMF group than in the azathioprine group, with an unadjusted hazard rate for MMF of 1.69. Both groups had similar adverse event rates [75]. Therefore, azathioprine is preferred over MMF for maintenance therapy in AAV.

References

1. Jennette JC. Rapidly progressive crescentic glomerulonephritis. Kidney Int. 2003;63(3):1164–77.
2. Bell ET. A clinical and pathological study of subacute and chronic glomerulonephritis, including lipoid nephrosis. Am J Pathol. 1938;14(6):691–736.5.
3. Ellis A. Natural history of Bright's disease. Clinical, histological and experimental observations. Lancet. 1942;239(6176):34–6.
4. Duncan DA, Drummond KN, Michael AF, Vernier RL. Pulmonary hemorrhage and glomerulonephritis. Report of six cases and study of the renal lesion by the fluorescent antibody technique and electron microscopy. Ann Intern Med. 1965;62:920–38.
5. Sturgill BC, Westervelt FB. Immunofluorescence studies in a case of Goodpasture's syndrome. JAMA. 1965;194(8):914–6.

6. Bacani RA, Velasquez F, Kanter A, Pirani CL, Pollak VE. Rapidly progressive (nonstreptococcal) glomerulonephritis. Ann Intern Med. 1968;69(3):463–85.
7. Martinez JS, Kohler PF. Variant "Goodpasture's syndrome"? The need for immunologic criteria in rapidly progressive glomerulonephritis and hemorrhagic pneumonitis. Ann Intern Med. 1971;75(1):67–76.
8. Whitworth JA, Morel-Maroger L, Mignon F, Richet G. The significance of extracapillary proliferation. Clinicopathological review of 60 patients. Nephron. 1976;16(1):1–19.
9. Stilmant MM, Bolton WK, Sturgill BC, Schmitt GW, Couser WG. Crescentic glomerulonephritis without immune deposits: clinicopathologic features. Kidney Int. 1979;15(2):184–95.
10. Cunningham 3rd RJ, Gilfoil M, Cavallo T, Brouhard BH, Travis LB, Berger M, et al. Rapidly progressive glomerulonephritis in children: a report of thirteen cases and a review of the literature. Pediatr Res. 1980;14(2):128–32.
11. Davies DJ, Moran JE, Niall JF, Ryan GB. Segmental necrotising glomerulonephritis with antineutrophil antibody: possible arbovirus aetiology? Br Med J (Clin Res Ed). 1982;285(6342):606.
12. Croker BP, Lee T, Gunnells JC. Clinical and pathologic features of polyarteritis nodosa and its renal-limited variant: primary crescentic and necrotizing glomerulonephritis. Hum Pathol. 1987;18(1):38–44.
13. Chen KT. Renal-limited polyarteritis nodosa. Hum Pathol. 1987;18(10):1074–5.
14. Jennette JC, Falk RJ. The pathology of vasculitis involving the kidney. Am J Kidney Dis. 1994;24(1):130–41.
15. Feehally J, Wheeler DC, Wallis J, Jones S, Lockwood CM, Savage CO. A case of microscopic polyarteritis associated with antineutrophil cytoplasmic antibodies. Clin Nephrol. 1987;27(4):214–5.
16. Walters MD, Savage CO, Dillon MJ, Lockwood CM, Barratt TM. Antineutrophil cytoplasm antibody in crescentic glomerulonephritis. Arch Dis Child. 1988;63(7):814–7.
17. Falk RJ, Jennette JC. Anti-neutrophil cytoplasmic autoantibodies with specificity for myeloperoxidase in patients with systemic vasculitis and idiopathic necrotizing and crescentic glomerulonephritis. N Engl J Med. 1988;318(25):1651–7.
18. Goldschmeding R, van der Schoot CE, ten Bokkel Huinink D, Hack CE, van den Ende ME, Kallenberg CG, et al. Wegener's granulomatosis autoantibodies identify a novel diisopropylfluorophosphate-binding protein in the lysosomes of normal human neutrophils. J Clin Invest. 1989;84(5):1577–87.
19. Charles LA, Falk RJ, Jennette JC. Reactivity of anti-neutrophil cytoplasmic autoantibodies with HL-60 cells. Clin Immunol Immunopathol. 1989;53(2 Pt 1):243–53.
20. Hogan SL, Nachman PH, Wilkman AS, Jennette JC, Falk RJ. Prognostic markers in patients with antineutrophil cytoplasmic autoantibody-associated microscopic polyangiitis and glomerulonephritis. J Am Soc Nephrol. 1996;7(1):23–32.
21. Hauer HA, Bajema IM, van Houwelingen HC, Ferrario F, Noël LH, Waldherr R, et al. Renal histology in ANCA-associated vasculitis: differences between diagnostic and serologic subgroups. Kidney Int. 2002;61(1):80–9.
22. Vizjak A, Rott T, Koselj-Kajtna M, Rozman B, Kaplan-Pavlovcic S, Ferluga D. Histologic and immunohistologic study and clinical presentation of ANCA-associated glomerulonephritis with correlation to ANCA antigen specificity. Am J Kidney Dis. 2003;41(3):539–49.
23. Haas M, Eustace JA. Immune complex deposits in ANCA-associated crescentic glomerulonephritis: a study of 126 cases. Kidney Int. 2004;65(6):2145–52.
24. Jennette JC, Falk RJ, Bacon PA, Basu N, Cid MC, Ferrario F, et al. 2012 Revised International Chapel Hill Consensus Conference Nomenclature of Vasculitides. Arthritis Rheum. 2013;65(1):1–11.
25. Berden AE, Ferrario F, Hagen EC, Jayne DR, Jennette JC, Joh K, et al. Histopathologic classification of ANCA-associated glomerulonephritis. J Am Soc Nephrol. 2010;21(10):1628–36.
26. Eleftheriou D, Dillon MJ, Tullus K, Marks SD, Pilkington CA, Roebuck DJ, et al. Systemic polyarteritis nodosa in the young: a single-center experience over thirty-two years. Arthritis Rheum. 2013;65(9):2476–85.
27. Falk RJ, Jennette JC. ANCA small-vessel vasculitis. J Am Soc Nephrol. 1997;8(2):314–22.
28. Ozen S, Ruperto N, Dillon MJ, Bagga A, Barron K, Davin JC, et al. EULAR/PReS endorsed consensus criteria for the classification of childhood vasculitides. Ann Rheum Dis. 2006;65(7):936–41.
29. Falk RJ, Terrell RS, Charles LA, Jennette JC. Antineutrophil cytoplasmic autoantibodies induce neutrophils to degranulate and produce oxygen radicals in vitro. Proc Natl Acad Sci U S A. 1990;87(11):4115–9.
30. Charles LA, Caldas ML, Falk RJ, Terrell RS, Jennette JC. Antibodies against granule proteins activate neutrophils in vitro. J Leukoc Biol. 1991;50(6):539–46.
31. Ewert BH, Jennette JC, Falk RJ. Anti-myeloperoxidase antibodies stimulate neutrophils to damage human endothelial cells. Kidney Int. 1992;41(2):375–83.
32. Johnson PA, Alexander HD, McMillan SA, Maxwell AP. Up-regulation of the endothelial cell adhesion molecule intercellular adhesion molecule-1 (ICAM-1) by autoantibodies in autoimmune vasculitis. Clin Exp Immunol. 1997;108(2):234–42.
33. Rarok AA, Limburg PC, Kallenberg CG. Neutrophil-activating potential of antineutrophil cytoplasm autoantibodies. J Leukoc Biol. 2003;74(1):3–15.
34. Schreiber A, Pham CT, Hu Y, Schneider W, Luft FC, Kettritz R. Neutrophil serine proteases promote IL-1β generation and injury in necrotizing crescentic glomerulonephritis. J Am Soc Nephrol. 2012;23(3):470–82.
35. Schlieben DJ, Korbet SM, Kimura RE, Schwartz MM, Lewis EJ. Pulmonary-renal syndrome in a newborn with placental transmission of ANCAs. Am J Kidney Dis. 2005;45(4):758–61.

36. van Paassen P, Tervaert JW, Heeringa P. Mechanisms of vasculitis: how pauci-immune is ANCA-associated renal vasculitis? Nephron Exp Nephrol. 2007;105(1):e10–6.

37. Kain R, Matsui K, Exner M, Binder S, Schaffner G, Sommer EM, et al. A novel class of autoantigens of anti-neutrophil cytoplasmic antibodies in necrotizing and crescentic glomerulonephritis: the lysosomal membrane glycoprotein h-lamp-2 in neutrophil granulocytes and a related membrane protein in glomerular endothelial cells. J Exp Med. 1995;181(2):585–97.

38. Kain R, Exner M, Brandes R, Ziebermayr R, Cunningham D, Alderson CA, et al. Molecular mimicry in pauci-immune focal necrotizing glomerulonephritis. Nat Med. 2008;14(10):1088–96.

39. Kain R, Tadema H, McKinney EF, Benharkou A, Brandes R, Peschel A, et al. High prevalence of autoantibodies to hLAMP-2 in anti-neutrophil cytoplasmic antibody-associated vasculitis. J Am Soc Nephrol. 2012;23(3):556–66.

40. Brinkmann V, Reichard U, Goosmann C, Fauler B, Uhlemann Y, Weiss DS, et al. Neutrophil extracellular traps kill bacteria. Science. 2004;303(5663):1532–5.

41. Kessenbrock K, Krumbholz M, Schönermarck U, Back W, Gross WL, Werb Z, et al. Netting neutrophils in autoimmune small-vessel vasculitis. Nat Med. 2009;15(6):623–5.

42. Knight A, Sandin S, Askling J. Risks and relative risks of Wegener's granulomatosis among close relatives of patients with the disease. Arthritis Rheum. 2008;58(1):302–7.

43. Willcocks LC, Lyons PA, Rees AJ, Smith KG. The contribution of genetic variation and infection to the pathogenesis of ANCA-associated systemic vasculitis. Arthritis Res Ther. 2010;12(1):202.

44. Heckmann M, Holle JU, Arning L, Knaup S, Hellmich B, Nothnagel M, et al. The Wegener's granulomatosis quantitative trait locus on chromosome 6p21.3 as characterised by tagSNP genotyping. Ann Rheum Dis. 2008;67(7):972–9.

45. Audrain MA, Sesboüé R, Baranger TA, Elliott J, Testa A, Martin JP, et al. Analysis of anti-neutrophil cytoplasmic antibodies (ANCA): frequency and specificity in a sample of 191 homozygous (PiZZ) alpha1-antitrypsin-deficient subjects. Nephrol Dial Transplant. 2001;16(1):39–44.

46. Lyons PA, Rayner TF, Trivedi S, Holle JU, Watts RA, Jayne DR, et al. Genetically distinct subsets within ANCA-associated vasculitis. N Engl J Med. 2012;367(3):214–23.

47. McCormic RV. Periarteritis occurring during propylthyourasil treatment. JAMA. 1950;144(17):1453–4.

48. Dolman KM, Gans RO, Vervaat TJ, Zevenbergen G, Maingay D, Nikkels RE, et al. Vasculitis and antineutrophil cytoplasmic autoantibodies associated with propylthiouracil therapy. Lancet. 1993;342(8872):651–2.

49. Vogt BA, Kim Y, Jennette JC, Falk RJ, Burke BA, Sinaiko A. Antineutrophil cytoplasmic autoantibody-positive crescentic glomerulonephritis as a complication of treatment with propylthiouracil in children. J Pediatr. 1994;124(6):986–8.

50. Fujieda M, Hattori M, Kurayama H, Koitabashi Y, Members and Coworkers of the Japanese Society for Pediatric Nephrology. Clinical features and outcomes in children with antineutrophil cytoplasmic autoantibody-positive glomerulonephritis associated with propylthiouracil treatment. J Am Soc Nephrol. 2002;13(2):437–45.

51. Wang C, Gou SJ, Xu PC, Zhao MH, Chen M. Epitope analysis of anti-myeloperoxidase antibodies in propylthiouracil-induced antineutrophil cytoplasmic antibody-associated vasculitis. Arthritis Res Ther. 2013;15(6):R196.

52. Yu F, Chen M, Gao Y, Wang SX, Zou WZ, Zhao MH, et al. Clinical and pathological features of renal involvement in propylthiouracil-associated ANCA-positive vasculitis. Am J Kidney Dis. 2007;49(5):607–14.

53. Hogan SL, Cooper GS, Savitz DA, Nylander-French LA, Parks CG, Chin H, et al. Association of silica exposure with anti-neutrophil cytoplasmic autoantibody small-vessel vasculitis: a population-based, case-control study. Clin J Am Soc Nephrol. 2007;2(2):290–9.

54. Stegeman CA, Tervaert JW, Sluiter WJ, Manson WL, de Jong PE, Kallenberg CG. Association of chronic nasal carriage of Staphylococcus aureus and higher relapse rates in Wegener granulomatosis. Ann Intern Med. 1994;120(1):12–7.

55. Gendelman S, Zeft A, Spalding SJ. Childhood-onset eosinophilic granulomatosis with polyangiitis (formerly Churg-Strauss syndrome): a contemporary single-center cohort. J Rheumatol. 2013;40(6):929–35.

56. Vanoni F, Bettinelli A, Keller F, Bianchetti MG, Simonetti GD. Vasculitides associated with IgG antineutrophil cytoplasmic autoantibodies in childhood. Pediatr Nephrol. 2010;25(2):205–12.

57. Hattori M, Kurayama H, Koitabashi Y, Japanese Society for Pediatric Nephrology. Antineutrophil cytoplasmic autoantibody-associated glomerulonephritis in children. J Am Soc Nephrol. 2001;12(7):1493–500.

58. Eleftheriou D, Dillon MJ, Brogan PA. Advances in childhood vasculitis. Curr Opin Rheumatol. 2009;21(4):411–8.

59. Tullus K, Marks SD. Vasculitis in children and adolescents: clinical presentation, etiopathogenesis, and treatment. Paediatr Drugs. 2009;11(6):375–80.

60. Radhakrishnan J, Cattran DC. The KDIGO practice guideline on glomerulonephritis: reading between the (guide)lines – application to the individual patient. Kidney Int. 2012;82(8):840–56.

61. Jayne D, Rasmussen N, Andrassy K, Bacon P, Tervaert JW, Dadoniex, et al. A randomized trial of maintenance therapy for vasculitis associated with antineutrophil cytoplasmic autoantibodies. N Engl J Med. 2003;349(1):36–44.

62. Nachman PH, Hogan SL, Jennette JC, Falk RJ. Treatment response and relapse in antineutrophil cytoplasmic autoantibody-associated microscopic

polyangiitis and glomerulonephritis. J Am Soc Nephrol. 1996;7(1):33–9.

63. Yu F, Huang JP, Zou WZ, Zhao MH. The clinical features of anti-neutrophil cytoplasmic antibody-associated systemic vasculitis in Chinese children. Pediatr Nephrol. 2006;21(4):497–502.

64. Siomou E, Tramma D, Bowen C, Milford DV. ANCA-associated glomerulonephritis/systemic vasculitis in childhood: clinical features-outcome. Pediatr Nephrol. 2012;27(10):1911–20.

65. Jayne DR, Gaskin G, Rasmussen N, Abramowicz D, Ferrario F, Guillevin L, et al. Randomized trial of plasma exchange or high-dosage methylprednisolone as adjunctive therapy for severe renal vasculitis. J Am Soc Nephrol. 2007;18(7):2180–8.

66. de Groot K, Harper L, Jayne DR, Flores Suarez LF, Gregorini G, Gross WL, et al. Pulse versus daily oral cyclophosphamide for induction of remission in antineutrophil cytoplasmic antibody-associated vasculitis: a randomized trial. Ann Intern Med. 2009;150(10):670–80.

67. Walters GD, Willis NS, Craig JC. Interventions for renal vasculitis in adults. A systematic review. BMC Nephrol. 2010;11:12.

68. Jones RB, Tervaert JW, Hauser T, Lugmani R, Morgan MD, Peh CA, et al. Rituximab versus cyclophosphamide in ANCA-associated renal vasculitis. N Engl J Med. 2010;363(3):211–20.

69. Stone JH, Merkel PA, Spiera R, Seo P, Langford CA, Hoffman GS, et al. Rituximab versus cyclophosphamide for ANCA-associated vasculitis. N Engl J Med. 2010;363(3):221–32.

70. Specks U, Merkel PA, Seo P, Spiera R, Langford CA, Hoffman GS, et al. Efficacy of remission-induction regimens for ANCA-associated vasculitis. N Engl J Med. 2013;369(5):417–27.

71. Glöckner WM, Sieberth HG, Wichmann HE, Backes E, Bambauer R, Boesken WH, et al. Plasma exchange and immunosuppression in rapidly progressive glomerulonephritis: a controlled, multi-center study. Clin Nephrol. 1988;29(1):1–8.

72. Cole E, Cattran D, Magil A, Greenwood C, Churchill D, Sutton D, et al. A prospective randomized trial of plasma exchange as additive therapy in idiopathic crescentic glomerulonephritis. The Canadian Apheresis Study Group. Am J Kidney Dis. 1992;20(3):261–9.

73. Walsh M, Catapano F, Szpirt W, Thorlund K, Bruchfeld A, Guillevin L, et al. Plasma exchange for renal vasculitis and idiopathic rapidly progressive glomerulonephritis: a meta-analysis. Am J Kidney Dis. 2011;57(4):566–74.

74. Westman KW, Bygren PG, Olsson H, Ranstam J, Wieslander J. Relapse rate, renal survival, and cancer morbidity in patients with Wegener's granulomatosis or microscopic polyangiitis with renal involvement. J Am Soc Nephrol. 1998;9(5):842–52.

75. Hiemstra TF, Walsh M, Mahr A, Savage CO, de Groot K, Harper L, et al. Mycophenolate mofetil vs azathioprine for remission maintenance in antineutrophil cytoplasmic antibody-associated vasculitis: a randomized controlled trial. JAMA. 2010;304(21):2381–8.

Lupus Nephritis

28

Stephen D. Marks and Kjell Tullus

Introduction

Systemic lupus erythematosus (SLE) is a lifelong, life-limiting, multisystem, autoimmune disorder, which is episodic in nature with a broad spectrum of clinical and immunological manifestations. SLE is characterised by widespread inflammation of blood vessels and connective tissues affecting the skin, joints, kidneys, heart, lungs, nervous and other systems. There is a higher rate and more severe organ involvement in children than in adults (especially with respect to haematological and renal disease) [1–4]. Renal involvement with biopsy-proven lupus nephritis occurs in up to 80 % of all cases of juvenile-onset SLE and is a major determinant of the prognosis, which improved with the introduction of corticosteroids and cyclophosphamide. We now also have an increasing armamentarium of immunosuppressive agents that can be used to treat active disease. However, there is still a significant morbidity and mortality for severe disease with considerable physical and psychosocial morbidity due to the variable, and often progressive, clinical course of juvenile-onset SLE. This results from both the sequelae of disease activity and the side-effects of medications, including the infectious risks from over-immunosuppression, and longer-term risks with accelerated atherosclerosis [5]. At least 4 of 11 American College of Rheumatology classification criteria for SLE gives 95 % sensitivity and 96 % specificity in clinical practice (Table 28.1) [6, 7].

Epidemiology

Juvenile-onset SLE accounts for up to 20 % of all SLE cases, with epidemiological studies demonstrating a minimum incidence in a paediatric population of 0.28 per 100,000 children at risk per year [8] with a prevalence in children and adults from various epidemiological studies of between 12.0 and 50.8 per 100,000 [9–16]. However, SLE has been reported to be common in children from China, Hong Kong and Taiwan and three times more frequent in Afro-Caribbean than Caucasian children [17, 18]. In addition, the prevalence and severity of renal and neuropsychiatric lupus is increased in Afro-Caribbean children [19]. In the United Kingdom, Asian and Afro-Caribbean children are over six times likely to be affected when compared to Caucasian children [20]. SLE is more prevalent in females of childbearing age possibly due to the hormonal influences, and is commoner over the age of 10 years [21, 22].

S.D. Marks (✉) • K. Tullus
Department of Pediatric Nephrology,
Great Ormond Street Hospital for Children
NHS Foundation Trust, Great Ormond Street,
London WC1N 3JH, UK
e-mail: stephen.marks@gosh.nhs.uk;
kjell.tullus@gosh.nhs.uk

© Springer-Verlag Berlin Heidelberg 2016
D.F. Geary, F. Schaefer (eds.), *Pediatric Kidney Disease*, DOI 10.1007/978-3-662-52972-0_28

Table 28.1 American College of Rheumatology Criteria for classification of SLE

1. Malar rash
2. Discoid rash
3. Photosensitivity
4. Oral ulcers
5. Arthritis
6. Serositis
Pleuritis
Pericarditis
7. Renal disorder
Proteinuria (>0.5 g/day) or persistently 3+
Red blood cell casts
8. Neurological disorder
Seizures
Psychosis (after excluding other causes)
9. Hematological disorder
Hemolytic anemia
Leucopenia (<4 × 10^9/l on two occasions)
Lymphopenia (<1.5 × 10^9/l on two occasions)
Thromobocytopenia (<100 × 10^9/l)
10. Immunological disorder
Elevated anti-double stranded DNA
Elevated anti-Smith antibodies
Positive antiphospholipid antibodies (previously lupus erythematosus cell tests or false positive *Treponema pallidum* immobilisation/Venereal Disease Reference Laboratory)
11. Elevated anti-nuclear antibodies (after exclusion of drug-induced lupus)

Etiopathogenesis

SLE is a multifactorial disorder with multigenic inheritance and various environmental factors implicated in its etiopathogenesis with abnormal regulation of cell-mediated and humoral immunity that lead to tissue damage. The developing immune system is immature compared to adults and the heterogeneity of the clinical manifestations probably reflects the complexity of the disease pathogenesis.

The immune system in SLE is characterised by a complex interplay between overactive B cells, abnormally activated T cells and antigen-presenting cells which lead to the production of an array of inflammatory cytokines, apoptotic cells, diverse autoantibodies and immune complexes. They in turn activate effector cells and the complement system leading to tissue injury and damage; these are the hallmarks of the clinical manifestations [23]. Moreover, several autoantibodies against cell wall components or circulating proteins can produce specific disease manifestations. However, it is interesting that some healthy children have positive ANA titres and that 88 % of adult SLE patients have autoantibodies (including ANA, anti-dsDNA and anti-Smith) present up to 9.4 years before SLE is ever diagnosed [24]. It is generally assumed that anti-dsDNA antibodies play an important role in the pathogenesis of LN. This is because an increase in anti-dsDNA titre often precedes onset of renal disease, immune deposits are present in glomeruli and eluates of glomeruli are enriched for anti-dsDNA. However, the classical concept of deposition of DNA-anti-DNA complexes inciting glomerular inflammation is questionable as free, naked, DNA is not present in the circulation and injection of these complexes hardly leads to glomerular localisation. The pathogenicity of anti-DNA has been proven with circulating immune complexes, in situ immune complexes, direct binding to renal and non-renal antigens, penetration into cells, stimulation of cytokines in the form of immune complexes. However, there are pathogenic and non-pathogenic anti-DNA antibodies and current assays do not distinguish these classes.

Genomic and gene expression studies in patients with SLE have revealed novel gene mutations and cytokine alterations that may explain many of the features of the disease as well as the genetic susceptibility. There is a familial incidence of SLE in 12–15 % of cases with a 10–20-fold increased risk of developing the disease if a sibling is affected compared to the general population (prevalence increases from 0.4 % of populations up to 3.5 % if there is a first degree relative with SLE) [10]. The concordance rate of SLE in monozygous twins is 24 % compared with 2 % in heterozygous pairs highlighting the importance of genetic (including HLA haplotypes, complement components and Fcγ receptor polymorphisms) and environmental factors in the aetiology of SLE [25–28]. The genetics of SLE is not fully understood with many susceptible loci, as there is a complex, multifactorial inheritance with associated environmental factors. Genetic linkage studies using microsatellite markers and single nucleotide polymorphisms have identified at least seven loci displaying significant linkage to SLE, including 1q23 (FcγRIIA, FcγRIIB, FcγRIIIA), 1q25-31, 1q41-42, 2q35-37, 4p16-15.2, 6p11-21 (MHC haplotypes), and 16q12.

Complement activation is involved in tissue damage with initial murine lupus models and later human studies revealing homozygous deficiencies of the components of the classical complement pathway (C1q, C1r, C1s, C2 and C4) predispose to the development of SLE. The complement system is an important part of the immune system which when dysregulated can result in the development of SLE, which occurs in 75 % and 90 % of patients with complete deficiencies of C4 and C1q respectively [29]. Although initially, anti-C1q was neither specific nor sensitive for SLE, in vitro testing has shown that anti-C1q is pathogenic in conjunction with complement-fixing antibodies and immune complexes with an increased prevalence of LN. Anti-C1q auto-antibodies are strongly associated with renal involvement in SLE and deposit in glomeruli together with C1q [30]. Anti-C1q antibodies are especially pathogenic in patients with SLE as they induce overt renal disease in the context of glomerular immune complex disease [31].

There are profound alterations in the B cell compartments of both children and adults with SLE [32, 33] with characteristic hypergammaglobulinemia and increased serum autoantibody titres, explaining why B cell depletion may be an effective therapy [34, 35]. In addition to autoantibodies and immune complexes, autoreactive T cells cause tissue damage in SLE with evidence of alterations in human SLE T cell signalling molecules and loss of self-tolerance [36]. Compared to healthy T cells, there are increased and accelerated signalling responses in T cells from patients with SLE with hyperreactivity to antigenic triggers, which may be due to genetic influences [37, 38]. Many cytokines including interferon and interleukins (IL-6, IL10, IL12 (p40) and IL-18), which are elevated in the serum of SLE patients correlate with disease activity [39].

The increase in autoantigens in SLE may be due to impaired immune complex clearance and apoptosis. There is evidence of defective clearance of apoptotic cells in some SLE patients, due to the genetic deficiency of molecules, including complement component deficiencies, with autoantigens undergoing structural modifications during the process of apoptosis that may induce immunogenicity [40].

The development of SLE may be attributable to genetic susceptibility with changes in the hormonal milieu, environmental, pharmaceutical and toxic agents (including crystalline silica, solvents and pesticides) [41]. However, there is also an association with infectious conditions influencing the developing immune system of children who develop SLE, including Epstein-Barr virus [42, 43].

Clinical Presentation

There is a varied clinical presentation of juvenile-onset SLE, although typically there are non-specific symptoms of being generally unwell with lethargy, aches, pains, episodic fever, anorexia, nausea and weight loss with a typical butterfly rash over a period of a few weeks or months. Most organ systems can be involved (Table 28.2) [44] although unusual presentations are sometimes encountered, which is why SLE has been called one of the great mimickers [45].

The majority of children with SLE present during their adolescence. From one of the largest cohort of 201 children with SLE from Toronto, Canada, 6 children (3 %) presented before the age of 6 years, 41 (20 %) between 6 and 10 years,

Table 28.2 Presenting symptoms of SLE

Malaise, weight loss, growth retardation	96 %
Cutaneous abnormalities	96 %
Hematological abnormalities	91 %
Fever	84 %
Lupus nephritis	84 %
Musculoskeletal complaints	82 %
Pleural/pulmonary disease	67 %
Hepatosplenomegaly and/or lymphadenopathy	58 %
Neurological disease	49 %
Other disease manifestations (including cardiac, ocular, gastro-intestinal, Raynaud's phenomenon)	13– 38 %

Used with permission of Springer Science + Business Media from Cameron [44]

62 (31%) between 11 and 13 years and 92 [46] between 14 and 18 years of age [46]. There was a female predominance of 80% with a slightly higher proportion of male patients than later in adulthood.

Lupus Nephritis

Up to 60–80% of children have some renal involvement close to the onset of the disease [44]. In a 1994 review of the presentation of lupus nephritis from different studies involving 208 children, 55% presented with nephrotic syndrome and 43% with proteinuria of lesser degrees (Table 28.3). Most children have microscopic haematuria while few (1.4%) presented with macroscopic haematuria. Fifty percent of the children have impaired renal function at onset while only 1.4% have acute kidney injury requiring renal replacement therapy. A small proportion will present with a rapidly progressive glomerulonephritis with biopsy-proven crescentic glomerulonephritis. Hypertension was found in 40% of children.

Other Organ Systems

Dermatological

The butterfly or malar rash is the classical rash over the cheeks and nose with photosensitivity to sunlight. However, other kinds of rashes can be present including maculopapular or purpuric rashes, livedo reticularis and urticaria. Hair loss and brown discolouration of the nails are rather common findings.

Table 28.3 Presenting features of lupus nephritis

Nephrotic syndrome (>3 g/day)	55%
Proteinuria (<3 g/day)	43%
Macroscopic haematuria	1.4%
Microscopic haematuria	79%
Hypertension	40%
Reduced GFR (<80 mls/min/1.73 m^2)	50%
Acute renal failure	1.4%

Used with permission of Springer Science + Business Media from Cameron [44]

Cerebral

Neurological symptoms, including headache, seizures and mood disorders are among the most severe that are found in SLE. The psychiatric symptoms can range from fatigue and depression to frank psychosis with hallucinations. Poor academic achievement is a common problem of multifactorial origin that is important to address in these children.

Haematological

Coombs' positive haemolytic anaemia, leucopenia, thrombocytopenia and pancytopenia are common findings in children with SLE. Erythrocyte sedimentation rate (ESR) is markedly raised in most children with SLE while high C-reactive protein (CRP) is found in only a small minority. Therefore, CRP can be helpful in differentiating between flares of disease activity of SLE or an infectious complication, such as septicaemia due to the disease itself and/or treatment.

Rheumatological

Generalised pain involving the musculo-skeletal system is a very common finding in SLE patients with severe arthritis less common than a milder arthritis or arthralgia. In particular, bone pain can also occur as a complication of corticosteroid treatment.

Other Organs

All serous membranes including pleura and pericardium are frequently affected. Hepatosplenomegaly and lymphadenopathy are commonly found in some children. Growth delay is often seen in children, partly related to pubertal delay. Primary and secondary amenorrhoea are manifestations of SLE and lupus nephritis, but also complications of high doses of cyclophosphamide treatment.

Antiphospholipid Syndrome

Antiphospholipid syndrome (APS) with anticardiolipin antibodies and/or lupus anticoagulant are found in 65% of children with SLE [47]. Patients with APS are prone to developing both venous and arterial thrombosis. APS is an independent risk factor for more severe renal disease due to microangiopathy in the kidneys and may require treatment as outlined below.

Classification Criteria

The American College of Rheumatology (ACR) classification criteria are utilised in classifying and not diagnosing patients with SLE (Table 28.1). The diagnosis of SLE is made in typical cases with classical organ involvement, elevated autoantibodies and hypocomplementaemia. However, in some cases, the initial diagnosis is more difficult due to the evolution of disease and these cases may not initially fulfil the criteria developed by ACR which have been refined for children [6, 7]. They consist of 11 different criteria of which four should be fulfilled for the diagnosis of SLE; however, meeting these criteria is not sufficient for a diagnosis of SLE because many children with other diseases can also formally match a number of these criteria.

The Systemic Lupus International Collaborating Clinics (SLICC) classification criteria for SLE was published in 2012 [48] where patients are classified if they have biopsy-proven lupus nephritis with either positive ANA or anti-dsDNA antibodies or at least four criteria (at least one clinical [acute and chronic cutaneous lupus, oral or nasal ulceration, non-scarring alopecia, arthritis, serositis, renal, neurologic, haemolytic anaemia, leucopenia and thrombocytopenia] and one laboratory [ANA, anti-dsDNA, anti-Smith, anti-phospholipid antibodies, hypocomplementaemia (C3, C4, CH50) and Direct Coombs' test (which is not counted if haemolytic anaemia is present)] criteria and this has now been validated in children [49].

Disease Activity Scoring Systems

There are various disease activity and damage scoring systems, which are very helpful in monitoring disease activity and damage in children and adolescents with SLE with respect to both clinical long-term follow-up and scientific studies. Scales of indices of disease activity continue to evolve and include SLEDAI (Systemic Lupus Erythematosus Disease Activity Index), SLAM (Systemic Lupus Activity Measure) and ECLAM (European Consensus Lupus Activity Measure). The British Isles Lupus Activity Assessment Group (BILAG) index is another scoring system that can be used and has been evaluated in children [50]. The BILAG index is based on the principle of the physician's intention to treat and is a clinical measure of disease activity in SLE patients which has been validated to be reliable, comprehensive and sensitive to change. It was developed to report disease activity in eight different systems (general, mucocutaneous, neurological, musculoskeletal, cardio-respiratory, vasculitis, renal and haematological), which differentiates it from other lupus activity indices.

Investigations

The initial investigations of a child with suspected SLE include haematological, biochemical and immunological investigations. Further investigations are warranted depending on organ involvement so a percutaneous renal biopsy and imaging of relevant organ systems are often required.

Blood Investigations

The initial blood test should include a full blood count with a blood film, erythrocyte sedimentation rate (ESR) and reticulocyte count. Anaemia, leucopenia and thrombocytopenia are common findings during active disease that normally improve when the disease gets under control. The leucocyte count, in particular the neutrophil count, should be monitored during active immunosuppressive treatment as the presence of neutropenia influences the doses of immunosuppressive therapies. However, lymphopenia is often seen with treatment and is mostly regarded as a "desired" side-effect which can sometimes be a marker of the effectiveness of treatment. ESR is a marker of disease activity, which can be clinically useful, although it is not uncommon for it to be markedly elevated even during clinical and serological remission. A coagulation screen and a direct Coombs' test should be performed to look for evidence of haemolysis.

The biochemistry profile should include estimation of renal function with plasma creatinine and urea, serum electrolytes, bone, thyroid and liver function tests (including serum albumin), pancreatic enzymes and C-reactive protein (where sepsis is clinically suspected). It is useful to calculate the estimated glomerular filtration rate using the Schwartz formula [51].

Immunology Testing

There is evidence of immune dysregulation in almost all children with SLE with positive immunological tests and anti-nuclear antibodies (ANA). ANA can sometimes be a non-specific finding but the use of anti-double-stranded DNA (dsDNA) and the extractable nuclear antibodies (ENA) and anti-C1q increases the specificity (Table 28.4). The pathogenic significance of these antibodies is debated and they can be found in serum sometimes several years before the development of symptoms [24]. However, it is clear that dsDNA and anti-C1q can be used to monitor disease activity as a marker of improvement or a pending flare of disease activity. Anti-C1q antibodies have also been shown to predict more severe renal involvement [52].

Complement C3 and C4, is mostly reduced during the active phases of disease and can also be used as useful markers of disease activity.

Table 28.4 Auto-antibodies in patients with lupus nephritis

	Frequency	Specificity	Association with disease activity
Anti-dsDNA	40–90%	High	Yes
Anti-SSA/Ro	35%	Low	No
Anti-SSB/La	15%	Low	No
Anti-Sm	5–30%	High	No
Anti-C1q	80–100%	High	Yes

Key: *dsDNA* double stranded DNA, *Anti SSA/Ro* anti-Sjögren's syndrome A, *Anti SSB/La* anti-Sjögren's syndrome B, *Anti Sm* Anti Smith, *Anti C1q* Anti-complement factor C1q

Anticardiolipin antibodies and lupus anticoagulant should be regularly monitored. Hypergammaglobulinaemia is a feature of SLE and it is useful to monitor serum immunoglobulins. It is controversial whether hypogammaglobulinaemia should be supplemented. We do not routinely administer substitutive intravenous immunoglobulin in children treated with B-lymphocyte depletion therapies (rituximab). B-lymphocyte counts should be monitored in children treated with rituximab by measuring the number of CD19 positive cells.

Urine Investigations

Urine testing should be regularly monitored in all children with SLE with urinalysis by dipstick performed for haematuria and proteinuria and laboratory evaluation of albuminuria or proteinuria. Urine microscopy is also helpful in looking for red blood cells and casts during the acute phase of lupus nephritis. Some standardised measurement of proteinuria or albuminuria should be regularly followed, which in most centres is carried out by analysing an early morning spot urine sample relating the urine excretion of protein or albumin to the urine levels of creatinine. Evidence of tubular dysfunction may help to identify lupus nephritis prior to the onset of albuminuria by measuring NAG (N-acetyl-beta-D-glucosaminidase):creatinine ratio, RBP (retinol binding protein):creatinine ratio or other tubular markers [53].

Other Investigations

It is important to base treatment decisions on the histopathology of percutaneous renal biopsies as it has been shown that the severity of the renal involvement sometimes is difficult to predict from clinical symptoms and signs. Estimated or formal measurements of glomerular filtration rate should be performed when there is a clinical suspicion of impaired renal function. Pulmonary function tests, electrocardiography, echocardiography and chest X-rays are important investigations in selected children. Cerebral imaging is advocated in children with neuropsychiatric evidence of cerebral lupus.

Follow-Up

Each child should at every clinic visit have a full clinical evaluation including weight, height and a disease activity score (as above). They should have their blood pressure monitored and their urine tested for proteinuria and haematuria. Regular blood tests should include full blood count, ESR and CRP, renal and liver function tests, electrolytes, complement C3 and C4 and autoantibodies including dsDNA. Fasting blood lipids including cholesterol, triglycerides, HDL, LDL and VLDL should be monitored at least once a year. Bone density should be measured in children with long-term daily corticosteroid therapy on an annual basis.

Histological Classification of Lupus Nephritis

The histological classification of lupus nephritis (LN) was initially formatted in 1975 by the World Health Organisation (WHO) and modified in 1982 and 1995. It describes the spectrum of LN as the type and extent of renal lesion and provides information on the immunosuppression required and prognosis. There was a revision of this classification by the International Society of Nephrology (ISN) and Renal Pathology Society (RPS) Working Group after their consensus conference in 2002 in order to standardise definitions, emphasise clinically relevant lesions, and encourage uniform and reproducible reporting between centres (Table 28.5) [54, 55]. This new classification facilitates clinical management by increased comprehension of the aetiopathogenesis of SLE and guides the clinician with treatment decisions, protocols and clinical research. However, there is widespread variation of the timing, type and distribution of histological lesions, including immune-complex mediated vasculitis, fibrinoid necrosis, inflammatory cell infiltrate and collagen sclerosis.

Table 28.5 International Society of Nephrology and Renal Pathology Society Working Group (ISN/RPS) revised histopathological classification of lupus nephritis

1. **Minimal mesangial lupus nephritis (LN)**

Normal glomeruli by LM, but mesangial immune deposits by IF

2. **Mesangial proliferative lupus nephritis (LN)**

Purely mesangial hypercellularity of any degree or mesangial matrix expansion by LM with mesangial immune deposits, with none or few, isolated subepithelial or subendothelial deposits by IF or EM not visible by LM

3. **Focal lupus nephritis (LN)**

Active or inactive focal (<50% involved glomeruli), segmental or global endo- or extracapillary GN, typically with focal, subendothelial immune deposits, with or without focal or diffuse mesangial alterations

III (A) Active focal proliferative LN

III (A/C) Active and sclerotic focal proliferative LN

III (C) Inactive sclerotic focal LN

* Indicate the proportion of glomeruli with active and with sclerotic lesions

* Indicate the proportion of glomeruli with fibrinoid necrosis and/or cellular crescents

4. **Diffuse segmental (IV-S) or global (IV-G) LN**

Active or inactive diffuse (50% or more involved glomeruli), segmental or global endo- or extracapillary GN with diffuse subendothelial immune deposits, with or without mesangial alterations. This class is divided into diffuse segmental (IV-S) when at least 50% of the involved glomeruli have segmental lesions, and diffuse global (IV-G) when at least 50% of the involved glomeruli have global lesions

IV (A) Active diffuse segmental or global proliferative LN

IV (A/C) Diffuse segmental or global proliferative and sclerotic LN

IV (C) Diffuse segmental or global sclerotic LN

* Indicate the proportion of glomeruli with active and with sclerotic lesions

* Indicate the proportion of glomeruli with fibrinoid necrosis and/or cellular crescents

5. **Membranous lupus nephritis**

Numerous global or segmental subepithelial immune deposits or their morphologic sequelae by LM and IF or EM with or without mesangial alterations

May occur in combination with III or IV in which case both will be diagnosed. May show advanced sclerosis

6. **Advanced sclerotic LN**

90% or more glomeruli globally sclerosed without residual activity

Classes I and II denote purely mesangial involvement (I, mesangial immune deposits without mesangial hypercellularity; II, mesangial immune deposits with mesangial expansion and hypercellularity), Class III for focal glomerulonephritis (involving less than 50 % of total number of glomeruli) with subdivisions for active and chronic lesions, Class IV for diffuse glomerulonephritis (involving at least 50 % of total number of glomeruli with examples in Figs. 28.1, 28.2a–d, and 28.3a–d) either with segmental (class IV-S) or global (class IV-G) involvement, and also with subdivisions for active and chronic lesions, Class V for membranous lupus nephritis (combinations of membranous and proliferative glomerulonephritis (i.e., Class III and V or Class IV and V) should be reported individually in the diagnostic line) and Class VI for advanced sclerosing lesions (which now for the first time categorically states that at least 90 % of glomeruli need to be globally sclerosed without residual activity). In addition, the new ISN/RPS classification includes overlap cases (see Fig. 28.4a–d

for an example of mixed Class IV and Class V lupus nephritis).

The histopathological features of LN includes the delineation of active and chronic histological lesions, which has been extensively reported in the various classification systems (Table 28.6) [57].

The active glomerular and tubulointerstitial lesions, which are potentially reversible and are scored up to 24 (with 12 denoting poor renal prognosis), include endocapillary hypercellularity, fibrinoid necrosis, karyorrhexis, cellular crescents, hyaline thrombi, wire loops (subendothelial deposits), haematoxylin bodies, leucocyte infiltratation and tubulo-interstitial disease with tubular atrophy and mononuclear cell infiltration. The chronic lesions are irreversible and include glomerular sclerosis, fibrous crescents, fibrous adhesions, extramembranous deposits, and tubulo-interstitial disease with interstitial fibrosis and tubular atrophy.

The clinicopathological correlation of LN has been evaluated in both adults and children

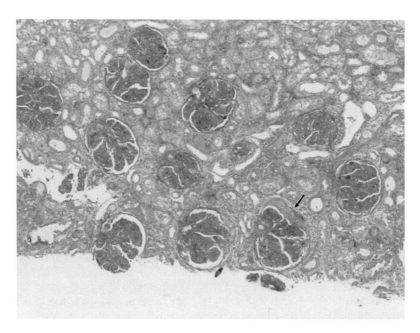

Fig. 28.1 Photomicrograph of a case of lupus nephritis demonstrating predominant diffuse endocapillary proliferative change with scattered superimposed extracapillary proliferative lesions (*Arrow*), Lupus nephritis Class IV-G (A/C) (PAS, original magnification ×100) (Used with permission of Taylor & Francis from Marks et al. [56])

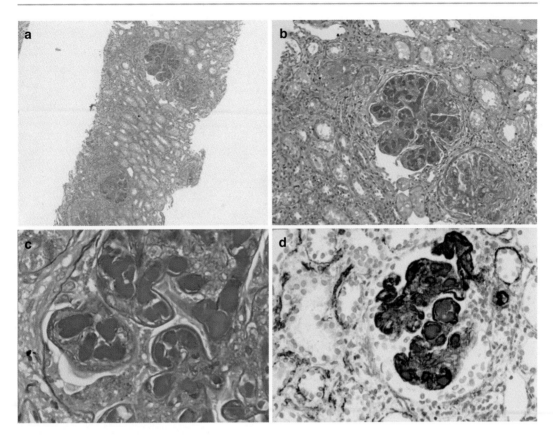

Fig. 28.2 Photomicrographs of a case of lupus nephritis presenting as apparent acute renal failure, demonstrating diffuse endocapillary proliferative change with scattered crescent formation (**a, b**) and extensive subendothelial deposits visualised as wire-loop and hyaline drop lesions (**b, c**). Immunostaining revealed a characteristic 'fullhouse' pattern of immunoglobulin and complement deposition. (**d**) Lupus nephritis Class IV-G (**a**) (PAS and immunostain, original magnifications ×40–400) (Used with permission of Taylor & Francis from Marks et al. [56])

according to different histopathological classifications. The largest adult series investigating the clinicopathological outcomes according to the new ISN/RPS classification of LN followed 60 Japanese subjects for 1–366 (mean 187) months (Fig. 28.5) [58]. The primary outcome was defined as developing end-stage kidney disease (ESKD) with secondary outcome as patients' death and/or ESKD. The primary and secondary outcomes of all subjects were 82 % and 78 % at 10 years, and 80 % and 73 % at 20 years, respectively. The primary outcome of subjects with nephrotic syndrome (n = 21) was statistically poorer (p = 0.0007) with the mean time of 50 % renal survival of 200 ± 29 months as compared to that of subjects without nephrotic syndrome (n = 39).

In comparison with adult-onset SLE, there are usually less patients in the series of childhood cases of LN. There have been larger series investigating clinicopathological outcomes of 39–67 children according to the WHO classification [59] and the new ISN/RPS classification of LN [60], which provide evidence that up to half of children with LN will have the most severe class (Class IV or diffuse LN). The new classification demonstrated that the subgroup of diffuse global sclerosing (IV-G(C)) LN was associated with the worst clinical outcome [60].

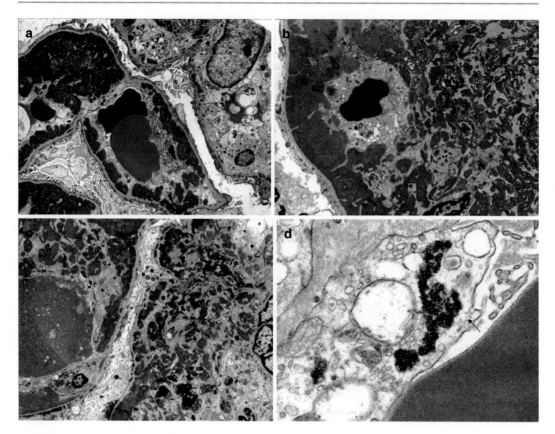

Fig. 28.3 Electronmicrographs of lupus nephritis demonstrating extensive mesangial and paramesangial electron dense deposits in association with massive subendothelial deposits (**a–c**) (**a**) corresponds to the case in Fig. 28.1 and (**b, c**) correspond to the case in Fig. 28.2). In addition, some cases may demonstrate the presence of tubuloreticular inclusions. (**d**) (Used with permission of Taylor & Francis from Marks et al. [56])

Treatment

The optimal treatment of children and adolescents with SLE is provided by a multi-disciplinary team of health professionals, including a paediatric rheumatologist, paediatric nephrologist and other paediatric specialists, with a dedicated specialist nurse and members of a psychosocial team.

Drug Treatment

The treatment of lupus with or without nephritis is based on evaluation of the severity of the disease. The treatment should be individually tailored depending on the presenting symptoms and severity of renal involvement, with emphasis on renal dysfunction and the degree of proteinuria. In all cases with suspected renal involvement, the histopathological grading of the renal biopsy is very helpful in deciding further treatment. Other potentially life-threatening symptoms, such as cerebral lupus should also be taken into consideration when deciding on the initial treatment. Most treatments have common or potential side-effects, which need to be considered for the individual child.

The treatment of juvenile-onset SLE is not based on large randomised controlled trials, but there is an increasing number of studies in adult patients and published clinical experience in children. The recommendations below describe the most commonly used protocols for treating children with SLE. Two recent consensus reports on the treatment of paediatric lupus have been published [61, 62]. The armamentarium of immunosuppressive agents is presently developing quickly

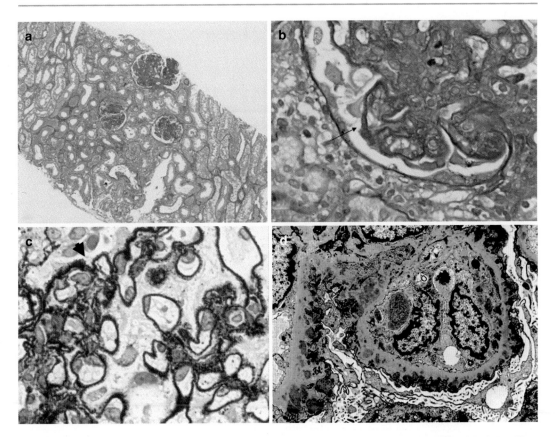

Fig. 28.4 Photomicrographs of a case of lupus nephritis presenting with nephrotic syndrome demonstrating diffuse endocapillary proliferative change with subendothelial deposits ((**a**, **b**) PAS, original magnifications ×40 and 400 respectively). In addition some glomeruli show florid 'spike' formation on silver staining ((**c**) PAMS, original magnification ×400) with mesangial, subendothelial and subepithelial deposits on ultrastructural examination (**d**). Lupus nephritis, mixed Class IV and Class V changes (Used with permission of Taylor & Francis from Marks et al. [56])

Table 28.6 Activity and chronicity indices of lupus nephritis

	Activity index	Chronicity index
Glomerular	Endocapillary hypercellularity Fibrinoid necrosis Karyorrhexis Cellular crescents Hyaline thrombi Wire loops (subendothelial deposits) Haematoxylic bodies Leucocyte infiltratation	Glomerular sclerosis Fibrous crescents Fibrous adhesions Extramembranous deposits
Tubulointerstitial	Mononuclear cell infiltration	Interstitial fibrosis
	Tubular necrosis	Tubular atrophy

with new drugs being introduced [63], so guidelines may change in the not too distant future.

Traditionally treatment has been divided into induction therapy to gain control of acute disease and maintenance therapy to maintain control over the disease. This is a helpful approach but it is not an uncommon clinical situation that a flare of disease activity is difficult to define.

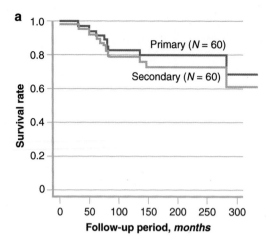

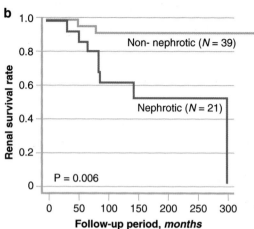

Fig. 28.5 Prognosis of lupus nephritis. The primary (ESKD) and secondary (patients' death and/or ESKD) outcomes (a) of 60 Japanese adult lupus nephritis subjects with and without nephrotic syndrome (b) at mean follow-up of 187 months (Used with permission of Nature Publishing Group from Yokoyama et al. [58])

Severe Multisystem Disease with or Without Nephritis (ISN/RPG Class III–V)

Induction Therapy

A common presentation to the nephrologist is a child that over a few weeks or months has developed generalised symptoms and at assessment by his or her local medical team is found to have an acute nephritic and/or nephrotic syndrome with a suspicion of SLE that is later confirmed by serology. It is important in cases with significant renal disease to commence treatment early without unnecessary delay to protect the kidneys from developing chronic damage.

The mainstay of induction treatment is based on corticosteroids and an immunosuppressive agent (Table 28.7). Historically, this used to be cyclophosphamide but is now more commonly, mycophenolate mofetil (MMF). For children with active disease, including severe renal dysfunction, B-lymphocyte depletion therapy with intravenous rituximab is often added [35, 64]. In children with a crescentic glomerulonephritis, we and others have mostly added plasma exchange to the treatment.

Corticosteroids

Intravenous pulses of methylprednisolone should be given during three consecutive days

Table 28.7 Induction therapy of ISN/RPS Class III, IV and V lupus nephritis

Methylprednisolone (intravenous) pulses × 3	600–1000 mg/m^2 (maximum 1 g)
Prednisolone (oral)	1–2 mg/kg/day (maximum 60–80 mg/day with rapid weaning)
[a]Mycophenolate mofetil	Start dose of 250 mg/day to a maximum of 40 mg/kg/day (or 2–3 g/day) in two divided doses
In severe cases or if not responding to the above:	
Plasma exchange	Daily for 5–10 days
Rituximab	See protocol in text

[a]Induction therapy with cyclophosphamide or azathioprine are alternatives in selected cases

(600–1000 mg/m^2) with a maximum of 1 g, infused over at least 30 min. In severe cases, these pulses may need to be repeated.

The methylprednisolone pulses will be followed by high doses of oral prednisolone (1–2 mg/kg/day to a maximum dose 60–80 mg/day). This high dose is dictated by the severity of the clinical situation but should be weaned down to a dose of 0.5 mg/kg/day within 6–8 weeks. This treatment will inevitably result in Cushingoid side effects, which can be debilitating for adolescents (such as fluid and water retention with increased appetite and weight gain with rounded facies, striae and growth delay). Other important side-effects include mood changes, hypertension, steroid-induced diabetes mellitus, osteoporosis and osteopenia. Therefore, for long-term adherence to therapy, it is very important to reduce the corticosteroid dose as quickly as the clinical situation allows in order to minimise these side-effects.

Mycophenolate Mofetil (MMF)

There is now solid evidence from recent studies that MMF in adult patients is equally good for induction therapy as cyclophosphamide. The first study to show this was in 42 adult patients from Hong Kong treated with 12 months of oral MMF therapy or 6 months of cyclophosphamide followed by 6 months of azathioprine. Both groups responded equally well to the treatment but there were significantly more side-effects in the cyclophosphamide group [65].

The Aspreva Lupus Management Study (ALMS), the largest study on the treatment of SLE with MMF, included 370 patients with Class III, IV and V lupus nephritis [66]. It consisted of two treatment stages: one 24 week induction phase and subsequently, a 3 year study of the maintenance phase. In the induction study, the 370 patients were randomised to either MMF (target dose 3 g/day) or intravenous cyclophosphamide (iv CyC) given as monthly pulses of 500–1000 mg/m^2. All patients received prednisolone tapered from a maximum dose of 60 mg/day. The response to treatment was defined as achieving the primary efficacy endpoint which was decrease in urine protein:creatinine ratio to below 3 mg/mg if baseline ≥3 mg/mg or by 50% if baseline <3 mg/mg *and* stabilisation (±25%) or improvement of serum creatinine. The ALMS study showed no difference between MMF and CyC: 56% and 53% of patients in the two groups respectively, responded to treatment. There was also no significant difference in the rate of side-effects.

In a further publication it was shown that the therapeutic response varied with race, in that black and Hispanic patients responded better to MMF (60%) compared to CyC (39%), p=0.03 [67]. The authors have also looked separately at patients with ISN/RPS Class V lupus nephritis (i.e., a membranous pattern on the kidney biopsy) and again no differences were found between the MMF and CyC treated groups [68].

A recent meta-analysis comparing MMF and CyC as induction treatment has been published [69]. Four trials with 668 patients were included and no difference in clinical efficacy was found between the two drugs with the overall RR (relative risk) for renal remission being 0.67 (95% CI 0.35–1.28). However, there was significantly less alopecia (RR 5.77; 95% CI 1.56–21.38) and amenorrhoea (RR 6.64; 95% CI 2.00–22.07) with MMF but no other side effects were significantly different.

There are no randomised controlled studies on the use of MMF in juvenile-onset SLE. We published one of the largest case series with 31 children and adolescents that were treated with MMF either initially or converted from azathioprine [70]. Seventy-three per cent of the treated children showed a response to the drug without any recorded major side-effects. MMF should now be regarded as part of the standard treatment for children with severe lupus.

The main problems with MMF are the gastrointestinal side-effects with abdominal pain and diarrhoea. These can mostly be avoided by slowly increasing the dose. A normal starting dose is 1 g/day in two divided doses up to a final dose of 2–3 g/day. If gastrointestinal side-effects are a continuing problem then the daily dose may be divided three or even four times a day.

Cyclophosphamide

Intravenous pulses of cyclophosphamide have been the most important steroid-sparing agents in achieving remission in severe SLE and lupus nephritis. However, this treatment has substantial short and long-term side effects, including nausea (which can be alleviated with routine use of ondansetron), alopecia, haemorrhagic cystitis and infectious risks of septicaemia due to neutropenia. Many girls develop amenorrhoea and with high doses, there is a risk for developing infertility. The modified National Institute of Health protocol of iv CyC (500–1000 mg/m^2 with dose reduction in renal failure) can be administered as monthly pulses for 6 months. It is important to keep the child well hydrated and to give MESNA to protect the child from developing haemorrhagic cystitis.

Controlled studies in adult patients show that intravenous cyclophosphamide gives significantly more side-effects, including severe infections compared to both oral azathioprine or MMF [65, 71–73]. Therefore, it is important to closely monitor the total white cell, neutrophil and lymphocyte counts with the nadir usually occurring around 7–10 days after the infusion. Subsequent doses may need to be reduced based on haematological side effects.

There is a long-term increased risk for developing malignancies and for infertility. Up to 14 % of cyclophosphamide treated patients younger than 41 years have premature ovarian failure, which is a common consequence of cyclophosphamide treatment. Cyclophosphamide is thus a drug that still has a place in the treatment of lupus nephritis but it is gradually being replaced by other drugs.

Rituximab

Rituximab is a humanised anti-CD20 antibody that was designed for treatment of B-cell lymphoma and in adults has been increasingly used for B-cell depletion therapy in autoimmune diseases such as rheumatoid arthritis or SLE [34]. We have used intravenous rituximab in over a hundred children with SLE or vasculitis and published the results of our first children [35, 74]. Our patients have shown very good responses to the treatment and have not experienced any severe side effects.

A relatively large randomised placebo controlled study of intravenous rituximab, called the LUNAR trial has been performed in 144 adult patients with ISN/RPS Class III or IV lupus nephritis [75]. The primary endpoint was the renal response at week 52. A complete response was normalisation of serum creatinine, no red-cells (<5/hpf) in the urine and a urine protein creatinine ratio of <1.0 mg/mg.

Only 31 % of patients in the placebo group and 25 % of the rituximab treated patient fulfilled these very strict criteria for a complete response. The patients that showed no response to the treatment were 43 % in the rituximab and 54 % in the placebo group (p=0.18). There were more serious side-effects in the placebo group, 74/100 patient years vs. 43/100 patient years in the rituximab group. Greater improvements of complement levels (p=0.025) and antibodies to dsDNA (p=0.007) were recorded in the rituximab group compared to placebo [76].

The negative result of this study was surprising, but several potential reasons have been put forward. Rituximab was given in addition to other treatments that in normal circumstances would have been regarded as sufficient. In addition, the endpoints were quite strict and difficult to fulfil. There are plans for further studies on rituximab with different designs. This study along with another randomised study in lupus patients without renal involvement (the EXPLORER trial) [77] have not shown any severe side-effect profiles.

A further large case series on 164 adult patients with biopsy proven lupus nephritis showed a complete response, partial response and no response in about a third of the treated patients [78]. This together with the paediatric case series that show a good therapeutic response means that we continue to recommend the use of rituximab in certain situations, which include severe life-threatening disease and those patients with active disease despite standard treatment.

Different protocols have been used and our protocol involves two administrations of intravenous rituximab as an infusion of 750 mg/m^2 (rounded up to the nearest 100 mg with a maximum dose of 1 g) with 14 days in between. In addition, an intravenous dose of 100 mg methylprednisolone is given immediately prior to the rituximab infusion.

Plasma Exchange

We advocate the use of plasmapheresis in very severe and refractory cases of SLE with cerebral lupus and/or crescentic glomerulonephritis in which five to ten plasma exchanges seem to

Table 28.8 Maintenance therapy of lupus nephritis

Prednisolone (oral)	10–15 mg alternate or every day
Azathioprine (oral)	2–2.5 mg/kg once daily
Alternatively,	
Mycophenolate mofetil (oral)	Start dose of 250 mg/day to a maximum of 40 mg/kg/day (or 2–3 g/day) in two divided doses
Hydroxychloroquine (oral)	4–6 mg/kg/day
	Normal dose 200 mg once daily

be useful in acutely improving some patients [64]. However, this is a controversial area and a controlled trial in adult patients with severe lupus nephritis could not confirm any benefits from adding plasma exchange to the standard treatment of methylprednisolone and cyclophosphamide [79], which was confirmed in a meta-analysis [80].

Intravenous Immunoglobulin

Intravenous immunoglobulin (at a dose of 2 g/kg to a maximum of 70 g) can be useful particularly in children with severe haematological disease. Some children benefit from regular infusions, which can be administered repeatedly (such as every 6 weeks).

Maintenance Therapy

All cases of severe lupus require maintenance therapy for a long period of time, although the length of treatment is not well defined. We advocate maintenance therapy for at least 2–3 years and possibly indefinitely in many cases, especially those with active lupus nephritis.

Corticosteroids

After the initial rather rapid reduction of the oral corticosteroid, the prednisolone dose should be continuously weaned down more slowly. The clinical response will decide how quickly the dose can be reduced. Long-term treatment with corticosteroids for several years is often needed, although there are quite different approaches on preferred maintenance dose. Our opinion is that it is very important to reduce the dose as quickly as

possible. This is important to reduce side-effects, but also to improve compliance. Teenagers do not like the Cushingoid appearance they develop with corticosteroids so some stop taking their medications when the acute symptoms have abided. This can lead to non-compliance also with the other treatments. Our goal is to aim for an alternate day treatment at a dose in the order of 10–15 mg every other day or if possible to discontinue corticosteroids completely. These doses of prednisolone should allow the child to grow normally [81].

Mycophenolate Mofetil

Mycophenolate mofetil (MMF) is most likely the best choice for long-term maintenance therapy. After the 24 week induction part of the ALMS trial, 227 patients were randomised to 3 years of maintenance therapy with MMF (2 g/day) or azathioprine (2 mg/kg/day) [82]. In this study, MMF was shown to be superior to azathioprine with respect to the primary end-point, time to treatment failure; hazard ratio 0.44 (95 % CI 0.25–0.77; p=0.003). Treatment failure occurred in 16 % of the patients in the MMF group and 32 % in the azathioprine group. Serious adverse events occurred in 24 % of patients treated with MMF compared to 33 % treated with azathioprine and the withdrawal due to adverse events was significantly higher in the azathioprine group (40 % versus 25 %; p=0.02) [83].

MMF was also compared to azathioprine in the MAINTAIN trial [84]. In this study, 105 patients were treated with similar doses of azathioprine and MMF as in the maintenance phase of ALMS. There was a tendency to fewer renal flares in the MMF group but the number of patients was not high enough for this to achieve statistical significance.

Azathioprine

Azathioprine at a dose of 2–2.5 mg/kg/day has for a long time been first line maintenance therapy and has a generally favourable side-effect profile. In the comparison of azathioprine or mycophenolate mofetil used as maintenance therapy, see above, MMF was shown to be better than azathioprine [83, 84].

Hydroxychloroquine

The use of antimalarial drugs (such as hydroxy-chloroquine at a dose of 4–6 mg/kg/day) should be considered for all lupus patients. It is especially helpful in children with marked skin and/or lung disease, lethargy and arthritis. Hydroxychloroquine also seems to reduce blood lipids and possibly the risk for later atherosclerosis. A high dose of 10 mg/kg has been used in lung disease up to a total maximum dose of 400 mg/day.

Treatment of Antiphospholipid Syndrome (APS)

Treatment for APS includes reducing lupus disease activity and appropriate anticoagulation treatment (such as life-long aspirin or warfarin if severe thrombo-embolic disease).

General Renal Management

As outlined in other parts of this book, general renal care is important in all children with renal impairment. This includes monitoring and treatment of hypertension and proteinuria. It is important to continuously evaluate renal function of these children with estimated GFR and if appropriate a formal GFR measurement. Supportive treatment of chronic kidney disease is needed in some of these children.

General Management

Sun Protection

All children with SLE and especially those with active skin disease should be advised to always use appropriate sunscreen and protect themselves from the sun.

Immunisations

Children with SLE, treated with immunosuppressive drugs, should avoid immunisation with live vaccines. Vaccination with killed vaccines should be carefully considered as they might induce a flare of the disease and also might not be as effective as they normally would be. In the United Kingdom and in other countries, pneumococcal vaccinations are recommended for all patients likely to be on corticosteroids for more than a month.

Management of Infection

Children on immunosuppressive treatment are more susceptible to severe infections than other children and it should be emphasised to the parents and the children that they should seek medical advice early in the case of fever or symptoms of an infection.

Prognosis

In the era before treatment became available the prognosis of patients with SLE was very poor with very few patients with a severe nephritis surviving more than 2 years [85]. The introduction of corticosteroids and immunosuppressive treatment with cyclophosphamide and azathioprine has made a huge impact on the long-term prognosis. In a long-term follow-up study (mean of 11 years) of 67 patients with lupus nephritis from a single centre, 6% [4] children died and 9% [6] developed ESKD [59]. From the same centre with a follow-up (mean 9 years), there was a 97% survival of 201 children with SLE [46].

The acute and short to medium term mortality from SLE is now caused both by active disease and complications to the treatment. In recent years it has also become evident that patients with SLE face another important threat to their long-term survival with increased atherosclerosis.

Disease Related Complications and Mortality

Data compiled by Professor Cameron comparing outcomes from 1965 to 1979 and 1980–1991 showed that some 40% of the mortality in children with lupus nephritis was due to renal failure and infections, respectively, while the remaining 20% were caused by active disease in other organs (mainly the brain but also the lungs and heart) [44]. The proportion of children dying from their renal failure is now most likely lower with increasing use of effective therapies, although the prognostic factors for developing renal failure remain the same (male gender, non-Caucasian race, nephrotic syndrome at onset and severity of disease on renal biopsy [59]).

Treatment Related Complications and Mortality

In recent studies infections have been the main cause of death therefore suggesting that the most important short term goal is to find therapies which are as good as current treatments but with fewer side effects. Recent comparative studies in adults showed that cyclophosphamide treatment was associated with significantly more severe infections compared to treatment with azathioprine or MMF [65, 71–73]. This emphasises the importance of monitoring white cell and neutrophil counts during therapy and early treatment of infectious complications. However, infections can sometimes be difficult to differentiate from a flare of disease activity, especially in children who are in ESKD on renal replacement therapy. CRP can be used as a helpful tool in these situations as very few patients even with active lupus have raised CRP levels [44] while most children with septicaemia do.

Severe viral infections, in particular with varicella zoster virus are seen, and children exposed to the virus or with early symptoms of varicella (or more often herpes zoster virus) should be treated with aciclovir therapy to reduce the risk of generalised infection.

Growth failure is a major problem in children with lupus, which can be related to the inflammatory disease or a complication of corticosteroid treatment. Sometimes it can be difficult to differentiate between them and this is a controversial area but it is our opinion that ongoing inflammation more often causes the growth failure than the treatment with low corticosteroid doses. Therefore, increasing immunosuppression rather than reducing treatment is often more beneficial for the growth of these children.

SLE patients have an increased risk of osteoporosis partly caused by their long-term treatment with steroids [86]. Treatment with calcium and vitamin D is advocated from some centres, but unfortunately it seems as if the beneficial effects from that treatment only persist during the treatment itself [87]. However, an increased nutritional calcium intake does seem to be able to improve bone accretion over a longer time [88]. It is recommended that children with SLE should be monitored with regular bone density scans.

Children on long-term immunosuppressive treatment are regarded to have an increased risk for developing malignancies, in particular skin cancers and lymphoma and should be advised to use sun protection. Bladder cancer has been reported to be associated with the use of cyclophosphamide in children with SLE [89]. A 10 year follow up of a very large cohort of 1000 adult lupus patients found that 23 developed malignancies with breast and uterine cancers being the most common [90]. Therefore, the risk of malignancy does not seem to be excessive.

Active lupus often causes amenorrhoea and delayed puberty, whereas treatment with cyclophosphamide can also reduce fertility. A study of 39 women younger than 40 years old showed that 12.5 % (2 out of 16) receiving seven intravenous doses of cyclophosphamide developed sustained amenorrhoea compared to 39 % (9 out of 23) receiving 15 or more doses (with a higher risk in women older than 25 years) [91].

Thrombosis

In the aforementioned 10-year follow up of 1000 adult patients, 9.2 % [92] developed thrombosis and of the 68 patients who died, 26.5 % had a thrombotic event. This is more commonly occurring in children with antiphospholipid syndrome. A 10-year follow-up of 149 children with SLE from Toronto showed that 24 were positive for lupus anticoagulant and that 13 of them experienced 21 thrombo-embolic events [93]. The authors emphasised the need to treat this subgroup of children with life-long anticoagulation.

Cardiovascular Disease

A Swedish register study on 4737 patients with SLE from 1964 to 1994 showed a 16-fold increased risk of death from cardiovascular diseases [92]. Therefore, it is our new challenge to try to prevent atherosclerosis and to improve our patients' long-term survival. This increased risk for cardiovascular death is multifactorial and includes classical risk factors, such as hypertension, hyperlipidaemia and corticosteroid treatment and disease-related risk factors such as proteinuria, vasculitis, low-grade systemic inflammation, antiphospholipid syndrome and elevated levels of homocysteine [94].

Carotid plaque and coronary artery calcifications are significantly increased in lupus patients [95, 96]. The prevention of increased atherosclerosis includes good control of inflammation, aggressive treatment of any hypertension and proteinuria and efforts to prevent steroid-induced obesity. A randomised placebo controlled study on treatment with atorvastatin could not be shown to reduce progression of the surrogate marker for atherosclerosis carotid intima-media thickness [97]. The active treatment did, however, reduce levels of high sensitivity CRP and total cholesterol and low-density lipoprotein. A secondary analysis suggested that atorvastatin reduced atherosclerosis progression in paediatric lupus patients with higher CRP values [98]. Hydroxycholoroquine has been shown to have a beneficial influence on the cardiovascular risk profile [99].

Adherence to Treatment

One important prognostic factor in children with lupus nephritis, as in all our children with chronic kidney disease, is compliance with treatment, especially during puberty. Non-adherence in adolescents is a common reason for relapse of symptoms and sometimes an acute presentation with renal failure after initially successful treatment. In such serious clinical situations, we would advocate the use of intravenous therapies (with cyclophosphamide or mainly rituximab treatment, which can be given at six-monthly intervals irrespective of peripheral CD19 counts) instead of oral treatments to ensure adherence and disease control.

Renal Replacement Therapy

The gold standard therapy for patients with ESKD due to lupus nephritis is that of other conditions with renal transplantation, especially as they seem to do equally well compared to matched controls with less than 10 % recurrence of lupus nephritis and similar long-term patient and renal allograft survival [100]. It is advisable that patients should be in remission for 6 months prior to transplantation and that immunosuppression should be standard, unless immunological concerns. However, it should be noted that the risk for thrombo-embolic complications was higher in the SLE group. Patients with SLE can have peritoneal and/or haemodialysis prior to transplantation, but in view of hypocomplementaemia and immunosuppression, clinicians should be wary of clinical presentation of flare of disease activity (which can be difficult to diagnose) versus infectious complications. Patients on peritoneal dialysis presenting with peritonitis should be treated with intravenous and intraperitoneal antibiotics.

Conclusion

The prognosis for children with SLE has over the last decades improved with most children now able to look forward to long lives without debilitating symptoms. However, the first important challenge for the future is to find ways to minimise treatment related mortality and morbidity. This has made us use less cyclophosphamide which has been replaced by other less toxic drugs mainly MMF. Rituximab is also used in many centres in severe cases but further studies are needed to fully delineate its role. Another important challenge is to find ways to reduce the burden of future premature cardiovascular disease in these children.

References

1. Brunner HI, Silverman ED, To T, Bombardier C, Feldman BM. Risk factors for damage in childhood-onset systemic lupus erythematosus: cumulative disease activity and medication use predict disease damage. Arthritis Rheum. 2002;46(2):436–44.
2. Jimenez S, Cervera R, Font J, Ingelmo M. The epidemiology of systemic lupus erythematosus. Clin Rev Allergy Immunol. 2003;25(1):3–12.
3. Rood MJ, ten Cate R, Suijlekom-Smit LW, den Ouden EJ, Ouwerkerk FE, Breedveld FC, et al. Childhood-onset systemic lupus erythematosus: clinical presentation and prognosis in 31 patients. Scand J Rheumatol. 1999;28(4):222–6.
4. Tucker LB, Menon S, Schaller JG, Isenberg DA. Adult- and childhood-onset systemic lupus erythematosus: a comparison of onset, clinical features, serology, and outcome. Br J Rheumatol. 1995;34(9):866–72.
5. Schanberg LE, Sandborg C. Dyslipoproteinemia and premature atherosclerosis in pediatric systemic lupus erythematosus. Curr Rheumatol Rep. 2004;6(6):425–33.
6. Hochberg MC. Updating the American College of Rheumatology revised criteria for the classification of systemic lupus erythematosus. Arthritis Rheum. 1997;40(9):1725.
7. Tan EM, Cohen AS, Fries JF, Masi AT, McShane DJ, Rothfield NF, et al. The 1982 revised criteria for the classification of systemic lupus erythematosus. Arthritis Rheum. 1982;25(11):1271–7.
8. Malleson PN, Fung MY, Rosenberg AM. The incidence of pediatric rheumatic diseases: results from the Canadian Pediatric Rheumatology Association Disease Registry. J Rheumatol. 1996;23(11):1981–7.
9. Fessel WJ. Systemic lupus erythematosus in the community. Incidence, prevalence, outcome, and first symptoms; the high prevalence in black women. Arch Intern Med. 1974;134(6):1027–35.
10. Hochberg MC. Prevalence of systemic lupus erythematosus in England and Wales, 1981–2. Ann Rheum Dis. 1987;46(9):664–6.
11. Hochberg MC. Systemic lupus erythematosus. Rheum Dis Clin N Am. 1990;16(3):617–39.
12. Hopkinson ND, Doherty M, Powell RJ. The prevalence and incidence of systemic lupus erythematosus in Nottingham, UK, 1989–1990. Br J Rheumatol. 1993;32(2):110–5.
13. Hopkinson ND, Doherty M, Powell RJ. Clinical features and race-specific incidence/prevalence rates of systemic lupus erythematosus in a geographically complete cohort of patients. Ann Rheum Dis. 1994;53(10):675–80.
14. Johnson AE, Gordon C, Palmer RG, Bacon PA. The prevalence and incidence of systemic lupus erythematosus in Birmingham, England. Relationship to ethnicity and country of birth. Arthritis Rheum. 1995;38(4):551–8.
15. Nived O, Sturfelt G, Wollheim F. Systemic lupus erythematosus in an adult population in southern Sweden: incidence, prevalence and validity of ARA revised classification criteria. Br J Rheumatol. 1985;24(2):147–54.
16. Siegel M, Lee SL. The epidemiology of systemic lupus erythematosus. Semin Arthritis Rheum. 1973;3(1):1–54.
17. Citera G, Wilson WA. Ethnic and geographic perspectives in SLE. Lupus. 1993;2(6):351–3.
18. Symmons DP. Frequency of lupus in people of African origin. Lupus. 1995;4(3):176–8.
19. Vyas S, Hidalgo G, Baqi N, Von Gizyki H, Singh A. Outcome in African-American children of neuropsychiatric lupus and lupus nephritis. Pediatr Nephrol. 2002;17(1):45–9.
20. Gardner-Medwin JM, Dolezalova P, Cummins C, Southwood TR. Incidence of Henoch-Schonlein purpura, Kawasaki disease, and rare vasculitides in children of different ethnic origins. Lancet. 2002;360(9341):1197–202.
21. Lahita RG. Sex hormones and systemic lupus erythematosus. Rheum Dis Clin N Am. 2000;26(4):951–68.
22. McMurray RW. Sex hormones in the pathogenesis of systemic lupus erythematosus. Front Biosci. 2001;6:E193–206.
23. Kyttaris VC, Katsiari CG, Juang YT, Tsokos GC. New insights into the pathogenesis of systemic lupus erythematosus. Curr Rheumatol Rep. 2005;7(6):469–75.
24. Arbuckle MR, McClain MT, Rubertone MV, Scofield RH, Dennis GJ, James JA, et al. Development of autoantibodies before the clinical onset of systemic lupus erythematosus. N Engl J Med. 2003;349(16):1526–33.
25. Deapen D, Escalante A, Weinrib L, Horwitz D, Bachman B, Roy-Burman P, et al. A revised estimate of twin concordance in systemic lupus erythematosus. Arthritis Rheum. 1992;35(3):311–8.
26. Kelly JA, Moser KL, Harley JB. The genetics of systemic lupus erythematosus: putting the pieces together. Genes Immun. 2002;3 Suppl 1:S71–85.
27. Manderson AP, Botto M, Walport MJ. The role of complement in the development of systemic lupus erythematosus. Annu Rev Immunol. 2004;22:431–56.
28. Tsao BP. The genetics of human systemic lupus erythematosus. Trends Immunol. 2003;24(11):595–602.
29. Pickering MC, Botto M, Taylor PR, Lachmann PJ, Walport MJ. Systemic lupus erythematosus, complement deficiency, and apoptosis. Adv Immunol. 2000;76:227–324.
30. Seelen MA, Trouw LA, Daha MR. Diagnostic and prognostic significance of anti-C1q antibodies in systemic lupus erythematosus. Curr Opin Nephrol Hypertens. 2003;12(6):619–24.
31. Trouw LA, Groeneveld TW, Seelen MA, Duijs JM, Bajema IM, Prins FA, et al. Anti-C1q autoantibodies deposit in glomeruli but are only pathogenic in com-

bination with glomerular C1q-containing immune complexes. J Clin Invest. 2004;114(5):679–88.

32. Odendahl M, Jacobi A, Hansen A, Feist E, Hiepe F, Burmester GR, et al. Disturbed peripheral B lymphocyte homeostasis in systemic lupus erythematosus. J Immunol. 2000;165(10):5970–9.

33. Tangye SG, Liu YJ, Aversa G, Phillips JH, de Vries JE. Identification of functional human splenic memory B cells by expression of CD148 and CD27. J Exp Med. 1998;188(9):1691–703.

34. Leandro MJ, Cambridge G, Edwards JC, Ehrenstein MR, Isenberg DA. B-cell depletion in the treatment of patients with systemic lupus erythematosus: a longitudinal analysis of 24 patients. Rheumatology (Oxford). 2005;44(12):1542–5.

35. Marks SD, Patey S, Brogan PA, Hasson N, Pilkington C, Woo P, et al. B lymphocyte depletion therapy in children with refractory systemic lupus erythematosus. Arthritis Rheum. 2005;52(10):3168–74.

36. Shlomchik MJ, Craft JE, Mamula MJ. From T to B and back again: positive feedback in systemic autoimmune disease. Nat Rev Immunol. 2001;1(2):147–53.

37. Tsokos GC, Nambiar MP, Tenbrock K, Juang YT. Rewiring the T-cell: signaling defects and novel prospects for the treatment of SLE. Trends Immunol. 2003;24(5):259–63.

38. Tsokos GC, Mitchell JP, Juang YT. T cell abnormalities in human and mouse lupus: intrinsic and extrinsic. Curr Opin Rheumatol. 2003;15(5):542–7.

39. Grondal G, Gunnarsson I, Ronnelid J, Rogberg S, Klareskog L, Lundberg I. Cytokine production, serum levels and disease activity in systemic lupus erythematosus. Clin Exp Rheumatol. 2000;18(5):565–70.

40. Casciola-Rosen L, Andrade F, Ulanet D, Wong WB, Rosen A. Cleavage by granzyme B is strongly predictive of autoantigen status: implications for initiation of autoimmunity. J Exp Med. 1999;190(6):815–26.

41. Cooper GS, Parks CG. Occupational and environmental exposures as risk factors for systemic lupus erythematosus. Curr Rheumatol Rep. 2004;6(5): 367–74.

42. Incaprera M, Rindi L, Bazzichi A, Garzelli C. Potential role of the Epstein-Barr virus in systemic lupus erythematosus autoimmunity. Clin Exp Rheumatol. 1998;16(3):289–94.

43. Moon UY, Park SJ, Oh ST, Kim WU, Park SH, Lee SH, et al. Patients with systemic lupus erythematosus have abnormally elevated Epstein-Barr virus load in blood. Arthritis Res Ther. 2004;6(4):R295–302.

44. Cameron JS. Lupus nephritis in childhood and adolescence. Pediatr Nephrol. 1994;8(2):230–49.

45. Iqbal S, Sher MR, Good RA, Cawkwell GD. Diversity in presenting manifestations of systemic lupus erythematosus in children. J Pediatr. 1999;135(4):500–5.

46. Marks SD, Hiraki L, Hagelberg S, Silverman ED, Hebert D. Age-related renal prognosis of childhood-onset SLE. Pediatr Nephrol. 2002;17(9):C107.

47. Lee T, von Scheven E, Sandborg C. Systemic lupus erythematosus and antiphospholipid syndrome in children and adolescents. Curr Opin Rheumatol. 2001;13(5):415–21.

48. Petri M, Orbai AM, Alarcon GS, Gordon C, Merrill JT, Fortin PR, et al. Derivation and validation of the Systemic Lupus International Collaborating Clinics classification criteria for systemic lupus erythematosus. Arthritis Rheum. 2012;64(8):2677–86.

49. Sag E, Tartaglione A, Batu ED, Ravelli A, Khalil SM, Marks SD, et al. Performance of the new SLICC classification criteria in childhood systemic lupus erythematosus: a multicentre study. Clin Exp Rheumatol. 2014;32(3):440–4.

50. Marks SD, Pilkington C, Woo P, Dillon MJ. The use of the British Isles Lupus Assessment Group (BILAG) index as a valid tool in assessing disease activity in childhood-onset systemic lupus erythematosus. Rheumatology (Oxford). 2004;43(9): 1186–9.

51. Schwartz GJ, Munoz A, Schneider MF, Mak RH, Kaskel F, Warady BA, et al. New equations to estimate GFR in children with CKD. J Am Soc Nephrol. 2009;20(3):629–37.

52. Marto N, Bertolaccini ML, Calabuig E, Hughes GR, Khamashta MA. Anti-C1q antibodies in nephritis: correlation between titres and renal disease activity and positive predictive value in systemic lupus erythematosus. Ann Rheum Dis. 2005;64(3):444–8.

53. Marks SD, Shah V, Pilkington C, Woo P, Dillon MJ. Renal tubular dysfunction in children with systemic lupus erythematosus. Pediatr Nephrol. 2005;20(2):141–8.

54. Weening JJ, D'Agati VD, Schwartz MM, Seshan SV, Alpers CE, Appel GB, et al. The classification of glomerulonephritis in systemic lupus erythematosus revisited. Kidney Int. 2004;65(2):521–30.

55. Weening JJ, D'Agati VD, Schwartz MM, Seshan SV, Alpers CE, Appel GB, et al. The classification of glomerulonephritis in systemic lupus erythematosus revisited. J Am Soc Nephrol. 2004;15(2):241–50.

56. Marks SD, Tullus K, Sebire NJ. Currrent Issues in pediatric lupus nephritis: role of revised histopathological classification. Fetal Pediatr Pathol. 2006;25(6):297–309.

57. Austin III HA, Muenz LR, Joyce KM, Antonovych TA, Kullick ME, Klippel JH, et al. Prognostic factors in lupus nephritis. Contribution of renal histologic data. Am J Med. 1983;75(3):382–91.

58. Yokoyama H, Wada T, Hara A, Yamahana J, Nakaya I, Kobayashi M, et al. The outcome and a new ISN/RPS 2003 classification of lupus nephritis in Japanese. Kidney Int. 2004;66(6):2382–8.

59. Hagelberg S, Lee Y, Bargman J, Mah G, Schneider R, Laskin C, et al. Longterm followup of childhood lupus nephritis. J Rheumatol. 2002;29(12): 2635–42.

60. Marks SD, Sebire NJ, Pilkington C, Tullus K. Clinicopathological correlations of paediatric lupus nephritis. Pediatr Nephrol. 2007;22(1):77–83.

61. Bertsias GK, Tektonidou M, Amoura Z, Aringer M, Bajema I, Berden JH, et al. Joint European League Against Rheumatism and European Renal Association-European Dialysis and Transplant Association (EULAR/ERA-EDTA) recommendations for the management of adult and paediatric lupus nephritis. Ann Rheum Dis. 2012;71(11):1771–82.

62. Mina R, von Scheven E, Ardoin SP, Eberhard BA, Punaro M, Ilowite N, et al. Consensus treatment plans for induction therapy of newly diagnosed proliferative lupus nephritis in juvenile systemic lupus erythematosus. Arthritis Care Res (Hoboken). 2012;64(3):375–83.

63. Tullus K. New developments in the treatment of systemic lupus erythematosus. Pediatr Nephrol. 2012;27(5):727–32.

64. Wright EC, Tullus K, Dillon MJ. Retrospective study of plasma exchange in children with systemic lupus erythematosus. Pediatr Nephrol. 2004;19(10): 1108–14.

65. Chan TM, Li FK, Tang CS, Wong RW, Fang GX, Ji YL, et al. Efficacy of mycophenolate mofetil in patients with diffuse proliferative lupus nephritis. Hong Kong-Guangzhou Nephrology Study Group. N Engl J Med. 2000;343(16):1156–62.

66. Appel GB, Contreras G, Dooley MA, Ginzler EM, Isenberg D, Jayne D, et al. Mycophenolate mofetil versus cyclophosphamide for induction treatment of lupus nephritis. J Am Soc Nephrol. 2009;20(5): 1103–12.

67. Isenberg D, Appel GB, Contreras G, Dooley MA, Ginzler EM, Jayne D, et al. Influence of race/ethnicity on response to lupus nephritis treatment: the ALMS study. Rheumatology (Oxford). 2010;49(1):128–40.

68. Radhakrishnan J, Moutzouris DA, Ginzler EM, Solomons N, Siempos II, Appel GB. Mycophenolate mofetil and intravenous cyclophosphamide are similar as induction therapy for class V lupus nephritis. Kidney Int. 2010;77(2):152–60.

69. Touma Z, Gladman DD, Urowitz MB, Beyene J, Uleryk EM, Shah PS. Mycophenolate mofetil for induction treatment of lupus nephritis: a systematic review and metaanalysis. J Rheumatol. 2011;38(1): 69–78.

70. Kazyra I, Pilkington C, Marks SD, Tullus K. Mycophenolate mofetil treatment in children and adolescents with lupus. Arch Dis Child. 2010;95(12):1059–61.

71. Chan TM, Tse KC, Tang CS, Mok MY, Li FK. Long-term study of mycophenolate mofetil as continuous induction and maintenance treatment for diffuse proliferative lupus nephritis. J Am Soc Nephrol. 2005;16(4):1076–84.

72. Contreras G, Pardo V, Leclercq B, Lenz O, Tozman E, O'Nan P, et al. Sequential therapies for proliferative lupus nephritis. N Engl J Med. 2004;350(10):971–80.

73. Ginzler EM, Dooley MA, Aranow C, Kim MY, Buyon J, Merrill JT, et al. Mycophenolate mofetil or intravenous cyclophosphamide for lupus nephritis. N Engl J Med. 2005;353(21):2219–28.

74. Marks SD, Tullus K. Successful outcomes with rituximab therapy for refractory childhood systemic lupus erythematosus. Pediatr Nephrol. 2006;21(4): 598–9.

75. Rovin BH, Furie R, Latinis K, Looney RJ, Fervenza FC, Sanchez-Guerrero J, et al. Efficacy and safety of rituximab in patients with active proliferative lupus nephritis: the lupus nephritis assessment with rituximab (LUNAR) study. Arthritis Rheum. 2012;64(4):1215–26.

76. Furie R, Rovin B, Appel G, Kamen D, Fervenza F, Spindler A, et al. Effect of rituximab on anti-double-stranded DNA antibody and C3 levels and relationship to response: results from the LUNAR trial. 9th International Congress on Systemic Lupus Erythematosus, Vancouver, June 24–27, Poster PO2 E 22 2010.

77. Merrill JT, Neuwelt CM, Wallace DJ, Shanahan JC, Latinis KM, Oates JC, et al. Efficacy and safety of rituximab in moderately-to-severely active systemic lupus erythematosus: the randomized, double-blind, phase II/III systemic lupus erythematosus evaluation of rituximab trial. Arthritis Rheum. 2010;62(1):222–33.

78. Diaz-Lagares C, Croca S, Sangle S, Vital EM, Catapano F, Martinez-Berriotxoa A, et al. Efficacy of rituximab in 164 patients with biopsy-proven lupus nephritis: pooled data from European cohorts. Autoimmun Rev. 2012;11(5):357–64.

79. Lewis EJ, Hunsicker LG, Lan SP, Rohde RD, Lachin JM. A controlled trial of plasmapheresis therapy in severe lupus nephritis. The Lupus Nephritis Collaborative Study Group. N Engl J Med. 1992; 326(21):1373–9.

80. Flanc RS, Roberts MA, Strippoli GF, Chadban SJ, Kerr PG, Atkins RC. Treatment for lupus nephritis. Cochrane Database Syst Rev. 2004;(1):CD002922.

81. Simmonds J, Trompeter R, Calvert T, Tullus K. Does long-term steroid use influence long-term growth? Pediatr Nephrol. 2005;20:C107.

82. Wofsy D, Appel GB, Dooley M, Ginzler E, Isenberg D, Jayne D, et al. Aspreva lupus management study ALMS) maintenance results. 9th International Congress on Systemic Lupus Erythematosus, Vancouver, June 24–27, Poster PO2 E23 2010.

83. Dooley MA, Jayne D, Ginzler EM, Isenberg D, Olsen NJ, Wofsy D, et al. Mycophenolate versus azathioprine as maintenance therapy for lupus nephritis. N Engl J Med. 2011;365(20):1886–95.

84. Houssiau FA, D'Cruz D, Sangle S, Remy P, Vasconcelos C, Petrovic R, et al. Azathioprine versus mycophenolate mofetil for long-term immunosuppression in lupus nephritis: results from the MAINTAIN Nephritis Trial. Ann Rheum Dis. 2010;69(12):2083–9.

85. Zetterstrom R, Berglund G. Systemic lupus erythematosus in childhood; a clinical study. Acta Paediatr. 1956;45(2):189–204.

86. Lee C, Ramsey-Goldman R. Bone health and systemic lupus erythematosus. Curr Rheumatol Rep. 2005;7(6):482–9.

87. Lee WT, Leung SS, Leung DM, Cheng JC. A follow-up study on the effects of calcium-supplement withdrawal and puberty on bone acquisition of children. Am J Clin Nutr. 1996;64(1):71–7.

88. Stark LJ, Davis AM, Janicke DM, Mackner LM, Hommel KA, Bean JA, et al. A randomized clinical trial of dietary calcium to improve bone accretion in children with juvenile rheumatoid arthritis. J Pediatr. 2006;148(4):501–7.

89. Alivizatos G, Dimopoulou I, Mitropoulos D, Dimopoulos AM, Koufakis I, Lykourinas M. Bladder cancer in a young girl with systemic lupus erythematosus treated with cyclophosphamide. Acta Urol Belg. 1991;59(1):133–7.

90. Cervera R, Khamashta MA, Font J, Sebastiani GD, Gil A, Lavilla P, et al. Morbidity and mortality in systemic lupus erythematosus during a 10-year period: a comparison of early and late manifestations in a cohort of 1,000 patients. Medicine (Baltimore). 2003;82(5):299–308.

91. Langevitz P, Klein L, Pras M, Many A. The effect of cyclophosphamide pulses on fertility in patients with lupus nephritis. Am J Reprod Immunol. 1992;28(3–4):157–8.

92. Bjornadal L, Baecklund E, Yin L, Granath F, Klareskog L, Ekbom A. Decreasing mortality in patients with rheumatoid arthritis: results from a large population based cohort in Sweden, 1964–95. J Rheumatol. 2002;29(5):906–12.

93. Levy DM, Massicotte MP, Harvey E, Hebert D, Silverman ED. Thromboembolism in paediatric lupus patients. Lupus. 2003;12(10):741–6.

94. Barsalou J, Bradley TJ, Silverman ED. Cardiovascular risk in pediatric-onset rheumatological diseases. Arthritis Res Ther. 2013;15(3):212.

95. Asanuma Y, Oeser A, Shintani AK, Turner E, Olsen N, Fazio S, et al. Premature coronary-artery atherosclerosis in systemic lupus erythematosus. N Engl J Med. 2003;349(25):2407–15.

96. Roman MJ, Shanker BA, Davis A, Lockshin MD, Sammaritano L, Simantov R, et al. Prevalence and correlates of accelerated atherosclerosis in systemic lupus erythematosus. N Engl J Med. 2003;349(25):2399–406.

97. Schanberg LE, Sandborg C, Barnhart HX, Ardoin SP, Yow E, Evans GW, et al. Use of atorvastatin in systemic lupus erythematosus in children and adolescents. Arthritis Rheum. 2012;64(1):285–96.

98. Ardoin SP, Schanberg LE, Sandborg CI, Barnhart HX, Evans GW, Yow E, et al. Secondary analysis of APPLE study suggests atorvastatin may reduce atherosclerosis progression in pubertal lupus patients with higher C reactive protein. Ann Rheum Dis. 2014;73(3):557–66.

99. Wallace DJ, Metzger AL, Stecher VJ, Turnbull BA, Kern PA. Cholesterol-lowering effect of hydroxychloroquine in patients with rheumatic disease: reversal of deleterious effects of steroids on lipids. Am J Med. 1990;89(3):322–6.

100. Moroni G, Tantardini F, Gallelli B, Quaglini S, Banfi G, Poli F, et al. The long-term prognosis of renal transplantation in patients with lupus nephritis. Am J Kidney Dis. 2005;45(5):903–11.

Jae Il Shin

Abbreviations

ACE	Angiotensin converting enzyme
ACR	American College of Rheumatology
ANCA	Anti-neutrophil cytoplasmic antibody
ARB	Angiotensin receptor blockers
CKD	Chronic kidney disease
ECP	Eosinophil cationic protein
ESRD	End stage renal disease
EULAR	European League Against Rheumatism
HLA	Human leukocyte antigen
HSP	Henoch-Schönlein purpura
HSPN	Henoch-Schönlein purpura nephritis
IgA	Immunoglobulin A
IgAN	IgA nephropathy
IL	Interleukin
ISKDC	International Study of Kidney Disease in Children
KDIGO	Kidney Disease Improving Global Outcome
MBL	Mannose-binding lectin
MP	Methylprednisolone
PRES	Paediatric Rheumatology European Society
RAS	Renin angiotensin system
RCTs	Randomized controlled trials
TGF	Transforming growth factor
TNF	Tumor necrosis factor
vWF	von Willebrand factor

J.I. Shin
Department of Pediatrics, Severance Children's
Hospital, Institute of Kidney Disease Research,
Yonsei University College of Medicine,
Yonsei-Ro 50, Seodaemun-Ku, C.P.O. Box 8044,
Seoul 120-752, South Korea
e-mail: shinji@yuhs.ac

Introduction

Henoch-Schönlein purpura (HSP) was first described by William Heberden [1], a London physician, in 1801 and was named after the description of the clinical entity characterized by purpura and joint pain by Johann Schönlein in 1837 [2] and of the frequent association of gastrointestinal symptoms and kidney involvement by Edouard Henoch in 1874 [3]. HSP is the most common form of IgA-mediated systemic vasculitis in children; it mainly affects the skin, joints, gastrointestinal tract and kidney. HSP is usually self-limited in 1–4 weeks, but relapses can occur. The overall prognosis of HSP is favorable, but the long-term prognosis is dependent on the degree of renal involvement [4, 5].

Diagnostic Criteria

The American College of Rheumatology (ACR) proposed in 1990 that the presence of any two or more of the following criteria was required for the diagnosis of HSP: (1) an age of less than 20 years at disease onset, (2) palpable purpura, (3) acute abdominal pain, and (4) biopsy showing granulocytes in the walls of small arterioles or venules [6]. In 2005, the diagnostic criteria for HSP were modified by the European League Against Rheumatism/Paediatric Rheumatology European Society (EULAR/PRES) [7]. In this new diagnostic system, the age criterion was deleted, "predominant IgA deposition" was included in the definition of the "biopsy" criterion, and arthritis and renal involvement were added as independent criteria [7]. Therefore, HSP is diagnosed as follows: palpable purpura (mandatory criterion) in the presence of at least one of the following four features: (1) diffuse abdominal pain, (2) any biopsy showing predominant IgA deposition, (3) arthritis or arthralgia (acute, any joint), and (4) renal involvement (any hematuria and/or proteinuria) [7]. Skin biopsy is rarely performed to diagnose HSP, but may be necessary in doubtful cases such as isolated purpura or atypical characteristics to differentiate from leukocytoclastic vasculitis. The latter will show no IgA deposits [7, 8].

Epidemiology

The prevalence of HSP varies from 3.0/100,000 to 26.7/100,000 children [9, 10]. HSP is more common in preschool aged children and in males and there seems to be an increased frequency in autumn and winter. The pathogenesis of HSP is unclear, but it is considered as a complex disease caused by various genetic and triggering environmental factors [9]. Although the exact etiology of HSP is still obscure, it is often preceded by an upper respiratory tract infection 1–3 weeks prior to the onset of symptoms. Various infectious agents, such as parvovirus B19, hepatitis B and C virus, adenovirus, Group A β-hemolytic streptococcus, staphylococcus aureus, and mycoplasma, and various drugs, vaccinations, cancers, insect bites or exposure to cold weather have been reported as triggering factors for HSP [9, 10]. Familial cases of HSP have also been reported [11].

Clinical Findings

Skin

Palpable purpura is the most common finding, but petechiae, maculae, papulae, urticaria, ecchymosis or bullae can also occur. Skin lesions are generally distributed symmetrically over the extensor surfaces of the lower legs (gravity or pressure-dependent areas) and arms and buttocks, but trunk, face, eyelids, earlobes and genitalia can also be involved [12]. In young children, edema of scalp and hands or feet can be observed. The skin rash usually resolves within 1–2 weeks, but persistent purpura (>4 weeks) or relapsing rashes are observed in about 25 % of children with HSP, and may be associated with the occurrence and severity of renal involvement [13–15].

Joints

Joint symptoms can occur in about 80 % of children with HSP and large joints of the lower extremities, such as ankle and knee, are usually affected [12, 16]. Joint pain is a frequent finding and periarticular swelling and tenderness, usually without synovial fluid effusion, may be present. Joint symptoms resolve with time without any deformity or erosions [12].

Gastrointestinal Tract

Gastrointestinal involvement is reported in about 50–70 % of children with HSP and is usually presented with diffuse abdominal pain, which can be increased after meals, and nausea, vomiting, and bloody stools such as melaena and hematochezia [12, 16, 17]. Gastrointestinal symptoms are caused by bowel wall edema and submucosal hemorrhage due to vasculitis. Severe gastrointestinal complications can occur as intussusception, bowel infarction, gangrene or bowel perforation, duodenal obstruction and massive gastrointestinal hemorrhage requiring blood transfusion, appendicitis, pancreatitis, hydrops of the gall bladder, protein losing enteropathy and formation of the fistula or strictures.

Other Nonrenal Organ Involvement

Although rare, HSP can be complicated by various nonrenal manifestations, such as neurologic symptoms (obtundation, seizure, paresis, cortical blindness, chorea, ataxia and cranial or peripheral neuropathy), urologic manifestations (orchitis, epididymitis, and stenosing ureteritis, presenting as renal colic), carditis, myositis or intramuscular bleeding, pulmonary hemorrhage, and anterior uveitis [18]. Because some of these manifestations can be rapidly fatal, close observation and monitoring of affected patients is important.

Kidney

The incidence of renal involvement in HSP varies from 20 to 80 % in published case series [13–15]. Renal involvement includes isolated haematuria (14 %), isolated proteinuria (9 %), both hematuria and proteinuria (56 %), nephrotic-range proteinuria (20 %) and nephrotic-nephritic syndrome (1 %) [15]. Hypertension may develop at the onset of disease or during recovery, even in the condition of normal or minimal urinary abnormalities [19]. The first urinary abnormalities are detected within 4 weeks of disease onset in 80 % of children with HSP and within the next 2 months in the remainder, although a small number of patients present with urinary abnormalities several months later or as the initial feature [20]. Minor urinary abnormalities usually resolve with time, whereas severe renal involvement such as nephrotic syndrome and acute nephritic syndrome, can progress to chronic kidney disease. In a systematic review of 1133 children with HSP observed in 12 studies, the overall incidence of long-term renal impairment (as defined by persistent nephrotic syndrome, nephritis, or hypertension) was 1.8 %. Permanent renal impairment occurred in none of the 65.8 % children with normal urinalysis during the acute disease, in 1.6 % of the 26.9 % with isolated haematuria and/or proteinuria, and in 19.5 % of the 7.2 % patients initially presenting with nephritic or nephrotic syndrome [20].

Risk Factors for Renal Involvement

Some authors reported that an older age at onset, persistent purpura (>4 weeks), severe abdominal symptoms, decreased factor XIII (fibrin stabilizing factor) activity and a relapsing disease pattern to be significant risk factors for renal involvement in children with HSP and these factors were linked to each other and all indicated a severe disease course [13–15]. Also, persistent purpura, severe abdominal symptoms, and relapse were associated with the development of significant proteinuria [14].

Atypical Presentation

HSP is diagnosed clinically, but atypical presentation often causes difficulties in the diagnosis of HSP. Gastrointestinal symptoms precede the cutaneous rash in about 25 % of children with HSP [17] and joint symptoms or scrotal pain may precede the skin rash [16, 17]. In addition, some diseases such as systemic lupus erythematosus, microscopic polyangiitis or Crohn's disease can mimic HSP [21]. Since atypical presentation of HSP can lead to an incorrect diagnosis causing unnecessary therapies and procedures (e.g., appendectomy) and unfavorable outcomes, it is important to include HSP in the list of differential diagnoses, although diagnostic ascertainment can be very difficult in those settings.

Laboratory and Radiologic Investigations

Because HSP is diagnosed clinically, there is no specific diagnostic test for HSP. Recommended initial investigations are complete blood count for checking anemia or leukocytosis, erythrocyte sedimentation rate for evaluating inflammation, clotting profile for excluding other bleeding disorders, biochemical profile for evaluating renal failure or hypoalbuminemia, anti-streptolysin O titer, urine dipstick and protein/creatinine ratio for evaluating renal involvement and screening for sepsis (e.g., blood culture for meningococcemia), if diagnosis is unclear and purpura is present [22]. Antinuclear antibodies, double-stranded DNA, antineutrophil cytoplasmic antibody (ANCA), complements (C3 and C4) and immunoglobulins (IgG, IgA and IgM) may also be necessary to differentiate HSP from other vasculitis or overlapping diseases.

HSP has a bleeding tendency due to abnormal platelet aggregation, decreased factor XIII levels by vasculitic process and increased von Willebrand factor (vWF) levels by endothelial injury despite normal platelet count and clotting factors [23, 24]. Plasma D-dimer levels can be increased [24]. A stool test for occult blood can be used to detect gastrointestinal hemorrhage.

Serum IgA levels (mostly IgA1) are increased in 50 % of children with HSP and IgA-rheumatoid factor, IgA-containing immune complexes, IgA-fibronectin aggregates and cryoglobulins have been found [25, 26]. Serum IgE and eosinophil cationic protein (ECP) levels can be elevated [27, 28] and C3, C4, and CH50 levels are occasionally decreased in the acute stage of disease [29]. ANCAs (c-ANCA and p-ANCA) are generally negative in HSP except some cases [30, 31], but IgA-ANCA has been detected in the acute stage of disease [32, 33] and antiphospholipid antibodies may be positive [34].

Imaging studies may be necessary to detect complications of HSP according to the symptoms [22]. Chest and abdominal X-ray can be done to detect pulmonary involvement or ileus or perforation of gastrointestinal tract in HSP. Renal ultrasound can detect increased echogenicity of kidneys or hydronephrosis and abdominal ultrasound can detect thickened bowel wall or intussusception [22].

Renal Histopathologic Findings

Light Microscopy Findings

The light microscopic findings of HSPN are characterized by mesangial proliferative glomerulonephritis with varying degrees of mesangial hypercellularity (Fig. 29.1a), seg-mental sclerosis (Fig. 29.1b) and crescents (Fig. 29.1c), similar to the predominant findings in IgA nephropathy (IgAN) [35, 36]. These glomerular changes are usually graded by the percentage of crescents involved according to the ISKDC classification system (Table 29.1) [37]. Crescents are reportedly much more common in HSPN than in IgAN [25] and are frequently seen in association with capillary wall destruction and endocapillary cell proliferation by subendothelial immune deposits of IgA and complement [38]. Crescents are classified as cellular, fibrocellular and fibrous. Crescents are cellular at the onset of the disease and evolve with time towards a fibrous phenotype, causing global glomerulosclerosis (Fig. 29.1d).

Because the ISKDC grading does not include tubulointerstitial changes and other various histologic features in HSPN, some authors have used histopathologic scoring systems, such as activity and chronicity scores [39, 40]. Acute changes include mesangial matrix increase, mesangial hypercellularity, endothelial swelling, hyalinosis, basement membrane adhesion to Bowman's capsule, glomerular lobulations, glomerular neutrophils, fibrinoid necrosis, nuclear debris, interstitial vasculitis with leukocytoclastic reaction, tubular damage, interstitial edema and interstitial mononuclear infiltrate [39]. Chronic changes include interstitial fibrosis and tubular atrophy (Fig. 29.5), fibrous crescents, global sclerosis and vascular hyalinosis and intimal hyperplasia [39]. The degree of tubulointerstitial lesions is correlated with the glomerular pathology [35].

Immunofluorescence Findings

Granular deposits of IgA (predominantly IgA1) in mesangial areas are characteristic of HSPN (Fig. 29.2a). The IgA deposits are diffuse in contrast to the frequent focal and segmental changes of glomeruli. C3 (Fig. 29.2b) and the alternative complement pathway components are frequently found, but the factors of classic complement pathway, such as C1q and C4, are rarely detected [38, 41].

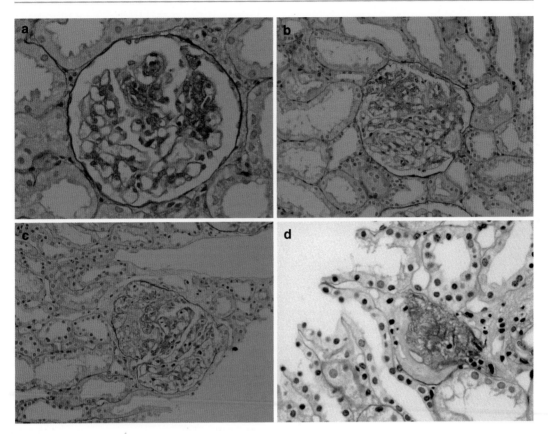

Fig. 29.1 Light microscopy findings in Henoch Schönlein purpura nephritis. (**a**) Mild mesangial cell proliferation (PAS, ×400). (**b**) Glomerulus with segmental sclerosis (PAS, ×200). (**c**) Glomerulus with cellular crescent (PAS, ×200). (**d**) Glomerulus with global sclerosis (PAS, ×400)

Table 29.1 The classification of the ISKDC in Henoch-Schönlein purpura nephritis

Grade I		Minimal alterations
Grade II		Mesangial proliferation without crescents
Grade III	IIIa	Focal mesangial proliferation or sclerosis with <50 % crescents
	IIIb	Diffuse mesangial proliferation or sclerosis with <50 % crescents
Grade IV	IVa	Focal mesangial proliferation or sclerosis with 50–75 % crescents
	IVb	Diffuse mesangial proliferation or sclerosis with 50–75 % crescents
Grade V	Va	Focal mesangial proliferation or sclerosis with >75 % crescents
	Vb	Diffuse mesangial proliferation or sclerosis with >75 % crescents
Grade VI		Membranoproliferative glomerulonephritis

IgA and C3 can be deposited in arterioles and capillary walls [25, 36, 38]. The deposits of IgG or IgM are less frequently detected [38, 42]. Glomerular fibrin deposits (Fig. 29.2c) are more frequently found in HSPN than in IgAN [25, 38] and are associated with the formation of crescents.

Electron Microscopy Findings

Electron-dense deposits are mainly found in mesangial areas (Fig. 29.3a), but the deposits can be detected in subendothelial areas (Fig. 29.3b) and rarely, hump-like deposits are found in subepithelial areas [25, 35, 41]. There are varying degrees of foot process effacement of visceral epithelial cells, depending on the degree of glomerular injury [25, 35, 41].

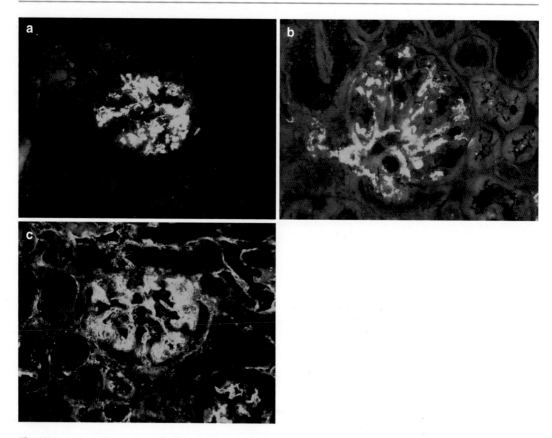

Fig. 29.2 Immunofluorescence findings in Henoch Schönlein purpura nephritis. (**a**) Mesangial IgA deposition (×100). (**b**) Mesangial C3 deposition (×200). (**c**) Mesangial fibrinogen deposition (×100)

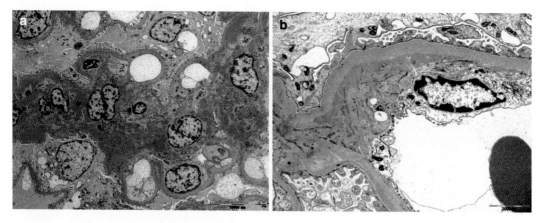

Fig. 29.3 Electron microscopy findings in Henoch Schönlein purpura nephritis. (**a**) Electron dense deposits in mesangial areas (×3000). (**b**) Electron-dense deposits in subendothelial areas (×10,000)

Clinicopathologic Correlations

In general a good correlation between the severity of renal involvement and pathologic grading is observed in HSPN and the severity of proteinuria at onset is a significant determinant of renal pathologic findings such as crescent formation, endocapillary proliferation, and tubular atrophy

[43]. Proteinuria is also correlated with the ISKDC grade [44]; however, even mild to moderate proteinuria may be associated with severe morphological changes [44]. Hence, renal biopsy may be indicated not only in patients with nephrotic syndrome, but also in those with mild proteinuria.

Although there are few reports on follow-up renal biopsies in HSPN, there is also a generally good correlation between the clinical course and histopathologic changes [45]. HSPN children who achieve clinical remission show a decrease in IgA deposits and regression of mesangial proliferation or crescents on follow-up renal biopsy, while those who have persistent nephritis demonstrate severe histologic findings with chronic lesions [45]. However, some reports emphasized that abnormal renal histologic findings can persist despite clinical remission [46, 47]. Algoet et al. reported that renal histologic findings were normal only in one of the four patients who had achieved complete clinical remission 5–9 years after the onset of HSP [46]. Shin et al. also showed persistent histologic abnormalities in all patients of a HSPN cohort after immunosuppressive treatment regardless of clinical improvement, suggesting the kidneys were not completely healed even in those with clinical remission [47].

Risk Factors for Poor Prognosis

The clinical presentation at the onset of HSPN is predictive of long-term outcome [20]. The risk of progression to chronic kidney disease (CKD) was highest in HSP children who presented with nephritic-nephrotic syndrome (45–50 %) followed by those with nephrotic syndrome (up to 40 %), acute nephritic syndrome (up to 15 %), hematuria and non-nephrotic proteinuria (5–15 %) and microscopic hematuria with or without minimal proteinuria (<5 %) [20, 48]. In a systematic review, the risk of long-term renal impairment was 12 times higher in HSPN patients with nephritic or nephrotic syndrome than in those with only abnormal urinalysis, and was 2.5 times higher in females than males [20]. Additional information is provided by very-long

term outcome studies of HSPN [49, 50]. Revisiting a cohort of HSP patients at an average of 23 years after first manifestation, Goldstein et al. observed highly unpredictable late outcomes; 7 of 78 patients with normal urinalysis or apparent complete recovery showed active renal disease or ESRD at long-term [49]. Ronkainen et al. also showed that even patients with mild renal symptoms at the onset of HSP carry a risk for severe long-term complications [50].

Also, the clinical course during follow-up may be important to predict the prognosis [48, 51, 52]. Bunchman et al. showed that a creatinine clearance <70 mL/min/1.73 m^2 3 years after onset predicted progression to ESRD, whereas a clearance >125 mL/min/1.73 m^2 predicted normal renal function at 10-year follow-up [51]. Coppo et al. demonstrated that the risk for progression was related to increasing mean proteinuria levels during follow-up in both children and adults with HSPN [52].

Histopathological lesions related to poor prognosis are a high grade of ISKDC, crescents of >50 % of glomeruli, glomerular sclerosis or tubulointerstitial changes [48, 53, 54]. However, the initial renal biopsy may not predict the outcome of HSPN since patients with mild histopathological disease activity (ISKDC II–III) usually receive less aggressive immunosuppressive therapy [55]. Therefore, some investigators suggested that serial biopsies might be helpful to establish the ultimate outcome in HSPN patients with renal flare-ups [46]. A younger age at onset was an independent determinant of histological regression. The activity index at the follow-up renal biopsy correlated positively with changes in mesangial IgA deposits and the chronicity index at the follow-up biopsy correlated positively with the time immunosuppressive therapy was started [47]. Also, one report suggested that the serum IgA/C3 ratio might be a useful marker for predicting serial histologic lesions of HSPN, because it correlated with the severity of renal pathology and clinical outcome in children with severe HSPN [56].

Schärer et al. in a comprehensive multivariate analysis demonstrated that initial renal insufficiency, nephrotic syndrome, and the severity of histological alterations (as defined by the perentage of glomeruli with crescents) are significant independent predictors of progressive renal failure in patients with HSPN [54].

From a systematic review of 12 unselected HSP populations it was recommended that if urinalysis is normal at presentation, monitoring can be limited to 6 months in patients with persistently normal urine findings [20]. However, the recommended duration of follow-up remains controversial since in individual children with normal urinalysis at onset renal involvement may still develop after several years [49, 50].

Pathogenesis

While the full pathogenesis of HSP remains to be elucidated, abnormalities of IgA play an important role. HSP develops as a consequence of leukocytoclastic vasculitis due to IgA deposition in the wall of capillaries and post capillary venules of various organs including skin or gastrointestinal tract and in mesangium of the kidney [10, 12, 21]. Genetic predisposition, activation of complements, various cytokines and autoantibodies and coagulation abnormalities are also involved in the pathogenesis of HSP [21].

Genetic Predisposition

Although HSP occurs mostly as sporadic cases, familial clustering has been reported [11]. Various candidate genes and genetic polymorphisms have been associated with the risk for HSP or HSPN [21]; human leukocyte antigen (HLA-A, B, B35, DRB1, DQA1), cytokines (interleukin (IL)-1ß, IL-1 receptor antagonist, IL-18, transforming growth factor (TGF)-ß), adhesion molecules (P-selectin, intracellular adhesion molecule-1), cytotoxic T-lymphocyte antigen 4, the MEFV gene (encoding pyrin, an important active member of the inflammasome), the renin-angiotensin system genes (angiotensin converting enzyme, angiotensinogen) and the C1GALT1 gene (encoding ß 1,3-galactosyltransferase, an

important role in the glycosylation of the IgA1 hinge region).

Abnormalities of IgA

Elevated serum levels of IgA, principally IgA1, and circulating IgA-containing immune complexes are observed in patients with HSPN [57, 58]. One study reported that the number of IgA-producing cells was increased in HSP, but not in other forms of leukocytoclastic vasculitis [59]. Both increased IgA synthesis and decreased clearance have been involved in the pathogenesis of HSPN [25]. It has been hypothesized that production of polymeric IgA by the mucosal immune system in response to various mucosally presented antigens [60] may be increased and the reticuloendothelial system function impaired in the pathogenesis of HSP [61]. Also, all patients with HSP have IgA1-circulating immune complexes of small molecular mass, while only those with nephritis have additional large-molecular-mass IgA1-IgG-containing circulating immune complexes [58].

There are two subclasses of IgA (IgA1 and IgA2) and ~90 % of serum IgA is IgA1. IgA1 and IgA2 differ structurally in the hinge region of the heavy chain. IgA1 has a proline-rich hinge region composed of five to six O-linked glycosylation sites in contrast to IgA2 and an abnormal glycosylation of the IgA1 hinge region would occur in the context of a deficiency of galactose and/or sialic acid [21, 57]. Such an aberrantly glycosylated IgA1 is prone to cause IgA aggregation and may change IgA1 structure, modifying interactions with IgA receptors and matrix proteins, leading to mesangial deposition of IgA1 [21, 57]. Although no confirmed genetic loci for HSP have been identified to date, it was recently reported that aberrant glycosylation of IgA1 is inherited in both pediatric IgAN and HSPN [62]. However, Kiryluk et al. reported that an increase of the poorly galactosylated IgA1 O-glycoforms levels may be insufficient in itself to cause IgAN or HSPN, because first-degree relatives had high serum levels of poorly galactosylated IgA1

O-glycoforms without any signs of either IgAN or HSPN [62]. They suggested that a "second hit" such as the formation of glycan-specific IgG (and IgA) antibodies, which could form large circulating immune complexes prone to deposition, might be required to develop overt disease [62].

Activation of Complement

Activation of complement, mainly of the alternative pathway, has been known as an important mechanism of tissue injury in HSP. Complement components are found in skin and glomeruli, and breakdown products of complement in plasma [29, 63, 64]. C4A and C4B deficiencies have been described in patients with HSPN [65] and glomerular deposition of C3 and properdin has been reported in 75–100 % of patients with HSPN [66]. Recently, activation of the lectin pathway of complement has also been demonstrated in patients with HSPN, which might contribute to the development of advanced glomerular injury and extended urinary abnormalities in HSPN [64]. The lectin pathway is initiated by mannose-binding lectin (MBL) and MBL also forms complexes with MBL-associated serine proteases (MASP-1, MASP-2 and MASP-3) [64]. Hisano et al. reported that MBL/MASP-1 might be associated with glomerular deposition of fibrinogen [64].

Activation of Eosinophils

Activation of eosinophils has also been proposed to play a role in the pathogenesis of HSPN [27, 28]. Elevated plasma IgE levels were more commonly found in patients with HSPN [27] and serum eosinophil cationic protein (ECP) levels were significantly higher in children with HSP than in those with IgAN or healthy controls [28]. Davin et al. speculated that the IgA-containing immune complexes could enhance IgE production locally by stimulation of the dermal and intestinal mast cells and deposition of IgA immune complexes was further enhanced by a subsequent increase in local capillary permeability [27].

Cytokines and Coagulation Abnormalities

Several proinflammatory cytokines including tumor necrosis factor (TNF)-α, IL-1β, IL-2, IL-6, IL-8, IL-17, TGF-β, and vascular endothelial growth factor have been reported to be involved in the development of HSP. They are likely to be secreted by vascular endothelial cells, thus initiating and propagating the inflammatory reaction [21].

Circulating immune complexes can cause vascular endothelial injury and coagulation abnormalities in HSP and plasma vWF levels are elevated at the acute stage of HSP [24]. Factor XIII activity can also be decreased at the acute stage of HSP, possibly due to a specific degradation of factor XIII by proteolytic enzymes from inflammatory cells [23].

Mesangial Proliferation and Crescent Formation

Once IgA-containing complexes are deposited in glomerular mesangium, various components of IgA-containing complexes, such as Fcα and Fcγ fragments, fibronectin, or C3b, can bind to their receptors on the surface of mesangial cells and trigger proliferation of mesangial cells, production of extracellular matrix and synthesis of cytokines, such as monocyte chemoattractant protein-1 and IL-8, recruiting neutrophils and monocytes [25, 36, 67–71]. Other cytokines (TNF-α, IL-1, IL-6 and TGF-β) involved in the pathogenesis of HSP can also stimulate mesangial cells [69–71].

In addition, local complement activation and intraglomerular coagulation by mesangial fibrin deposition can destruct the glomerular basement membrane and attraction of macrophages and proliferation of cytokine-induced epithelial cells in the Bowman's space can disrupt capsular integrity, leading to interstitial fibroblast infiltration in the Bowman's space, causing crescent formation [25, 36, 38, 72].

Treatment

Prevention of Nephritis in HSP

Corticosteroids are commonly administered in the acute stage of HSP to reduce the severity and duration of abdominal pain or arthralgia [73]. A number of retrospective studies, randomized controlled trials (RCTs), systematic review and meta-analyses have addressed the use of corticosteroids for preventing nephritis, with conflicting results [48, 73–76]. A recent well conducted randomized, double-blind, placebo-controlled trial showed no benefit of prednisone (4-week treatment) in preventing the development of nephritis in HSP, but observed more rapid resolution of nephritis [73]. These results might be due to the reduction of mesangial proliferation and crescent formation by prednisone [77]. In addition, another recent randomized, double-blind, placebo-controlled trial reported that early 2-week treatment with prednisolone did not reduce the prevalence of proteinuria 12 months after disease onset in children with HSP [74]. Based on this evidence, the Kidney Disease Improving Global Outcome (KDIGO) guidelines recommend not using corticosteroids to prevent HSP nephritis [78].

Although the general use of prednisone to prevent nephritis is not supported, HSP patients with extrarenal symptoms might benefit from early treatment. Some HSP patients cannot tolerate oral medications due to abdominal pain; in these initial intravenous followed by oral steroid therapy could be a useful and effective therapeutic strategy [79].

Treatment of HSPN

Treatment of HSPN should be aimed to prevent long-term renal morbidity in patients at risk, but there have been few RCTs to establish the beneficial treatment due to the rarity of severe HSPN. Therefore, the treatment of HSPN still remains controversial.

The KDIGO Guidelines and Therapeutic Considerations in Pediatric HSPN

The KDIGO initiative recently published guidelines on the treatment of HSPN [78]. The guidelines suggest that HSPN children with persistent proteinuria of >0.5–1 g/day/1.73 m^2 should be treated with angiotensin converting enzyme (ACE) inhibitors or angiotensin receptor blockers (ARB), and children with GFR >50 ml/min/1.73 m^2 and persistent proteinuria >1 g/day/1.73 m^2 after a trial of RAS blockade should receive a 6-month course of corticosteroids (same as for IgAN). For cases with >50 % crescents on biopsy, the guidelines recommend steroids and cyclophosphamide. If plasma creatinine is >500 μmol/L, oral prednisone should be preceded by three methylprednisolone (MP) pulses with additional plasma exchange. These guidelines were applied identically as for crescentic IgAN and ANCA vasculitis, independently of the patient's age, both for children and adults with HSPN [78]. However, some experts in pediatric nephrology pointed out that the KDIGO guidelines might run the risk of delaying the initiation of effective treatment and increasing the long-term risk of CKD due to under treatment of HSPN [80]. They argued that (1) whereas the guidelines suggested for adults and children with HSPN are only based on randomized controlled trials performed in adults with IgAN, HSPN and IgAN are different diseases and have different outcomes in spite of similarities; (2) it is very important to treat initial episodes adequately without delay in HSPN, and following the KDIGO guideline might delay a potentially more effective treatment, increase the risk of CKD progression in patients with ISKDC grade IIIa and cause a higher cumulative exposure to immunosuppressive therapy; (3) cyclophosphamide was ineffective in the treatment of HSPN in the randomized controlled pediatric trials of the ISKDC; and (4) the guideline does not suggest addition of immunosuppressive drugs to steroids in patients with <50 % crescentic glomeruli even in the presence of nephrotic syndrome and/or deterioration of GFR, but more aggressive treatments, such as MP pulses, other immunosuppressive drugs or plasma exchange, may be required in these patients [80].

In addition, several aspects regarding the treatment of HSPN deserve attention. Firstly, the highly heterogenous spontaneous evolution of HSPN should be considered. Many children with even severe proteinuria at onset achieve spontaneous remission, whereas some children presenting with mild proteinuria develop severe renal pathology and progress to renal failure in the long run [44, 81]. Secondly, the choice of therapy should be driven by the purpose of treatment. In most glomerular diseases, proteinuria reduction is accepted as an adequate surrogate marker of renal disease remission [82]. In HSPN, however, some long-term studies have shown that clinical remission may not uniformly translate into a favorable long-term outcome [49, 50]. One study showed a discrepancy between clinical remission and histological improvement [47]. Therefore, it may be important to induce histological regression in addition to reduction of proteinuria in treating severe HSPN. Thirdly, it should be considered whether treatment will be based on clinical presentation or renal pathology in HSPN. Ronkainen et al. reported that the first renal biopsy did not predict the outcome of HSPN. The outcome of patients with ISKDC grades II–III was worse than of those with grades IV–V, probably because the latter received more aggressive immunosuppressive treatments. The authors suggested that the treatment of HSPN should be based on clinical presentation rather than biopsy findings [55].

Indications for Renal Biopsy

Although clear outcome-based indications for renal biopsy in HSPN have not been established, it is usually recommended in patients with (1) nephrotic syndrome, (2) nephritic syndrome, (3) decreased renal function, (4) nephrotic-range proteinuria, and (5) non-nephrotic proteinuria persisting for more than 3 months [22]. Although the indication of renal biopsy in HSPN with persistent mild to moderate proteinuria may be controversial, Halling et al. argued that it should be enforced since

severe morphological changes are found in some of these patients [44]. Also, the interval between disease onset and the time of renal biopsy may impact on histopathological findings; the fraction of crescents may increase markedly within days in patients with active disease [39, 80]. Repeat renal biopsies should be considered in patients showing aggravation of renal symptoms or poor response to treatment [80].

Treatment of Mild or Moderately Severe HSPN

Patients with mild HSPN, such as microscopic hematuria or gross hematuria of short duration, generally do not require any medications.

In HSPN children with persistent proteinuria of 0.5–1 g/day/1.73 m^2, the KDIGO guidelines recommend the use of ACE inhibitors or ARB [78]. In a study of 31 patients with moderately severe HSPN (ISKDC grade I–III and serum albumin >2.5 g/dl), proteinuria was reduced efficiently by RAS blockers except a single case of a clinical relapse at 1 year [83]. Davin and Coppo suggested that the use of RAS blockers should be appropriate in cases lacking acute inflammation and crescentic lesions, whereas delaying effective anti-inflammatory treatment may be detrimental in patients with acute inflammatory glomerular lesions [80]. Recent studies showed that 9 of 13 patients with mild to moderate proteinuria had severe morphological changes and 18 % of patients with mild proteinuria at onset showed a poor prognosis [44, 81]. Hence, a rational therapeutic approach could be as follows: in patients with non-nephrotic, normoalbuminemic proteinuria early in the course of HSPN, monotherapy with a RAS blocker may be applied for 1–2 months and the further course observed. In patients with non-nephrotic proteinuria and mildly decreased serum albumin levels at onset of HSPN, combined oral steroids and RAS blockade may be used for 1–2 months. In patients with persistent (>2–3 months) non-nephrotic proteinuria and/or decreased serum albumin levels during the course of HSPN despite these treatments, renal biopsy should be performed and more potent anti-inflammatory treatments considered in the light of the histopathological findings. These may include MP pulses, azathioprine/ mycophenolate mofetil (MMF) or a calcineurin inhibitor, in addition to oral steroids and RAS blockade. The beneficial effect of alternative treatments such as fish oil, rifampin or tonsillectomy on moderately severe HSPN has not been established to date [48, 84].

Treatment of Severe HSPN

Although the definitions of severe nephritis in HSPN may differ among studies, it generally includes nephrotic syndrome, acute nephritic syndrome, nephrotic range proteinuria (>40 mg/ m^2/h) or proteinuria >1 g/day and histopathological lesions exceeding ISKDC grade IIIa [50]. Treatment of severe HSPN remains controversial due to a paucity of RCTs [48, 84, 85]. Most published work relies on retrospective analyses of small cohorts with heterogenous disease severity. However, there is consensus that intense initial therapy is indicated in severe HSPN, considering a 15 % overall long-term CKD risk and well documented unfavorable outcomes of untreated patients, reduced CKD risk following intense treatment and worse outcomes with delayed treatment [86–89].

Oral steroids have been shown to be ineffective in severe nephritis [5, 87, 88]. Niaudet et al. suggested that intravenous MP pulses should be started early in the course of severe HSPN before the crescents become fibrous, because renal scarring by extensive glomerular damage during the acute episode may be irreversible and lead to progressive CKD [88]. Hence, in patients with very severe HSPN, intravenous MP pulses should be initiated immediately. Oral steroids can be applied and tapered following the MP pulses. Also, RAS blockers can be used as an add-on therapy concurrently as a nephroprotective, proteinuria-minimizing therapy [80].

An RCT performed by the ISKDC showed no differences in outcome between oral cyclophosphamide (90 mg/m^2/day for 42 days) and supportive therapy in children with severe HSPN [90], although retrospective case series had suggested a beneficial effect of this therapy

[91, 92]. A recent placebo-controlled prospective study comparing cyclophosphamide plus prednisone to prednisone alone demonstrated the lack of efficacy of cyclophosphamide also in adults with HSPN [93]. In view of these negative results and the potential side effects of the drug, cyclophosphamide is not recommended in severe HSPN [80].

Another randomized clinical trial in a limited number of children suggested that cyclosporin A may not be inferior to intravenous MP pulses in children with severe HSPN. Resolution of nephrotic-range proteinuria was achieved within 3 months in all 11 cyclosporin-treated patients, while it was not achieved with the initial treatment of MP pulses in 6 of the 13 due to slower response [94]. Additional immunosuppressive treatment was necessary in none of the cyclosporin-treated patients, but in six patients treated with MP pulses [94]. Repeat renal biopsy findings performed after 2-year follow-up showed similar improvement in both treatment arms [94].

Hence, at the current state of knowledge, calcineurin inhibition appears as an alternative first choice or follow-up therapy in patients who do not respond rapidly to intravenous MP pulses. MMF or azathioprine may also be used, although the claim of efficacy for these drugs is based exclusively on non-randomized or uncontrolled studies [39, 40, 95–102]. Administration of azathioprine and cyclosporin was associated with histological regression with reduced IgA deposits in severe HSPN [40, 97, 98].

Persistence of urinary abnormalities is an ominous sign in severe HSPN [40, 52]. Hence, in patients with persistent gross proteinuria after initial intensive therapy, a follow-up renal biopsy may be needed to assess the histopathological effects of initial treatment, in particular regarding the extent and acute vs. chronic nature of the remaining renal lesions. If persistent active histological lesions are found, adjustment of the immunosuppressive therapy should be considered. Although rare, in chronically persistent severe HSPN resistant to azathioprine late remission was anecdotally induced by switching to cyclosporin or MP pulses [103, 104]. RAS blocker monotherapy is a valid approach in cases of persisting proteinuria with a high chronicity index at the follow-up renal biopsy [80]. On the other hand, it should be emphasized that proteinuria can resolve spontaneously years after discontinuation of immunosuppression in patients with severe HSPN [40, 98].

In patients presenting with impaired renal function with rapidly progressive course or crescentic HSPN affecting more than 50 % of glomeruli (ISKDC IV and V), several intensive therapies have been suggested, emphasizing that early treatment was important in achieving successful outcome [54, 87–89, 105–112]. Plasmapheresis has been attempted as the treatment of rapidly progressive HSPN to remove circulating immune complexes, immunoglobulins and mediators of inflammation and it has been used either alone or with other immunosuppressive drugs [54, 89, 105–108]. Hattori et al. reported that plasmapheresis as the sole therapy was effective in improving the prognosis of patients with rapidly progressive HSPN, particularly if instituted early in the course of the disease [89]. Schärer et al. suggested that plasmapheresis might delay the rate of progression, albeit not prevent eventual ESRD in children with crescentic HSPN [54] (Fig. 29.4). Therefore, plasmapheresis can be applied promptly in patients who have nephritic and nephrotic syndrome and progressive renal

function impairment associated with ISKDC IV or V, and in those who are resistant to steroids and other immunosuppressive drugs.

In addition, multiple combinations of several drugs, including cyclophosphamide, have been tried in the setting of rapidly progressive HSPN, although cyclophosphamide was not effective in treating severe HSPN [109–112]. Öner et al. reported a beneficial effect of triple therapy (MP pulses, cyclophosphamide, dipyridamole) on 12 patients with rapidly progressive HSPN [109] and Iijima et al. also suggested the efficacy of a polypragmatic approach with multiple combined therapies (MP pulses, cyclophosphamide, heparin/warfarin, dipyridamole) in 14 patients with rapidly progressive HSPN (ISKDC IV or V) [110].

It has been speculated that fibrinolytic urokinase treatment might decrease crescent formation by reducing glomerular fibrin deposition [72, 111, 112]. Kawasaki et al. found methylprednisolone/urokinase pulse therapy (MUPT, MP pulses, urokinase, heparin/warfarin, dipyridamole) effective in patients with rapidly progressive HSPN [111]. Addition of cyclophosphamide to MUPT was more effective than MUPT in the treatment of rapidly progressive HSPN [112].

The experimental nature of these therapeutic approaches should be emphasized. The relative efficacy of individual and combined elements of treatment in severe and rapidly progressive HSPN

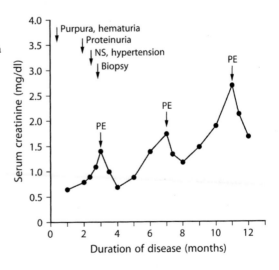

Fig. 29.4 Change in serum creatinine in a 12 year-old girl with rapidly progressive Henoch-Schönlein purpura nephritis with nephrotic syndrome (*NS*) treated by plasma exchange (*PE*) (Used with permission of Springer Science + Business Media from Schärer et al. [54])

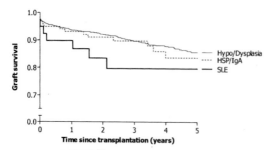

Fig. 29.5 Kidney allograft survival for patients with Henoch Schönlein Purpura/IgA nephropathy (HSP/IgA) relative to patients with renal hypo/dysplasia and systemic lupus erythematosus (SLE) (Used with permission of Oxford University Press from Van Stralen et al. [116])

awaits demonstration in RCTs with strict inclusion criteria and standardized treatment protocols.

Special Conditions

Renal Transplantation

HSPN may recur after renal transplantation. In 1994, the risk of clinical recurrence was 35 % and the risk of graft loss due to recurrence 11 % at 5 years after renal transplantation [113]. A recent study showed lower post-transplant HSPN recurrence rates than previously reported and the risk of graft loss related to recurrence was 2.5 % and 7.5 % at 5 and 10 years, respectively [114]. Although the risk of graft failure due to recurrence of underlying disease is increased in HSPN, the diagnosis of HSP does not impact overall renal allograft survival [115, 116] (Fig. 29.5). Histologic recurrence is more frequently observed on routine renal biopsies but often does not cause clinical consequences [117]. The severity of HSPN at presentation and the types of immunosuppression after renal transplantation did not affect the risk of HSPN recurrence [114, 116].

Pregnancy

Women with a history of HSP during childhood may be at increased risk for renal complications during pregnancy [22, 50, 118]. Ronkainen et al.

reported that 16 (70 %) of 23 pregnancies were complicated by hypertension, proteinuria, or both and 5 (56 %) of the 9 women with complicated pregnancies had a poor renal outcome [50]. Therefore, close monitoring during pregnancy is recommended in women with a history of childhood HSP.

References

1. Heberden W. Commentaria di morboriana: historia and curatione. London: Payne; 1801.
2. Schönlein JL. Allgemeine und specielle pathologie und therapie. Würtzberg: Etlinger; 1832.
3. Henoch EH. Verhandlungen arztlicher gesellschaffen. Berliner Klinische Wochenschrift. 1868;5:517–30.
4. Koskimies O, Mir S, Rapola J, Vilska J. Henoch-Schönlein nephritis: long-term prognosis of unselected patients. Arch Dis Child. 1981;56(6):482–4.
5. Meadow SR, Glasgow EF, White RH, Moncrieff MW, Cameron JS, Ogg CS. Schönlein-Henoch nephritis. Q J Med. 1972;41(163):241–58.
6. Mills JA, Michel BA, Bloch DA, Calabrese LH, Hunder GG, Arend WP, et al. The American College of Rheumatology 1990 criteria for the classification of Henoch-Schönlein purpura. Arthritis Rheum. 1990;33(8):1114–21.
7. Ozen S, Ruperto N, Dillon MJ, Bagga A, Barron K, Davin JC, et al. EULAR/PReS endorsed consensus criteria for the classification of childhood vasculitides. Ann Rheum Dis. 2006;65(7):936–41.
8. Ozen S, Pistorio A, Iusan SM, Bakkaloglu A, Herlin T, Brik R, et al. EULAR/PRINTO/PRES criteria for Henoch-Schönlein purpura, childhood polyarteritis nodosa, childhood Wegener granulomatosis and childhood Takayasu arteritis: Ankara 2008. Part II: final classification criteria. Ann Rheum Dis. 2010;69(5):798–806.
9. Nielsen HE. Epidemiology of Schönlein-Henoch purpura. Acta Paediatr Scand. 1988;77(1):125–31.
10. Piram M, Mahr A. Epidemiology of immunoglobulin A vasculitis (Henoch-Schönlein): current state of knowledge. Curr Opin Rheumatol. 2013;25(2):171–8.
11. Shin JI, Lee JS. Familial clustering of Henoch-Schönlein purpura or IgA nephropathy: genetic background or environmental triggers? Pediatr Dermatol. 2008;25(6):651.
12. Tizard EJ, Hamilton-Ayres MJ. Henoch Schonlein purpura. Arch Dis Child Educ Pract Ed. 2008;93(1):1–8.
13. Kaku Y, Nohara K, Honda S. Renal involvement in Henoch-Schönlein purpura: a multivariate analysis of prognostic factors. Kidney Int. 1998;53(6):1755–9.
14. Shin JI, Park JM, Shin YH, Hwang DH, Kim JH, Lee JS. Predictive factors for nephritis, relapse, and

significant proteinuria in childhood Henoch-Schönlein purpura. Scand J Rheumatol. 2006;35(1):56–60.

15. Jauhola O, Ronkainen J, Koskimies O, Ala-Houhala M, Arikoski P, Hölttä T, et al. Renal manifestations of Henoch-Schonlein purpura in a 6-month prospective study of 223 children. Arch Dis Child. 2010;95(11):877–82.

16. Saulsbury FT. Henoch-Schönlein Purpura in children. Report of 100 patients and review of the literature. Medicine (Baltimore). 1999;78(6):395–409.

17. Chang WL, Yang YH, Lin YT, Chiang BL. Gastrointestinal manifestations in Henoch-Schönlein purpura: a review of 261 patients. Acta Paediatr. 2004;93(11):1427–31.

18. Saulsbury FT. Clinical update: Henoch-Schönlein purpura. Lancet. 2007;369(9566):976–8.

19. Nussinovitch N, Elishkevitz K, Volovitz B, Nussinovitch M. Hypertension as a late sequela of Henoch-Schönlein purpura. Clin Pediatr (Phila). 2005;44(6):543–7.

20. Narchi H. Risk of long term renal impairment and duration of follow up recommended for Henoch-Schonlein purpura with normal or minimal urinary findings: a systematic review. Arch Dis Child. 2005;90(9):916–20.

21. Park SJ, Suh JS, Lee JH, Lee JW, Kim SH, Han KH, et al. Advances in our understanding of the pathogenesis of Henoch-Schönlein purpura and the implications for improving its diagnosis. Expert Rev Clin Immunol. 2013;9(12):1223–38.

22. McCarthy HJ, Tizard EJ. Clinical practice: diagnosis and management of Henoch-Schönlein purpura. Eur J Pediatr. 2010;169(6):643–50.

23. Henriksson P, Hedner U, Nilsson IM. Factor XIII (fibrin stabilising factor) in Henoch-Schönlein's purpura. Acta Paediatr Scand. 1977;66(3):273–7.

24. a. Yilmaz D, Kavakli K, Ozkayin N. The elevated markers of hypercoagulability in children with Henoch-Schönlein purpura. Pediatr Hematol Oncol. 2005;22(1):41–8; b. Culic S, Jakl R, Metlicic V, Paukovic-Sekulic B, Resic B, Culic V, et al. Platelet function analysis in children with Schönlein-Henoch syndrome. Arch Med Res. 2001;32(4):268–72.

25. Davin JC, Ten Berge IJ, Weening JJ. What is the difference between IgA nephropathy and Henoch-Schönlein purpura nephritis? Kidney Int. 2001;59(3):823–34.

26. Saulsbury FT. The role of IgA1 rheumatoid factor in the formation of IgA-containing immune complexes in Henoch-Schönlein purpura. J Clin Lab Immunol. 1987;23(3):123–7.

27. Davin JC, Pierard G, Dechenne C, Grossman D, Nagy J, Quacoe M, et al. Possible pathogenic role of IgE in Henoch-Schönlein purpura. Pediatr Nephrol. 1994;8(2):169–71.

28. Namgoong MK, Lim BK, Kim JS. Eosinophil cationic protein in Henoch-Schönlein purpura and in IgA nephropathy. Pediatr Nephrol. 1997;11:703–6.

29. Motoyama O, Iitaka K. Henoch-Schonlein purpura with hypocomplementemia in children. Pediatr Int. 2005;47(1):39–42.

30. Robson WL, Leung AK, Woodman RC. The absence of anti-neutrophil cytoplasmic antibodies in patients with Henoch-Schönlein purpura. Pediatr Nephrol. 1994;8(3):295–8.

31. Choi JN, Shin JI, Lee JS, Kim HS. Antineutrophil cytoplasmic antibody in Korean children with Henoch-Schönlein purpura. J Korean Soc Pediatr Nephrol. 2008;12(2):164–9.

32. Saulsbury FT, Kirkpatrick PR, Bolton WK. IgA antineutrophil cytoplasmic antibody in Henoch-Schönlein purpura. Am J Nephrol. 1991;11(4):295–300.

33. Ozaltin F, Bakkaloglu A, Ozen S, Topaloglu R, Kavak U, Kalyoncu M, et al. The significance of IgA class of antineutrophil cytoplasmic antibodies (ANCA) in childhood Henoch-Schönlein purpura. Clin Rheumatol. 2004;23:426–9.

34. Shin JI, Lee JS, Kim HS. Lupus anticoagulant and IgM anti-phospholipid antibodies in Korean children with Henoch-Schonlein purpura. Scand J Rheumatol. 2009;38(1):73–4.

35. Rai A, Nast C, Adler S. Henoch-Schönlein purpura nephritis. J Am Soc Nephrol. 1999;10:2637–44.

36. Davin JC. Henoch-Schonlein purpura nephritis: pathophysiology, treatment, and future strategy. Clin J Am Soc Nephrol. 2011;6:679–89.

37. Counahan R, Winterborn MH, White RH, Heaton JM, Meadow SR, Bluett NH, et al. Prognosis of Henoch-Schönlein nephritis in children. Br Med J. 1977;2(6078):11–4.

38. Emancipator SN. Primary and secondary forms of IgA nephritis and Schönlein-Henoch syndrome. In: Heptinstall RH, editor. Pathology of the kidney. London: Little Brown; 1993.

39. Foster BJ, Bernard C, Drummond KN, Sharma AK. Effective therapy for severe Henoch-Schonlein purpura nephritis with prednisone and azathioprine: a clinical and histopathologic study. J Pediatr. 2000;136(3):370–5.

40. Shin JI, Park JM, Shin YH, Kim JH, Lee JS, Kim PK, et al. Can azathioprine and steroids alter the progression of severe Henoch-Schönlein nephritis in children? Pediatr Nephrol. 2005;20(8):1087–92.

41. Urizar RE, Michael A, Sisson S, Vernier RL. Anaphylactoid purpura. II. Immunofluorescent and electron microscopic studies of the glomerular lesions. Lab Invest. 1968;19(4):437–50.

42. Sinniah R, Feng PH, Chen BT. Henoch-Schoenlein syndrome: a clinical and morphological study of renal biopsies. Clin Nephrol. 1978;9(6):219–28.

43. Nickavar A, Mehrazma M, Lahouti A. Clinicopathologic correlations in Henoch-Schonlein nephritis. Iran J Kidney Dis. 2012;6(6):437–40.

44. Halling SF, Söderberg MP, Berg UB. Henoch Schönlein nephritis: clinical findings related to renal function and morphology. Pediatr Nephrol. 2005;20(1):46–51.

45. Niaudet P, Levy M, Broyer M, Habib R. Clinicopathologic correlations in severe forms of

Henoch-Schönlein purpura nephritis based on repeat biopsies. Contrib Nephrol. 1984;40:250–4.

46. Algoet C, Proesmans W. Renal biopsy 2–9 years after Henoch Schönlein purpura. Pediatr Nephrol. 2003;18(5):471–3.

47. Shin JI, Park JM, Kim JH, Lee JS, Jeong HJ. Factors affecting histological regression of crescentic Henoch-Schönlein nephritis in children. Pediatr Nephrol. 2006;21(1):54–9.

48. Bogdanović R. Henoch-Schönlein purpura nephritis in children: risk factors, prevention and treatment. Acta Paediatr. 2009;98(12):1882–9.

49. Goldstein AR, White RH, Akuse R, Chantler C. Long-term follow-up of childhood Henoch-Schönlein nephritis. Lancet. 1992;339(8788):280–2.

50. Ronkainen J, Nuutinen M, Koskimies O. The adult kidney 24 years after childhood Henoch-Schönlein purpura: a retrospective cohort study. Lancet. 2002;360(9334):666–70.

51. Bunchman TE, Mauer SM, Sibley RK, Vernier RL. Anaphylactoid purpura: characteristics of 16 patients who progressed to renal failure. Pediatr Nephrol. 1988;2(4):393–7.

52. Coppo R, Andrulli S, Amore A, Gianoglio B, Conti G, Peruzzi L, et al. Predictors of outcome in Henoch-Schönlein nephritis in children and adults. Am J Kidney Dis. 2006;47(6):993–1003.

53. Kawasaki Y, Suzuki J, Sakai N, Nemoto K, Nozawa R, Suzuki S, et al. Clinical and pathological features of children with Henoch-Schoenlein purpura nephritis: risk factors associated with poor prognosis. Clin Nephrol. 2003;60(3):153–60.

54. Schärer K, Krmar R, Querfeld U, Ruder H, Waldherr R, Schaefer F. Clinical outcome of Schönlein-Henoch purpura nephritis in children. Pediatr Nephrol. 1999;13:816–23.

55. Ronkainen J, Ala-Houhala M, Huttunen NP, Jahnukainen T, Koskimies O, Ormälä T, et al. Outcome of Henoch-Schoenlein nephritis with nephrotic-range proteinuria. Clin Nephrol. 2003;60(2):80–4.

56. Shin JI, Park JM, Shin YH, Lee JS, Jeong HJ, Kim HS. Serum IgA/C3 ratio may be a useful marker of disease activity in severe Henoch-Schönlein nephritis. Nephron Clin Pract. 2005;101(2):c72–8.

57. Coppo R, Basolo B, Piccoli G, Mazzucco G, Bulzomì MR, Roccatello D, et al. IgA1 and IgA2 immune complexes in primary IgA nephropathy and Henoch-Schönlein nephritis. Clin Exp Immunol. 1984;57(3):583–90.

58. Levinsky RJ, Barratt TM. IgA immune complexes in Henoch-Schönlein purpura. Lancet. 1979;2(8152):1100–3.

59. Casanueva B, Rodriguez-Valverde V, Luceño A. Circulating IgA producing cells in the differential diagnosis of Henoch-Schönlein purpura. J Rheumatol. 1988;15(8):1229–33.

60. Allen A, Harper S, Feehally J. Origin and structure of pathogenic IgA in IgA nephropathy. Biochem Soc Trans. 1997;25(2):486–90.

61. Davin JC, Vandenbroeck MC, Foidart JB, Mahieu PR. Sequential measurements of the reticuloendothelial system function in Henoch-Schönlein disease of childhood. Correlations with various immunological parameters. Acta Paediatr Scand. 1985;74(2):201–6.

62. Kiryluk K, Moldoveanu Z, Sanders JT, Eison TM, Suzuki H, Julian BA, et al. Aberrant glycosylation of IgA1 is inherited in both pediatric IgA nephropathy and Henoch-Schönlein purpura nephritis. Kidney Int. 2011;80(1):79–87.

63. Garcia-Fuentes M, Martin A, Chantler C, Williams DG. Serum complement components in Henoch-Schönlein purpura. Arch Dis Child. 1978;53(5):417–9.

64. Hisano S, Matsushita M, Fujita T, Iwasaki H. Activation of the lectin complement pathway in Henoch-Schönlein purpura nephritis. Am J Kidney Dis. 2005;45(2):295–302.

65. Ault BH, Stapleton FB, Rivas ML, Waldo FB, Roy 3rd S, McLean RH, et al. Association of Henoch-Schönlein purpura glomerulonephritis with C4B deficiency. J Pediatr. 1990;117(5):753–5.

66. Evans DJ, Williams DG, Peters DK, Sissons JG, Boulton-Jones JM, Ogg CS, et al. Glomerular deposition of properdin in Henoch-Schönlein syndrome and idiopathic focal nephritis. Br Med J. 1973;3(5875):326–8.

67. Davies M. The mesangial cell: a tissue culture view. Kidney Int. 1994;45(2):320–7.

68. Oortwijn BD, Roos A, Royle L, van Gijlswijk-Janssen DJ, Faber-Krol MC, Eijgenraam JW, et al. Differential glycosylation of polymeric and monomeric IgA: a possible role in glomerular inflammation in IgA nephropathy. J Am Soc Nephrol. 2006;17(12):3529–39.

69. Chen A, Chen WP, Sheu LF, Lin CY. Pathogenesis of IgA nephropathy: in vitro activation of human mesangial cells by IgA immune complex leads to cytokine secretion. J Pathol. 1994;173(2):119–26.

70. Gómez-Guerrero C, López-Armada MJ, González E, Egido J. Soluble IgA and IgG aggregates are catabolized by cultured rat mesangial cells and induce production of TNF-alpha and IL-6, and proliferation. J Immunol. 1994;153(11):5247–55.

71. López-Armada MJ, Gómez-Guerrero C, Egido J. Receptors for immune complexes activate gene expression and synthesis of matrix proteins in cultured rat and human mesangial cells: role of TGF-beta. J Immunol. 1996;157(5):2136–42.

72. Shin JI, Park JM, Shin YH, Lee JS, Jeong HJ. Role of mesangial fibrinogen deposition in the pathogenesis of crescentic Henoch-Schonlein nephritis in children. J Clin Pathol. 2005;58(11):1147–51.

73. Ronkainen J, Koskimies O, Ala-Houhala M, Antikainen M, Merenmies J, Rajantie J, et al. Early prednisone therapy in Henoch-Schönlein purpura: a randomized, double-blind, placebo-controlled trial. J Pediatr. 2006;149(2):241–7.

74. Dudley J, Smith G, Llewelyn-Edwards A, Bayliss K, Pike K, Tizard J. Randomised, double-blind, placebo-controlled trial to determine whether steroids reduce the incidence and severity of nephropathy in Henoch-Schonlein Purpura (HSP). Arch Dis Child. 2013;98(10):756–63.

75. Weiss PF, Feinstein JA, Luan X, Burnham JM, Feudtner C. Effects of corticosteroid on Henoch-Schönlein purpura: a systematic review. Pediatrics. 2007;120(5):1079–87.

76. Chartapisak W, Opastirakul S, Hodson EM, Willis NS, Craig JC. Interventions for preventing and treating kidney disease in Henoch-Schönlein Purpura (HSP). Cochrane Database Syst Rev. 2009;(3):CD005128.

77. Shin JI, Lee JS. Can corticosteroid therapy alter the course of nephritis in children with Henoch-Schönlein purpura? Nat Clin Pract Rheumatol. 2008;4(3):126–7.

78. KDIGO guidelines on glomerulonephritis. Henoch-Schönlein purpura nephritis. Kidney Int Suppl. 2012;2(2):218–20.

79. Shin JI, Lee SJ, Lee JS, Kim KH. Intravenous dexamethasone followed by oral prednisolone versus oral prednisolone in the treatment of childhood Henoch-Schönlein purpura. Rheumatol Int. 2011;31(11):1429–32.

80. Davin JC, Coppo R. Pitfalls in recommending evidence-based guidelines for a protean disease like Henoch-Schönlein purpura nephritis. Pediatr Nephrol. 2013;28(10):1897–903.

81. Edström Halling S, Söderberg MP, Berg UB. Predictors of outcome in Henoch-Schönlein nephritis. Pediatr Nephrol. 2010;25(6):1101–8.

82. Ruggenenti P, Schieppati A, Remuzzi G. Progression, remission, regression of chronic renal diseases. Lancet. 2001;357(9268):1601–8.

83. Ninchoji T, Kaito H, Nozu K, Hashimura Y, Kanda K, Kamioka I, et al. Treatment strategies for Henoch-Schönlein purpura nephritis by histological and clinical severity. Pediatr Nephrol. 2011;26(4):563–9.

84. Zaffanello M, Brugnara M, Franchini M. Therapy for children with Henoch-Schonlein purpura nephritis: a systematic review. Scientific World Journal. 2007;7:20–30.

85. Zaffanello M, Fanos V. Treatment-based literature of Henoch-Schönlein purpura nephritis in childhood. Pediatr Nephrol. 2009;24(10):1901–11.

86. Levy M, Broyer M, Arsan A, Levy-Bentolila D, Habib R. Anaphylactoid purpura nephritis in childhood: natural history and immunopathology. Adv Nephrol Necker Hosp. 1976;6:183–228.

87. Andersen RF, Rubak S, Jespersen B, Rittig S. Early high-dose immunosuppression in Henoch-Schönlein nephrotic syndrome may improve outcome. Scand J Urol Nephrol. 2009;43(5):409–15.

88. Niaudet P, Habib R. Methylprednisolone pulse therapy in the treatment of severe forms of Schönlein-Henoch nephritis. Pediatr Nephrol. 1998;12(3):238–43.

89. Hattori M, Ito K, Konomoto T, Kawaguchi H, Yoshioka T, Khono M. Plasmapheresis as the sole therapy for rapidly progressive Henoch-Schönlein purpura nephritis in children. Am J Kidney Dis. 1999;33(3):427–33.

90. Tarshish P, Bernstein J, Edelmann Jr CM. Henoch-Schönlein purpura nephritis: course of disease and efficacy of cyclophosphamide. Pediatr Nephrol. 2004;19(1):51–6.

91. Flynn JT, Smoyer WE, Bunchman TE, Kershaw DB, Sedman AB. Treatment of Henoch-Schönlein Purpura glomerulonephritis in children with high-dose corticosteroids plus oral cyclophosphamide. Am J Nephrol. 2001;21(2):128–33.

92. Tanaka H, Suzuki K, Nakahata T, Ito E, Waga S. Early treatment with oral immunosuppressants in severe proteinuric purpura nephritis. Pediatr Nephrol. 2003;18(4):347–50.

93. Pillebout E, Alberti C, Guillevin L, Ouslimani A, Thervet E, CESAR study group. Addition of cyclophosphamide to steroids provides no benefit compared with steroids alone in treating adult patients with severe Henoch Schönlein purpura. Kidney Int. 2010;78(5):495–502.

94. Jauhola O, Ronkainen J, Autio-Harmainen H, Koskimies O, Ala-Houhala M, Arikoski P, et al. Cyclosporine A vs. methylprednisolone for Henoch-Schönlein nephritis: a randomized trial. Pediatr Nephrol. 2011;26(12):2159–66.

95. Bergstein J, Leiser J, Andreoli SP. Response of crescentic Henoch-Schoenlein purpura nephritis to corticosteroid and azathioprine therapy. Clin Nephrol. 1998;49:9–14.

96. Singh S, Devidayal, Kumar L, Joshi K, Minz RW, Datta U. Severe Henoch-Schönlein nephritis: resolution with azathioprine and steroids. Rheumatol Int. 2002;22:133–7.

97. Ronkainen J, Autio-Harmainen H, Nuutinen M. Cyclosporin A for the treatment of severe Henoch-Schönlein glomerulonephritis. Pediatr Nephrol. 2003;18:1138–42.

98. Shin JI, Park JM, Shin YH, Kim JH, Kim PK, Lee JS, et al. Cyclosporin A therapy for severe Henoch-Schönlein nephritis with nephrotic syndrome. Pediatr Nephrol. 2005;20:1093–7.

99. Shin JI, Park JM, Shin YH, Kim JH, Lee JS, Jeong HJ. Henoch-Schönlein purpura nephritis with nephrotic-range proteinuria: histological regression possibly associated with cyclosporin A and steroid treatment. Scand J Rheumatol. 2005;34:392–5.

100. Park JM, Won SC, Shin JI, Yim H, Pai KS. Cyclosporin A therapy for Henoch-Schönlein nephritis with nephrotic-range proteinuria. Pediatr Nephrol. 2011;26(3):411–7.

101. Du Y, Hou L, Zhao C, Han M, Wu Y. Treatment of children with Henoch-Schönlein purpura nephritis with mycophenolate mofetil. Pediatr Nephrol. 2012;27(5):765–71.

102. Ren P, Han F, Chen L, Xu Y, Wang Y, Chen J. The combination of mycophenolate mofetil with corticosteroids induces remission of Henoch-Schönlein purpura nephritis. Am J Nephrol. 2012;36(3):271–7.

103. Shin JI, Park JM, Lee JS, Kim JH, Kim PK, Jeong HJ. Successful use of cyclosporin A in severe Schönlein-Henoch nephritis resistant to both methylprednisolone pulse and azathioprine. Clin Rheumatol. 2006;25:759–60.

104. Shin JI, Park JM, Kim JH, Lee JS, Jeong HJ. Methylprednisolone pulse therapy by the Tune-Mendoza protocol in a child with severe Henoch-Schönlein nephritis. Scand J Rheumatol. 2006;35:162–3.

105. Kauffmann RH, Houwert DA. Plasmapheresis in rapidly progressive Henoch-Schoenlein glomerulonephritis and the effect on circulating IgA immune complexes. Clin Nephrol. 1981;16:155–60.

106. Gianviti A, Trompeter RS, Barratt TM, Lythgoe MF, Dillon MJ. Retrospective study of plasma exchange in patients with idiopathic rapidly progressive glomerulonephritis and vasculitis. Arch Dis Child. 1996;75:186–90.

107. Kawasaki Y, Suzuki J, Murai M, Takahashi A, Isome M, Nozawa R, et al. Plasmapheresis therapy for rapidly progressive Henoch-Schönlein nephritis. Pediatr Nephrol. 2004;19(8):920–3.

108. Shenoy M, Ognjanovic MV, Coulthard MG. Treating severe Henoch-Schönlein and IgA nephritis with plasmapheresis alone. Pediatr Nephrol. 2007;22:1167–71.

109. Oner A, Tinaztepe K, Erdogan O. The effect of triple therapy on rapidly progressive type of Henoch-Schönlein nephritis. Pediatr Nephrol. 1995;9:6–10.

110. Iijima K, Ito-Kariya S, Nakamura H, Yoshikawa N. Multiple combined therapy for severe Henoch-Schönlein nephritis in children. Pediatr Nephrol. 1998;12:244–8.

111. Kawasaki Y, Suzuki J, Nozawa R, Suzuki S, Suzuki H. Efficacy of methylprednisolone and urokinase pulse therapy for severe Henoch-Schönlein nephritis. Pediatrics. 2003;111:785–9.

112. Kawasaki Y, Suzuki J, Suzuki H. Efficacy of methylprednisolone and urokinase pulse therapy combined with or without cyclophosphamide in severe Henoch-Schoenlein nephritis: a clinical and histopathological study. Nephrol Dial Transplant. 2004;19:858–64.

113. Meulders Q, Pirson Y, Cosyns JP, Squifflet JP, van Ypersele de Strihou C. Course of Henoch-Schönlein nephritis after renal transplantation. Report on ten patients and review of the literature. Transplantation. 1994;58(11):1179–86.

114. Kanaan N, Mourad G, Thervet E, Peeters P, Hourmant M, Vanrenterghem Y, et al. Recurrence and graft loss after kidney transplantation for Henoch-Schönlein purpura nephritis: a multicenter analysis. Clin J Am Soc Nephrol. 2011;6(7):1768–72.

115. Samuel JP, Bell CS, Molony DA, Braun MC. Long-term outcome of renal transplantation patients with Henoch-Schonlein purpura. Clin J Am Soc Nephrol. 2011;6(8):2034–40.

116. Van Stralen KJ, Verrina E, Belingheri M, Dudley J, Dusek J, Grenda R, Macher MA, Puretic Z, Rubic J, Rudaitis S, Rudin C, Schaefer F, Jager KJ, ESPN/ERA-EDTA Registry. Impact of graft loss among kidney diseases with a high risk of post-transplant recurrence in the paediatric population. Nephrol Dial Transplant. 2013;28:1031–8.

117. Thervet E, Aouizerate J, Noel LH, Brocheriou I, Martinez F, Mamzer MF, et al. Histologic recurrence of Henoch-Schonlein purpura nephropathy after renal transplantation on routine allograft biopsy. Transplantation. 2011;92(8):907–12.

118. Tayabali S, Andersen K, Yoong W. Diagnosis and management of Henoch-Schönlein purpura in pregnancy: a review of the literature. Arch Gynecol Obstet. 2012;286:825–9.

Verna Yiu, Rungrote Natesirinilkul, and Leonardo R. Brandão

Hemostasis

Hemostasis constitutes a physiologic response of the human body regulated by the dynamic equilibrium between pro-coagulant and natural anticoagulant mechanisms. An inherited and/or acquired defect in any of those pro- or anticoagulant forces may "tip the clotting balance", resulting in either bleeding or clotting.

Endothelial cells are one of the major components of the hemostatic system, covering the vascular structures and having a primordial anticoagulant role when the body is in a "steady state." However, after an endothelial injury occurs, a process entitled primary hemostasis ensues, where platelets play a major role towards thrombus formation particularly under high shear stress forces (e.g., arterial circulatory component). Secondly, in conjunction with the now activated platelets and their newly exposed negatively charged phospholipid (PL) membranes, the coagulation factors that are circulating in a non-active state are activated in sequence to promote the formation of an insoluble thrombus, which will ultimately anchor the platelet plug to the newly formed wound site, preventing excessive bleeding. The integration of the steps summarized above is part of the novel accepted model that integrates the hemostatic response, entitled the "cellular model" of the coagulation cascade [1]. The mechanisms of the second wave, called secondary hemostasis, are counterbalanced by the progressively increased activation of different natural anticoagulant pathways, which will ultimately tailor down the formation of insoluble thrombus in an attempt to restrain its growth to the wound site. Additionally, the fibrinolytic system will also help contain the newly formed thrombus to the wound site, by promoting a local thrombolytic effect to digest thrombus formed in excess (Fig. 30.1). Moreover, non-coagulation components in blood, such as red blood cells (RBC) and white blood cells (WBC), are also found to have a contributory role in the hemostatic system. Understanding normal hemostasis is helpful and necessary to explain the pathophysiology of hemorrhage and thrombosis in patients with renal diseases.

V. Yiu (✉)
Pediatric Nephrology, Alberta Health Services/
University of Alberta, 14-030 Seventh Street Plaza
North Tower, 10030-107 St, Edmonton,
Alberta T5J 3E4, Canada
e-mail: verna.yiu@ualberta.ca

R. Natesirinilkul
Department of Pediatrics, Faculty of Medicine,
Chiang Mai University Hospital, 110 Intawaroros
Road, Chiang Mai 50200, Thailand
e-mail: rungrote.n@cmu.ac.th

L.R. Brandão
Department of Pediatrics, The Hospital for Sick
Children, 555 University Avenue, 10th Floor,
Black Wing, Room 10412, Toronto M5G 1X8,
ON, Canada
e-mail: leonardo.brandao@sickkids.ca

© Springer-Verlag Berlin Heidelberg 2016
D.F. Geary, F. Schaefer (eds.), *Pediatric Kidney Disease*, DOI 10.1007/978-3-662-52972-0_30

Primary Hemostasis

Vessel Wall

When a vessel wall is damaged, many different pro-coagulant components of the hemostatic system are activated to generate a clot. The release of cytokines leading to vasoconstriction and activation of the local endothelial cells occurs immediately after injury. This process is a result of the neurogenic reflex when endothelin, a vasoconstrictive agent, is released from endothelial cells in a process that sustains hemostasis for an initial short period of time [2]. Additionally, serotonin, a substance which is released from dense granules of activated platelets, and thromboxane A2 (TXA2), a derivative of platelet membrane PL metabolism, stimulate smooth muscles of the vessel wall and augment the process of vasoconstriction [3].

Endothelium

Endothelial cells have a great influence on hemostasis because of their interaction with all parts of the hemostatic system. Endothelial cells produce several important substances directly or indirectly related to the hemostatic processes, as follows: [2, 3]

- Vasoactive substances:
  - Nitric oxide (NO) and prostacyclin (PGI2) which are both potent vasodilators
  - Heparan sulfates, a group of "heparin-like" compounds that prevent the initiation phase of the coagulation cascade
- Pro-coagulant activation:
  - Von Willebrand factor (VWF)
  - Coagulation cascade: tissue factor (TF) and factor VIII (FVIII)
- Anticoagulation mechanisms:

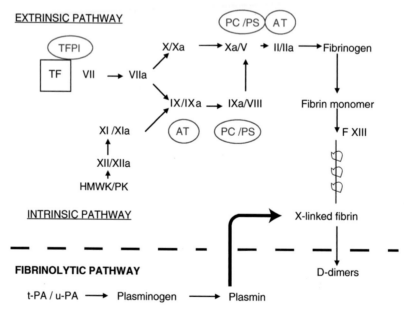

Fig. 30.1 The coagulation cascade and the fibrinolytic pathway. *Red*: natural coagulation inhibitors; *black*: procoagulant system: *bold*: fibrinolytic pathway. Abbreviations: *PC* protein C, *PS* protein S, *AT* antithrombin, *TFPI* tissue factor pathway inhibitor, *TF* tissue factor, *VII* factor VII, *VIIa* activated factor VII, *X* factor X, *Xa* activated factor X, *V* factor V, *II* prothrombin, *IIa* thrombin, *IX* factor IX, *IXa* activated factor IX, *FXIII* factor XIII, *XII* factor XII, *XIIa* activated factor XII, *HMWK* high molecular weight kininogen, *PK* pre-kalikrein, *X-linked* cross linked, *t-PA* tissue plasminogen activator, *u-PA* urokinase

(a) Natural anticoagulant pathways, as follows:
  – Protein C (PC)/protein S (PS)/thrombomodulin (TM)/ endothelial protein C receptor (EPCR)
  – Tissue factor pathway inhibitor (TFPI)
(b) Fibrinolytic system:
  – Tissue-type plasminogen activator (t-PA) and urinary type plasminogen activator (u-PA)
  – Plasminogen activator inhibitor type 1 (PAI-1)

In addition, the disruption of endothelial cells at the site of vascular injury exposes subendothelial matrix, which is an activator of platelets and of the coagulation system [3–5].

Platelets

Platelets are disc-like, anucleated cells generated by megakaryocytes in the bone marrow that have a major role in primary hemostasis. After the exposure of subendothelial matrix, circulating platelets adhere to the injured site in a process called "platelet adhesion." This first step of platelet activation results from the interaction between several glycoprotein (GP) complexes expressed by the platelet surface (e.g., GP Ib/IX/V, GP Ia/IIa and GP VI), with the subendothelial matrix. For instance, the complex named GP Ib/IX/V interacts with VWF under high shear conditions as the VWF molecule unfolds, exposing the domains which will bind to the GP complex expressed by the platelet membrane, promoting the platelet to vessel wall interaction that leads to adherence of platelets to subendothelial matrix. In addition, GP Ia/IIa and GP VI adhere directly to collagen fibers in subendothelial matrix [5, 6].

After platelet adhesion, platelet activation occurs rapidly. During this process, the many pro-coagulant substances contained within platelet granules are released, including calcium (Ca^{++}) and ADP from dense granules, FV, FXI, FXIII, VWF, platelet factor-4 (PF4) and other substances from alpha granules, all ultimately leading to further activation of other platelets. During this second step of platelet activation, platelets also change their shapes by remodeling their platelet cytoskeleton, to fully spread with pseudopodia and expose important platelet membrane PL, phosphatidylserine and phosphatidylethanolamine [4]. This process further increases the amount of activated platelet surface area, which is necessary for the next step of secondary hemostasis [4, 7].

The major platelet GP activated during this step is GP IIb/IIIa, which works with fibrinogen under low shear flow and VWF under high shear flow, to promote platelet-platelet interactions, also known as platelet aggregation. Several agonists, such as ADP, collagen, arachidonic acid and thrombin at the damaged vessel wall, also play a role on specific receptors in this process [4, 5].

Secondary Hemostasis

The secondary hemostatic wave combines serial proteolytic reactions to activate coagulation proteins (e.g., coagulation factors), culminating in the formation of an insoluble fibrin clot (Fig. 30.1). Postulated in 1964, the original waterfall cascade model of coagulation is still helpful to explain the in vitro phenomenon evaluated by screening coagulation tests, namely the prothrombin time (PT) for the extrinsic pathway and the activated partial thromboplastin time (APTT) for the intrinsic pathway of the coagulation cascade [7, 8]. Coagulation factors are most often synthesized in the liver, and can be classified by their functions into a few distinct groups as follows: contact factors (include prekallikrein, high-molecular-weight kininogen, FXII and FXI), extrinsic tenase complex (comprises TF and activated FVIIa), intrinsic tenase complex (consists of both FVIIIa and FIXa), prothrombinase complex (includes FXa and FVa), thrombin (FIIa) (activates fibrinogen and FXIII, which stabilizes fibrin), and fibrinogen and factor XIII (FXIII) which work together to form a fibrin clot.

Anticoagulation System

There are three major systems of proteins that counteract the coagulation system by inactivating coagulation proteins.

(a) *Antithrombin (AT)* inhibits mainly FIIa and FXa. In addition, it also inactivates FIXa, FXIa and FXIIa. The liver synthesizes AT, which potentiates unfractionated heparin anticoagulant power by 1000-fold.
(b) *TFPI* inactivates the extrinsic tenase complex. TFPI is released from endothelial cells and platelets.
(c) *PC, PS and TM* work together to inhibit FVa and FVIIIa. After being released from endothelium and activated by thrombin, TM combines with TM receptor and EPCR to form a complex with PC. Then activated PC (APC) is released from the complex and works with PS to inhibit target factors. Both PC and PS are vitamin K-dependent enzymes and synthesized by the liver [2, 7].

Fibrinolytic System

The fibrinolytic system is a complex system that lyses or "digests" fibrinogen and non-cross linked and cross-linked fibrin. There are many proteins involved in the fibrinolytic system [9] and these include:

(a) *Plasminogen, t-PA and u-PA* work together to lyse a clot.
(b) α_2-*antiplasmin* (α_2-*AP*) is synthesized in the liver and inactivates plasmin by forming a 1:1 ratio complex.
(c) α_2-*macroglobulin* (α_2-*M*) is a four-polypeptide protease that can inhibit plasmin and tPA.
(d) *Thrombin-activitable fibrinolytic inhibitor (TAFI)* is synthesized by the liver and activated by thrombin and plasmin. It inhibits fibrinolysis by cleaving some parts of fibrin, which prevent fibrin degradation by plasmin.

The final products of fibrinolysis are called fibrin degradation products (FDP), which consists of different-sized lysed fibrin-derived fragments.

One of the FDP- laboratory tests, which is commonly used in clinical practice, is called D-dimer.

Other Components

(a) *Red Blood Cells (RBCs)*: in normal blood flow conditions, RBCs circulate in the central part of the flow within vessels while platelets flow along the vessel wall [4]. This blood rheology facilitates platelets to reach injured sites quicker. Patients with decreased red cell mass lose this mechanism, potentially having an impaired platelet function. Nonetheless, hemolytic anemias may cause a hypercoagulable state leading to an increased risk for thromboembolic events (TEs) by other mechanisms [10].
(b) *White Blood Cells (WBCs)*: an extremely high number of WBC causes hyperviscosity of the blood and can result in thromboembolism in leukemic patients. In addition, monocytes can be activated and express TF in some specific conditions, contributing to clot formation [11].

Age-Appropriate Development of Hemostasis (Developmental Hemostasis)

The development of hemostasis evolves from the fetal period, starting at 10 weeks of gestational age. The late doctor Maureen Andrew and her colleagues were among the many leaders of research in this field of hemostasis [12, 13]. Their work has provided a clearer understanding of the pathophysiology of bleeding and clotting disorders in neonates and children.

Primary Hemostasis

(a) Vessel wall and endothelial cells: increased levels of glycoaminoglycans in vessel walls of neonates promote antithrombotic property by working with AT, while increased levels of VWF and large VWF multimers from endothelial cells counteract this effect [14].

(b) Platelets: there is no difference in terms of platelet numbers between normal neonates and children. Conversely, the platelet count in preterm neonates can be lower than term neonates due to several factors. Platelets in full-term neonates express a lower quantity of specific receptors on the platelet surface. The response to several agonists may also be less pronounced in comparison to the response found in adult platelets. However, this laboratory finding suggestive of a likely platelet function defect is counterbalanced by a higher red cell mass, mean corpuscular volume (MCV), higher circulating VWF level and a higher proportion of large VWF multimers [15].

Secondary Hemostasis

At birth, the levels of vitamin K-dependent factors (prothrombin, FVII, FIX and FX), contact factors and FV are lower than the ones measured in adults. In contrast, FVIII, VWF and TF levels are higher than that of adults during the first 6 months of life, subsequently decreasing [12, 13, 16, 17]. The levels of fibrinogen and FXIII are similar from birth to adulthood [12, 16, 17]. However, a study of endogenous thrombin potential (ETP) showed almost two-time higher levels in adults compared to children aged less than 5 years [17].

Anticoagulation System

At birth, the levels of AT and TFPI are lower than circulating adult levels. The same finding applies for PC and PS [12, 16, 17]. PS gradually increases to adult levels at 6 months of age whereas for PC, circulating levels reach adult values only after the age of 11 years of age [13].

Thrombolytic System

The levels of plasmin, PAI-1 and α_2-AP are lower at birth than in adults. In contrast, t-PA and α_2-M are much higher than in adults. Most of the fibrinolytic proteins reach adult levels within 5 days of life, except plasminogen, which increases to adult levels at 6 months of age, and α_2-M, which is still elevated until the second to third decade of life. The level of u-PA measured in neonates remains controversial [8, 12].

Ultimately, normal neonates and infants do not bleed spontaneously when challenged during birth despite their distinct platelet-related laboratory testing results. Likewise, despite having lower circulating levels of many of the natural anticoagulant pathways, neonates, infants, and children have an incidence of thrombosis that is much lower than the one reported in adults [18]. Moreover, venous thrombotic events in neonates and infants are almost invariably provoked. This contrast between laboratory and clinical findings highlights some of the limitations of current laboratory testing, as well as the yet unraveled aspects of developmental hemostasis.

Bleeding in Renal Disease

Uremic Coagulopathy

The association between uremia and bleeding was first described in 1764 by GB Morgagni. In 1836, R. Bright published on 100 cases of patients with albuminous urine and again, noted the connection between purpura and uremia. The observation that bleeding in uremic patients occurs despite having normal clotting factors led to the supposition that the primary abnormality must be within the platelet system [19]. Despite many theories and suppositions, the exact etiology of uremic coagulopathy remains poorly understood.

Clinical Manifestations

The occurrence of bleeding in uremia is twofold higher in those with chronic kidney disease (CKD) and has been reported in many locales [19–21]. This includes potential bleeding in the areas of the skin and mucosa, the gastrointestinal tract, the retroperitoneum, ocular tissues, genitourinary system, and intracranium. There are potential risks of bleeding during surgery or postoperatively, from venipuncture sites, and renal biopsy sites. Pleural and pericardial hemorrhagic effusions have also been described. Most of these reports have been in the adult population with only a few scattered reports of bleeding risks in uremic children [19]. Whether the adult risks of bleeding can be extrapolated to children is a question that is still unknown.

Pathogenesis

Studies have measured the levels and function of coagulation factors in chronic renal failure and results have been found to be normal [22]. From these data, it is assumed that platelets in the uremic state are primarily responsible for the bleeding risk in chronic renal failure. When placed into normal plasma, uremic platelets demonstrate normal function implying that causative factors are present in the surrounding uremic plasma. However, research has found that there are both intrinsic and extrinsic platelet abnormalities that result in the uremic coagulopathy.

Intrinsic Platelet Abnormalities

In chronic kidney disease (CKD) and uremia, the content of ADP and serotonin is reduced in the platelet granules. This is felt to be either an acquired storage pool defect or a defect in secretory mechanisms [22]. Cyclic adenosine monophosphate (cAMP) has been reported to be increased in CKD, which can affect the mobilization of calcium in response to stimulus and ultimately, platelet activation. It may be through an imbalance between ADP, serotonin and cAMP that results in platelet activation defects. Other defects include low levels of GP Ib/V/IX in association with elevated levels of glycocalicin, a proteolytic byproduct released by GP Ib/V/IX when damaged on the platelet surface [23]. Thromboxane A2 levels, generated from free arachidonic acid, have also been found to be low in uremia and result in poor platelet adhesion and aggregation [24].

Platelet contractility defects may be another factor contributing to platelet dysfunction by reducing its mobility and secretory capacity [25]. In uremic states, platelets have deficient cytoskeletal proteins, such as α-actin and tropomyosin, with the abnormalities becoming more pronounced after activation by thrombin.

Platelet: Vessel Wall Abnormalities

Levels of VWF and fibrinogen have been documented to be normal in uremic states [21, 22]. There is normal surface expression of the platelet receptor GP Ib/V/IX although the total levels of GP Ib/V/IX have been found to be suboptimal [23]. It has also been shown that there is impaired binding of VWF to GP 1b/V/IX and that this interaction reduction results in lower levels of TXA2 and ADP, both necessary to stabilize hemostatic plugs [26]. Another noted abnormality is reduced binding capacity of VWF and fibrinogen to GP IIb/IIIa resulting in reduced platelet adhesion to injured endothelium. This may be secondary to receptor blockade by fibrinogen, or through substances that are dialyzable as dialysis improves this anomaly.

Other extrinsic factors that might come into play include platelets and prostaglandins [27–29]. Anemia in CKD may influence platelet function through changes in laminar blood flow, as previously noted. A reduction in hematocrit can change platelet travel from where it is normally at the periphery of a blood vessel to the central part where erythrocytes traverse. Reduced contact with vessel wall results in stimulation of platelet ADP release and activation of PGI-1, which reduces platelet activity. Prostaglandin-I2 (PGI2) is a vasodilator released by endothelial cells and inhibits platelet function through its action on adenylyl cyclase and its modulating effects on cAMP and calcium mobilization within platelets. Although several studies have shown increased production of PGI2 in endothelium of uremic models, blockage of PGI2 production does not result in improved coagulation thereby suggesting that there are other factors that are involved in platelet dysfunction in renal failure. Vasoactive substances like Nitric Oxide are increased in CKD, which can further inhibit platelet function.

Circulating uremic toxins may also play a role in uremic coagulopathy. Substances such as urea, creatinine, phenol, phenolic acids or guanidino-succinic acid (GSA) have all been investigated for their potential effects on platelet function [23]. Phenolic acid impairs primary aggregation of platelets to ADP. And GSA has been found to inhibit the second wave of ADP-induced platelet aggregation. This is further supported by the observation that dialysis can improve or partially correct these defects.

Finally, platelet number and volume are both reduced in uremia [29]. Platelet numbers are lower in uremia when compared to healthy controls although they are rarely less than 80×10^9/L. The reduction in platelet volume can further reduce the amount of circulating platelet mass resulting in ineffectual platelet contact with injured endothelium.

Treatment

Treatment for uremic coagulopathy in the past was based on its ability to correct or normalize the prolonged bleeding time (BT) observed in uremic patients. However, BT has no in vivo correlation with risk of bleeding so that treatment should only be directed towards active cases of bleeding in the setting of uremia. Treatments utilized include dialysis, erythropoietin, desmopressin (DDAVP), estrogens, and cryoprecipitate [26, 27, 30, 31]. DDAVP should be the first line of therapy in a bleeding uremic patient [26]. Discussion here will focus around the use of DDAVP in settings where there is a significant history of clinical bleeding.

DDAVP was first utilized for its anti-diuretic properties until it was discovered in the 1970s to have hemostatic properties [32]. Infusions of DDAVP have been found to increase VWF, factor VIII coagulant activity, ristocetin co-factor and tissue plasminogen activator. The rise of coagula-

tion factors is rapid, likely related to release of endogenous reserves rather than new synthesis. DDAVP may also promote the glycoprotein transmembrane proteins including VWF and GP IIb/IIIa.

Administration of DDAVP

- Administered via intravenous, subcutaneous, or intranasal.
- The maximal effect on clotting factor levels occurs at 30 min lasting up to 6 h with an intravenous dose of 0.3 µg/kg (to a maximum of 20 µg/dose infused in 20–50 ml of normal saline over 15–30 min).
- With subcutaneous dosing, the levels peak at 1–2 h.
- For intranasal administration, a dose of 300 µg is comparable to 0.2 µg/kg intravenous dose (one single spray in one nostril (150 µg) if <12 years/50 k; 1 puff per nostril (300 µg) if ≥12 years/50 k)
- Adverse effects of DDAVP include: facial flushing, headache, hypotension, tachycardia, water retention, hyponatremia and seizures (uncommon but higher incidence in children less than 5 years of age). Hypotonic solutions should be administered with caution in children who have received DDAVP.
- DDAVP should not be used in children <3 years, or in cases of polydipsia, unstable angina or severe cases of congestive heart failure because of its antidiuretic effects.

Conjugated Estrogens have been reported to improve the BT in uremia by increasing platelet responsiveness [30]. There have been no reports of its use in children although adult studies recommend a dosage of 0.6 mg/kg/day given intravenously daily for 4–5 days. Effects start within 6 h and can last for up to 2 weeks after an intravenous course. It can also be given as an oral dose but the effect is shorter lasting up to 5 days. Side effects include hypertension, fluid retention and raised liver transaminases.

Cryoprecipitate is rich in factor VIII, vWF, fibrinogen and factor XIII but carries with it the risks of blood borne infections and anaphylaxis.

Clotting in Renal Disease

Nephrotic Syndrome

Hemostasis and Nephrotic Syndrome

Nephrotic syndrome (NS) is a hypercoagulable state with an increased predisposition to the development of thromboembolic events [33–38] Its prevalence is highest in the adult population with membranous nephropathy and is estimated at 37%. In pediatrics, where the commonest cause of nephrotic syndrome is minimal change lesion, the prevalence is much less frequent with the majority of studies noting it to be less than 10% (range between 0.8% to as high as 28%). It has been suggested that pediatric cases of thromboembolism in the setting of nephrotic syndrome are more likely to be associated with secondary causes of NS, is more severe, and associated with a poorer prognosis as compared with an adult counterpart. In both age groups, thromboembolic events tend to occur early in the course of disease (usually <3 months from onset).

Thrombotic Manifestations of Nephrotic Syndrome

Both venous and arterial thrombosis cases have been reported in the pediatric age group [33, 35, 38, 39]. Commonly affected areas for venous thrombosis include: deep leg veins, inferior vena cava, superior vena cava, hepatic veins, sagittal sinus, and sinovenous vessels. Arterial thromboses are also more common in nephrotic children and can involve any artery including femoral, mesenteric and intracardiac areas. Pulmonary vascular clots can occur both as a spontaneous in situ phenomenon and as a consequence of an embolic event.

Pathogenesis

The prothrombotic tendencies in nephrotic patients have been attributed to a number of factors including state of hydration and hyperviscosity, imbalance between clotting factors and thrombophilic proteins, increase in platelets and platelet activation, abnormalities of the fibrinolytic system and use of medications [34, 36].

Antithrombin (AT) is an endogenous anticoagulant that was first documented to be low in NS in 1976 and has since been confirmed in subsequent studies [33–35]. In these studies, AT had a strong correlation with plasma albumin levels and a negative correlation with urinary protein excretion suggesting that one of the mechanisms resulting in low AT levels is due to its loss in the urine [40]. Subsequent remission of the nephrotic syndrome results in normalization of AT levels. Data on other in vivo anticoagulants have not been conclusive although the majority of studies suggest that Protein C, Protein S, and Tissue Factor Pathway Inhibitor are all elevated during acute nephrotic relapses [33, 38, 41–43]. This might exert a protective effect against clotting and might explain why in children, the episodes of thromboembolic events, are less frequent when compared to adult nephrotic patients.

Platelets have been found to be higher in numbers and more active in nephrotic children. Studies suggest improved platelet availability due to their higher numbers and increased exposure of the normally albumin bound arachidonic acid leading to thromboxane A2 activation and subsequent platelet aggregation [38, 44]. Hyperlipidemia may also promote platelet aggregation, based on the simple observation that treatment with lipid lowering agents improves platelet hyperaggregability in nephrotics [45].

The fibrinolytic system is also speculated to influence the risk of thromboembolic events in NS. Lower levels of plasminogen and tissue-type plasminogen activator (tPA) results in diminished fibrinolytic activity. This may be accentuated by hypoalbuminemia where albumin is a cofactor for binding plasminogen to fibrin [33, 38].

Finally, use of corticosteroids for the management of childhood nephritic syndrome has been reported to be associated with hypercoagulability [46, 47]. Mechanisms responsible include increase in coagulation factors and reduction in fibrinolysis.

Antiphospholipid Antibody Syndrome (APS)

Antiphospholipid antibody syndrome (APS) is a form of acquired autoimmune thrombophilia, which has the following clinical manifestations: arterial and venous thrombosis, including renal artery and vein, recurrent fetal loss, thrombocytopenia and neurologic complications. These autoantibodies have been labeled lupus anticoagulant (LA), anticardiolipin antibody (ACLA) and anti-β2 glycoprotein 1 (β2-GP1) and bind to plasma proteins (β2-GP1, prothrombin, protein C, protein S or annexin V) on negatively charged phospholipids. These proteins have been associated with the development of thrombosis due to a number of different prothrombotic mechanisms [48, 49].

Primary APS is rare in children [50, 51]. However, secondary APS occurs in children with systemic lupus erythematosus (SLE) with a prevalence of ACLA of 9–87 % and LA 11–62 % [51, 52]. There is a higher prevalence of thrombosis in children with LA. APS has also been recently described in children with Henoch Schonlein Purpura with and without central nervous system involvement [53–55]. If a patient with APS, with or without SLE develops a thrombosis, anticoagulant therapy should be initiated in the absence of contraindications. Treatment may include thrombectomy (arterial thrombosis), fibrinolysis (if potential loss of life, organ such as kidney, or limb), and anticoagulation (see Treatment of Thrombosis). If the APA continues to be present on laboratory testing separated by 6 weeks, strong consideration should be given to continuing anticoagulation until the APA is negative [56]. There are data to suggest that thromboprophylaxis studies in children with APLA and SLE may be warranted [57, 58]. The data are inconclusive therefore no definitive recommendations can be made for thromboprophylaxis.

Renal Artery Thrombosis

In neonates, renal artery thrombosis (RAT) occurs as a result of umbilical arterial cannulation (UAC) with the incidence of symptomatic cases low in the range of 1–3 % [59]. In older children, RAT is most commonly associated with renal transplant and occurs at the site of vascular anastomosis. It has also recently been reported in patients placed on ventricular assist devices [60]. The incidence of RAT associated with renal transplantation as estimated from the North American Pediatric Renal Transplant Cooperative Study (NAPRTCS) at approximately 3 %, with recent estimates due to advanced immunosuppressive therapy being as low as 1 % [61]. Previous analyses of the NAPRTCS identified the following risk factors for renal artery thrombosis in a graft: cadaver donor source, peritoneal dialysis, in excess of five pre transplant blood transfusions, cold ischemia time >24 h, type of immunosuppression, and prior renal transplant [61–64]. There are no studies on the treatment of renal artery thrombosis determining the safety and efficacy of embolectomy, fibrinolysis or anticoagulation. If renal artery thrombosis associated with renal transplant is diagnosed, embolectomy or fibrinolytic/anticoagulation therapy should be considered in the absence of contraindications (bleeding) to attempt to save the graft [65].

Renal Vein Thrombosis

Although renal vein thrombosis (RVT) is the most common non-catheter related thrombosis in the newborn period, few long term outcome studies have been carried out [66–71]. Most renal vein thromboses present in the first month (with 70 % presenting in the first week of life). It affects twice as many males with a left sided predominance. The clinical features of renal vein thrombosis are variable and include hematuria, oliguria-anuria, hypertension, decreased renal function, palpable flank mass, thrombocytopenia and abnormal. Doppler ultrasound may show a decrease in amplitude or absence of venous signal, abnormal flow patterns in a number of renal venous branches or evidence of venous collateral development. The etiology of renal vein thrombosis in most cases is unknown. There is speculation about decreased levels of naturally occurring anticoagulants and fibrinolytic compounds leading to the thrombotic event [71]. Risk factors reported for the development of renal vein thrombosis include prematurity, maternal diabetes mellitus (either type 1 or gestational), pathologic states associated with thrombosis (eg, shock, dehydration perinatal asphyxia, polycythemia, cyanotic heart disease), sepsis, umbilical venous catheterization, conjoined twins, and inherited prothrombotic abnormalities [69, 72, 73]. However, the prevalence of these disorders has not been studied in a cohort of patients with neonatal renal vein thrombosis.

The sequelae of renal vein thrombosis reported in the literature include death (5%), glomerular disease (3–100%), tubular dysfunction (9–47%), hypertension (9–100%), and evidence of renal scarring or atrophy (27–100) [66–71]. Performance of multicentre, randomized clinical trials is urgently required to investigate the safety and efficacy of treatment for renal vein thrombosis and to determine the long term outcomes.

Hemolytic Uremic Syndrome and Coagulation

Although this topic is reviewed in detail elsewhere in this book, because HUS is a procoagulant state, it is pertinent to review this feature of the disease here. Thrombotic microangiopathy (TMA) consists of two clinical entities: hemolytic uremic syndrome (HUS) and thrombotic thrombocytopenic purpura (TTP). Both share a common underlying pathophysiology of endothelial cell wall injury, fibrin and platelet deposition, and subsequent hemolysis. The HUS triad of hemolytic anemia, thrombocytopenia and renal involvement underscore the primary abnormality with this entity, which is related to a procoagulant state initiated by endothelial injury [72]. In the presence of shiga toxin, up-regulation occurs of the chemokine stromal cell-derived factor-1 (SDF-1), which is found in kidney, spleen, lung, liver, brain, heart and muscle. This chemokine activates a pathway that enhances platelet activation induced by thrombin thereby resulting in platelet aggregation [73, 74]. Shiga toxin has also been found to inhibit prostacyclin production and increase thromboxane A2 release from endothelial cells thereby favoring platelet aggregation. Inhibition of SDF01 normalized platelets in vivo and prevented formation of platelet strings [75].

The procoagulant state of HUS is evidenced by the clinical manifestations of the formation of microthrombi throughout the systemic circulation. Subclinical thrombogenesis occurs even prior to the onset of HUS with elevation of markers of thrombin activation (increase in prothrombin fragments $1+2$ and thrombin-antithrombin complexes) [73]. In the normal state, levels of thrombin activation markers are negligible. Tissue factor (TF), expressed on mononuclear and endothelial cells and an initiator of the coagulation cascade leading to thrombin generation, has been found to be upregulated by shiga toxin. Blockade of thrombin activity with lepirudin prevented lethal shiga toxin effects in greyhounds suggesting that shiga toxin may mediate injury via thrombin activation.

The thrombocytopenia in HUS is also intertwined in this process and is due to a consumptive process with platelet deposition in the microthrombi [74]. The platelets are activated with degranulation as evidenced by reduction in intracellular levels of β-thromboglobulin and impaired aggregation in vitro. Other evidence of platelet activation includes increase in platelet microparticles and platelet derived factors including platelet factor-4, β-thromboglobulin, and P-selectin. The resultant effect is the formation of platelet aggregates through binding of fibrinogen leading to thrombus formation.

Fibrinolysis has been suggested to be depressed in the setting of HUS adding to the prothrombotic state in HUS [73, 74]. However, studies are conflicting as to whether indications of this, such as elevated levels of plasminogen activator inhibitor type 1 (PAI-1), support this finding [75].

Finally, other evidence of vascular and complement activation includes increases in the following: terminal complement complex, Fas-ligand and soluble Fas, interleukin-1 receptor antagonist, transforming growth factor, platelet activating factor, degraded VWF multimers and numerous plasma factors as previously noted [75, 76]. All of these changes support an enhanced thrombogenic state.

Diagnosis of Thromboembolism (TE)

Deep vein thrombosis (DVT) and pulmonary embolism (PE) are the two major categories of venous thrombotic events (VTE), both notably prevalent in the adult population [77]. In the USA alone, approximately 160,000–240,000 cases of DVT are diagnosed every year [78]. In children, VTE was initially thought to be extremely rare. However, VTE is now recognized as "a new epidemic pediatric condition," particularly in the hospital setting [79, 80].

Importantly, thrombotic events in children are also associated with a significant thrombus-related morbidity and mortality, and affect children with a variety of underlying conditions [81]. For example, patients with nephrotic syndrome are at increased risk of developing DVT, particularly renal vein thrombosis (RVT), as well as PE [40, 82]. Renal vein thrombosis can be associated with several clinical complications including chronic renal tubular dysfunction and hypertension [83], whereas PE has an associated mortality rate of approximately 9% [84]. Therefore, prompt investigation of children either under clinical suspicion or at risk for VTE development is vital to decrease VTE-related short and long-term complications.

Deep vein thrombosis can present with symptoms such as pain or swelling of the affected limb [85]. However, thrombotic events in children are commonly not accompanied by signs and symptoms, given that they are usually secondary to the placement of a central venous catheter (CVC) [86]. In those instances, their clinical presentation usually occurs in a sub-acute manner, when partial obstruction of the venous territory caused by the CVC and thrombus is counterbalanced by collateral vessel development. Moreover, CVC-related DVT in children is very prevalent in the upper venous system, where the mild findings of limb swelling can also be interpreted as line-related infection, leading to under-recognition of those events. Hence, to diagnose VTE in children, imaging studies are required. A summary of the various imaging modalities used for the diagnosis of VTE in children is listed in Table 30.1.

The most common radiological modality utilised to diagnose DVT, the ultrasound Doppler (USD), is a very sensitive method for the detection of lower limb DVT. However, this imaging modality is not so sensitive for the diagnosis of upper limb DVT in children, especially for events located within the intrathoracic territory, as USD relies on vessel compressibility to confirm the presence of an intraluminal thrombus [87]. Therefore, a composite of USD and venogram has been suggested as the best way to diagnosed upper extremity DVT in children. The role of computerized tomography (CT) and magnetic resonance imaging (MRI) to diagnose upper extremity DVT in children is currently evolving.

Besides imaging studies, laboratory biomarkers have also been used in the management of adults with VTE. Most commonly, D-dimer has been the test used to rule out thrombotic events. To further improve the use of D-dimer testing in clinical practice, clinical predictive rules were also instituted. Their development allowed patients to be stratified into low, moderate or high clinical suspicion groups, which in conjunction to laboratory testing further improved the positive and negative pre-imaging predictive values of D-dimers.

In general, the sensitivity of D-dimer for the diagnosis of VTE in adult patients is around 90% [94] and the specificity, around 49–78% [95, 96]. For example, a normal D-dimer testing may have a negative predictive value as high as 99% to exclude VTE in patients who have a low pretest clinical likelihood [96]. On the other hand, the low sensitivity of D-dimer testing for the diagnosis of VTE may be due to the fact that D-dimer levels are usually influenced by several factors, particularly underlying diseases such as recent major surgery, trauma, cancer, pregnancy, disseminated intravascular coagulation (DIC) and end-stage liver diseases [97, 98].

The three most comprehensive pediatric studies to date have shown controversial results

Table 30.1 Summary of imaging studies for diagnosis of TE

Types of TE	Imaging	Advantages	Disadvantages
Deep vein thrombosis of limbs [75, 85–88]	Venography	Gold standard, ability to quantify venous obstruction and identify collateral veins	Invasive procedure, technical experience, cost, contrast media- related side effects, exposure to radiation, inter-radiologist interpretation discrepancy (up to 16%)
	Doppler ultrasound Sensitivity 94% and specificity 98% (adults)	Noninvasive procedure, readily available, possible for bedside evaluation	Inter-variation between operators, difficulty to test in patients with obesity, edema, trauma, burns and casts, less sensitive for upper limb DVT especially for intrathoracic vessels
	CT venography sensitivity 100% and specificity 96% (adults)	Minimally invasive procedure, less radiation exposure, well tolerate contrast media	High technical demand, cost, not readily available, radiation and contrast exposure
	MR venography sensitivity 100% and specificity 96–100% (adults)	Minimally invasive procedure, well tolerate contrast media than CT	High technical demands, cost, not readily available, requirement for anesthesia in young children
Pulmonary embolism [77, 85–89]	Pulmonary angiography	Gold standard	Same as venography for DVT of limbs; mortality of ~1% in adults
	Ventilation/perfusion (V/Q) scan sensitivity 31% and specificity 97% for high-probability scan (adults)	Less radiation exposure	Not convenient for young children due to the requirement of cooperation of patients
	CT pulmonary angiography sensitivity 69% and specificity 69% (adults)	Same as CT venography for DVT of limbs	Same as CT venography for DVT of limbs
	MR pulmonary angiography sensitivity 78% and specificity 99% (adults)	Same as MR venography for DVT of limbs	Same as MR venography for DVT of limbs
	Echocardiography for RV free wall hypokinesis sensitivity 77% and specificity 94% (adults)	Same as ultrasound for DVT of limbs	Unable to detect mild degree of PE, same as ultrasound for DVT of limbs
Renal vein thrombosis [85, 86, 89, 90]	Ultrasound high sensitivity	Same as ultrasound for DVT of limbs	Inter-variation between operators, bowel gas obscuring abdominal findings
	CT venography sensitivity almost 100% and specificity almost 100% (adults)	Findings not affected by bowel gas, same as CT venography for DVT of limbs	Same as CT venography for DVT of limbs
	MR venography sensitivity 94–96% and specificity 100% (adults)	Findings not affected by bowel gas, same as MR venography for DVT of limbs	Same as MR venography for DVT of limbs
Portal vein thrombosis [85, 86, 91–93]	Doppler ultrasound sensitivity 70–90%, specificity 99% and negative predictive value 98% (adults)	Same as ultrasound for DVT of limbs	Same as ultrasound of renal vein thrombosis
	CT venography	Able to show varices and hepatic parenchyma, same as CT venography for renal vein thrombosis	Same as CT venography for DVT of limbs
	MR venography	Able to show varices and hepatic parenchyma, same as MR venography for renal vein thrombosis	Same as MR venography for DVT of limbs

Data from: Young [85] and Monagle [86]

CT computerized tomography, *DVT* deep vein thrombosis, *MR* magnetic resonance

regarding the performance of D-dimer testing as a diagnostic tool for DVT in children. A retrospective chart review at John Hopkins University evaluated children with suspected VTE that had both imaging and D-dimer testing done within 72 h of imaging. The researchers identified 33 patients; 26 diagnosed with acute VTE, 6 unchanged chronic VTE, and 1 without VTE. D-dimer levels were significantly higher in patients with acute VTE compared to the remaining patients (77 % sensitivity; 71 % specificity) [99]. Conversely, another study at Boston Children's Hospital evaluated 132 patients referred for computerized tomography (CT) pulmonary angiography to rule out PE who also had D-dimer levels drawn: 88 % of the patients with PE and 87 % of those without PE had a positive D-dimer result, thus showing that D-dimer positivity did not show a significant relationship with the presence of PE [100]. The third study examined the role of the Wells score, which has been validated for the stratification of adults at risk to develop PE, as a potential tool to risk stratify children investigated for PE. The Wells score used in combination to D-dimer testing did not differentiate children with or without PE [101], illustrating that pediatric-specific tools will be required to improve the use of D-dimer in the pediatric population.

Thrombophilia Work Up

Thrombus formation results from a dynamic balance between pro- and anticoagulant forces; more specifically, from several different pro- and anticoagulant factors involved in the generation or inhibition of thrombin formation.

Thrombophilia refers to conditions, either inherited or acquired, that increase the risk of thrombus formation. Patients identified with an inherited or acquired thrombophilia may be predisposed to sustain a thrombotic event. However, having one isolated thrombophilia trait rarely leads to an immediate VTE.

A little more than a decade ago, the International Society of Thrombosis and Haemostasis (ISTH) published a position statement suggesting that thrombophilia investigation should occur in a stratified manner (e.g., first tier, second tier and

third tier tests) in all pediatric patients with an objectively documented VTE. Nevertheless, the epidemiology of VTE in children has evolved demonstrating that underlying conditions and/or acquired risk factors other than thrombophilia are usually present in children with VTE, rendering the role of thrombophilia as a potential causal risk factor less relevant [102].

We now understand that with rare exceptions, the practice of submitting children recently diagnosed with VTE to laboratory investigation to find an abnormality in the patients' blood that might aggravate the risk of VTE is controversial and, in most instances, not justified. Moreover, acute VTE may also affect the circulating levels of many of the natural anticoagulant factors [e.g., protein C (PC), protein S (PS), antithrombin (AT, formerly known as ATIII)], adding to the reasoning of why thrombophilia should not be part of an initial VTE diagnosis [102]. Furthermore, except in extremely rare instances, thrombophilia work up results do not change the choice of antithrombotic intensity or duration [103, 104]. Those rare instances include newborns with purpura fulminans, as its recognition requires prompt PC or PS replacement in addition to anticoagulation [103]. Similarly, children with unprovoked VTE who may have higher recurrent rates than provoked VTE, particularly if associated to lupus anticoagulant antibodies, PC, PS or AT deficiencies [105], may also benefit from an initial laboratory work up [103].

The recent results revealed by a meta-analysis enumerating the respective thrombotic risk for first onset and recurrent VTE of the most common thrombophilia traits in children [105, 106] are summarized in Table 30.2.

Treatment

When a patient is diagnosed with VTE, treatment with antithrombotic agents, including antiplatelet, anticoagulant or thrombolytic agents is usually considered. The goal of using anticoagulant drugs is to prevent progression of acute TE, whereas in thrombolytic therapy the goal is to lyse the thrombus in cases where the patient has a life-, limb-, or organ-threatening condition.

Table 30.2 The summary of thrombophilic risks in children

Thrombophilic risks	Prevalence in the general population [107]	OR (95 % CI) for first onset VTE in children [106]	OR (95 % CI) for recurrent VTE in children [106]	Acquired conditions related to abnormal thrombophilic tests [102]
Congenital thrombophilic risks				
Antithrombin deficiency – AT activity[a]	0.02 %	8.73 (3.12–24.42)	3.37 (1.57–7.20)	Acute thrombosis, nephrotic syndrome, complex congenital heart disease, L-asparaginase therapy, liver disease, heparin therapy
Protein C deficiency – PC activity[a]	0.2 %	7.75 (4.48–13.38)	2.53 (1.30–4.92)	Acute thrombosis, nephrotic syndrome, complex congenital heart disease, liver disease, warfarin therapy
Protein S deficiency – total and free PS antigen[a]	0.03–0.3 %	5.77 (3.07–10.85)	3.76 (1.57–7.20)	Acute thrombosis, nephrotic syndrome, complex congenital heart disease, liver disease, warfarin therapy, inflammation, pregnancy
Factor V Leiden (G1691A) – genetic test[a]	3–7 %	3.56 (2.57–4.93)	0.77 (0.40–1.45)	–
Prothrombin G20210A – genetic test[a]	0.7–4 %	2.63 (1.61–4.29)	2.15 (1.12–4.10)	–
Lipoprotein (a)[a]	–	4.50 (3.19–6.35)	0.84 (0.50–1.40)	Inflammation, nephrotic syndrome
Acquired thrombophilic risks				
Antiphospholipid antibodies (persistent)[b] [31] – lupus anticoagulant[a] – anticardiolipin antibodies[a] – anti beta-2 glycoprotein I antibodies [31]	1–8 % 5 % 3.4 %	4.9 (2.20–10.90)	–	Infection

AT antithrombin, *CI* confidence interval, *OR* odds ratio, *PC* protein C, *PS* protein S
[a]Level I laboratory testing for thrombophilia in pediatric patients on behalf of the Subcommittee for Perinatal and Pediatric Thrombosis of the Scientific and Standardization Committee of the International Society of Thrombosis and Haemostasis (ISTH) [108]
[b]Persistent means that at least one of the three tests was positive twice with at least 12 weeks between the repeated testing

The guidelines of antithrombotic treatment in children published by the American College of Chest Physician [103] and the British Committee for Standard in Haematology [104] are the main available references regarding anticoagulant therapy in children. However, most recommendations are not based on randomized controlled trials due to the limitation in the number of studies in children. A summary of those recommenda-tions related to the most commonly used agents is included herein:

- *Unfractionated heparin (UFH) or heparin* is a glycosaminoglycan which forms a complex with AT, enhancing the inhibitory effect of AT against both activated factors X (FXa) and factor II (FIIa, e.g., thrombin) [109]. Moreover, this complex can also inhibit FIXa,

Table 30.3 Unfractionated heparin dosing

Loading dose: 50–75 units/kg, IV, over 10 min					
Maintenance dose:			≤1 year of age: 28 units/kg/h		
			>1 year of age: 20 units/kg/h		
aPTT (seconds)	Anti-Xa (units/mL)	Bolus (Units/kg)	HOLD (minutes)	Rate change	Repeat aPTT
<50	<0.1	50	0	Increase 10%	4 h
50–59	0.1–0.34	0	0	Increase 10%	4 h
60–85	0.35–0.7	0	0	0	24 h
86–95	0.71–0.89	0	0	Decrease 10%	4 h
96–120	0.9–1.20	0	30	Decrease 10%	4 h
>120	>1.20	0	60	Decrease 10%	4 h

FXIa and FXIIa [110]. Due to higher volume of distribution and physiologically low AT in infants [103, 104], the dose of heparin required for anticoagulation in infants is higher than the one required in children aged more than 1 year (Table 30.3). The anticoagulant effects of heparin can be monitored by laboratory assays such as the activated partial thromboplastin time (aPTT) or the anti-FXa assay [105]. Because of its short half-life, around 30 min in children, heparin is rapidly cleared from the body after discontinuation and its effect can be fully reversed by protamine sulfate [111].

• *Low molecular weight heparin (LMWH)*: this class of heparinoids is derived from unfractionated heparin after it is chemically fragmented into smaller molecular sizes. Whereas UFH contains polysaccharide chains from 5 to 40 kDa with at least 18 repeats of pentasaccharide sequences that bind to antithrombin, conferring on the molecule its most potent anticoagulant effects (e.g., protease activity inhibition of activated coagulation factors II (FII, thrombin) and FX [anti-IIa and anti-Xa inhibition]), LMWH has chains with an average molecular weight between 4 and 5 kDa that still contain enough pentasaccharide sequences to retain anti-IIa and anti-Xa activity, depending on the LMWH length [109]. Overall, because of its reduced molecular size LMWH inhibits FXa more effectively than thrombin. Similar to what occurs with unfractionated heparin, the dose requirements for LMWH in children are also age-appropriate (Tables 30.4 and 30.5). Infants younger than 2 months need higher doses in comparison to children more than 2 months of age. Because the kidney excretes LMWH, patients who have poor renal function should be monitored with the anti-FXa assay carefully to prevent drug retention [109]. While there are several formulations of LMWH available, Enoxaparin is the one most commonly used in pediatric patients. Unlike heparin, LMWH effect is only partially reversed by protamine sulfate [111].

• *Warfarin* is an oral vitamin-K antagonist that inhibits the carboxylation of the vitamin K-dependent factors II (FII), FVII, FIX and FX by blocking the activity of the enzyme vitamin K epoxide reductase complex subunit 1 (VKORC1) in the vitamin K cycle [112]. Therefore, the production of carboxylated factors, which are the active forms of these coagulation proteins, is subsequently depleted. The effect of warfarin effect can be reversed by vitamin K. To date, oral vitamin K inhibitors constitute the only class of oral anticoagulants widely used in children (Table 30.6). However, there are limitations for using warfarin in children; the drug level, which is monitored by international normalization ratio (INR), can be affected by many food and other drugs, it takes a longer time than heparin or LMWH for patients to reach a therapeutic drug level, no liquid preparation is available, and its use is not recommended in infants [103, 104].

The summary of conventional anticoagulation in children is shown in Table 30.7.

Table 30.4 Low Molecular Weight (LMWH – Enoxaparin) dosing

	Age ≤2 months	Age >2 months-18 years
Initial treatment dose	1.75 mg/kg/dose SC q12h	1 mg/kg/dose SQ q 12 h
Initial prophylactic dose	0.75 mg/kg/dose SC q12h	0.5 mg/kg/dose SQ q12h
	or 1.5 mg/kg/dose SQ q24h	or 1 mg/kg/dose SC q24h

Table 30.5 Low Molecular Weight (LMWH – enoxaparin) adjustment

Anti-Xa (units/kg)	HOLD	Dose change	Repeat anti-Xa
<0.35	No	Increase 25 %	4 h post next dose
0.35–0.49	No	Increase 10 %	4 h post next dose
0.5–1.0	No	0	1×/week; 4 h post morning dose
1.01–1.5	No	Decrease 20 %	4 h post morning dose
1.6–2.0	3 h	Decrease 30 %	Trough level prior to next dose; and then
			4 h post morning dose
>2.0	Yes (until level <0.5)	Decrease 40 %	Trough level prior to next dose, until
			Level <0.5, and then 4 h post
			Morning dose

Table 30.6 Warfarin loading doses (days 2–4)

	0.2 mg/kg PO, qday; maximum 5 mg
Loading dose:	0.1 mg/kg; with liver dysfunction, Fontan procedure, or severe renal impairment
INR	1.1–1.3	Repeat initial loading dose
INR	1.4–3.0	50 % of initial loading dose
INR	3.1–3.5	25 % of initial loading dose
INR	>3.5	Hold until INR <3.5, then restart at 50 % less than previous dose

Two additional major groups of anticoagulants have been launched in current adult practice: direct thrombin inhibitors (DTI, parenteral: lepirudin, bivalirudin and argatroban) and direct FXa inhibitors (parenteral: danaparoid and fondaparinux).

New oral anticoagulants (NOAC), including the DTIs; ximelagratan and dabigatran etexilate and the anti-Xa inhibitors; apixaban, rivaroxaban and edoxaban, whose use has been approved in adult patients, are still under investigation for their use in children. Currently, their pediatric use has been restricted to phase I-II studies.

Regarding the use of NOAC in children, they are indicated mostly in the event of an extremely rare complication named heparin-induced thrombocytopenia (HIT) [113]. Disadvantages of these new drugs consist of their route of administration (injection or infusion), and the lack of specific antidote in the event of a bleeding complication [111].

Lepirudin, bivalirubin, argatroban, and danaparoid can be used for children requiring hemodialysis who develop HIT, but most of the doses have been extrapolated from the adult literature. There are only a few pediatric studies including children on hemodialysis or continuous renal replacement therapy with HIT [114–119]. The available pediatric doses that have been reported derive mostly from children undergoing surgery under cardiopulmonary bypass (CPB) who had also been diagnosed with HIT [120–125]. Whereas danaparoid has been used in these patients, fondaparinux does not seem to be a good option due to potential accumulation of the drug [126]; moreover, there are some case reports of HIT associated with fondaparinux in adults [127–129]. The summary of new anticoagulants available for treatment of HIT in children requiring hemodialysis is shown in Table 30.8.

Thrombolytic therapy is used in instances when an immediate thrombus lysis is required, such as life-, limb- or organ threatening scenarios. Pulmonary embolism accompanied by hypotension (massive PE), extensive or progressive DVT of a lower limb, bilateral RVT, or failure of treatment with conventional anticoagulants are examples of pediatric cases when this therapy should be considered [130, 131]. Tissue plasminogen activator (tPA) has been the drug of choice

Table 30.7 Conventional anticoagulant in children

	Heparin	Enoxaparin	Warfarin
Route of administration	Intravenous	Subcutaneous	Oral
Treatment dose	Bolus 75–100 units/kg/ dose then Age less than 1 year 28 units/kg/dose Age 1 year and more 20 units/kg/dose	Age less than 2 months 1.75 mg/kg/dose Age 2 months and more 1 mg/kg/dose	0.2 mg/kg/dose
Administration interval for treatment dose	Bolus followed by continuous infusion	Every 12 h	Once daily
Target range	Anti-FXa for heparin 0.35–0.70 U/ml APTT which correlates to anti-FXa at therapeutic level	Anti-FXa for Enoxaparin 0.5–1.0 U/ml	INR 2.0–3.0
Half-life	30 min	6 h	42 h
Anti-thrombin dependence	Yes	Yes	No
Antidote	Protamine	Protamine (partial)	Vitamin K
Elimination	Renal	Renal	Liver
Bleeding risk	1.5–24 %	0.8–5 % (major bleeding)	0.05–12.2 %/year (major bleeding)
Other complications	HIT (0.3–1.0 %) Osteoporosis (rare)	No report of HIT and osteoporosis in children	Warfarin induced skin necrosis (0.01–0.1 %) Hair loss (rare) Tracheal calcification (rare)

Data from Chalmers et al. [103]; Paul et al. [104]; and Young [111]

HIT heparin-induced thrombocytopenia which is suspected when patients who receive heparin and develop thrombocytopenia within 5–10 days after heparin treatment with new episode or progression of TE

Table 30.8 New anticoagulants that can be used in for treatment of HIT in children requiring hemodialysis

	Lepirudin [120, 121]	Bivalirudin [120, 122, 123]	Argatroban [120, 123–125]	Danaparoid [119, 120]
Route of administration	Intravenous	Intravenous	Intravenous	Intravenous
Treatment dose	Loading dose 0.1–0.4 mg/kg, then 0.1–0.15 mg/kg/h	Loading dose 0.5–1.0 mg/kg, then continuous infusion 2.5 mg/kg/h	Loading dose 75–250 µg/kg, then continuous infusion with 0.1–24 µg/kg/ min (average dose 1–5 µg/kg/min)	1000 U plus 30 U/kg in patients aged <10 years and 1500 plus 30 U/kg in patients aged 10–17 years, then subsequent dose adjusted by anti-Xa
Half-life	40–90 min	25–34 min	39–60 min	Approximately 25 h
Target range	APTT ratio 1.5–2.5 times of baseline	ACT >200–400 s or APTT ratio 1.5–2 times of baseline	ACT >200–400 s or APTT ratio 1.5–2 times of baseline	Anti-Xa <0.3 U/ml pre-dialysis If anti-Xa 0.3–0.5 U/ml, then decrease dose by 250 U If anti-Xa >0.5 U/ml, then hold next dose
Elimination	Renal	Intravascular proteolysis	Liver	Renal
Antidote	None	None	None	None

in children [130]. However, the risk of major bleeding can be as high as 11–18 % and intracerebral hemorrhage has been reported in up to 1.5 % of pediatric patients who receive this therapy. Therefore, some patients might not be ideal candidates for this type of treatment. Contraindications for thrombolytic therapy include any type of previous operation within 10 days prior to therapy, severe asphyxia within 7 days prior to therapy, an invasive procedure within 3 days of therapy, seizures within 48 h of therapy, preterm newborns with gestational age less than 32 weeks and patients who are bleeding and are unable to maintain platelet count >50–100×10^9/L and fibrinogen >1.0 g/L [130, 131]. Again, tPA is the recommended agent by the American College of Chest Physician and the British Committee for Standard in Haematology [103, 104] to be used for thrombolytic therapy in neonates and children.

In brief, there are two methods to administer thrombolytic therapy in children: systemic thrombolysis and catheter-directed thrombolysis. Two types of dosage of systemic thrombolysis have been published in children: high dose tPA, with doses ranging between 0.1 and 0.6 mg/kg/h for 6 h, and low dose tPA, with doses ranging between 0.01 and 0.06 mg/kg/h for 4–48 h. Even though lower doses have been claimed to have a lower incidence of therapy-associated bleeding [130, 131], the American College of Chest Physician recommends a dose of 0.5 mg/kg/h for 6 h [104].

As to catheter-directed tPA therapy, there have been no randomized trials and very few prospective pediatric series in children [132]. Even though the risk of major bleeding is potentially smaller and the efficacy higher in patients who are treated with this modality (dose reduction of tPA to 0.015–0.2 mg/kg/h), there have been no comparisons regarding efficacy and safety in children [130, 131]. Currently, the use of catheter-directed thrombolysis in children depends on center availability, local protocol, and level of complexity of care delivered.

In summary, in the last decade, there have been tremendous progresses in the recognition and care of children afflicted by VTE, which includes children with renal underlying conditions. Further prospective collaborative studies are required to continue to move the field forward.

Conclusion

Children with renal disease may have disordered hemostasis resulting in a risk of either bleeding or clotting. Normal hemostasis in children must be understood by the clinician in order to determine whether, in a child with renal disease, therapeutic intervention to prevent abnormal bleeding or clotting is prudent. Unfortunately, there are few properly designed studies in children with renal disease providing guidelines for best practice relating to diagnosis and treatment of disordered hemostasis. These studies are urgently required to optimize care for this complicated group of children.

Acknowledgment We would like to acknowledge the past contributions of Dr. Patricia Massicotte and Mary Bauman for their work in authoring the previous edition chapter for which some was utilized for this current chapter.

References

1. Mann KG. Thrombin generation in hemorrhage control and vascular occlusion. Circulation. 2011; 124:225–35.
2. Israels LG, Israels ED. Endothelium. In: Israels LG, Israels ED, editors. Mechanisms in hematology. 3rd ed. Concord: Core Health Service; 2002. p. 393–402.
3. Israels S, Israels ED. Platelet structure and function. In: Israels LG, Israels ED, editors. Mechanisms in hematology. 3rd ed. Concord: Core Health Service; 2002. p. 369–92.
4. Hoffman M. Remodeling the blood coagulation cascade. J Thromb Thrombolysis. 2003;16:17–20.
5. Rumbaut RE, Thiagarajan P. Platelet adhesion to vascular wall. In: Granger DN, Granger J, editors. Platelet-vessel wall interactions in hemostasis and thrombosis. 1st ed. San Rafael: Morgan & Claypool Life Sciences; 2010. p. 13–22.
6. Adams RL, Bird RJ. Review article: coagulation cascade and therapeutics update: relevance to nephrology. Part 1: overview of coagulation, thrombophilias and history of anticoagulants. Nephrology (Carlton). 2009;14:462–70.
7. Davie EW. A brief historical review of the waterfall/cascade of blood coagulation. J Biol Chem. 2003;278:50819–32.

8. Renne T, Schmaier AH, Nichel KF, Blomback M, Maas C. In vivo roles of factor XII. Blood. 2012;120:496–303.

9. Albisetti M. The fibrinolytic system in children. Semin Thromb Hemost. 2003;29:339–48.

10. Mosesson MW. Fibrinogen and fibrin structure and functions. J Thromb Haemost. 2005;3:1894–904.

11. Ataga KI. Hypercoagulability and thrombotic complications in hemolytic anemias. Haematologica. 2009;94(11):1481–4.

12. Andrew M, Paes B, Milner R, Johnston M, Mitchell L, Tollefsen DM, et al. Development of the human coagulation system in the healthy premature infant. Blood. 1988;72(5):1651–7.

13. Andrew M, Vegh P, Johnston M, Bowker J, Ofosu F, Mitchell L. Maturation of the hemostatic system during childhood. Blood. 1992;80(8):1998–2005.

14. Van Cott EM, Grabowski EF. Vascular hemostasis in flowing blood in children. Semin Thromb Hemost. 1998;24(6):583–90.

15. Sola-Visner M. Platelets in the neonatal period: developmental differences in platelet production, function, and hemostasis and the potential impact of therapies. Hematol Am Soc Hematol Educ Program. 2012;2012:506–11.

16. Kuhle S, Male C, Mitchell L. Developmental hemostasis: pro- and anticoagulant systems during childhood. Semin Thromb Hemost. 2003;29(4):329–38.

17. Moagle P, Barnes C, Ignjatovic V, Furmedge J, Newall F, Chan A, et al. Developmental haemostasis. Impact for clinical haemostasis laboratories. Thromb Haemost. 2006;95(2):362–72.

18. Rosendaal FR. Thrombosis in the young: epidemiology and risk factors. A focus on venous thrombosis. Thromb Haemost. 1997;78(1):1–6.

19. Davidovich E, Schwarz Z, Davidovitch E, Eidelman E, Bimstein E. Oral findings and periodontal status in children, adolescents and young adults suffering from renal failure. J Clin Periodontol. 2005;32:1076–82.

20. Parikh AM, Spencer FA, Lessard D, et al. Venous thromboembolism in patients with reduced estimated GFR: a population based perspective. Am J Kidney Dis. 2011;58:746–55.

21. Pavord S, Myers B. Bleeding and thrombotic complications of kidney disease. Blood Rev. 2011;25:271–8.

22. Casonato A, Pontara E, Vertolli UP, et al. Plasma and platelet von Willebrand factor abnormalities in patients with uremia: lack of correlation with uremic bleeding. Clin Appl Thromb Hemost. 2001;7:81–6.

23. Kaw D, Malhotra D. Platelet dysfunction and end-stage renal disease. Sem Dial. 2006;19:317–22.

24. Mezzano D, Tagle R, Panes D, Perez M, Downey P, Munoz B, Aranda E, Biarja F, Thambo S, Gonzaez F, Mezzano S, Perreira J. Hemostatic disorder of uremia: the platelet defect, main determinant of prolonged bleeding time, is correlated with indices of activation of coagulation and fibrinolysis. Thromb Haemost. 1996;76:312–21.

25. DiMinno G, Martinez J, McKean ML, DeLaRosa J, Burke JF, Murphy S. Platelet dysfunction in uremia: multifaceted defect partially corrected by dialysis. Am J Med. 1985;79:552–9.

26. Escolar G, Diaz-Ricart M, Cases A. Uremic platelet dysfunction: past and present. Curr Hematol Rep. 2005;4:359–67.

27. Hedges SJ, Dehoney SB, Hooper JS, et al. Evidence-based treatment recommendations for uremic bleeding. Nat Clin Pract Nephrol. 2007;3:138–53.

28. Leung N. Hematologic manifestations of kidney disease. Sem Hematol. 2013;50:207–15.

29. Gaarder A, Jonsen J, Laland S, et al. Adenosine diphosphate in red cells as a factor in the adhesiveness of human blood platelets. Nature. 1961;192:531–2.

30. Sloan JA, Schiff MJ. Beneficial effect of low dose transdermal estrogen on bleeding tome and clinical bleeding in uremia. Am J Kidney Dis. 1995;26:22–6.

31. Cases A, Escolar G, Reverter JC, Ordinas A, Lopez-Pedret J, Revert L, Castillo R. Recombinant human erythropoietin treatment improves platelet function in uremic patients. Kidney Int. 1992;42:668–72.

32. Lethagen S. Desmopressin and hemostasis. Ann Hematol. 1994;69:173–80.

33. Singhal R, Brimble KS. Thromboembolic complications in the nephrotic syndrome: pathophysiology and clinical management. Thromb Res. 2006;118:397–407.

34. Mehls O, Andrassy K, Koderisch J, Herzog U, Ritz E. Hemostasis and thromboembolism in children with NS: differences from adults. J Pediatr. 1987;110:862–7.

35. Hoyer PF, Gonda S, Barthels M, Krohn HP, Brodehl J. Thromboembolic complications in children with nephrotic syndrome: risk and incidence. Acta Paediatr Scand. 1986;75:804–10.

36. Citak A, Emre S, Şirin A, Bilge I, Nayr A. Hemostatic problems and thromboembolic complications in nephrotic children. Pediatr Nephrol. 2000;14:138–42.

37. Lilova MI, Velkovski IG, Topalov IB. Thromboembolic complications in children with nephrotic syndrome in Bulgaria (1974–1996). Pediatr Nephrol. 2000;15:74–8.

38. Barbanu B, Gigante A, Amoroso A, Ciani R. Thrombosis in nephrotic syndrome. Semin Thromb Hemost. 2013;39:469–76.

39. Kerlin BA, Blatt NB, Fuh B, Zhao S, Lehman A, Blanhong C, Mahan JD, Smoyer WE. Epidemiology and risk factors for thromboembolic complications of childhood nephritic syndrome: a Midwest Pediatric Nephrology Consortium (MWPNC) Study. J Pediatr. 2009;155:105–10.

40. Suri D, Ahluwalia J, Saxena AK, Sodhi KS, Singh P, Mittal BR, Das R, Rawat A, Singh S. Thromboembolic complications in childhood nephrotic syndrome: a clinical profile. Clin Exp Nephrol. 2014;18(5):803–13.

41. Elidrissy ATH, Abdurrahman MB, Bahakim HM, Jones MD, Gader AMA. Haemostatic measurements in childhood nephrotic syndrome. Eur J Pediatr. 1991;150:378.

42. al-Mugeiren MM, Gader AM, al-Rasheed SA, Bahakim HM, al-Monnen AK, al-Salloum A. Coagulopathy of childhood nephrotic syndrome – a reappraisal of the role of natural anticoagulants and fibrinolysis. Haemostasis. 1996;26:304–10.

43. Yermiaku T, Shalev H, Landau D, Dvilansky A. Protein C and protein S in pediatric nephrotic patients. Sangre (Barc). 1996;41:155–7.

44. Anand NK, Chand G, Talib VH, Chellani H, Pande J. Hemostatic profile in nephrotic syndrome. Indian Pediatr. 1996;33:1005–12.

45. Yashiro M, Muso E, Shio H, Sasayana S. Amelioration of hypercholesterolaemia by HMG-CoA Reductase Inhibitor (Pravastatin) improved platelet hyperaggregability in nephritic patients. Nephrol Dial Transplant. 1994;9:1842–3.

46. Patrassi GM, Sartori MT, Livi U, et al. Impairment of fibrinolytic potential in long-term steroid treatment after heart transplantion. Transplantation. 1997;64:1610–3.

47. Llach F. Hypercoagulability, renal vein thrombosis and other thrombotic complications of nephrotic syndrome. Kidney Int. 1985;28:429–39.

48. Robertson B, Greaves M. Antiphospholipid syndrome: an evolving story. Blood Rev. 2006;20(4):201–12.

49. Mineo C, Shaul PW. New insights into the molecular basis of the Antiphospholipid Syndrome. Drug Discov Today Dis Mech. 2011;8:e47–52.

50. Berman H, Rodriguez-Pinto I, Cervera R, Gregory S, de Meis E, Ewerton Maia Rodrigues C, Emi Aikawa N, Freire de Carvalho J, Springer J, Niedzwiecki M, Espinoza D, On behalf of the Catastrophic Registry Project Group. (European Forum on Antiphospholipid Antibodies) Pediatric Catastrophic Antiphospholipi Antibody Syndrome: descriptive analysis of 45 patients from the "CAPS Registry". Autoimmun Rev. 2014;13:157–62.

51. Falcini F. Vascular and connective tissue diseases in the paediatric world. Lupus. 2004;13(2):77–84.

52. Lee T, von Scheven E, Sandborg C. Systemic lupus erythematosus and antiphospholipid syndrome in children and adolescents. Curr Opin Rheumatol. 2001;13(5):415–21.

53. Zhang H, Huang J. Henoch-Schonlein Purpura associated with antiphospholipid syndrome. Pediatr Nephrol. 2010;25:377–8.

54. Monastiri K, Selmi H, Tabarki B, Yacoub M, Mahjoub T, Essoussi AS. Primary antiphospholipid syndrome presenting as complicated Henoch Schŏnlein purpura. Arch Dis Child. 2002;86:132–3.

55. Liu A, Zhang H. Detection of antiphospholipid antibody in children with Henoch Schŏnlein purpura and central nervous system involvement. Pediatr Neurol. 2012;47:167–70.

56. Levine JS, Branch DW, Rauch J. The antiphospholipid syndrome.[see comment]. N Engl J Med. 2002;346(10):752–63.

57. Berube C, Mitchell L, Silverman E, et al. The relationship of antiphospholipid antibodies to thromboembolic events in pediatric patients with systemic lupus erythematosus: a cross-sectional study. Pediatr Res. 1998;44(3):351–6.

58. Sharma M, Carpenter S. Thromboprophylaxis in a pediatric hospital. Curr Prob Pediatr Adolesc Health Care. 2013;43:177–82.

59. Selbert J, Northington FJ, Miers JF, Taylor BJ. Aortic thrombosis after umbilical artery catheterization in neonates: prevalence of complications on long term follow-up. Am J Roentgenol. 1991;156:567–9.

60. Poudel A, Neiberger R. Enlarged and echogenic kidneys while on a pediatric ventricular assist device. J Extra Corpor Technol. 2013;45:248–50.

61. Smith JM, Stablein D, Singh A, Harmon W, McDonald RA. Decreased risk of renal allograft thrombosis associated with interleukin-2 receptor antagonists: a report of the NAPRTCS. Am J Transplant. 2006;6(3):585–8.

62. Harmon WE, Stablein D, Alexander SR, Tejani A. Graft thrombosis in pediatric renal transplant recipients. A report of the North American Pediatric Renal Transplant Cooperative Study. Transplantation. 1991;51(2):406–12.

63. Massicotte-Nolan P, Glofcheski DJ, Kruuv J, Lepock JR. Relationship between hyperthermic cell killing and protein denaturation by alcohols. Radiat Res. 1981;87(2):284–99.

64. Proesmans W, van de Wijdeven P, Van Geet C. Thrombophilia in neonatal renal venous and arterial thrombosis. Pediatr Nephrol. 2005;20(2):241–2.

65. Monagle P, Chan A, Massicotte P, Chalmers E, Michelson AD. Antithrombotic therapy in children: the Seventh ACCP Conference on Antithrombotic and Thrombolytic Therapy. Chest. 2004;126(3 Suppl):645S–87.

66. Goldenberg NA. Long-term outcomes of venous thrombosis in children. Curr Opin Hematol. 2005; 12(5):370–6.

67. Marks SD, Massicotte MP, Steele BT, et al. Neonatal renal venous thrombosis: clinical outcomes and prevalence of prothrombotic disorders. J Pediatr. 2005;146(6):811–6.

68. Winyard PJD, Bharucha T, De Bruyn R, et al. Perinatal renal venous thrombosis: presenting renal length predicts outcome. Arch Dis Child Fetal Neonatal Ed. 2006;91(4):F273–8.

69. Brandão LR, Simpson EA, Lau KK. Neonatal renal vein thrombosis. Sem Fetal Neo Med. 2011;16: 323–8.

70. Kosch A, Kuwertz-Broking E, Heller C, Kurnik K, Schobess R, Nowak-Gottl U. Renal venous thrombosis in neonates: prothrombotic risk factors and long-term follow-up. Blood. 2004;104(5):1356–60.

71. Kuhle S, Massicotte P, Chan A, Mitchell L. A case series of 72 neonates with renal vein thrombosis. Data from the 1-800-NO-CLOTS Registry. Thromb Haemost. 2004;92(4):729–33.

72. Chandler WL, Jolacic S, Boster DR, Ciol MA, Williams GD, Watkins SL, Igarashi T, Tarr

PI. Prothrombotic coagulation abnormalities preceding hemolytic uremic syndrome. N Engl J Med. 2002;346:23–32.

73. Karpman D, Papadopoulou D, Nilssen K, Sjogren AC, Mikaelsson C, Lethagen S. Platelet activation by Shiga toxin and circulating factors as a pathogenetic mechanism in hemolytic uremic syndrome. Blood. 2001;97:3100–8.

74. Petruzziello-Pellegrini TN, Yuen DA, Page AV, Patel S, Soltyk AM, Matouk CC, Wong DK, Turgeon PJ, Fish JE, Ho JJ, et al. The CXCR4/CXCR7/SDF-1 pathway contributes to the pathogenesis of shiga toxin-associated hemolytic uremic syndrome in humans and mice. J Clin Invest. 2012;122:759–96.

75. VanGeet C, Proesmans W, Arnout J, Vermylen J, Dederck PJ. Activation of both coagulation and fibrinolysis in childhood hemolytic uremic syndrome. Kidney Int. 1998;54:1324–30.

76. Tarr PI. Basic fibroblast growth factor and shiga toxin-0157:H7-associated hemolytic uremic syndrome. J Am Soc Nephrol. 2003;13:817–20.

77. Goldhaber SZ, Bounameaux H. Pulmonary embolism and deep vein thrombosis. Lancet. 2012;379 (9828):1835–46.

78. Grosse SD. Incidence-based cost estimates require population-based incidence data. A critique of Mahan et al. Thromb Haemost. 2012;107(1):192–3.

79. Raffini L, Huang YS, Witmer C, Feudtner C. Dramatic increase in venous thromboembolism in children's hospitals in the United States from 2001 to 2007. Pediatrics. 2009;124(4):1001–8.

80. Anderson Jr FA, Wheeler HB, Goldberg RJ, Hosmer DW, Patwardhan NA, Jovanovic B, et al. A population-based perspective of the hospital incidence and case-fatality rates of deep vein thrombosis and pulmonary embolism. The Worcester DVT Study. Arch Intern Med. 1991;151(5):933–8.

81. Monagle P, Adams M, Mahoney M, Ali K, Barnard D, Bernstein M, et al. Outcome of pediatric thromboembolic disease: a report from the Canadian Childhood Thrombophilia Registry. Pediatr Res. 2000;47(6):763–6.

82. Zaffanello M, Franchini M. Thromboembolism in childhood nephrotic syndrome: a rare but serious complication. Hematology. 2007;12(1):69–73.

83. Lau KK, Stoffman JM, Williams S, McCusker P, Brandão L, Patel S, et al; Canadian Pediatric Thrombosis and Hemostasis Network. Neonatal renal vein thrombosis: review of the English-language literature between 1992 and 2006. Pediatrics. 2007;120(5):e1278–84.

84. Biss TT, Brandão LR, Kahr WH, Chan AK, Williams S. Clinical features and outcome of pulmonary embolism in children. Br J Haematol. 2008;142(5):808–18.

85. Young G. Diagnosis and treatment of thrombosis in children: general principles. Pediatr Blood Cancer. 2006;46(5):540–6.

86. Monagle P. Diagnosis and management of deep venous thrombosis and pulmonary embolism in neonates and children. Semin Thromb Hemost. 2012;38: 683–90.

87. Male C, Kuhle S, Mitchell L. Diagnosis of venous thromboembolism in children. Semin Thromb Hemost. 2003;29:377–90.

88. Huisman MV, Klok FA. Diagnostic management of acute deep vein thrombosis and pulmonary embolism. J Thromb Haemost. 2013;11:412–22.

89. Brandão LR, Labarque V, Diab Y, Williams S, Manson DE. Pulmonary embolism in children. Semin Thromb Hemost. 2011;37:772–85.

90. Zhang LJ, Wu X, Yang GF, Tang CX, Luo S, Zhou CS, Ji XM, Lu GM. Three-dimensional contrast-enhanced magnetic resonance venography for detection of renal vein thrombosis: comparison with multidetector CT venography. Acta Radiol. 2013;54:1125–31.

91. Williams S, Chan AK. Neonatal portal vein thrombosis: diagnosis and management. Semin Fetal Neonatal Med. 2011;16:329–39.

92. Parikh S, Shat R, Kapoor P. Portal vein thrombosis. Am J Med. 2010;123:111–9.

93. Rodriguez-Luna H, Vargas HE. Portal vein thrombosis. Curr Treat Options Gastroenterol. 2007;10: 435–43.

94. Brill-Edwards P, Lee A. D-dimer testing in the diagnosis of acute venous thromboembolism. Thromb Haemost. 1999;82:688–94.

95. Wells P, Anderson D. The diagnosis and treatment of venous thromboembolism. Hematol Am Soc Hematol Educ Program. 2013;22013:457–63.

96. Yamaki T, Nozaki M, Sakurai H, Kikuchi Y, Soejima K, Kono T, et al. Combined use of pretest clinical probability score and latex agglutination D-dimer testing for excluding acute deep vein thrombosis. J Vasc Surg. 2009;50:1099–105.

97. Hunt BJ. Bleeding and coagulopathies in critical care. N Engl J Med. 2014;370:847–59.

98. Stein PD, Hull RD, Patel KC, Olson RE, Ghali WA, Brant R, et al. D-dimer for the exclusion of acute venous thrombosis and pulmonary embolism: a systematic review. Ann Intern Med. 2004;140:589–602.

99. Strousse JJ, Tamma P, Kickler TS, Takemoto CM. D-dimer for the diagnosis of venous thromboembolism in children. Am J Hematol. 2009;84:62–3.

100. Lee EY, Tse SK, Zurakowski D, Johnson VM, Lee NJ, Tracy DA, et al. Children suspected of having pulmonary embolism: multidetector CT pulmonary angiography-thromboembolic risk factors and implications for appropriate use. Radiology. 2012;262:242–51.

101. Biss TT, Brandão L, Kahr WH, Chan AK, Williams S. Clinical probability score and D-dimer estimation lack utility in the diagnosis of childhood pulmonary embolism. J Thromb Haemost. 2008;7:1633–8.

102. Raffini L. Thrombophilia in children: who to test, how, when and why? Hematol Am Soc Hematol Educ Program. 2008;2008:228–35.

103. Chalmers EA, Ganesen VJ, Liesner R, Maroo S, Nokes TJC, Saunders D, et al. British Committee for Standard in Haematology. Guideline on the investigation, management and prevention of venous thrombosis in children. Br J Haematol. 2011;154: 196–207.

104. Paul M, Chan AK, Goldenberg NA, Ichord RN, Journeycake JM, Nowak-Gottl U, American College of Chest Physicians. Antithrombotic therapy in neonates and children: antithrombotic therapy and prevention of thrombosis, 9th ed: American College of chest physicians evidence-based clinical practice guidelines. Chest. 2012;141 Suppl 2:e735s–801s.

105. Kenet G, Aronis S, Berkun Y, Bonduel M, Chan A, Goldenberg NA, et al. Impact of persistent antiphospholipid antibodies on risk of incident symptomatic thromboembolism in children: a systematic review and meta-analysis. Semin Thromb Hemost. 2011;37:802–9.

106. Young G, Albisetti M, Bonduel M, Brandão L, Chan A, Friedrichs F, et al. Impact of inherited thrombophilia on venous thromboembolism in children: a systematic review and meta-analysis of observational studies. Circulation. 2008;118:1373–82.

107. Middeldorp S. Is thrombophilia testing useful? Hematol Am Soc Hematol Educ Program. 2011; 2011:150–5.

108. Manco-Johnson MJ, Grabowski EF, Hellgreen M, Kemahli AS, Massicotte MP, Muntean W, et al. Laboratory testing for thrombophilia in pediatric patients. On behalf of the Subcommittee for Perinatal and Pediatric Thrombosis of the Scientific and Standardization Committee of the International Society of Thrombosis and Haemostasis (ISTH). Thromb Haemost. 2002;88(1):155–6.

109. Davenport A. Review article: low-molecular-weight heparin as an alternative anticoagulant to unfractionated heparin for routine outpatient haemodialysis treatments. Nephrology (Carlton). 2009;14(5): 455–61.

110. Garcia DA, Baglin TP, Weitz JI, Samama MM, American College of Chest Physicians. Parenteral anticoagulants: antithrombotic therapy and prevention of thrombosis, 9th ed: American College of chest physicians evidence-based clinical practice guidelines. Chest. 2012;141(2 Suppl):e24S–43.

111. Young G. New anticoagulants in children: a review of recent studies and a look to future. Thromb Res. 2011;127(2):70–4.

112. Vear SI, Stein CM, Ho RH. Warfarin pharmacogenomics in children. Pediatr Blood Cancer. 2013;60(9):1402–7.

113. Avila ML, Shah V, Brandão LR. Systematic review on heparin-induced thrombocytopenia in children: a call to action. J Thromb Haemost. 2013;11(4): 660–9.

114. Gay BE, Räz HR, Schmid HR, Beer JH. Long-term application of lepirudin on chronic haemodialysis over 34 months after heparin-induced thrombocytopenia. Nephrol Dial Transplant. 2007;22(6):1790–1.

115. Gajra A, Vajpayee N, Smith A, Poiesz BJ, Narsipur S. Lepirudin for anticoagulation in patients with heparin-induced thrombocytopenia treated with continuous renal replacement therapy. Am J Hematol. 2007;82(5):391–3.

116. Tsu LV, Dager WE. Bivalirudin dosing adjustments for reduced renal function with or without hemodialysis in the management of heparin-induced thrombocytopenia. Ann Pharmacother. 2011;45(10): 1185–92.

117. Delhaye C, Maluenda G, Wakabayashi K, Ben-Dor I, Collins SD, Syed AI, et al. Safety and in-hospital outcomes of bivalirudin use in dialysis patients undergoing percutaneous coronary intervention. Am J Cardiol. 2010;105(3):297–301.

118. Link A, Girndt M, Selejan S, Mathes A, Böhm M, Rensing H. Argatroban for anticoagulation in continuous renal replacement therapy. Crit Care Med. 2009;37(1):105–10.

119. Neuhaus TJ, Goetschel P, Schmugge M, Leumann E. Heparin-induced thrombocytopenia type II on hemodialysis: switch to danaparoid. Pediatr Nephrol. 2000;14(8–9):713–6.

120. Chan VH, Monagle P, Massicotte P, Chan AK. Novel paediatric anticoagulants: a review of the current literature. Blood Coagul Fibrinolysis. 2010;21(2): 144–51.

121. Knoderer CA, Knoderer HM, Turrentine MW, Kumar M. Lepirudin anticoagulation for heparin-induced thrombocytopenia after cardiac surgery in a pediatric patient. Pharmacotherapy. 2006;26(5): 709–12.

122. Gates R, Yost P, Parker B. The use of bivalirudin for cardiopulmonary bypass anticoagulation in pediatric heparin-induced thrombocytopenia patients. Artif Organs. 2010;34(8):667–9.

123. Almond CS, Harrington J, Thiagarajan R, Duncan CN, LaPierre R, Halwick D, et al. Successful use of bivalirudin for cardiac transplantation in a child with heparin-induced thrombocytopenia. J Heart Lung Transplant. 2006;25(11):1376–9.

124. Young G, Boshkov LK, Sullivan JE, Raffini LJ, Cox DS, Boyle DA, et al. Argatroban therapy in pediatric patients requiring nonheparin anticoagulation: an open-label, safety, efficacy, and pharmacokinetic study. Pediatr Blood Cancer. 2011;56(7):1103–9.

125. Potter KE, Raj A, Sullivan JE. Argatroban for anticoagulation in pediatric patients with heparin-induced thrombocytopenia requiring extracorporeal life support. J Pediatr Hematol Oncol. 2007;29(4): 265–8.

126. Sharathkumar AA, Crandall C, Lin JJ, Pipe S. Treatment of thrombosis with fondaparinux (Arixtra) in a patient with end-stage renal disease receiving hemodialysis therapy. J Pediatr Hematol Oncol. 2007;29(8):581–4.

127. Pistulli R, Oberle V, Figulla HR, Yilmaz A, Pfeifer R. Fondaparinux cross-reacts with heparin antibodies in vitro in a patient with fondaparinux-related thrombocytopenia. Blood Coagul Fibrinolysis. 2011;22(1):76–8.

128. Warkentin TE, Maurer BT, Aster RH. Heparin-induced thrombocytopenia associated with fondaparinux. N Engl J Med. 2007;356(25):2653–4.

129. Rota E, Bazzan M, Fantino G. Fondaparinux-related thrombocytopenia in a previous low-molecular-weight heparin (LMWH)-induced heparin induced thrombocytopenia (HIT). Thromb Haemost. 2008; 99(4):779–81.

130. Albisetti M. Thrombolytic therapy in children. Thromb Res. 2006;118(1):95–105.

131. Williams MD. Thrombolysis in children. Br J Haematol. 2009;148(1):26–36.

132. Goldenberg NA, Branchford B, Wang M, Ray Jr C, Durham JD, Manco-Johnson MJ. Percutaneous mechanical and pharmacomechanical thrombolysis for occlusive deep vein thrombosis of the proximal limb in adolescent subjects: findings from an institution-based prospective inception cohort study of pediatric venous thromboembolism. J Vasc Interv Radiol. 2011;22(2):121–32.

Part VII

Renal Tubular Disorders

Differential Diagnosis and Management of Fluid, Electrolyte and Acid-Base Disorders

31

Mario G. Bianchetti, Giacomo D. Simonetti, Sebastiano A.G. Lava, and Alberto Bettinelli[†]

Introduction

In this chapter, the disturbances involving fluid, electrolyte and acid-base balance will be addressed in different sections that deal with water, salt, K^+, acid-base, Ca^{++}, Mg^{++}, and phosphate. This traditional presentation is didactically relevant. It is worth mentioning, however, that more than one disturbance in fluid, electrolyte and acid-base homeostasis often concurrently occurs in the same subject.

In general, the etiology of fluid, electrolyte and acid-base disorders is straightforward, since the most commonly occurring causes are easily recognized on clinical grounds. In some cases, however, the cause is not readily apparent, and a comprehensive systematic approach is recommended. The diagnostic approach to initially unexplained "isolated" disturbances involving the fluid, electrolyte and the acid-base balance should include both very careful history and clinical examination as well as the concurrent assessment of an extended "electrolyte spectrum." In the setting of initially unclassified and apparently "isolated" disturbances involving the fluid, electrolyte and acid-base balance, the concomitant measurement in blood of pH, pCO_2, HCO_3^-, Na^+, K^+, Cl^-, Ca^{++} (either total or ionized), Mg^{++}, inorganic phosphate, alkaline phosphatase, total protein level (or albumin), uric acid, urea and creatinine is advised.

Water and Salt

Body Fluid Compartments

Water accounts for $\approx$50–75 % of the body mass. The most significant determinants of the wide range in water content are age and gender: (a) the water content of a newborn, an adolescent and an elderly man are $\approx$75 %, $\approx$60 % and $\approx$50 %; (b) after puberty males generally have 2–10 % higher water content than females (Fig. 31.1). The intracellular compartment contains about two-third of the total body water and the remaining is held in the extracellular compartment. The solute composition of the intracellular and extracellular fluid differs considerably because the sodium pump (= Na^+-K^+-ATPase) maintains K^+ in a primarily intracellular and Na^+ in a primarily extracellular location.

[†]Author was deceased at the time of publication.

Alberto Bettinelli renowned scientist, meticulous teacher, and especially compassionate pediatric kidney disease specialist, passed away on August 15, 2014, just a few weeks after his sixtieth birthday. It is with affection and gratitude that we dedicate this chapter to this unforgettable friend and partner, with whom we shared many moments of our life. We all miss him very much.

M.G. Bianchetti (✉)
G.D. Simonetti • S.A.G. Lava
Department of Pediatrics, Ospedale San Giovanni, Bellinzona, Switzerland
e-mail: mario.bianchetti@pediatrician.ch; giacomo.simonetti@eoc.ch; sebastiano.lava@bluewin.ch

© Springer-Verlag Berlin Heidelberg 2016
D.F. Geary, F. Schaefer (eds.), *Pediatric Kidney Disease*, DOI 10.1007/978-3-662-52972-0_31

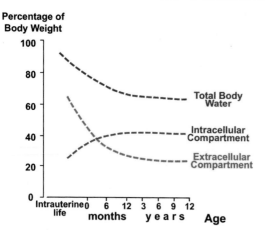

Fig. 31.1 Influence of age on the subdivision of total body water, intracellular fluid and extracellular fluid. For clinical purposes, "the rule of 3" is suggested: (1) total body water makes up 2/3 of the body mass; (2) the intracellular compartment contains 2/3 of the total body water; (3) the extracellular compartment is further subdivided into the interstitial and the intravascular compartments (blood volume), which contain 2/3 and 1/3 of the extracellular fluid, respectively

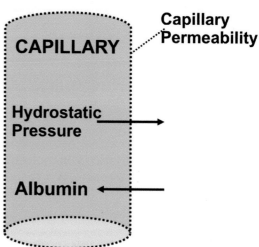

Fig. 31.2 Distribution of ultrafiltrate across the capillary membrane. The barrel-shaped structure represents a capillary. A high hydrostatic pressure or increased capillary permeability causes fluid to leave the vascular space. By contrast, an increased intravascular albumin concentration (and, therefore, an increased oncotic pressure) causes fluid to enter the vascular space

Consequently, K^+ largely determines the intracellular and Na^+ the extracellular compartment [1–4]. The extracellular compartment is further subdivided into the interstitial and the total intravascular compartments (total blood volume), which contain $\approx 2/3$ and $\approx 1/3$ of the extracellular fluid [1–4], respectively (the transcellular fluid compartment, which comprises the digestive, cerebrospinal, intraocular, pleural, peritoneal and synovial fluids, will not be further addressed in this review).

The size of the total intravascular compartment is determined by the overall size of the extracellular fluid compartment and by the Starling forces: they control the partition of fluids between intravascular and interstitial compartments across the capillary membrane that is crossed by salts like Na^+Cl^- and by glucose but not by blood proteins (especially albumin). Three major forces control the distribution of fluids across the capillary membrane (Fig. 31.2):

1. The hydrostatic pressure, which causes fluids to leave the vascular space;
2. The higher concentration of proteins in the intravascular compartment as compared with that in interstitial fluid, which causes fluids to

enter the vascular space. This force, which is called oncotic pressure, is due both to the concentration gradient of albumin (blood proteins other than albumin account for 50 % of the weight of proteins in blood but only for 25 % of the oncotic pressure) as well to the fact that albumin is anionic and therefore attracts cations (largely Na^+) into the vascular compartment (Gibbs-Donnan effect; Fig. 31.3);
3. Capillary permeability, which is a further modulator of the distribution of fluids across the capillary membrane.

Effective Circulating Volume

The total intravascular compartment is subdivided into the effective ($\approx$ arterial) and the ineffective ($\approx$ venous) compartment. Effective circulating volume denotes the part of the total intravascular compartment that is in the arterial system and is effectively perfusing the tissues. The effective circulating volume is biologically more relevant than the total intravascular (respectively the ineffective) compartment and usually varies directly with the

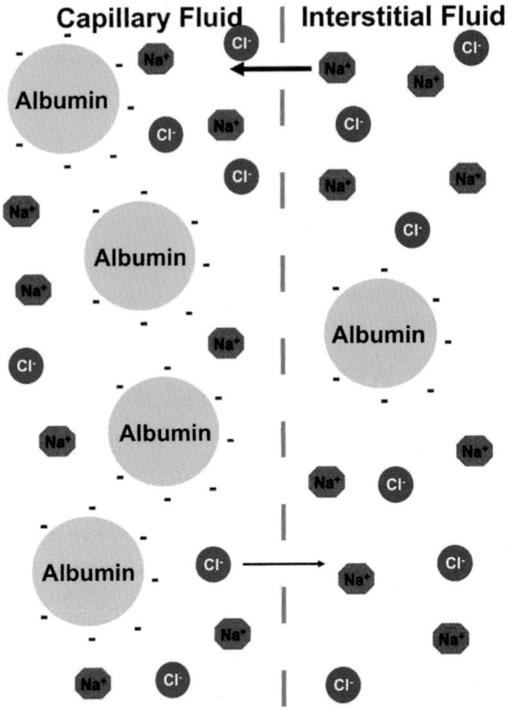

Fig. 31.3 The Gibbs-Donnan effect. There is a difference in the concentration of anionic albumin, which is impermeant, between the vascular (albumin approximately 40 g/L) and the interstitial (albumin approximately 10 g/L) compartments. The negative charges of albumin "attract" cations (largely Na^+) into the vascular compartment and "repell" anions (Cl^- and HCO_3^-) out. Because the concentration of Na^+ exceeds that of Cl^- and HCO_3^-, "attraction" outweighs "repulsion". Consequently, the Gibbs-Donnan effect increases the vascular compartment. The dashed line, which represents the capillary bed separating the intravascular and interstitial spaces, is freely permeable to Na^+, K^+, Cl^-, and glucose

extracellular fluid volume. As a result, the regulation of extracellular fluid balance (by alterations in urinary Na^+ excretion) and the maintenance of the effective circulating volume are intimately related. Na^+ loading will tend to produce volume expansion, whereas Na^+-loss (e.g., due to vomiting, diarrhea, or diuretic therapy) will lead to volume depletion. The body responds to changes in effective circulating volume in two steps:

1. The change is sensed by the volume receptors that are located in the cardiopulmonary circulation, in the carotid sinuses and aortic arch, and in the kidney;

2. These receptors activate effectors that restore normovolemia by varying vascular resistance, cardiac output, and renal water and salt excretion. In brief, the non-renal receptors primarily govern the activity of the sympathetic nervous system and natriuretic peptides, whereas the renal receptors affect volume balance by modulating the renin-angiotensin II-aldosterone system [1–4].

In some settings the effective circulating volume is independent of the extracellular fluid volume. For example, among patients with heart failure the extracellular fluid volume is increased but these patients are effectively volume depleted due to the low volume of blood pumped by the heart [1–4].

Blood Osmolality: Measurement of Sodium

Osmolality is the concentration of all solutes in a given weight of water (the similar concept of osmolarity denotes the concentration of all of the solutes in a given volume of water). The total (or true) blood osmolality is equal to the sum of the osmolalities of the individual solutes in blood. Most of the osmoles in blood are Na^+ salts, with lesser contributions from other ions, glucose, and urea. However, under normal circumstances, the osmotic effect of the ions in blood can usually be estimated as two times the Na^+ concentration. *Blood osmolality* (in mosm/kg H_2O) can be measured directly (via determination of freezing point depression) or estimated from circulating Na^+, glucose and urea (in mmol/L[1]) as follows [3–9]:

$$\left(Na^+ \times 2\right) + glucose + urea$$

The *effective blood osmolality*, known colloquially as blood tonicity, is a further clinically significant entity, which denotes the concentration of solutes impermeable to cell membranes

---

[1]To obtain glucose in mmol/L divide glucose in mg/dL by 18. To obtain urea in mmol/L divide urea nitrogen in mg/dL by 2.8 or urea in mg/dL by 6.0.

(Na$^+$, glucose, mannitol) and are therefore restricted to the extracellular compartment (osmoreceptors sense effective blood osmolality rather than the total blood osmolality). These solutes are effective because they create osmotic pressure gradients across cell membranes leading to movement of water from the intracellular to the extracellular compartment. Solutes that are permeable to cell membranes (urea, ethanol, methanol) are ineffective solutes because they do not generate osmotic pressure gradients across cell membranes and therefore are not associated with such water shifts. Glucose is a unique solute because, at normal concentrations in blood, it is actively taken up by cells and therefore acts as an ineffective solute, but under conditions of impaired cellular uptake (like diabetes mellitus) it becomes an effective extracellular solute.

Since no direct measurement of effective blood osmolality (which is biologically more important than the total or true blood osmolality) is possible, the following equations are used to calculate this entity [3–9]:

$$\left(Na^+ \times 2\right) + glucose\, measured\, total$$
$$blood\, osmolality - urea$$

Although strictly speaking, a Na$^+$ concentration outside the range of 135–145 mmol/L denotes dysnatremia, clinically relevant hypo- or hypernatremia is mostly defined as a concentration outside the range of 130–150 mmol/L [3, 4].

Dehydration and Extracellular Fluid Volume Depletion

Although dehydration semantically and in general usage means loss of water, in physiology and medicine the term denotes both a loss of water and salt. Depending on the type of pathophysiologic process, water and salts (primarily Na$^+$Cl$^-$) may be lost in physiologic proportion or lost disparately, with each type producing a somewhat different clinical picture, designated as normotonic (mostly isonatremic), hypertonic (mostly hypernatremic), or hypotonic (always hyponatremic) dehydration. Dehydration develops when

fluids are lost from the extracellular space at a rate exceeding intake. The most common sites for extracellular fluid loss are:

1. The intestinal tract (diarrhea, vomiting, or bleeding);
2. The skin (fever, excessive sweating or burns); and
3. The urine (osmotic diuresis, diuretic therapy, diabetes insipidus, or salt losing renal tubular disorders). More rarely, dehydration results from prolonged inadequate intake without excessive losses [3–9].

The risk for dehydration is high in children and especially infants for the following causes:

1. Infants and children are more susceptible to infectious diarrhea and vomiting than adults;
2. There is a higher proportional turnover of body fluids in infants compared to adults (it is estimated that the daily fluid intake and outgo, as a proportion of extracellular fluid, is in infancy more than three times that of an adult, Fig. 31.4);
3. Young children do not communicate their need for fluids or do not independently access fluids to replenish volume losses.

Dehydration reduces the effective circulating volume, therefore impairing tissue perfusion. If not rapidly corrected, ischemic end-organ damage occurs.

Three groups of symptoms and signs occur in dehydration:

(a) Those related to the manner in which fluids loss occurs (including diarrhea, vomiting or polyuria);
(b) Those related to the electrolyte and acid-base imbalances that sometimes accompany dehydration; and
(c) Those directly due to dehydration.

The following discussion will focus on the third group.

When assessing a child with a tendency towards dehydration, the clinician needs to

Daily Fluid Intake and Outgo

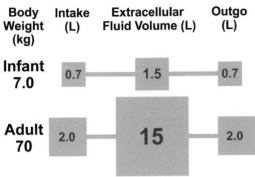

Body Weight (kg)	Intake (L)	Extracellular Fluid Volume (L)	Outgo (L)
Infant 7.0	0.7	1.5	0.7
Adult 70	2.0	15	2.0

Fig. 31.4 Fluid turnover in infancy and adulthood. There is a proportionally greater turnover of fluids and solutes in infants and children as compared with adults. The figure depicts fluid intake, extracellular fluid volume and fluid outgo (diuresis and perspiratio insensibilis) in a healthy 6-month-old infant weighing 7.0 kg (input represents ≈50% of extracellular fluid volume) and in a healthy adult weighing 70 kg (input represents ≈15% of extracellular fluid volume)

Table 31.1 "4-item 8-point rating scale" clinical dehydration scale

Characteristic	Score		
	0	1	2
General appearance	Normal	Thirsty, restless or lethargic but irritable when touched	Drowsy, limp, cold, or sweaty; comatose or not
Eyes	Normal	Slightly sunken	Very sunken
Mucous membranes (tongue)	Moist	Sticky	Dry
Tears	Tears	Decreased tears	Absent tears

The score consists of four clinical items, which may be summed for a total score ranging from 0 to 8. The final three categories are no or minimal dehydration (<3%; score of 0), mild dehydration (3% to <6% dehydration; score of 1–4), and moderate to severe dehydration (≥6% dehydration; score of 5–8)

address the degree of extracellular fluid volume depletion. More rarely the clinician will address the laboratory testing and the type of fluid lost (extracellular or intracellular fluid).

Degree of Dehydration

It is crucial to correctly assess the degree of dehydration since severe extracellular fluid volume depletion calls for rapid isotonic fluid resuscitation. Dehydration is most objectively measured as a change in weight from baseline (acute loss of body weight reflects the loss of fluid, not lean body mass; thus, a 1.3 kg weight loss reflects the loss of 1.3 l of fluid). In most cases, however, an accurate recent weight is unavailable.

As a result, a pertinent history and a number of findings on physical examination are used to help assess dehydration. Skin turgor, sometimes referred to as skin elasticity, is a sign commonly used to assess the degree of hydration (the skin on the back of the hand, lower arm, or abdomen is grasped between two fingers, held for a few seconds and then released: skin with normal turgor snaps rapidly back to its normal position but skin with decreased turgor remains elevated and returns slowly to its normal position). However, decreased skin turgor is a late sign in dehydra-

tion that is associated with moderate or, more frequently, severe dehydration. Like decreased skin turgor, arterial hypotension is a late sign in hypovolemia (in children with minimal to mild dehydration blood pressure is often slightly increased). Symptoms and signs of dehydration include dry mucous membranes, sunken eyes, reduced urine output, a sunken fontanelle, delayed capillary refill, deep respiration with or without increased respiratory rate, and tachycardia. Several attempts have been made to determine a measure of dehydration by using combinations of clinical findings. In children ≤4 years of age with a diagnosis of acute diarrhea or vomiting, four clinical items (a. general appearance, b. eyes, c. mucous membranes, and d. tears), which may be summed for a total score ranging from 0 to 8 [10], accurately estimate dehydration (Table 31.1).

Laboratory Testing and the Type of Fluid Lost

Laboratory testing can confirm the presence of dehydration. The fractional clearance of $Na^\pm$ (which measures the amount of filtered Na^+ that is excreted in the urine)

$$\frac{Urinary\,Na^+ \times Circulating\,Creatinine}{Circulating\,Na^+ \times Urinary\,Creatinine}$$

is $<0.5 \times 10^{-2}$ (or $<0.5\%$) and the urine spot Na$^\pm$ concentration <30 mmol/L (unless the disease underlying dehydration is renal).

Furthermore, in dehydration, the urine is concentrated with an osmolality >450 mosm/kg H$_2$O. The urinary concentration is measured with an osmometer or fairly estimated, in the absence of proteinuria and glucosuria, from the specific gravity, as determined by refractometry (dipstick assessment of specific gravity is unreliable), as follows:

$$\left(specific\,gravity - 1000\right) \times 40$$

Furthermore, laboratory testing can detect associated electrolyte and acid-base abnormalities but determination of circulating electrolytes and acid-base balance is typically limited to children requiring intravenous fluids. These children are more severely volume depleted and are therefore at greater risk for dyselectrolytemias. Laboratory testing is less useful for assessing the degree of volume depletion.

Bicarbonatemia ≤ 17.0 mmol/L is considered by some a useful laboratory test to assess dehydration.

The *blood urea* level might be a further good biochemical marker of dehydration because it reflects both the decreased glomerular filtration rate and the enhanced Na$^+$ and water reabsorption in the proximal tubule. Unfortunately this test is of limited usefulness since it can be increased by other factors such as bleeding or tissue breakdown (on the other side the rise can be minimized by a concomitant decrease in protein intake).

The serum Na$^+$ concentration varies with the relative loss of solute to water. Changes in Na$^+$ concentration play a pivotal role in deciding the type of fluid depletion (Fig. 31.5):

- Hyponatremic (and hypotonic) dehydration: The development of hyponatremia reflects net solute loss in excess of water loss. This does not occur directly, as fluid losses such as diarrhea are not hypertonic. Usually solute and water are lost in proportion, but water is taken in and retained in the context of hypovolemia-induced secretion of anti-diuretic hormone. Since body water shifts from extracellular fluid to cells under these circumstances, signs of dehydration easily become profound.
- Normonatremic (and isotonic) dehydration: In this setting, solute is lost in proportion to water loss.
- Hypernatremic (and hypertonic) dehydration: This setting reflects water loss in excess of solute loss. Since body water shifts from intracellular to extracellular fluid under these circumstances, these children have less signs of dehydration for any given amount of fluid loss than do children with normonatremic (or normotonic) dehydration and especially those with hyponatremic dehydration.

Dysnatremia

Consequences, Symptoms, and Diagnostic Work Up

Under normal conditions, blood Na$^+$ concentration is maintained within the narrow range of 135–145 mmol/L despite great variations in water and salt intake. Na$^+$ and its accompanying anions Cl$^-$ and HCO$_3^-$ account for 90% of the extracellular effective osmolality. The main determinant of the Na$^+$ concentration is the plasma water content, itself determined by water intake (thirst or habit), "insensible" losses (such as metabolic water and sweat), and urinary dilution. The last of these is under most circumstances crucial and predominantly determined by anti-diuretic hormone. In response to this hormone, concentrated urine is produced. Dysnatremias produce central nervous system dysfunction. While hyponatremia may induce brain swelling, hypernatremia may induce brain shrinkage, yet the clinical features elicited by opposite changes in tonicity are remarkably similar [3–9].

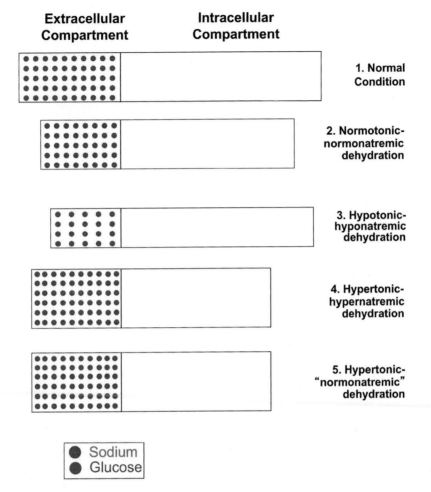

Fig. 31.5 Extracellular and intracellular compartments in children with dehydration. Normally, the extracellular compartment makes up approximately 20 % and the intracellular 40 % of the body weight (*panel 1* of the figure). The *second, third* and *fourth panels* depict the relationship between extracellular and intracellular compartment in three children with dehydration in the context of an acute diarrheal disease: dehydration is normotonic-normonatremic in the first (*panel 2*), hypotonic-hyponatremic (mainly extracellular fluid losses) in the second (*panel 3*), and hypernatremic (mainly intracellular fluid losses) in the third child (*panel 4*). The *lower panel* depicts the relationship between extracellular and intracellular compartment (mainly intracellular fluid losses) in a child with dehydration in the context of diabetic ketoacidosis (hypertonic-"normonatremic" dehydration; the *brackets* indicate that in the context of diabetic ketoacidosis the concentration of circulating sodium is normal or even reduced). In each panel the *red circles* denote sodium and *blue circles* impermeable solutes that do not move freely across cell membranes (in the present example glucose). For reasons of simplicity, no symbols are given for potassium, the main intracellular cation

Hyponatremia

Hyoponatremia is classified (Fig. 31.6) according to the extracellular fluid volume status, as either "hypovolemic" (= depletional) or "normo-hypervolemic" (= dilutional). Vasopressin is released both in children with low effective circulating volume, the most common cause of hyponatremia in everyday clinical practice, as well as in those with normo-hypervolemic hyponatremia. In hypovolemic hyponatremia, vasopressin release is triggered by the low effective arterial blood volume (this condition is also referred to as "syndrome of appropriate antidiuresis"). In dilutional hyponatremia, the primary defect is a euvolemic, inappropriate

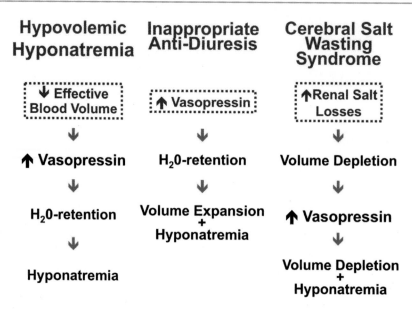

Fig. 31.6 Extracellular fluid volume status in children with hyponatremia. Hyoponatremia is classified according to the extracellular fluid volume status, as either hypovolemic (= depletional) or normo- hypervolemic (= dilutional). In most cases (*left panel*) hyponatremia results from a low effective arterial blood volume and is termed hypovolemic hyponatremia (the term appropriate anti-diuresis is sometimes used in this circumstance). The true syndrome of inappropriate anti-diuresis results from persistently high levels of vasopressin or, more rarely, activation of its renal receptor (*middle panel*). Cerebral salt-wasting syndrome is a further form of hyponatremia that sometimes develops in patients with intracranial disorders (*right panel*). In this condition, renal salt-wasting is the primary defect, which is followed by volume depletion leading to a secondary rise in vasopressin

increase in circulating vasopressin levels (this condition is also termed "syndrome of inappropriate anti-diuresis").

Assessing the cause of hyponatremia may be straightforward if an obvious cause is present (for example in the setting of vomiting or diarrhea) or in the presence of a clinically evident extracellular fluid volume depletion [3–5, 8, 9]. Sometimes, however, assessing the volume status and distinguishing hypovolemic from normo- hypervolemic hyponatremia may not be straightforward. In such cases, the urine spot Na^+ and the fractional Na^+ clearance are helpful, as patients with dilutional hyponatremia have a urinary $Na^+ >30$ mmol/L (and fractional Na^+ clearance $>0.5\%$), whereas those with extracellular fluid volume depletion (unless the source is renal) will have a urinary $Na^+ <30$ mmol/L (and fractional Na^+ clearance $<0.5\%$). Since effective blood osmolality is mostly low in hyponatremia, and urine is less than maximally dilute (inappropriately concentrated), blood and urine osmolalities, although usually measured, are rarely discriminant.

A decrease in Na^+ concentration and effective blood osmolality causes movement of water into brain cells and results in cellular swelling and raised intracranial pressure. Nausea and malaise are typically seen when the Na^+ level acutely falls $<125–130$ mmol/L. Headache, lethargy, restlessness, and disorientation follow, as its concentration falls $<115–120$ mmol/L. With severe and rapidly evolving hyponatremia, seizure, coma, permanent brain damage, respiratory arrest, brain stem herniation, and death may occur. In more gradually evolving hyponatremia, the brain self regulates to prevent swelling over hours to days by transport of, firstly, Na^+, Cl^-, and K^+ and, later, solutes like glutamate, taurine, myoinositol, and glutamine from intracellular to extracellular compartments. This induces water loss and ameliorates brain swelling, and hence leads to few symptoms in subacute and chronic hyponatremia.

Evaluating the Cause

In normovolemic subjects, the primary defense against developing hyponatremia is the ability to dilute urine and excrete free-water [3–5, 8, 9]. Rarely is excess ingestion of free-water alone the cause of hyponatremia. It is also rare to develop hyponatremia from excess urinary Na^+ losses in the absence of free-water ingestion. In order for hyponatremia to develop both a relative excess of free-water as well as an underlying condition that impairs the ability to excrete free-water are typically required. Renal water handling is primarily under the control of vasopressin, which is released from the posterior pituitary and impairs water diuresis by increasing the permeability to water in the collecting tubule.

There are osmotic, hemodynamic and non-hemodynamic stimuli for release of vasopressin. In most cases, hyponatremia develops when the body attempts to preserve the extracellular fluid volume at the expense of circulating Na^+ (therefore, a hemodynamic stimulus for vasopressin production overrides an inhibitory effect of hyponatremia). However, there are further stimuli for production of vasopressin in hospitalized children that make virtually any hospitalized patient at risk for hyponatremia (Table 31.2).

Some specific causes of hypotonic hyponatremia deserve further discussion.

Hospital-acquired hyponatremia is most often seen in the postoperative period or in association with a reduced effective circulating volume. Postoperative hyponatremia is a serious problem in children, which sometimes is caused by a combination of nonosmotic stimuli for release of anti-diuretic hormone, such as pain, nausea, stress, narcotics, and edema-forming conditions. Subclinical depletion of the effective blood volume and administration of hypotonic fluids are currently considered the most important causes of postoperative hyponatremia.

More rarely, hospital-acquired hyponatremia is seen in association with the syndrome of inappropriate anti-diuresis, which is caused either by elevated activity of vasopressin or, less commonly, by hyperfunction of its renal (= V2) receptor, independently of increased effective blood osmolality and hemodynamic stimulus

Table 31.2 Causes of hypotonic hyponatremia in childhood

Extracellular fluid volume reduced	Extracellular fluid volume normal or increased
Intestinal salt loss	Increased body water
Diarrheal dehydration	Parenteral hypotonic solutions
Vomiting, gastric suction	Exercise-associated hyponatermia
Fistulae	Habitual (and psychogenic) polydipsia
Laxative abuse	
Transcutaneous salt loss	Non osmolar release of antidiuretic hormones[a]
Cystic fibrosis	Cardiac failure
Endurance sport	Sever liver disease (mostly cirrhosis)
	Nephrotic syndrome
	Glucocorticoid deficiency
	Drugs causing renal water retention
	[Hypothyroidism][b]
Renal sodium loss	Syndrome of inappropriate anti-diuresis
Mineralocorticoid deficiency (or resistance)	Classic syndrome of inappropriate secretion of antidiuretic hormone
Diuretics	
Salt wasting renal failure	Hereditary nephrogenic inappropriate antidiuresis
Salt wasting tubulopathies (including Bartter syndromes, Gitelman syndrome, and De Toni-Debré–Fanconi syndrome)	
Cerebral salt wasting	
Perioperative (e.g., preoperative fasting, vomiting, third space losses)	Reduced renal water loss
	Chronic renal failure
	Oliguric acute renal failure

[a]Effective arterial blood volume mostly reduced
[b]Evidence supporting this association rather poor

(i.e., reduced effective circulating volume). It is currently assumed that this condition results not only from dilution of the blood by free-water but also from inappropriate natriuresis. The syndrome of inappropriate anti-diuresis (Fig. 31.6) should be suspected in any child with hyponatremic hypotonia, a urine osmolality >100 mosmol/kg H_2O, a normal fractional Na^+ clearance (>0.5 %), low normal or reduced uric acid level, low blood urea level and normal acid-base and K^+ balance. The longstanding assumption that hypontremia associated with meningitis or respiratory infections is caused by inappropriate anti-diuresis is not substantiated by reports that adequately assessed the volume status (Fig. 31.7).

Desmopressin, a synthetic analogue of the natural anti-diuretic hormone, is used in central diabetes insipidus, in some bleeding disorders, in diagnostic urine concentration testing and especially in primary nocturnal enuresis with nocturnal polyuria. Desmopressin is generally regarded as a safe drug and adverse effects are uncommon. Nonetheless, hyponatremic water intoxication leading to convulsions has been reported as a rare side effect of desmopressin therapy in enuretic children. This complication mostly develops in subjects managed with the intranasal formulation ≲14 days after starting the medication, following excess fluid intake and during intercurrent illnesses (Table 31.3).

Male infants have been described with hypo-natremia and laboratory features consistent with release of vasopressin but who had no measurable circulating levels of this hormone. This rare condition results from gain-of-function mutations of the X-linked receptor gene that mediates the renal response to vasopressin, resulting in persistent activation of the receptor. The condition, which has been termed *hereditary nephrogenic syndrome of inappropriate anti-diuresis*, represents a kind of mirror image of the X-linked nephrogenic diabetes insipidus, the result of loss-of-function genetic defects in the aforementioned renal receptor.

Cerebral salt wasting syndrome is a peculiar form of depletional hyponatremia that sometimes occurs in patients with cerebral disease (Fig. 31.7). It mimics the syndrome of inappropriate anti-diuresis, except that salt-wasting is the primary defect with the ensuing volume depletion leading to a secondary release of vasopressin. Salt wasting of central origin might result from increased secretion of a natriuretic peptide with subsequent suppression of aldosterone synthesis. The distinction between cerebral salt wasting and inappropriate activity of vasopressin

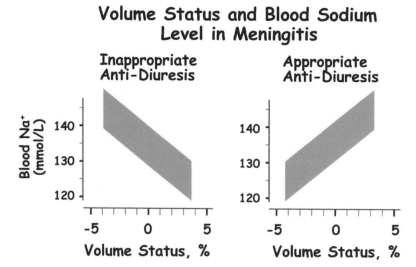

Fig. 31.7 Relationship between state of hydration and circulating sodium in acute meningitis and respiratory infectious diseases. It has been traditionally assumed that hyponatremia in this setting results from inappropriate

anti-diuresis (*left panel*). Data from the literature suggest that hyponatremia is due to appropriate, volume-dependent anti-diuresis (*right panel*)

Table 31.3 Drug-induced hyponatremia

Diuretics (thiazides more commonly than loop diuretics)
Drugs blocking the renin-angiotensin-aldosterone system (converting enzyme inhibitors, sartans or renin inhibitors)
Other drugs
↑ **water permeability of the renal collecting tubule**: arginine-vasopressin, vasopressin analogues like desmopressin and oxytocin
↑ **antidiuretic hormone release**, ↑ **antidiuretic hormone action**: carbamazepine, lamotrigine, valproate, barbiturates, antidiabetic drugs (chlorpropamide, tolbutamide), clofibrate, colchicine, nicotine, vincristine, cyclophosphamide
↓ **synthesis of prostaglandins**: nonsteroidal anti-inflammatory drugs including salicylates, paracetamol
Mechanism unknown: haloperidol, tricyclic antidepressants, selective serotonin-reuptake inhibitors, monoamine oxidase inhibitors, narcotics like morphine

Used with permission of BMJ Publishing Group from Haycock [8]

is not always simple since the true volume status is sometimes difficult to ascertain.

Endurance athletes sometimes replace their dilute but Na^+-containing sweat losses with excessive amounts of severely hypotonic solutions: the net effect is a reduction in the circulating Na^+ level. The effect is likely compounded by a reduced renal function during exercise (such individuals may also be taking non-steroidal anti-inflammatory drugs, which can impair the excretion of free water).

A tendency towards low normal blood Na^+ level is sometimes seen in children who drink excessively and present with polyuria and polydipsia. Usually the problem is simply one of habit, particularly in infants who are attached to a bottle (= *habitual polydipsia*). Rarely, in childhood, polydipsia is a symptom of significant psychopathology (= *psychogenic polydipsia*).

Diuretics (thiazides more frequently than loop diuretics) and drugs that block the renin-angiotensin-aldosterone system (converting enzyme inhibitors, sartans or renin inhibitors) make up a common cause of hyponatremia (Table 31.3). More rarely, other drugs sometimes cause renal retention of fluids and therefore dilutional hyponatremia.

Hypernatremia

Hypernatremia reflects a net water loss or a hypertonic Na^+ gain, with inevitable hypertonicity [3–7]. Severe symptoms are usually evident only with acute and large increases in Na^+ concentrations ≥ 160 mmol/L. Importantly, the sensation of thirst protecting against the tendency towards hypernatemia is absent or reduced in patients with altered mental status or with hypothalamic lesions and in infancy.

The cause of hypernatremia is almost always evident from the history. Determination of urine osmolality in relation to the effective blood osmolality and the urine Na^+ concentration helps if the cause is unclear. Patients with diabetes insipidus present with polyuria and polydipsia (and not hypernatremia unless thirst sensation is impaired). Central diabetes insipidus and nephrogenic diabetes insipidus may be differentiated by the response to water deprivation (failure to concentrate urine) followed by desmopressin, causing concentration of urine uniquely in patients with central diabetes insipidus.

Non-specific symptoms such as anorexia, muscle weakness, restlessness, nausea, and vomiting tend to occur early. More serious signs follow, with altered mental status, lethargy, irritability, stupor, or coma. Acute brain shrinkage can induce vascular rupture, with cerebral bleeding and subarachnoid hemorrhage.

Evaluating the Cause

Two mechanisms protect against developing hypernatremia ($Na^+ > 145$ mmol/L) or increased effective blood osmolality: the ability to release vasopressin (and therefore to concentrate urine) and a powerful thirst mechanism. Release of vasopressin occurs when the effective blood osmolality exceeds 275–280 mosmol/kg H_2O and results in maximally concentrated urine when the effective blood osmolality exceeds 290–295 mosmol/kg H_2O. Thirst, the second line of defense, provides a further protection against hypernatremia and increased effective

Table 31.4 Causes of hypernatremia in childhood

Hypovolemic	Normovolemic	Hypervolemic
Inadequate intake	**Hypodypsia** (essential hypernatremia)	**Inappropriate intravenous fluids** (e.g., hypertonic saline, NaHCO$_3$)
Breast feeding hypernatremia	**Hyperventilation**	**Salt poisoning** (accidental, deliberate)
Poor access to water	Fever	**Primary aldosteronism** (and other conditions that cause low-renin hypertension)
Altered thirst perception (uncosciousness, mental impairment)		
Intestinal salt loss (diarrheal dehydration)		
Renal water and salt loss		
Postobstructive polyuria		
Diuretics		
Diabetes insipidus (either primary or, more rarely, secondary[a])		
Medullary renal damage		

[a]Secondary nephrogenic diabetes insipidus may develop as a complication of inherited renal diseases such as nephropathic cystinosis, Bartter and Gitelman syndromes and nephronophthisis

osmolality. If the thirst mechanism is intact and there is unrestricted access to free-water, it is rare to develop sustained hypernatremia from either excess Na$^+$ ingestion or a renal concentrating defect (Table 31.4). Hypernatremia is primarily a hospital-acquired condition occurring in children who have restricted access to fluids. Most children with hypernatremia are debilitated by an acute or chronic disease, have neurological impairment, are critically ill or are born premature. Hypernatremia in the intensive care setting is common as these children are typically either intubated or moribund, and often are fluid restricted, receive large amounts of Na$^+$ as blood products or have renal concentrating defects from diuretics or renal dysfunction. The majority of hypernatremia results from the failure to administer sufficient free-water to children who are unable to care for themselves and have restricted access to fluids.

Two special causes of hypernatremia deserve some further discussion.

- A frequent cause of hypernatremia in the outpatient setting is currently *breastfeeding-associated hypernatremia*, which should more properly be labeled "not-enough-breastfeeding-associated hypernatremia". This condition occurs between days 7 and 15 in otherwise healthy term or near-term newborns of first-time mothers who are exclusively breast-fed. In all cases feeding had been difficult to establish and the volume of milk ingested was likely to have been low. The underlying problem is water deficiency: Na$^+$ concentration raises predominantly as a result of low volume intake and a loss of water, demonstrating that inadequate feeding is the cause of hypernatremic dehydration. Monitoring postnatal weight loss provides an objective assessment of the adequacy of nutritional intake allowing targeted support to those infants who fail to thrive or demonstrate excessive weight loss ($\geq 10\%$ of birth weight).

- Diarrhea or vomiting are a further reason of hypernatremia in the outpatient setting, but are much less common than in the past, presumably due to the advent of low solute infant formulas and the increased use and availability of oral rehydration solutions.

Management

The discussion will exclusively focus on some features of parenteral hydration, and the management of hyponatremia with V2 anti-diuretic hormone receptor antagonists [3–9].

Maintenance and Perioperative Fluids

Intravenous maintenance fluids are designed to provide water and electrolyte requirements in a fasting patient. The prescription for intravenous maintenance fluids was originally described by Holliday (Table 31.5), who rationalized a daily H_2O requirement of 1700–1800 mL/m² body surface area and the addition of 3 and 2 mmol/kg body weight of Na^+ and K^+ respectively (approximating the electrolyte requirements and urinary excretion in healthy infants). This is the basis for the traditional recommendation that hypotonic intravenous maintenance solutions are ideal for children. This approach has been recently questioned because of the potential for these hypotonic solutions to cause hyponatremia. Surgical patients appear the subgroup of children with highest risk to develop severe hyponatremia with the use of hypotonic intravenous solutions, likely because they tend to be hypovolemic. Furthermore, traditional maintenance fluid recommendations may be much greater than actual water needs in children at risk of hyponatremia.

Most authors currently suggest (Table 31.5) that hyponatremia should be prevented by a) using isotonic (usually normal saline, which contains NaCl 9 g/L) or near isotonic (usually Ringer's lactate) solutions and b) reducing by ≈20 % the daily volume of maintenance fluid to 1400–1500 mL/m² body surface area. Considering the potential for hypoglycemia in infancy, normal saline in 5 % glucose in water (which contains glucose 50 g/L) is considered the safest fluid composition for most children.

Dehydration

Oral rehydration therapy is currently the treatment of choice for children with minimal, mild or moderate dehydration due to diarrheal diseases. However, in the practice of pediatric emergency medicine, intravenous rehydration is a commonly used intervention for these children.

Treatment approaches to parenteral rehydration in the hospitalized child vary. There are numerous ways to estimate the degree of

Table 31.5 Intravenous maintenance fluids designed to provide water and electrolyte requirements in a fasting patient

	Holliday's recommendation	Current suggestion
Solution	5 % dextrose in water supplemented with NaCl 3 mmol/kg body weight daily	Isotonic saline and 5 % dextrose in water
Amount (mL/m² body surface area[a] daily)	1700–1800	1400–1500
Clinical practice	100 mL/kg body weight for a child weighing less than 10 kg[b] + 50 mL/kg for each additional kg up to 20 kg + 20-[25] mL/kg for each kg in excess of 20 kg	80 mL/kg body weight for a child weighing less than 10 kg[b] + 40 mL/kg for each additional kg up to 20 kg + 15-[20] mL/kg for each kg in excess of 20 kg

Both the recommendation originally described by Holliday and the most recent recommendation are given. The addition of KCl 2 mmol/kg body weight is also recommended

[a]The Mosteller's formula may be used to calculate the body surface area (in m²):
$$\sqrt{\frac{height\,(cm) \times body\,wight\,(kg)}{3600}}$$

[b]In children weighing ≤5.0 kg the daily parenteral water requirement is 120 mL/kg body weight

dehydration (the "4-item 8-point rating scale" is currently widely recommended; Table 31.1), to calculate fluid and electrolyte deficits, and to deliver the deficits to the patient. The aim of treatment is generally to accomplish rapid full repletion within ≤6 h. In many children with mild to moderate dehydration, especially those resistant to initial oral rehydration therapy, and in children with severe dehydration, intravenous isotonic (or near isotonic) crystalloid solutions such as normal saline or lactate Ringer's are administered as repeated boluses of 10–20 mL/kg body weight (administered over 20–60 min). This procedure has recently been challenged by the results of a large randomized clinical trial in African children with severe dehydration due to septic shock, in which higher mortality was observed in patients receiving aggressive fluid resuscitation (single bolus of 20–40 ml/kg) as compared to children with no bolus administration [11]. Hence, fluid boluses may be contraindicated in patients with septic hemodynamic dysregulation.

In children with diarrhea or vomiting, reduced carbohydrate intake leads to free fatty acid breakdown, excess ketones, and an increased likelihood of continued nausea and vomiting. Consequently, some authorities have suggested the use of a glucose containing normal solution (mostly the aforementioned normal saline in 5 % glucose in water), which will stimulate insulin release, reduce free fatty acid breakdown, and therefore reduce treatment failure due to persisting nausea and vomiting (owing to hyperketonemia).

The child with hypovolemic circulatory shock presents with (a) increased heart rate and weak peripheral pulses, (b) cold, pale and diaphoretic skin, and (c) delayed capillary refill. The initial management recommended by the American Academy of Pediatrics includes the administration of a high concentration of O_2 (ensuring that 100 % of the available arterial hemoglobin is oxygenated) and fluid resuscitation by isotonic crystalloid fluid boluses at a maximum total dose of 60 mL/kg body weight. Common errors in the child with hypovolemic circulatory shock secondary to a diarrheal disease are delayed or inadequate (i.e., with hypotonic crystalloid solution) fluid resuscitation.

Children with hypernatremic dehydration are also hydrated parenterally with isotonic crystalloid solutions until diagnosis of the dyselectrolytemia, followed by slightly hypotonic solutions (e.g., half-saline) in order to slowly correct the circulating Na^+ concentration (abruptly correcting hypernatremia using a Na^+ free glucose solution creates an increased risk of brain edema; Fig. 31.8). In acute dysnatremic dehydration, Na^+ should be corrected slowly at a rate not exceeding 0.5 mmol/L per hour (or more than by 12 mmol/L per day). Subacute or chronic hypernatremia should be corrected even more slowly.

Hydration in Infectious Diseases Associated with a Tendency Towards Hyponatremia

Fluid restriction has been widely advocated in the initial management of infectious diseases such as meningitis, pneumonia or bronchiolitis, which are often associated with a low Na^+ level. However, there is no evidence that fluid restriction is useful. Furthermore, hyponatremia results from appropriate, volume-dependent antidiuresis in these disease conditions. In clinical practice, initial restoration of the intravascular space with an isotonic crystalloid followed by isotonic maintenance fluids 1400–1500 mL/m^2 body surface area per day (Table 31.5, right panel) are currently advised. In cases presenting with overt hyponatremia frequent monitoring of electrolytes is also required with adjustments to be made according to laboratory findings.

Normo/Hypervolemic Hyponatremia

Normo- or hypervolemic hyponatremia is managed primarily by restricting water intake. An alternative may be the use of vasopressin receptor antagonists. There are three receptors for vasopressin: the $V1_a$ receptors that mediate vasoconstriction, the $V1_b$ receptors that mediate adrenocorticotropin release, and the V2 receptors that mediate the anti-diuretic response. Vaptans, oral V2 receptor antagonists, have recently been approved for the management of normovolemic and hypervolemic hyponatremia: these agents produce a selective water diuresis (without affecting Na^+ and K^+ excretion) that raises the circulating Na^+ level. Little information on these "aquaretics" is currently available in children; pediatric clinical trials are currently underway.

Vaptans do not correct hyponatremia in patients affected with nephrogenic syndrome of inappropriate childhood anti-diuresis. In these patients, a way to enhance water excretion is the oral administration of urea (dosage in adults: 30 g/day). This regimen, which may be effective because it causes simultaneously water diuresis and renal Na^+ retention, is well tolerated, and has been used chronically in pediatric outpatients.

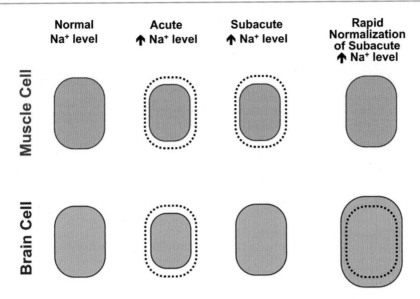

Fig. 31.8 Cell volume in acute or subacute hypernatremia and after rapid correction of hypernatremia. When hypernatremia develops acutely, all cells are reduced in size (the degree of cell volume reduction reflects the degree of hypernatremia). When hypernatremia is present for 36–48 h or more (= subacute hypernatremia), cell volume reduction persists in most cells, including muscle cells (*upper panel*). However, brain cells and red blood cells tend to restore their normal cell volume (*lower panel*). A rapid normalization of sodium level in children affected with subacute or chronic hypernatremia pathologically increases the volume of brain cells (and red blood cells). Swelling of cells, which does not have serious consequences when it occurs in most organs, may have damaging consequences when it occurs in the brain (*lower panel, right*)

Potassium

Balance

Most (98 %) of the K^+ in the body (40–50 mmol/kg) is within cells. The maintenance of distribution of K^+ across cells is largely dependent on the activity of the sodium pump (= Na^+-K^+-ATPase). In healthy humans the extracellular K^+ concentration is maintained between 3.5 and 5.0 mmol/L. K^+ balance, like that of other ions, is a function of intake and urinary excretion. In adults, the daily K^+ intake averages 0.5–2 mmol/kg body weight (Fig. 31.9). The homeostasis goal of the adult is to remain in zero K^+ balance. Thus, ≈90–95 % of the typical daily intake of 1 mmol/kg is ultimately eliminated from the body in the urine (the residual 5–10 % is lost through the stool). Infants maintain a positive K^+ balance (the estimated requirement for growth is 1.2 mmol/day during the first 3 months of life, 0.8 mmol/day up to 1 year and 0.4 mmol/day thereafter).

The net accretion of K^+ ensures the availability of adequate substrate for incorporation into cells newly formed during periods of somatic growth. Postnatal growth is associated with an increase in total body K^+ from ≈8 mmol/cm body height at birth to >14 mmol/cm body height by 18 years of age. The rate of accretion of body K^+ per kg body weight in the infant is more rapid than in the older child, reflecting both an increase in cell number and K^+ concentration, at least in skeletal muscle, with advancing age [11–13].

Regulation of Circulating Potassium

Circulating K^+ concentration is regulated by the total body K^+ content, which depends upon (a) the external balance, i.e. the difference between intake and excretion in the urine, feces and sweat, and (b) the internal balance, which represents the relative distribution of K^+ between the intracellular and the extracellular spaces [11–13].

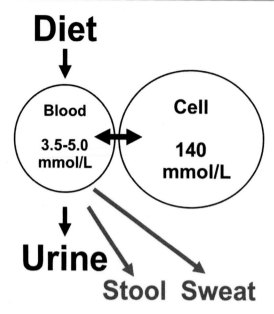

Diet

Blood

3.5-5.0 mmol/L

Cell

140 mmol/L

Urine

Stool Sweat

Fig. 31.9 Major factors governing the homeostasis of potassium. Most of the potassium in the body resides within cells. The maintenance of distribution of potassium across cells is largely dependent on the activity of the sodium pump. Potassium balance, like that of other ions, is a function of intake and urinary excretion. Since only small amounts of potassium are normally lost in the sweat and in the stool, they are depicted in a different color. However, substantial intestinal potassium and therefore potassium depletion can be seen with vomiting, diarrhea or other intestinal disease conditions or when sweat production is chronically increased

External (Renal) Potassium Homeostasis

Virtually all regulation of urinary K^+ excretion and therefore of external K^+ homeostasis occurs in the *renal cortical collecting tubule*. Indeed almost all of the filtered K^+ is reabsorbed in the proximal tubule and the loop of Henle, so that <10 % of the filtered load is delivered to the cortical collecting tubule. This tubular segment adjusts the external homeostasis of K^+ by modulating its secretion.

The major physiologic regulators of K^+ secretion within the cortical collecting tubule are "hyperkalemia" and aldosterone, which act in concert to promote the tubular secretion and therefore the urinary excretion of this ion.

Increasing the flow rate traversing the cortical collecting tubule is a further factor that may increase the K^+ excretion. This response is most prominent in the presence of hyperkalemia, since the concurrent elevations in aldosterone and circulating K^+ concentration produce a high level of K^+ secretion within the cortical collecting tubule.

Internal Potassium Homeostasis

The main modulators of the distribution of K^+ between the intracellular and the extracellular spaces are insulin, the sympathetic nervous system (via β_2-adrenergic receptors) and the acid-base balance.

Prenatal and Neonatal Potassium Balance

During fetal life K^+ is actively transported across the placenta from the mother to the fetus (indeed, the fetal K^+ concentration is maintained at levels ≥ 5.0 mmol/L even in the face of maternal K^+ deficiency). The tendency to retain K^+ early in postnatal life is reflected by the observation that infants, especially premature newborns, tend to have higher circulating K^+ levels than children. Furthermore, in infancy the ability to increase urinary K^+ excretion is blunted (see: non-oliguric hyperkalaemia of the premature infant).

Symptoms, Signs, and Consequences of Hypokalemia and Hyperkalemia

Excess or deficient K^+ in the extracellular space impairs cardiovascular, neuromuscular, renal and endocrine-metabolic body functions [12, 13]. The most dangerous clinical consequence of these dyselectrolytemias is the predisposition to life-threatening cardiac arrhythmias. The manifestations of hypokalemia are outlined in Table 31.6, those of hyperkalemia in Table 31.7.

The severity of hypokalemic manifestations is proportionate to the degree and duration of hypokalemia and symptoms generally do not become manifest until the K^+ concentration is below 2.5–3.0 mmol/L. Hypokalemia causes characteristic electrocardiographic changes

Table 31.6 Body functions impaired by hypokalemia

Cardiovascular abnormalities
Cardiac arrhythmias (prolonged QT-interval, premature atrial and ventricular beats, sinus bradycardia, paroxysmal atrial or junctional tachycardia, atrioventricular block, and ventricular tachycardia or fibrillation)
Increased systemic vascular resistance
Neuromuscular disturbances
Skeletal muscle weakness (usually beginning with the lower extremities and progressing to the trunk and upper extremities; sometimes involvement of the respiratory muscles)
Muscle cramps, rhabdomyolysis
Smooth muscle dysfunction (intestinal and urinary system)
Renal effects
Decreased urinary concentrating ability (decreased expression of the antidiuretic hormone-sensitive water channel aquaporin-2)
Increased renal ammonium production (and therefore ↑ generation of HCO_3^-)
Hypokalemic nephropathy[a] (interstitial fibrosis, tubular atrophy, cyst formation in the renal medulla).
Endocrine and metabolic effects
Negative nitrogen balance (causing growth retardation)
Glucose intolerance (with tendency towards diabetes mellitus)
Decreased aldosterone release (direct adrenal action), increased renin secretion
Hepatic encephalopathy (in susceptible individuals)

[a]Following prolonged hypokalemia

Table 31.7 Body functions impaired by hyperkalemia

Cardiovascular abnormalities
Cardiac arrhythmias (ventricular fibrillation or standstill are the most severe consequences)
Reduced systemic vascular resistance
Neuromuscular disturbances
Skeletal muscle weakness (usually beginning with the lower extremities and progressing to the trunk and upper extremities; rarely involvement of the respiratory muscles)
Smooth muscle dysfunction (intestinal and urinary system)
Renal effects
Reduced renal ammonium production (and therefore reduced generation of HCO_3^-)
Endocrine and metabolic effects
Increased aldosterone release (direct adrenal action), reduced renin secretion

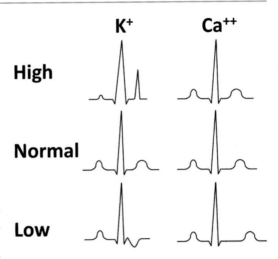

Fig. 31.10 Diagram illustrating some electrocardiographic consequences of hyperkalemia, hypokalemia, hypercalcemia and hypocalcemia. The electrocardiographic changes of hyperkalemia include tall and "peaked" T waves, QRS widening and, at very high K^+ concentrations, ventricular arrhythmias (not shown). Hypokalemia produces a decreased amplitude of the T wave and an increased amplitude of U waves, which occur at the end of the T wave. Hypercalcemia manifests with a shortened, hypocalcemia with a prolonged QT interval

(Fig. 31.10): depression of the ST segment, a decreased amplitude of the T wave, and an increased amplitude of U waves which occur at the end of the T wave.

There are very few symptoms or signs of hyperkalemia, and these tend to occur only with very high levels. Symptoms generally do not become manifest until the K^+ concentration exceeds 7.0 mmol/L, unless the rise in concentration has been very rapid. Hyperkalemia produces the following elecrocardiographic changes: peaked T wave with shortened QT interval is the first change, followed by progressive lengthening of the PR interval and QRS duration. The severity of hyperkalemia is classified as follows: (a) mild: K^+ between 5.1 and 6.0 mmol/L and absent or equivocal electrocardiographic changes; (b) moderate: K^+ between 6.1 and 7.0 mmol/L and definite eletrocardiographic changes in reploarization ("peaked" T waves); (c) severe: K^+ ≥7.1 mmol/L and severe definite eletrocardiographic changes including atrial standstill, advanced atrio-ventricular heart block, QRS widening or ventricular arrhythmia (usually associated with weakness of skeletal muscle). The electrocardiographic signs of hyperkalemia are given in Fig. 31.10.

Evaluating the Causes of Hypokalemia and Hyperkalemia (Diagnostic Tests)

The following tests have been developed to evaluate and distinguish the various causes of hypo- or hyperkalemia in childhood [11–13]:

1. The transtubular K^+ concentration gradient, colloquially referred to as TTKG, measures the K^+ secretion within the cortical collecting tubule and represents an estimate of the aldosterone activity. This parameter can be easily calculated assuming a. that the urine osmolality at the end of the cortical collecting tubule is similar to that of blood, and b. that no K^+ secretion or reabsorption takes place in the medullary collecting tubule. If these assumptions are accurate, then the K^+ concentration in the final urine will rise above that in the cortical collecting tubule due to reabsorption of water in the medullary collecting duct. This effect can be accounted for by dividing the urine K^+ concentration by the ratio of the urine to blood osmolality. If, for example, this ratio is 2, then 50 % of the water leaving the cortical collecting tubule has been reabsorbed in the medulla, thereby doubling the luminal K^+ concentration. This parameter is calculated as follows:

$$\frac{Urinary\,K^+ \big/ Urinary\,Osmolality}{Blood\,Osmolality \big/ Circulating\,K^+}$$

Blood osmolality (in mosm/kg) can be measured with an osmometer or very reasonably estimated from circulating Na^+, glucose, and urea (in mmol/l) as follows: $\left(Na^+ \times 2\right) + glucose + urea$. On the other hand, urinary osmolality (in mmol/kg H_2O) can be measured with an osmometer or

estimated, in the absence of proteinuria and glucosuria, from the specific gravity, as determined by refractometry, as follows: (specific gravity – 1000) ×40.

2. The fractional clearance of K^+ (which measures the amount of filtered K^+ that is excreted in the urine)

$$\frac{Urinary\,K^+ \times Circulating\,Creatinine}{Circulating\,K^+ \times Urinary\,Creatinine}$$

and the molar urinary potassium/creatinine ratio (mol/mol)

$$\frac{Urinary\,K^+}{Urinary\,Creatinine}$$

are two further frequently used tests, which are strongly correlated.

3. The fractional clearance of Cl^- (which measures the amount of filtered Cl^- that is excreted in the urine)

$$\frac{Urinary\,Cl^- \times Circulating\,Creatinine}{Circulating\,Cl^- \times Urinary\,Creatinine}$$

and especially the molar urinary chloride/creatinine ratio (mol/mol; see above)

$$\frac{Urinary\,Cl^-}{Urinary\,Creatinine}$$

are two further, closely correlated tests that have been suggested.

The molar urinary potassium/creatinine and the urinary chloride/creatinine indices are based on a near-constant creatinine excretion rate and consequently have a limited significance in patients with a very low body mass index.

4. The 24-h K^+-excretion is a further useful diagnostic test. The use of this traditional diagnostic test is not generally advised considering that 24-h urine collections are troublesome and difficult to obtain (and often imprecise) in children who are not hospitalized, are not practical in a medical emergency, and almost impossible without

invasive techniques such as bladder catheterization in infants.

In our experience the following two urinary tests are useful to distinguish the various causes of hypokalemia and hyperkalemia:

- In normotensive children with hypokalemia the transtubular K^+ gradient and the urinary potassium/creatinine ratio (and perhaps the fractional clearance of K^+) easily help distinguish hypokalemia due to a short-term shift of the ion into cells (transtubular K^+ gradient <2.5; urinary potassium/creatinine <2.5 mol/mol) from hypokalemia resulting from a deficit of this ion, including renal K^+ losing conditions and hypokalemia complicating intestinal diseases (in patients experiencing diarrhea secondary hyperaldosteronism caused by circulating volume depletion leads to an increased urine K^+ excretion).
- In normotensive children with hypokalemia and metabolic alkalosis the urinary excretion of Cl^- helps distinguish renal (urinary chloride/creatinine ratio >10 mol/mol) from non-renal causes (urinary chloride/creatinine ratio <10 mol/mol), as explained in the section on metabolic alkalosis. It has sometimes been incorrectly assumed that, when hypokalemia occurs in the context of non-renal conditions, the fractional clearance of K^+, the molar urinary potassium/creatinine ratio and the 24 h K^+-excretion are very low, allowing discrimination of non-renal and renal conditions. However, in most children with non-renal hypokalemia extracellular volume depletion is present also, leading to secondary activation of the renin-angiotensin II-aldosterone system, and therefore to an increased urinary K^+ excretion. As a consequence, the urinary K^+ excretion sometimes does not discriminate between non-renal and renal conditions associated with hypokalemia.

In hyperkalemia the molar urinary potassium/creatinine ratio and the transtubular K^+ gradient help distinguish impaired from unimpaired urinary K^+ excretion. In subjects with unimpaired urinary K^+ excretion the molar urinary potassium/creatinine ratio is expected to be >20 mol/mol, the transtubular K^+ gradient >7.

Hypokalemia

The clinician evaluating a child with hypokalemia (<3.5 mmol/l) should consider five groups of causes [12–17]: (a) spurious hypokalemia; (b) redistribution; (c) true K^+ depletion due to non-renal (mostly intestinal) conditions; (d) true K^+ depletion due to renal conditions; and (e) hypokalemia associated with an expanded "effective" circulating volume and therefore with systemic hypertension due to enhanced mineralocorticoid activity (Table 31.8).

The total K^+ stores are reduced only in subjects with hypokalemia due to non-renal or renal conditions. On the other side, the body K^+ content is normal in children with spurious hypokalemia, in those with an increased shift of K^+ into cells and in those with hypokalemia associated with an expanded "effective" circulating volume.

Occasionally, metabolically active cells take up K^+ after blood has been drawn and before it has been tested in the laboratory. This condition, which has been called *spurious hypokalemia*, has been noted in patients with acute myeloid leukemia associated with a very high white blood cell count and in hot weather. The problem of spurious hypokalemia, which is much less common than spurious hyperkalaemia, can be avoided if plasma (or serum) is rapidly separated from the cells or if the blood is stored at 4 °C.

Normal total body K^+ content with hypokalemia results from an *increased shift of this ion into cells*. Metabolic alkalosis, increased endogenous secretion or exogenous administration of insulin, sympathetic activation and exogenous administration of β_2-adrenergic receptors are the main causes of hypokalemia caused by cellular uptake of K^+. Hypokalemic periodic paralysis is an uncommon form of hypokalemia resulting from an increased shift of K^+ into cells, which is characterized by recurrent episodes of hypokalemia (associated with hypophosphatemia and mild hypomagnesemia) and muscular weakness or

Table 31.8 Causes of hypokalemia

Spurious hypokalemia (cells take up potassium after blood has been drawn)
Hypokalemia associated with normal or low blood pressure
Increased shift of potassium into cells (total body K⁺ content normal)
Activation of β_2-adrenergic receptors
Endogenous: stress, hypothermia
Exogenous: β_2-adrenergic agonists (e.g., albuterol), xanthines
Hormones
Insulin
Endogenous: anabolism (e.g., refeeding syndrome)
Exogenous: treatment of diabetic ketoacidosis
Aldosterone (possibly)
Alkalosis (metabolic)
Rare causes
Hypokalemic periodic paralysis
Congenital (autosomal dominant inheritance)
Complicating thyrotoxicosis (particularly in Chinese males)
Barium-induced hypokalemia, acute chloroquine intoxication
Maturation of red cell precursors after treatment of megaloblastic anemia with vitamin B_{12} or folic acid
Paraneoplastic hypokalemia secondary to increased cell synthesis in acute myeloid leukemia[a]
True potassium depletion (= total K⁺ body content reduced)
Extrarenal "conditions"
Prolonged poor potassium intake, protein-energy malnutrition
Gastrointestinal conditions
Gastric (associated with alkalosis): vomiting, nasogastric suction
Small bowel
Associated with acidosis: biliary drainage, intestinal fistula, malabsorption, diarrhea (including diarrhea associated with HIV-infection), radiation enteropathy
Associated with alkalosis: congenital chloride diarrhea
Large bowel
Associated with acidosis: uretero-sigmoidoscopy
Acid-base balance unpredictable: bowel cleansing agents, laxatives, clay ingestion, potassium binding resin ingestion
Sweating, full thickness burns
Cystic fibrosis
Dialysis
Renal "conditions"
Tubulointerstitial nephritis, post-obstructive diuresis, recovery from acute renal failure
With metabolic acidosis: renal tubular acidosis (type I or II), carbonic anhydrase inhibitors (e.g., acetazolamide and topiramate), amphotericin B, outdated tetracyclines
With metabolic alkalosis
Inherited conditions: Bartter syndromes, Gitelman syndrome and related syndromes
Acquired conditions: normotensive primary aldosteronism, loop and thiazide diuretics, high dose antibiotics (penicillin, naficillin, ampicillin, carbenicillin, ticarcillin), magnesium depletion
Acid-base balance unpredictable: cetuximab

Hypokalemia associated with high blood pressure (often associated with metabolic alkalosis; total K⁺ body content normal)

Low renin: primary aldosteronism (either hyperplasia or adenoma), apparent mineralocorticoid excess (= defect in 11-β-hydroxysteroid-dehydrogenase), Liddle syndrome (congenitally increased function of the collecting tubule sodium channels), dexamethasone-responsive aldosteronism (synthesis of aldosterone promoted not only by renin but also by adrenocorticotropin), congenital adrenal hyperplasia (11-β-hydroxylase or 17-α-hydroxylase deficiency), Cushing disease, exogenous mineralocorticoids, licorice-ingestion (=11-β-hydroxysteroid-dehydrogenase blockade)
Normal or high renin: renal artery stenosis, malignant hypertension, renin producing tumor

[a]The pathogenic mechanism includes also hyperkaluresis due to activation of the renin-angiotensin II system

paralysis that occurs primarily in males of Asian descent. The hypokalemic episodes are precipitated by rest after exercise, a carbohydrate meal or the administration of insulin or β-adrenergic agonists (e.g., epinephrine).

The K⁺ stores may be depleted when *dietary K⁺ is very low* and therefore fails to counterbalance the obligatory K⁺ losses and, in infancy and childhood, the required K⁺ accretion. Since the kidney is able to lower K⁺ excretion to very low figures in the presence of K⁺ depletion, decreased intake alone will cause hypokalemia only in rare cases. However, it contributes to the severity of K⁺ depletion when another problem is superimposed. Under normal circumstances the net fluid loss from the skin and the gastrointestinal tract is small, therefore preventing the development of K⁺ depletion. Sometimes, however, in cases such as prolonged exertion in hot, dry environment, in cystic fibrosis (in these patients sweat contains large amounts of Na⁺, K⁺ and Cl⁻), and especially in the context of various gastrointestinal conditions (Table 31.8) K⁺ loss occurs. In most of these cases extracellular volume depletion is present also, leading to secondary activation of the renin-angiotensin II-aldosterone system, and further worsening the K⁺ deficiency. It has even been noted that in some patients with diarrheal states an increased urinary K⁺ excretion plays a more important role than intestinal losses in the development of K⁺ deficiency. Hypokalemia is mostly associated with metabolic alkalosis after poor dietary K⁺ intake, in the context of "upper" gastrointestinal conditions or in conditions associated with increased sweating and with acidosis in "lower" gastrointestinal conditions. Finally, *renal*

K⁺ losses occur either associated with acidosis or, more frequently, with alkalosis.

Excessive mineralocorticoid activity is the main cause of hypokalemia associated with metabolic alkalosis and arterial hypertension. The underlying mechanism will be discussed elsewhere.

Clinical Work Up

The clue to the diagnosis of spurious hypokalemia is a normal electrocardiogram without the characteristic changes (Fig. 31.10). Considering that the great majority of children with true hypokalemia have either a gastrointestinal condition or take drugs associated with renal K⁺ wasting, the causes of hypokalemia can almost always be discerned clinically. When the data obtained from the clinical history fail to establish a presumptive diagnosis, the following simple steps are suggested:

- Repeated measurement of blood pressure;
- Concurrent determination of the acid-base balance, Na⁺, Cl⁻, Ca⁺⁺, Mg⁺⁺, inorganic phosphate, alkaline phosphatase, uric acid, and especially urea and creatinine; In normotensive subjects the molar urinary potassium/creatinine ratio distinguishes hypokalemia due to a short-term shift of K⁺ into cells (ratio <2.5 mol/mol) from hypokalemia resulting from a deficit of the ion;
- In normotensive subjects with hypokalemia and metabolic alkalosis the urinary chloride/creatinine ratio discriminates renal (ratio >10 mol/mol) from non-renal causes (ratio <10 mol/mol).

Management

Considering the numerous origins of hypokalemia, this section will focus exclusively on the urgency and the mode of substitution in patients with normotensive hypokalemia [15–17].

The urgency for substitution is dictated by following factors:

1. Conditions that increase the likelihood of dangerous cardiac arrhythmias;
2. The possibility that K^+ will shift into cells (e.g., during recovery from diabetic ketoacidosis);
3. Severe muscle weakness in a child who must intensively hyperventilate because of metabolic acidosis,
4. Magnitude of the ongoing K^+ losses (e.g., during severe diarrhea); and
5. Degree of hypokalemia.

Potassium Preparations

- Potassium chloride: preferred in metabolic alkalosis due to diuretic therapy or vomiting;
- Potassium citrate or potassium bicarbonate: prescribed in hypokalemia and metabolic acidosis (typically renal tubular acidosis);
- Potassium phosphate: administered in the recovery from diabetic ketoacidosis, in subjects at risk of refeeding syndrome and during total parenteral nutrition.

The concurrent intravenous administration of K^+Cl^- with glucose or bicarbonate is not advised in patients with severe hypokalemia, because glucose and bicarbonate cause a shift of K^+ into cells and transiently reduce circulating K^+ concentration. Route of administration is as follows: The safest way to administer K^+ is by mouth. Intestinal conditions that limit intake or absorption of K^+, severe hypokalemia (<2.5 mmol/L), characteristic electrocardiogram abnormalities (with or without cardiac arrhythmias) or respiratory muscle weakness and an anticipated shift of K^+ into cells mandate intravenous substitution.

Intravenous K⁺Cl⁻

Bolus of K^+Cl^- is recommended exclusively in very severe degree of hypokalemia and abnormal electrocardiogram. The aim will be to raise K^+ to 3.0 mmol/l in 1–2 min.[2] The amount of intravenous K^+Cl^- (in mmol) will be chosen from measured K^+ (in mmol/l) and body weight (in kg) using the formula: $(3.0 - \text{measured } K^+) \times \text{body weight} \times 0.04$. Following this bolus, the rate of infusion of K^+ should be reduced to 0.015 mmol/kg body weight per minute, and measurement of K^+ concentration should be repeated each 5–10 min.

N.B.: The K^+Cl^- supplementation should be minimal if hypokalemia is due exclusively to an abnormal distribution of the K^+ stores (e.g., exogenous administration of β_2-adrenergic receptors or hypokalemic periodic paralysis).

In conditions demanding intravenous K^+ but without any acute emergency the rate of infused K^+ should not exceed 0.5–1.0 mmol/kg body weight hourly. Furthermore the K^+ concentration in intravenous solutions should be less than 60 mmol/L for use in peripheral veins because higher concentrations lead to local discomfort, venous spasm and sclerosis.

Parenteral supplemental K^+ administration is the most common cause of severe hyperkalemia. Consequently, the safest route to give K^+ is by mouth. A traditional approach to minimizing hypokalemia is to ensure adequate dietary K^+ intake (unfortunately the K^+ contained in foods that have a high K^+ content is almost entirely coupled with phosphate rather than with Cl^- and therefore is not effective in repairing K^+-loss associated with Cl^--depletion, including use of diuretics, vomiting or nasogastric drainage). In most circumstances, oral replacement with K^+Cl^- (1–3 mmol/kg body weight daily in divided doses) is effective in correcting hypokalemia.

---

[2]The basis for this decision is as follows: the total blood volume approximates 7% of body weight (this volume circulates each minute, cardiac output being at least 70 mL/min/kg body weight) and plasma volume 60% of blood volume, i.e. approximately 4% of body weight. Consequently a 50.0-kg adolescent with a very severe hypokalemia of 1.5 mmol/L will be given $(3.0-1.5) \times 50 \times 0.04 = 3.0$ mmol of K^+Cl^- in 1–2 min. Considering that infused K^+ will mix with interstitial fluid (approximately three to four times the plasma volume) before reaching cell membrane, there will be a much smaller increase in K^+ concentration near cell membranes.

Table 31.9 Causes of hyperkalemia (drugs associated with hyperkalemia appear in Table 31.10)

Spurious hyperkalemia (potassium movement out of the cells during or after blood has been drawn)
Mechanical trauma during venipuncture
Hereditary spherocytosis
Familial pseudohyperkalemia
True hyperkalemia
Increased potassium load[a]
Increased shift of potassium out of cells
Normal anion gap metabolic acidosis
Insulin deficiency
Extracellular hypertonicity
Increased tissue catabolism (severe hemolysis, rhabdomyolysis, tumor lysis syndrome, immediately after cardiac surgery)
Severe exercise
Familial hyperkalemic periodic paralysis (= Gamstorp disease)
Hyperkalaemia of the premature infant
Impaired renal potassium excretion
Global renal failure: acute or chronic
Hyperreninemic hypoaldosteronism: adrenal insufficiency (= Addison disease), salt-losing congenital adrenal hyperplasia (21-hydroxylase deficiency)
Hyporeninemic hypoaldosteronism: idiopathic, complicating acute glomerulonephritis or mild-to-moderate renal failure)
Pseudohypoaldosteronism
Type 1 (cortical collecting tubule)
Primary
Autosomal recessive[b]: reduced sodium channel activity
Autosomal dominant: mutations in the gene for the mineralocorticoid receptor, phenotype mild and transient
Secondary: complicating obstructive uropathy (with or without urinary tract infection), systemic lupus erythematosus, sickle cell disease, renal transplantation, renal amyloidosis
Type 2 (= Familial hyperkalemic hypertension or Gordon syndrome[c])

[a]Not a cause of hyperkalemia, unless very acute (and important) or occurring in subjects with impaired potassium excretion (due, for example, to underlying kidney disease)
[b]Autosomal recessive pseudohypoaldosteronism type 1 is opposite to Liddle syndrome
[c]The clinical phenotype of Gordon syndrome is opposite to Gitelman syndrome

Hyperkalemia

The clinician evaluating a child with hyperkalemia (>5.5 mmol/L) will initially consider the possible diagnosis of *spurious hyperkalemia* (Table 31.9) [12–14, 18–20]. The term refers to those conditions in which the elevation in the measured K^+ is due to K^+ movement out of the cells during or after the blood specimen has been drawn. The major cause of this common problem is mechanical trauma during venipuncture, resulting in the release of K^+ from red cells and a characteristic reddish tint of the serum (or plasma) due to the release of hemoglobin. A normal electrocardiogram without the characteristic signs (Fig. 31.10) is the initial clue to this diagnosis.

In very rare instances, however, red serum (or red plasma) represents severe intravascular hemolysis rather than a hemolyzed specimen. Furthermore spurious hyperkalemia can also occur in hereditary spherocytosis and in familial pseudohyperkalemia, a rare autosomal dominant disorder recognized as a laboratory artifact. In the circulation, the Na^+ and K^+ content of red cells is normal. However, the measured plasma or serum K^+ concentration is elevated because of an abnormally high rate of efflux of K^+ from the red cells when the temperature is lowered below 22 °C. The in vitro K^+ efflux can be reversed by incubation at 37 °C. K^+ also moves out of white cells and platelets after clotting has occurred. Thus, the serum K^+ concentration normally exceeds the true value in the plasma by 0.1–0.5 mmol/L. Although in normal individuals this difference is clinically insignificant, the measured serum K^+ concentration may be as high as 9 mmol/L in patients with marked leukocytosis or thrombocytosis. Spurious hyperkalemia is suspected whenever there is no apparent cause for the elevation in the serum K^+ concentration in an asymptomatic patient.

True hyperkalemia (Table 31.9) occurs rarely in healthy subjects, because cellular and urinary adaptations prevent substantial extracellular K^+ accumulation. Furthermore, the efficiency of K^+ handling is increased if K^+ intake is enhanced, thereby tolerating what might be a fatal K^+ load. These observations lead to the following conclusions concerning the development of hyperkalemia:

1. *Increasing K⁺ load* is not a cause of hyperkalemia, unless very acute or occurring in a patient with impaired urinary K⁺ excretion. In special conditions, acute hyperkalemia can be induced (primarily in infants because of their small size) by the intravenous administration of unusual large doses of K⁺ or the use of stored blood for transfusions.

2. The net *release of K⁺ from the cells* can cause a transient elevation in the circulating K⁺ concentration (in the presence of normal or even low total body K⁺ stores). Four causes of hyperkalemia resulting from release of the ion from cells will be discussed: (a) extracellular hypertonicity; (b) tumor lysis syndrome; (c) hyperkalemic familial periodic paralysis; and (d) non-oliguric hyperkalaemia of the premature infant.

   An *elevated extracellular tonicity* results in water movement from the cells into the extracellular fluid. This is linked with K⁺ movement out of the cells by two mechanisms. First, the loss of water raises the intracellular K⁺ level, creating a gradient for passive K⁺ exit. Second, the friction forces between water and solute result in K⁺ being carried along with water. Hypertonicity-induced hyperkalemia occurs in hyperglycemia, in hypernatremia, and following administration of mannitol.

   The phenotype of acute *tumor lysis syndrome* is opposite to refeeding syndrome. The term denotes the metabolic abnormalities that occur either spontaneously or immediately after initiation of cytotoxic therapy in neoplastic disorders. The findings include hyperuricemia, hyperkalemia, hyperphosphatemia, hypocalcemia (due to precipitation of calcium phosphate), and acute renal failure. The syndrome has been noted in children with a tumor characterized by rapid cell turnover such as lymphomas (particularly non-Hodgkin lymphoma) and some leukemias.

   The distinction between spontaneous tumor lysis syndrome and that noted during therapy is the lack of hyperphosphatemia in the spontaneous form. It has been suggested that rapidly growing tumors with high cell turnover rates lead to high uric acid levels through rapid nucleoprotein turnover but the tumors reutilize released phosphorus for synthesis of new tumor cells. In contrast, the acute increase in uric acid levels associated with chemotherapy is due to cell destruction; in this setting, there are no new cancer cells to reutilize the released phosphate.

   Hyperkalemic familial periodic paralysis, or Gamstorp disease, is a rare inherited autosomal dominant disease that causes patients to experience episodes of flaccid weakness[3] associated with increased K⁺ levels. In this syndrome, hyperkalemia occurs with increased K⁺ intake, cold weather, exercise or at rest. The attacks of paralysis, however, are not always linked with hyperkalemia.

   Non-oliguric hyperkalemia (>6.5 mmol/L) of the premature infant is a common and serious condition. The features are a rapid rise of K⁺ concentration to excessively high values at 24 h after birth, a tendency towards cardiac arrhythmia, and occurrence only within 72 h after birth exclusively in premature infants. This peculiar condition mainly results from a K⁺ loss from the intra- into the extracellular space. Moreover, renal K⁺ excretion that is dependent on both glomerular filtration rate and urinary output is slightly decreased in this setting. Finally, aldosterone unresponsiveness, rather than a decreased concentration of aldosterone, also contributes to the degree of hyperkalemia. However, since there is no significant K⁺ intake during the first days of life of premature infants, even total absence of renal K⁺ excretion cannot increase K⁺ concentration, if there is no intra- to extracellular K⁺ shift.

3. Persistent hyperkalemia requires an *impaired urinary K⁺ excretion* (the total body K⁺ stores are increased in this condition). Two factors

---

[3]Please note that hyperkalemic skeletal muscle paralysis can occur in hyperkalemia of any cause, not only in this rare inherited disorder.

modulate renal K^+ homeostasis in the cortical collecting tubule: "hyperkalemia" and aldosterone, which act in concert to promote the tubular secretion and therefore the excretion of K^+, and the flow rate traversing the cortical collecting tubule. Consequently, a decreased aldosterone release or effect or a decreased renal tubular flow rate are the major conditions impairing urinary K^+ excretion.

Any cause of *decreased aldosterone release or effect* can diminish the efficiency of K^+ secretion and lead to hyperkalemia. The ensuing tendency towards hyperkalemia directly stimulates K^+ secretion, partially overcoming the relative absence of aldosterone. The net effect is that the rise in the K^+ concentration is generally small in patients with normal renal function, but can be clinically important in the presence of underlying renal insufficiency or with multiple insults.

The ability to maintain K^+ excretion at near normal levels is habitually preserved in advanced renal disease as long as both aldosterone secretion and distal flow are maintained. Thus, hyperkalemia generally develops in oliguria or in the presence of an additional problem including high K^+ diet, increased tissue breakdown or reduced aldosterone bioactivity. Impaired cell uptake of K^+ also contributes to the development of hyperkalemia in advanced renal failure. *Decreased distal tubular flow* rate due to marked effective volume depletion, as in heart failure or "salt-losing" nephropathy, can also induce hyperkalemia.

Acute and chronic renal failure, the most recognized causes of impaired urinary K^+ excretion, will be discussed elsewhere (Chapters in Parts 10 and 12 in this book). Hyperkalemia and a tendency towards hyponatremia and metabolic acidosis characteristically occur in children with hyperreninemic hypoaldosteronism (including classic congenital adrenal hyperplasia), hyporeninemic hypoaldosteronism, and end-organ resistance to aldosterone, mostly referred to as pseudohypoaldosteronism. In North-America, Japan, and most European countries neonatal screening (measurement of 17-hydroxy-hydroxyprogesterone in filter paper blood) iden-tifies children affected by classic congenital adrenal hyperplasia due to 21-hydroxylase deficiency before salt-losing crises with hyperkalemia develop. Consequently in these countries classic congenital adrenal hyperplasia is nowadays an uncommon cause of hyperkalemia. In our experience, secondary type 1 pseudohypoaldosteronism is, together with advanced renal failure, a common cause of true hyperkalemia, at least in infancy. Secondary type 1 pseudohypoaldosteronism develops in infants with urinary tract infections, in infants (but not older children) with urinary tract anomalies (either obstructive or vesicoureteral reflux), and especially in infants with both urinary tract infections and urinary tract anomalies.

Finally, the syndrome of (acquired) *hyporeninemic hypoaldosteronism*, which is characterized by mild hyperkalemia and metabolic acidosis, is due to diminished renin release and, subsequently, decreased angiotensin II and aldosterone production. The syndrome, which mostly occurs in subjects with mild renal failure, has been first reported in subjects with overt diabetic kidney disease and has been occasionally noted in children with acute glomerulonephritis or mild-to-moderate chronic renal failure.

Prescribed medications, over-the-counter drugs, and nutritional supplements may disrupt K^+ balance and promote the development of hyperkalemia, as shown in Table 31.10. Although most of these products are well tolerated, drug-induced hyperkalemia may develop in subjects with underlying renal impairment or other abnormalities in K^+ handling. Their hyperkalemic action is less evident in children than in elderly subjects.

Clinical Work Up

The clue to the diagnosis of spurious hyperkalemia, the most common cause of elevated K^+ levels in clinically asymptomatic infants and children, is a normal electrocardiogram without the characteristic changes.

Considering that the great majority of children with true hyperkalemia have renal failure (either

Table 31.10 Drugs that have been associated with hyperkalemia

Medication	Mechanism of action
Increased K+ input	K+ ingestion or infusion
K+ supplements (and salt substitutes)	
Nutritional and herbal supplements	
Stored packed red blood cells	
Potassium containing penicillins	
Transcellular K+ shifts	
β-adrenergic receptor antagonists	↓ β₂-driven K+ uptake
Intravenous amino acids (Lysine,	↑ K+ release from cells
Arginine, Aminocaproic acid)	
Succinylcholine	Depolarized cell membranes
Digoxin intoxication	↓ Na+-pump
Impaired renal excretion	
Potassium sparing diuretics	
Spironolactone, eplerenone	Aldosterone antagonists
Triamterene, amiloride	Na+ channels blocked (collecting tubule)
Trimethoprim[a], pentamidine	Na+ channels blocked (collecting tubule)
Nonsteroidal anti-inflammatory drugs	↓ Aldosterone synthesis, ↓ glomerular filtration rate, ↓ renal blood flow
Blockers of the renin-angiotensin II-aldosterone system (converting enzyme inhibitors, angiotensin II-antagonists, renin inhibitors)	↓ Aldosterone synthesis
Heparins (both unfractionated and low molecular weight heparins)	↓ Aldosterone synthesis
Calcineurin inhibitors (e.g., cyclosporine and tacrolimus)	↓ Aldosterone synthesis, ↓ Na+-pump, ↓ K+-channels

Data from Alfonzo [41]; and Hollander-Rodriguez and Calvert [42]
[a]Including cotrimoxazole, the fixed combination of trimethoprim with sulfomethoxazole

acute or chronic), secondary type 1 pseudohypoaldosteronism or take drugs that can cause hyperkalemia, the cause of hyperkaemia can mostly be discerned clinically. When the data obtained from the clinical history fail to establish a presumptive diagnosis, the following simple steps are suggested [12–14, 18–20]:

- Repeated measurement of blood pressure;
- Concurrent determination of the acid-base balance, Na+, Cl−, Ca++, Mg++, inorganic phosphate, alkaline phosphatase, uric acid, and especially urea and creatinine;
- In subjects with true hyperkalemia unrelated to an impaired urinary K+ excretion the expected molar urinary potassium/creatinine ratio is >20 mol/mol and the transtubular potassium gradient >10.

Management

Because many conditions account for true hyperkalemia, there is no universal therapy for this dyselectrolytemia. The following measures deserve consideration upon recognition of hyperkalemia with increased total body K+ stores:

1. Interruption of excessive dietary K+ intake;
2. Discontinuation of drugs that may cause hyperkalemia;
3. Increasing renal K+ excretion (for this purpose children without end-stage renal failure or physical signs of fluid overload must have substantial salt intake[4] via oral or parenteral routes; the use of a loop diuretic, less frequently four thiazide diuretic, also increases renal K+ excretion);
4. Increasing gastrointestinal K+ excretion using cation exchange resins; and
5. Institution of dialysis in children with end-stage renal failure.

[4]A low salt intake and extracellular fluid volume depletion are the most commonly observed contributing factors in the development of hyperkalemia in children with renal failure. In patients with a salt-retaining disease, proper management is achieved by avoiding severe restriction of dietary salt while concurrently administering diuretics.

Table 31.11 Currently recommended emergency interventions for severe hyperkalemia (≥7.1 mmol/L) with electrocardiogram abnormalities

Medication	Dosage	Onset (minutes)	Length of effect (hours)	Comments – cautions
Nebulized albuterol	10–20 mg (diluted in 4 mL of saline) over 10 min	15–30	4–6	May increase heart rate
Intravenous albuterol	10 µg/kg body weight over 15 min	15–30	4–6	May increase heart rate
Glucose and insulin	Glucose 0.5–1.0 g/kg body weight and Insulin 0.1 U/kg body weight intravenously over 15 min	15–30	4–6	Tendency towards hyopoglycemia (monitor blood glucose level)
Intravenous calcium	4.5–9.0 mg/kg body weight over 1–3 min	Immediate	0.5–1	Does not lower potassium level

Albuterol and intravenous glucose (with insulin) lowers extracellular potassium level by driving potassium into cells, while calcium directly antagonizes the membrane actions of hyperkalemia but does not modify extracellular potassium concentration. None of these interventions modify the total body potassium content

Emergencies

Because of the serious deleterious cardiac effects, severe hyperkalemia (≥7.1 mmol/L) with electrocardiographic abnormalities requires emergency intervention. The following measures, which are listed according to their rapidity of action, have been recommended:

- Intravenous Ca^{++}, which directly antagonizes the membrane actions of hyperkalemia;
- Intravenous insulin (and glucose), which lowers extracellular K^+ level by driving K^+ into cell;
- Intravenous or nebulised β_2-adrenergic agonists, which, like insulin, drive K^+ into cells; and
- Intravenous $NaHCO_3$, which results in H^+ ion release from cells (as part of the buffering reaction), a change that is accompanied by K^+ movement into cells to preserve electroneutrality.
- Intravenous loop-diuretics

Available data indicate:

1. That nebulized (or inhaled) albuterol, a β_2-adrenergic agonist, or intravenous insulin (and glucose) are the best supported recommendations (the effect on K^+ is more pronounced in adults patients given nebulized albuterol than in those given intravenous albuterol, but these data

likely do not apply for small children who might not inhale correctly);
2. That their combination may be more effective than either alone;
3. That although there are no properly conducted studies assessing the efficacy of Ca^{++}, there remains little doubt of its effectiveness in treating arrhythmias; and
4. That evidence for the use of intravenous $NaHCO_3$ is equivocal. For practical purposes, the emergency interventions given in Table 31.11 are advised.

Acid-Base Balance

Maintenance of acid-base balance within narrow limits (i.e. pH 7.00–7.30 within the cell depending on the cell type and tissue of origin and pH 7.35–7.45 in extracellular fluids) is a crucial function of the living organism, largely because of its effects on body proteins. The "pCO2-HCO_3^--pH"-based approach, popularized by Relman and Schwartz in the 1960s, relies upon the definition of pH in blood as a function of the ratio between the partial pressure of carbon dioxide (pCO_2; mm Hg or kPa) and the bicarbonate (HCO_3^-; mmol/L or meq/L) concentration, as

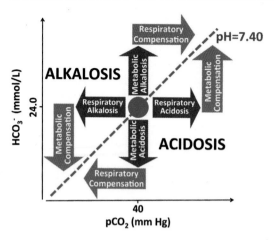

Fig. 31.11 Common sense diagram depicting the four primary disturbances of acid-base balance with the expected compensation. There are four primary disturbances (*red arrows*) of acid-base balance. Since ventilation modulates pCO_2, any disturbance in pH that results from a primary change in pCO_2 is called respiratory acid-base disorder: retention of CO_2 leads to a reduction in pH (<7.35) called respiratory acidosis, while a fall in pCO_2 leads to a rise in pH (>7.45) called respiratory alkalosis. On the other side, primary changes in the HCO_3^- concentration are called metabolic acid-base disorders: a primary reduction in HCO_3^- is termed metabolic acidosis and a primary increase in HCO_3^- is called metabolic alkalosis. Since blood pH is determined by the ratio between HCO_3^- and pCO_2, and not either one alone, primary respiratory (primary changes in pCO_2) disturbances invoke compensatory metabolic (secondary changes in HCO_3^-) responses (*green arrows*), and primary metabolic (primary changes in HCO_3^-) disturbances elicit compensatory respiratory (secondary changes in pCO_2) responses (*green arrows*)

Table 31.12 Predicted compensations to simple primary acid-base disturbances

Disorder	Primary change	Compensatory response
Metabolic acidosis	↓ HCO_3^-	↓ pCO_2 by 1.3[c] mm Hg for↓1.0mmol/L[d]inHCO_3^-
Metabolic alkalosis	↑ HCO_3^-	↑ pCO_2 by 0.6[c] mm Hg for↑1.0mmol/L[d]inHCO_3^-
Respiratory acidosis	↑ pCO_2	
Acute		↑ 1.0 mmol/L[a] in HCO_3^- for ↑ 10 mmHg[b] in pCO_2
Chronic		↑ 3.5 mmol/L[a] in HCO_3^- for ↑ 10 mmHg[b] in pCO_2
Respiratory alkalosis	↓ pCO_2	
Acute		↓ 2.0 mmol/L[a] in HCO_3^- for ↓ 10 mmHg[b] in pCO_2
Chronic		↓ 5.0 mmol/L[a] in HCO_3^- for ↓ 10 mmHg[b] in pCO_2

Data from: Whittier and Rutecki [43]; and from Laski and Kurtzman [44]
[a]Range approximately ± 2.0 mmol/L
[b]From 40 mmHg
[c]Range approximately ± 3 mmHg
[d]From 25 mmol/L

indicated by the (simplified) Henderson-Hasselbalch equation [21, 22]:

$$pH = pK + \frac{HCO_3^-}{pCO_2}$$

Arterial blood is the standard sample for the determination of acid-base balance but arterial blood sampling, which is often painful and hazardous, is often unavailable in childhood. In this age group, acid-base balance is mostly assessed in arterialized capillary blood samples (from the finger pulp following hand warming during ≥10 min or the earlobe following spreading the lobe with a vasodilating cream during ≥10 min) or in venous blood samples. Normal values for peripheral venous blood differ from those of

arterial blood due to the uptake and buffering of metabolically produced CO_2 in the capillary circulation. If a tourniquet is used to facilitate phlebotomy, it should be released about one minute before blood is drawn to avoid changes induced by ischemia. The peripheral venous pH range is ≈0.02–0.04 pH units lower than in arterial blood, the pCO_2 ≈3–8 mmHg higher and the HCO_3^- concentration ≈1–2 mmol/L higher. Automated blood gas analyzers measure pH and pCO_2, while the HCO_3^- concentration is calculated from the Henderson-Hasselbalch equation. Most currently available blood gas analyzers determine circulating L-lactate as well (the assay does not detect D-lactate). Abnormalities of blood pH result from a deviation in circulating bicarbonate (HCO_3^-; mmol/L) or in partial pressure of carbon dioxide (pCO_2; mm Hg).[5] There are four primary

---

[5]To obtain SI units (kPa) divide by 7.5.

disturbances of acid-base balance (Fig. 31.11). Since alveolar ventilation regulates pCO_2, any disturbance in pH that results from a primary change in pCO_2 is called respiratory acid-base disorder: retention of CO_2 leads to a reduction in pH (<7.35) called respiratory acidosis, a fall in pCO_2 leads to a rise in pH (>7.45) called respiratory alkalosis. On the other side, primary changes in the concentration of HCO_3^- are called metabolic acid-base disorders: a primary reduction in HCO_3^- is termed metabolic acidosis and a primary increase in HCO_3^- is called metabolic alkalosis.

Blood pH is determined by the ratio between HCO_3^- and pCO_2, not either one alone. Thus, primary respiratory disturbances (primary changes in pCO_2) invoke compensatory metabolic responses (secondary changes in HCO_3^-), and primary metabolic disturbances (primary changes in HCO_3^-) elicit compensatory respiratory responses (secondary changes in pCO_2). For instance, metabolic acidosis due to an increase in endogenous acids (e.g., ketoacidosis) lowers extracellular fluid HCO_3^- and decreases extracellular pH. This stimulates the medullary chemoreceptors to increase the ventilation in an attempt to return the ratio of HCO_3^- to pCO_2, and thus pH, towards normal. The physiologic metabolic and respiratory compensations to simple primary acid-base disturbances can be guessed from the relationships displayed in Table 31.12.

"Base excess" and "standard HCO_3^-" are in vitro generated parameters of the acid-base balance that are of little value and often even misleading [21, 22].

Systemic Effects of Metabolic Acid-Base Abnormalities

The systemic effects of acid-base abnormalities will be briefly addressed below [20, 21].

Respiratory System

Primary metabolic acid-base balance disturbances (primary changes in HCO_3^-) elicit compensatory respiratory responses (secondary changes in pCO_2). Metabolic acidosis (=primary reduction in HCO_3^-) stimulates the ventilation to correct the ratio of HCO_3^- to pCO_2, and thus pH, towards normal (Fig. 31.11). The rise in ventilation occurs within minutes but may take several hours to reach its fullest expression. The increase is more the result of increased tidal volume than respiratory rate. This degree of hyperventilation, called Kussmaul respiration, may cause some dyspnea and be appreciated on physical examination. In a child with simple metabolic acidosis the pCO_2 is expected to decrease by 1.3 mmHg for each mmol per liter decrease in HCO_3^- (Table 31.12), reaching a minimum of 10–15 mmHg. Thus, a patient with metabolic acidosis and HCO_3^- of 16.0 mmol/L would be expected to have a pCO_2 of ≈30 mmHg, i.e. between 27 and 33 mmHg. Values for pCO_2 <27 or >33 mmHg define a mixed disturbance (metabolic acidosis and respiratory alkalosis or metabolic acidosis and respiratory acidosis, respectively).

Primary metabolic alkalosis (= primary increase in HCO_3^-) may lead to compensatory hypoventilation and consequent CO_2 retention. Uncomplicated metabolic alkalosis is usually not associated with profound alveolar hypoventilation. Metabolic alkalosis should be repaired before surgery (e.g., before pyloromyotomy in infantile hypertrophic pyloric stenosis) because this acid-base abnormality predisposes to respiratory depression in the immediate postoperative course. In these patients, postoperative respiratory depression is common, possibly as a result of persisting cerebrospinal fluid alkalosis.

Potassium Balance

There are major interactions between the internal K^+ balance and acute metabolic acid-base changes. In patients with normal anion gap metabolic acidosis the excess hydrogen ions are buffered in the cell and electroneutrality is maintained by movements of intracellular K^+ into the extracellular fluid. Interestingly, metabolic acidosis is much less likely to raise the extracellular K^+ concentration in patients with high anion gap acidosis like L-lactate acidosis or ketoacidosis. The underlying mechanisms are briefly explained in Fig. 31.12 (upper panel). For similar reasons,

Metabolic Acidosis

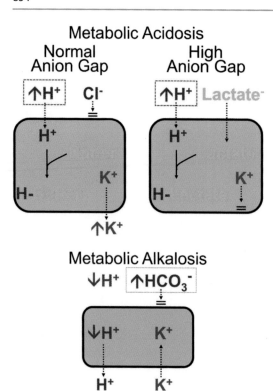

Normal Anion Gap

High Anion Gap

Metabolic Alkalosis

Fig. 31.12 Effect of metabolic acidosis or alkalosis on circulating potassium level. Both in normal (= hyperchloremic) and high (= normochloremic) anion gap metabolic acidosis some extracellular H⁺ shifts into the intracellular fluid volume (the squares denote the cell membrane). In normal anion gap (*left upper panel*) metabolic acidosis, Cl⁻ remains largely in the extracellular fluid volume. On the contrary, in high anion gap (*right upper panel*) metabolic acidosis (e.g., L-lactate acidosis) some organic anions enter the intracellular fluid. Hence, a tendency towards hyperkalemia, the consequence of a shift of K⁺ from the intracellular to the extracellular fluid volume, occurs almost exclusively in normal anion gap metabolic acidosis only. Please note that hyperkalemia is followed by a stimulated aldosterone release and results in the urinary excretion of the extra K⁺. No tendency towards hyperkalemia occurs in respiratory acidosis. In metabolic alkalosis (*lower panel*) some intracellular H⁺ shifts into the extracellular fluid volume. Hence, a tendency towards hypokalemia, the consequence of a shift of K⁺ from the extracellular to the intracellular fluid volume, occurs. No tendency towards hypokalemia occurs in respiratory alkalosis

some tendency towards hypokalemia is noted in metabolic alkalosis (Fig. 31.12, lower panel). Respiratory acidosis and alkalosis do not significantly modulate K⁺ balance.

Effect of Alkalemia on the Concentration of Ionized Calcium and Magnesium in Blood

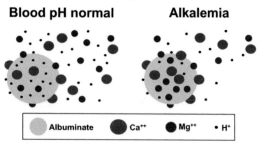

Blood pH normal **Alkalemia**

Albuminate Ca⁺⁺ Mg⁺⁺ • H⁺

Fig. 31.13 Effect of Alkalemia on the concentration of ionized calcium and magnesium in blood. In the context of alkalemia (e.g., hyperventilation) blood H⁺ concentration decreases. As a consequence, freely ionized calcium and magnesium concentrations decrease. The opposite is observed in the context of acidemia

Ca⁺⁺ (and Mg⁺⁺) Balance

Acid-base disorders affect circulating Ca^{++}, Mg^{++}, inorganic phosphate, and K⁺. Acidemia increases calcium phosphate dissociation, increasing free (ionized) Ca^{++}. Acidemia also allows greater dissociation of Ca^{++} and Mg++ from plasma protein. The effect of acidosis on Ca^{++} salt dissociation extends to bone. Alkalemia might increase calcium phosphate precipitation and lowers ionized Ca^{++} and Mg^{++} (the underlying mechanisms are explained in Fig. 31.13).

Hemoglobin Oxygen Affinity

Blood pH alters hemoglobin oxygen binding and tissue oxygen delivery. Acidemia decreases hemoglobin oxygen affinity, shifts the oxygen dissociation curve "to the right" and increases tissue delivery of oxygen (Bohr effect). On the contrary, alkalemia shifts the curve to the left, increasing the oxygen binding to hemoglobin and tending to decrease tissue delivery.

Cardiovascular System

Acidemia impairs cardiovascular function in four ways: (a) it depresses vascular tone; (b) it alters the release of, and the response to, catecholamines; (c), it depresses myocardial contractility inducing diastolic dysfunction; and (d) it induces arrhythmias (in mild to moderate acidemia, increased catecholamines produce sinus tachycardia; when acidemia is severe, vagal activity increases and bradycardia ensues; there is also an increased risk of ventricular fibrillation). Alkalemia exerts fewer effects on the cardiovascular system. The predominant clinical problem is an increase in myocardial irritability. Alkalemia reduces the free Ca^{++} and Mg^{++} inside the cell and out, and most alkalemic patients are also hypokalemic. Changes in both ions contribute to the increased potential for arrhythmias.

Alkalemia has significant effects on vascular tone in the cerebral circulation: hypocarbia constricts the cerebral vasculature as indicated by the fact that subjects with respiratory alkalosis develop lightheadedness and lack of mental acuity, but coma does not occur.

Central Nervous System

Acidosis and alkalosis impair central and peripheral nervous system function. Alkalemia increases seizure activity. If pH is $\geq$7.60, seizures may occur in the absence of an underlying epileptic diathesis. Acidosis depresses the central nervous system (this most frequently occurs in respiratory acidosis). Early signs of impairment include tremors, myoclonic jerks, and clonic movement disorders. At pH $\leq$7.10, there is generalized depression of neuronal excitability. Central effects of severe hypercarbia include lethargy and stupor at pCO_2 60 mmHg or more, coma occurs at pCO_2 $\geq$90 mmHg. Metabolic acidosis causes central nervous system depression less commonly. Fewer than 10% of diabetics with ketoacidosis develop coma (hyperosmolarity and the presence of acetoacetate may be more important than acidosis per se).

Metabolism

A final aspect of acid-base pathophysiology is the effect of pH on metabolism. The most often cited example of pH control of enzyme activity is the pH regulation of phosphofructokinase, which catalyzes a rate-controlling step in carbohydrate metabolism. Glycolysis terminates in lactic and pyruvic acid; and accumulation of these acids reduces pH. This is but one example of pH feedback. Most enzymes operate most effectively at a specific optimum pH. As pH varies from the optimum, enzyme activity changes. The integrated

response of the individual enzyme alterations may serve to maintain or restore normal pH.

Metabolic Acidosis

Primary hypobicarbonatemia and, therefore, metabolic acidosis mostly occurs when endogenous acids are produced faster than they can be excreted, when HCO_3^- is lost from the body, or when exogenous acids are administered [21–25].

The main laboratory tool in metabolic acidosis is the calculation of the blood anion gap (Fig. 31.14), the difference between the major measured cations (Na^+ and K^+; mmol/L) and the major measured anions (bicarbonate and Cl^-; mmol/L) by means of the equation:

$$\left(Na^+ + K^+\right) - \left(Cl^- + HCO_3^-\right)$$

Because electroneutrality must be maintained, the anion gap results from the difference between the unmeasured anions (primarily albumin, which is largely responsible for the normal anion gap, but also phosphate, sulfate, and organic anions such as lactate) and the remaining cations (Ca^{++} and Mg^{++}).

The calculation of blood anion gap (reference: $\leq$18 mmol/L[6]) allows separation of the two major types of metabolic acidosis: one type has an increased anion gap (>18 mmol/L; high anion gap metabolic acidosis) and the other does not (normal anion gap metabolic acidosis or hyperchloremic metabolic acidosis), as shown in Fig. 31.14 and Table 31.13.

High Anion Gap Metabolic Acidosis

The HCO_3^- deficit observed in high anion gap metabolic acidosis results from retention of fixed acids, which deplete HCO_3^- stores by releasing their protons. Two mechanisms lead to this form of metabolic acidosis (Fig. 31.14 and Table 31.13):

---

[6]The blood anion gap sometimes does not include the blood concentration of K^+: $Na^+ - (HCO_3^- + Cl^-)$. The approximate upper value of this anion gap is lower by 4 mmol/L: 14 mmol/L.

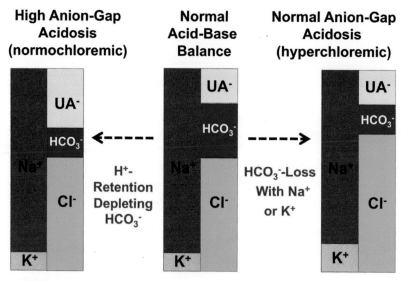

High Anion-Gap Acidosis (normochloremic)   **Normal Acid-Base Balance**   **Normal Anion-Gap Acidosis (hyperchloremic)**

H⁺-Retention Depleting HCO₃⁻

HCO₃⁻-Loss With Na⁺ or K⁺

UA⁻ = unmeasured anions = (Na⁺ + K⁺) - (Cl⁻ + HCO₃⁻)

Fig. 31.14 High anion gap (= normochloremic) and normal anion gap (= hyperchloremic) metabolic acidosis. Calculation of the blood anion gap, the difference between the major measured cations (Na⁺ and K⁺; mmol/L) and the major measured anions (HCO₃⁻ and Cl⁻; mmol/L), is a crucial laboratory diagnostic tool in patients with metabolic acidosis. The blood anion gap separates two major types of metabolic acidosis. High anion gap (= normochloremic) metabolic acidosis results from retention of fixed acids, which deplete HCO₃⁻ stores by releasing their protons (most cases develop following excessive endogenous or exogenous acid load). Most cases of normal anion gap (= hyperchloremic) metabolic acidosis result from an intestinal or a renal loss of HCO₃⁻ (accompanied either by Na⁺ or K⁺). The figure also emphasizes the tendency towards hyperkalemia (the result of a K⁺-shift from the intracellular to the extracellular fluid volume) in normal anion gap (hyperchloremic) metabolic acidosis (as explained in Fig. 31.11)

1. Excessive acid load (endogenous or exogenous) overwhelming the normal capacity to decompose or excrete the acid; and
2. Diminished capacity to excrete the normal load of fixed acids in the context of renal failure.

In health, the blood anion gap is predominantly due to the net negative charge of albumin. Abnormally low serum albumin levels influence acid-base interpretation as calculated by the anion gap: e.g., in a patient with increased production of endogenous acids, elevation of the anion gap may be masked by concurrent hypoalbuminemia. In this condition the anion gap corrected for albumin may be calculated by means of the following formula (albumin in g/L):

$$\left(Na^{+}+K^{+}\right)-\left(Cl^{-}+HCO_{3}^{-}\right)+\frac{1}{4}\left(40-Albumin\right)$$

Considering that many currently available blood gas analyzers determine circulating L-lactate, the determination of the albumin and lactate corrected anion gap has been recently suggested (upper reference: 15 mmol/L):

$$\left(Na^{+}+K^{+}\right)-\left(Cl^{-}+HCO_{3}^{-}+Lactate\right)+$$
$$\frac{1}{4}\left(40-Albumin\right)$$

Normal Anion Gap Metabolic Acidosis (Hyperchloremic)

This form of metabolic acidosis develops (Fig. 31.14 and Table 31.13) (a) from a primary loss of HCO₃⁻, (b) from the failure to replenish HCO₃⁻ stores depleted by the daily production of fixed acids (H⁺: 1–3 mmol/kg body weight) in subjects with normal glomerular filtration rate or (c) from the administration of exogenous acids (including the rapid administration of large

Table 31.13 Causes of metabolic acidosis

Metabolic acidosis with increased anion gap
Excessive acid load
Endogenous sources of acid (due to abnormal metabolism of substrates)
Ketoacidosis (largely β-hydroxybutyric acid)
Congenital organic acidemias (e.g., methylmalonic acidemia and propionic acidemia)
L-lactate acidosis
Type A (impaired tissue oxygenation; e.g., sepsis, hypovolemia, cardiac failure)
Type B (altered metabolism of L-lactate with normal tissue oxygenation in the context of a mitochondrial impairment)
Inherited metabolic diseases: either altered production of glucose from lactate or altered degradation of pyruvate
Thiamine deficiency
Drugs (e.g., biguanides, antiretroviral agents)
Toxins (e.g., ethanol)
Chronic diseases (mostly hepatic)
Overproduction of organic acids in the gastrointestinal tract (D-lactate)
Conversion of alcohols (methanol, ethylene glycol) to acids and poisonous aldehydes
Defective renal excretion of acids due to generalized renal failure ("uremic acidosis")
Metabolic acidosis with normal anion gap
Losses of bicarbonate HCO$_3^-$
Intestinal: diarrhea, surgical drainage of the intestinal tract, gastrointestinal fistulas resulting in losses of fluid rich in HCO$_3^-$, patients whose ureters have been attached to the intestinal tract (the alkali of intestinal secretion is lost by titration with acid urine)
Urinary: carbonic anhydrase inhibitors (e.g., acetazolamide), proximal renal tubular acidosis (= type 2)
Failure to replenish HCO$_3^-$ stores depleted by the daily production of fixed acids
Distal renal tubular acidosis (either classic, also called type 1, or type 4)
Diminished mineralocorticoid (or glucocorticoid) activity (adrenal insufficiency, selective hypoaldosteronism, aldosterone resistance)
Administration of potassium sparing diuretics (spironolactone, eplerenone, amiloride, triamterene)
Exogenous infusions
Amino acids like L-arginine and L-lysine (during parenteral nutrition)
HCl or NH$_4$Cl
Rapid administration of normal saline solution (= "dilutional" metabolic acidosis)

volumes of normal saline solution and other Cl$^-$ rich fluids).

The following factors account for the metabolic acidosis that is observed after administration of normal saline solution, which is called "dilutional" (or "chloride overload") acidosis:

1. Volume expansion, which results from infusion of normal saline, reduces the renal threshold for HCO$_3^-$ leading to bicarbonaturia;
2. The infusion of normal saline with a Na$^+$ level almost identical to that of blood results in a relatively stable Na$^+$ level in blood.

By contrast, the concentration of Cl$^-$ in the infused solution, which is much higher than that of normal blood, leads to progressive hyperchloremia and hypobicarbonatemia.

Urine Net Charge

The kidney prevents the development of metabolic acidosis by modulating the HCO$_3^-$ concentration in blood. This is done by (a) preventing loss of large amounts of filtered HCO$_3^-$ (primarily a task of the proximal tubule, which may reclaim the filtered HCO$_3^-$) and (b) generating HCO$_3^-$ (primarily a task of the distal tubule). The main mechanism by which the distal tubule generates HCO$_3^-$ is the conversion of glutamine to NH$_4^+$, which is excreted in the urine, plus HCO$_3^-$, which is added to the blood. As a consequence, the urinary NH$_4^+$ excretion reflects the renal HCO$_3^-$ generation, and the renal NH$_4^+$ excretion can be equated with HCO$_3^-$ regeneration on a 1:1 basis. In a child with normal anion gap metabolic acidosis and normal renal mechanisms of acidification a very low urinary concentration of HCO$_3^-$ and, more importantly, a large concentration of NH$_4^+$ will result. The measurement of these parameters, which is complicated by the need to avoid significant changes in urine composition after voiding,[7] is usually unavailable in clinical practice. In the context of metabolic acidosis, a urinary pH significantly <6.2 indicates a very low

---

[7]The changes are due to bacterial overgrowth, especially at room temperature, as well as to open exposure to the atmosphere, which produces gas loss.

urinary concentration of HCO_3^- and argues against an altered renal mechanisms of urinary acidification. Furthermore, and more importantly, the crucial concept of urinary net charge or urine anion gap[8] (which results from urinary Na^+, K^+ and Cl^-) was developed as an indirect assessment of urinary NH_4^+ concentration. Usually, because ammonium (an unmeasured cation) accompanies Cl^- in the context of metabolic acidosis, the concentration of Cl^- should be greater than the sum of Na^+ and K^+, and the net charge negative ($Na^+ + K^+ < Cl^-$). A positive net charge ($Na^+ + K^+ > Cl^-$) indicates impaired ammonium secretion and, therefore, impaired distal acidification of renal tubule. For instance, in the aforementioned context of metabolic acidosis with normal renal mechanisms of acidification (e.g. a child with normal anion gap metabolic acidosis due to mild diarrhea) the enhanced urinary NH_4^+ excretion will result in a large urinary level of urinary NH_4Cl and consequently the measured urinary cations (= $Na^+ + K^+$) will have a concentration lower than that of the measured anion Cl^-: $Na^+ + K^+ < Cl^-$. On the contrary, in a child with an impaired renal acidification, the urine net charge will be as follows: $Na^+ + K^+ > Cl^-$ (Table 31.14).

When the urine net charge is positive ($Na^+ + K^+ > Cl^-$) and it is unclear whether increased excretion of unmeasured anions is responsible, the urinary NH_4^+ concentration can be estimated from calculation of the urine osmolal gap (Table 31.14). This calculation requires measurement of the urine osmolality (in mosm/kg) and the urine Na^+, K^+, urea, and, if the dipstick is positive, glucose concentrations[9] (in mmol/L). In the context of metabolic acidosis, an estimated urinary NH_4^+ concentration of <20 mmol/L indicates an impaired NH_4^+ excretion.

Metabolic Acidosis During the First Months of Life

During the first months of life bicarbonatemia is lower by 2–4 mmol/L than in older children, and

Table 31.14 Indirect assessment of urinary excretion of NH_4^+ by means of the urinary net charge in subjects with normal anion gap metabolic acidosis

Distal acidification of the renal tubule	Urinary NH_4^+	Urinary net charge
Normal	↑ NH_4^+	$Na^+ + K^+ < Cl^-$
Impaired	↓ NH_4^+	$Na^+ + K^+ > Cl^{-a}$

[a]The urine osmolal charge is a more precise estimate of the urinary NH_4^+ concentration in this setting:

$$\frac{\text{Measured Osmolality} - \left[2 \times (Na + K) + Urea + Glucose \right]}{2}$$

it is even lower in preterm infants. This is the consequence of a lower renal threshold for bicarbonate. In addition, in preterm infants and in growing children the daily production of H^+ is higher by 50–100 % than that noted in adults (this is mainly explained by the fact that the growing skeleton releases 20 mmol of H^+ for each 1 g of Ca^{++} that is incorporated). The clinical implications of these data are that, as compared with older children, newborns and infants have a relatively limited capacity to compensate for hypobicarbonatemia. In this age the tendency towards metabolic acidosis is compensated for by the large intake of milk, whose alkali content is high. Infants are therefore more prone to develop metabolic acidosis in conditions associated with a decreased milk intake.

Symptoms, Signs, and Consequences

The signs and symptoms of acute metabolic acidosis include:

1. High respiratory rate (in young children and infants, the increase in depth of respiration, as observed in classic Kussmaul type deep breathing, may not be as apparent as in adults and the response to metabolic acidosis may be tachypnea alone);
2. Abdominal pain and vomiting;
3. Irritability and lethargy.

The gastrointestinal absorption and excretion of dietary base plays a major role in acid-base homeostasis in infants in whom the predominantly milk-based diet supplies a considerable

---

[8]The term urine anion gap is a misnomer for what should have been named urine cation gap.

[9]The obtain urea and glucose in mmol/L divide blood urea nitrogen (in mg/dL) by 2.8 and glucose (in mg/dL) by 18.

amount of alkali. Infants are therefore more vulnerable to developing metabolic acidosis in illnesses associated with decreased milk intake.

Since an excessive chronic acid burden interferes with Ca^{++} deposition in the bone and Ca^{++} intestinal absorption, metabolic acidosis of any form can impair growth in children. Other signs and symptoms are abdominal pain, vomiting, irritability, lethargy, seizures and coma. However, the latter manifestations are primarily due to the underlying disease (e.g., organic acidemias or hyperosmolality in diabetic ketoacidosis) and not primarily to the acidosis itself.

Clinical Work Up

The causes of metabolic acidosis, which appear in Table 31.13, can almost always be discerned clinically. A careful history and physical examination and the determination of the blood anion gap direct an accurate evaluation. For the initial diagnostic approach to metabolic acidosis of unknown origin the following initial steps are taken [21–25]:

- Confirm the diagnosis of metabolic acidosis
- Confirm that the respiratory response is appropriate
- Distinguish high from normal anion gap metabolic acidosis:
  - Normal anion gap: consider intestinal loss of HCO_3^-
  - High anion gap: assess urinary ketones, blood glucose and blood L-lactate

The major causes of high anion gap acidosis are L-lactate acidosis, which results from impaired tissue oxygenation (type A acidosis) or from an altered metabolism of L-lactate with normal tissue oxygenation in the context of a mitochondrial impairment (type B acidosis), diabetic ketoacidosis, which mainly results from the accumulation of ß-hydroxybutyrate, and "uremic" metabolic acidosis, which is characterized by the accumulation of phosphate, sulfate, and organic anions.

In children, normal anion gap metabolic acidosis mostly results from intestinal bicarbonate losses due to diarrhea. Renal bicarbonate wasting is much less common. In children with normal anion gap acidosis but without history of diarrhea, the concurrent determination of urinary Na^+, K^+, Cl^- will provide information on the renal mechanisms of acidification.

Sometimes there is overlap between the causes of a normal and high anion gap metabolic acidosis. Diarrhea, for example, is most often associated with a normal anion gap. However, severe diarrhea and hypovolemia can result in an increase in the anion gap due to hypoperfusion-induced lactic acidosis and starvation ketosis.

Management

The management of metabolic acidosis includes the following four points:

1. Emergency measures: Avoidance of further production of H^+ including measures to ensure a proper airway, adequate peripheral perfusion and O_2 delivery. For instance, in a child with type A L-lactate acidosis in the context of severe dehydration, delivery of O_2 and the rapid administration of normal saline will regenerate adenosine triphosphate. On the other hand, in a child with accidental methanol intoxication the administration of ethanol might stop the production of toxins leading to acidosis.
2. Increasing pH level by lowering the pCO_2, ensuring an adequate degree of hyperventilation, if necessary by mechanical ventilation.
3. Correction of the underlying condition. For example, the administration of insulin, in addition to normal saline, in diabetic ketoacidosis.
4. Administration of $NaHCO_3$. The use of $NaHCO_3$ is controversial considering the possible benefits (a. metabolic advantage of faster glycolysis with better availability of adenosine triphopsphate in vital organs; b. improved cardiac action) and the risks (a. extracellular fluid volume expansion; b. tendency towards hypernatremia; c. development of hypokalemia and hypocalcemia; d. worsening of intracellular acidosis) The following guidelines have been suggested for administration of $NaHCO_3$:

Table 31.15 Conditions associating metabolic acidosis and potassium depletion

Condition	Basis of potassium depletion
Classic distal renal tubular acidosis	Renal loss
Diarrhea	Renal and intestinal loss
Diabetic ketoacidosis	Renal loss (osmotic diuresis)[a]

[a]Circulating potassium is often initially normal in diabetic ketoacidosis

- Diabetic ketoacidosis: $NaHCO_3$ should be considered when hyperkalemia persists despite insulin therapy, when acidemia worsens despite insulin therapy (suggesting insulin resistance as a result of acidemia) and perhaps when HCO_3^- is <5.0 mmol/L. We are very reluctant to use bicarbonate in diabetic ketoacidosis because the administration of $NaHCO_3$ is a risk factor for cerebral edema.
- Type A L-lactate metabolic acidosis: In this form of acidosis the primary effort should be directed at improving delivery of O_2. $NaHCO_3$ should be given when HCO_3^- is <5.0 mmol/L.

Since the "HCO_3^- space" is ≈ 0.5 L/kg body weight the dose of $NaHCO_3$ in severe metabolic acidosis may be calculated from body weight (in kg), current blood HCO_3^-, and desired blood HCO_3^- (both in mmol/l), using the equation:

$$\text{Body weight} \times 0.5 \left(\text{desired HCO}_3^- - \text{current HCO}_3^-\right)$$

Hence, a child weighing 20 kg with a severe hypobicarbonatemia of 3.5 mmol/L will be given 40 mmol of $NaHCO_3$ over several minutes (i.e. 2.0 mmol/kg body weight) if the "desired" blood HCO_3^- level is 7.5 mmol/L. In most cases, however, the initial dosage of $NaHCO_3$ is 1.0 mmol/kg body weight, a dosage that is expected to increase blood HCO_3^- by 2.0 mmol/L.

Correction of metabolic acidosis tends to decrease circulating K^+ level. Hence, one must avoid a severe degree of hypokalemia when $NaHCO_3$ is given. K^+ depletion and metabolic acidosis are associated in three settings: classic distal renal tubular acidosis, acute diarrheal disease and diabetic ketoacidosis, as shown in Table 31.15.

The management of renal tubular acidosis will be discussed in Chap. 36, that of uremic acidosis in the chapters in the sections devoted to renal replacement therapy.

Metabolic Alkalosis

Primary hyperbicarbonatemia and, therefore, alkalemia, are the hallmarks of metabolic alkalosis [20, 22, 26, 27]. In this peculiar acid-base disorder (Table 31.16) hyperbicarbonatemia, alkalemia and the compensatory hypoventilation (resulting in a rise of the pCO_2) are almost always associated with hypokalemia (see: systemic effects of acid-base abnormalities).

With the constraints of electroneutrality, the ways to add HCO_3^- to extracellular space are loss of the anion Cl^- or retention of Na^+. Hence circulating HCO_3^- may be raised either (1) associated with a normal or contracted "effective" circulating volume (blood pressure normal or low) or with (2) an expanded "effective" circulating volume (blood pressure increased).

Metabolic Alkalosis Associated with Normal or Contracted "Effective" Circulating Volume (Unaccompanied Cl^- Deficiency Syndrome or Normotensive Hypokalemic Metabolic Alkalosis) = Chloride Depletion Metabolic Alkalosis

In this clinical-laboratory entity Cl^- is lost from the extracellular space "not accompanied" by the major cations Na^+ and K^+ but "accompanied" by H^+ or NH_4^+. Since a loss of H^+ or NH_4^+ is equivalent to a gain of HCO_3^-, the final effect is loss of Cl^- and gain of HCO_3^-.

Two further steps complete the development of metabolic alkalosis:

- "Extra" HCO_3^-, which is filtered by the kidney, is mostly reabsorbed and only a little HCO_3^- is excreted;
- Contraction of the circulating volume activates the renin-angiotensin II-aldosterone system resulting in urinary K^+ excretion, which further aggravates hyperbicarbonatemia.

Secondary hyperaldosteronism resulting in urinary K^+ excretion is the main cause of hypokalemia that accompanies this form of metabolic alkalosis.

This clinical-laboratory entity, termed in the past volume contraction hypokalemic alkalosis, is currently termed Cl^- depletion hypokalemic alkalosis because balance and clearance studies indicate that Cl^- repletion in the face of persisting alkali loading, volume contraction, and K^+ and Na^+ depletion repairs alkalosis. During the first months of life metabolic alkalosis is often not associated with hypokalemia (alternatively it is associated with mild hypokalemia) because the ability of the kidney to excrete K^+ is reduced early in life.

Maternal Cl^- depletion, deficient Cl^- intake, gastrointestinal Cl^- losses, cutaneous Cl^- losses in the setting of cystic fibrosis, diuretics and renal tubular disturbances are the most

Table 31.16 Causes of metabolic alkalosis (linked with hypokalemia)

Associated with normal (or contracted) "effective" circulating volume (and therefore with normal or even low blood pressure)
(a) Nonrenal causes (low urine chloride excretion: chloride/creatinine <10 mol/mol)
Intestinal causes
Low dietary chloride intake (e.g., soybean formula with a low chloride content in infancy, "tea and toast diet")
Loss of gastric secretions (vomiting, nasogastric suction)
Posthypercapnia
Congenital chloridodiarrhea (uncommon), villous adenoma (uncommon)
Cutaneous cause
Cystic fibrosis
Excessive sweating (uncommon, associated with low dietary chloride intake)
"Posthypercapnia" (= posthypercapnic alkalosis)
Refeeding syndrome
Transient neonatal metabolic alkalosis in infants of mothers affected by chloride deficiency (eating disorders associated with chloride deficiency, Bartter syndromes, Gitelman syndrome)
(b) Renal causes (high urine chloride excretion: chloride/creatinine >>10 mol/mol)
Primary chloride losing tubulopathies (Bartter syndromes, Gitelman syndrome)
Secondary chloride losing tubulopathies (some cases of chronic cisplatin tubulopathy)
Current diuretic use (including surreptitious use)[a]
Associated with an expanded "effective" circulating volume (and therefore with high blood pressure)
Enhanced mineralocorticoid activity
Primary aldosteronism (either hyperplasia or adenoma)
Apparent mineralocorticoid excess (= defect in 11-β-hydroxysteroid-dehydrogenase), Liddle syndrome (congenitally increased function of the collecting tubule sodium channels), dexamethasone-responsive aldosteronism (synthesis of aldosterone promoted not only by renin but also by adrenocorticotropin), congenital adrenal hyperplasia (11-β-hydroxylase or 17-α-hydroxylase deficiency), Cushing disease
Secondary hyperaldosteronism (including renal artery stenosis, malignant hypertension, and renin producing tumor)
Exogenous mineralocorticoids, licorice-ingestion (=11-β-hydroxysteroid-dehydrogenase blockade)
Reduced renal function plus a source of HCO_3^-: alkali ingestion, ingestion of ion-exchange resin plus nonreabsorbable alkali

[a]The urinary chloride excretion is low in subjects with remote use of diuretics

important causes of normotensive hypokalemic metabolic alkalosis (Table 31.16). The urinary excretion of chloride is low in patients with non-renal and normal or high in subjects with renal causes of this peculiar form of metabolic alkalosis. In our experience the determination of the molar urinary chloride/creatinine ratio in spot urine samples from patients with normotensive metabolic alkalosis distinguishes between renal (urinary chloride/creatinine ratio largely >10 mol/mol) and non-renal causes (urinary chloride/creatinine ratio <10 mol/mol). In clinical practice this simple parameter is useful in patients in whom the etiology of metabolic alkalosis with normal or low normal blood pressure is not obtainable from the history. Please note that the urinary chloride/creatinine ratio is also usually >10 mol/mol in patients with metabolic alkalosis associated with expanded effective circulating volume (see below).

Posthypercapnic Alkalosis (Posthypercapnia)

Chronic respiratory acidosis is associated with a compensatory hyperbicarbonatemia. In those patients with a tendency towards a contracted circulating volume when pCO_2 falls to normal, there will be a stimulus for persistently increased HCO_3^- levels and hypokalemia. In addition, a rapid correction of chronic respiratory acidosis (e.g., mechanical ventilation) results in an acute rise in cerebral pH that can produce serious neurologic sequelae or even death. Consequently, pCO_2 should be lowered slowly and carefully in chronic hypercapnia.

Metabolic Alkalosis Associated with an Expanded "Effective" Circulating Volume (= Hypertensive Metabolic Alkalosis)

The second way to add HCO_3^- to the circulating volume and preserving electroneutrality is to retain HCO_3^- along with Na^+, therefore expanding the extracellular fluid volume and increasing blood pressure. Obviously, to retain extra Na^+ (along with HCO_3^-) "permission" of the kidney will be required.

The mechanisms for renal retention of Na^+ and HCO_3^- include either (1) an enhanced reabsorption of filtered HCO_3^- or (2) a reduced glomerular filtration rate plus a source of HCO_3^- (e.g., the ingestion of large amounts of milk and the absorbable antacid $CaCO_3$).

Excessive mineralocorticoid activity is the main cause of metabolic alkalosis associated with hypokalemia and expanded circulating volume. The corresponding causes appear in Table 31.16.

Symptoms, Signs, and Consequences

There are no specific diagnostic symptoms or signs of metabolic alkalosis [14, 21, 22, 26, 27]. Physical examination may reveal neuromuscolar irritability, such as tetany or hyperactive reflexes. These signs will be more pronounced if hypocalcemia is an accompanying feature, since the ionized Ca^{++} concentration decreases as pH rises. The symptoms and signs of accompanying hypokalemia have been discussed above.

It is recognized that in children with both normal (or contracted) and expanded circulating volume and metabolic alkalosis the assessment of the fluid volume status by physical examination and history may be quite inaccurate. This assumption is supported by the experience in infantile hypertrophic pyloric stenosis where the clinical assessment of the fluid volume status may be quite inaccurate, and the severity of metabolic alkalosis helps to define the amount of fluid replacement required.

Management

The most frequent causes of hypokalemic metabolic alkalosis associated with a normal or contracted "effective" circulating volume include intestinal (mostly gastric) or cutaneous fluid losses, and excessive diuretic therapy. These forms of metabolic alkalosis are termed "chloride responsive," because they are reversed by the oral intravenous administration of Na^+Cl^-, K^+Cl^- and water. Many institutions hydrate infants with hypertrophic pyloric stenosis with a "near isotonic" parenteral solution containing glucose 5 % (=50 g/L), Na^+Cl^- 80–90 mmol/L and K^+Cl^- 20–30 mmol/L until correction of the acid-base and K^+ balance. The initial parenteral repair consists of a normal saline solution at least in children with both hypokalemic alkalosis and rather severe hyponatremia (≤ 120 mmol/L).

Occasionally, severe metabolic alkalosis is additionally treated with (i) a carbonic anhydrase inhibitor like acetazolamide, which induces bicarbonaturia accompanied by Na^+- and K^+-losses, (ii) with NH_4Cl, or (iii) with HCl (through a central venous line). Finally, hemodialysis (or hemofiltration) with a low dialysate HCO_3^- in association with saline infusion has been advised for the treatment of severe metabolic alkalosis in advanced kidney disease.

The management of the causes of hypertensive hypokalemic metabolic alkalosis will be discussed elsewhere.

In "chloride responsive" metabolic alkalosis the oral administration of K+ with any anion other than Cl^- (e.g., citrate) prevents the correction of alkalosis.

Respiratory Acid-Base Disturbances

These acid-base disorders will not be discussed in this textbook of clinical nephrology with the exception of Table 31.17, which depicts the main causes.

Calcium

Balance

A 70 kg man contains one kg of Ca^{++} (=25 mol), 99 % of which resides in the skeleton in the form of hydroxyapatite and 1 % of which is found in soft tissues and the extracellular space. Since Ca^{++} plays a crucial role in neuromuscular function, blood coagulation, and intracellular signaling, circulating Ca^{++} concentrations are maintained within a tight physiologic range. The Ca^{++} (and phosphate) homeostasis involves intestinal, bone, and renal function. Regulation of intestinal function is important because, in contrast to the complete absorption of dietary Na^+, K^+ and Cl^-, that of Ca^{++} (like Mg^{++} and phos-

Table 31.17 Causes of respiratory acidosis (hypoventilation) and alkalosis (hyperventilation)

Respiratory acidosis (hypoventilation)
Central nervous system (patient does not breathe)
Cerebral
Posthypoxic brain damage
Cerebral trauma
Intracranial disease
Psychotropic drugs
Brain stem
Brain stem herniation
Encephalitis
Central sleep apnea
Severe metabolic alkalosis
Sedative or narcotic drugs
Upper airway reflexes
Bulbar palsy
Anterior horn cell lesion (including Guillan-Barré and poliomyelitis)
Disruption of airways
Peripheral disorders (patient cannot breathe)
Respiratory muscle disease
Myasthenia, Guillain-Barré syndrome, myopathy, muscular dystrophy
Muscle fatigue or paralysis (including hypokalemic paralysis)
Airway and pulmonary disease
Interstitial lung disease (including lung fibrosis)
Obstructive disease (including upper airway obstruction, asthma, bronchiolitis, cystic fibrosis)
Obstructive sleep apnea
Obesity, kyphoscoliosis
Respiratory alkalosis (hyperventilation)
Hypoxia: intrinsic pulmonary disease, high altitude, congestive heart failure, cyanotic congenital heart disease
Pulmonary receptor stimulation: pneumonia, asthma, interstitial lung disease, pulmonary edema, pulmonary thromboembolism
Drugs: salicylates, niketamide, catecholamines, theophylline, progesterone
Central nervous disorders: subarachnoid hemorrhage, Cheyne-Stokes respiration, primary hyperventilation syndrome
Miscellaneous: panic attacks with hyperventilation (rare before puberty), fever, sepsis, recovery from metabolic acidosis

phate) is incomplete. This limitation is due both to the requirement for vitamin D and to the formation of insoluble salts in the intestinal lumen, such as calcium phosphate, calcium oxalate, and magnesium phosphate.

A normal adult ingests $\approx$1000 mg (=25 mmol) of Ca^{++} per day, of which $\approx$40–50 % may be absorbed. However, 300 mg (approximately 8 mmol) of Ca^{++} from digestive secretions is lost in the stool, resulting in the net absorption of no more than 10–20 %. In the steady state, this amount of Ca^{++} is excreted in the urine. Within the blood Ca^{++}, $\approx$40 % is bound to albumin, 15 % is complexed with citrate, sulfate, or phosphate, and 45 % exists as the physiologically important ionized form [28–30].

Considering that a large proportion of circulating Ca^{++} is bound to albumin, the determination of albumin (or the direct measurement of ionized Ca^{++}) is essential to the diagnosis of true hypocalcemia or hypercalcemia. The following simple formula [28–30] may be used for correction of total calcium to account for albumin binding:

$$\text{measured}\,Ca^{2+}\left[mmol\,/\,L\right]+\frac{40-\text{albumin}\left[g\,/\,L\right]}{40}$$

Although only a small fraction of the total body Ca^{++} is located in the plasma, it is the blood level of ionized Ca^{++} that is under control of calciotropic hormones:

- *Vitamin D*
- *Parathyroid hormone* and
- *The Ca^{++}-sensing receptor*. This receptor, which is found on the cell surface of tissues such as the parathyroid gland, kidney, and bone, detects hypocalcemia and leads to enhanced secretion of parathyroid hormone. Summarizing the process briefly, a fall in circulating Ca^{++} in normal subjects leads to a compensatory increase in parathyroid hormone secretion, which returns the Ca^{++} level to normal by two major actions: increased Ca^{++} release from bone and stimulated production of 1,25-dihydroxyvitamin D, the active metabolite of vitamin D, resulting in an increase in intestinal Ca^{++} absorption [28–30].

- *Parathyroid hormone related peptide* is a further calciotropic hormone with the following identified actions: (i) During pregnancy, Ca^{++} is transferred from the maternal circulation to the fetus by a pump regulated by this hormone; (ii) Parathyroid hormone related peptide levels are elevated during lactation and contribute substantially to the movement of Ca^{++} from the maternal skeleton to the mammary glands; (iii) Finally, this peptide is involved in the pathogenesis of hypercalcemia of malignancies [28–30].

Hypocalcemia

Non-neonatal Hypocalcemia

Symptoms and Signs

Symptoms and signs of hypocalcemia, which is often asymptomatic, result from neuromuscular, ocular, ectodermal, dental, gastrointestinal, cardiovascular, skeletal or endocrine dysfunctions, and are related to the severity and chronicity of the hypocalcemia (Table 31.18). Hypocalcemia manifests with a prolonged QT interval on standard electrocardiogram (Fig. 31.10). However, some signs and symptoms are unique to chronic hypoparathyroidism and not hypocalcemia: these include candidiasis and dysmorphic changes in **A**utoimmune **P**oly**E**ndocrinopathy-**C**andidiasis-**E**ctodermal **D**ystrophy (=APECED-association). Among the symptoms of hypocalcemia, tetany, papilledema and seizures may occur in patients who develop hypocalcemia acutely. By comparison, ectodermal and dental changes, cataracts, basal ganglia calcification, and extrapyramidal disorders are features of chronic hypocalcemia and are common in hypoparathyroidism [28–31].

Causes

Deficiency or impaired function of (a) parathyroid hormone, (b) vitamin D or (c) Ca^{++}-sensing receptor are major causes of reduced blood level of ionized Ca^{++}. Because bone Ca^{++} stores are so large, the major reason for hypocalcemia is decreased bone resorption. Sometimes acute

Table 31.18 Clinical signs and symptoms of hypocalcemia

Neuromuscular
Tetany
Sensory dysfunction: circumoral and acral paresthesias
Muscular dysfunction
Stiffness, myalgia, muscle spasms and cramps
Forced adduction of the thumb, flexion of the metacarpophalangeal joints and wrists, and extension of the fingers
Laryngismus stridulus (spasm of respiratory muscles and of glottis causing dyspnea)
Autonomic dysfunction: diaphoresis, bronchospasm, biliary colic
Trousseau sign: inflation of a sphygmomanometer above systolic blood pressure for 3–4 min induces a carpal spasm
Chvostek sign: ipsilateral tapping of the facial nerve just anterior to the ear followed by contraction of the facial muscles (the complete sign is contraction of corner of the mouth, the nose and the eye; contraction of the corner of the mouth alone often occurs in normal subjects)
Myopathy: generalized muscle weakness and wasting with normal creatine kinase (myopathy represents more a feature of vitamin D deficiency than hypocalcemia per se; elevated parathyroid hormone level or hypophosphatemia may contribute to the myopathy)
Extrapyramidal disorders: Bradykinetic movement disorders, sometimes dystonia, hemiballismus, choreoathetosis, oculogyric crises
Convulsions (generalized or partial)
Mental retardation, psychosis
Ocular
Cataract (rarely keratoconjunctivitis)
Papilledema (often associated with benign intracranial hypertension; rarely optic neuritis is present)
Ectodermal (especially in the context of severe, chronic hypocalcemia)
Dry scaly skin
Hyperpigmentation, dermatitis, eczema, and psoriasis
Course, brittle, and sparse hair with patchy alopecia
Brittle nails, with characteristic transverse grooves
Candidiasis: usually as a component of <u>A</u>utoimmune <u>P</u>oly<u>E</u>ndocrinopathy-<u>C</u>andidiasis-<u>E</u>ctodermal <u>D</u>ystrophy (= APECED-association)
Dental (dental hypoplasia, failure of tooth eruption, defective enamel and root formation, and abraded carious teeth)
Gastrointestinal
Loose stools (steatorrhea due to impaired pancreatic secretion)
Gastric achlorhydria
Cardiovascular
Systemic hypotension, decreased myocardial function, congestive heart failure
Prolonged QT interval on standard electrocardiogram with tendency towards cardiac arrhythmias (clinically relevant if hypocalcemia is associated with hypokalemia and hypomagnesemia)
Skeletal
Rachitic findings
Delayed closure of the fontanelles
Parietal and frontal bossing
Craniotabes
Rachitic rosary: enlargement of the costochondral junction visible as beeding along the anterolateral aspects of the chest
Harrison sulcus caused by the muscular pull of the diaphragmatic attachments to the lower ribs
Enlargement and bowing of the distal radius, ulna, tibia and fibula

(continued)

Table 31.18 (continued)

Progressive lateral bowing of the femur and tibia
Children with hypoparathyroidism: increased bone mineral density, osteosclerosis and thickening of the calvarium
Children with pseudohypoparathyroidism: Albright's hereditary osteodystrophy, osteitis fibrosa cystica (due to normal skeletal responsiveness to parathyroid hormone)
Endocrine manifestations
Impaired insulin release
Hypothyroidism, prolactin deficiency, and ovarian failure associated with polyglandular autoimmune syndromes

events such as hyperphosphatemia, can produce hypocalcemia even though the regulatory systems are intact. The main causes of hypocalcaemia include vitamin D deficiency, Ca^{++} deficiency, impaired vitamin D metabolism, impaired parathyroid hormone action (secondary to end organ resistance), reduced production of parathyroid hormone, and abnormal Ca^{++}-sensing receptor or impaired renal function (Table 31.19).

Diagnostic Work Up

Hypocalcemia is a rather common clinical problem, the cause of which can very often be determined from the history (as with a breast-fed infant not receiving any supplementation of vitamin D presenting with non-febrile generalized convulsions, enlargement of the costochondral junction along the anterolateral aspects of the chest and enlargement of the wrist). In some cases, however, the underlying condition is not readily apparent. A detailed history documenting diet, lifestyle, family, and drug history, as well as development and hearing is important. The examination should include an assessment of skin, nails, teeth, and the skeleton, as well as the cardiovascular system. A comprehensive range of investigations should be performed at baseline, which has been divided into first and second line (Table 31.20). The objective of assessing urine Ca^{++} excretion is to establish whether the molar urine calcium/creatinine is inappropriately high in the presence of hypocalcemia. Reference values for urine calcium/creatinine ratio in young children are not well defined and will vary according to factors such as diet. The upper limits of normal urine Ca^{++} excretion in healthy children appear in the footnote of Table 31.20. Renal phosphate handling may be abnormal despite a

blood phosphate within the quoted laboratory normal range, and should be assessed in more detail by determining the tubular maximum reabsorption threshold of phosphate (see section on Phosphate).

Checking biochemistry of the parents and possibly siblings is crucial when inherited diseases such as hypocalcaemic hypercalciuria and hypophosphataemic rickets are suspected. It is also important to measure maternal Ca^{++} and vitamin D levels in the case of hypocalcaemia in infancy because of the link with maternal vitamin D deficiency and hyperparathyroidism. Maternal hyperparathyroidism is linked with adverse pregnancy outcome and causes transient hypocalcemia in the newborn because the fetal parathyroids are suppressed following exposure to high Ca^{++} levels in utero. An autoantibody screen including adrenal, parathyroid, smooth muscle and microsomal antibodies is useful in cases of isolated hypoparathyroidism and where APECED-association is suspected. Renal ultrasound scan looking for evidence of nephrocalcinosis or renal dysplasia is also often advised.

The biochemical picture of hypocalcemia can be categorized according to the presence of undetectable, normal or high levels of circulating parathyroid hormone, an approach that reflects the underlying pathophysiology [31].

Undetectable or low levels of this hormone in the hypocalcemic child suggest hypoparathyroidism (Table 31.19). Aplasia or hypoplasia of the parathyroids is most commonly due to the DiGeorge syndrome associated with deletion of chromosome 22q11. A similar phenotype including hypoparathyroidism has also been associated with deletions of chromosome 10p, while the HDR-association (**H**ypoparathyroidism,

Table 31.19 Causes of hypocalcemia in infants and children

Parathyroid hormone level low
Abnormal production of parathyroid hormone
Magnesium deficiency[a]
Following neck surgery
Hypoparathyroidism (autosomal recessive, autosomal dominant, or X linked)
Di George anomaly (=22q11 deletions), 10p13 deletion, Hall-Hittner or CHARGE-association (=Coloboma, Heart anomaly, Choanal Atresia, mental Retardation, Genital hypoplasia, and Ear anomalies), HDR-association (= Hypoparathyroidism, Deafness, Renal dysplasia)
Autoimmune PolyEndocrinopathy-Candidiasis-Ectodermal Dystrophy (= APECED-association)
Infiltrative lesions such as Wilson's disease and thalassemia
Mitochondrial diseases (e.g. Kearns Sayre syndrome)
Altered "set point" (calcium sensing receptor activating mutations)
Parathyroid hormone level high
Hypovitaminosis D, calcium deficiency, impaired vitamin D metabolism
Hypovitaminosis D
Reduced vitamin D intake or production in the skin
Decreased intestinal absorption (e.g. celiac disease and cystic fibrosis)
Calcium deficiency
Impaired vitamin D "metabolism"
Severe liver disease
Drugs that "inactivate" vitamin D: anticonvulsants (phenobarbital, phenytoin, carbamazepine oxcarbazepine), antimicrobials (isoniazid and rifampicin), antiretroviral drugs
Enzyme deficiency: defects of the 1-α-hydroxylase gene (= vitamin D dependent rickets type I)
End organ resistance to vitamin D (= vitamin D dependent rickets type II)
Signaling defects: pseudohypoparathyroidisms
Renal failure, osteopetrosis, excessive fluoride intake

Data from: Carmeliet et al. [29]; Used with permission of BMJ Publishing Group from Singh et al. [31]
[a]Severe chronic magnesium deficiency (≤0.45 mmol/L) causes hypocalcaemia by impairing parathyroid hormone secretion as well as parathyroid hormone action

Table 31.20 First and second line investigations in childhood hypocalcemia when the cause cannot be determined from the history and clinical examination

First line investigations	Second line investigations
Blood values	
Phosphate[a], Magnesium	Autoantibody screen
Alkaline Phosphatase	Family evaluation
Na$^+$, K$^+$, HCO$_3^-$, Creatinine	Maternal Vitamin D-status
Parathyroid Hormone	1,25-hydroxyvitamin D
25-Hydroxyvitamin D	Genetic studies (e.g. 22q11 deletion)
Urinary values	
Urinalysis (for glucose, protein and pH)	
Calcium[b], Phosphate[a], Creatinine	
Imaging	
Hand and wrist radiograph	Renal ultrasound
Skull radiograph	

Used with permission of BMJ Publishing Group from Singh et al. [31]
[a]Calculate the maximal tubular reabsorption of phosphate as indicated in the section on phosphate
[b]The upper limit of normal for urine calcium/creatinine in healthy children is 2.20 mol/mol (or 0.81 mg/mg) in infants aged 6–12 months, 1.50 mol/mol (or 0.56 mg/mg) in infants aged 13–24 months, 1.40 mol/mol (or 0.50 mg/mg) in infants aged 25–36 months, 1.10 mol/mol (or 0.41 mg/mg) in children aged 3–5 years, 0.80 mol/mol (or 0.30 mg/mg) in children aged 5–7 years and 0.70 mol/mol (or 0.25 mg/mg) in older children

hormone gene are rare. Diseases such as APECED can present with hypoparathyroidism in the absence of the two other major manifestations, which are candidiasis and adrenal failure. There should be a high index of suspicion for this disease in all cases of hypoparathyroidism presenting in children older than 4 years. Children with APECED may have other "minor" features such as malabsorption, gallstones, hepatitis, dysplastic nails and teeth. Screening should be considered in the siblings of affected individuals. Mitochondrial disease is a rare cause of hypoparathyroidism but is not usually an isolated finding.

Detectable parathyroid hormone values (low-normal or normal) in an asymptomatic individual raise the possibility of hypocalcemic

Deafness, and Renal dysplasia) is due to defects in the GATA3 gene. Defects in the parathyroid

hypercalciuria, an abnormality of the Ca^{++}-sensing receptor which can be assessed in more detail by determining urinary Ca^{++} excretion. This parameter is typically low in longstanding hypoparathyroidism, and a relatively high urine Ca^{++} excretion (molar urinary calcium/creatinine ratio ≥ 0.30) suggests hypocalcemic hypercalciuria. This abnormality is due to activating mutations of the Ca^{++}-sensing receptor with downshift of the setpoint for Ca^{++} responsive parathyroid hormone release. Mg^{++} levels are low in this disorder because the Ca^{++}-sensing receptor also detects this cation. Interestingly, the biochemical picture of hypocalcemic hypercalciuria sometimes resembles Bartter syndromes and includes hypokalemia and hyperbicarbonatemia.

If blood creatinine is normal, thereby excluding renal insufficiency, then increased parathyroid hormone levels point towards a diagnosis of rickets[10] or pseudohypoparathyroidism. Vitamin D deficiency is still prevalent in the Western world. High-risk groups include families, where the maternal and child diet may be low in Ca^{++} and vitamin D and where exposure to sunlight can be limited. The diagnosis of Fanconi-De Toni-Debré syndrome should be considered in any hypocalcemic child with persistent glycosuria, phosphaturia, and acidosis. Pseudohypoparathyroidism is a heterogeneous disorder that results from signaling defects of the cell surface receptors. Patients may become hypocalcemic despite a compensatory increase in parathyroid hormone concentration, and may have other endocrine problems, such as primary hypothyroidism and hypogonadism that are also manifestations of an abnormal signaling mechanism. Some patients are overweight and mentally retarded.

Neonatal Hypocalcemia

Hypocalcemia is a common metabolic problem in newborns. During pregnancy, Ca^{++} is transferred from the maternal circulation to the fetus by a pump regulated by parathyroid hormone-related peptide. This process results in higher blood Ca^{++} in the fetus than in the mother and leads to fetal hypercalcemia, with total Ca^{++} level of ≈ 2.50–2.75 mmol/L in umbilical cord blood [28–31].

The cessation of placental transfer of Ca^{++} at birth is followed by a fall in total blood Ca^{++} concentration to ≈ 2.00–2.25 mmol/L and ionized Ca^{++} to ≈ 1.10–1.35 mmol/L at 24 h. Ca^{++} subsequently rises, reaching levels seen in older children and adults by 2 weeks of age.

The definition of hypocalcemia depends upon birth weight: (a) in term infants or premature infants >1.50 kg birth weight, hypocalcemia is defined as a total Ca^{++} concentration <2.00 mmol/L or a ionized fraction <1.10 mmol/L; (b) premature infants with birth weight <1.50 kg are hypocalcemic if they have a total Ca^{++} concentration <1.75 mmol/L or a ionized fraction of <1.00 mmol/L [28–31].

Symptoms and Signs

Neonatal hypocalcemia is usually asymptomatic. Among those who become symptomatic, the characteristic sign is increased neuromuscular irritability. Such infants are jittery and often have muscle jerking. Generalized or partial clonic seizures can occur. Rare presentations include inspiratory stridor caused by laryngospasm, wheezing caused by bronchospasm or vomiting possibly resulting from pylorospasm [28–31].

Causes

The causes of neonatal hypocalcemia are classified by the timing of onset. Hypocalcemia is considered to be early when it occurs in the first 2–3 days after birth.

Early Neonatal Hypocalcemia

Early hypocalcemia is an exaggeration of the normal decline in Ca^{++} concentration after birth. It occurs commonly in premature infants, in infants of diabetic mothers, and after perinatal asphyxia or intrauterine growth restriction:

- Prematurity: One-third of premature infants and the majority of very-low-birth-weight infants develop hypocalcemia during the first 2 days after birth. Multiple factors contribute

---

[10]In hypophosphataemic rickets, circulating parathyroid hormone and calcium are usually normal.

to the fall. They include hypoalbuminemia and factors that lower both total and ionized Ca^{++}, such as reduced intake of Ca^{++} because of low intake of milk, possible impaired response to parathyroid hormone, increased calcitonin and increased urinary Ca^{++} losses.

- Infants of diabetic mothers: Hypocalcemia occurs in 10–20 % of infants of diabetic mothers. The lowest concentration typically occurs between 24 and 72 h after birth and often is associated with hyperphosphatemia. Hypocalcemia is caused by lower parathyroid hormone concentrations after birth in this condition compared to normal infants. Hypoparathyroidism is likely related to intrauterine hypercalcemia suppressing the fetal parathyroid glands. Concurrent hypomagnesemia is a further contributing factor.
- Birth asphyxia: Infants with birth asphyxia frequently have hypocalcemia and hyperphosphatemia. Possible mechanisms include increased phosphate load caused by tissue catabolism, decreased intake due to delayed initiation of feedings, renal insufficiency, acidosis, and increased serum calcitonin concentration.
- Intrauterine growth restriction: Hypocalcemia occurs with increased frequency in infants with intrauterine growth restriction. The mechanism is thought to involve decreased transfer of Ca^{++} across the placenta.

Late Neonatal Hypocalcemia

Late hypocalcemia develops after the second or third day after birth. It typically occurs at the end of the first week. Here are the scenarios:

- Hypoparathyroidism: Hypoparathyroidism associated with excess phosphorus intake is the most common cause of late neonatal hypocalcemia. Hypoparathyroidism often occurs as part of a syndrome, including DiGeorge syndrome or, more rarely, mitochondrial cytopathies.
- Maternal hyperparathyroidism: Infants born to mothers with hyperparathyroidism frequently have hypocalcemia. The mechanism is related to increased transplacental Ca^{++}

transport caused by maternal hypercalcemia, which results in excessive fetal hypercalcemia that inhibits fetal and neonatal parathyroid secretion. Affected infants typically develop increased neuromuscular irritability in the first 3 weeks after birth, but they can present later.

- Hypomagnesemia: Hypomagnesemia causes resistance to parathyroid hormone and impairs its secretion, both of which can result in hypocalcemia. The most common etiology in newborns is transient hypomagnesemia, although rare disorders of intestinal or renal tubular Mg^{++} transport can occur.
- Other causes: Critically ill or premature infants are exposed to many therapeutic interventions that may cause transient hypocalcemia including bicarbonate infusion resulting in metabolic alkalosis, transfusion with citrated blood or infusion of lipids leading to formation of Ca^{++} complexes and decreased ionized Ca^{++}. Finally, mild hypocalcemia has been associated with phototherapy. Other rare causes include acute renal failure of any cause, usually associated with hyperphosphatemia, any disorder of vitamin D metabolism and rotavirus infections.
- High phosphate intake: Intake of excess phosphate is an historically important cause of late hypocalcemia that was seen in term infants fed bovine milk or a formula with a high phosphorus concentration. It has been postulated that the high phosphorus levels antagonize parathyroid hormone or may produce increased Ca^{++} and phosphorus deposition in bones. Symptomatic infants typically present with tetany or seizures at 5–10 days of age. Severe hyperphosphatemia and hypocalcemia also can be caused by phosphate enemas.

Hypercalcemia

Signs and Symptoms

Hypercalcemia is more difficult to diagnose than hypocalcemia because of the nonspecific nature of symptoms and signs (Table 31.21). Hypercalcemia manifests with a shortened QT interval on electrocardiogram (Fig. 31.10). Major

Table 31.21 Symptoms and signs of hypercalcemia

General
Weakness
Depression
Anorexia
Central nervous system
Impaired concentration
Increased sleep requirement
Altered state of consciousness
Mental retardation
Polydypsia (and polyuria)
Muscular: weakness
Ocular
Palpebral calcification
Band keratopathy
Conjunctival calcification
Dermal: Pruritus and skin calcifications
Gastrointestinal
Constipation
Anorexia, nausea, vomiting
Pancreatitis
Peptic ulcer
Cardiovascular
Shortened QT interval on standard electrocardiogram[a]
Arterial hypertension
Skeletal: joint pain (pseudogout)
Renal dysfunction
Altered urinary concentration ability with polyuria and polydypsia
Nephrolithiasis, nephrocalcinosis, renal failure
Distal renal tubular acidosis

[a]Without any major tendency towards cardiac arrhythmias (arrhythmias and ST-segment elevation mimicking myocardial infarction has been reported exclusively in patients with total Ca^{++} >3.50 mmol/L)

symptoms include sekeletal pain, fatigue, anorexia, nausea and vomiting, and particularly important are polyuria and polydipsia. Changes in behavior and frank psychiatric disorders may also be a result of hypercalcemia. The extent of symptoms and signs is a function of both the degree of hypercalcemia and the rate of onset of the elevation in the blood concentration. Thus, a rather severe hypercalcemia of 3.50 mmol/L is asymptomatic when it develops chronically, while an acute rise to these values may cause marked changes in sensorium. It is worthy of

mention, however, that symptoms and signs associated with hypercalcemia may be due to the elevation in the Ca^{++} concentration but also to the underlying disease [28–30, 32, 33].

Causes

Hypercalcemia results when the entry of Ca^{++} into the circulation exceeds the excretion of Ca^{++} into the urine or deposition in bone. Since the major sources of Ca^{++} are the bone and the intestinal tract, hypercalcemia mostly results from increased bone resorption or from increased intestinal absorption. In some cases, however, multiple sites are involved in the development of hypercalcemia. The great majority of adult patients with elevated Ca^{++} level will be found to have either *primary hyperparathyroidism or malignancy* (this form of hypercalcemia is thought in many instances to be caused by secretion of parathyroid hormone related peptide), although the differential diagnosis is much longer. For these other causes of hypercalcemia, which include *vitamin D (or A) intoxication, sarcoidosis, tuberculosis, some fungal infections, thyreotoxicosis, Addison's disease, milk-alkali syndrome (= calcium-alkali syndrome)* related to the prescription of Ca^{++}, absorbable alkali and vitamin D supplements), treatment with *thiazides or lithium carbonate, familial hypocalciuric hypercalcemia, prolonged immobilization* in subjects with high skeletal turnover (including adolescents) and the recovery phase of *rhabdomyolysis*, the use of the mnemonic VITAMINS TRAPS (Table 31.22) has been suggested. Children present with hypercalcemia less frequently than adults, but the causes that are common in adults are also common in children. Young children and infants, however, present with hypercalcemia in association with some rather rare conditions seen almost exclusively in that population. *Idiopathic infantile hypercalcemia* is characterized by an increased sensitivity to vitamin D. It is the consequence of loss of function mutations in the gene that encodes the enzymatic system responsible for the inactivation of 25-hydroxyvitamin D, resulting in its decreased conversion into inactive metabolites [28–30, 32, 33].

Table 31.22 Causes of hypercalcemia (note that some causes of hypercalcemia are given twice)

Classical causes (Mnemonic VITAMINS TRAP)
<u>V</u>itamin D and vitamin A
<u>I</u>mmobilization
<u>T</u>hyrotoxicosis
<u>A</u>ddison's disease
<u>M</u>ilk-alkali syndrome (= calcium-alkali syndrome)
<u>I</u>nflammatory disorders (granulomatous diseases with excessive production of calcitriol)
<u>N</u>eoplastic-related disease[a]
<u>S</u>arcoidosis
<u>T</u>hiazides[b] and other drugs
<u>R</u>habdomyolysis (recovery phase)
<u>AIDS</u>
<u>P</u>arathyroid disease[a] (including familial hypocalciuric hypercalcemia), <u>p</u>arenteral nutrition

Hypercalcemia associated with elevated calcitriol (1,25-dihydroxyvitamin D₃)
Sarcoidosis
Acute granulomatous pneumonia, lipoid pneumonia
Tuberculosis (and other mycobacterial infections)
Wegener's granulomatosis
Crohn's disease
Hepatic granulomatosis
Talc and silicone granulomatosis
Cat scratch disease
Neonatal subcutaneous fat necrosis

Hypercalcemia associated with elevated parathyroid hormone related peptide
Hypercalcemia of malignancy
Some benign tumors (ovary, kidney, pheochromcytoma)
Systemic lupus erythematosus
HIV-associated lymphadenopathy
Massive mammary hyperplasia
During late pregnancy and lactation in hypoparathyroidism

Drugs associated with the development of hypercalcemia
Common: calcium, vitamin D, vitamin A, lithium, thiazides[b] (e.g., hydrochlorothiazide, chlortalidone)
Less common: theophyllin (toxic doses), recombinant growth hormone, foscarnet, hepatitis B vaccination, manganese toxicity, omeprazole

Rare causes of hypercalcemia with an unknown underlying mechanism
Infections: nocardiosis, brucellosis, cytomegaloviric infection (in AIDS), berylliosis
Juvenile idiopathic arthritis

Table 31.22 (continued)

Advanced chronic liver disease

Rare causes of hypercalcemia in infancy and young children
Reduced function of the calcium-sensing receptor
Deactivating mutations
Heterozygous: familial hypocalciuric hypercalcemia
Homozygous: severe neonatal hyperparathyroidism
Autoantibodies directed at the calcium-sensing receptor
Congenital hyperparathyroidism
Idiopathic infantile hypercalcemia
Jansens metaphyseal chondrodysplasia[c]
Williams-Beuren syndrome
Down syndrome
Hypophosphatasia
Congenital lactase deficiency
Phosphate depletion in severe prematurity
Renal tubular acidosis
Primary hyperoxaluria
Neonatal subcutaneous fat necrosis

[a]Malignancy and primary hyperparathyroidism account for 80–90 % of cases of hypercalcemia in adulthood
[b]Although thiazides are frequently cited as a cause of hypercalcemia, it is more usual that they bring mild pre-existing hypercalcemia to light
[c]Consequence of a constitutive activation of the parathyroid hormone receptor

Diagnostic Work Up

The causes of hypercalcemia are often discerned clinically. Clinical history (calcium-alkali syndrome, which replaces the traditional term of milk-alkali syndrome, is currently a cause of hypercalcemia that results from the widespread use of over-the-counter Ca^{++} and vitamin D supplements), physical examination and rather simple laboratory data (circulating phosphate and creatinine; urinary Ca^{++}, phosphate and creatinine) and chest x-ray (looking for sarcoidosis) provide the correct diagnosis in many cases.

Step 1: Assess Clinical and Simple Laboratory Data

Clinical history and physical examination are useful in establishing the diagnosis of hypercalcemia induced by immobilization, medication or thyreotoxicosis, and the diagnosis of "syndromic" hypercalcemia, including Williams-Beuren syndrome, Down syndrome and Jansens metaphyseal chondrodysplasia. Measurement of the serum phosphate concentration and urinary Ca^{++} excretion also may be helpful in selected cases: hyperparathyroidism and the humoral hypercalcemia of malignancy induced by secretion of parathyroid hormone related peptide often present with hypophosphatemia resulting from inhibition of renal proximal tubular phosphate reabsorption. In comparison, the serum phosphate concentration is normal or elevated in granulomatous diseases, vitamin D intoxication, immobilization, thyrotoxicosis and metastatic bone disease. Calciuria is usually raised or high-normal in hyperparathyroidism and hypercalcemia of malignancy. Two conditions lead to relative hypocalciuria: thiazides, which directly enhance active reabsorption of Ca^{++} in the distal tubule, and familial hypocalciuric hypercalcemia, in which the fractional excretion of Ca^{++} is often <1.0 % (further clues to the possible presence of this disorder are a family history of hypercalcemia and few if any hypercalcemic symptoms).

Step 2: Analyze Parathyroid Hormone Level

An elevated parathyroid hormone concentration indicates the presence of primary hyperparathyroidism or a patient taking lithium. Ten to 20 % of patients with primary hyperparathyroidism have a parathyroid hormone concentration in the upper end of the normal range: such a "normal" level, which indicates that the secretion is not suppressed, is virtually diagnostic of primary hyperparathyroidism, since it is still inappropriately high considering the presence of hypercalcemia. A low or low-normal parathyroid hormone level is consistent with all other non-parathyroid hormone-induced causes of hypercalcemia.

Step 3: Analyze Vitamin D Metabolites

The levels of vitamin D metabolites 25-hydroxyvitamin D and 1,25-dihydroxyvitamin D are assessed if there is no obvious malignancy and parathyroid hormone levels are not elevated. An elevated 25-hydroxyvitamin D is indicative of either vitamin D intoxication or idiopathic infantile

hypercalcemia. On the other hand, increased 1,25-dihydroxyvitamin D may be induced by direct intake of this metabolite or non-renal production in granulomatous diseases or lymphoma.

Management

The degree of hypercalcemia and the rate of rise of Ca^{++} level habitually determine symptoms and urgency of treatment [32, 33]:

- Asymptomatic or mildly symptomatic hypercalcemia (total Ca^{++} <3.00 mmol/) does not require immediate treatment. Similarly, Ca^{++} of 3.00–3.50 mmol/L is often well-tolerated chronically, and may not require urgent treatment. (However, an acute rise to these concentrations may cause marked sensorium changes, which require more urgent measures.)
- Total Ca^{++} concentration >3.50 mmol/L requires immediate treatment, regardless of symptoms.

The nonsurgical management of childhood hypercalcemia includes following points:

1. Avoidance of the cause. For example, removal of exogenous vitamin D and Ca^{++} in children with vitamin D intoxication, calcium-alkali syndrome or idiopathic infantile hypercalcemia.
2. Specific management. Steroids inhibit the effects of vitamin D and are particularly effective in hypercalcemia secondary to granulomatous diseases. The bisphosphonates, which inhibit skeletal Ca^{++} release, are effective in hypercalcemia that results from excessive bone resorption of any cause (including among others hypercalcemia of malignancy, hypercalcemia associated with neonatal subcutaneous fat necrosis and vitamin D intoxication). Pharmacologic doses of calcitonin reduce the Ca^{++} levels by decreasing bone resorption. The effect of calcitonin, which is limited to the first 48 h, is most beneficial in subjects with total Ca^{++} >3.50 mmol/L when combined with a bisphosphonate and administration of saline.
3. Normal saline, administered at a rapid rate (initially 2800–3000 ml/m^2 body surface area

daily), corrects possible volume depletion due to hypercalcemia-induced renal salt wasting and promotes renal Ca^{++} excretion. The loop diuretic furosemide is no longer recommended with the exception of cases with volume overload.

Magnesium

Balance

A 70 kg man contains $\approx$1 mol of Mg^{++}. About half of it is present in bone tissue, the other half in soft tissue, whereas no more than 1–2 % of the total body Mg^{++} is present in extracellular fluids. Intracellular Mg^{++} serves as cofactor for many enzymes that produce and store energy via hydrolysis of adenosine triphosphate [30, 34, 35].

In healthy humans the total circulating Mg^{++} concentration is maintained within narrow limits and ranges between 0.75 and 1.00 mmol/L.[11] Approximately 1/4 of circulating Mg^{++} is bound to albumin. For the remaining 3/4 of circulating Mg^{++} $\approx$10 % is complexed to inorganic phosphate, citrate and other compounds, while 90 % ($\approx$2/3 of total circulating Mg^{++}) is in the form of free ion.

Mg^{++} balance, like that of other ions, is a function of intake and urinary excretion. In adults the daily Mg^{++} intake averages 0.23–0.28 mmol/kg (5.6–6.8 mg/kg) body weight. About 1/3 of this Mg^{++} is absorbed. In healthy adults there is no net gain or loss of Mg^{++} from bone so that balance is achieved by the urinary excretion of the 0.06–0.08 mmol/kg (1.5–1.9 mg/kg) body weight.

Only 15–25 % of filtered Mg^{++} is reabsorbed in the proximal tubule and 5–10 % in the distal tubule. The major site of Mg^{++} transport is the thick ascending limb of the loop of Henle where 60–70 % of the filtered load is reabsorbed [30, 34, 35].

With negative Mg^{++} balance, the initial loss comes primarily from the extracellular fluid

(equilibration with bone stores begins after several weeks). Thus, circulating Mg^{++} falls rapidly with negative Mg^{++} balance, leading to a conspicuous decrease in Mg^{++} excretion unless urinary Mg^{++} wasting is present. The fractional clearance of Mg^{++}, which is 3–5 % in healthy subjects ingesting a normal diet, can fall to <0.5 % with Mg^{++} depletion due to non-renal losses. This parameter is calculated from the following equation:

$$\frac{Urinary\,Mg^{++} \times Circulating\,Creatinine}{Circulating\,Mg^{++} \times Urinary\,Creatinine}$$

There is no protection against hypermagnesemia with loss of renal function. In this setting, high intake leads to extracellular Mg^{++} retention.

Hypomagnesemia

Hypomagnesemia, which is not rare, results either from intestinal (including dietary insufficiency) or renal losses (Table 31.23). In the presence of hypomagnesemia the healthy kidney lowers Mg^{++} excretion to very low values. Hence, the diagnosis of hypomagnesemia caused by intestinal Mg^{++} losses (or low dietary Mg^{++} intake) is established by the demonstration of low urinary excretion of Mg^{++}. Conversely the diagnosis of hypomagnesemia caused by renal losses is established by the demonstration of inappropriately high (= "normal") urinary Mg^{++} excretion [30, 34, 35].

Decreased Intake, Poor Intestinal Absorption or Intestinal Loss

Intestinal secretory losses, which contain some Mg^{++} are continuous and not regulated. Although the obligatory losses are not large, marked dietary deprivation can lead to progressive Mg^{++} depletion. Mg^{++} loss will also occur when the intestinal secretions are incompletely reabsorbed as with most disorders of the small bowel, including acute or chronic diarrhea, malabsorption and steatorrhea, and small bowel bypass surgery. Prolonged use of a proton pump inhibitors is an increasingly recognized cause of hypomagnesemia (these drugs interfere with the transport of

---

[11] Circulating magnesium levels can be reported in mmol/L, meq/L, mg/dL or mg/L. The valence of magnesium is 2 and its molecular mass 24.3; therefore 0.50 mmol/L is equivalent to 1.00 meq/L, 1.22 mg/dL and 12.2 mg/L.

Table 31.23 Causes of hypomagnesemia

Decreased magnesium intake and intestinal losses
Dietary deprivation
Small bowel disorders, including acute or chronic diarrhea, malabsorption and steatorrhea, and small bowel bypass surgery
Acute pancreatitis
Paunier disease[a] (= hypomagnesemia with secondary hypocalcemia)
Management with proton-pump inhibitors
Renal losses
Primary renal magnesium wasting diseases
Drugs
Loop and thiazide-type diuretics
Drugs other than diuretics (aminoglycoside antibiotics, amphotericin B, cisplatin, pentamidine, cyclosporine, tacrolimus, foscarnet, cetuximab[b])
Volume expansion
Hypercalcemia
Miscellaneous: recovery from acute tubular necrosis, following renal transplantation and during a postobstructive diuresis
Further causes
Alcohol
Refeeding syndrome
Diabetes mellitus
Following surgery
"Hungry bone syndrome" following parathyroidectomy for hyperparathyroidism
Neonatal hypomagnesemia
Maternal hypomagnesemia
Intrauterine growth retardation

[a]Often combined with impaired renal magnesium conservation
[b]A monoclonal antibody against the epithelial growth factor receptor

this ion across the intestinal wall). Hypomagnesemia can also be seen in acute pancreatitis (saponification of Mg^{++} and Ca^{++} in necrotic fat is the underlying mechanism). Paunier disease or hypomagnesemia with secondary hypocalcemia is a very rare defect of intestinal Mg^{++} resorption (usually combined with impaired renal Mg^{++} conservation), which presents early in infancy with hypocalcemia responsive to Mg^{++} administration. The disease is caused by a loss of function mutation in an ion channel of the transient receptor potential gene family called TRPM6 [34, 35].

Renal Losses

Urinary Mg^{++} losses can be induced by different mechanisms:

- *Primary renal Mg^{++} wasting*: these disorders are discussed in Chap. 34.
- *Drugs*: Both loop and thiazide diuretics can inhibit net Mg^{++} reabsorption, while the K^+-sparing diuretics may lower excretion of Mg^{++}. The degree of hypomagnesemia induced by the loop and thiazide diuretics is generally mild, in part because the associated volume contraction will tend to increase proximal Na^+, water, and Mg^{++} reabsorption. Many further drugs can also produce urinary Mg^{++} wasting, as depicted in Table 31.23.
- *Volume expansion*: Expansion of the extracellular fluid volume can decrease passive Mg^{++} transport. Mild hypomagnesemia may ensue if this is sustained.
- *Hypercalcemia*: Ca^{++} and Mg^{++} seem to compete for transport in the thick ascending limb of the loop of Henle. The increased filtered Ca^{++} load in hypercalcemic states will deliver more Ca^{++} to the loop; the ensuing rise in Ca^{++} reabsorption will diminish that of Mg^{++}.
- *Miscellaneous*: Mg^{++} wasting can be seen as part of the tubular dysfunction seen with recovery from acute tubular necrosis, following renal transplantation and during a postobstructive diuresis.
- *Alcohol*: Excessive urinary excretion of Mg^{++} is common in alcoholic patients. Dietary deficiency, acute pancreatitis, diarrhea and refeeding also contribute to hypomagnesemia in these patients.

Further Causes

- Hypomagnesemia, together with hypophosphatemia, hypokalemia and increasing extracellular fluid volume, occurs in the context of refeeding syndrome (See: hypophosphatemia).
- Hypomagnesemia sometimes occurs in diabetes mellitus and is related in part to the degree of hyperglycemia.
- Hypomagnesemia can be seen following surgery, at least in part due to chelation by circulating free fatty acids.

- Hypomagnesemia can occur as part of the "hungry bone" syndrome in which there is increased Mg^{++} uptake by renewing bone following parathyroidectomy (for hyperparathyroidism).

Neonatal Hypomagnesemia

Like in older children, in newborns hypomagnesemia may result from decreased Mg^{++} intake, intestinal losses or renal losses. However, two peculiar causes of neonatal hypomagnesemia deserve consideration: maternal hypomagnesemia and intrauterine growth retardation:

- *Maternal hypomagnesemia*: Neonatal hypomagnesemia secondary to maternal hypomagnesemia is a recognized feature of maternal diabetes mellitus. However, maternal hypomagnesemia from any cause has been associated with neonatal hypomagnesemia.
- *Intrauterine growth retardation*: Hypomagnesemia sometimes occurs in infants whose birth weight is small in relation to their gestational age. Circulating Mg^{++} is normally low for the first 3–5 days of life.

Symptoms, Signs, and Consequences
Mg^{++} depletion is often associated with two biochemical abnormalities: (1) hypokalemia and (2) hypocalcemia. As a result, it is often difficult to ascribe specific manifestations solely to hypomagnesemia. The typical signs and symptoms of Mg^{++} depletion include tetany, positive Chvostek, Trousseau and Lust signs, or generalized convulsions. Generalized weakness and anorexia sometimes also occur. In addition, Mg^{++} depletion can induce ventricular arrhythmias, particularly during myocardial ischemia or cardiopulmonary bypass [30, 34, 35].

Hypokalemia

Hypokalemia, mostly accompanied by metabolic alkalosis, is common in hypomagnesemia. This association is in part due to underlying disorders

that cause both Mg^{++} and K^+ loss, such as diuretic therapy and diarrhea. There is also evidence that concomitant Mg^{++} depletion aggravates hypokalemia and renders it refractory to treatment by potassium because Mg^{++} depletion increasing distal K^+ secretion, as depicted in Fig. 31.15 [34, 35].

Hypocalcemia

Hypocalcemia is the classical sign of severe hypomagnesemia (≤ 0.50 mmol/L). The following factors account for this tendency [30, 34, 35]:

- Inappropriately low circulating *parathyroid hormone* secretion;

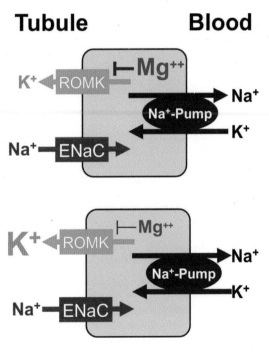

Fig. 31.15 Renal mechanism underlying hypokalemia in Mg^{++} depletion. In the distal nephron K^+ is taken up into cells across the basolateral membrane via Na^+ pump (*blue oval*) and secreted into luminal fluid via the apical ROMK K^+ channels (*red rectangle*). Na^+ is reabsorbed via epithelial Na^+ channels (ENaC, *green rectangle*). Intracellular Mg^{++} inhibits the ROMK K^+ channels and decreases K^+-secretion (*upper panel*). A decrease in intracellular Mg^{++} releases the Mg^{++}-mediated inhibition of ROMK K^+ channels, increases K^+-secretion (*lower panel*) and results in hypokalemia that is refractory to treatment by K^+. ROMK denotes renal outer medullary K^+ channel

- Inappropriately low *1,25-dihydroxyvitamin D*, the active metabolite of vitamin D;
- Bone resistance to *parathyroid hormone* (hypomagnesemia interferes with G protein activation in response to parathyroid hormone, thereby minimizing the stimulation of adenylate cyclase).

Repletion

Repletion of Mg^{++} is controversial in asymptomatic (mostly mild) hypomagnesemia. Oral repletion using lactate, oxide, pidolate or chloride salts is usually preferred. Because of the laxative effect of oral Mg^{++}, the amounts administered must be tailored to the individual patients (0.30 mmol/kg body weight of Mg^{++} per day in divided doses results in diarrhea in $\approx 10\%$ of patients). The parenteral route is preferred in critically ill patients but the exact dosage is poorly understood. For true emergencies (e.g., generalized convulsions or ventricular arrhythmias) Mg^{++} is administered (either as sulphate or as chloride) intravenously over 1–2 min in a dosage of 0.15–0.20 mmol/kg body weight[12] (repeated if no response 5–10 min later). In subjects with moderate to severe but rather oligosymptomatic Mg^{++} deficiency the mentioned dose is given over 4–6 h until circulating Mg^{++} returns to normal.

Inorganic Phosphate

Balance

In a 70 kg man, the body phosphate content amounts to $\approx 1\%$ of the body weight, or 700 g (=23 mol). 85% is contained in the bone tissue and teeth, 14% in the soft tissues, and the remaining 1% in extracellular fluids [36].

In the blood phosphate is found both as organic as well as inorganic salt but clinical laboratories measure the inorganic form. Of the circulating inorganic phosphate, $\approx 10\%$ is bound to

---

[12]Approximately 3.5–4.5 mg/kg body weight of elemental magnesium.

Table 31.24 Fasting values for circulating inorganic phosphate, fractional phosphate excretion and maximal tubular phosphate reabsorption in infancy and childhood

Age	Blood inorganic phosphate mmol/L[a]	Fractional phosphate excretion 10^{-2}	Maximal tubular reabsorption of phosphate mmol/L[a]
0–3 months	1.62–2.40	11.9–38.7	1.02–2.00
4–6 months	1.78–2.21	3.50–34.9	1.27–1.88
6–12 months	1.38–2.15	10.3–20.0	1.13–1.86
1–2 years	1.32–1.93	5.50–23.3	1.05–1.74
3–4 years	1.02–1.92	≤ 18.4	0.90–1.78
5–6 years	1.13–1.73	0.60–15.0	1.02–1.62
7–8 years	1.06–1.80	≤ 16.8	0.98–1.64
9–10 years	1.13–1.70	1.80–14.1	1.00–1.58
11–12 years	1.04–1.79	1.80–12.1	0.97–1.65
13–15 years	0.97–1.80	≤ 12.6	0.91–1.68

Used with permission of Springer Science + Business Media from Brodehl [37]
[a]To obtain traditional units (mg/dL) multiply by 3.1

protein, 5% is complexed with Ca^{++}, Mg^{++} or Na^+ and 85% exists as ionized phosphate. The normal blood concentration of inorganic phosphate is highest during the neonatal period and early childhood and declines thereafter (Table 31.24) because infants and children retain phosphate avidly. There is a mean diurnal variation in concentration of phosphate of ≈ 0.20 mmol/L (≈ 0.6 mg/dl) with a nadir at 11.00, subsequently rising to a plateau at 16.00 h and peaking in the early night.

The average diet of a 70 kg man provides 800–1500 mg (25–50 mmol) phosphate daily. As much as two-thirds of the dietary phosphate is absorbed in the gut but intestinal secretion, mainly in saliva and bile acids, adds 200 mg (6 mmol) of phosphate into the intestinal lumen daily. Under steady-state conditions, the kidney is the most important modulator of the blood phosphate level, ensuring that urinary phosphate output is equivalent to the net phosphate absorption from the intestine. Phosphate is freely filtered across the glomerulus, and 80–90% of the phosphate is reabsorbed by the renal tubules (mostly in the proximal tubule) in subjects aged 6 months or more (Table 31.24). The renal tubular handling of phosphate is best expressed as fractional excretion of phosphate or, more precisely, as maximal tubular reabsorption of phosphate, which clarifies the relationship between circulating phosphate and urinary phosphate excretion. The fractional clearance of phosphate, the tubular phosphate reabsorption and the maximal tubular phosphate reabsorption are easily calculated, following an overnight fast, from plasma (P_{Ph}) and urinary (U_{Ph}) phosphate, and plasma (P_{Cr}) and urinary (U_{Cr}) creatinine, as follows [37]:

$$\text{Fractional excretion} = \frac{U_{Ph} \times P_{Cr}}{P_{Ph} \times U_{Cr}}$$

$$\text{Tubular phospate reabsorption} = 1 - \frac{U_{Ph} \times P_{Cr}}{P_{Ph} \times U_{Cr}}$$

$$\text{Maximal reabsorption} = P_{Ph} - \left(\frac{U_{Ph} \times P_{Cr}}{U_{Cr}} \right)$$

The reference values [36] for the fractional excretion of phosphate and the maximal tubular reabsorption of phosphate are age dependent and appear in Table 31.24 and Fig. 31.16.

Three groups of hormonal factors regulate phosphate homeostasis [36]:

1. *1,25-dihydroxyvitamin D* stimulates the intestinal phosphate absorption;
2. *Parathyroid hormone* decreases the renal tubular reabsorption and causes phosphaturia.
3. *"Phosphatonins"* are phosphaturic factors other than parathyroid hormone. *Fibroblast growth factor 23* is currently considered the most important phosphatonin.

Hypophosphatemia

Hypophosphatemia does not necessarily mean phosphate depletion since it can occur in the presence of a low, normal, or high total body phosphate. On the other hand, phosphate depletion may exist with normal, low, or elevated levels of blood phosphate.

The normal phosphate level in adolescents and adults ranges between 0.97 and 1.80 mmol/L (2.9–5.4 mg/dL). In this age group, hypophosphatemia

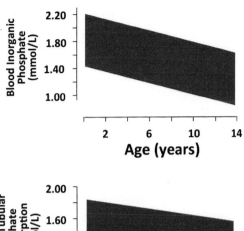

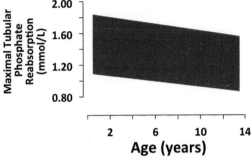

Fig. 31.16 Influence of age on fasting blood inorganic phosphate and maximal tubular reabsorption of phosphate. Blood inorganic phosphate and maximal tubular reabsorption of phosphate measured in infants, children and adolescents (Used with permission of Springer Science + Business Media from Brodehl [37])

is arbitrarily divided into moderate cases (phosphate 0.32–0.65 mmol/L or 0.96–1.95 mg/dL) and severe cases (phosphate <0.32 mmol/L or <0.96 mg/dL). There are three major mechanisms by which hypophosphatemia can occur: (1) low dietary intake or poor intestinal absorption, (2) internal redistribution, and (3) increased urinary loss. In patients with hypophosphatemia caused by decreased intestinal absorption or internal redistribution the fractional excretion of phosphate and the maximal tubular reabsorption of phosphate are normal (Table 31.25). On the contrary, these parameters are inappropriately altered in patients with increased urinary loss [38–40].

Low Dietary Intake or Poor Intestinal Absorption

Given the fact that phosphate is ubiquitous in foods, the development of deficiency would be anticipated only in severe cases of malnutrition or in very-low-birth weight infants at the time of

Table 31.25 Causes of hypophosphatemia

With normal maximal tubular phosphate reabsorption and fractional excretion of phosphate
Low dietary intake or poor intestinal absorption
Low dietary intake: severe malnutrition, very-low-birthweight infants
Poor absorption: steatorrhea, chronic diarrhea, use of phosphate binders
Internal redistribution
Refeeding syndrome in malnutrition (including diabetic ketoacidosis treated with insulin)
Respiratory alkalosis
Hungry bone syndrome after parathyroidectomy
With increased maximal tubular phosphate reabsorption and fractional excretion of phosphate
Hyperparathyroidism
De Toni-Debré–Fanconi syndrome (= general impairment of the proximal tubule)[a]
Gitelman syndrome and Bartter syndromes[b]
Hypophosphatemic rickets[c]
After kidney transplantation (= posttransplant hypophosphatemia)

[a]Various drugs may cause an incomplete or, more rarely, a complete form of De Toni-Debré–Fanconi syndrome with hypophosphatemia, including paracetamol poisoning and treatment with ifosfamide, valproic acid, the iron chelator deferasirox or ß$_2$-adrenoreceptors (e.g., albuterol)
[b]Hypophosphatemia is rather mild in these post-proximal tubular disorders
[c]At least in part explained by increased activity of fibroblast growth factor 23

rapid postnatal growth. If phosphate restriction is severe and prolonged, or if intestinal absorption is reduced by the chronic use of phosphate binders, then the constant intestinal loss may induce phosphate depletion.

Internal Redistribution

In the majority of cases, an acute shift in phosphate from the extracellular to the intracellular compartment is primarily responsible for lowering phosphatemia. The most frequent cause is refeeding syndrome, a recognized and potentially fatal condition that occurs when previously malnourished patients are fed. The fluid and electrolyte abnormalities noted in the refeeding syndrome and those noted in severe diabetic ketoacidosis following the administration of insulin therapy are similar.

Patients who are malnourished develop a total body depletion of phosphate, Mg^{++} and K^+. Nonetheless, their blood levels are maintained by redistribution from the intracellular space. The delivery of glucose as part of a feeding strategy causes a huge increase in the circulating insulin level that induces a rapid uptake of glucose, K^+, phosphate and Mg^{++} into cells. The blood concentration of these metabolites falls dramatically. In addition, the body begins to retain fluid, and the extracellular space expands. Although hypophosphatemia is the predominant feature of the syndrome, rapid falls in K^+ and Mg^{++} levels, together with some tendency towards metabolic alkalosis, predispose to cardiac arrhythmias, while extracellular space expansion can precipitate acute heart failure in patients with cardiovascular disease. The most effective way to treat refeeding syndrome is to be aware of it. One should start feeding slowly and aggressively supplement and monitor phosphate, K^+ and Mg^{++} for 4 days after feeding is started.

Another cause of hypophosphatemia in hospitalized patients is respiratory alkalosis. Severe hyperventilation can be seen in patients with anxiety, pain, sepsis, and in patients during mechanical ventilation. The fall in carbon dioxide will result in a similar change in the cell because carbon dioxide readily diffuses across cell membranes. The elevated pH stimulates the glycolysis, leading to an accelerated production of phosphorylated metabolites and a rapid shift of phosphate into the cells.

The hungry bone syndrome, characterized by massive deposition of Ca^{++} and phosphate in the bone, can occur after parathyroidectomy for long-standing hyperparathyroidism (both primary and secondary).

Urinary Loss

In hyperparathyroidism, both primary and secondary, there is an increased urinary loss of phosphate. Fanconi-De Toni-Debré syndrome is characterized by a general impairment of the proximal tubule leading to urinary loss of compounds normally reabsorbed by the proximal tubule. It results in hypophosphatemia, glucosuria, hyperaminoaciduria, uricosuria, and hyperbicarbonaturia (causing renal tubular acidosis). The urinary phosphate excretion is also increased in patients with hereditary hypophosphatemic rickets and tumor-induced osteomalacia and rickets, as discussed in Chap. 32. Recent data demonstrate a mild tendency the urinary loss of phosphate in Gitelman and Bartter syndromes. Following kidney transplant, hypophosphatemia has been described in the absence of both hyperparathyroidism and other signs of proximal tubule dysfunction.

Symptoms, Signs, and Consequences

Phosphate depletion can cause a variety of symptoms and signs [36, 38–40]. Two major mechanisms are responsible for these symptoms: (a) decrease in intracellular adenosine triphosphate and (b) in diphosphoglycerate. In adults, hypophosphatemia is symptomatic when the phosphate level is <0.35 mmol/L. Hypophosphatemia may be asymptomatic under certain clinical situations: patients recovering from diabetic ketoacidosis and patients with prolonged hyperventilation are usually asymptomatic because often there is not real phosphate depletion. The clinical features of phosphate depletion appear in Table 31.26.

Management

Hypophosphatemia does not automatically mean that replacement with phosphate is indicated. To determine whether treatment is indicated it is necessary to establish the cause of the hypophosphatemia, in which the history and the clinical setting are important. The identification and treatment of the primary cause usually leads to normalization of the circulating phosphate level. As an example, the hypophosphatemia found in patients with diabetic ketoacidosis will usually correct spontaneously with normal dietary intake. However, replacement therapy is needed in patients with hypophosphatemia in combination with evidence of renal or gastrointestinal phosphate loss, the presence of underlying risk factors, and particularly if there are the clinical manifestations described above [40].

The safest mode of therapy is oral. Cow's milk is a good phosphate source: it contains 1 g

Table 31.26 Symptoms, signs and consequences of phosphate depletion

Skeletal muscle and bone: proximal myopathy, rhabdomyolysis[a]
Cardiovascular system: impaired myocardial contractility
Respiratory system: respiratory failure (and failed weaning)
Neurological system: paresthesias, tremors, seizures, features resembling Guillain-Barré syndrome or Wernicke encephalopathy
Hematological system: hemolysis, impaired granulocyte chemotaxis and phagocytosis causing Gram-negative sepsis, altered platelet function and thrombocytopenia

[a]In patients with rhabdomyolysis hypophosphatemia can be masked by the release of phosphate from the injured muscle

(32 mmol) elemental phosphate per L. Alternatively, oral preparations in the form of sodium phosphate or potassium phosphate can be used. The average adult patient requires 1–2 g (32–64 mmol) phosphate per day for 7–10 days to replenish body stores. An important side effect of oral supplementation is diarrhea.

Intravenous phosphate, usually 2.5–5.0 mg/kg (0.08–0.16 mmol/kg) over 6 h is given in symptomatic patients, who cannot take milk or tablets. More aggressive repletion with phosphate has been advocated but the magnitude of the response is unpredictable (close monitoring of phosphate level is crucial). Side effects of intravenous phosphate repletion are hypocalcemia, metastatic calcification, hyperkalemia associated with K^+-containing supplements, volume excess, hypernatremia, metabolic acidosis, and hyperphosphatemia.

Hyperphosphatemia

Spurious or artefactual hyperphosphatemia has been observed if hemolysis occurs during the collection or processing of blood samples. Spurious hyperphosphatemia due to interference with analytical methods occurs in patients with hyperglobulinemia, hyperlipidemia or hyperbilirubinemia and following contamination with

Table 31.27 Causes of hyperphosphatemia

Artifactual or spurious
Increased phosphate load (with normal fractional excretion of phosphate and normal maximal tubular phosphate reabsorption)
High dietary intake or increased intestinal absorption
Newborns and infants fed cow's milk (rather than breast milk or adapted formula milk)
Parenteral administration of phosphate salts
Large amounts of phosphate-containing laxatives, phosphate enemas[a]
Vitamin D intoxication
Internal redistribution
Tumor lysis syndrome (before treatment and after initiation of cytotoxic therapy)
Rhabdomyolysis
Lactic and ketoacidosis (or severe hyperglycemia alone)[b], including severe dehydration in the context of acute diarrhea
Decreased renal phosphate excretion
Reduced renal function (either acute or chronic)
Increased renal tubular phosphate reabsorption (= decreased fractional phosphate excretion and increased maximal tubular phosphate reabsorption)
Hypoparathyroidism (and pseudohypoparathyroidism)
Acromegaly
Drugs: growth hormone, bisphosponates, dipyridamole
Idiopathic childhood nephrotic syndrome
Familial hyperphosphatemic tumoral calcinosis

[a]The danger of hyperphosphatemia secondary to phosphate enema is especially high in children less than 2 years of age
[b]Metabolic acidosis blunts glycolysis and therefore cellular phosphate utilization. In addition, tissue hypoxia or insulin deficiency also play a crucial role

heparinized saline from indwelling catheters. True hyperphosphatemia indicates either an increased phosphate load or a decreased renal phosphate excretion, as shown in Table 31.27. High dietary ingestion of phosphate alone rarely causes hyperphosphatemia with the exception of newborns and infants fed cow's milk, whose phosphate content is six times greater than human milk [36].

Acutely or chronically impaired renal function plays at least a partial role in most instances of hyperphosphatemia, including physiologically low glomerular filtration rate to explain the inability of the neonate to eliminate excess phosphate, mild renal insufficiency (due to volume contraction secondary to diarrhea) in subjects ingesting large amounts of phosphate-containing laxatives or mild to moderate tubulointerstitial injury secondary to intrarenal accumulation of uric acid in tumor lysis syndrome (see "hyperkalemia").

Familial hyperphosphatemic tumoral calcinosis is a recessive disorder characterized by hyperphosphatemia due to an increased maximal tubular phosphate reabsorption. Affected subjects present with extra-articular soft tissue deposition of calcium phosphate. This very rare disease (a kind of mirror image of some forms of hypophosphatemic rickets) results from inactivating mutations that lead to deficiency of circulating fibrolast growth factor 23 [36].

References

1. Moritz ML, Ayus JC. Disorders of water metabolism in children: hyponatremia and hypernatremia. Pediatr Rev. 2002;23:371–80.
2. Moritz ML, Ayus JC. Preventing neurological complications from dysnatremias in children. Pediatr Nephrol. 2005;20:1687–700.
3. Bianchetti MG, Simonetti GD, Bettinelli A. Body fluids and salt metabolism – part I. Ital J Pediatr. 2009;35:36.
4. Peruzzo M, Milani GP, Garzoni L, Longoni L, Simonetti GD, Bettinelli A, Fossali EF, Bianchetti MG. Body fluids and salt metabolism – part II. Ital J Pediatr. 2010;36:78.
5. Reynolds RM, Padfield PL, Seckl JR. Disorders of sodium balance. BMJ. 2006;332:702–5.
6. Sam R, Feizi I. Understanding hypernatremia. Am J Nephrol. 2012;36:97–104.
7. Haycock GB. Hypernatraemia: diagnosis and management. Arch Dis Child Educ Pract Ed. 2006;91:8–13.
8. Haycock GB. Hyponatraemia: diagnosis and management. Arch Dis Child Educ Pract Ed. 2006;91:37–41.
9. Ball SG. How I, approach hyponatraemia. Clin Med. 2013;13:291–5.
10. Bailey B, Gravel J, Goldman RD, Friedman JN, Parkin PC. External validation of the clinical dehydration scale for children with acute gastroenteritis. Acad Emerg Med. 2010;17:583–8.
11. Maitland K, Kiguli S, Opoka RO, Engoru C, Olupot-Olupot P, Akech SO, et al. Mortality after fluid bolus in African children with severe infection. N Engl J Med. 2011;364:2483–95.

12. Daly K, Farrington E. Hypokalemia and hyperkalemia in infants and children: pathophysiology and treatment. J Pediatr Health Care. 2013;27:486–96.
13. Dussol B. Equilibre potassique, hypokaliémie et hyperkaliémie. Nephrol Ther. 2010;6:180–99.
14. Jain G, Ong S, Warnock DG. Genetic disorders of potassium homeostasis. Semin Nephrol. 2013;33:300–9.
15. Greenlee M, Wingo CS, McDonough AA, Youn JH, Kone BC. Narrative review: evolving concepts in potassium homeostasis and hypokalemia. Ann Intern Med. 2009;150:619–25. Erratum in: Ann Intern Med. 2009;151:143–4.
16. Palmer BF. A physiologic-based approach to the evaluation of a patient with hypokalemia. Am J Kidney Dis. 2010;56:1184–90.
17. Unwin RJ, Luft FC, Shirley DG. Pathophysiology and management of hypokalemia: a clinical perspective. Nat Rev Nephrol. 2011;7:75–84.
18. Nyirenda MJ, Tang JI, Padfield PL, Seckl JR. Hyperkalaemia. BMJ. 2009;339:1019–24.
19. Lehnhardt A, Kemper MJ. Pathogenesis, diagnosis and management of hyperkalemia. Pediatr Nephrol. 2011;26:377–84.
20. Masilamani K, van der Voort J. The management of acute hyperkalaemia in neonates and children. Arch Dis Child. 2012;97:376–80.
21. Adrogué HJ, Gennari FJ, Galla JH, Madias NE. Assessing acid-base disorders. Kidney Int. 2009;76:1239–47.
22. Carmody JB, Norwood VF. A clinical approach to paediatric acid-base disorders. Postgrad Med J. 2012;88:143–51.
23. Kraut JA, Madias NE. Metabolic acidosis: pathophysiology, diagnosis and management. Nat Rev Nephrol. 2010;6:274–85.
24. Morris CG, Low J. Metabolic acidosis in the critically ill: part 1.Classification and pathophysiology. Anaesthesia. 2008;63:294–301.
25. Morris CG, Low J. Metabolic acidosis in the critically ill: part 2.Causes and treatment. Anaesthesia. 2008;63:396–411.
26. Gennari FJ. Pathophysiology of metabolic alkalosis: a new classification based on the centrality of stimulated collecting duct ion transport. Am J Kidney Dis. 2011;58:626–36.
27. Luke RG, Galla JH. It is chloride depletion alkalosis, not contraction alkalosis. J Am Soc Nephrol. 2012;23:204–7.
28. Allgrove J. Disorders of calcium metabolism. Curr Paediatr. 2003;13:529–35.
29. Carmeliet G, Van Cromphaut S, Daci E, Maes C, Bouillon R. Disorders of calcium homeostasis. Best Pract Res Clin Endocrinol Metab. 2003;17:529–46.
30. Hoorn EJ, Zietse R. Disorders of calcium and magnesium balance: a physiology-based approach. Pediatr Nephrol. 2013;28:1195–206.
31. Singh J, Moghal N, Pearce SH, Cheetham T. The investigation of hypocalcaemia and rickets. Arch Dis Child. 2003;88:403–7.
32. Inzucchi SE. Understanding hypercalcemia – its metabolic basis, signs, and symptoms. Postgrad Med. 2004;115:69–70. 73–6.
33. Jacobs TP, Bilezikian JP. Clinical review: rare causes of hypercalcemia. J Clin Endocrinol Metab. 2005;90:6316–22.
34. Alexander RT, Hoenderop JG, Bindels RJ. Molecular determinants of magnesium homeostasis: insights from human disease. J Am Soc Nephrol. 2008;19:1451–8.
35. Dimke H, Monnens L, Hoenderop JG, Bindels RJ. Evaluation of hypomagnesemia: lessons from disorders of tubular transport. Am J Kidney Dis. 2013;62:377–83.
36. Goretti M, Penido MG, Alon US. Phosphate homeostasis and its role in bone health. Pediatr Nephrol. 2012;27:2039–48.
37. Brodehl J. Assessment and interpretation of the tubular threshold for phosphate in infants and children. Pediatr Nephrol. 1994;8:645.
38. Gaasbeek A, Meinders AE. Hypophosphatemia: an update on its etiology and treatment. Am J Med. 2005;118:1094–101.
39. Amanzadeh J, Reilly Jr RF. Hypophosphatemia: an evidence-based approach to its clinical consequences and management. Nat Clin Pract Nephrol. 2006;2:136–48.
40. Ritz E, Haxsen V, Zeier M. Disorders of phosphate metabolism – pathomechanisms and management of hypophosphataemic disorders. Best Pract Res Clin Endocrinol Metab. 2003;17:547–58.
41. Alfonzo AV, Isles C, Geddes C, Deighan C. Potassium disorders—clinical spectrum and emergency management. Resuscitation. 2006;70:10–25.
42. Hollander-Rodriguez JC, Calvert Jr JF. Hyperkalemia. Am Fam Phys. 2006;73:283–90.
43. Whittier WL, Rutecki GW. Primer on clinical acid-base problem solving. Dis Mon. 2004;50:122–62.
44. Laski ME, Kurtzman NA. Acid-base disorders in medicine. Dis Mon. 1996;42:51–125.

Renal Fanconi Syndromes and Other Proximal Tubular Disorders

Detlef Bockenhauer and Robert Kleta

Introduction

Fanconi first described the concept that defective renal proximal tubule reabsorption of solutes might contribute to "non-nephrotic glycosuric dwarfing with hypophosphataemic rickets in early childhood" [1]. Rickets and albuminuria secondary to kidney disease was described some 50 years previously but attributed to a disorder of adolescence [2]. Fanconi's first case presented at 3 months with rickets and recurrent fevers. She had glycosuria and albuminuria and progressed to terminal renal failure by 5 years of age. At autopsy the renal tubule cells appeared filled with crystals, which were thought to be cystine. In subsequent reports, Debré, de Toni and Fanconi all described series of children with rickets, glycosuria and albuminuria [3–5]. In acknowledgment of this pioneering work, we now refer to this symptom constellation as Fanconi-Debre-deToni syndrome, or just short as "renal Fanconi syndrome" (RFS). The presentation, course and outcome of the described children, however, varied markedly. This reflects that RFS is not a uniform entity, but a diagnosis of proximal tubular dysfunction, which can be due to a variety of different causes (Tables 32.1 and 32.2). RFS can be isolated or in the context of multiorgan disorders, congenital or acquired, transient or permanent, associated with progression to end-stage kidney disease (ESKD) or with stable kidney function throughout. Moreover, it can differ in the extent and severity of tubular dysfunction. Severe and generalized proximal tubular dysfunction is seen in cystinosis whilst many children with, e.g., Dent disease or Lowe syndrome may have no clinically significant disturbance of phosphate and bicarbonate transport [39]. Indeed, there is some debate at what point proximal tubular dysfunction can be called RFS [40].

Here, we use the term RFS to include disorders with dysfunction of multiple proximal tubular pathways, but recognize that not every transport system need be affected. This clinical and biochemical heterogeneity is likely to arise from the multiple mechanisms involved in proximal tubular transport, reflecting not only the bulk of solute and water reabsorption but also the re-uptake of proteins, amino acids, vitamins, cytokines and many other substances. RFS do not therefore have a common and single pathogenetic basis but reflect the interplay of a number of different biochemical processes. Identification of the underlying etiology is therefore of utmost importance, as it informs management and prognosis.

D. Bockenhauer (✉) • R. Kleta
UCL Centre for Nephrology, Great Ormond Street Hospital for Children, Rowland Hill Street, London NW3 2PF, UK
e-mail: d.bockenhauer@ucl.ac.uk; r.kleta@ucl.ac.uk

© Springer-Verlag Berlin Heidelberg 2016
D.F. Geary, F. Schaefer (eds.), *Pediatric Kidney Disease*, DOI 10.1007/978-3-662-52972-0_32

Table 32.1 Congenital causes of Fanconi syndrome by age of onset

Onset	Disorder	Associated features	Diagnostic test
Neonatal	Galactosemia	Liver dysfunction, jaundice, encephalopathy, sepsis	Red cell galactose 1-phosphate uridyl transferase
	Mitochondrial disorders	Usually multisystem dysfunction (brain, muscle, liver, heart)	Lactate/pyruvate (plasma lactate may be normal due to urinary losses), muscle enzymology
	Tyrosinemia	Poor growth, hepatic enlargement and dysfunction	Plasma amino acids, urine organic acids (succinylacetone)
Infancy	Fructosemia	Rapid onset after fructose ingestion, vomiting, hypoglycemia, hepatomegaly	Hepatic fructose-1-phosphate aldolase B
	Cystinosis	Poor growth, vomiting, rickets ± corneal cystine crystals	Leukocyte cystine concentration, Mutation analysis (*CTNS*)
	Fanconi Bickel syndrome	Failure to thrive, hepatomegaly, hypoglycemia rickets, severe glycosuria, galactosuria	Mutation analysis (*GLUT2*)
	Lowe's syndrome	Males (X-linked), cataracts, hypotonia, developmental delay	Clinical and molecular genetic diagnosis (*OCRL*)
Childhood	Cystinosis	As above	
	Dent disease	Males (X-linked), hypercalciuria, nephrocalcinosis	Molecular diagnosis (*CLCN5*, *OCRL*)
	Wilson's disease	Hepatic and neurological disease, Kayser-Fleischer rings	Copper, coeruloplasmin

Used with permission of Oxford University Press from van't Hoff [6]

Clinical Features

The presenting clinical features of RFS are usually failure-to-thrive and rickets, although patients with RFS in the context of a systemic disorder may first be identified via the extra-renal manifestations, such as the cataracts in Lowe syndrome, or myopathy in mitochondrial cytopathies.

The failure-to-thrive is presumably due to the high volume losses, with patients preoccupied with drinking, rather than caloric intake. Some patients exhibit features of a secondary nephrogenic diabetes insipidus, further compounding the water losses from impaired proximal reabsorption [41, 42].

Rickets is the consequence of renal phosphate losses (see below) as well as impaired proximal hydroxylation of vitamin D. The critical step in the formation of 1,25 OH-cholecaliferol is mitochondrial 1α-hydroxylation in the proximal tubule. For this to occur, cholecalciferol, bound to its carrier vitamin D-binding protein (a low-molecular weight protein) needs to be reabsorbed from the tubular lumen, a process impaired in RFS [43].

Biochemical Abnormalities

Excessive urinary levels of a wide range of solutes and substances normally reabsorbed in the proximal tubule are the biochemical hallmarks of RFS.

Proteinuria

Proteinuria is made up of albumin, low molecular weight proteins and tubular enzymes, such as

Table 32.2 Acquired causes of the renal Fanconi syndrome

Drugs and toxins
Anti-cancer drugs
Ifosfamide (see text)
Streptozocin [7, 8]
Antibiotics
Aminoglycoside (see text)
Expired tetracyclines [9, 10]
Anti-retrovirals
Adefovir/Cidofovir/Tenofovir [11–15]
ddI [16, 17]
Heavy metals
Lead poisoning [18]
Cadmium [19]
Sodium valproate [20]
Aristolochic acid (Chinese herb nephropathy) [21–23]
Toluene/glue sniffing [24]
Fumaric acid [25]
Suramin [26]
Paraquat [27]
L-Lysine [28]
Renal disorders
Tubulointerstitial nephritis [29]
Membranous nephropathy with anti-tubular basement antibodies [30–38]

retinol binding protein (RBP), α-1 microglobulin, β-2 microglobulin, N-acetylglucoseaminidase, alanine aminopeptidase. The urinary level of these very sensitive markers of proximal tubular dysfunction is markedly elevated in RFS [44, 45]. Albuminuria precedes glomerular dysfunction, present in some but not all forms, in Fanconi syndrome and whilst elevated, does not reach nephrotic range proteinuria [46]. This reflects the amount of filtered albumin – requiring tubular reabsorption -, which has been estimated at 0.4–1 g albumin per 1.73 m² per day [47, 48]. The total amount of protein loss can be variable, reflecting potential concomitant glomerular dysfunction and the degree of impairment of reabsorption. In a family with autosomal dominant isolated RFS without apparent glomerular dysfunction the total amount was roughly 1 g per day in affected adults [49]. It is important to remember that urine dipsticks primarily detect larger proteins including albumin and thus can miss the mostly low-molecular weight proteinuria of RFS. Tubular proteinuria may be seen in some forms of nephrotic syndrome, reflecting associated tubulointerstitial damage [50, 51].

Aminoaciduria

The aminoaciduria seen in RFS is generalized and its pattern is influenced by plasma values, so that in rare situations of severe protein malnutrition, aminoaciduria as analyzed on thin-layer chromatography, may be recorded as "normal" or "mild" [44]. Quantitative analysis by ion-exchange chromatography should be used to determine the degree and specific nature of aminoaciduria.

Organic Aciduria

Organic acids, including citrate and uric acid, are also exclusively reabsorbed in the proximal tubule and excretion is thus increased in RFS [52]. Consequently, patients with RFS typically have hyperuricosuria with hypouricemia, as well as hypercitraturia [53]. Moreover, transport of drugs, such as probenecid, furosemide or penicillin, can be affected, potentially altering pharmacokinetics [54]. The increased excretion of lactate can lead to normalization of plasma lactate levels in mitochondrial cytopathies, resulting in another potential diagnostic pitfall [55].

Glycosuria

Renal glycosuria in RFS reflects the impaired ability for glucose reabsorption, so that glycosuria occurs with normal blood glucose levels. As RFS is typically associated with marked polyuria, the urinary glucose concentration may be less than the 5 mmol/l detected by dipsticks [39]. Formal laboratory measurement, ideally of a 24-h urine collection, should thus be used to detect and quantify glycosuria. Normally, less than 1.5 mmol (300 mg)/day/1.73 m² are excreted [56].

Renal Tubular Acidosis

Since the proximal tubule is the key site for bicarbonate reabsorption, bicarbonaturia is a typical feature of RFS with a consequent metabolic acidosis (Chap. 36). The degree to which the threshold for reabsorption is reduced is variable, according to the underlying cause of RFS. In severe acidosis, filtered bicarbonate is reduced to a level below the threshold for proximal reabsorption and urine pH falls below 5.3 if distal acidification is intact. The hyperchloremic metabolic acidosis contributes to loss of skeletal calcium and consequent hypercalciuria and requires treatment with large doses of alkali.

Phosphaturia

Renal phosphate wasting with secondary hypophosphatemia is another hallmark of proximal tubular dysfunction, leading to rickets or bone disease. Urine phosphate handling is usually assessed as the tubular reabsorption (TRP), the complement to the fractional excretion of phosphate (FEP). Thus it is calculated as: TRP [%] = 100 − FEP [%]. Usually, a TRP >70 % is considered normal; however, this can be misleading. If plasma phosphate is close to or below the threshold of tubular phosphate reabsorption, TRP may be misleadingly "normal". To account for the filtered load, urinary phosphate excretion is best assessed using the tubular threshold concentration for phosphate excretion, corrected for glomerular filtration rate (TmP/GFR) [57]. It is calculated as follows: TmP/GFR = (Phosphate plasma − Phosphate urine/Creatinine urine × Creatinine plasma). Normal values are age-dependent and listed in Table 32.3.

Hypercalciuria

Approximately 70 % of filtered calcium is reabsorbed in the proximal tubule and, consequently hypercalciuria is another characteristic of renal Fanconi syndrome. It is further compounded by

Table 32.3 Normal age-specific values for TmP/GFR

Age	mmol/L
<1 month	1.48–3.43
1–3 months	1.48–3.30
4–6 months	1.15–2.60
7 months–2 years	1.10–2.70
2–4 years	1.04–2.79
4–6 years	1.05–2.60
6–8 years	1.26–2.35
8–10 years	1.10–2.31
10–12 years	1.15–2.58
12–15 years	1.18–2.09
>15 years	0.80–1.35

Data from References [58–60]

the acidosis-mediated calcium release from bone (see above). Nephrocalcinosis and stone formation can ensue, but interestingly is rather uncommon. Presumably, the polyuria inherent in Fanconi syndrome is protective against these complications, as may be the increased luminal concentration of citrate (see section "Organic Aciduria") [61].

Hypokalemia

Potassium, like almost all other electrolytes, is predominantly reabsorbed in the proximal tubule, making hypokalemia another typical feature. It can further be compounded by hyperaldosteronism if electrolyte and fluid losses result in volume contraction [62–64].

Other Substances

Carnitine is reabsorbed in the proximal tubule and is therefore lost in excess in RFS. Low plasma carnitine concentrations have been reported in children with cystinosis and tyrosinemia [65, 66] leading to plasma and muscle deficiencies of carnitine, which could contribute to the myopathy in these disorders. Moreover, losses of vitamins, carrier proteins and chemokines have all been described in RFS [46, 67].

Pathogenesis

The variation in etiology, manifestations and severity of RFS make it unlikely that there is a single common pathogenetic mechanism. Most studies of the pathogenesis have, of necessity, focused on one biochemical pathway. However, in vivo, it is more likely that a number of inter-linked biochemical processes are disrupted in a variable manner.

Disruption of Energy Production

The high transport activity of the proximal tubule requires a large amount of energy. Thus, disruption of the energy supply is an obvious etiology of RFS. Consequently, it is not surprising that RFS is a frequent complication of mitochondrial cytopathies [55]. Further insight was recently provided by genetic investigations in a family with autosomal dominant RFS, which identified a mutation in a peroxisomal enzyme that caused misrouting to the mitochondria, where it disrupted fatty acid oxidation [68]. This highlighted the dependence of the proximal tubule on mitochondrial fatty acid oxidation, rather than glucose metabolism [69, 70].

Mitochondrial dysfunction has also been implicated in the development of RFS in cystinosis (Chap. 40). Similar studies have been undertaken in models of tyrosinemia, which is associated with excessive accumulation of succinylacetone (SA). SA reduced sodium-dependent uptake of sugar and amino acids across rat brush border membranes [71] and intra-peritoneal injection of SA to rats led to development of RFS [72]. SA inhibits sodium-dependent phosphate transport by brush border membrane vesicles, decreases ATP production and inhibits mitochondrial respiration [73]. Administration of maleic acid, used to create an animal model of RFS, causes a reduction in ATP and phosphate concentrations, NaK ATPase activity and coenzyme A [74].

Glutathione Depletion

Another line of investigation has emphasized the role of glutathione (GSH) in the pathogenesis of RFS. GSH has a number of key cellular roles including post-translational protein modification, xenobiotic detoxification and it acts as a major antioxidant. These studies have mainly focused on cystinosis (Chap. 40), but deficiency of GSH has also been implicated in other forms of the RFS. Ifosfamide toxicity which leads to RFS, may be mediated by its interaction with γ-glutamyl transpeptidase, a precursor of GSH synthesis, and by hepatic metabolism to chloroacetaldehyde [75]. Incubation of chloroacetaldehyde with isolated human renal proximal tubules was associated with depletion of GSH, coenzyme A, acetyl-coenzyme A and ATP [76]. Wistar rats injected with ifosfamide develop RFS, associated with GSH depletion which is attenuated by treatment with melatonin [76]. Addition of ochratoxin A, the presumed toxin causing RFS in Balkan Endemic Nephropathy, to rat proximal tubular cells causes an elevation of reactive oxygen species and depletion of cellular GSH [77]. However, newer data point towards an ifosfamide specific renal proximal tubular uptake and metabolism as being causative for the specific side effect of RFS [78].

Reduced Activity of Cotransporters

Increased solute excretion in RFS could result from reduced expression or activity of sodium-coupled cotransporters, which mediate proximal tubular reabsorption. In the animal maleic acid model of RFS, decreased NaPi2a mRNA expression and consequent reduced NaPi2a protein were observed [79].

Mice lacking hepatocyte nuclear factor 1 alpha (HNF1α), a transcription factor expressed in liver, pancreas, kidney and intestine, develop RFS, abnormal bile metabolism and diabetes [80]. HNF1α −/− mice had reduced expression of sodium-coupled transporters for glucose (SGLT2) and phosphate (NaPi1 and NaPi4) but normal levels of NaPi2a, the major phosphate transporter [81]. Recently, two siblings with a homozygous mutation in *SLC34A1*, the gene encoding NaPi2A, were reported who suffered from proximal tubular dysfunction [82]. It is yet to be clarified, how exactly this specific defect in proximal tubular phosphate transport causes a more generalized proximal tubular dysfunction.

Disruption of the Endocytic Pathway (Megalin/Cubilin)

An important task of the proximal tubule is to reabsorb filtered proteins, including peptide hormones, as well as small carrier proteins binding fat-soluble vitamins and trace elements. Therefore, by reabsorbing filtered proteins the proximal tubule actively participates in the homeostasis of hormones, trace elements and vitamins. In addition, some lipoproteins, such as apolipoprotein A-I and A-IV are also reabsorbed in the proximal tubule [83]. Reabsorption of the vast majority of filtered proteins is mediated by two endocytic receptors: megalin and cubilin (reviewed in [84–86]). These receptors contain several protein-binding domains and protrude from the microvilli, which make up the brush border of the proximal tubule, into the tubular lumen. Once a protein is attached, the receptor-ligand complex moves towards the base of the microvilli into clathrin-coated pits, which then bud off into the cytoplasm to form endosomes (see Fig. 32.1). Subsequently, the receptors are recycled back to the membrane to mediate further uptake. The fate of the protein ligands is different: most are degraded by acid hydrolysis after fusion of the endosome to a lysosome, while others, such as vitamins, are released back into the blood circulation across the basolateral membrane. In this fashion, the megalin/cubilin complex assumes a role in the regulation of several hormonal pathways, the importance of which becomes apparent, when considering, for instance, calcium-regulation: Megalin competes with the PTH receptor for the binding of filtered PTH and renders it non-functional by endocytosis and subsequent delivery to a lysosome for degradation [88]. In contrast, megalin/cubilin facilitates activation of Vitamin D by binding of filtered 25-OH vitamin D-Vitamin D binding protein and thus allowing uptake into the proximal tubule cell and activation by 1α-hydroxylase [43, 89].

Megalin is a large transmembrane protein belonging to the family of low-density lipoprotein receptors and was originally identified as the target of antibodies causing Heymann nephritis in rats [90]. It is expressed in epithelial cells of a variety of other tissues active in endocytosis [87]. Megalin-deficient mice mostly die in utero, but those that survive indeed show Fanconi-type low-molecular weight proteinuria, confirming the central role of megalin in endocytosis in the proximal tubule [91]. Interestingly, mutations in *LRP2*, the gene encoding megalin, were recently identified as the cause of Donnai-Barrow syndrome [92]. Donnai-Barrow syndrome is characterized by facial and ocular anomalies, sensorineural hearing loss and proteinuria. However, whilst these patients have, as expected, low-molecular weight proteinuria, there is no generalized proximal tubular dysfunction [93].

Cubilin is a peripheral membrane protein and is dependent on megalin to initiate endocytosis after ligand binding. These two proteins are co-expressed in proximal tubule and along the endocytic pathway and work in tandem to mediate protein uptake [85, 86]. Cubulin is otherwise known as the intrinsic factor-vitamin B12 receptor [94]. Loss-of-function mutations are associated with juvenile megaloblastic anemia or Imerslund-Graesbeck disease [95, 96]. The anemia is caused by deficient intestinal endocytosis of intrinsic factor-vitamin B12. In addition, some of these patients also have a selective low-molecular weight proteinuria that identifies those proteins requiring cubilin for endocytosis, such as albumin, transferrin, immunoglobulin light chains and $\alpha 1$- and $\beta 2$-microglobulin [97]. Recently, two siblings with nephrotic range proteinuria were found to have homozygous mutations in cubilin [98]. Yet, as with megalin, mutations in humans are not associated with complete RFS.

Decreased expression of both megalin and cubilin at the brush border has been described in a mouse model of Dent disease. Concurrently, decreased levels of megalin have been found in the

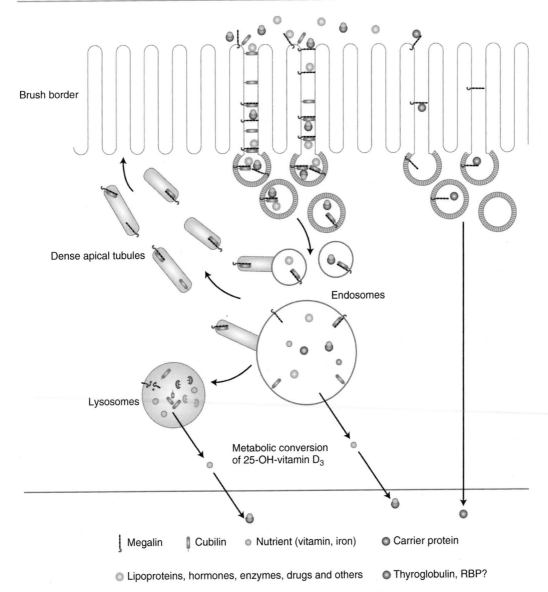

Fig. 32.1 Role of Megalin and Cubilin in proximal tubular transport. The receptors Megalin and Cubilin stick out from the brush border into the lumen of the proximal tubule. Once bound to a ligand (such as LMWP, nutrients etc.), the complex is endocytosed and ligand and receptor are separated by the low pH in the endosomes. The receptors are subsequently recycled to the membrane (Used with permission of Nature Publishing Group from Christensen and Birn [87])

urine of patients with Dent disease and Lowe syndrome, suggesting defective trafficking of the receptors as the basis of the low-molecular weight proteinuria seen in affected patients [99, 100]. The loss of vitamins, hormones and trace elements associated with endocytic dysfunction may explain some of the clinical heterogeneity seen in RFS.

Primary Renal Fanconi Syndrome

Sometimes, Fanconi syndrome appears in patients without an identified cause. The majority of these primary or idiopathic cases occur in adulthood, but some have also been reported in children [101]. A small number of cases occur in families and different modes of inheritance have been reported [49, 102–106]. Amongst the families with autosomal-dominant inheritance two distinct forms are recognized: Fanconi syndrome with early renal failure and one form with preserved GFR into advanced age. For the latter one, an underlying genetic basis has recently been identified: misrouting of an enzyme from the peroxisome to the mitochondria, where it is hypothesized to interfere with fatty acid oxidation [68]. An autosomal recessive form of an incomplete RFS has been attributed to loss-of-function mutations in the phosphate transporter NaPi2a (SLC34A1) [82].

Treatment of these primary forms is symptomatic and in those with kidney failure, transplantation is an option.

Cystinosis

Nephropathic cystinosis, the most common cause of RFS in children, is covered in Chap. 40.

Tyrosinemia

The tyrosinemias are a group of disorders affecting the metabolism of tyrosine. The most severe one is tyrosinemia type 1, due to a defect in the enzyme fumarylacetoacetate hydrolase. Severity of clinical symptoms is variable but typically includes hepatic dysfunction with progression to cirrhosis and risk of hepatic cancer, as well as a porphyria-like neuropathy. In addition, patients develop a severe Fanconi syndrome and chronic renal impairment can eventually ensue. The enzymatic defect in tyrosinemia leads to an accumulation of succinylacetone, which is thought to cause the symptoms. In experimental models succinylacetone inhibits transport in the proximal tubule, potentially by inhibition of mitochondrial function [71–73]. In addition, it inhibits porphobilinogen synthetase, which may explain the porphyria-like neuropathy [107]. Further evidence for the pathogenic role of succinylacetone comes from the discovery that blockade of tyrosine metabolism further upstream effectively

remedies the symptoms of tyrosinemia: mice deleted for the gene encoding fumarylacetoacetate hydrolase die in the neonatal period, but are rescued by the additional deletion of the 4-OH-phenylpyruvate dioxygenase (HPD) gene (the basis for tyrosinemia type 3) which prevents the accumulation of succinylacetone [108]. Similarly, administration of nitisinone, a blocker of HPD effectively prevents and even reverses the symptoms of tyrosimemia in the vast majority of patients [109]. Consequently, nitisinone is now the first line therapy for tyrosinemia together with a tyrosine- and phenylalanine-restricted diet [110]. In the roughly 10 % of patients where this fails, liver transplantation is an option. However, even though transplantation corrects the enzymatic defect in the liver, elevated levels of succinylacetone are still found in the urine of these patients and some of them have persisting tubular defects [111, 112].

Mitochondrial Cytopathies

The proximal tubule has a high energy requirement in order to reabsorb the bulk of filtered solutes. Cellular energy is provided in the form of ATP, produced by the respiratory chain in mitochondria. Therefore, proximal tubular cells are rich in mitochondria and it is not surprising that the proximal tubule is particularly susceptible to mitochondrial dysfunction. Indeed, Fanconi syndrome is the most common renal manifestation of mitochondrial cytopathies. The clinical manifestations of mitochondrial disorders are highly variable, but those with Fanconi syndrome typically have severe multi-organ involvement and present during infancy [55]. Neuromuscular manifestations usually predominate and the prognosis is often poor. Mitochondrial DNA mutations are inherited through the maternal line, as mitochondria derive from the maternal egg. An egg contains several mitochondria, each carrying their own DNA. Mutations in mitochondrial DNA can therefore be present in some mitochondria, but not in others within the same cell, a state termed heteroplasmy. Depending on the number of mitochondria with mutations passed on during cell division the ratio of mutated to healthy mito-chondria can be highly variable within different tissues and cells, which may explain some of the clinical variability. However, the majority of genes encoding the respiratory chain enzymes are encoded in the nuclear genome and mutations in these genes are typically inherited in autosomal-recessive fashion and affect all mito-chondria uniformly.

An initial investigation in suspected mito-chondrial cytopathies is typically to determine the ratio of lactate to pyruvate in the serum. However, in patients with Fanconi syndrome, this ratio is often normal, due to the grossly increased loss of organic acids in the urine [55]. Therefore, measurement of activity of respiratory chain enzymes should be performed in those patients with high suspicion of a mitochondrial cytopathy. Renal histology is typically non-specific, show-ing tubular damage, but may show giant mito-chondria [113, 114]. Some forms of mitochondrial cytopathies can be improved by supplementation with certain vitamins, especially those with a deficiency in the coenzyme Q10 [115]. Otherwise, no definitive treatment exists and management is only supportive for the renal manifestations.

Fanconi-Bickel-Syndrome

Fanconi-Bickel-syndrome is a rare autosomal-recessive glycogen-storage disease, caused by mutations in the gene *SLC2A2* encoding the glu-cose transporter GLUT2 [116, 117]. Patients typically present in infancy with hepatomegaly, failure-to-thrive and renal Fanconi-syndrome with excessive glucosuria [118]. GLUT2 is expressed in liver, intestine, pancreatic β-cells and proximal tubule cells. In hepatocytes, the transporter facilitates glucose uptake, as well as release. The impaired release leads to hepato-megaly and hypoglycemia during fasting, while the defective uptake causes post-prandial hyper-glycemia. In the pancreas, it leads to impaired glucose sensing and insulin release [118, 119]. In the kidney, GLUT2 localizes to the basolateral membrane of the proximal tubule, easily explain-ing the excessive glucosuria, which has been

reported to exceed 300 g per day [120] The renal Fanconi syndrome is less well understood, but may be due to impaired mitochondrial function [121]. Interestingly, *GLUT2*-deleted mice repro-duce the hepatic and pancreatic phenotype and also have glucosuria, but a RFS has not been reported [119]. The mouse model is therefore not helpful in understanding the mechanisms respon-sible for the RFS.

Mutations in *SLC2A2* associated with Fanconi-Bickel are typically severe, expected to completely abrogate GLUT2 function, although mutations with a milder phenotype with only mild glycosuria and LMWP have recently been described [122]. Interestingly, some heterozy-gote carriers of *SLC2A2* mutations can have iso-lated renal glucosuria and some milder recessive mutations, associated only with glucosuria and LMWP have also been described [122, 123].

Treatment consists of frequent feedings of slowly absorbed carbohydrates, as well as replacement of renal losses of water and solutes [124].

Fructose Intolerance

Fructose intolerance is due to a deficiency in the enzyme fructose-1-phosphate aldolase B, also simply called aldolase. Affected infants typically become symptomatic at weaning, with the intro-duction of fructose-containing food, such as fruits and vegetables. Patients develop nausea, vomiting and diarrhea and can progress to hypo-glycemia, convulsions and shock. Proximal tubule dysfunction develops and is most obvious in the form of a renal tubular acidosis, which is compounded by accumulation of lactic acid in the blood. The mechanism of cellular dysfunc-tion is thought to be intracellular phosphate depletion due to phosphorylation of accumulat-ing fructose. Phosphate is required for the gener-ation of the cellular fuel ATP [125]. Moreover, a direct association between aldolase and the vacu-olar proton pump V-H⁺-ATPase has been shown [126]. This pump is involved in bicarbonate reab-sorption in the proximal tubule, as well as acid secretion in the distal tubule and an inhibition by defective aldolase may explain the pronounced acidosis seen in patients. Treatment consists of a fructose-free diet, which completely reverses the renal symptoms.

Galactosemia

A reversible and incomplete form of proximal tubular dysfunction can be seen in infants with classical galactosemia, an autosomal-recessive disorder due to loss-of-function of the enzyme galactose-1-phosphate uridyl transferase [127]. This is a key enzyme for the conversion of galactose to glucose. Affected infants typically present with failure-to-thrive and develop vomiting, diarrhea and jaundice after ingestion of galactose-containing feeds. Untreated, hepatomegaly with progression to cirrhosis, cataracts and mental retardation develop. Renal manifestation are aminoaciduria, albuminuria, acidosis and galactosuria, the latter due to the elevated blood galactose levels [128]. The mechanism of tubular dysfunction is unclear, but may be related to intracellular depletion of free phosphate, due to phosphorylation of the accumulating galactose.

The diagnosis is made by increased blood galactose levels and confirmed by demonstration of enzyme deficiency. Importantly, the Fanconi syndrome is completely reversible with treatment, which is the elimination of galactose from the diet.

ARC-Syndrome

The combination of arthrogryposis, renal dysfunction and cholestasis is a rare autosomal recessive disorder, due to mutations in genes encoding vacuolar sorting protein involved in intracellular transport, including *VPS33B and VIPAR* [129, 130]. Affected neonates are identified by their contractures, conjugated hyperbilirubinemia and severe failure to thrive. In addition, giant platelets with a bleeding diathesis are observed. Renal manifestations include severe proximal tubular dysfunction, but nephrocalcinosis, nephrogenic diabetes insipidus and dysplasia

have also been described [131]. No specific treatment exists and the prognosis is poor with patients typically dying in their first year of life [129, 131–134]. However, milder forms have been described [135].

Membranous Nephropathy with Anti-proximal Tubule Basement Membrane Antibodies

Several reports exist about an association between membranous nephropathy and RFS [30–38, 136]. In most cases, antibodies have been found directed against the basement membrane of the proximal tubule. In some cases, pulmonary symptoms associated with anti-alveolar basement membrane antibodies are also present [34]. Most likely the antibodies are directed against an antigen expressed in the glomerulus, as well, explaining the combination of glomerular and proximal tubular dysfunction. In two families the syndrome has been linked to a region on the X-chromosome, but no gene has yet been identified [36].

Dent Disease

Clinical Features

Dent disease is an X-linked recessive proximal tubulopathy, characterized by low-molecular weight proteinuria (LMWP) and hypercalciuria with nephrocalcinosis and nephrolithiasis, as well as progressive renal failure [137]. Patients may also have aminoaciduria, glucosuria and phosphaturia, consistent with generalized proximal tubular dysfunction. It was first described as hypercalciuric rickets by Dent and Friedman [138]. Clinical manifestations can vary enormously and once an underlying gene, *CLCN5*, was identified in 1996, it was realized that mutations in the same gene also caused related tubulopathies, previously thought to be distinct, namely X-linked recessive nephrolithiasis and Japanese idiopathic low-molecular-weight proteinuria [139–145]. Patients typically manifest with complications of hypercalciuria, such as hematuria, nephrocalcinosis or stones. Progression to ESKD is rare in childhood. Women very rarely can be affected, probably due to skewed X-chromosome inactivation [146]. The diagnosis is made by the presence of hypercalciuria and low-molecular weight proteinuria (see section "Proteinuria") and typically a family history on the maternal side. Renal histology is non-specific, showing features of interstitial nephritis and calcium deposits and is thus not useful in establishing the diagnosis.

Genetics

The first gene identified to underlie Dent disease was *CLCN5*, encoding a proton-chloride antiporter expressed in the proximal tubule and especially on late endosomes and lysosomes [139]. Mutations in this gene are identified in approximately 60% of patients with a clinical diagnosis of Dent disease. A second gene, *OCRL*, encoding a phosphatidylinositol 4,5-bisphosphate 5-phosphatase, was identified later and mutations in this gene are found in approximately 15% of patients [147]. These patients are often referred to as having Dent2 disease, to distinguish them from CLCN5-based Dent disease. In the remaining approximately 25% of patients, no mutation in either gene is found, indicating that other genes may be responsible.

The identification of *OCRL* underlying Dent disease was surprising, as this gene also underlies Lowe syndrome, which besides renal proximal tubular dysfunction includes cataracts and developmental delay (see below). A genotype-phenotype effect has been hypothesized, as frameshift, splice site and nonsense mutations in *OCRL* causing Dent disease all cluster in exons 1–7, whereas those associated with Lowe syndrome mostly localize to the exons further downstream [148]. Use of potential alternate start codons in exons 7 and 8, which maintain the *OCRL* frame and, presumably, some functionality, could explain the milder phenotype in Dent

disease. However, this hypothesis cannot explain, why some missense mutations in OCRL are associated with multiorgan disease (the Lowe phenotype) in some patients and predominant kidney involvement (the Dent phenotype) in others [148].

Pathophysiology

Whilst the identification of underlying genes has provided great insights, the pathogenesis of Dent disease is still incompletely understood. *CLCN5* clearly plays an important part in endocytosis in the proximal tubule. It is highly expressed in endosomes and lysosomes, where it co-localizes with endocytosed proteins [149]. *CLCN5* is likely to provide an electric shunt in the lysosome that neutralizes the electrical gradient otherwise created by the H^+-ATPase, to allow its efficient operation. However, *CLCN5* is not a voltage-gated chloride channel, as initially described, but in fact a Cl^-/H^+ antiporter, which thus would remove protons from the lysosomal lumen [150, 151]. However, the net effect of CLCN5 function still appears to favor lysosomal acidification, as loss of function of *CLCN5* has been shown to impair this process in mice and recently also in human proximal tubular cells [149, 152]. Initially, the LMWP was thought to be a consequence of the impaired lysosomal function, but there is evidence for a role of CLCN5 beyond the lysosome. CLCN5 is also expressed at the apical surface of proximal tubule cells, where it is important in the assembly of the endocytic complex containing megalin and cubilin (see above) [99, 153–155]. Indeed, megalin and cubilin expression at the brush border is dramatically reduced in *CLCN5*-deleted mice, as is the excretion of megalin in the urine in Dent patients and the mouse model [99, 100]. Therefore, the proteinuria seen in this disease likely reflects impaired receptor-mediated endocytosis [152]. This is consistent also with the involvement of OCRL in endocytosis (see "Lowe Syndrome", below). Indeed, the renal phenotype of Lowe syndrome strongly resembles that of Dent disease [39] and proteomic analysis of the urine of patients with Dent disease shows a similar pattern as in Lowe syndrome, suggesting that *CLCN5* and *OCRL* may participate in similar endocytic pathways [156]. Potentially, in patients with Dent2 disease, other PIP$_2$ 5-phosphatases can compensate for the loss of *OCRL* except with respect to endocytosis and hypercalciuria. Redundancy in PIP$_2$ 5-phosphatases is suggested by the fact that *OCRL*-deleted mice do not show any clinical phenotype [157]. Interestingly, children with Dent2 disease frequently have some extra-renal manifestations in the form of elevated plasma levels of LDH and CK and poorer growth [158]. In addition, mild developmental delay is noted in some patients and it has been suggested that Dent2 disease is just a milder form of Lowe syndrome [159].

The hypercalciuria of Dent disease is poorly understood. One hypothesis is based on altered endocytosis of PTH and vitamin D-binding protein and a subsequently altered balance of calciotropic hormones [160]. Others propose a more direct role of CLCN5 in calcium handling by the kidney and bone [161, 162]. This discrepancy may in part be due to the fact that there are two different mouse strains with deleted *CLCN5* function, one of which has LMWP but no hypercalciuria [149].

Treatment

Treatment is mainly symptomatic and includes a large fluid intake to dilute urinary calcium and 1α-OH vitamin D supplementation, to normalize PTH levels, so as to treat or prevent rickets. This needs to be monitored carefully, as excessive supplementation would worsen the hypercalciuria. Citrate supplementation has been helpful in a mouse model of the disease [163]. Thiazide diuretics have been shown to reduce calcium excretion and thus reduce the stone-forming risk in Dent disease [164] but are sometimes poorly tolerated. This is interesting, as thiazides are thought to enhance calcium reabsorption in the proximal tubule, the segment affected in these patients [165].

Lowe Syndrome

Clinical Features

Lowe syndrome (oculo-cerebro-renal syndrome) was first described in 1952 as a clinical entity comprising "organic aciduria, decreased renal ammonia production, hydrophthalmus and mental retardation" [166]. Severity of symptoms varies, but in its complete form, patients are profoundly hypotonic with absent reflexes, have severe mental impairment, congenital cataracts, glaucoma and a renal Fanconi syndrome [167, 168]. There is often a delay in establishing the diagnosis and the renal manifestations can be minimal in early years but gross LMWP is characteristic [44]. Most patients first present to the ophthalmologist due to congenital cataracts [169, 170]. In addition, about 50 % of patients suffer from cataracts [171]. Interestingly, individual patients with OCRL mutations and brain and kidney involvement, but without cataracts, have been described recently further blurring the distinction between Dent2 disease and Lowe syndrome [148, 172, 173].

Motor development is typically delayed and most patients do not achieve independent walking before 3 years of age. Mental impairment can be very variable, but in one study most patients had IQ measured around 50, yet with 25 % in the normal range (>70). Seizures have been reported in about a third of patients [174]. Brain imaging, if performed, may show white matter changes, cerebral atrophy or periventricular cysts [175–177]. Behavioral abnormalities in the form of temper tantrums, negativism and obsessive behavior are another typical feature that can be extremely difficult for the families [178, 179].

The renal phenotype, as discussed above, is predominated by LMWP and hypercalciuria, but can involve more generalized proximal dysfunction, such as a metabolic acidosis and phosphate wasting [39]. Hypercalciuria is presumably due to impaired proximal reabsorption, but may be compounded by increased intestinal absorption, which OCRL may be involved in regulating [180]. Associated with the hypercalciuria is nephrocalcinosis/lithiasis with is seen in about two thirds of Lowe patients.

Renal histology is non-specific, showing some distortion of proximal tubular architecture and later also glomerular changes [181]. Most patients exhibit a slow progression of renal insufficiency with ESKD typically reported during the fourth and fifth decade of life [182, 183]. Estimating the GFR in children with Lowe syndrome from serum creatinine with the Schwartz-Haycock formula exceeds formal GFR measurement by approximately 65 %, probably due to the low muscle mass of these patients [39].

In addition to the manifestations in eyes, brain and kidneys, other clinical symptoms can occur. These include:

- platelet dysfunction with increased bleeding risk [184]
- a debilitating arthropathy [185]
- growth failure [167], which is independent of GFR [159]
- skeletal abnormalities, such as kyphosis, scoliosis, joint hypermobility and hip dislocation [186]. Some of these features may be secondary to the neurological features, such as the muscular hypotonia
- dental abnormalities, such as eruption and dental cysts [187]
- dermal cysts [188]

Genetics

The gene underlying Lowe syndrome was cloned in 1992 and named OCRL [189].

Mutations are identified in approximately 80–90 % of cases suspected of Lowe syndrome and in one study roughly one third of these occurred de novo [148]. About two thirds of mutations in patients diagnosed with Lowe syndrome are nonsense, frameshift and splice site changes, the remainder missense plus a few gross deletions. The presence of lens opacities has been suggested to identify female mutation carriers, although the reported sensitivity is variable [44, 170, 190–193].

Pathophysiology

Since identification of the underlying gene, much progress has been made towards understanding the pathophysiology. The OCRL protein contains several functional domains, including a phosphatidylinositol 4,5-bisphosphate (PIP_2) 5-phosphatase located in the Golgi apparatus. Impairment of this phosphatase function results in elevated cellular levels of PIP_2. PIP_2 levels affect vesicle trafficking at the Golgi [194] and may also account for alterations in the actin cytoskeleton seen in fibroblasts from patients with Lowe's syndrome [195], resulting in altered endosomal membrane trafficking [196] (Fig. 32.2). Besides, the phosphatase domain, the OCRL protein also contains several other domains that are important for endosomal trafficking via protein-protein interactions, including an N-terminal PH (pleckstrin homology) domain, an ASH (ASPM-SPD2-Hydin) domain, and a C-terminal RhoGAP (Rho GTPase activating) domain [198]. Missense mutations within the RhoGAP domain were identified in some patients with Lowe syndrome, highlighting its importance for OCRL function [199].

Beyond the role in endocytosis, intracellular trafficking and regulation of the actin skeleton, OCRL has also been implicated in a wide range of cellular processes, including cell migration, cell polarity, cell-cell interaction, cytokinesis, mitochondrial function and cilia formation. Indeed, it has been suggested that Lowe syndrome could be considered a mitochondrial cytopathy [200] or, more recently, a ciliopathy [201]. It remains to be determined to what degree these multiple mechanisms are clinically relevant and contribute to the variable phenotype associated with OCRL mutations.

Treatment

There is no specific treatment of Lowe syndrome and thus, treatment is symptomatic. Supplementation of electrolytes, alkali and vitamin D is based on biochemistries, and vitamin D is usually needed in 1-alfa hydroxylated forms. Oversupplementation could worsen the

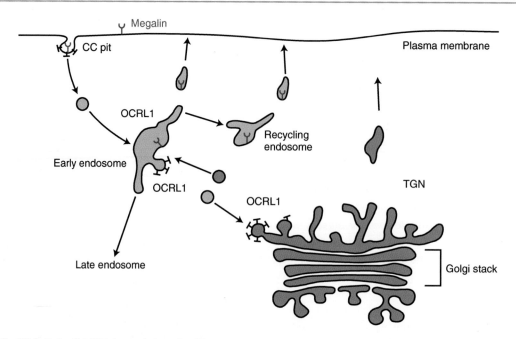

Fig. 32.2 Role of OCRL in regulation of traffic between apical membrane, endosomes and the trans-Golgi network. OCRL is present in clathrin-coated pits (CC) on the apical membrane of proximal tubular epithelial cells, early endosomes and the trans-Golgi network (TGN) (Used with permission of John Wiley and Sons from Lowe [197])

hypercalciuria, so monitoring parathyroid hormone (PTH) and calcium levels is advised. Nutritional support with tube-feeding is often helpful in the more severely affected patients.

The bleeding diathesis from the platelet dysfunction may be ameliorated with tranexamic acid and this should be considered prior to elective surgeries.

Cataract surgery is usually required early on, but vision is nevertheless typically impaired and rarely better than 20/70 [202]. Anti-epileptic drugs can help in those patients suffering from recurrent seizures [176].

Acquired RFS

Many exogenous causes of RFS have been reported and are listed in Table 32.2. The mechanism of tubular damage is often unclear, although mitochondrial dysfunction has been implicated in some forms (see below).

Treatment, aside from supportive measures, is always the removal of the offending agent, which typically reverses the symptoms. Except for those compounds, where blood levels can be measured (such as lead or aminoglycosides), no specific diagnostic tests exist. Thus, the diagnosis is typically made through suspicion of an exogenous cause and its subsequent removal.

Chemotherapeutic Agents

Ifosfamide is the chemotherapeutic agent most commonly associated with RFS, which is seen in up to 10 % of patients. Risk factors include total dose, reduced renal mass, young age or the combination with other nephrotoxic agents, such as cisplatin [203–207]. Symptoms typically reverse within weeks after cessation of the drug, but in some cases persist for several years and chronic impaired kidney function is possible [208, 209].

Antibiotics and Antiretrovirals

Aminoglycosides are well known for their nephrotoxic side effects. In a small percentage of patients they can also induce RFS. In fact, aminoaciduria has been proposed as a highly sensitive marker for aminoglycoside-induced renal injury, at least in the rat model [210]. The mechanism of damage is thought to be mitochondrial dysfunction: aminoglycosides target bacterial ribosomes where they induce faulty protein synthesis and since mitochondrial ribosomes bear structural resemblances to those of bacteria, they are vulnerable to the toxicity [211]. The risk appears to be related to the dosage and length of treatment and symptoms typically reverse after cessation of the drug (reviewed in [212]).

With the advent of retroviral treatment, tenofovir has become an increasingly common cause of RFS, although rarely seen in children as risk factor for tenofovir toxicity include older age, pre-existing kidney disease and low body mass [11, 213]. The exact mechanism is unclear, but includes mitochochondrial dysfunction.

Treatment

Specific therapy of Fanconi syndromes depends on the underlying cause. The renal features of galactosemia and hereditary fructose intolerance are reversed by appropriate dietary therapy. Removal of the causative toxin or drug usually ameliorates the tubulopathy although some drugs (e.g., ifosfamide) can cause long-term dysfunction. Nitisinone (NTBC (2-(2-nitro-4-trifluoromethylbenzoyl)-1,3-cyclohexanedione)), reverses the Fanconi syndrome in tyrosinemia (see above). Otherwise, treatment of RFS is mainly supportive. In severe cases, rehydration initially with 0.9 % saline and careful electrolyte correction is necessary and can be hazardous. Historically, fatalities occurred during rehydration with glucose-containing solutions, which exacerbated the profound hypokalemia. Rapid correction of acidosis can precipitate hypocalcemic seizures, the "hungry bone" phenomenon [214]. Once stabilized, many patients require large doses of alkali (3–20 mmol/kg/day), to be prescribed in the form of sodium or potassium bicarbonate or citrate, or as a compound preparation (e.g., polycitra). Citrate may be advantageous, as a large proportion of patients

are prone to hypercalciuria and subsequent development of nephrocalcinosis. Supplements of sodium chloride may also be needed. For some children, provision of all the above supplements fails to correct the biochemical disturbances and growth failure persists. Indomethacin or an alternative non-steroidal anti-inflammatory agent may be helpful in such cases [215]. Carnitine supplements have been used to correct the plasma and muscle carnitine deficiencies that can occur due to renal losses. Hypophosphataemic rickets requires treatment with phosphate supplementation and 1α-calcidol or calcitriol.

Acknowledgment Dr. William van't Hoff, who co-authored this chapter in the first edition.

References

1. Fanconi G. Die nicht diabetischen Glykosurien und Hyperglyklaemien des aelteren Kindes. Jahrb Kinderheilkunde. 1931;133:257–300.
2. Lucas RC. On a form of late rickets associated with albuminuria. Rickets of adolescence. Lancet. 1883;1:993–4.
3. de Toni G. Remarks on the relationship between renal rickets (renal dwarfism) and renal diabetes. Acta Pediatr. 1933;16:479–84.
4. Debre R, Marie J, Cleret F, Messimy R. Rachitisme tardif coexistant avec une Nephrite chronique et une Glycosurie. Arch Med Enfants. 1934;37:597–606.
5. Fanconi G. Der nephrotisch-glykosurische Zwergwuchs mit hypophosphataemischer Rachitis. Dtsch Med Wochenschr. 1936;62:1169–71.
6. van't Hoff W. Renal tubular disorders. In: Postlethwaite RJ, editor. Clinical paediatric nephrology. 3rd ed. New York: Oxford University Press; 2003. p. 103–12.
7. Kintzel PE. Anticancer drug-induced kidney disorders. Drug Saf. 2001;24(1):19–38.
8. Sadoff L. Nephrotoxicity of streptozotocin (NSC-85998). Cancer Chemother Rep. 1970;54(6):457–9.
9. Montoliu J, Carrera M, Darnell A, Revert L. Lactic acidosis and Fanconi's syndrome due to degraded tetracycline. Br Med J (Clin Res Ed). 1981;283(6306):1576–7.
10. Cleveland WW, Adams WC, Mann JB, Nyhan WL. Acquired fanconi syndrome following degraded tetracycline. J Pediatr. 1965;66:333–42.
11. Hall AM. Update on tenofovir toxicity in the kidney. Pediatr Nephrol. 2013;28(7):1011–23.
12. Izzedine H, Hulot JS, Villard E, Goyenvalle C, Dominguez S, Ghosn J, et al. Association between ABCC2 gene haplotypes and tenofovir-induced

proximal tubulopathy. J Infect Dis. 2006;194(11):1481–91.

13. Earle KE, Seneviratne T, Shaker J, Shoback D. Fanconi's syndrome in HIV+ adults: report of three cases and literature review. J Bone Miner Res. 2004;19(5):714–21.

14. Verhelst D, Monge M, Meynard JL, Fouqueray B, Mougenot B, Girard PM, et al. Fanconi syndrome and renal failure induced by tenofovir: a first case report. Am J Kidney Dis. 2002;40(6):1331–3.

15. Vittecoq D, Dumitrescu L, Beaufils H, Deray G. Fanconi syndrome associated with cidofovir therapy. Antimicrob Agents Chemother. 1997;41(8): 1846.

16. Izzedine H, Launay-Vacher V, Deray G. Fanconi syndrome associated with didanosine therapy. Aids. 2005;19(8):844–5.

17. Crowther MA, Callaghan W, Hodsman AB, Mackie ID. Dideoxyinosine-associated nephrotoxicity. Aids. 1993;7(1):131–2.

18. Chisolm Jr JJ, Harrison HC, Eberlein WR, Harrison HE. Amino-aciduria, hypophosphatemia, and rickets in lead poisoning; study of a case. AMA Am J Dis Child. 1955;89(2):159–68.

19. Kazantzis G, Flynn FV, Spowage JS, Trott DG. Renal tubular malfunction and pulmonary emphysema in cadmium pigment workers. Q J Med. 1963;32:165–92.

20. Lande MB, Kim MS, Bartlett C, Guay-Woodford LM. Reversible Fanconi syndrome associated with valproate therapy. J Pediatr. 1993;123(2):320–2.

21. Hong YT, Fu LS, Chung LH, Hung SC, Huang YT, Chi CS. Fanconi's syndrome, interstitial fibrosis and renal failure by aristolochic acid in Chinese herbs. Pediatr Nephrol. 2006;21(4):577–9.

22. Lee S, Lee T, Lee B, Choi H, Yang M, Ihm CG, et al. Fanconi's syndrome and subsequent progressive renal failure caused by a Chinese herb containing aristolochic acid. Nephrology (Carlton). 2004;9(3):126–9.

23. Yang SS, Chu P, Lin YF, Chen A, Lin SH. Aristolochic acid-induced Fanconi's syndrome and nephropathy presenting as hypokalemic paralysis. Am J Kidney Dis. 2002;39(3), E14.

24. Moss AH, Gabow PA, Kaehny WD, Goodman SI, Haut LL. Fanconi's syndrome and distal renal tubular acidosis after glue sniffing. Ann Intern Med. 1980;92(1):69–70.

25. Raschka C, Koch HJ. Longterm treatment of psoriasis using fumaric acid preparations can be associated with severe proximal tubular damage. Hum Exp Toxicol. 1999;18(12):738–9.

26. Rago RP, Miles JM, Sufit RL, Spriggs DR, Wilding G. Suramin-induced weakness from hypophosphatemia and mitochondrial myopathy. Association of suramin with mitochondrial toxicity in humans. Cancer. 1994;73(7):1954–9.

27. Gil HW, Yang JO, Lee EY, Hong SY. Paraquat-induced Fanconi syndrome. Nephrology (Carlton). 2005;10(5):430–2.

28. Lo JC, Chertow GM, Rennke H, Seifter JL. Fanconi's syndrome and tubulointerstitial nephritis in association with L-lysine ingestion. Am J Kidney Dis. 1996;28(4):614–7.

29. Igarashi T, Kawato H, Kamoshita S, Nosaka K, Seiya K, Hayakawa H. Acute tubulointerstitial nephritis with uveitis syndrome presenting as multiple tubular dysfunction including Fanconi's syndrome. Pediatr Nephrol. 1992;6(6):547–9.

30. Shenoy M, Krishnan R, Moghal N. Childhood membranous nephropathy in association with interstitial nephritis and Fanconi syndrome. Pediatr Nephrol. 2006;21(3):441.

31. Dumas R, Dumas ML, Baldet P, Bascoul S. Membranous glomerulonephritis in two brothers associated in one with tubulo-interstitial disease, Fanconi syndrome and anti-TBM antibodies (author's transl). Arch Fr Pediatr. 1982;39(2):75–8.

32. Griswold WR, Krous HF, Reznik V, Lemire J, Wilson NW, Bastian J, et al. The syndrome of autoimmune interstitial nephritis and membranous nephropathy. Pediatr Nephrol. 1997;11(6):699–702.

33. Katz A, Fish AJ, Santamaria P, Nevins TE, Kim Y, Butkowski RJ. Role of antibodies to tubulointerstitial nephritis antigen in human anti-tubular basement membrane nephritis associated with membranous nephropathy. Am J Med. 1992;93(6):691–8.

34. Levy M, Gagnadoux MF, Beziau A, Habib R. Membranous glomerulonephritis associated with anti-tubular and anti-alveolar basement membrane antibodies. Clin Nephrol. 1978;10(4):158–65.

35. Makker SP, Widstrom R, Huang J. Membranous nephropathy, interstitial nephritis, and Fanconi syndrome – glomerular antigen. Pediatr Nephrol. 1996;10(1):7–13.

36. Tay AH, Ren EC, Murugasu B, Sim SK, Tan PH, Cohen AH, et al. Membranous nephropathy with anti-tubular basement membrane antibody may be X-linked. Pediatr Nephrol. 2000;14(8–9):747–53.

37. Wood EG, Brouhard BH, Travis LB, Cavallo T, Lynch RE. Membranous glomerulonephropathy with tubular dysfunction and linear tubular basement membrane IgG deposition. J Pediatr. 1982;101(3):414–7.

38. Yagame M, Tomino Y, Miura M, Suga T, Nomoto Y, Sakai H. An adult case of Fanconi's syndrome associated with membranous nephropathy. Tokai J Exp Clin Med. 1986;11(2):101–6.

39. Bockenhauer D, Bokenkamp A, van't Hoff W, Levtchenko E, Kist-van Holthe JE, Tasic V, et al. Renal phenotype in Lowe syndrome: a selective proximal tubular dysfunction. Clin J Am Soc Nephrol. 2008;3(5):1430–6.

40. Kleta R. Fanconi or not Fanconi? Lowe syndrome revisited. Clin J Am Soc Nephrol. 2008;3(5):1244–5.

41. Bockenhauer D, van't Hoff W, Dattani M, Lehnhardt A, Subtirelu M, Hildebrandt F, et al. Secondary nephrogenic diabetes insipidus as a complication of inherited renal diseases. Nephron Physiol. 2010;116(4):23–9.

42. Bockenhauer D, Bichet DG. Inherited secondary nephrogenic diabetes insipidus: concentrating on humans. Am J Physiol Renal Physiol. 2013;304(8):F1037–42.

43. Nykjaer A, Dragun D, Walther D, Vorum H, Jacobsen C, Herz J, et al. An endocytic pathway essential for renal uptake and activation of the steroid 25-(OH) vitamin D3. Cell. 1999;96(4):507–15.

44. Laube GF, Russell-Eggitt IM, van't Hoff WG. Early proximal tubular dysfunction in Lowe's syndrome. Arch Dis Child. 2004;89(5):479–80.

45. Norden AG, Scheinman SJ, Deschodt-Lanckman MM, Lapsley M, Nortier JL, Thakker RV, et al. Tubular proteinuria defined by a study of Dent's (CLCN5 mutation) and other tubular diseases. Kidney Int. 2000;57(1):240–9.

46. Norden AG, Lapsley M, Lee PJ, Pusey CD, Scheinman SJ, Tam FW, et al. Glomerular protein sieving and implications for renal failure in Fanconi syndrome. Kidney Int. 2001;60(5):1885–92.

47. Birn H, Christensen EI. Renal albumin absorption in physiology and pathology. Kidney Int. 2006;69(3):440–9.

48. Mogensen CE, Solling. Studies on renal tubular protein reabsorption: partial and near complete inhibition by certain amino acids. Scand J Clin Lab Invest. 1977;37(6):477–86.

49. Tolaymat A, Sakarcan A, Neiberger R. Idiopathic Fanconi syndrome in a family. Part I. Clinical aspects. J Am Soc Nephrol. 1992;2(8):1310–7.

50. Bazzi C, Petrini C, Rizza V, Arrigo G, D'Amico G. A modern approach to selectivity of proteinuria and tubulointerstitial damage in nephrotic syndrome. Kidney Int. 2000;58(4):1732–41.

51. Valles P, Peralta M, Carrizo L, Martin L, Principi I, Gonzalez A, et al. Follow-up of steroid-resistant nephrotic syndrome: tubular proteinuria and enzymuria. Pediatr Nephrol. 2000;15(3–4):252–8.

52. Cogan MG. Disorders of proximal nephron function. Am J Med. 1982;72(2):275–88.

53. Unwin RJ, Capasso G, Shirley DG. An overview of divalent cation and citrate handling by the kidney. Nephron Physiol. 2004;98(2):15–20.

54. Roch-Ramel F. Renal transport of organic anions. Curr Opin Nephrol Hypertens. 1998;7(5):517–24.

55. Niaudet P, Rotig A. Renal involvement in mitochondrial cytopathies. Pediatr Nephrol. 1996;10(3):368–73.

56. Elsas LJ, Rosenberg LE. Familial renal glycosuria: a genetic reappraisal of hexose transport by kidney and intestine. J Clin Invest. 1969;48(10):1845–54.

57. Walton RJ, Bijvoet OL. Nomogram for derivation of renal threshold phosphate concentration. Lancet. 1975;2(7929):309–10.

58. Kruse K, Kracht U, Gopfert G. Renal threshold phosphate concentration (TmPO4/GFR). Arch Dis Child. 1982;57(3):217–23.

59. Bistarakis L, Voskaki I, Lambadaridis J, Sereti H, Sbyrakis S. Renal handling of phosphate in the first six months of life. Arch Dis Child. 1986;61(7):677–81.

60. Shaw NJ, Wheeldon J, Brocklebank JT. Indices of intact serum parathyroid hormone and renal excretion of calcium, phosphate, and magnesium. Arch Dis Child. 1990;65(11):1208–11.

61. Pajor AM. Citrate transport by the kidney and intestine. Semin Nephrol. 1999;19(2):195–200.

62. Houston IB, Boichis H, Edelmann Jr CM. Fanconi syndrome with renal sodium wasting and metabolic alkalosis. Am J Med. 1968;44(4):638–46.

63. Lemire J, Kaplan BS. The various renal manifestations of the nephropathic form of cystinosis. Am J Nephrol. 1984;4(2):81–5.

64. Yildiz B, Durmus-Aydogdu S, Kural N, Bildirici K, Basmak H, Yarar C. A patient with cystinosis presenting transient features of Bartter syndrome. Turk J Pediatr. 2006;48(3):260–2.

65. Gahl WA, Bernardini IM, Dalakas MC, Markello TC, Krasnewich DM, Charnas LR. Muscle carnitine repletion by long-term carnitine supplementation in nephropathic cystinosis. Pediatr Res. 1993;34(2):115–9.

66. Nissenkorn A, Korman SH, Vardi O, Levine A, Katzir Z, Ballin A, et al. Carnitine-deficient myopathy as a presentation of tyrosinemia type I. J Child Neurol. 2001;16(9):642–4.

67. Moestrup SK, Verroust PJ. Megalin- and cubilin-mediated endocytosis of protein-bound vitamins, lipids, and hormones in polarized epithelia. Annu Rev Nutr. 2001;21:407–28.

68. Klootwijk ED, Reichold M, Helip-Wooley A, Tolaymat A, Broeker C, Robinette SL, et al. Mistargeting of peroxisomal EHHADH and inherited renal Fanconi's syndrome. N Engl J Med. 2014;370(2):129–38.

69. Schmidt U, Dubach UC, Guder WG, Funk B, Paris K. Metabolic patterns in various structures of the rat nephron. The distribution of enzymes of carbohydrate metabolism. Curr Probl Clin Biochem. 1975;4:22–32.

70. Balaban RS, Mandel LJ. Metabolic substrate utilization by rabbit proximal tubule. An NADH fluorescence study. Am J Physiol. 1988;254(3 Pt 2):F407–16.

71. Spencer PD, Medow MS, Moses LC, Roth KS. Effects of succinylacetone on the uptake of sugars and amino acids by brush border vesicles. Kidney Int. 1988;34(5):671–7.

72. Wyss PA, Boynton SB, Chu J, Spencer RF, Roth KS. Physiological basis for an animal model of the renal Fanconi syndrome: use of succinylacetone in the rat. Clin Sci (Lond). 1992;83(1):81–7.

73. Roth KS, Carter BE, Higgins ES. Succinylacetone effects on renal tubular phosphate metabolism: a model for experimental renal Fanconi syndrome. Proc Soc Exp Biol Med. 1991;196(4):428–31.

74. Eiam-ong S, Spohn M, Kurtzman NA, Sabatini S. Insights into the biochemical mechanism of

maleic acid-induced Fanconi syndrome. Kidney Int. 1995;48(5):1542–8.

75. Rossi R, Kleta R, Ehrich JH. Renal involvement in children with malignancies. Pediatr Nephrol. 1999;13(2):153–62.

76. Sener G, Sehirli O, Yegen BC, Cetinel S, Gedik N, Sakarcan A. Melatonin attenuates ifosfamide-induced Fanconi syndrome in rats. J Pineal Res. 2004;37(1):17–25.

77. Schwerdt G, Freudinger R, Mildenberger S, Silbernagl S, Gekle M. The nephrotoxin ochratoxin A induces apoptosis in cultured human proximal tubule cells. Cell Biol Toxicol. 1999;15(6):405–15.

78. Ciarimboli G, Holle SK, Vollenbrocker B, Hagos Y, Reuter S, Burckhardt G, et al. New clues for nephrotoxicity induced by ifosfamide: preferential renal uptake via the human organic cation transporter 2. Mol Pharm. 2011;8(1):270–9.

79. Haviv YS, Wald H, Levi M, Dranitzki-Elhalel M, Popovtzer MM. Late-onset downregulation of NaPi-2 in experimental Fanconi syndrome. Pediatr Nephrol. 2001;16(5):412–6.

80. Pontoglio M, Barra J, Hadchouel M, Doyen A, Kress C, Bach JP, et al. Hepatocyte nuclear factor 1 inactivation results in hepatic dysfunction, phenylketonuria, and renal Fanconi syndrome. Cell. 1996;84(4):575–85.

81. Cheret C, Doyen A, Yaniv M, Pontoglio M. Hepatocyte nuclear factor 1 alpha controls renal expression of the Npt1-Npt4 anionic transporter locus. J Mol Biol. 2002;322(5):929–41.

82. Magen D, Berger L, Coady MJ, Ilivitzki A, Militianu D, Tieder M, et al. A loss-of-function mutation in NaPi-IIa and renal Fanconi's syndrome. N Engl J Med. 2010;362(12):1102–9.

83. Graversen JH, Castro G, Kandoussi A, Nielsen H, Christensen EI, Norden A, et al. A pivotal role of the human kidney in catabolism of HDL protein components apolipoprotein A-I and A-IV but not of A-II. Lipids. 2008;43(5):467–70.

84. Vormann J. Magnesium: nutrition and metabolism. Mol Asp Med. 2003;24(1–3):27–37.

85. Verroust PJ, Birn H, Nielsen R, Kozyraki R, Christensen EI. The tandem endocytic receptors megalin and cubilin are important proteins in renal pathology. Kidney Int. 2002;62(3):745–56.

86. Christensen EI, Gburek J. Protein reabsorption in renal proximal tubule-function and dysfunction in kidney pathophysiology. Pediatr Nephrol. 2004;19(7):714–21.

87. Christensen EI, Birn H. Megalin and cubilin: multifunctional endocytic receptors. Nat Rev Mol Cell Biol. 2002;3(4):256–66.

88. Hilpert J, Nykjaer A, Jacobsen C, Wallukat G, Nielsen R, Moestrup SK, et al. Megalin antagonizes activation of the parathyroid hormone receptor. J Biol Chem. 1999;274(9):5620–5.

89. Nykjaer A, Fyfe JC, Kozyraki R, Leheste JR, Jacobsen C, Nielsen MS, et al. Cubilin dysfunction causes abnormal metabolism of the steroid hormone

25(OH) vitamin D(3). Proc Natl Acad Sci U S A. 2001;98(24):13895–900.

90. Raychowdhury R, Niles JL, McCluskey RT, Smith JA. Autoimmune target in Heymann nephritis is a glycoprotein with homology to the LDL receptor. Science. 1989;244(4909):1163–5.

91. Leheste JR, Rolinski B, Vorum H, Hilpert J, Nykjaer A, Jacobsen C, et al. Megalin knockout mice as an animal model of low molecular weight proteinuria. Am J Pathol. 1999;155(4):1361–70.

92. Kantarci S, Al-Gazali L, Hill RS, Donnai D, Black GC, Bieth E, et al. Mutations in LRP2, which encodes the multiligand receptor megalin, cause Donnai-Barrow and facio-oculo-acoustico-renal syndromes. Nat Genet. 2007;39(8):957–9.

93. Storm T, Tranebjaerg L, Frykholm C, Birn H, Verroust PJ, Neveus T, et al. Renal phenotypic investigations of megalin-deficient patients: novel insights into tubular proteinuria and albumin filtration. Nephrol Dial Transplant. 2013;28(3): 585–91.

94. Moestrup SK, Kozyraki R, Kristiansen M, Kaysen JH, Rasmussen HH, Brault D, et al. The intrinsic factor-vitamin B12 receptor and target of teratogenic antibodies is a megalin-binding peripheral membrane protein with homology to developmental proteins. J Biol Chem. 1998;273(9):5235–42.

95. Imerslund O. Idiopathic chronic megaloblastic anemia in children. Acta Paediatr Suppl. 1960;49 Suppl 119:1–115.

96. Grasbeck R, Gordin R, Kantero I, Kuhlback B. Selective vitamin B12 malabsorption and proteinuria in young people. A syndrome. Acta Med Scand. 1960;167:289–96.

97. Wahlstedt-Froberg V, Pettersson T, Aminoff M, Dugue B, Grasbeck R. Proteinuria in cubilin-deficient patients with selective vitamin B12 malabsorption. Pediatr Nephrol. 2003;18(5):417–21.

98. Ovunc B, Otto EA, Vega-Warner V, Saisawat P, Ashraf S, Ramaswami G, et al. Exome sequencing reveals cubilin mutation as a single-gene cause of proteinuria. J Am Soc Nephrol. 2011;22(10):1815–20.

99. Christensen EI, Devuyst O, Dom G, Nielsen R, Van der Smissen P, Verroust P, et al. Loss of chloride channel ClC-5 impairs endocytosis by defective trafficking of megalin and cubilin in kidney proximal tubules. Proc Natl Acad Sci U S A. 2003;100(14):8472–7.

100. Norden AG, Lapsley M, Igarashi T, Kelleher CL, Lee PJ, Matsuyama T, et al. Urinary megalin deficiency implicates abnormal tubular endocytic function in Fanconi syndrome. J Am Soc Nephrol. 2002;13(1):125–33.

101. Haffner D, Weinfurth A, Seidel C, Manz F, Schmidt H, Waldherr R, et al. Body growth in primary de Toni-Debre-Fanconi syndrome. Pediatr Nephrol. 1997;11(1):40–5.

102. Friedman AL, Trygstad CW, Chesney RW. Autosomal dominant Fanconi syndrome with

early renal failure. Am J Med Genet. 1978;2(3):225–32.

103. Neimann N, Pierson M, Marchal C, Rauber G, Grignon G. Familial glomerulo-tubular nephropathy with the de Toni-Debre-Fanconi syndrome. Arch Fr Pediatr. 1968;25(1):43–69.

104. Tieder M, Arie R, Modai D, Samuel R, Weissgarten J, Liberman UA. Elevated serum 1,25-dihydroxyvitamin D concentrations in siblings with primary Fanconi's syndrome. N Engl J Med. 1988;319(13):845–9.

105. Patrick A, Cameron JS, Ogg CS. A family with a dominant form of idiopathic Fanconi syndrome leading to renal failure in adult life. Clin Nephrol. 1981;16(6):289–92.

106. Wen SF, Friedman AL, Oberley TD. Two case studies from a family with primary Fanconi syndrome. Am J Kidney Dis. 1989;13(3):240–6.

107. Sassa S, Kappas A. Hereditary tyrosinemia and the heme biosynthetic pathway. Profound inhibition of delta-aminolevulinic acid dehydratase activity by succinylacetone. J Clin Invest. 1983;71(3): 625–34.

108. Endo F, Sun MS. Tyrosinaemia type I and apoptosis of hepatocytes and renal tubular cells. J Inherit Metab Dis. 2002;25(3):227–34.

109. Holme E, Lindstedt S. Tyrosinaemia type I and NTBC (2-(2-nitro-4-trifluoromethylbenzoyl)-1,3-cyclohexanedione). J Inherit Metab Dis. 1998;21(5):507–17.

110. McKiernan PJ. Nitisinone in the treatment of hereditary tyrosinaemia type 1. Drugs. 2006;66(6): 743–50.

111. Tuchman M, Freese DK, Sharp HL, Ramnaraine ML, Ascher N, Bloomer JR. Contribution of extra-hepatic tissues to biochemical abnormalities in hereditary tyrosinemia type I: study of three patients after liver transplantation. J Pediatr. 1987;110(3):399–403.

112. Pierik LJ, van Spronsen FJ, Bijleveld CM, van Dael CM. Renal function in tyrosinaemia type I after liver transplantation: a long-term follow-up. J Inherit Metab Dis. 2005;28(6):871–6.

113. Thorner PS, Balfe JW, Becker LE, Baumal R. Abnormal mitochondria on a renal biopsy from a case of mitochondrial myopathy. Pediatr Pathol. 1985;4(1–2):25–35.

114. Hall AM, Unwin RJ. The not so 'mighty chondrion': emergence of renal diseases due to mitochondrial dysfunction. Nephron Physiol. 2007;105(1):1–10.

115. Montini G, Malaventura C, Salviati L. Early coenzyme Q10 supplementation in primary coenzyme Q10 deficiency. N Engl J Med. 2008;358(26): 2849–50.

116. Peduto A, Spada M, Alluto A, La Dolcetta M, Ponzone A, Santer R. A novel mutation in the GLUT2 gene in a patient with Fanconi-Bickel syndrome detected by neonatal screening for galactosaemia. J Inherit Metab Dis. 2004;27(2): 279–80.

117. Santer R, Calado J. Familial renal glucosuria and SGLT2: from a mendelian trait to a therapeutic target. Clin J Am Soc Nephrol. 2010;5(1):133–41.

118. Santer R, Schneppenheim R, Suter D, Schaub J, Steinmann B. Fanconi-Bickel syndrome – the original patient and his natural history, historical steps leading to the primary defect, and a review of the literature. Eur J Pediatr. 1998;157(10):783–97.

119. Guillam MT, Hummler E, Schaerer E, Yeh JI, Birnbaum MJ, Beermann F, et al. Early diabetes and abnormal postnatal pancreatic islet development in mice lacking Glut-2. Nat Genet. 1997;17(3):327–30.

120. Brivet M, Moatti N, Corriat A, Lemonnier A, Odievre M. Defective galactose oxidation in a patient with glycogen storage disease and Fanconi syndrome. Pediatr Res. 1983;17(2):157–61.

121. Odievre MH, Lombes A, Dessemme P, Santer R, Brivet M, Chevallier B, et al. A secondary respiratory chain defect in a patient with Fanconi-Bickel syndrome. J Inherit Metab Dis. 2002;25(5):379–84.

122. Grunert SC, Schwab KO, Pohl M, Sass JO, Santer R. Fanconi-Bickel syndrome: GLUT2 mutations associated with a mild phenotype. Mol Genet Metab. 2012;105(3):433–7.

123. Sakamoto O, Ogawa E, Ohura T, Igarashi Y, Matsubara Y, Narisawa K, et al. Mutation analysis of the GLUT2 gene in patients with Fanconi-Bickel syndrome. Pediatr Res. 2000;48(5):586–9.

124. Lee PJ, Van't Hoff WG, Leonard JV. Catch-up growth in Fanconi-Bickel syndrome with uncooked cornstarch. J Inherit Metab Dis. 1995;18(2):153–6.

125. Morris Jr RC, Nigon K, Reed EB. Evidence that the severity of depletion of inorganic phosphate determines the severity of the disturbance of adenine nucleotide metabolism in the liver and renal cortex of the fructose-loaded rat. J Clin Invest. 1978;61(1):209–20.

126. Lu M, Holliday LS, Zhang L, Dunn Jr WA, Gluck SL. Interaction between aldolase and vacuolar H+-ATPase: evidence for direct coupling of glycolysis to the ATP-hydrolyzing proton pump. J Biol Chem. 2001;276(32):30407–13.

127. Reichardt JK, Woo SL. Molecular basis of galactosemia: mutations and polymorphisms in the gene encoding human galactose-1-phosphate uridylyltransferase. Proc Natl Acad Sci U S A. 1991;88(7):2633–7.

128. Golberg L, Holzel A, Komrower GM, Schwarz V. A clinical and biochemical study of galactosaemia; a possible explanation of the nature of the biochemical lesion. Arch Dis Child. 1956;31(158):254–64.

129. Gissen P, Johnson CA, Morgan NV, Stapelbroek JM, Forshew T, Cooper WN, et al. Mutations in VPS33B, encoding a regulator of SNARE-dependent membrane fusion, cause arthrogryposis-renal dysfunction-cholestasis (ARC) syndrome. Nat Genet. 2004;36(4):400–4.

130. Cullinane AR, Straatman-Iwanowska A, Zaucker A, Wakabayashi Y, Bruce CK, Luo G, et al. Mutations

in VIPAR cause an arthrogryposis, renal dysfunction and cholestasis syndrome phenotype with defects in epithelial polarization. Nat Genet. 2010;42(4):303–12.

131. Eastham KM, McKiernan PJ, Milford DV, Ramani P, Wyllie J, van't Hoff W, et al. ARC syndrome: an expanding range of phenotypes. Arch Dis Child. 2001;85(5):415–20.

132. Horslen SP, Quarrell OW, Tanner MS. Liver histology in the arthrogryposis multiplex congenita, renal dysfunction, and cholestasis (ARC) syndrome: report of three new cases and review. J Med Genet. 1994;31(1):62–4.

133. Di Rocco M, Callea F, Pollice B, Faraci M, Campiani F, Borrone C. Arthrogryposis, renal dysfunction and cholestasis syndrome: report of five patients from three Italian families. Eur J Pediatr. 1995;154(10):835–9.

134. Gissen P, Tee L, Johnson CA, Genin E, Caliebe A, Chitayat D, et al. Clinical and molecular genetic features of ARC syndrome. Hum Genet. 2006;120(3):396–409.

135. Smith H, Galmes R, Gogolina E, Straatman-Iwanowska A, Reay K, Banushi B, et al. Associations among genotype, clinical phenotype, and intracellular localization of trafficking proteins in ARC syndrome. Hum Mutat. 2012;33(12):1656–64.

136. Kazama I, Matsubara M, Michimata M, Suzuki M, Hatano R, Sato H, et al. Adult onset Fanconi syndrome: extensive tubulo-interstitial lesions and glomerulopathy in the early stage of Chinese herbs nephropathy. Clin Exp Nephrol. 2004;8(3):283–7.

137. Wrong OM, Norden AG, Feest TG. Dent's disease; a familial proximal renal tubular syndrome with low-molecular-weight proteinuria, hypercalciuria, nephrocalcinosis, metabolic bone disease, progressive renal failure and a marked male predominance. QJM. 1994;87(8):473–93.

138. Dent CE, Friedman M. Hypercalcuric rickets associated with renal tubular damage. Arch Dis Child. 1964;39:240–9.

139. Lloyd SE, Pearce SH, Fisher SE, Steinmeyer K, Schwappach B, Scheinman SJ, et al. A common molecular basis for three inherited kidney stone diseases. Nature. 1996;379(6564):445–9.

140. Igarashi T, Inatomi J, Ohara T, Kuwahara T, Shimadzu M, Thakker RV. Clinical and genetic studies of CLCN5 mutations in Japanese families with Dent's disease. Kidney Int. 2000;58(2):520–7.

141. Thakker RV. Pathogenesis of Dent's disease and related syndromes of X-linked nephrolithiasis. Kidney Int. 2000;57(3):787–93.

142. Scheinman SJ, Cox JP, Lloyd SE, Pearce SH, Salenger PV, Hoopes RR, et al. Isolated hypercalciuria with mutation in CLCN5: relevance to idiopathic hypercalciuria. Kidney Int. 2000;57(1):232–9.

143. Langlois V, Bernard C, Scheinman SJ, Thakker RV, Cox JP, Goodyer PR. Clinical features of X-linked nephrolithiasis in childhood. Pediatr Nephrol. 1998;12(8):625–9.

144. Akuta N, Lloyd SE, Igarashi T, Shiraga H, Matsuyama T, Yokoro S, et al. Mutations of CLCN5 in Japanese children with idiopathic low molecular weight proteinuria, hypercalciuria and nephrocalcinosis. Kidney Int. 1997;52(4):911–6.

145. Lloyd SE, Pearce SH, Gunther W, Kawaguchi H, Igarashi T, Jentsch TJ, et al. Idiopathic low molecular weight proteinuria associated with hypercalciuric nephrocalcinosis in Japanese children is due to mutations of the renal chloride channel (CLCN5). J Clin Invest. 1997;99(5):967–74.

146. Hoopes Jr RR, Hueber PA, Reid Jr RJ, Braden GL, Goodyer PR, Melnyk AR, et al. CLCN5 chloride-channel mutations in six new North American families with X-linked nephrolithiasis. Kidney Int. 1998;54(3):698–705.

147. Hoopes Jr RR, Shrimpton AE, Knohl SJ, Hueber P, Hoppe B, Matyus J, et al. Dent disease with mutations in OCRL1. Am J Hum Genet. 2005;76(2):260–7.

148. Hichri H, Rendu J, Monnier N, Coutton C, Dorseuil O, Poussou RV, et al. From Lowe syndrome to Dent disease: correlations between mutations of the OCRL1 gene and clinical and biochemical phenotypes. Hum Mutat. 2011;32(4):379–88.

149. Piwon N, Gunther W, Schwake M, Bosl MR, Jentsch TJ. ClC-5 Cl- -channel disruption impairs endocytosis in a mouse model for Dent's disease. Nature. 2000;408(6810):369–73.

150. Scheel O, Zdebik AA, Lourdel S, Jentsch TJ. Voltage-dependent electrogenic chloride/proton exchange by endosomal CLC proteins. Nature. 2005;436(7049):424–7.

151. Accardi A, Miller C. Secondary active transport mediated by a prokaryotic homologue of ClC Cl-channels. Nature. 2004;427(6977):803–7.

152. Gorvin CM, Wilmer MJ, Piret SE, Harding B, van den Heuvel LP, Wrong O, et al. Receptor-mediated endocytosis and endosomal acidification is impaired in proximal tubule epithelial cells of Dent disease patients. Proc Natl Acad Sci U S A. 2013;110(17):7014–9.

153. Wang Y, Cai H, Cebotaru L, Hryciw DH, Weinman EJ, Donowitz M, et al. ClC-5: role in endocytosis in the proximal tubule. Am J Physiol Ren Physiol. 2005;289(4):F850–62.

154. Hryciw DH, Ekberg J, Ferguson C, Lee A, Wang D, Parton RG, et al. Regulation of albumin endocytosis by PSD95/Dlg/ZO-1 (PDZ) scaffolds. Interaction of Na+-H+ exchange regulatory factor-2 with ClC-5. J Biol Chem. 2006;281(23):16068–77.

155. Hryciw DH, Ekberg J, Pollock CA, Poronnik P. ClC-5: a chloride channel with multiple roles in renal tubular albumin uptake. Int J Biochem Cell Biol. 2006;38(7):1036–42.

156. Norden AG, Sharratt P, Cutillas PR, Cramer R, Gardner SC, Unwin RJ. Quantitative amino acid and proteomic analysis: very low excretion of polypeptides >750 Da in normal urine. Kidney Int. 2004;66(5):1994–2003.

157. Janne PA, Suchy SF, Bernard D, MacDonald M, Crawley J, Grinberg A, et al. Functional overlap between murine Inpp5b and Ocrl1 may explain why deficiency of the murine ortholog for OCRL1 does not cause Lowe syndrome in mice. J Clin Invest. 1998;101(10):2042–53.

158. Utsch B, Bokenkamp A, Benz MR, Besbas N, Dotsch J, Franke I, Frund S, Gok F, Hoppe B, Karle S, Kuwertz-Broking E, Laube G, Neb M, Nuutinen M, Ozaltin F, Rascher W, Ring T, Tasic V, van Wijk JA, Ludwig M. Novel OCRL1 mutations in patients with the phenotype of Dent disease. Am J Kidney Dis. 2006;48(6):942–56.

159. Bokenkamp A, Bockenhauer D, Cheong HI, Hoppe B, Tasic V, Unwin R, et al. Dent-2 disease: a mild variant of Lowe syndrome. J Pediatr. 2009;155(1):94–9.

160. Gunther W, Piwon N, Jentsch TJ. The ClC-5 chloride channel knock-out mouse – an animal model for Dent's disease. Pflugers Arch. 2003;445(4):456–62.

161. Silva IV, Cebotaru V, Wang H, Wang XT, Wang SS, Guo G, et al. The ClC-5 knockout mouse model of Dent's disease has renal hypercalciuria and increased bone turnover. J Bone Miner Res. 2003;18(4):615–23.

162. Devuyst O, Jouret F, Auzanneau C, Courtoy PJ. Chloride channels and endocytosis: new insights from Dent's disease and ClC-5 knockout mice. Nephron Physiol. 2005;99(3):69–73.

163. Cebotaru V, Kaul S, Devuyst O, Cai H, Racusen L, Guggino WB, et al. High citrate diet delays progression of renal insufficiency in the ClC-5 knockout mouse model of Dent's disease. Kidney Int. 2005;68(2):642–52.

164. Raja KA, Schurman S, D'Mello RG, Blowey D, Goodyer P, Van Why S, et al. Responsiveness of hypercalciuria to thiazide in Dent's disease. J Am Soc Nephrol. 2002;13(12):2938–44.

165. Nijenhuis T, Vallon V, van der Kemp AW, Loffing J, Hoenderop JG, Bindels RJ. Enhanced passive Ca2+ reabsorption and reduced Mg2+ channel abundance explains thiazide-induced hypocalciuria and hypomagnesemia. J Clin Invest. 2005;115(6):1651–8.

166. Lowe CU, Terrey M, Mac LE. Organic-aciduria, decreased renal ammonia production, hydrophthalmos, and mental retardation; a clinical entity. AMA Am J Dis Child. 1952;83(2):164–84.

167. Charnas LR, Bernardini I, Rader D, Hoeg JM, Gahl WA. Clinical and laboratory findings in the oculo-cerebrorenal syndrome of Lowe, with special reference to growth and renal function. N Engl J Med. 1991;324(19):1318–25.

168. Abbassi V, Lowe CU, Calcagno PL. Oculo-cerebro-renal syndrome. A review. Am J Dis Child. 1968;115(2):145–68.

169. Loi M. Lowe syndrome. Orphanet J Rare Dis. 2006;1:16.

170. Roschinger W, Muntau AC, Rudolph G, Roscher AA, Kammerer S. Carrier assessment in families with lowe oculocerebrorenal syndrome: novel mutations in the OCRL1 gene and correlation of direct DNA diagnosis with ocular examination. Mol Genet Metab. 2000;69(3):213–22.

171. Walton DS, Katsavounidou G, Lowe CU. Glaucoma with the oculocerebrorenal syndrome of Lowe. J Glaucoma. 2005;14(3):181–5.

172. Keilhauer CN, Gal A, Sold JE, Zimmermann J, Netzer KO, Schramm L. Clinical findings in a patient with Lowe syndrome and a splice site mutation in the OCRL1 gene. Klin Monbl Augenheilkd. 2007;224(3):207–9.

173. Pasternack SM, Bockenhauer D, Refke M, Tasic V, Draaken M, Conrad C, et al. A premature termination mutation in a patient with Lowe syndrome without congenital cataracts: dropping the "O" in OCRL. Klin Padiatr. 2013;225(1):29–33.

174. Recker F, Reutter H, Ludwig M. Lowe syndrome/Dent-2 disease: a comprehensive review of known and novel aspects. J Pediatr Genet. 2013;02(02):053–68.

175. Charnas L, Bernar J, Pezeshkpour GH, Dalakas M, Harper GS, Gahl WA. MRI findings and peripheral neuropathy in Lowe's syndrome. Neuropediatrics. 1988;19(1):7–9.

176. Ono J, Harada K, Mano T, Yamamoto T, Okada S. MR findings and neurologic manifestations in Lowe oculocerebrorenal syndrome. Pediatr Neurol. 1996;14(2):162–4.

177. Schneider JF, Boltshauser E, Neuhaus TJ, Rauscher C, Martin E. MRI and proton spectroscopy in Lowe syndrome. Neuropediatrics. 2001;32(1):45–8.

178. Kenworthy L, Charnas L. Evidence for a discrete behavioral phenotype in the oculocerebrorenal syndrome of Lowe. Am J Med Genet. 1995;59(3):283–90.

179. Kenworthy L, Park T, Charnas LR. Cognitive and behavioral profile of the oculocerebrorenal syndrome of Lowe. Am J Med Genet. 1993;46(3):297–303.

180. Wu G, Zhang W, Na T, Jing H, Wu H, Peng JB. Suppression of intestinal calcium entry channel TRPV6 by OCRL, a lipid phosphatase associated with Lowe syndrome and Dent disease. Am J Physiol Cell Physiol. 2012;302(10):C1479–91.

181. Witzleben CL, Schoen EJ, Tu WH, McDonald LW. Progressive morphologic renal changes in the oculo-cerebro-renal syndrome of Lowe. Am J Med. 1968;44(2):319–24.

182. Tricot L, Yahiaoui Y, Teixeira L, Benabdallah L, Rothschild E, Juquel JP, et al. End-stage renal failure in Lowe syndrome. Nephrol Dial Transplant. 2003;18(9):1923–5.

183. Schramm L, Gal A, Zimmermann J, Netzer KO, Heidbreder E, Lopau K, et al. Advanced renal insufficiency in a 34-year-old man with Lowe syndrome. Am J Kidney Dis. 2004;43(3):538–43.

184. Lasne D, Baujat G, Mirault T, Lunardi J, Grelac F, Egot M, et al. Bleeding disorders in Lowe syndrome patients: evidence for a link between OCRL mutations and primary haemostasis disorders. Br J Haematol. 2010;150(6):685–8.

185. Athreya BH, Schumacher HR, Getz HD, Norman ME, Borden S, Witzleben CL. Arthropathy of Lowe's (oculocerebrorenal) syndrome. Arthritis Rheum. 1983;26(6):728–35.

186. Holtgrewe JL, Kalen V. Orthopedic manifestations of the Lowe (oculocerebrorenal) syndrome. J Pediatr Orthop. 1986;6(2):165–71.

187. Rodrigues Santos MT, Watanabe MM, Manzano FS, Lopes CH, Masiero D. Oculocerebrorenal Lowe syndrome: a literature review and two case reports. Spec Care Dent: Off Publ Am Assoc Hosp Dent, Acad Dent Handicap, Am Soc Geriatr Dent. 2007;27(3):108–11.

188. Won JH, Lee MJ, Park JS, Chung H, Kim JK, Shim JS. Multiple epidermal cysts in lowe syndrome. Ann Dermatol. 2010;22(4):444–6.

189. Attree O, Olivos IM, Okabe I, Bailey LC, Nelson DL, Lewis RA, et al. The Lowe's oculocerebrorenal syndrome gene encodes a protein highly homologous to inositol polyphosphate-5-phosphatase. Nature. 1992;358(6383):239–42.

190. Lin T, Lewis RA, Nussbaum RL. Molecular confirmation of carriers for Lowe syndrome. Ophthalmology. 1999;106(1):119–22.

191. Brown N, Gardner RJ. Lowe syndrome: identification of the carrier state. Birth Defects Orig Artic Ser. 1976;12(3):579–95.

192. Delleman JW, Bleeker-Wagemakers EM, van Veelen AW. Opacities of the lens indicating carrier status in the oculo-cerebro-renal (Lowe) syndrome. J Pediatr Ophthalmol. 1977;14(4):205–12.

193. Cibis GW, Waeltermann JM, Whitcraft CT, Tripathi RC, Harris DJ. Lenticular opacities in carriers of Lowe's syndrome. Ophthalmology. 1986;93(8):1041–5.

194. Dressman MA, Olivos-Glander IM, Nussbaum RL, Suchy SF. Ocrl1, a PtdIns(4,5)P(2) 5-phosphatase, is localized to the trans-Golgi network of fibroblasts and epithelial cells. J Histochem Cytochem. 2000;48(2):179–90.

195. Suchy SF, Nussbaum RL. The deficiency of PIP2 5-phosphatase in Lowe syndrome affects actin polymerization. Am J Hum Genet. 2002;71(6):1420–7.

196. Apodaca G. Endocytic traffic in polarized epithelial cells: role of the actin and microtubule cytoskeleton. Traffic. 2001;2(3):149–59.

197. Lowe M. Structure and function of the Lowe syndrome protein OCRL1. Traffic. 2005;6(9):711–9.

198. Pirruccello M, De Camilli P. Inositol 5-phosphatases: insights from the Lowe syndrome protein OCRL. Trends Biochem Sci. 2012;37(4):134–43.

199. McCrea HJ, Paradise S, Tomasini L, Addis M, Melis MA, De Matteis MA, et al. All known patient mutations in the ASH-RhoGAP domains of OCRL affect targeting and APPL1 binding. Biochem Biophys Res Commun. 2008;369(2):493–9.

200. Gobernado JM, Lousa M, Gimeno A, Gonsalvez M. Mitochondrial defects in Lowe's oculocerebrorenal syndrome. Arch Neurol. 1984;41(2):208–9.

201. Madhivanan K, Mukherjee D, Aguilar RC. Lowe syndrome: Between primary cilia assembly and Rac1-mediated membrane remodeling. Commun Integr Biol. 2012;5(6):641–4.

202. Kruger SJ, Wilson Jr ME, Hutchinson AK, Peterseim MM, Bartholomew LR, Saunders RA. Cataracts and glaucoma in patients with oculocerebrorenal syndrome. Arch Ophthalmol. 2003;121(9):1234–7.

203. Rossi R, Pleyer J, Schafers P, Kuhn N, Kleta R, Deufel T, et al. Development of ifosfamide-induced nephrotoxicity: prospective follow-up in 75 patients. Med Pediatr Oncol. 1999;32(3):177–82.

204. Rossi R, Ehrich JH. Partial and complete de Toni-Debre-Fanconi syndrome after ifosfamide chemotherapy of childhood malignancy. Eur J Clin Pharmacol. 1993;44 Suppl 1:S43–5.

205. Loebstein R, Koren G. Ifosfamide-induced nephrotoxicity in children: critical review of predictive risk factors. Pediatrics. 1998;101(6), E8.

206. Skinner R, Pearson AD, English MW, Price L, Wyllie RA, Coulthard MG, et al. Cisplatin dose rate as a risk factor for nephrotoxicity in children. Br J Cancer. 1998;77(10):1677–82.

207. Skinner R, Pearson AD, English MW, Price L, Wyllie RA, Coulthard MG, et al. Risk factors for ifosfamide nephrotoxicity in children. Lancet. 1996;348(9027):578–80.

208. Loebstein R, Atanackovic G, Bishai R, Wolpin J, Khattak S, Hashemi G, et al. Risk factors for long-term outcome of ifosfamide-induced nephrotoxicity in children. J Clin Pharmacol. 1999;39(5):454–61.

209. Skinner R, Cotterill SJ, Stevens MC. Risk factors for nephrotoxicity after ifosfamide treatment in children: a UKCCSG Late Effects Group study. United Kingdom Children's Cancer Study Group. Br J Cancer. 2000;82(10):1636–45.

210. Macpherson NA, Moscarello MA, Goldberg DM. Aminoaciduria is an earlier index of renal tubular damage than conventional renal disease markers in the gentamicin-rat model of acute renal failure. Clin Invest Med. 1991;14(2):101–10.

211. Spahn CM, Prescott CD. Throwing a spanner in the works: antibiotics and the translation apparatus. J Mol Med. 1996;74(8):423–39.

212. Izzedine H, Launay-Vacher V, Isnard-Bagnis C, Deray G. Drug-induced Fanconi's syndrome. Am J Kidney Dis. 2003;41(2):292–309.

213. Hall AM, Hendry BM, Nitsch D, Connolly JO. Tenofovir-associated kidney toxicity in HIV-infected patients: a review of the evidence. Am J Kidney Dis: Off J Nat Kidney Found. 2011;57(5):773–80.

214. Frisch LS, Mimouni F. Hypomagnesemia following correction of metabolic acidosis: a case of hungry bones. J Am Coll Nutr. 1993;12(6):710–3.

215. Haycock GB, Al-Dahhan J, Mak RH, Chantler C. Effect of indomethacin on clinical progress and renal function in cystinosis. Arch Dis Child. 1982;57(12):934–9.

Bartter-, Gitelman-, and Related Syndromes

33

Siegfried Waldegger and Martin Konrad

Abbreviations

aBS	Antenatal Bartter syndrome
ACE	Angiotensin converting enzyme
ASDN	Aldosterone sensitive distal nephron
AVP	Arginine vasopressin
BS	Bartter syndrome
BSND	Bartter syndrome with sensorineural deafness
CaSR	Calcium-sensing receptor
cBS	Classic Bartter syndrome
CD	Collecting duct
ClC-K	Chloride channel – kidney specific
CNT	Connecting tubule
COX	Cyclooxygenase
DCT	Distal convoluted tubule
EAST	Epilepsy-ataxia-sensorineural deafness-tubulopathy syndrome
ECF	Extracellular fluid
ENaC	Epithelial sodium channel
GS	Gitelman syndrome
NCCT	Sodium-chloride-cotransporter
NKCC2	Sodium-potassium-2chloride-cotransporter
NO	Nitric oxide
NSAID	Nonsteroidal anti-inflammatory drug
PGE$_2$	Prostaglandin E$_2$
PHA-I	Pseudohypoaldosteronism type I
RAAS	Renin angiontensin aldosterone system
ROMK	Renal outer medullary potassium channel
TAL	Thick ascending limb
TGF	Tubuloglomerular feedback
TRPM6	Transient receptor potential cation channel subfamily M, member 6

S. Waldegger (✉)
Department of Pediatrics, University Hospital Innsbruck, Anichstr. 35, Innsbruck 6020, Austria
e-mail: siegfried.waldegger@tirol-kliniken.at

M. Konrad
General Pediatrics, University Children's Hospital Muenster, Waldeyerstrasse 22, Muenster 48149, Germany
e-mail: konradma@uni-muenster.de

Basic Principles of Ion Transport in the TAL and the Early DCT

With respect to their role in sodium reabsorption, the TAL and early DCT form a functional unit that separates tubular sodium chloride from water. Compared to sodium reabsorption in the other nephron segments, which occurs via sodium hydrogen exchange or by sodium channels in the proximal nephron and in the ASDN, respectively, TAL and early DCT sodium transport is accomplished primarily by the active reabsorption of sodium together with chloride from the tubular fluid. These nephron segments are relatively water-tight and thus prevent osmotically driven absorptive flow of water. About 30 % of the total

© Springer-Verlag Berlin Heidelberg 2016
D.F. Geary, F. Schaefer (eds.), *Pediatric Kidney Disease*, DOI 10.1007/978-3-662-52972-0_33

sodium load provided by glomerular filtration is absorbed along the TAL and – via counter current multiplication – contribute to medullary interstitial hypertonicity. TAL sodium reabsorption thus not only accounts for the – in quantitative terms – most important mechanism of sodium retention (apart from the proximal nephron, which reabsorbs about 60 % of the filtered sodium load), but also generates the osmotic driving force for water reabsorption along the CD. For this reason, disturbances in TAL salt reabsorption result in both salt-wasting and severely reduced urinary concentrating capacity (i.e., water loss). In contrast, DCT mediated salt reabsorption accounts for only about 5 % of the filtered sodium load and does not contribute to the urinary concentrating mechanisms. Impaired DCT salt reabsorption therefore does not interfere with urinary concentrating capability, although the accompanying saluresis indirectly increases renal water excretion even with normal urine osmolalities.

Transepithelial sodium chloride reabsorption in the TAL and DCT is driven by secondary active transport processes that depend on a low intracellular sodium concentration maintained by active extrusion of sodium by the basolateral sodium-potassium-ATPase (sodium pump). By far the majority of TAL sodium reabsorption depends upon the operation of the furosemide-sensitive sodium-potassium-chloride cotransporter (NKCC2) with about half of the sodium taking the transcellular route and half taking a paracellular route by cation-selective intercellular pathways (Fig. 33.1a). Potassium that enters the TAL cell by sodium-potassium-chloride cotransport (one potassium ion being transported with one sodium and two chloride ions) recycles back to the tubular urine through ROMK type potassium channels (Renal Outer Medulla K channels). This not only guarantees proper activity of NKCC2-mediated transport along the entire length of the TAL by replenishment of urinary potassium that otherwise would rapidly decrease along the TAL through reabsorption by NKCC2. Even more important, luminal potassium secretion in addition establishes a lumen-positive transepithelial voltage gradient that provides – in terms of energy recovery – a low-priced driving force for paracellular transport of cations like sodium, calcium, and magnesium. The essential functions of the TAL thus not only include the reabsorption of sodium chloride but also that of magnesium and calcium. Noteworthy, all of the TAL chloride reabsorption occurs by the transcellular route. Overall parity of sodium (with ~50 % transcellular and ~50 % paracellular) and chloride (100 % transcellular) reabsorption is due to the stoichiometry of the apical NKCC2 cotransporter that transports two chloride ions for each sodium ion (Fig. 33.1a).

Taken together, the initial step of transcellular sodium chloride and paracellular sodium transport across the TAL epithelium critically depends on the proper activity of NKCC2 and ROMK.

In contrast to the TAL, sodium chloride reabsorption in the DCT occurs almost exclusively by the transcellular route (Fig. 33.1b). Luminal sodium chloride uptake is mediated by the electroneutral thiazide-sensitive sodium chloride cotransporter NCCT that is structurally related to the NKCC2 protein, but transports one sodium ion together with one chloride ion without potassium. A relevant apical potassium conductance seems not to exist in early DCT cells, that instead express TRPM6 cation channels that permit apical magnesium entry. Inhibition of NCCT transport by long term administration of thiazides or by genetic ablation in animal models has been shown to reduce the number of DCT cells, which might explain impaired renal magnesium reabsorption with consequent hypomagnesemia observed in human diseases caused by impaired NCCT mediated transport.

DCT and TAL cells differ with respect to the apical entry step for sodium chloride; however, as mentioned above, basolateral sodium release in both cell types is accounted for by the sodium pump. Moreover, epithelial cells in TAL and early DCT share similar pathways for basolateral chloride exit. In both cell types two highly homologous ClC-K type chloride channel proteins (ClC-Ka and ClC-Kb) associate with their beta subunit barttin to form a basolateral chloride conductance, which accounts for the release of the majority of reabsorbed chloride ions (Fig. 33.1a,b).

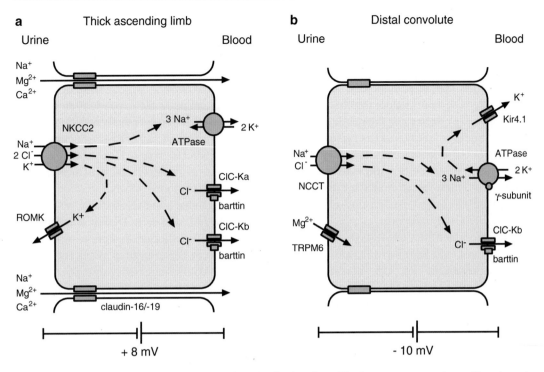

Fig. 33.1 Mechanisms of sodium reabsorption along the distal nephron. The key transport proteins and ion channels are shown for the thick ascending limb (**a**) and the distal convolute (**b**). For details, please see text

Taken together, NCCT mediates early DCT cell sodium chloride uptake and ClC-K channels in association with barttin account for basolateral chloride release.

In the transition zone between the TAL and DCT a plaque of closely packed epithelial cells morphologically different from TAL- and DCT-cells forms the *macula densa*. Together with closely adjacent extraglomerular mesangial cells and granular cells of the afferent arterioles appendant to the same nephron, these specialized tubular cells assemble the juxtaglomerular apparatus. *Macula densa* cells serve an important function in coupling renal hemodynamics with tubular reabsorption in that they monitor the sodium chloride concentration of the tubular fluid. Via paracrine signalling molecules like prostaglandin E_2 (PGE_2), ATP, adenosin, and NO, the *macula densa* provides a feed-back mechanism, which adapts glomerular filtration to tubular reabsorption (tubuloglomerular feedback, TGF). In case of an increased sodium chloride concentration at the *macula densa* the TGF induces afferent arte-

riole vasoconstriction and decreases renin release, whereas a decreased *macula densa* sodium chloride concentration dilates the afferent arteriole and increases renin release. To sense the tubular sodium chloride concentration the *macula densa* takes advantage of essentially the same repertoire of transport proteins as found in salt-reabsorbing TAL cells. Via apical sodium chloride uptake (NKCC2 and ROMK) and basolateral chloride release (ClC-K and barttin) changes in luminal sodium chloride concentration are translated in alterations of basolateral transmembrane voltage. This again results from recycling of potassium into the tubular lumen, which guarantees an asymmetric – hence electrogenic – transcellular transport of sodium chloride, which results in basolateral membrane depolarization. This in turn regulates among other processes voltage-sensitive calcium entry, which triggers a series of intracellular signalling events eventually resulting in the release of the above mentioned paracrine signals. Owing to these combined functions in transepithelial transport and sensing of tubular sodium chloride, impaired activity of one of the participating proteins not only results in salt-wasting due to reduced TAL salt-reabsorbing capacity, but also abrogates the TGF as an important safety valve, which otherwise would reduce the filtered sodium chloride load by decreasing glomerular filtration. In fact, blinding of the *macula densa* for the tubular sodium chloride concentration with resultant disinhibition of glomerular filtration might constitute the single most important mechanism underlying the severe salt-wasting observed in impaired TAL salt transport.

Taken together, NKCC2, ROMK, ClC-K chloride channels, and barttin participate in the salt sensing-mechanism of the *macula densa*. Impaired function of one of these proteins affects the TGF and prevents adjustment of glomerular filtration with tubular salt-reabsorbing capacity, which further aggravates renal salt wasting [1].

Hypokalemic Salt-Wasting Tubular Disorders

With the exception of the medullary collecting duct that is primarily responsible for the reabsorption of water, reabsorption of sodium chloride from the glomerular filtrate at least in quantitative terms constitutes the key function of all nephron segments. Given the normal daily amount of 170 l of glomerular filtrate produced by adult kidneys, at a normal plasma sodium concentration of 140 mmol/l and plasma chloride concentration of 105 mmol/l the filtered load of sodium and chloride per 24 h amounts to 23.8 mols (about 550 g) and 17.9 mols (about 630 g), respectively. Healthy kidneys manage the reabsorption of more than 99 % of the filtered load, with about 60 % by the proximal tubule, 30 % by the TAL, 5 % by the early DCT, and the remainder by the aldosterone-sensitive distal nephron (ASDN). Impairment of sodium transport in any of these nephron segments causes a permanent reduction in extracellular fluid volume, which in turn causes compensatory activation of sodium conserving mechanisms, i.e., stimulation of renin secretion and aldosterone

synthesis. Accordingly, with intact ASDN function, the primary symptoms of renal salt-wasting like hypovolemia with tendency for reduced arterial blood pressure mix with those of secondary hyperaldosteronism, which increases ASDN sodium retention at the expense of an increased potassium excretion eventually resulting in hypokalemia. In case of renal salt-wasting, hypokalemia thus indicates proper function of the ASDN and points to the involvement of nephron segments upstream to the ASDN.

As mentioned above, sodium reabsorption along the TAL and early DCT is coupled to the reabsorption of chloride. Sodium-wasting caused by defects in these nephron segments hence is accompanied by decreased reabsorption of chloride. Unlike sodium, which at least partially may be recovered by increased reabsorption along the ASDN, chloride irretrievably gets lost with the urine. Accordingly, the urinary chloride-loss exceeds that of sodium and for the sake of electroneutrality has to be balanced by other cations like ammonium or potassium. Loss of ammonium, the main carrier of protons in the urine, results in metabolic alkalosis, potassium loss in addition aggravates hypokalemia caused by secondary hyperaldosteronism. For this reason, hypochloremia with metabolic alkalosis, in addition to severe hypokalemia characterizes salt-wasting due to defects along the TAL and early DCT.

Finally, sodium reabsorption along the proximal tubule via the sodium proton exchanger and the carboanhydrase is indirectly coupled to the reabsorption of bicarbonate. Proximal tubular salt-wasting thus – in addition to hypokalemia – is accompanied by urinary loss of bicarbonate resulting in hyperchloremic metabolic acidosis.

Taken together, in the state of renal salt-wasting the determination of plasma potassium, chloride, and bicarbonate concentrations allows for the rapid assessment of the affected nephron segment. Of note, in this context the determination of the plasma sodium concentration is not very helpful, since changes in plasma sodium – the more or less exclusive extracellular cation accounting for plasma osmolality – reflects disturbances in the osmoregulation (i.e., water balance) rather than in the regulation of sodium balance.

Apart from more general disturbances of proximal tubular function which among other transport processes affect proximal tubular sodium reabsorption (as seen in Fanconi syndrome), no hereditary defects specifically affecting the proximal tubular sodium proton exchanger have been described in humans. By contrast, several genetic defects affect sodium chloride transport along the TAL and DCT and will be the focus of the following section.

Renal Salt-Wasting with Hypokalemia and Hypochloremic Metabolic Alkalosis

Historical Overview and Nomenclature

In 1957, two pediatricians described an infant with congenital hypokalemic alkalosis, failure to thrive, dehydration, and hyposthenuria, who finally died at the age of 7.5 months [2]. Some years later, two patients with normotensive hyperaldosteronism, hyperplasia of the juxtaglomerular apparatus, metabolic alkalosis and severe renal potassium wasting were characterized by the endocrinologist Frederic Bartter [3]. Other features of this syndrome were increased activity of the renin-angiotensin system and a relative vascular resistance to the pressor effect of exogeneously applied angiotensin II. Following these original reports, hundreds of such Bartter syndrome (BS) cases have been described. While all shared the findings of hypokalemia and hypochloremic alkalosis, patients differed with respect to age of onset, severity of symptoms, degree of growth retardation, urinary concentration capacity, magnitude of urinary excretion of potassium and prostaglandins, presence of hypomagnesemia, and extents of urinary calcium excretion.

Gitelman and colleagues pointed to the susceptibility to carpopedal spasms and tetany in three BS cases [4]. Tetany was attributed to low plasma magnesium levels secondary to impaired renal conservation of magnesium. Further examination of these patients in addition revealed low urinary calcium excretion [5]. Consequently, the association of hypocalciuria with renal magnesium-wasting was regarded as a hallmark to separate the then defined Gitelman syndrome (GS) from other forms of BS [6]. Interestingly, both patients in Bartter's original report displayed positive Chvostek's sign and carpopedal spasms. Indeed, in a review of the original observations described by Bartter et al., one of the coauthors conceded that the majority of patients seen by both endocrinologists perfectly matched the later description of Gitelman [7].

Phenotypic homogeneity of BS was challenged even more seriously when the pediatricians Fanconi and McCredie described high urinary calcium excretion and medullary nephrocalcinosis in preterm infants initially suspected of having BS [8, 9]. Descriptions of this variant in the literature became more frequent in the 1980s, most likely because advances in neonatal medicine resulted in higher survival rates of extremely preterm born babies. The neonatologist Ohlsson finally described the antenatal history with maternal polyhydramnios, which likely predisposed to premature birth [10]. Immediately after birth, profound polyuria put such patients at great risk for life-threatening dehydration. Contraction of the extracellular fluid (ECF) volume is accompanied by markedly elevated renal and extrarenal prostaglandin E_2 (PGE_2) production. Treatment with prostaglandin synthesis inhibitors effectively reduced polyuria, ameliorated hypokalemia, and improved growth. To emphasize the obviously critical role of PGE_2 in the pathogenesis of this distinct tubular disorder, Seyberth coined the term hyperprostaglandin E syndrome [11, 12]. Another variant of this severe, prenatal-onset salt-wasting disorder was first described in a Bedouin family. It differs from the above mentioned antenatal variant of BS by the presence of sensorineural deafness, absence of medullary nephrocalcinosis, and slowly deteriorating renal function [13].

Taken together, renal salt-wasting syndromes associated with hypokalemia and hypochloremic metabolic alkalosis (frequently subsumed as "Bartter syndrome" in a broader sense) present with marked clinical variability. Severe, early onset forms (antenatal Bartter syndrome, aBS) with symptoms directly arising from profound salt-wasting with extracellular volume depletion contrast with mild, late onset forms primarily characterized by the features of secondary hyperaldosteronism (Gitelman syndrome, GS). In between these two extremes, the Bartter syndrome sensu stricto (classic Bartter syndrome, cBS) presents as a disorder with intermediate severity. Variable extents of extracellular volume depletion and secondary electrolyte disturbances contribute to a rather variable disease phenotype, which in its extremes may mimic aBS or GS.

This classification based on clinical criteria was enriched by clarification of the underlying genetic defects which all follow an autosomal recessive mode of inheritance. As disclosed by molecular genetic analyses, aBS results from disturbed salt reabsorption along the TAL due to defects either in NKCC2 [14], ROMK [15], Barttin [16], or both, ClC-Ka and ClC-Kb [17]. The cBS is caused by dysfunction of ClC-Kb [18], which impairs salt transport to some extent along the TAL and in particular along the DCT. A pure defect of salt reabsorption in the DCT due to dysfunction of NCCT finally results in GS [19]. Unfortunately, a frequently used classification merely based on molecular genetic criteria, which simply follows the chronology of the identification of the genetic defects, does not accommodate a more easily understood functional classification. According to this molecular genetic classification, Bartter syndrome type I (BS I) refers to a defect of NKKC2 (gene name *SLC12A1*), BS II of ROMK (*KCNJ1*), BS III of ClC-Kb (*CLCNKB*), and BS IV of Barttin (*BSND*). GS, owing to disturbed NCCT (*SLC12A3*) function, despite its apparent relatedness to this group of disorders was not included in this classification. Instead, Bartter syndrome type V (BS V) was suggested for some gain-of-function mutations of the Calcium-Sensing-Receptor (CaSR), which, however, cause autosomal dominant hypocalcemia with variable degrees of renal salt-wasting explained by the inhibitory effect of CaSR-activation on salt-transport along the TAL [20–22]. The autosomal

dominant mode of inheritance and the clinically more relevant hypocalcemia are features not compatible with Bartter syndrome and make the designation BS V rather impractical. We therefore will not consider BS V in the following sections.

Another facet of the clinical and genetic heterogeneity of inherited renal salt wasting disorders emerged in 2009, when a new autosomal recessive clinical syndrome characterized by epilepsy, ataxia, sensorineural deafness and renal salt wasting with/without mental retardation was described under the acronyms EAST or SeSAME syndrome [23, 24]. EAST/SeSAME syndrome is caused by loss of function mutations in the *KCNJ10* gene encoding the inwardly-rectifying potassium channel Kir4.1 [23, 24]. The renal tubular defect disturbs the reabsorption of sodium chloride in the DCT and thus symptoms closely resemble GS with hypokalemic alkalosis, hypomagnesemia and hypocalciuria.

Taken together, renal salt-wasting with hypokalemia and hypochloremic metabolic alkalosis becomes manifest in four clinically defined syndromes: aBS, cBS, GS, and EAST syndrome. From a functional point of view, aBS arises from sodium chloride transport defects of the TAL. cBS combines features of weak TAL-defects with disturbed DCT function, whereas GS and EAST syndrome reflect pure DCT dysfunction.

Genetic Disorders of the TAL, the Antenatal Bartter Syndrome

Furosemide-Sensitive Na-K-2Cl-Cotransporter (NKCC2)

Disruption of sodium chloride reabsorption in the TAL due to inactivating mutations of the *SLC12A1* gene which encodes NKCC2 causes antenatal BS, a severe disorder with onset in utero. Within the second trimester, fetal polyuria leads to increasing maternal polyhydramnios. Chloride concentration in the amniotic fluid is elevated up to 118 mmol/l [25, 26]. Untreated, premature delivery occurs around 32 weeks of gestation. The most striking abnormality of the newborns is profound polyuria. With adequate fluid replacement, daily urinary outputs can easily exceed half of the body weight of the newborn (>20 ml/kg/h). Despite ECF volume contraction and presence of high AVP levels, urine osmolality hardly approaches that of plasma, indicating a severe renal concentrating defect. Salt reabsorption along the TAL segment is also critical for urine dilution, which explains that urine osmolality on the other hand typically does not decrease below 160 mosmol/kg. Some preserved ability to dilute urine might be explained by an adaptive increase of salt reabsorption in the DCT which functions as the most distal portion of the diluting segment. This moderate hyposthenuria clearly separates NKCC2-deficient patients from polyuric patients with nephrogenic diabetes insipidus, who typically display urine osmolalities below 100 mosmol/kg.

Within the first months of life, nearly all patients develop medullary nephrocalcinosis in parallel with persistently high urinary calcium excretion. Amazingly, conservation of magnesium is not affected to a similar extent and NKCC2-deficient patients usually do not develop hypomagnesemia. This is even more surprising given that mutations in either CLDN16 or CLDN19 which both encode tight junction proteins that mediate paracellular transport of divalent cations along the TAL, invariably cause both hypercalciuria and hypermagnesiuria with subsequent hypomagnesemia [27, 28]. With respect to magnesium transport, the difference between both disorders might be explained by an upregulation of magnesium reabsorption parallel to a compensatory increase of sodium chloride reabsorption in DCT cells in case of a NKCC2 defect [29].

Renal Outer-Medullary Potassium Channel (ROMK)

ROMK-deficient patients due to mutations in the KCNJ1 gene similarly show a history of maternal polyhydramnios, prematurity with median age of gestation of 33 weeks, vasopressin-insensitive polyuria, isosthenuria, and hypercalciuria with secondary nephrocalcinosis. As in the case of NKCC2 dysfunction, the severity of the symptoms argues for a complete defect of sodium

chloride reabsorption along the TAL. The mechanism of RAAS activation is virtually identical to that proposed for NKCC2-deficient patients. However, despite the presence of high plasma aldosterone levels, ROMK-deficient patients exhibit transient hyperkalemia in the first days of life [30]. The simultaneous appearance of hyperkalemia and hyponatremia resembles the clinical picture of mineralocorticoid-deficiency (which, however, shows low aldosterone levels) or that of pseudohypoaldosteronism type I (PHA-I; high aldosterone levels). Indeed, several published cases of PHA-I turned out to be misdiagnosed and subsequent genetic analysis revealed ROMK mutations as the underlying defect [31]. The severity of initial hyperkalemia decreases with gestational age [32]. Hyperkalemia may be attributed to the additional role of ROMK in the cortical collecting duct (CCD) where it participates in the process of potassium secretion. Although less pronounced as compared to NKCC2-deficiency, the majority of ROMK-deficient patients develop hypokalemia in the later course of the disease. The transient nature of hyperkalemia may be explained by the upregulation of alternative pathways for potassium secretion in the CCD.

The Chloride Channel (ClC-K) Beta-Subunit Barttin

In 2001, a new player in the process of salt reabsorption along the TAL and DCT was identified – the ClC-K channel beta-subunit barttin. Discovery of barttin was accomplished by linkage analysis of a very rare variant of tubular salt-wasting associated with sensorineural deafness. By a positional cloning strategy, a novel gene, BSND, was identified and inactivating mutations were found in affected individuals [16]. Because the gene product, barttin, had no homology to any known protein, its physiologic function remained unclear until its role as an essential beta-subunit of the ClC-K channels was demonstrated [33, 34].

Two ClC-K isoforms of the CLC family of chloride channels are highly expressed along the distal nephron, with ClC-Ka being primarily expressed in the thin ascending limb and decreasing expression levels along the adjacent distal nephron. Its close homologue, ClC-Kb, is predominantly expressed in the DCT. Along the TAL, both channel isoforms are equally expressed. Barttin, which is found in all ClC-K expressing nephron segments, is essential for proper ClC-K channel function in that it facilitates the transport of ClC-K channels to the cell surface and modulates biophysical properties of the assembled channel complex.

In affected individuals, the Barttin defect seems to completely disrupt chloride exit across the basolateral membrane in TAL as well as DCT cells. Accordingly, patients display the severest salt-wasting kidney disorder described so far. As with defects of NKCC2 and ROMK, the first symptom of a Barttin defect is maternal polyhydramnios due to fetal polyuria beginning at approximately 22 weeks of gestation. Again, polyhydramnios accounts for preterm labor and extreme prematurity. Postnatally, patients are at high risk of volume depletion. Plasma chloride levels fall to approximately 80 mmol/l; a further decrease usually can be avoided by close laboratory monitoring and rapid intervention. Polyuria again is resistant to vasopressin and urine osmolalities range between 200 and 400 mOsmol/kg.

Unlike patients with loss-of-function mutations of ROMK and NKCC2, Barttin-deficient patients exhibit only transitory hypercalciuria [35]. Medullary nephrocalcinosis is absent, yet progressive renal failure is common with histologic signs of pronounced tissue damage like glomerular sclerosis, tubular atrophy, and mononuclear infiltration. The mechanisms underlying the deterioration of renal function are not yet understood. The lack of hypercalciuria, however, may be explained by disturbed sodium chloride reabsorption along the DCT. Isolated DCT dysfunction as seen in GS (see below) or after long-term inhibition of NCCT-mediated transport by thiazides is known to induce hypocalciuria. This effect might counter-balance the hypercalciuric effect of TAL-dysfunction in case of a combined impairment of salt reabsorption along the TAL and DCT. In contrast to calcium, the renal conservation of magnesium is severely impaired, leading to pronounced hypomagnesemia. This might be explained by the disruption of both magnesium reabsorption pathways, the paracellular one in the TAL and the transcellular one in the DCT, respectively.

Barttin defects are invariably associated with sensorineurinal deafness. Elucidation of the pathogenesis of this rare disorder has provided a deeper insight into the mechanisms of potassium rich endolymph secretion in the inner ear: Marginal cells of the *stria vascularis* contribute to the endolymph formation by apical potassium secretion. Transcellular potassium transport is mediated by the furosemide-sensitive Na-K-2Cl-cotransporter type 1 (NKCC1) ensuring basolateral potassium entry into the marginal cells. Voltage-dependent potassium channels mediate apical potassium secretion into the endolymph. Proper function of NKCC1 requires basolateral recycling of chloride. Deafness associated with Barttin defects suggests that this recycling is enabled by the ClC-K/barttin channel complex.

A Digenic Disorder: The ClC-Ka/b Phenotype

The concept of the physiologic role of Barttin as a common beta-subunit of ClC-K channels was substantiated by the description of patients harbouring inactivating mutations in both the ClC-Ka and ClC-Kb chloride channels, respectively [17, 36]. The clinical symptoms resulting from this digenic disease are indistinguishable from those of Barttin-deficient patients. This observation not only proves the concept of the functional interaction of barttin with both ClC-K isoforms but also excludes important other functions of Barttin not related to ClC-K channel interaction.

Disorders of the DCT, Classic Bartter Syndrome, Gitelman Syndrome, and EAST Syndrome

The Basolateral Chloride Channel ClC-Kb

In the context of a normal ClC-Ka function, an isolated defect of ClC-Kb which is encoded by the *CLCNKB* gene leads to a more variable phenotype. Several studies have indicated that the clinical variability is not related to a certain type of mutation [37, 38]. Even the most deleterious mutation, which implies the absence of the complete *CLCNKB* gene and which affects nearly 50% of patients, can cause varying degrees of disease severity. Features of tubular dysfunction distal from the TAL predominate, suggesting a major role of ClC-Kb along the DCT. Although TAL salt transport can be impaired to a variable extent, its function is never completely perturbed. Obviously, alternative routes of basolateral chloride exit can be recruited in the TAL segment, most likely via ClC-Ka.

With respect to renal function, the neonatal period in ClC-Kb-deficient patients usually passes without major problems. Maternal polyhydramnios is observed in only one fourth of the patients and usually is mild. Accordingly, duration of pregnancy is not substantially shortened. More than half of the patients are diagnosed within the first year of life. Symptoms at initial presentation include failure to thrive, dehydration, muscular hypotonia, and lethargy. Laboratory examination typically reveals low plasma chloride concentrations (down to 60 mmol/l), decreased plasma sodium concentration, and severe hypokalemic alkalosis. At first presentation, electrolyte derangement is usually more pronounced as compared to the other variants of BS. However, because renal salt wasting progresses slowly and polyuria may be absent, medical consultation may be delayed. Plasma renin activity is greatly increased, whereas plasma aldosterone concentration is only slightly elevated. This discrepancy might be attributed to negative feed-back regulation of aldosterone incretion by hypokalemia and alkalosis. Therefore, normal or slightly elevated aldosterone levels under conditions of profound hypokalemic alkalosis are in fact inappropriately low.

Urinary concentrating ability is preserved at least to a certain extent and a number of patients achieve urinary osmolalities above 700 mosmol/kg in morning urine samples. Because renal medullary interstitial hypertonicity is critically dependent on sodium chloride reabsorption in the TAL, the ability to concentrate urine above 700 mosmol/kg indicates nearly intact TAL function despite of ClC-Kb deficiency. Moreover, the integrity of TAL function is also reflected by the finding that hypercalciuria is not a typical feature of ClC-Kb dysfunction and – if present – occurs only temporarily. The majority of patients exhibit normal or even low urinary calcium excretion. Accordingly, medullary nephrocalcinosis – a hallmark of pure TAL dysfunction – is rare. The plasma magnesium concentration gradually decreases over time owing to impaired renal magnesium conservation, as is observed in other forms of abnormal DCT function. Accordingly, several ClC-Kb deficient patients exhibit both hypomagnesemia and hypocalciuria, a constellation which usually is thought to be highly indicative for an NCCT-defect. ClC-Kb deficiency thus may mimic GS.

The symptoms associated with defects of ClC-Kb largely parallel the disease phenotype reported in Bartter's original description. Therefore, patients with mutations in *CLCNKB* are referred to as cBS. The ethnic origin of Bartter's first patients supports this idea. Both were African Americans, and among this racial group only *CLCNKB* mutations have been identified to date. It has also been suggested that African Americans were affected from BS more frequently and to suffer from a more severe course of the disease. In a study in five African American patients with ClC-Kb mutations, two of them had a history of polyhydramnios which elicited extreme prematurity [39].

Thiazide-Sensitive NaCl- Cotransporter (NCCT)

DCT epithelia contain two cell types: early DCT cells (DCT1) which express the NCCT as its predominant apical sodium entry pathway, and further distal residing late DCT cells (DCT2), which express the epithelial sodium channel (ENaC) as the main pathway for apical sodium reabsorption. Both sodium entry pathways are inducible by aldosterone. Early DCT and late DCT cells probably also differ with respect to their function in divalent cation transport.

Genetic defects in *SLC12A3* encoding NCCT result in only mild renal salt wasting. Initial presentation frequently occurs at school age or later with the characteristic symptoms being muscular weakness, cramps, fatigue, and dwarfism. Not uncommonly, patients are diagnosed accidentally while seeking medical consultation because of growth retardation, constipation or enuresis. Whereas a history of salt craving is common, urinary concentrating ability typically is preserved. Laboratory examination shows a typical constellation of metabolic alkalosis, low normal chloride levels, hypokalemia, and hypomagnesemia, urine analysis shows hypocalciuria. Family studies revealed that electrolyte imbalances are present from infancy, although most of the affected infants displayed no obvious clinical signs. Of note, the combination of hypokalemia and hypomagnesemia exerts an exceptionally unfavorable effect on cardiac excitability, which puts these patients at high risk for cardiac arrhythmia.

The pathognomonic feature of GS is the dissociation of renal calcium and magnesium handling, with low urinary calcium and high urinary magnesium levels. Subsequent hypomagnesemia causes neuromuscular irritability and tetany. Decreased renal calcium elimination together with magnesium deficiency favors deposition of mineral calcium as demonstrated by increased bone density as well as chondrocalcinosis. Although the combination of hypomagnesemia and hypocalciuria is typical for GS, it is neither a specific nor universal finding. Clinical observations in GS patients disclosed intra- and inter-individual variations in urinary calcium concentrations which can be attributed to gender, age-related conditions of bone metabolism, intake of magnesium supplements, changes in diuresis and urinary osmolality, respectively. Likewise, hypomagnesemia might not be present from the beginning. Because less than one percent of total body magnesium is circulating in the blood, renal magnesium loss can be balanced temporarily by magnesium release from bone and muscle stores as well as by an increase of intestinal magnesium reabsorption. Accordingly, the strict definition of hypomagnesemia with coincident hypocalciuria in order to separate GS from cBS appears arbitrary.

The mechanisms compromising distal magnesium reabsorption and favoring reabsorption of calcium are not yet completely understood. The occasional co-existence of hypomagnesemia and hypocalciuria in ClC-Kb deficient patients indicates that this phenomenon is not restricted to NCCT defects but is rather a consequence of impaired transcellular sodium chloride reabsorption along the early DCT. It is tempting to speculate, that with a functional defect of early DCT cells, which in addition to sodium chloride normally reabsorb magnesium by apical TRPM6 magnesium channels, these cells are replaced by late DCT cells, which reabsorb sodium via ENaC channels and calcium via epithelial calcium channels (TRPV5). Accordingly, reabsorption of magnesium would decrease and that of calcium increase. Moreover, other phenomena like for example the redistribution of renal tubular sodium chloride reabsorption to more proximal nephron segments (proximal tubule and TAL) might contribute to alterations in renal calcium and magnesium handling.

Kir4.1 Potassium Channel (KCNJ10, EAST/SeSAME Syndrome)

In 2009, a newly described autosomal recessive clinical syndrome characterized by epilepsy, ataxia, sensorineural deafness and renal salt wasting with/without mental retardation was described under the acronyms EAST or SeSAME syndrome [23, 24]. EAST/SeSAME syndrome is caused by loss of function mutations in the *KCNJ10* gene encoding the inwardly-rectifying potassium channel Kir4.1 [23, 24]. The expression pattern of Kir4.1 fits the disease phenotype with high expression levels in brain, the stria vascularis of the inner ear, and in the distal nephron, especially in the DCT. Here, Kir4.1 is localized at the basolateral membrane of DCT cells where it is thought to function in collaboration with the Na^+K^+-ATPase as it might allow for a recycling of potassium ions entering the tubular cells in countermove for the extruded sodium [24]. Loss of Kir4.1 function most likely leads to a depolarization of the basolateral membrane and thereby to a reduction of the driving force for basolateral anion channels as well as sodium-coupled exchangers. By this mechanism, Kir4.1 defects could also affect the putative Na^+/Mg^{2+} exchanger and possibly explain the magnesium wasting observed in EAST/SeSAME syndrome. Moreover, it could be demonstrated that lack of Kir4.1 decreases basolateral chloride conductance and results is a diminished expression of NCCT in the apical membrane [40]. These results could explain the salt loss observed in EAST/SeSAME patients. Interestingly, the renal phenotype of Kir4.1 knockout mice had not been thoroughly studied until the description of the human disease [41]. However, the reevaluation of Kir4.1 knockout mice clearly demonstrated renal salt wasting leading to significant growth retardation [23].

Patients usually present early in infancy with generalized tonic-clonic seizures, speech and motor delay, as well as severe ataxia leading to an inability to walk, intention tremor, and dysdiadochokinesis. In addition they exhibit a severe hearing impairment. Renal salt wasting may develop or be recognized only later during the course of the disease [42]. Closely resembling GS, the renal phenotype includes the combination of hypokalemic alkalosis, hypomagnesemia and hypocalciuria.

A summary of the most important clinical features and the ordinary age of disease manifestation is given in Table 33.1.

Treatment

As with other hereditary diseases the desirable correction of the primary genetic defects is not yet feasible. In the case of salt-wasting kidney disorders, however, the correction of secondary phenomena like increased renal prostaglandin synthesis or disturbed electrolyte homeostasis have been part of treatment virtually from the first description of the diseases. To the present, the cornerstones in the treatment of renal salt-wasting are non-steroidal anti-inflammatory drugs (NSAID) and long-term electrolyte substitution [1].

In aBS, inhibition of renal and systemic prostaglandin synthesis leads to reduced urinary prostaglandin E_2 (PGE_2) excretion, dramatically decreases polyuria, converts hyposthenuria to isosthenuria, reduces hypercalciuria, and stimulates catch up growth [11, 12, 32]. Maintenance of euvolemia in the immediate postnatal period by meticulous replacement of renal fluid and salt loss is of central importance before starting NSAID therapy, which might precipitate acute renal failure if extracellular volume is depleted. There is long standing experience with the unselective cyclooxygenase (COX) inhibitor indomethacin which is started at 0.05 mg/kg per day and may be gradually increased to 1.5 mg/kg per day according to its effects on urinary output, renal PGE_2-synthesis and blood aldosterone levels. However, the potential benefit of indomethacin in preterm infants and neonates should be weighted against potential risks of severe gastrointestinal complications, e.g., ulcers, perforation and necrotizing enterocolitis [43, 44]. In particular, indomethacin therapy of newborns with ROMK defects may be complicated by oliguric renal failure and severe hyperkalemia. At any age, ROMK-deficient patients are particularly sensitive to indomethacin, with doses well below 1 mg/kg/day sufficient to maintain normal plasma potassium levels.

Gastrointestinal side effects like gastritis and peptic ulcers are also the main drawbacks of longterm indomethacin therapy. These might be reduced by the use of COX-2 specific inhibitors, which show a comparable effect on renal salt wasting but adversely affect blood pressure [45]. A convincing explanation for these unsurpassed effects of NSAIDs is still missing although a reduction of glomerular filtration and blockage of an aberrant tubulo-glomerular feedback certainly are important contributors. Despite these beneficial effects of NSAIDs, lifelong substitution of potassium chloride usually is required to prevent life-threatening episodes of hypokalemia. Additional potassium supplementation is more often required for NKCC2-deficient than ROMK-deficient patients [1, 32]. In single patients, treatment with a potassium-sparing diuretic (e.g., spironolactone) has been shown to effectively increase serum potassium levels. Also ACE inhibitors have been used in a few patients with

Table 33.1 Age at manifestation and leading symptoms of genetically defined renal salt wasting disorders

	NKCC2	ROMK	Barttin	ClC-Kb	NCCT	Kir4.1
Phenotype	Antenatal Bartter syndrome	Antenatal Bartter syndrome	BSND	Classic Bartter syndrome	Gitelman syndrome	EAST/SeSAME syndrome
Polyhydramnios	+++	+++	+++	+	−	−
Age at first manifestation	Perinatal	Perinatal	Perinatal	0–5 years	>5 years	Infancy
Leading symptoms	Polyuria	Polyuria	Polyuria	Hypokalemia	Hypokalemia	Ataxia
	Hypochloremia	Hypochloremia	Hypochloremia	Hypochloremia	Hypomagnesemia	Deafness
	Alkalosis	Alkalosis	Alkalosis	Alkalosis	Alkalosis	Hypokalemia
	Hypokalemia	Initially hyperkalemia, later hypokalemia	Hypokalemia	Failure to thrive	Hypocalciuria	Hypomagnesemia
	Nephrocalcinosis	Nephrocalcinosis	Deafness		Growth retardation	Alkalosis
						Hypocalciuria

success but should be used with caution because ACE inhibitors could impair the compensatory mechanisms for sodium reabsorption in the more distal nephron. Thiazides should not be used to reduce hypercalciuria, since they interfere with compensatory mechanisms in the DCT and further aggravate salt and fluid losses.

Patients with BSND are managed primarily with intravenous fluids in neonatal intensive care units. In contrast to other forms of aBS, and despite high levels of urinary PGE_2, the effect of indomethacin on growth and correction of electrolyte disorders is rather poor [35, 46]. Hypokalemic metabolic alkalosis persists despite high doses of sodium chloride and potassium chloride supplementation [35]. In a single patient, combined therapy with indomethacin and captopril was needed to discontinue intravenous fluids and improve weight gain [47]. A pre-emptive nephrectomy for refractory electrolyte and fluid losses and persistent failure to thrive, followed by peritoneal dialysis and successful renal transplantation has been reported in a 1-year old child with BSND [48].

Patients with cBS are typically treated with NSAIDs. Indomethacin is the most frequently used drug, usually started within the first years of life at doses ranging from 1 to 2.5 mg/kg/day. Potassium supplementation (usually KCl, 1–3 mmol/kg/day) is mandatory in cBS, as hypokalemia is often severe at presentation and is not fully corrected by indomethacin (D89). If potassium chloride alone fails to correct hypokalemia, then addition of spironolactone (1–1.5 mg/kg/day) is recommended. ACE-inhibitors should be given with caution because of the risk of hypotension. Magnesium supplementation should be added when hypomagnesemia is present, but the correction is typically difficult [32].

In patients with GS, unrestricted salt intake and magnesium and potassium supplementations are the main therapeutic measures. Magnesium supplementation should be considered first, since magnesium repletion will facilitate potassium repletion and reduce the risk of tetany and other complications related to hypomagnesemia [49, 50]. All types of magnesium salts are effective, but their bioavailability is variable. Magnesium chloride, magnesium lactate and magnesium aspartate show higher bioavailability [49]. Magnesium chloride is recommended since it will also correct the urinary loss of chloride. The dose of magnesium must be adjusted individually in three to four daily administrations, with diarrhea being the limiting factor. In addition to magnesium, high doses of oral potassium chloride supplements (up to 10 mmol/kg/day in children) may be required [51]. Importantly, magnesium and potassium supplementation results in a catchup growth [52, 53]. Spironolactone or amiloride can be useful, both to increase serum potassium levels in patients resistant to potassium chloride supplements and to treat magnesium depletion that is worsened by elevated aldosterone levels [54]. Both drugs should be started cautiously to avoid hypotension. Patients should not be denied their usual salt craving, particularly if they practice regular physical activity. Following the pathophysiology with salt loss distal to the *macula densa* and thus not involving disturbances of the tubuloglomerular feedback, prostaglandin inhibitors are less frequently used in GS, since urinary PGE_2 levels are usually normal. However, in a recent controlled, randomized crossover study, Blanchard et al. demonstrated that indomethacin in GS effectively increases potassium levels. In this study, it was even more effective than amiloride or eplerenone [55]. Considering the occurrence of prolonged QT interval in up to half GS patients [56, 57], QT-prolonging medications should be used with caution.

Although GS adversely affects the quality of life [58], information about the long-term outcome of these patients are lacking. Renal function and growth appear to be normal, provided lifelong supplementation. Progression to renal failure is extremely rare in GS: only two patients with GS who developed end-stage renal disease have been reported [59, 60].

Conclusion

Parallel loss of sodium and chloride from disturbed renal tubular function is the basis of several distinct diseases, which differ with respect to the degree of ECV-contraction and secondary electrolyte derangements. Common features of all combined sodium chloride transport defects are hypokalemia, hypochloremia, and metabolic alkalosis. Clarification of the underlying genetic defects has contributed greatly to understanding the contribution of the affected proteins to renal salt transport.

References

1. Jeck N, Schlingmann KP, Reinalter SC, Komhoff M, Peters M, Waldegger S, Seyberth HW. Salt handling in the distal nephron: lessons learned from inherited human disorders. Am J Physiol Regul Integr Comp Physiol. 2005;288:R782–95.
2. Rosenbaum P, Hughes M. Persistent, probably congenital, hypokalemic metabolic alkalosis with hyaline degeneration of renal tubules and normal urinary aldosterone. Am J Dis Child. 1957;94:560.
3. Bartter FC, Pronove P, Gill Jr JR, Maccardle RC. Hyperplasia of the juxtaglomerular complex with hyperaldosteronism and hypokalemic alkalosis. A new syndrome. Am J Med. 1962;33:811–28.
4. Gitelman HJ, Graham JB, Welt LG. A new familial disorder characterized by hypokalemia and hypomagnesemia. Trans Assoc Am Phys. 1966;79:221–35.
5. Rodriguez-Soriano J, Vallo A, Garcia-Fuentes M. Hypomagnesaemia of hereditary renal origin. Pediatr Nephrol. 1987;1:465–72.
6. Bettinelli A, Bianchetti MG, Girardin E, Caringella A, Cecconi M, Appiani AC, Pavanello L, Gastaldi R, Isimbaldi C, Lama G, et al. Use of calcium excretion values to distinguish two forms of primary renal tubular hypokalemic alkalosis: Bartter and Gitelman syndromes. J Pediatr. 1992;120:38–43.
7. Bartter FC, Pronove P, Gill Jr JR, MacCardle RC. Hyperplasia of the juxtaglomerular complex with hyperaldosteronism and hypokalemic alkalosis. A new syndrome. J Am Soc Nephrol. 1962;9:516–28.
8. Fanconi A, Schachenmann G, Nussli R, Prader A. Chronic hypokalaemia with growth retardation, normotensive hyperrenin-hyperaldosteronism ("Bartter's syndrome"), and hypercalciuria. Report of two cases with emphasis on natural history and on catch-up growth during treatment. Helv Paediatr Acta. 1971;26:144–63.
9. McCredie DA, Blair-West JR, Scoggins BA, Shipman R. Potassium-losing nephropathy of childhood. Med J Aust. 1971;1:129–35.
10. Ohlsson A, Sieck U, Cumming W, Akhtar M, Serenius F. A variant of Bartter's syndrome. Bartter's syndrome associated with hydramnios, prematurity, hypercalciuria and nephrocalcinosis. Acta Paediatr Scand. 1984;73:868–74.
11. Seyberth HW, Koniger SJ, Rascher W, Kuhl PG, Schweer H. Role of prostaglandins in hyperprostaglandin E syndrome and in selected renal tubular disorders. Pediatr Nephrol. 1987;1:491–7.
12. Seyberth HW, Rascher W, Schweer H, Kuhl PG, Mehls O, Scharer K. Congenital hypokalemia with hypercalciuria in preterm infants: a hyperprostaglandinuric tubular syndrome different from Bartter syndrome. J Pediatr. 1985;107:694–701.
13. Landau D, Shalev H, Ohaly M, Carmi R. Infantile variant of Bartter syndrome and sensorineural deafness: a new autosomal recessive disorder. Am J Med Genet. 1995;59:454–9.
14. Simon DB, Karet FE, Hamdan JM, DiPietro A, Sanjad SA, Lifton RP. Bartter's syndrome, hypokalaemic alkalosis with hypercalciuria, is caused by mutations in the Na-K-2Cl cotransporter NKCC2. Nat Genet. 1996;13:183–8.
15. Simon DB, Karet FE, Rodriguez-Soriano J, Hamdan JH, DiPietro A, Trachtman H, Sanjad SA, Lifton RP. Genetic heterogeneity of Bartter's syndrome revealed by mutations in the K+ channel, ROMK. Nat Genet. 1996;14:152–6.
16. Birkenhager R, Otto E, Schurmann MJ, Vollmer M, Ruf EM, Maier-Lutz I, Beekmann F, Fekete A, Omran H, Feldmann D, Milford DV, Jeck N, Konrad M, Landau D, Knoers NV, Antignac C, Sudbrak R, Kispert A, Hildebrandt F. Mutation of BSND causes Bartter syndrome with sensorineural deafness and kidney failure. Nat Genet. 2001;29:310–4.
17. Schlingmann KP, Konrad M, Jeck N, Waldegger P, Reinalter SC, Holder M, Seyberth HW, Waldegger S. Salt wasting and deafness resulting from mutations in two chloride channels. N Engl J Med. 2004;350:1314–9.
18. Simon DB, Bindra RS, Mansfield TA, Nelson-Williams C, Mendonca E, Stone R, Schurman S, Nayir A, Alpay H, Bakkaloglu A, Rodriguez-Soriano J, Morales JM, Sanjad SA, Taylor CM, Pilz D, Brem A, Trachtman H, Griswold W, Richard GA, John E, Lifton RP. Mutations in the chloride channel gene, CLCNKB, cause Bartter's syndrome type III. Nat Genet. 1997;17:171–8.
19. Simon DB, Nelson-Williams C, Bia MJ, Ellison D, Karet FE, Molina AM, Vaara I, Iwata F, Cushner HM, Koolen M, Gainza FJ, Gitelman HJ, Lifton RP. Gitelman's variant of Bartter's syndrome, inherited hypokalemic alkalosis, is caused by mutations in the thiazide sensitive Na-Cl cotransporter. Nat Genet. 1996;12:24–30.
20. Hebert SC. Bartter syndrome. Curr Opin Nephrol Hypertens. 2003;12:527–32.
21. Watanabe S, Fukumoto S, Chang H, Takeuchi Y, Hasegawa Y, Okazaki R, Chikatsu N, Fujita T. Association between activating mutations of calcium-sensing receptor and Bartter's syndrome. Lancet. 2002;360:692–4.
22. Vargas-Poussou R, Huang C, Hulin P, Houillier P, Jeunemaitre X, Paillard M, Planelles G, Dechaux M, Miller RT, Antignac C. Functional characterization of a calcium-sensing receptor mutation in severe autosomal dominant hypocalcemia with a Bartterlike syndrome. J Am Soc Nephrol. 2002;13:2259–66.

23. Bockenhauer D, Feather S, Stanescu HC, Bandulik S, Zdebik AA, Reichold M, Tobin J, Lieberer E, Sterner C, Landoure G, Arora R, Sirmanna T, Thompson D, Cross JH, van't Hoff W, Al Masri O, Tullus K, Yeung S, Anikster Y, Klootwijk E, Hubank M, Dillon MJ, Heitzmann D, Arcos-Burgos M, Knepper MA, Dobbie A, Gahl WA, Warth R, Sheridan E, Kleta R. Epilepsy, ataxia, sensorineural deafness, tubulopathy, and KCNJ10 mutations. N Engl J Med. 2009;360(19):1960–70.

24. Scholl UI, Choi M, Liu T, Ramaekers VT, Häusller MG, Grimmer J, Tobe SW, Farhi A, Nelson-Williams C, Lifton RP. Seizures, sensorineural deafness, ataxia, mental retardation, and electrolyte imbalance (SeSAME syndrome) caused by mutations in KCNJ10. Proc Natl Acad Sci U S A. 2009;106(14):5842–7.

25. Massa G, Proesmans W, Devlieger H, Vandenberghe K, Van Assche A, Eggermont E. Electrolyte composition of the amniotic fluid in Bartter syndrome. Eur J Obstet Gynecol Reprod Biol. 1987;24:335–40.

26. Proesmans W, Massa G, Vandenberghe K, Van Assche A. Prenatal diagnosis of Bartter syndrome. Lancet. 1987;1:394.

27. Simon DB, Lu Y, Choate KA, Velazquez H, Al-Sabban E, Praga M, Casari G, Bettinelli A, Colussi G, Rodriguez-Soriano J, McCredie D, Milford D, Sanjad S, Lifton RP. Paracellin-1, a renal tight junction protein required for paracellular Mg2+ resorption. Science. 1999;285:103–6.

28. Konrad M, Schaller A, Seelow D, Pandey AV, Waldegger S, Lesslauer A, Vitzthum H, Suzuki Y, Luk JM, Becker C, Schlingmann KP, Schmid M, Rodriguez-Soriano J, Ariceta G, Cano F, Enriquez R, Jueppner H, Bakkaloglu SA, Hediger MA, Gallati S, Neuhauss SCF, Nürnberg P, Weber S. Mutations in the tight-junction gene claudin 19 (CLDN19) are associated with renal magnesium wasting, renal failure, and severe ocular involvement. Am J Hum Genet. 2006;5:949–57.

29. Kamel KS, Oh MS, Halperin ML. Bartter's, Gitelman's, and Gordon's syndromes. From physiology to molecular biology and back, yet still some unanswered questions. Nephron. 2002;92 Suppl 1:18–27.

30. Jeck N, Derst C, Wischmeyer E, Ott H, Weber S, Rudin C, Seyberth HW, Daut J, Karschin A, Konrad M. Functional heterogeneity of ROMK mutations linked to hyperprostaglandin E syndrome. Kidney Int. 2001;59:1803–11.

31. Finer G, Shalev H, Birk OS, Galron D, Jeck N, Sinai-Treiman L, Landau D. Transient neonatal hyperkalemia in the antenatal (ROMK defective) Bartter syndrome. J Pediatr. 2003;142:318–23.

32. Peters M, Jeck N, Reinalter S, Leonhardt A, Tonshoff B, Klaus GG, Konrad M, Seyberth HW. Clinical presentation of genetically defined patients with hypokalemic salt-losing tubulopathies. Am J Med. 2002;112:183–90.

33. Estevez R, Boettger T, Stein V, Birkenhager R, Otto E, Hildebrandt F, Jentsch TJ. Barttin is a Cl- channel beta-subunit crucial for renal Cl- reabsorption and inner ear K+ secretion. Nature. 2001;414:558–61.

34. Waldegger S, Jeck N, Barth P, Peters M, Vitzthum H, Wolf K, Kurtz A, Konrad M, Seyberth HW. Barttin increases surface expression and changes current properties of ClC-K channels. Pflugers Arch. 2002;444:411–8.

35. Jeck N, Reinalter SC, Henne T, Marg W, Mallmann R, Pasel K, Vollmer M, Klaus G, Leonhardt A, Seyberth HW, Konrad M. Hypokalemic salt-losing tubulopathy with chronic renal failure and sensorineural deafness. Pediatrics. 2001;108, E5.

36. Nozu K, Inagaki T, Fu XJ, Nozu Y, Kaito H, Kanda K, Sekine T, Igarashi T, Nakanishi K, Yoshikawa N, Iijima K, Matsuo M. Molecular analysis of digenic inheritance in Bartter syndrome with sensorineural deafness. J Med Genet. 2008;45(3):182–6.

37. Konrad M, Vollmer M, Lemmink HH, van den Heuvel LP, Jeck N, Vargas-Poussou R, Lakings A, Ruf R, Deschenes G, Antignac C, Guay-Woodford L, Knoers NV, Seyberth HW, Feldmann D, Hildebrandt F. Mutations in the chloride channel gene CLCNKB as a cause of classic Bartter syndrome. J Am Soc Nephrol. 2000;11:1449–59.

38. Zelikovic I, Szargel R, Hawash A, Labay V, Hatib I, Cohen N, Nakhoul F. A novel mutation in the chloride channel gene, CLCNKB, as a cause of Gitelman and Bartter syndromes. Kidney Int. 2003;63:24–32.

39. Schurman SJ, Perlman SA, Sutphen R, Campos A, Garin EH, Cruz DN, Shoemaker LR. Genotype/phenotype observations in African Americans with Bartter syndrome. J Pediatr. 2001;139:105–10.

40. Zhang C, Wang L, Zhang J, Su XT, Lin DH, Scholl UI, Giebisch G, Lifton RP, Wang WH. KCNJ10 determines the expression of the apical Na-Cl cotransporter (NCC) in the early distal convoluted tubule (DCT1). Proc Natl Acad Sci U S A. 2014;111(32):11864–9.

41. Neusch C, Rozengurt N, Jacobs RE, Lester HA, Kofuji P. Kir4.1 potassium channel subunit is crucial for oligodendrocyte development and in vivo myelination. J Neurosci. 2001;21(15):5429–38.

42. Scholl UI, Dave HB, Lu M, Farhi A, Nelson-Williams C, Listmann JA, Lifton RP. SeSAME/EAST syndrome – phenotypic variability and delayed activity of the distal convoluted tubule. Pediatr Nephrol. 2012;27:2081–90.

43. Rodriguez-Soriano J. Bartter's syndrome comes of age. Pediatrics. 1999;103:663–4.

44. Vaisbich MH, Fujimura MD, Koch VH. Bartter syndrome: benefits and side effects of long-term treatment. Pediatr Nephrol. 2004;19:858–63.

45. Reinalter SC, Jeck N, Brochhausen C, Watzer B, Nüsing RM, Seyberth HW, Kömhoff M. Role of cyclooxygenase-2 in hyperprostaglandin E syndrome/antenatal Bartter syndrome. Kidney Int. 2002;62:253–60.

46. Shalev H, Ohali M, Kachko L, Landau D. The neonatal variant of Bartter syndrome and deafness: preservation of renal function. Pediatrics. 2003;112:628–33.

47. Zaffanello M, Taranta A, Palma A, Bettinelli A, Marseglia GL, Emma F. Type IV Bartter syndrome: report of two new cases. Pediatr Nephrol. 2006;21:766–70.

48. Chaudhuri A, Salvatierra Jr O, Alexander SR, Sarwal MM. Option of pre-emptive nephrectomy and renal transplantation for Bartter's syndrome. Pediatr Transplant. 2006;10:266–70.

49. Knoers NV. Gitelman syndrome. Adv Chronic Kidney Dis. 2006;13:148–54.

50. Rodríguez-Soriano J. Bartter and related syndromes: the puzzle is almost solved. Pediatr Nephrol. 1998;12:315–27.

51. Shaer AJ. Inherited primary renal tubular hypokalemic alkalosis: a review of Gitelman and Bartter syndromes. Am J Med Sci. 2001;322:316–32.

52. Riveira-Munoz E, Chang Q, Godefroid N, Hoenderop JG, Bindels RJ, Dahan K, Devuyst O, Belgian Network for Study of Gitelman Syndrome. Transcriptional and functional analyses of SLC12A3 mutations: new clues for the pathogenesis of Gitelman syndrome. J Am Soc Nephrol. 2007;18:1271–83.

53. Godefroid N, Riveira-Munoz E, Saint-Martin C, Nassogne MC, Dahan K, Devuyst O. A novel splicing mutation in SLC12A3 associated with Gitelman syndrome and idiopathic intracranial hypertension. Am J Kidney Dis. 2006;48:e73–9.

54. Colussi G, Rombolà G, De Ferrari ME, Macaluso M, Minetti L. Correction of hypokalemia with antialdosterone therapy in Gitelman's syndrome. Am J Nephrol. 1994;14:127–35.

55. Blanchard A, Vargas-Poussou R, Vallet M, Caumont-Prim A, Allard J, Desport E, Dubourg L, Monge M, Bergerot D, Baron S, Essig M, Bridoux F, Tack I, Azizi M. Indomethacin, amiloride, or eplerenone for traiting hypokalemia in Gitelman syndrome. J Am Soc Nephrol. 2015;26:468–75.

56. Bettinelli A, Tosetto C, Colussi G, Tommasini G, Edefonti A, Bianchetti MG. Electrocardiogram with prolonged QT interval in Gitelman disease. Kidney Int. 2002;62:580–4.

57. Foglia PE, Bettinelli A, Tosetto C, Cortesi C, Crosazzo L, Edefonti A, Bianchetti MG. Cardiac work up in primary renal hypokalaemia-hypomagnesaemia (Gitelman syndrome). Nephrol Dial Transplant. 2004;19:1398–402.

58. Cruz DN, Simon DB, Nelson-Williams C, Farhi A, Finberg K, Burleson L, Gill JR, Lifton RP. Mutations in the Na-Cl cotransporter reduce blood pressure in humans. Hypertension. 2001;37:1458–64.

59. Bonfante L, Davis PA, Spinello M, Antonello A, D'Angelo A, Semplicini A, Calò L. Chronic renal failure, end-stage renal disease, and peritoneal dialysis in Gitelman's syndrome. Am J Kidney Dis. 2001;38:165–8.

60. Calò LA, Marchini F, Davis PA, Rigotti P, Pagnin E, Semplicini A. Kidney transplant in Gitelman's syndrome. Report of the first case. J Nephrol. 2003;16:144–7.

Disorders of Calcium and Magnesium Metabolism

34

Martin Konrad and Karl Peter Schlingmann

Calcium Physiology

Approximately 1 kg of the adult human body consists of elemental Ca^{2+} of which 99 % are bound in bone. The extracellular fluid contains only ~1000 mg of Ca^{2+}. Following recommendations of national boards of nutrition 800–1200 mg of Ca^{2+} should be taken up daily with a normal diet [1]. The intestine reabsorbs approximately 25–33 % of the nutritional Ca^{2+} content [2]. In the kidney, ~800 mg of Ca^{2+} are filtered per day in the glomeruli of which 99 % are reabsorbed along the renal tubule. Only ~10 mg (~0.1 mg/kg/day) are excreted with the urine. In serum, ~50 % of Ca^{2+} are present in the free ionized form, ~35 % are protein-bound, and ~15 % are complexed to bicarbonate, citrate or phosphate. The physiological range for blood Ca^{2+} equals 1.1–1.35 mmol/L for free, ionized Ca^{2+} and 2.2–2.6 mmol/L for total Ca^{2+} (in the presence of physiological whole protein levels) [3]. Only the free, ionized fraction is responsible for the biological Ca^{2+} effects.

Blood Ca^{2+} levels are kept within a narrow physiological range by the concerted action of hormonal systems that control intestinal Ca^{2+} uptake, renal Ca^{2+} excretion, and Ca^{2+} transport in bone and soft tissues. The hormonal control systems comprise the parathyroid gland, active 1,25-$(OH)_2$-vitamin D_3, and the bone-derived, phosphaturic hormone FGF-23 [4]. All three systems are tightly linked and influence each other's activity. Parathyroid hormone (PTH) increases intestinal Ca^{2+} absorption and Ca^{2+} release from bone; it promotes renal Ca^{2+} reabsorption while stimulating renal phosphate excretion. In contrast, active 1,25-$(OH)_2$-vitamin D_3 promotes intestinal Ca^{2+} and phosphate absorption as well as renal Ca^{2+} and phosphate conservation, thereby ensuring sufficient Ca^{2+} and phosphate supply for bone mineralization. Finally, FGF-23 together with its co-factor klotho increases renal phosphate excretion by inhibiting proximal tubular phosphate reabsorption [5]. In addition, FGF-23 also negatively regulates Vitamin D by inhibiting its activation and promoting its degradation. The common aim of this hormonal interplay is to keep extracellular Ca^{2+} levels constant while supplying sufficient amounts of Ca^{2+} for soft tissues and bone mineralization.

Disturbances of Calcium Homeostasis

Disturbances in Ca^{2+} metabolism comprise states of Ca^{2+} deficiency as well as Ca^{2+} excess usually detected in the form of hypo- or hypercalcemia.

M. Konrad (✉) • K.P. Schlingmann
Department of General Pediatrics, University Children's Hospital Münster, Waldeyerstrasse 22, Münster 48149, Germany
e-mail: konradma@uni-muenster.de; karlpeter.schlingmann@ukmuenster.de

© Springer-Verlag Berlin Heidelberg 2016
D.F. Geary, F. Schaefer (eds.), *Pediatric Kidney Disease*, DOI 10.1007/978-3-662-52972-0_34

Whereas hypocalcemia represents a more common finding and is usually apparent by typical clinical signs and symptoms, hypercalcemia in infancy and childhood is a rare event and may remain unrecognized as clinical symptoms are rather unspecific. An overview on symptoms, causes, and the diagnostic work-up of pediatric hypocalcemia as well as hypercalcemia is provided in Chap. 31. Here, we focus on hereditary disorders of Ca^{2+} metabolism. These typically manifest with characteristic changes in serum and urine Ca^{2+} levels. As for acquired disorders of Ca^{2+} homeostasis, the diagnostic work-up, next to the parallel measurement of serum and urine electrolytes and creatinine, comprises the determination of PTH and vitamin D metabolites. Not only for the nephrologist, the assessment of urinary Ca^{2+} excretion rates provides an important information on inappropriate renal Ca^{2+} conservation in face of Ca^{2+} deficiency. Reference values for renal Ca^{2+} excretion in infants and children are provided in Table 34.1 [6]. Metz reviewed data available for infants and children, provided an age-dependent logarithmic equation, and proposed cut-offs for hypercalciuria [7]. For the definition of hypocalciuria (i.e., in patients with Gitelman syndrome, see below), Bianchetti et al. suggest to multiply the values for the 5th percentile by the factor of 3 [8].

Table 34.1 Reference ranges for urinary calcium excretion in children

Age (years)	Urinary Ca/Crea mg/mg (mol/mol)	
	5th percentile	95th percentile
0–1	0.03 (0.09)	0.81 (2.2)
1–2	0.03 (0.07)	0.56 (1.5)
2–3	0.02 (0.06)	0.50 (1.4)
3–5	0.02 (0.05)	0.41 (1.1)
5–7	0.01 (0.04)	0.30 (0.8)
7–10	0.01 (0.04)	0.25 (0.7)
10–14	0.01 (0.04)	0.24 (0.7)
14–17	0.01 (0.04)	0.24 (0.7)

Used with permission of Nature Publishing Group from Matos et al. [6]

Hypocalcemia

Following the approach outlined in Chap. 31 (Table 31.19), the etiology of Ca^{2+} deficiency and hypocalcemia can be divided into different entities according to the serum level of PTH [9]. Low levels of PTH indicate a primary dysfunction of the parathyroid gland with impaired or absent PTH production or release. Hereditary disorders involving an abnormal parathyroid gland function include primary hypoparathyroidism due to mutations in the *PTH* gene, due to DiGeorge syndrome caused by microdeletions on chromosome 22q11, or due to HDR syndrome (hypoparathyroidism, deafness, renal abnormalities) with underlying mutations in the transcription factor GATA3. Inappropriately low or normal levels of

PTH may point to an activating mutation in the *CASR* gene encoding the Ca^{2+} sensing-receptor (CaSR) causing autosomal-dominant hypocalcemia (ADH). This entity will be discussed in more detail below. It might be differentiated from the above mentioned disorders by determination of urinary Ca^{2+} excretion: In contrast to low urinary Ca^{2+} excretions found in primary forms of parathyroid dysfunction, urinary Ca^{2+} excretions are inappropriately high in face of hypocalcemia in patients with ADH. Elevated levels of PTH in the presence of a normal renal function are also found in acquired Ca^{2+}- and vitamin D-deficient rickets. Whereas hypocalcemia might also be an associated finding in renal Fanconi syndrome, it is rather uncommon in other disorders of the proximal tubule such as hypophosphatemic rickets, Dent's disease or Lowe syndrome. These disorders are all discussed in detail in Chap. 32.

A heterogeneous group of rare hereditary disorders leading to the common feature of PTH end-organ resistance and hypocalcemia despite elevated PTH serum levels is pseudohypoparathyroidism. Different genetic defects have been discovered as the underlying cause including loss of function mutations in the *GNAS* gene encoding the Gs-alpha isoform or methylation defects of the *GNAS* gene locus [10].

The extracellular Ca^{2+}/Mg^{2+}-sensing receptor (CaSR) plays an essential role in Ca^{2+} and Mg^{2+} homeostasis by influencing not only PTH secretion but also by directly regulating the rate of Ca^{2+} and Mg^{2+} reabsorption in the kidney.

More than 20 years after its first description [11], the precise role of the CaSR for divalent cation metabolism is still not fully understood. In the kidney, the CaSR is expressed at the basolateral membrane of epithelial cells of the distal nephron, predominantly in the TAL [12].

It is well established that changes in extracellular Ca^{2+} concentration influence the transport of salt, water, Ca^{2+}, and Mg^{2+} in the distal renal tubule. According to the traditional hypothesis, the CaSR is involved in all of these adaptations induced by changes in extracellular Ca^{2+}. However, this assumption has been challenged by recent experimental evidence that the renal CaSR specifically controls tubular Ca^{2+} and Mg^{2+} transport in the TAL, independent of PTH, whereas it does not significantly alter water or salt transport [13]. These novel findings appear to be important for our understanding of the pathophysiology of CaSR mutations described below.

Autosomal Dominant Hypoparathyroidism (OMIM #601198)

Autosomal dominant hypoparathyroidism (ADH) is caused by activating mutations in the *CASR* gene. Affected patients typically manifest during childhood with seizures or carpopedal spasms. Laboratory evaluation reveals the typical combination of hypocalcemia and low PTH levels. Serum Ca^{2+} levels are typically in a range of 1.50–1.75 mmol/L. In addition, many patients also exhibit moderate hypomagnesemia [14, 15]. Patients are often given the incorrect diagnosis of primary hypoparathyroidism on the basis of inappropriately low PTH levels. As indicated above, the differential diagnosis can be established by determination of urinary Ca^{2+} excretions, which are low in primary hypoparathyroidism whereas ADH patients exhibit increased renal Ca^{2+} excretions. The differentiation of ADH from primary hypoparathyroidism is of particular importance because treatment with vitamin D in ADH may result in a dramatic increase in hypercalciuria and the

occurrence of nephrocalcinosis and impairment of renal function. Therefore, therapy with vitamin D or Ca^{2+} supplementation should be reserved for symptomatic patients with the aim to maintain serum Ca^{2+} levels just sufficient for the relief of symptoms [15].

Activating *CASR* mutations lead to a lower setpoint of the receptor or an increased affinity for extracellular Ca^{2+} and Mg^{2+}. This inadequate activation by physiological extracellular Ca^{2+} and Mg^{2+} levels results in diminished PTH secretion in the parathyroid gland as well as a decreased reabsorption of both divalent cations mainly in the cTAL of the kidney tubule. A severe degree of hypocalcemia and hypomagnesemia is observed in patients with complete activation of the CaSR at physiologic serum Ca^{2+} and Mg^{2+} concentrations who also exhibit a Bartter-like phenotype [16]. In these patients, CaSR activation inhibits TAL mediated salt and divalent cation reabsorption to an extent that cannot be compensated in later nephron segments [16].

Hypercalcemia

In contrast to hypocalcemia, hypercalcemia represents a rather uncommon finding in infancy and childhood, but requires prompt diagnostic workup and targeted therapy [17, 18]. Hypercalcemia is defined as ionized Ca^{2+} levels above 1.35 mmol/L, usually with a concomitant elevation of total serum Ca^{2+} levels above 2.7 mmol/L. While most children with a mild degree of hypercalcemia remain asymptomatic, more severe hypercalcemia can lead to a serious clinical disease pattern that may even be life-threatening. Symptoms of hypercalcemia include failure to thrive, weight loss, dehydration, fever, muscular hypotonia, constipation, irritability, lethargy, and disturbed consciousness. Cardiovascular findings may comprise bradycardia, shortened QT interval, and arterial hypertension (Table 34.2).

An impairment of renal function by volume contraction can further limit renal Ca^{2+} elimination and therefore aggravate the excess in serum Ca^{2+} levels. On the other hand, the increase of renal Ca^{2+} excretion in hypercalcemic conditions

Table 34.2 Symptoms of acute hypercalcemia

Nervous system
Muscle weakness
Irritability/confusion
Somnolence, stupor, coma
Abnormal behaviour
Headaches
Gastrointestinal tract
Loss of appetite
Nausea/vomiting
Constipation
Abdominal cramping
Pancreatitis
Kidneys and urinary tract
Polyuria/ polydipsia
Dehydratation
Nephrocalcinosis
Nephro-/urolithiasis
Musculoskeletal system
Bone pain
Ectopic calcifications
Heart/cardiovascular system
Shortened QT-intervall
Cardiac arrhythmia
Arterial hypertension

Table 34.3 Evaluation of hypercalcemia in children

Laboratory tests	
Blood	Ionized and total calcium
	Sodium, potassium, chloride, magnesium, and phosphate
	Retention parameters
	Alkaline phosphatase
	Blood gases
	Intact parathyroid hormone (iPTH)
	Vitamin D metabolites (25-OH-D$_3$, 1,25-(OH)$_2$-D$_3$)
Optional	PTH-related peptide (PTHrP)
	Vitamin A
	Angiotensin converting enzyme (ACE)
	FISH (Williams-Beuren syndrome)
Urine	Calcium
	Creatinine
	– > calculation of Ca/creatinine ratio and tubular phosphate reabsorption
	Sodium, potassium, chloride, magnesium, and phosphate
Imaging studies	
	Ultrasound examination of kidneys and urinary tract
Optional	X-ray studies (long bones, thorax)
	Ultrasound of parathyroid glands
	Scintigraphy of parathyroid glands

is a risk factor for the development of nephrocalcinosis and stone formation.

The assessment of the patient's past medical history should comprise medications including over-the-counter vitamin preparations and family history with a focus on disturbances in Ca^{2+} metabolism, renal disease and urolithiasis.

The etiology of hypercalcemia in children and especially infants significantly differs from that in adulthood where primary hyperparathyroidism and malignancy represent the most common underlying causes [19]. In early life, the time at which symptoms occur may yield an important information on the underlying etiology, especially in infants rare hereditary disorders should be considered in the differential diagnosis [17].

The diagnostic work-up, next to a thorough medical history, therefore requires comprehensive laboratory testings including molecular genetics. Next to the parallel measurement of serum and urine electrolytes, the determination

of PTH and vitamin D metabolites represents the most important element. Potential diagnostic parameters are summarized in Table 34.3.

Inappropriately normal or elevated levels of PTH point to a primary defect in the parathyroid gland (Fig. 34.1). Next to primary hyperparathyroidism which is extremely rare in infancy and childhood, hypercalcemia caused by elevated PTH might be caused by a hereditary disorder of the CaSR. In contrast to dominant activating mutations as present in ADH (see above), inactivating mutations can be present in either heterozygous or homozygous/compound-heterozygous state leading to Familial Hypocalciuric Hypercalcemia (FHH) and Neonatal Severe Hyperparathyroidism (NSHPT), respectively (see below).

In face of an appropriate suppression of PTH, vitamin D metabolites should be evaluated. The determination of 25-OH-vitamin D$_3$ primarily helps to exclude overt vitamin D intoxication. While cut-off values vary in the literature, usually

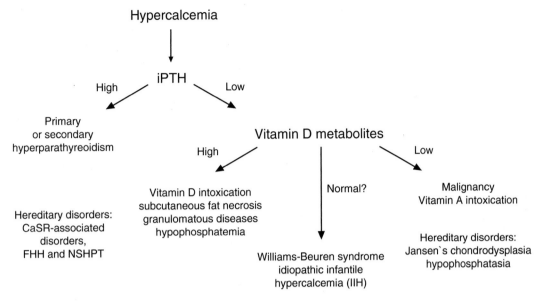

Hypercalcemia

iPTH

High — Primary or secondary hyperparathyreoidism

Low — Vitamin D metabolites

High — Vitamin D intoxication subcutaneous fat necrosis granulomatous diseases hypophosphatemia

Normal? — Williams-Beuren syndrome idiopathic infantile hypercalcemia (IIH)

Low — Malignancy Vitamin A intoxication

Hereditary disorders: CaSR-associated disorders, FHH and NSHPT

Hereditary disorders: Jansen's chondrodysplasia hypophosphatasia

Fig. 34.1 Diagnostic approach in hypercalcemia in childhood. Central diagnostic steps are the determination of parathyroid hormone (PTH) and vitamin D metabolites. Following this diagnostic approach, three major entities can be discerned: PTH-dependent hypercalcemia as present in primary hyperparathyroidism and in disorders due to inactivating mutation of the CaSR, vitamin D-induced hypercalcemia including idiopathic infantile hypercalcemia, and hypercalcemia due to third causes including also hypophosphatasia

levels above 200 ng/mL are regarded as toxic [20]. Besides, serum levels of active $1,25\text{-}(OH)_2$-vitamin D_3 are of critical importance for further diagnostic considerations (Fig. 34.1). Elevated levels are not only observed in vitamin D poisoning, but also in disorders with extra-renal expression of 1α-hydroxylase including granulomatous disease or subcutaneous fat necrosis. In these disorders, 1α-hydroxylase (CYP27B1) is expressed by monocytes and not, as in the kidney, regulated by serum Ca^{2+}, phosphate, PTH, and $1,25\text{-}(OH)_2$-vitamin D_3.

Until recently, two disease entities, namely Williams-Beuren syndrome and idiopathic infantile hypercalcemia, remained unclassifiable as measurement of vitamin D metabolites in affected patients had yielded contradictory results.

Acute therapeutic measures in hypercalcemic patients primarily aim at the lowering of serum Ca^{2+} levels into the reference range resulting in a rapid relief of clinical symptoms. For this purpose, different pharmacologic approaches have been considered (Table 34.4).

Before clarification of the underlying etiology, vitamin D supplements need to be stopped and, if adequate, a low-Ca^{2+} diet should be

Table 34.4 Therapy of hypercalcemia in children

General measures
Stop of vitamin D supplements
Calcium restriction in enteral and parenteral nutrition
Specific measures
Promotion of renal calcium excretion
Furosemide 0.5–1 mg/kg q.6 h
Inhibition of enteral calcium absorption/inhibition of vitamin D-conversion
Glucocorticoids, i.e., methylprednisolone ~1 mg/kg q.6 h
Sodium cellulose phosphate
Inhibition of calcium release from bone
Bisphosphonates, i.e., pamidronate 0.5–1 mg/kg over 4–6 h
Calcitonin 4–8 IU/kg
Inhibition of vitamin D-activation by 1α-hydroxylase
Imidazole derivates, i.e., ketoconazole 3–9 mg/kg per day
Hemodialysis/hemofiltration

implemented. Vigorous rehydration, usually performed via the intravenous route, is a central component of every therapeutic strategy.

Quantities up to twice the daily fluid requirements have been described. The pharmacologic treatment includes therapeutic measures to decrease Ca^{2+} absorption from the intestine, to promote renal Ca^{2+} excretion, as well as to inhibit Ca^{2+} release from bone. For the increase of renal Ca^{2+} elimination, loop diuretics such as furosemide, which inhibits passive paracellular Ca^{2+} reabsorption in the thick ascending limb by blocking active transcellular salt reabsorption, are widely used. A fast and effective approach to inhibit enteral Ca^{2+} absorption is the administration of glucocorticoids, i.e., prednisolone. Next to this intestinal effect, glucocorticoids also inhibit the conversion of 25-OH-vitamin D_3 into active 1,25-$(OH)_2$-vitamin D_3, an effect that is of special importance in vitamin D-mediated hypercalcemia. Sodium cellulose phosphate (SCP) is a non-absorbable cation exchange resin used for the removal of excess Ca^{2+} from the body [21]. It was initially used in patients with so-called absorptive hypercalciuria in order to decrease renal Ca^{2+} excretions and prevent stone formation [22]. In the acute phase of hypercalcemia calcitonin may be used because of its prompt and pronounced effect on serum Ca^{2+} levels; however, its therapeutic usefulness is limited by its short duration of action due to the development of end organ resistance. In the presence of intermediate to severe symptomatic hypercalcemia, bisphosphonates such as pamidronate are used [23]. If bisphosphonate therapy is considered, it is important to have the diagnostic work-up completed in advance to avoid misinterpretation of diagnostic tests for PTH and vitamin D metabolites. A class of drugs that are specifically used in vitamin D-mediated hypercalcemia are imidazole derivates such as ketoconazole [24]. Next to their antifungal effect they also inhibit mammalian cytochrome P450 enzymes. Via inhibition of 1 α-hydroxylase (CYP27B1) they are able to effectively lower serum levels of active 1,25-$(OH)_2$-vitamin D_3 and consecutively normalize serum Ca^{2+} levels. In patients with extremely high serum Ca^{2+} levels hemofiltration and hemodialysis have been performed with success [25].

Hypercalcemia with Inappropriately High PTH

Familial Hypocalciuric Hypercalcemia (OMIM #145980)/Neonatal Severe Hyperparathyroidism (OMIM #239200)

Familial hypocalciuric hypercalcemia (FHH) and neonatal severe hyperparathyroidism (NSHPT) result from inactivating mutations of the CaSR present in either heterozygous or homozygous (or compound heterozygous) state, respectively [26]. FHH patients normally present with mild to moderate hypercalcemia, accompanied by few if any symptoms and often do not require treatment (Table 34.8). Urinary excretion rates for Ca^{2+} and Mg^{2+} are markedly reduced and serum PTH levels are inappropriately high. In addition, affected individuals also show mild hypermagnesemia [27].

In contrast, NSHPT patients with two mutant CaSR alleles usually present in early infancy with polyuria and dehydration due to severe symptomatic hypercalcemia (Table 34.8). Unrecognized and untreated, hyperparathyroidism and hypercalcemia result in skeletal deformities, extraosseous calcifications, and also a severe neurodevelopmental deficit. Early treatment with partial-to-total parathyroidectomy therefore seems to be essential for outcome [28]. Data on serum Mg^{2+} in NSHPT are sparse. However, elevations to levels around 50 % above the reference range have been reported.

Hypercalcemia with Suppressed PTH and Inappropriately High 1,25-$(OH)_2$-Vitamin D_3

Idiopathic Infantile Hypercalcemia (OMIM #143880)

Idiopathic Infantile Hypercalcemia was first decribed in the 1950s after an epidemic occurrence in the United Kingdom [29, 30]. Affected infants clinically present with typical symptoms of severe hypercalcemia. Concomitant hypercalciuria typically leads to the development of early nephrocalcinosis (Table 34.8). The laboratory analysis reveals serum Ca^{2+} levels up to 5 mmol/L. Intact PTH is suppressed while levels of active $1,25\text{-}(OH)_2\text{-vitamin } D_3$ are usually elevated or in the upper normal range. Early, a connection to exogenous vitamin D was suspected as high doses of up to 4000 IU vitamin D per day were used in infants in the UK while there was no increased incidence at the same time in the US where traditionally lower doses of vitamin D supplements were used for the prevention of rickets. Later, similar observations were also made in other European countries, i.e., Poland [31]. Some children exhibited a complex phenotype that became later known as the Williams Beuren syndrome [32, 33]. However, most hypercalcemic infants did not have syndromic features and were considered to be affected by a milder variant of the syndrome that was termed idiopathic infantile hypercalcemia (IIH) [29, 30].

The pathophysiology of IIH remained unknown until the recent discovery of loss-of-function mutations in the vitamin D catabolizing enzyme 25-OH-vitamin D_3-24-hydroxylase (CYP24A1) [34]. CYP24A1 is responsible for several sequential degradation steps that convert active $1,25\text{-}(OH)_2\text{-vitamin } D_3$ into water soluble calcitroic acid [35, 36]. Loss-of-function mutations of *CYP24A1* lead to an accumulation and increased action of active $1,25\text{-}(OH)_2\text{-vitamin } D_3$. Functional studies *in vitro* demonstrated a complete loss of enzyme function for most of the identified *CYP24A1* mutations [34]. In addition to the genetic analysis of the *CYP24A1* gene, the determination of 24-hydroxylated vitamin D metabolites by liquid chromatography/mass spectrometry (LC/MS) represents a quick and reliable test in the diagnosis of the disease [37].

The critical role of a certain cumulative dose of exogenous vitamin D is underscored by the following observations: Under the most commonly used dose of 500 IU vitamin D_3 per day, symptoms usually develop after several months, most likely with an incomplete penetrance of the genetic trait. Higher doses of supplemental vitamin D most likely lead to an increased incidence of the disease in infancy and an earlier manifestation. Regimens using oral bolus doses of up to 600,000 IU provoke symptoms of acute vitamin D toxicity in infants with CYP24A1 deficiency while being tolerated well by healthy individuals [38]. Finally, omitting vitamin D supplementation in a genetically affected infant due to symptomatic disease in the older sibling was able to prevent hypercalcemic episodes and the development of nephrocalcinosis [34].

After diagnosis of symptomatic hypercalcemia with inappropriately high levels of $1,25\text{-}(OH)_2\text{-vitamin } D_3$, vitamin D prophylaxis is stopped and a low-Ca^{2+} diet is implemented. The restriction of dietary Ca^{2+} must be carefully monitored as it might lead to defective mineralization of bone as well as increased intestinal absorption of oxalate with subsequent risk of stone formation. Next to these specific therapeutic measures, vigorous intravenous rehydration and a repertory of strategies to reduce serum Ca^{2+} levels as described above are used.

Currently, it remains elusive why many of the affected individuals after acute treatment in infancy do not show recurrence of symptomatic hypercalcemia during later life. Potentially, compensatory mechanisms such as down-regulation of 1α-hydroxylase (CYP27B1) are able to prevent an excessive activation of vitamin D. However, suppressed PTH and inappropriately high $1,25\text{-}(OH)_2\text{-vitamin } D_3$ levels remain detectable for a long time during follow-up. Nephrocalcinosis persists, however does typically not result in an impairment of renal function. Interestingly, CYP24A1 mutations have also been identified in adult patients with mild hypercalcemia, nephrocalcinosis, and recurrent kidney stone disease [39–41]. Therefore, compound-heterozygous/homozygous or even heterozygous mutations in *CYP24A1* may represent a risk factor for the development of a wider spectrum of diseases associated with an increased action of vitamin D.

Magnesium Physiology

Mg^{2+} is the second most abundant intracellular cation in the body. As a cofactor for many enzymes, it is involved in energy metabolism and protein and nucleic acid synthesis. It also plays a critical role in the modulation of membrane transporters and in signal transduction. Under physiologic conditions, serum Mg^{2+} is maintained at almost constant levels. Homeostasis depends on the balance between intestinal absorption and renal excretion. Mg^{2+} deficiency can result from reduced dietary intake, intestinal malabsorption or renal loss. The control of body Mg^{2+} homeostasis primarily resides in the kidney tubules.

The daily dietary intake of Mg^{2+} varies substantially. Within physiologic ranges, diminished Mg^{2+} intake is balanced by enhanced Mg^{2+} absorption in the intestine and reduced renal excretion. These transport processes are regulated by metabolic and hormonal influences [42, 43]. The principal site of Mg^{2+} absorption is the small intestine, with smaller amounts being absorbed in the colon. Intestinal Mg^{2+} absorption occurs via two different pathways: a saturable active transcellular transport and a nonsaturable paracellular passive transport (Fig. 34.2a) [43, 44]. Saturation kinetics of the transcellular transport system are explained by the limited transport capacity of active transport. At low intraluminal concentrations Mg^{2+} is absorbed primarily via the active transcellular route and with rising concentrations via the paracellular pathway, yielding a curvilinear function for total absorption (Fig. 34.2b).

In the kidney, approximately 80 % of total serum Mg^{2+} is filtered in the glomeruli, of which more than 95 % is reabsorbed along the nephron. Mg^{2+} reabsorption differs in quantity and kinetics depending on the different nephron segments. Fifteen to 20 % are reabsorbed in the proximal tubule of the adult kidney. Interestingly, the premature kidney of the newborn is able to reabsorb up to 70 % of the filtered Mg^{2+} in this nephron segment [45].

From early childhood onward, the majority of Mg^{2+} (around 70 %) is reabsorbed in the loop of Henle, especially in the cortical thick ascending limb. Transport in this segment is passive and paracellular, driven by the lumen-positive transepithelial voltage (Fig. 34.2a). Although only 5–10 % of the filtered Mg^{2+} is reabsorbed in the distal convoluted tubule (DCT), this is the part of the nephron where the fine adjustment of renal

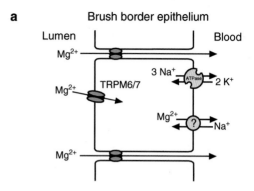

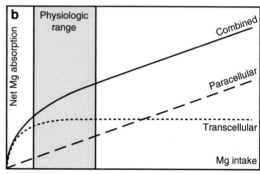

Fig. 34.2 Intestinal Mg^{2+} reabsorption. (**a**) Model of intestinal Mg^{2+} absorption via two independent pathways: passive absorption via the paracellular pathway and active, transcellular transport consisting of an apical entry through a putative Mg^{2+} channel and a basolateral exit mediated by a putative Na^+–coupled exchange. (**b**) Kinetics of intestinal Mg^{2+} absorption in humans. Paracellular transport linearly rising with intraluminal concentrations (*dotted line*) and saturable active transcellular transport (*dashed line*) together yield a curvilinear function for net Mg^{2+} absorption (*solid line*)

excretion is accomplished. The reabsorption rate in the DCT defines the final urinary Mg^{2+} excretion as there is no significant uptake of Mg^{2+} in the collecting duct. Mg^{2+} transport in this part of the nephron is an active transcellular process (Fig. 34.2b). The apical entry into DCT cells is mediated by a specific and regulated Mg^{2+} channel driven by a favorable transmembrane voltage [46]. The mechanism of basolateral transport into the interstitium is unknown. Here, Mg^{2+} has to be extruded against an unfavorable electrochemical gradient. Most physiologic studies favor a Na^+-dependent exchange mechanism [47]. Mg^{2+} entry into DCT cells appears to be the rate-limiting step and the site of regulation. Mg^{2+} transport in the distal tubule has been extensively reviewed by Dai et al. [46]. Finally, 3–5 % of the filtered Mg^{2+} is excreted in the urine.

Magnesium Depletion

Mg^{2+} depletion usually occurs secondary to another disease process or to a therapeutic agent. Some disorders that can be associated with Mg^{2+} depletion are summarized in Table 34.5 [48]. Mg^{2+} may be lost via the gastrointestinal tract, either by excessive loss of secreted fluids or impaired absorption of both dietary and endogenous Mg^{2+}. The Mg^{2+} content of upper intestinal tract fluids is approximately 0.5 mmol/L, and vomiting or nasogastric suction may contribute to Mg^{2+} depletion from loss of these fluids. The Mg^{2+} content of diarrheal fluids and fistulous drainage is much higher (up to 7.5 mmol/L), and, consequently, Mg^{2+} depletion is common in patients with acute or chronic diarrhea. Malabsorption syndromes such as celiac disease may also result in Mg^{2+} deficiency. Also acute severe pancreatitis may be associated with hypomagnesemia.

Excessive excretion of Mg^{2+} into the urine is another cause of Mg^{2+} depletion. Renal Mg^{2+} excretion is proportional to tubular fluid flow as well as to Na^+ and Ca^{2+} excretion. Therefore, both chronic intravenous fluid therapy with Na^+-containing fluids and disorders in which there is extracellular volume expansion may result in Mg^{2+} depletion. Hypercalcemia and hypercalciuria have been shown to decrease renal Mg^{2+} reabsorption and are probably the cause of excessive renal Mg^{2+} excretion and hypomagnesemia observed in many hypercalcemic states. A large variety of pharmacological agents also cause renal Mg^{2+} wasting and Mg^{2+} depletion (see below). Various renal diseases, e.g., chronic pyelonephritis or postobstructive nephropathy may also be accompanied by Mg^{2+} losses.

During infancy and childhood, a substantial proportion of patients receiving medical attention for signs of hypomagnesemia are affected by inherited renal disorders associated with Mg^{2+} wasting. In these disorders, hypomagnesemia may either be the leading symptom or may be part of a complex phenotype resulting from tubular

Table 34.5 Major causes of magnesium deficiency

Gastrointestinal disorders
Prolonged nasogastric suction/vomiting
Acute and chronic diarrhea
Malabsorption syndromes (e.g., celiac disease)
Extensive bowel resection
Intestinal and biliary fistulas
Acute hemorrhagic pancreatitis
Renal loss
Chronic parenteral fluid therapy
Osmotic diuresis (e.g., due to presence of glucose in diabetes mellitus)
Hypercalcemia
Drugs (e.g., diuretics, aminoglycosides, calcineurin inhibitors)
Alcohol
Metabolic acidosis
Renal diseases
Chronic pyelonephritis, interstitial nephritis, and glomerulonephritis
Polyuria after acute renal failure
Postobstructive nephropathy
Renal tubular acidosis
Renal transplantation
Inherited tubular diseases
Endocrine disorders
Hyperparathyroidism
Hyperthyroidism
Hyperaldosteronism
Syndrome of inappropriate secretion of antidiuretic hormone (SIADH)

dysfunction. Finally, Mg^{2+} wasting may be caused by endocrine disorders, e.g., by hyperparathyroidism because of the hypercalcemia or within the context of a SIADH state. In SIADH, Mg^{2+} losses are explained by the volume expansion.

Manifestations of Hypomagnesemia

Mg^{2+} deficiency and hypomagnesemia often remain asymptomatic. Clinical symptoms are mostly not very specific and Mg^{2+} deficiency is frequently associated with other electrolyte abnormalities. The biochemical and physiologic manifestations of severe Mg^{2+} depletion are summarized in Table 34.6.

Table 34.6 Major manifestations of magnesium depletion

Biochemical
Hypokalemia
Excessive renal potassium excretion
Decreased intracellular potassium
Hypocalcemia
Impaired parathyroid hormone (PTH) secretion
Renal and skeletal resistance to PTH
Resistance to vitamin D
Neuromuscular
Positive Chvostek's and Trousseau's sign
Spontaneous carpal-pedal spasm
Seizures
Vertigo, ataxia, nystagmus, athetoid and chorioform movements
Muscular weakness, tremor, fasciculation and wasting
Psychiatric: depression, psychosis
Cardiovascular
Electrocardiographic abnormalities
Prolonged PR- and QT-intervals
U-waves
Cardiac arrhythmia
Atrial tachycardia, fibrillations
"torsades de pointes"
Gastrointestinal
Nausea, vomiting
Anorexia

Hypokalemia

A common feature of Mg^{2+} depletion is hypokalemia [48]. During Mg^{2+} depletion there is loss of K^+ from the cell with intracellular K^+ depletion, which is enhanced due to the inability of the kidney to conserve K^+. Attempts to replete the K^+ deficit with K^+ therapy alone are not successful without simultaneous Mg^{2+} supplementation. This K^+ depletion may be a contributing cause of electrocardiographic findings and cardiac arrhythmia observed in Mg^{2+} deficiency.

Hypocalcemia

Hypocalcemia is a common finding in moderate to severe Mg^{2+} depletion and may be a major

contributing factor to the increased neuromuscular excitability often present in Mg^{2+}-depleted patients. The pathogenesis of hypocalcemia is multifactorial. Impaired PTH secretion appears to be a major factor in hypomagnesemia-induced hypocalcemia. Serum PTH concentrations are usually low in these patients, and Mg^{2+} administration will immediately stimulate PTH secretion. Patients with hypocalcemia due to Mg^{2+} depletion also exhibit both renal and skeletal resistance to exogenously administered PTH, as manifested by subnormal urinary cyclic AMP (cAMP) and phosphate excretion and a diminished calcemic response. All these effects are reversed following several days of Mg^{2+} therapy. The paradoxical inhibition of PTH secretion in patients with severe hypomagnesemia had already been described in the 1970s [49]. Later, the failure of the parathyroid gland to synthesize and secrete PTH has been attributed to a defect in g-protein signaling within parathyroid cells [50]. As a functional consequence, the intracellular signaling pathways responsible for Ca^{2+}-sensing Receptor (CaSR)-mediated inhibition of PTH secretion are enhanced including inositol phosphate generation and cAMP inhibition. Moreover, a defect in adenylate cyclase function has been postulated as Mg^{2+} is both an essential part of the substrate (Mg-ATP) as well as an important co-factor for catalytic activity [51].

Vitamin D metabolism and action may also be abnormal in hypocalcemic Mg^{2+}-deficient patients. Resistance to vitamin D therapy has been reported in such cases. This resistance may be due to impaired metabolism of vitamin D because plasma concentrations of 1,25-dihydroxyvitamin D_3 are low. Because PTH is a major stimulator of 1,25-dihydroxyvitamin D_3 synthesis, the impaired PTH secretion observed in hypomagnesemia and hypocalcemia may also be a cause of the impaired metabolism of vitamin D.

Neuromuscular Manifestations

Neuromuscular hyperexcitability may be the prominent complaint of patients with Mg^{2+} deficiency. Tetany and muscle cramps may be present. Generalized seizures may also occur. Other neuromuscular signs may include dizziness, disequilibrium, muscular tremor, wasting, and weakness [48]. Although hypocalcemia often contributes to the neurologic signs, hypomagnesemia without hypocalcemia has also been reported to result in neuromuscular hyperexcitability.

Cardiovascular Manifestations

Mg^{2+} depletion may also result in electrocardiographic abnormalities as well as in cardiac arrhythmias [52], which may be manifested by tachycardia, premature beats, or a totally irregular cardiac rhythm (fibrillation). Cardiac arrhythmia is also known to occur during K^+ depletion; therefore, the effect of Mg^{2+} deficiency on K^+ loss may be a contributing factor [48].

Clinical Assessment of Magnesium Deficiency

Although Mg^{2+} is an abundant cation in the body, more than 99 % of it are located either intracellularly or in the skeleton. The less than 1 % of total Mg^{2+} present in the body fluids is the most assessable for clinical testing, and the total serum Mg^{2+} concentration is the most widely used measure of Mg^{2+} status, although its limitations in reflecting Mg^{2+} deficiency are well recognized [53]. The reference range for normal total serum Mg^{2+} concentration is a subject of ongoing debate, but concentrations of 0.7–1.1 mmol/L are widely accepted. Because the measurement of serum Mg^{2+} concentration does not necessarily reflect the true total body Mg^{2+} content, it has been suggested that measurement of ionized serum Mg^{2+} or intracellular Mg^{2+} concentrations might provide more precise information on Mg^{2+} status. However, the relevance of such measurements to body Mg^{2+} stores has been questioned because the ionized serum Mg^{2+} and intracellular Mg^{2+} did not correlate with tissue Mg^{2+} and the correlation with the results of Mg^{2+} retention tests was contradictory [54–56]. The use of stable Mg^{2+} isotopes and muscle ^{31}P-nuclear magnetic resonance spectroscopy represent promising new methods for non-invasive estimation of body and/or tissue Mg^{2+} pools. However, they are not particularly suitable for routine measurements.

Hypomagnesemia develops late in the course of Mg^{2+} deficiency and intracellular Mg^{2+} depletion may be present despite normal serum Mg^{2+} levels. Due to the kidney's ability to sensitively adapt its Mg^{2+} transport rate to imminent deficiency, the urinary Mg^{2+} excretion rate is important in the assessment of the Mg^{2+} status. In hypomagnesemic patients, urinary Mg^{2+} excretion rates help to discern renal Mg^{2+} wasting from extrarenal losses. In the presence of hypomagnesemia, the 24-h Mg^{2+} excretion is expected to decrease below 1 mmol [57]. Mg^{2+}/creatinine ratios and fractional Mg^{2+} excretions have also been advocated as indicators of evolving Mg^{2+} deficiency [58, 59]. However, the interpretation of these results seems to be limited due to intra- and inter-individual variability [60, 61].

In patients at risk for Mg^{2+} deficiency but with normal serum Mg^{2+} levels, the Mg^{2+} status can be further evaluated by determining the amount of Mg^{2+} excreted in the urine following an intravenous infusion of Mg^{2+}. This procedure has been described as "parenteral Mg^{2+} loading test" and is still the gold standard for the evaluation of the body Mg^{2+} status [53, 55]. Normal subjects excrete at least 80 % of an intravenous Mg^{2+} load within 24 h, whereas patients with Mg^{2+} deficiency excrete much less. The Mg^{2+} loading test, however, requires normal renal handling of Mg^{2+}. A suggested work-flow for a diagnostic work-up in patients with suspected magnesium deficiency is provided in Fig. 34.3.

Acquired Hypomagnesemia

Cisplatin and Carboplatin

The cytostatic agent cisplatin and the newer antineoplastic drug, carboplatin, are widely used in various protocols for the therapy of solid tumors. Among different side effects, nephrotoxicity receives most attention as the major dose-limiting factor. Carboplatin has been reported to have less severe side effects than cisplatin [62–64].

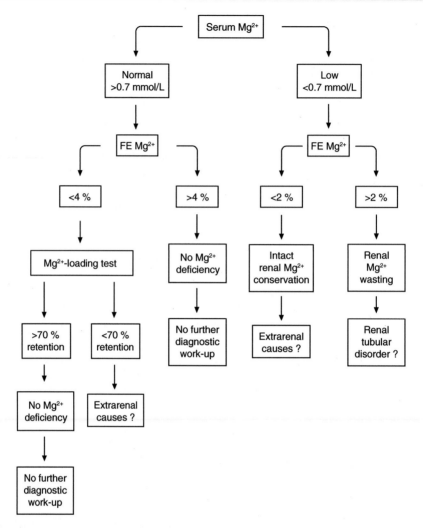

Fig. 34.3 Diagnostic work-up in patients with suspected magnesium deficiency. In face of hypomagnesemia, the determination of urinary Mg^{2+} excretions allows for a distinction between renal magnesium wasting and extrarenal losses. In normomagnesemic individuals with low urinary magnesium excretions, an increased retention of Mg^{2+} in the magnesium loading test might indicate magnesium deficiency. This test, however, requires an intact renal magnesium conservation process

Hypomagnesemia due to renal Mg^{2+} wasting is regularly observed in patients treated with cisplatin [63, 65]. The incidence of Mg^{2+} deficiency is greater than 30 % and even increases to over 70 % with longer cisplatin usage and greater accumulated doses. Interestingly, cisplatin-induced Mg^{2+} wasting is relatively selective [63]. Hypocalcemia and hypokalemia may be observed but only with prolonged and severe Mg^{2+} deficiency [66]. The influence of Mg^{2+} deficiency on PTH secretion and end-organ resistance is a pos-sible explanation for enhanced urinary Ca^{2+} excretion and diminished mobilization resulting in low plasma Ca^{2+} concentrations. The effects on K^+ balance are more difficult to explain. The hypokalemia observed with Mg^{2+} deficiency is refractory to K^+ supplementation. The effects of cisplatin may persist for months or years, long after the inorganic platinum has disappeared from the renal tissue [67, 68].

Recently, Ledeganck et al. demonstrated downregulation of EGF and TRPM6 in the DCT in a rat model of cisplatin-induced nephrotoxicity [69]. The nephrotoxicity could effectively be prevented by Mg^{2+} supplementation either during or even before cisplatin administration, demonstrating the close relationship between cisplatin-induced Mg^{2+} deficiency and nephrotoxicity [70].

Aminoglycosides

Aminoglycosides, such as gentamicin, induce renal impairment in up to 35 % patients dependent on the dose and duration of administration. In addition, aminoglycosides cause hypermagnesiuria and hypomagnesemia [71]. As many as 25 % of patients receiving gentamicin develop hypomagnesemia [71]. The hypermagnesiuric response occurs soon after the onset of therapy; it is dose-dependent and readily reversible upon withdrawal. As with adults, neonates also display an immediate increase of Ca^{2+} and Mg^{2+} excretion after gentamicin infusion [72, 73]. Mg^{2+} wasting is associated with hypercalciuria that may lead to diminished plasma Ca^{2+} concentrations. This would suggest that aminoglycosides affect renal Mg^{2+} and Ca^{2+} transport in the distal tubule where both are reabsorbed. The cellular mechanisms are not completely understood but hypermagnesiuria and hypercalciuria are observed in the absence of histopathological changes. Because gentamicin is a polyvalent cation it has been postulated that it may interfere with the function of the Ca^{2+}-sensing receptor CaSR [46, 74]. Activation of this receptor by polyvalent cations inhibits passive absorption of Mg^{2+} and Ca^{2+} in the loop of Henle and active hormone-mediated transport in the DCT leading to renal Mg^{2+} and Ca^{2+} wasting. The observation that gentamicin treatment results in an up-regulation of Ca^{2+} and Mg^{2+} transport proteins in the DCT, namely TRPV5, TRPM6 and calbindin-D28k, suggests that this adaptation represents an attempt to counter upstream losses, i.e., in the TAL [75]. This would be in accordance with the hypothesis that gentamicin affects Na^+ reabsorption in TAL leading to a reduced lumen-positive voltage and a subsequent reduction in Ca^{2+} and Mg^{2+} reabsorption.

Calcineurin Inhibitors

The calcineurin inhibitors cyclosporin A and tacrolimus (FK506) are widely prescribed as immunosuppressants to organ transplant recipients and in numerous immunologic disorders. Under this therapy, patients are at high risk of developing renal injury and hypertension. Tubular dysfunction with subsequent disturbance of mineral metabolism is another common side effect. Both drugs commonly lead to renal Mg^{2+} wasting and hypomagnesemia [76]. Unlike the other agents mentioned above, these drugs also cause modest hypercalcemia with hypercalciuria and hypokalemia [76]. The hypomagnesemic effect is probably attenuated by the fall in GFR and reduction in filtered Mg^{2+} but this defect appears to be specific for Mg^{2+}. Calcineurin inhibitor therapy is associated with an inappropriately high fractional excretion rate of Mg^{2+}, suggesting impaired passive reabsorption in the TAL or active Mg^{2+} transport in the DCT [77]. Cyclosporin A reduces claudin-16 expression in the TAL [78]. Moreover, tacrolimus downregulates specific Ca^{2+} and Mg^{2+} transport proteins in the DCT. In animals, tacrolimus induced a decrease in the expression of TRPV5, calbindin-D28k and TRPM6 [79]. These effects appeared to be specific as no morphologic features of tubular toxicity were observed. With respect to Mg^{2+} it is interesting to note that TRPM6 expression in the intestine was not changed upon tacrolimus administration. It is unknown whether these drugs act through their inhibitory effect on calcineurin, their intracellular receptor. It is speculated that FK506-binding proteins, which are known to bind and regulate the Ca^{2+}-permeable transient receptor potential-like (TRPL) cation channels might be involved because tacrolimus disrupts this binding [80].

In analogy, one might speculate that certain FK-binding proteins might modulate TRPV5 or TRPM6 expression or activity. Hypomagnesemia has been implicated as a contributor to the nephrotoxicity and arterial hypertension associated with calcineurin inhibitors. Mervaala et al. demonstrated that the adverse effects of cyclosporine

A in spontaneously hypertensive rats largely depend on dietary Na^+ and that these adverse effects can be prevented by Mg^{2+} supplementation [81]. Mg^{2+} supplementation also had a beneficial effect on cyclosporine A nephrotoxicity in a rat model [82].

EGF Receptor Antibodies

The EGF hormone axis has been implicated in renal Mg^{2+} handling by the identification of a homozygous mutation in the *EGF* gene in a family with isolated recessive hypomagnesemia (see below) [83]. The way for this discovery was paved by the observation that anticancer treatments with monoclonal antibodies against the EGF receptor (EGFR) resulted in renal Mg^{2+} wasting and hypomagnesemia [84]. Of note, patients treated with EGFR targeting antibodies (cetuximab, panitumumab) for colorectal cancer usually receive a combination therapy with platinum compounds potentially aggravating the effects on serum Mg^{2+} levels. A significant number of patients receiving such a chemotherapeutic regimen show decreasing serum Mg^{2+} concentrations over time [84, 85]. Twenty-four hour urine collections as well as Mg^{2+} loading tests in single patients demonstrated a defect in renal Mg^{2+} conservation [84]. Together with the genetic findings in patients with isolated recessive hypomagnesemia due to a pro-EGF mutation, these observations imply a selective effect of EGFR targeting on transcellular Mg^{2+} transport in the DCT. There, TRPM6 mediated Mg^{2+} uptake into DCT cells is stimulated by basolaterally secreted EGF via its receptor (EGFR) [83].

Proton-Pump Inhibitors (PPIs)

Over the last 20 years, PPIs for the reduction of gastric acidity have emerged to one of the most widely prescribed classes of drugs worldwide [86]. Due to the large number of patients, even rare side effects can be detected that potentially remain undiscovered during initial clinical trials. Symptomatic hypomagnesemia has been observed in a small but significant number of patients receiving PPIs [87]. It is well conceivable that in a substantially larger number of patients, the relationship between low serum Mg^{2+} levels and the use of PPIs remains unrecognized. A recent review summarizing the data from previous publications reveals severely lowered serum Mg^{2+} levels below 0.4 mmol/L with concomitant hypocalcemia, a laboratory constellation reminiscent of HSH due to TRPM6 defects [86]. The initial report on hypomagnesemia following PPI treatment had already described suppressed PTH levels during phases of severe hypomagnesemia as a probable cause of hypocalcemia (as in HSH) [87]. Although a number of patients additionally receive diuretics, this finding does not explain the profound degree of Mg^{2+} deficiency observed in patients receiving PPIs.

Data regarding urinary Mg^{2+} excretions in hypomagnesemic patients receiving PPIs are inconclusive. Fractional Mg^{2+} excretions were reported to be low in face of profound hypomagnesemia possibly pointing to an intact tubular Mg^{2+} reabsorption [87, 88]. However, as observed in HSH patients, a renal Mg^{2+} leak might only become apparent if serum Mg^{2+} levels reach a certain threshold. An alternative explanation could involve a disturbed intestinal reabsorption of Mg^{2+}. Unfortunately, the molecular link between proton-pump inhibition and hypomagnesemia still remains unclear. In regard of the severe degree of hypomagnesemia, possible molecular mechanisms include an inhibition of TRPM6 leading to a combined intestinal and renal defect, but also a disturbance of ATPases or ATPase-subunits other than gastric H^+-K^+-ATPase involved in epithelial Mg^{2+} transport.

In any case, it is recommended to monitor serum Mg^{2+} levels patients receiving PPIs, particularly those with concomitant cardiac disease and risk for arrhythmia. Contrariwise, attention should be drawn to the medication of patients clinically presenting with a hypomagnesemia with secondary hypocalcemia (HSH) phenotype (see below).

Miscellaneous Agents

A number of antibiotics, tuberculostatics, and antiviral drugs may result in renal Mg^{2+} wasting [71]. The cellular basis by which these agents lead to abnormal Mg^{2+} reabsorption is largely unknown. Many agents are associated with general cytotoxicity. Amphotericin B may lead to an acquired distal tubular acidosis which in turn reduces renal Mg^{2+} reabsorption. Pamidronate, used in the treatment of acute symptomatic hypercalcemia of various origin, has also been reported to cause transient hypomagnesemia. Again, the cellular mechanisms are difficult to predict since this drug is used in patients with hypercalcemia that may aggravate renal Mg^{2+} wasting [89].

Therapy of Hypomagnesemia

The substitution of Mg^{2+} in patients with hypomagnesemia is primarily aimed at the relief of clinical symptoms. Unfortunately, in patients with renal Mg^{2+} wasting, normal values for total serum Mg^{2+} are hardly achieved by oral substitution without considerable side effects, mainly resulting from the cathartic effects of Mg^{2+} salts.

The primary route of administration depends on the severity of the clinical findings. Acute intravenous infusion is usually reserved for patients with symptomatic hypomagnesemia, i.e., with cerebral convulsions or tetany [90]. Intravenous administration should be preferred to painful intramuscular injections, especially in children.

In neonates and children, the initial treatment usually consists of 25–50 mg Mg^{2+} sulphate (0.1–0.2 mmol Mg^{2+}) per kilogram body weight slowly given intravenously (over 20 min) (up to a maximum of 2 g Mg^{2+} sulphate, which is the adult dosage). This dose can be repeated every 6–8 h or can be followed by a continuous infusion of 100–200 mg Mg^{2+} sulphate (0.4–0.8 mmol Mg^{2+}) per kilogram body weight given over 24 h [91, 92].

In the presence of hypocalcemia, this regimen can be continued for 3–5 days. When Mg^{2+} is administered intravenously, Ca^{2+} gluconate (i.v.) should be available as an antidote. Control of blood pressure, heart rate, and respiration is important as well as a close monitoring of serum Mg^{2+} levels. Before administration, normal renal function has to be ascertained.

In asymptomatic hypomagnesemic or Mg^{2+}-deficient patients, oral replacement represents the preferred route of administration. Exact dosages required to correct Mg^{2+} deficiency are largely unknown. For the paediatric population, 10–20 mg Mg^{2+} (0.4–0.8 mmol) per kg body weight given three to four times a day has been recommended to correct hypomagnesemia [93]. However, in our personal experience, continuous administration of Mg^{2+}, for example dissolved in mineral water, has proven to be of advantage, as peak Mg^{2+} blood levels are avoided.

Solubility, intestinal absorption, and side effects greatly differ depending on the Mg^{2+} salt used for oral treatment. The bioavailability and pharmacokinetics of diverse Mg^{2+} salts have been reviewed [94]. Considering solubility, intestinal absorption and bioavailability, organic Mg^{2+} salts such as Mg^{2+} citrate or aspartate appear most suitable for oral replacement therapy. In addition, the laxative effect of these preparations seems to be less pronounced compared with inorganic Mg^{2+} salts.

In addition to replacement therapy, the use of certain diuretics has been proposed for the reduction of renal Mg^{2+} excretion. The aldosterone antagonist spironolactone, as well as K^+-sparing diuretics such as amiloride, exert Mg^{2+}-sparing effects [95, 96]. Studies in patients with hereditary Mg^{2+} wasting disorders showed a beneficial effect of these diuretics on renal Mg^{2+} excretions, serum Mg^{2+} levels, and clinical manifestations [97, 98].

Hereditary Disorders of Mg^{2+} Handling

Recent advances in molecular genetics of hereditary hypomagnesemia substantiated the role of a variety of genes and their encoded proteins in human epithelial Mg^{2+} transport (Table 34.7). The knowledge of underlying genetic defects helps to distinguish different clinical subtypes of hereditary disorders of Mg^{2+} homeostasis. By careful clinical observation and additional biochemical parameters, the different disease

Table 34.7 Inherited disorders of Ca^{2+} and Mg^{2+} handling

Disorder	OMIM #	Inheritance	Gene	Protein
Autosomal dominant hypoparathyroidism (ADH)	601198	AD	CASR	CaSR, Ca^{2+}/Mg^{2+} sensing receptor
Familial hypocalciuric hypercalcemia (FHH)	145980	AD	CASR	CaSR, Ca^{2+}/Mg^{2+} sensing receptor
Neonatal severe hyperparathyroidism (NSHPT)	239200	AR	CASR	CaSR, Ca^{2+}/Mg^{2+} sensing receptor
Idiopathic infantile hypercalcemia	143880	AR	CYP24A1	25-OH-vitamin D_3-24-hydroxylase
Familial hypomagnesemia with hypercalciuria/nephrocalcinosis (FHHNC)	248250	AR	CLDN16	Claudin-16 (paracellin-1), tight junction protein
Familial hypomagnesemia with hypercalciuria/nephrocalcinosis (FHHNC) and severe ocular involvement	248190	AR	CLDN19	Claudin-19, tight junction protein
Gitelman syndrome (GS)	263800	AR	SLC12A3	NCCT, NaCl cotransporter
EAST/SeSAME syndrome	612780	AR	KCNJ10	Kir4.1, basolateral potassium channel
Hypomagnesemia with secondary hypocalcemia (HSH)	602014	AR	TRPM6	TRPM6, putative ion channel
Isolated dominant hypomagnesemia (IDH)	154020	AD	FXYD2	γ-subunit of the Na^+-K^+-ATPase
	176260	AD	KCNA1	Kv1.1, apical potassium channel
Isolated recessive hypomagnesemia (IRH)	248250	AR	EGF	pro-EGF (epidermal growth factor)
Hypomagnesemia with impaired brain development	613882	AR, AD	CNNM2	ACDP2, CNNM2, Cyclin M2
HNF1β nephropathy	137920	AD	HNF1B	HNF1beta, transcription factor
Transient neonatal hyperphenylalaninemia	264070	AR	PCBD1	PCBD1, tetrahydrobioterin metabolism
Hypomagnesemia/metabolic syndrome	500005	mito	MTTI	Mitochondrial tRNA (Isoleucin)

entities can already be distinguished in many cases, even though there may be a considerable overlap in phenotypic characteristics (Table 34.8).

Familial Hypomagnesemia with Hypercalciuria and Nephrocalcinosis (OMIM #248250)

Familial hypomagnesemia with hypercalciuria and nephrocalcinosis (FHHNC) is an autosomal recessive disorder caused by mutations in two different members of the claudin gene family which encode tight junction proteins, namely claudin-16 and claudin-19 [99, 100]. Since its first description in the 1950s [101], more than 150 patients have been reported allowing a comprehensive characterization of the clinical spectrum [102–105]. Due to excessive renal Mg^{2+} and Ca^{2+} wasting, affected individuals almost uniformly develop the characteristic triad of hypomagnesemia, hypercalciuria, and nephrocalcinosis that gave the disease its name. Additional biochemical abnormalities include elevated PTH levels before the onset of chronic

Table 34.8 Clinical and biochemical characteristics of inherited Ca^{2+} and Mg^{2+} disorders

Disorder	Age at onset	Serum Mg^{2+}	Serum Ca^{2+}	Serum K^+	Blood pH	Urine Mg^{2+}	Urine Ca^{2+}	Nephro-calcinosis	Renal stones
Autosomal dominant hypoparathyroidism (ADH)	Infancy	↓	↓	N	N or ↓	↑	↑ – ↑↑	Yesᵃ	Yesᵃ
Familial hypocalciuric hypercalcemia (FHH)	Often asymptomatic	N to ↑	↑	N	N	↓	↓	No	?
Neonatal severe hyperparathyroidism (NSHPT)	Infancy	N to ↑	↑↑↑	N	N	↓	↓	No	?
Idiopathic infantile hypercalcemia	Infancy	N	↑↑↑	N	N	?	↑↑	Yes	Yes
Familial hypomagnesemia with hypercalciuria/ nephrocalcinosis (FHHNC)	Childhood	↓	N	N	N or ↓	↑↑	↑↑	Yes	Yes
Gitelman syndrome (GS)	Adolescence	↓	N	↓	↑	↑	↓	No	No
EAST/SeSAME syndrome	Infancy	↓	N	↓	↑	↑	↓	No	No
Hypomagnesemia with secondary hypocalcemia (HSH)	Infancy	↓↓↓	↓	N	N	↑	N	No	No
Isolated dominant hypomagnesemia (IDH)	Childhood	↓	N	N	N	↑	↓	No	No
Isolated recessive hypomagnesemia (IRH)	Childhood	↓	N	N	N	↑	N	No	No
Hypomagnesemia with impaired brain development	Infancy to adolescence	↓↓	N	N	N	↑	N	No	No
HNF1B nephropathy	Childhood	↓	N	N	N	↑	↓	No	No
Transient neonatal hyperphenylalaninemia	Adulthood	↓	N	N	N	↑	↓	No	No
Hypomagnesemia/metabolic syndrome	Adulthood	↓	N	↓	N	↑	↓	No	No

ᵃFrequent complication under therapy with Ca^{2+} and vitamin D

renal failure, hypocitraturia, and hyperuricemia. The majority of patients clinically present during early childhood with recurrent urinary tract infections, polyuria/polydipsia, nephrolithiasis, and/or failure to thrive. Clinical symptoms of severe hypomagnesemia such as seizures and muscular tetany are less common. The clinical course of FHHNC patients is often complicated by the development of chronic renal insufficiency early in life. A considerable number of patients exhibit a marked decline in GFR (<60 ml/min per 1.73 m^2) already at the time of diagnosis and about one third of patients develops ESRD during adolescence. Hypomagnesemia may completely disappear with the decline of GFR due to a reduction in filtered Mg^{2+} that limits urinary Mg^{2+} losses.

Whereas the renal phenotype is almost identical in carriers of *CLDN16* and *CLDN19* mutations, ocular involvement including severe myopia, nystagmus, or macular coloboma are observed only in patients with *CLDN19* mutations [100, 102, 104, 105].

In addition to oral Mg^{2+} supplementation, therapy aims at the reduction of Ca^{2+} excretion in order to prevent the progression of nephrocalcinosis and stone formation because the degree of renal calcifications has been correlated with progression of chronic renal failure [102]. In a short term study, thiazides have been demonstrated to effectively reduce urinary Ca^{2+} excretion in FHHNC patients [106]. However, these therapeutic strategies have not been shown yet to significantly influence the progression of renal failure. Supportive therapy is important for the protection of kidney function and should include provision of sufficient fluids and effective treatment of stone formation and bacterial colonization. As expected, renal transplantation is performed without evidence of recurrence of the disease because the primary defect resides in the kidney.

Based on clinical observations and clearance studies, it had been postulated that the primary defect in FHHNC was related to disturbed Mg^{2+} and Ca^{2+} reabsorption in the TAL [107]. In 1999, using a positional cloning approach, Simon et al. identified a new gene (*CLDN16*, formerly *PCLN1*) mutated in patients with FHHNC [99].

CLDN16 codes for claudin-16, a member of the claudin family. More than 20 claudins identified so far comprise a family of ~22 kD proteins with four transmembrane segments, two extracellular domains, and intracellular N- and C-termini. Claudins are crucial components of tight junctions and the individual composition of tight junctions strands with different claudin members confers the characteristic properties of different epithelia regarding paracellular permeability and/or transepithelial resistance. In this context, a crucial role has been attributed to the first extracellular domain of the claudin protein which is extremely variable in number and position of charged amino acid residues [108]. Individual charges have been shown to influence paracellular ion selectivity, suggesting that claudins positioned on opposing cells forming the paracellular pathway provide charge-selective pores within the tight junction barrier.

The majority of *CLDN16* mutations reported in FHHNC are simple missense mutations affecting the transmembrane domains and the extracellular loops with a particular clustering in the first extracellular loop which contains the ion selectivity filter. Within this domain, patients originating from Germany or Eastern European countries exhibit a common mutation (p.L151F) due to a founder effect [103]. As this mutation is present in approximately 50 % of mutant alleles, molecular diagnosis is greatly facilitated in patients originating from these countries. Defects in *Cldn16* have also been shown to underlie the development of a chronic interstitial nephritis in Japanese cattle that rapidly develop chronic renal failure shortly after birth [109]. Interestingly, affected animals show hypocalcemia but no hypomagnesemia, which might be explained by advanced renal failure present at the time of examination. The fact that, in contrast to the point mutations identified in human FHHNC, large deletions of *Cldn16* are responsible for the disease in cattle, might explain the more severe phenotype with early-onset renal failure. However, *Cldn16* knockout mice do not display renal failure during the first months of life [110].

In FHHNC patients, progressive renal failure is generally thought to more likely be a consequence of massive urinary Ca^{2+} wasting and nephrocalcinosis. A genotype-phenotype correlation exists inasmuch as the presence of *CLDN16* mutations leading to a complete loss-of-function on both alleles is associated with younger age at manifestation and a more rapid decline in renal function compared to patients with at least one allele with residual claudin-16 function [111].

Moreover, two independent studies describe a high incidence of hypercalciuria, nephrolithiasis and/or nephrocalcinosis in first degree relatives of FHHNC patients [102, 103]. A subsequent study also reported a tendency towards mild hypomagnesemia in family members with heterozygous *CLDN16* mutations [112]. Thus, one might speculate that *CLDN16* mutations could be involved in idiopathic hypercalciuric stone formation.

Finally, a homozygous *CLDN16* mutation (p.T303R) affecting the C-terminal PDZ domain has been identified in two families with isolated hypercalciuria and nephrocalcinosis without disturbances in renal Mg^{2+} handling [113]. Interestingly, the hypercalciuria disappeared during follow-up and urinary Ca^{2+} levels reached normal values beyond puberty.

Molecular genetic studies in FHHNC patients with severe ocular involvement lead to the identification of mutations in a second member of the claudin family, claudin-19 (encoded by *CLDN19*) [100]. Claudin-16 and claudin-19 colocalize at tight junctions of the TAL [100]. Tight-junction strands in this part of the renal tubule also express other members of the claudin family including claudin-3, claudin-10 and claudin-18. These other claudins are able to maintain the barrier function of the tight junction complex also in the absence of claudin-16 and -19; however, claudin-16 and -19 depleted tight junctions display a loss in cation permselectivity.

Gitelman Syndrome (OMIM #263800)

Gitelman syndrome (GS) is the most frequent inherited salt wasting disorder with an estimated prevalence of approximately 1:40,000 [114]. It is caused by mutations in the *SLC12A3* gene coding for the thiazide-sensitive NaCl cotransporter,

NCCT [115]. The NCCT is exclusively expressed at the apical membrane of the DCT where it reabsorbs approximately 5–10 % of the filtered NaCl. The cardinal biochemical features of GS are persistent hypokalemia and metabolic alkalosis together with hypomagnesemia and hypocalciuria [116, 117].

In their initial report, Gitelman et al. already pointed to the susceptibility to carpopedal spasms and tetany in three patients with suspected Bartter syndrome [116]. Tetany was attributed to low plasma Mg^{2+} levels secondary to impaired renal Mg^{2+} wasting. Further examination of these patients revealed low urinary Ca^{2+} excretion, which is rarely observed in hypomagnesemic states [107]. Consequently, the association of hypocalciuria with renal Mg^{2+} wasting was regarded as a hallmark to separate the newly defined GS from other forms of hypokalemic salt-losing tubular disorders (Bartter-like syndromes) [118]. The initial presentation of GS most frequently occurs at school age or later with the characteristic symptoms being muscular weakness, cramps, and fatigue [119]. Moreover, patients are frequently diagnosed accidentally while searching medical consultation because of growth retardation, constipation or enuresis. However, a thorough past medical history commonly reveals long-standing salt craving. Typically, urinary concentrating ability is not affected. Laboratory examination shows a typical constellation of metabolic alkalosis, low normal Cl^- levels, hypokalemia, and hypomagnesemia; urine analysis reveals hypocalciuria [8]. Family studies demonstrated that electrolyte imbalances are present from infancy on, although the affected infants displayed no obvious clinical signs [120].

Of note, the combination of hypokalemia and hypomagnesemia exerts an exceptionally unfavorable effect on cardiac excitability, which puts these patients at high risk for cardiac arrhythmia [121].

The pathognomonic feature of Gitelman syndrome is the dissociation of renal Ca^{2+} and Mg^{2+} handling, with low urinary Ca^{2+} and high urinary Mg^{2+} levels. Subsequent hypomagnesemia causes neuromuscular irritability and tetany. Decreased renal Ca^{2+} elimination together with Mg^{2+}

deficiency favors deposition of mineral Ca^{2+} as demonstrated by increased bone density as well as chondrocalcinosis [122].

Although the combination of hypomagnesemia and hypocalciuria is typical for NCCT-deficiency, it is neither a specific nor universal finding. Clinical observations in NCCT-deficient patients disclosed intra- and inter-individual variations in urinary Ca^{2+} concentrations which can be attributed to gender, age-related conditions of bone metabolism, intake of Mg^{2+} supplements, changes in diuresis and urinary osmolality, respectively. Likewise, hypomagnesemia might not be present from the beginning. Renal Mg^{2+} loss can be balanced temporarily by Mg^{2+} release from bone and muscle stores as well as by an increase of intestinal Mg^{2+} reabsorption. The mechanisms compromising distal Mg^{2+} reabsorption and favoring reabsorption of Ca^{2+} are not yet completely understood.

In contrast to TAL defects, disturbed salt reabsorption along the DCT does not affect the tubulo-glomerular feedback and thus is not associated with increased renal prostaglandin synthesis [123]. Accordingly, NSAIDs are of little benefit in Gitelman syndrome. Substitution of KCl and Mg^{2+} is therefore of prime importance in the treatment of this disorder. As pointed out above, avoidance of factors which in addition to hypokalemia and hypomagnesemia might affect cardiac excitability (in particular QT-time prolonging drugs) is mandatory to prevent life-threatening cardiac arrhythmia.

EAST/SeSAME Syndrome (OMIM #612780)

In 2009, a newly characterized clinical syndrome with autosomal recessive inheritance combining epilepsy, ataxia, sensorineural deafness and renal NaCl wasting with/without mental retardation was described under the acronyms EAST or SeSAME syndrome [124, 125]. Patients usually present early in infancy with generalized tonic–clonic seizures, speech and motor delay, as well as severe ataxia leading to an inability to walk,

intention tremor, and dysdiadochokinesis. In addition they exhibit a severe hearing impairment. Renal salt wasting is often recognized later during the course of the disease. Closely resembling GS, the renal phenotype includes the combination of hypokalemic alkalosis, hypomagnesaemia and hypocalciuria.

EAST/SeSAME syndrome is caused by loss-of-function mutations in the *KCNJ10* gene encoding the inwardly-rectifying K^+-channel Kir4.1 [124, 125]. The expression pattern of Kir4.1 fits to the disease phenotype with highest expression in brain, the stria vascularis of the inner ear, and in the distal nephron, especially in the DCT. Here, Kir4.1 is localized at the basolateral membrane of DCT cells and supposed to function in collaboration with Na^+-K^+-ATPase as it might allow for a recycling of K^+ ions entering the tubular cells in countermove for the extruded Na^+ [125]. Loss of Kir4.1 function most likely leads to a depolarization of the basolateral membrane and thereby to a reduction of the driving force for basolateral anion channels as well as sodium-coupled exchangers. By this mechanism, Kir4.1 defects could also affect the putative Na^+/Mg^{2+} exchanger and possibly explain the Mg^{2+} wasting observed in EAST/SeSAME syndrome. Interestingly, the renal phenotype of Kir4.1 knockout mice had not been thoroughly studied until the description of human disease [126]. The re-evaluation of Kir4.1 deficient mice, however, clearly demonstrated renal salt wasting leading to significant growth retardation [124].

Hypomagnesemia with Secondary Hypocalcemia (OMIM #602014)

Hypomagnesemia with secondary hypocalcemia (HSH) is a rare autosomal recessive disorder that manifests in early infancy with generalized seizures or other symptoms of increased neuromuscular excitability [127]. Biochemical abnormalities include extremely low serum Mg^{2+} (about 0.2 mmol/L) and low serum Ca^{2+} levels. The mechanism leading to hypocalcemia is still not completely understood but PTH levels in HSH patients were found to be inappropriately low. Already in the 1970s, severe hypomagnesemia was shown to result in an impaired synthesis and/or release of PTH [49]. Later, the failure of the parathyroid gland to synthesize and secrete parathyroid hormone was attributed to a defect in g-protein signaling within parathyroid cells required for CaSR-mediated stimulation of PTH release [50]. The hypocalcemia observed in HSH is resistant to treatment with Ca^{2+} or vitamin D. Relief of clinical symptoms, normocalcemia, and normalization of PTH levels are only achieved by administration of high doses of Mg^{2+} [128]. Delayed diagnosis or non-compliance with treatment can be fatal or result in permanent neurological damage.

Transport studies in HSH patients pointed to a primary defect in intestinal Mg^{2+} absorption [129, 130]. However, in some patients an additional renal leak for Mg^{2+} was suspected [131].

By linkage analysis, a gene locus (*HOMG1*) for HSH had been mapped to chromosome 9q22 in 1997 [132]. Later, two independent groups identified *TRPM6* at this locus and reported loss of function mutations as the underlying cause of HSH [133, 134]. To date, mutations in *TRPM6* have been identified in more than 40 families affected by HSH [133–137]. The mutational spectrum mainly comprises truncating mutations. In addition, a number of missense mutations have been described leading to the exchange of single amino acids [133, 135, 137, 138]. Functional data for a subset of these also indicate a complete loss-of-function which might therefore be considered a prerequisite for the development of the typical HSH phenotype.

TRPM6 encodes a member of the transient receptor potential (TRP) family of cation channels. Together with its close homologue TRPM7, TRPM6 displays the unique feature of a kinase domain of the atypical α-kinase family linked to an ion channel domain [139]. Before the discovery of TRPM6 mutations in HSH, TRPM7 had already been characterized as a Ca^{2+} and Mg^{2+} permeable ion channel regulated by Mg-ATP [140]. *TRPM6* mRNA shows a more restricted expression pattern than TRPM7 with highest lev-els along the intestine (duodenum, jejunum, ileum, colon) and the DCT of the kidney [133].

The detection of TRPM6 expression in the DCT confirms the hypothesis of an additional role of renal Mg^{2+} wasting for the pathogenesis of HSH [141]. This was also supported by intravenous Mg^{2+} loading tests in HSH patients, which disclosed a considerable renal Mg^{2+} leak albeit still being hypomagnesemic [134].

In the intestine, intraluminal Mg^{2+} concentrations and rates of Mg^{2+} absorption show a curvilinear relationship presumably reflecting two transport processes working in parallel: an active and saturable transcellular transport essential at low intraluminal Mg^{2+} concentrations and a passive paracellular Mg^{2+} absorption gaining importance at higher intraluminal Mg^{2+} concentrations [44]. The observation that in HSH patients the substitution of high oral doses of Mg^{2+} achieves at least subnormal serum Mg^{2+} levels supports this theory of two independent intestinal transport systems for Mg^{2+}. TRPM6 probably represents a molecular component of active transcellular Mg^{2+} transport. An increased intraluminal Mg^{2+} concentration (by increased oral intake) enables to compensate for the defect in active transcellular transport by increasing absorption via the passive paracellular pathway (Fig. 34.1).

The biophysical characterization of TRPM6 remains controversial. In general, functional ion channels of the TRP family are composed as tetramers, i.e., are consisting of four channel subunits at the cell surface. Initially, several groups failed to observe measurable currents upon heterologous expression of TRPM6 using different expression systems [142, 143]. Instead, they demonstrated the existence of functional heteromers with highly homologous TRPM7. Schmitz et al. further demonstrated that TRPM6 and TRPM7 are functionally non-redundant but specifically influence each other's biological activity. Furthermore, the authors showed that TRPM6 can phosphorylate TRPM7 and modulate the function of TRPM7 in a Mg^{2+}-dependent manner [143].

In contrast, Voets et al. succeeded in functionally expressing TRPM6 by using a specialized pCINeo/IRES-GFP vector allowing for the parallel, but non-covalent expression of GFP together with the ion channel protein [144]. They demonstrated that TRPM6, like TRPM7, was permeable for Mg^{2+} and Ca^{2+} and regulated by intracellular Mg^{2+} levels. Permeation characteristics with currents almost exclusively carried by divalent cations with a higher affinity for Mg^{2+} than Ca^{2+} supported the role of TRPM6 as the apical Mg^{2+} influx pathway [144]. Subsequently functional differences between TRPM6 monomers, TRPM6/7 heteromers, and TRPM7 monomers were demonstrated [145, 146].

Isolated Dominant Hypomagnesemia (OMIM #154020)

A first variant of isolated dominant hypomagnesemia (IDH) was described in 1999 in two related families by Meij et al. who discovered a mutation in the *FXYD2* gene on chromosome 11q23 encoding a γ-subunit of renal Na^+K^+-ATPase [147]. The original description of the phenotype had been published in the 1980s by Geven et al. [148].

The index patients of both families presented with seizures during childhood (at 7 and 13 years). Serum Mg^{2+} levels in the two girls at that time were ~0.4 mmol/L. One index patient was treated for seizures of unknown origin with antiepileptic drugs until her serum Mg^{2+} levels were evaluated in adolescence. At that time severe mental retardation was evident.

Systematic serum Mg^{2+} measurements performed in members of both families revealed low serum Mg^{2+} levels (~0.5 mmol/L) in numerous apparently healthy individuals. A ^{28}Mg-retention study in one index patient pointed to a primary renal defect while the intestinal Mg^{2+} absorption was preserved or even stimulated in compensation for renal losses [148]. In addition, urinary Ca^{2+} excretion rates were low in all hypomagnesemic family members, a finding reminiscent of GS. But in contrast to GS patients, no other associated biochemical abnormality was reported, especially no hypokalemic alkalosis.

The γ-subunit of Na^+K^+-ATPase encoded by *FXYD2* is a member of a family of small single transmembrane proteins which share the common amino acid motif F-X-Y-D. The FXYD proteins constitute regulatory, tissue-specific subunits of the Na^+K^+-ATPase. FXYD2 and another member, FXYD4, are highly expressed along the nephron displaying an alternating expression pattern [149]. The γ-subunit FXYD2 in turn comprises two isoforms (named γ-α and γ-β) that are differentially expressed along the nephron. Whereas the γ-α isoform is present predominantly in the proximal tubule, the expression of the γ-β isoform predominates in the distal nephron, especially in the DCT [150]. There, FXYD2 increases the apparent affinity of Na^+K^+-ATPase for ATP while decreasing its Na^+ affinity [151]. Thus, FXDY2 might provide a mechanism for balancing energy utilization and maintaining appropriate salt gradients.

Expression studies of the mutant G41R-γ-subunit in mammalian renal tubule cells revealed a dominant-negative effect of the mutation leading to a retention of the γ-subunit within the cell. The assumption of a dominant negative effect was substantiated by the observation that individuals with a large heterozygous deletion of chromosome 11q including the *FXYD2* gene exhibit normal serum Mg^{2+} levels [152].

Urinary Mg^{2+} wasting together with the expression pattern of the *FXYD2* gene point to defective transcellular Mg^{2+} reabsorption in the DCT in IDH patients. But how can a defect of Na^+K^+-ATPase modulation lead to impaired renal Mg^{2+} conservation? One possible explanation is based on changes in intracellular Na^+ and K^+ levels. Diminished intracellular K^+ might depolarize the apical membrane resulting in a decrease in Mg^{2+} uptake [147]. Alternatively, an increase in intracellular Na^+ could impair basolateral Mg^{2+} transport which is presumably achieved by a Na^+-coupled exchange mechanism. Another explanation is that the γ-subunit is not only involved in Na^+K^+-ATPase function but also an essential component of a yet unidentified ATP-dependent transport system specific for Mg^{2+}. Like for Ca^{2+}, both a specific Mg^{2+}-ATPase and a Na^+-coupled exchanger might exist. Further studies are needed to clarify this issue.

Isolated Dominant Hypomagnesemia (OMIM #176260)

Genetic heterogeneity in IDH was demonstrated by the identification of a heterozygous missense mutation in *KCNA1* encoding the voltage-gated potassium channel Kv1.1 in a large Brazilian family [153].

The clinical phenotype of affected patients includes muscle cramps, tetany, tremor, and muscle weakness starting during infancy. Laboratory analyses revealed a renal Mg^{2+} leak without alterations in renal Ca^{2+} handling. Previously, *KCNA1* mutations had already been identified in patients with episodic ataxia with myokymia (OMIM 160120), a neurologic disorder characterized by an intermittent appearance of incoordination and imbalance as well as myokymia, an involuntary, spontaneous, and localized trembling of muscles [154]. In addition to muscle cramps and tetany attributed to Mg^{2+} deficiency, these symptoms were also present in members of the aforementioned Brazilian kindred with hypomagnesaemia.

The identified *KCNA1* mutation (c.A763G) leads to a non-conservative amino acid exchange (p.N255D) in the encoded Kv1.1 K^+-channel. Functional voltage-gated K^+-channels of the KCNA family are composed of tetramers. Co-expression of the mutant p.N255D-Kv1.1 with wildtype channel subunits in HEK293 cells resulted in a significant reduction in current amplitudes compatible with a dominant-negative effect of the mutant. This dominant-negative effect rather seems to be the result of an impaired gating of the K^+-channel tetramer as trafficking to the plasma membrane is preserved [155].

Kv1.1 expression was demonstrated in kidney in the DCT, presumably at the apical membrane. As it is co-localized there with TRPM6, Glaudemans et al. proposed a model in which Kv1.1 allows for hyperpolarization of the apical membrane of DCT cells as a prerequisite for TRPM6-mediated Mg^{2+} entry (Fig. 34.4a,b).

Thereby, the authors, for the first time, linked Mg^{2+} reabsorption in the DCT to K^+ secretion and identified a new interdependence of renal Mg^{2+} and K^+ handling at the molecular level [153].

Isolated Recessive Hypomagnesemia (OMIM #248250)

Already in the 1980s, Geven et al. reported a form of isolated hypomagnesemia in a consanguineous family indicating autosomal recessive inheritance [156]. Two affected sisters presented in infancy with generalized seizures. Unfortunately, a late diagnosis resulted in neurodevelopmental deficits in both girls. A thorough clinical and laboratory workup at 4 and 8 years of age, respectively, revealed serum Mg^{2+} levels around 0.5–0.6 mmol/L with no other associated serum electrolyte abnormality. Of note, renal Ca^{2+} excretion rates were in the normal range. A ^{28}Mg-retention test in one patient indicated a primary defect in renal Mg^{2+} conservation [156].

Groenestege et al. were able to identify a homozygous missense mutation in the *EGF* gene leading to a nonconservative amino acid exchange in the encoded pro-EGF protein (pro-epidermal growth factor) in the two sisters [83]. In the kidney, co-expression with key proteins of transcellular Mg^{2+} reabsorption including TRPM6 in the DCT was demonstrated. Pro-EGF is a transmembrane protein that is inserted in both the luminal and basolateral membrane of polarized epithelia. After the soluble EGF peptide is cleaved, it is able to bind and activate specialized EGF receptors (EGFRs). In case of the DCT, these EGFRs are exclusively expressed at the basolateral membrane. Their activation was shown to lead to an increase in TRPM6 trafficking to the luminal membrane and increased Mg^{2+} reabsorption [157]. The mutation described in IRH (p.P1070L) disrupts the basolateral sorting motif in pro-EGF leading to a mistargeting of pro-EGF [83]. Therefore, the activation of basolateral EGFRs is compromised which ultimately causes the disturbance in active transcellular Mg^{2+} reabsorption. Despite acting in a paracrine fashion in the DCT,

Fig. 34.4 Mg²⁺ reabsorption in the distal tubule. (**a**) Mg²⁺ reabsorption in the thick ascending limb of Henle's loop. Paracellular reabsorption of Mg²⁺ and Ca²⁺ is driven by lumen-positive transcellular voltage generated by the transcellular reabsorption of NaCl. (**b**) Mg²⁺ reabsorption in the distal convoluted tubule. Mg²⁺ is actively reabsorbed via the transcellular pathway involving an apical entry step through a Mg²⁺-permeable ion channel (TRPM6) and a basolateral exit, presumably mediated by a Na⁺–coupled exchange mechanism. The molecular identity of the basolateral exchange is unknown

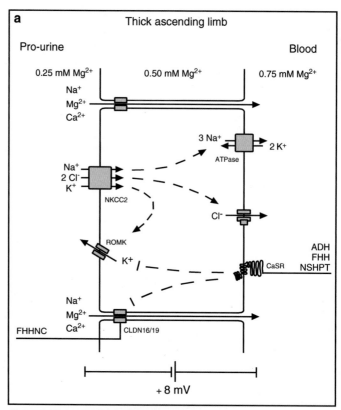

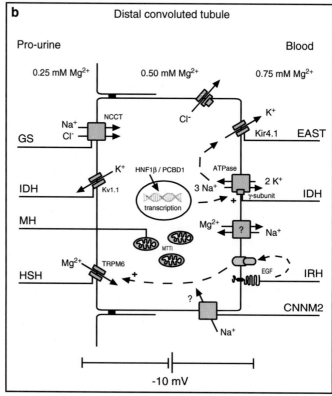

the authors speculate on a role of EGF as a first selectively acting magnesiotropic hormone [83].

Hypomagnesemia with Impaired Brain Development (OMIM # 613882)

Another form of hereditary Mg^{2+} wasting could be linked to mutations in *CNNM2* encoding the transmembrane protein CNNM2 or Cyclin M2 [158]. CNNM2 (originally termed ACDP2) had previously been identified by differential expression in a mouse DCT cell line under varying Mg^{2+} concentrations as well as by microarray analysis of the renal transcriptome in mice lacking claudin-16 [158, 159]. In addition, common variants in CNNM2 had been shown to be associated with serum Mg^{2+} levels in a genome-wide association study [160].

Stuiver et al. identified heterozygous *CNNM2* mutations in two families with IDH [158]. Clinical symptoms and age at manifestation were variable with symptoms ranging from seizures in early childhood to muscle weakness, vertigo and headache during adolescence. Other heterozygous carriers from both families even remained asymptomatic. Except for hypomagnesemia (serum Mg^{2+} of 0.36–0.51 mmol/L in symptomatic patients), no additional serum or urine electrolyte abnormalities were described. Whereas a truncating frame-shift mutation was identified in one of the described families, affected individuals of the second family were found to carry a missense mutation leading to a non-conservative amino acid exchange in CNNM2 [158]. The functional characterization of mutant CNNM2-p.T568I demonstrated that the protein trafficking in HEK293 cells was preserved. However, patch clamp analyses revealed a significant reduction in Mg^{2+}-sensitive, inwardly-rectifying Na^+ currents [158].

The phenotypic and genetic spectrum of CNNM2-associated disease was broadened by the identification of a recessive mutation in a family with parental consanguinity [161]. The two affected siblings exhibited hypomagnesemia (~0.5 mmol/L) and severe psychomotor retardation. MR imaging of the central nervous system in one of the patients revealed widened outer cerebrospinal liquor spaces as well as myelinization defects. Moreover, by screening a larger cohort of sporadic hypomagnesemia cases, the same study revealed four subjects with *de novo* heterozygous mutations [161]. The affected children presented in infancy with generalized convulsions and displayed significant intellectual disability.

Despite this clinical and genetic progress, the precise physiological function of CNNM2 still remains enigmatic. CNNM2 is ubiquitously expressed in mammalian tissues, most prominently in kidney, brain and lung [162, 163]. In the kidney, CNNM2 expression was demonstrated at the basolateral membrane of TAL and DCT.

Although CNNM2 had been proposed as a Mg^{2+} transporter according to overexpression studies in Xenopus oocytes [159]; Mg^{2+} transport could not be directly measured in mammalian cells using patch clamp analyses [158]. *In silico* modeling of CNNM2 protein domains identified a Mg^{2+}-ATP binding site suggesting a putative role in Mg^{2+}-sensing [163]. Using stable Mg^{2+} isotopes, an increase in cellular Mg^{2+} uptake was demonstrated after overexpression of CNNM2, an effect that was abrogated by the introduction of pathogenic mutations identified in hypomagnesemic patients [161]. Finally, CNNM2 function was studied in the zebrafish model. Here, knock-down of CNNM2 expression lead to a decrease in whole-body Mg^{2+} as well as developmental defects of the central nervous system in line with human disease. The zebrafish phenotype could be rescued by wildtype mammalian Cnnm2 but not by Cnnm2 with inserted human mutations, underlining the specificity of the knock-down approach [161]. Further studies will be needed to clarify if CNNM2 serves as a Mg^{2+}-sensor or whether it can actively transport Mg^{2+}.

HNF1B Nephropathy (OMIM# 137920)

Hepatocyte nuclear factor 1β (HNF1B) is a transcription factor critical for the development of the kidney and the pancreas. Heterozygous mutations in *HNF1B* were first implicated in a subtype of maturity-onset diabetes of the young (MODY5) [164]. Later, an association with developmental renal disease was reported. The renal phenotype is highly variable comprising enlarged hyperechogenic kidneys, multicystic kidney disease, renal agenesis, renal hypoplasia, cystic dysplasia, as well as hyperuricemic nephropathy. The association with both symptom complexes led to the term renal cysts and diabetes syndrome (RCAD) [165]. However, this denomination might be misleading because neither the renal cystic phenotype nor the diabetes are constant clinical findings [166]. For this reason, the new term HNF1B nephropathy has been introduced.

HNF1B mutations are present in heterozygous state, either inherited or de novo, and comprise point mutations as well as whole-gene deletions [167]. Interestingly, ~50% of patients present with hypomagnesemia due to impaired renal Mg^{2+} conservation [167, 168]. Renal Mg^{2+} wasting is accompanied by hypocalciuria indicating an involvement of the DCT.

The *HNF1B* gene encodes a transcription factor of the homeodomain-containing superfamily that regulates the expression of numerous renal genes including *FXYD2* (see above), which contains several HNF1B-binding sites in its promoter region [168]. In accordance with the phenotype and *in silico* data, Adalat et al. showed that HNF1B can induce the expression of FXYD2 *in vitro*. Therefore, defective FXYD2 transcription potentially represents a mechanism explaining renal Mg^{2+} wasting in patients with HNF1B mutations.

Transient Neonatal Hyperphenylalaninemia (OMIM# 264070)

Recently, renal Mg^{2+} wasting has been demonstrated in transient neonatal hyperphenylalaninemia due to recessive mutations in the *PCBD1* gene [169]. Affected patients develop hypomagnesemia and a MODY type diabetes in adulthood. Functional studies revealed that PCBD1 is an essential dimerization cofactor of HNF1B. Defective dimerization of PCBD1 with

HNF1B abrogated the HNF1B-mediated stimulation of *FXYD2* promoter activity in the DCT [169].

Mitochondrial Hypomagnesemia (OMIM #500005)

A mutation in the mitochondrial tRNA gene for Isoleucine, tRNA[Ile] or MTTI, has been discovered in a large Caucasian kindred [170]. An extensive clinical evaluation of this family was prompted after the discovery of hypomagnesemia in the index patient. Pedigree analysis was compatible with mitochondrial inheritance as the phenotype was exclusively transmitted by affected females. The phenotype included hypomagnesemia, hypercholesterolemia, and hypertension. Of the adults on the maternal lineage, the majority of offspring exhibited at least one of the mentioned symptoms, approximately half of the individuals showed a combination of two or more symptoms, and around 1/6 had all three features [170]. Serum Mg^{2+} levels of family members on the maternal lineage greatly varied ranging from ~0.8 to ~2.5 mg/dL (equivalent to ~0.3 to ~1.0 mmol/L) with approximately 50% of individuals being hypomagnesemic.

The hypomagnesemic individuals (serum Mg^{2+} <0.9 mmol/L) showed higher fractional excretions (median around 7.5%) than their normomagnesemic relatives on the maternal lineage (median around 3%), clearly pointing to renal Mg^{2+} wasting as causative for hypomagnesemia. Interestingly, hypomagnesemia was accompanied by decreased urinary Ca^{2+} levels, a finding pointing to the DCT as the affected tubular segment.

The mitochondrial mutation observed in the examined family affects the tRNA[Ile] gene MTTI. The observed nucleotide exchange occurs at the T-nucleotide directly adjacent to the anticodon triplet. This position is highly conserved among species and critical for codon-anticodon recognition. The functional consequences of the tRNA defect for mitochondrial function remain to be elucidated in detail. As ATP consumption along the tubule is highest in the DCT, the authors speculate on an impaired energy metabolism of DCT cells as a consequence of the mitochondrial defect which in turn could lead to disturbed transcellular Mg^{2+} reabsorption [170]. Further studies in these patients might help to better understand the mechanism of distal tubular Mg^{2+} wasting in this disease.

References

1. Committee to Review Dietary Reference Intakes for Vitamin D and Calcium, Institutes of Medicine. Dietary reference intakes for calcium and vitamin D. Washington, DC: The National Academies; 2011.
2. Gueguen L, Pointillart A. The bioavailability of dietary calcium. J Am Coll Nutr. 2000;19(2 Suppl):119s–36.
3. Moe SM. Confusion on the complexity of calcium balance. Semin Dial. 2010;23(5):492–7.
4. Martin A, David V, Quarles LD. Regulation and function of the FGF23/klotho endocrine pathways. Physiol Rev. 2012;92(1):131–55.
5. Kumar R, Tebben PJ, Thompson JR. Vitamin D and the kidney. Arch Biochem Biophys. 2012;523(1):77–86.
6. Matos V, van Melle G, Boulat O, et al. Urinary phosphate/creatinine, calcium/creatinine, and magnesium/creatinine ratios in a healthy pediatric population. J Pediatr. 1997;131(2):252–7.
7. Metz MP. Determining urinary calcium/creatinine cut-offs for the paediatric population using published data. Ann Clin Biochem. 2006;43(Pt 5):398–401.
8. Bianchetti MG, Edefonti A, Bettinelli A. The biochemical diagnosis of Gitelman disease and the definition of "hypocalciuria". Pediatr Nephrol. 2003;18(5):409–11.
9. Singh J, Moghal N, Pearce SH, et al. The investigation of hypocalcaemia and rickets. Arch Dis Child. 2003;88(5):403–7.
10. Bastepe M. Genetics and epigenetics of parathyroid hormone resistance. Endocr Dev. 2013;24:11–24.
11. Brown EM, Pollak M, Chou YH, et al. Cloning and functional characterization of extracellular Ca(2+)-sensing receptors from parathyroid and kidney. Bone. 1995;17(2 Suppl):7S–11.
12. Loupy A, Ramakrishnan SK, Wootla B, et al. PTH-independent regulation of blood calcium concentration by the calcium-sensing receptor. J Clin Invest. 2012;122(9):3355–67.
13. Houillier P. Calcium-sensing in the kidney. Curr Opin Nephrol Hypertens. 2013;22(5):566–71.
14. Pollak MR, Brown EM, Estep HL, et al. Autosomal dominant hypocalcaemia caused by a Ca(2+)-sensing receptor gene mutation. Nat Genet. 1994;8(3):303–7.
15. Pearce SH, Williamson C, Kifor O, et al. A familial syndrome of hypocalcemia with hypercalciuria due to mutations in the calcium-sensing receptor. N Engl J Med. 1996;335(15):1115–22.
16. Watanabe S, Fukumoto S, Chang H, et al. Association between activating mutations of calcium-sensing receptor and Bartter's syndrome. Lancet. 2002;360(9334):692–4.
17. Rodd C, Goodyer P. Hypercalcemia of the newborn: etiology, evaluation, and management. Pediatr Nephrol. 1999;13(6):542–7.
18. Davies JH. A practical approach to problems of hypercalcaemia. Endocr Dev. 2009;16:93–114.
19. Davies JH, Shaw NJ. Investigation and management of hypercalcaemia in children. Arch Dis Child. 2012;97(6):533–8.
20. Vieth R. The mechanisms of vitamin D toxicity. Bone Miner. 1990;11(3):267–72.
21. Mizusawa Y, Burke JR. Prednisolone and cellulose phosphate treatment in idiopathic infantile hypercalcaemia with nephrocalcinosis. J Paediatr Child Health. 1996;32(4):350–2.
22. Pak CY. Clinical pharmacology of sodium cellulose phosphate. J Clin Pharmacol. 1979;19(8–9 Pt 1):451–7.
23. Skalova S, Cerna L, Bayer M, et al. Intravenous pamidronate in the treatment of severe idiopathic infantile hypercalcemia. Iran J Kidney Dis. 2013;7(2):160–4.
24. Nguyen M, Boutignon H, Mallet E, et al. Infantile hypercalcemia and hypercalciuria: new insights into a vitamin D-dependent mechanism and response to ketoconazole treatment. J Pediatr. 2010;157(2):296–302.
25. Fencl F, Blahova K, Schlingmann KP, et al. Severe hypercalcemic crisis in an infant with idiopathic infantile hypercalcemia caused by mutation in CYP24A1 gene. Eur J Pediatr. 2013;172(1):45–9.
26. Pollak MR, Brown EM, Chou YH, et al. Mutations in the human Ca(2+)-sensing receptor gene cause familial hypocalciuric hypercalcemia and neonatal severe hyperparathyroidism. Cell. 1993;75(7):1297–303.
27. Marx SJ, Attie MF, Levine MA, et al. The hypocalciuric or benign variant of familial hypercalcemia: clinical and biochemical features in fifteen kindreds. Medicine (Baltimore). 1981;60(6):397–412.
28. Cole DE, Janicic N, Salisbury SR, et al. Neonatal severe hyperparathyroidism, secondary hyperparathyroidism, and familial hypocalciuric hypercalcemia: multiple different phenotypes associated with an inactivating Alu insertion mutation of the calcium-sensing receptor gene. Am J Med Genet. 1997;71(2):202–10.
29. Lightwood R, Stapleton T. Idiopathic hypercalcaemia in infants. Lancet. 1953;265(6779):255–6.
30. Fanconi G. Chronic disorders of calcium and phosphate metabolism in children. Schweiz Med Wochenschr. 1951;81(38):908–13.
31. Pronicka E, Rowińska E, Kulczycka H, et al. Persistent hypercalciuria and elevated 25-hydroxyvitamin D3 in children with infantile hypercalcaemia. Pediatr Nephrol. 1997;11(1):2–6.
32. Williams JC, Barratt-Boyes BG, Lowe JB. Supravalvular aortic stenosis. Circulation. 1961;24:1311–8.
33. Beuren AJ, Apitz J, Harmjanz D. Supravalvular aortic stenosis in association with mental retardation

and a certain facial appearance. Circulation. 1962; 26:1235–40.

34. Schlingmann KP, Kaufmann M, Weber S, et al. Mutations in CYP24A1 and idiopathic infantile hypercalcemia. N Engl J Med. 2011;365(5):410–21.

35. Makin G, Lohnes D, Byford V, et al. Target cell metabolism of 1,25-dihydroxyvitamin D3 to calcitroic acid. Evidence for a pathway in kidney and bone involving 24-oxidation. Biochem J. 1989; 262(1):173–80.

36. Reddy GS, Tserng KY. Calcitroic acid, end product of renal metabolism of 1,25-dihydroxyvitamin D3 through C-24 oxidation pathway. Biochemistry. 1989;28(4):1763–9.

37. Kaufmann M, Gallagher JC, Peacock M, et al. Clinical utility of simultaneous quantitation of 25-hydroxyvitamin D and 24,25-dihydroxyvitamin D by LC-MS/MS involving derivatization with DMEQ-TAD. J Clin Endocrinol Metab. 2014;99(7):2567–74.

38. Misselwitz J, Hesse V. Hypercalcemia following prophylactic vitamin D administration. Kinderarztl Prax. 1986;54(8):431–8.

39. Streeten EA, Zarbalian K, Damcott CM. CYP24A1 mutations in idiopathic infantile hypercalcemia. N Engl J Med. 2011;365(18):1741–2; author reply 1742–3.

40. Tebben PJ, Milliner DS, Horst RL, et al. Hypercalcemia, hypercalciuria, and elevated calcitriol concentrations with autosomal dominant transmission due to CYP24A1 mutations: effects of ketoconazole therapy. J Clin Endocrinol Metab. 2012;97(3):E423–7.

41. Nesterova G, Malicdan MC, Yasuda K, et al. 1,25-(OH)2D-24 hydroxylase (CYP24A1) deficiency as a cause of nephrolithiasis. Clin J Am Soc Nephrol. 2013;8(4):649–57.

42. Quamme GA, de Rouffignac C. Epithelial magnesium transport and regulation by the kidney. Front Biosci. 2000;5:D694–711.

43. Kerstan DQG. Physiology and pathophysiology of intestinal absorption of magnesium. In: Massry SG MH, Nishizawa Y, editors. Calcium in internal medicine. Surry: Springer-Verlag; 2002. p. 171–83.

44. Fine KD, Santa Ana CA, Porter JL, et al. Intestinal absorption of magnesium from food and supplements. J Clin Invest. 1991;88(2):396–402.

45. de Rouffignac C, Quamme G. Renal magnesium handling and its hormonal control. Physiol Rev. 1994;74(2):305–22.

46. Dai LJ, Ritchie G, Kerstan D, et al. Magnesium transport in the renal distal convoluted tubule. Physiol Rev. 2001;81(1):51–84.

47. Quamme GA. Renal magnesium handling: new insights in understanding old problems. Kidney Int. 1997;52(5):1180–95.

48. Whang R, Hampton EM, Whang DD. Magnesium homeostasis and clinical disorders of magnesium deficiency. Ann Pharmacother. 1994;28(2):220–6.

49. Anast CS, Mohs JM, Kaplan SL, et al. Evidence for parathyroid failure in magnesium deficiency. Science. 1972;177(4049):606–8.

50. Quitterer U, Hoffmann M, Freichel M, et al. Paradoxical block of parathormone secretion is mediated by increased activity of G alpha subunits. J Biol Chem. 2001;276(9):6763–9.

51. Zimmermann G, Zhou D, Taussig R. Mutations uncover a role for two magnesium ions in the catalytic mechanism of adenylyl cyclase. J Biol Chem. 1998;273(31):19650–5.

52. Hollifield JW. Magnesium depletion, diuretics, and arrhythmias. Am J Med. 1987;82(3a):30–7.

53. Elin RJ. Magnesium: the fifth but forgotten electrolyte. Am J Clin Pathol. 1994;102(5):616–22.

54. Arnold A, Tovey J, Mangat P, et al. Magnesium deficiency in critically ill patients. Anaesthesia. 1995;50(3):203–5.

55. Hébert P, Mehta N, Wang J, et al. Functional magnesium deficiency in critically ill patients identified using a magnesium-loading test. Crit Care Med. 1997;25(5):749–55.

56. Hashimoto Y, Nishimura Y, Maeda H, et al. Assessment of magnesium status in patients with bronchial asthma. J Asthma. 2000;37(6):489–96.

57. Sutton RA, Domrongkitchaiporn S. Abnormal renal magnesium handling. Miner Electrolyte Metab. 1993;19(4–5):232–40.

58. Elisaf M, Panteli K, Theodorou J, et al. Fractional excretion of magnesium in normal subjects and in patients with hypomagnesemia. Magnes Res. 1997;10(4):315–20.

59. Tang NL, Cran YK, Hui E, et al. Application of urine magnesium/creatinine ratio as an indicator for insufficient magnesium intake. Clin Biochem. 2000; 33(8):675–8.

60. Nicoll GW, Struthers AD, Fraser CG. Biological variation of urinary magnesium. Clin Chem. 1991;37(10 Pt 1):1794–5.

61. Djurhuus MS, Gram J, Petersen PH, et al. Biological variation of serum and urinary magnesium in apparently healthy males. Scand J Clin Lab Invest. 1995;55(6):549–58.

62. English MW, Skinner R, Pearson AD, et al. Dose-related nephrotoxicity of carboplatin in children. Br J Cancer. 1999;81(2):336–41.

63. Goren MP. Cisplatin nephrotoxicity affects magnesium and calcium metabolism. Med Pediatr Oncol. 2003;41(3):186–9.

64. Boulikas T, Vougiouka M. Recent clinical trials using cisplatin, carboplatin and their combination chemotherapy drugs (review). Oncol Rep. 2004;11(3):559–95.

65. Lajer H, Daugaard G. Cisplatin and hypomagnesemia. Cancer Treat Rev. 1999;25(1):47–58.

66. Mavichak V, Coppin CM, Wong NL, et al. Renal magnesium wasting and hypocalciuria in chronic cis-platinum nephropathy in man. Clin Sci (Lond). 1988;75(2):203–7.

67. Bianchetti MG, Kanaka C, Ridolfi-Lüthy A, et al. Persisting renotubular sequelae after cisplatin in children and adolescents. Am J Nephrol. 1991;11(2):127–30.

68. Markmann M, Rothman R, Reichman B, et al. Persistent hypomagnesemia following cisplatin chemotherapy in patients with ovarian cancer. J Cancer Res Clin Oncol. 1991;117(2):89–90.

69. Ledeganck KJ, Boulet GA, Bogers JJ, et al. The TRPM6/EGF pathway is downregulated in a rat model of cisplatin nephrotoxicity. PLoS ONE. 2013;8(2):e57016.

70. Yoshida T, Niho S, Toda M, et al. Protective effect of magnesium preloading on cisplatin-induced nephrotoxicity: a retrospective study. Jpn J Clin Oncol. 2014;44(4):346–54.

71. Shah GM, Kirschenbaum MA. Renal magnesium wasting associated with therapeutic agents. Miner Electrolyte Metab. 1991;17(1):58–64.

72. Elliott C, Newman N, Madan A. Gentamicin effects on urinary electrolyte excretion in healthy subjects. Clin Pharmacol Ther. 2000;67(1):16–21.

73. Giapros VI, Cholevas VI, Andronikou SK. Acute effects of gentamicin on urinary electrolyte excretion in neonates. Pediatr Nephrol. 2004;19(3):322–5.

74. Ward DT, McLarnon SJ, Riccardi D. Aminoglycosides increase intracellular calcium levels and ERK activity in proximal tubular OK cells expressing the extracellular calcium-sensing receptor. J Am Soc Nephrol. 2002;13(6):1481–9.

75. Lee CT, Chen HC, Ng HY, et al. Renal adaptation to gentamicin-induced mineral loss. Am J Nephrol. 2012;35(3):279–86.

76. Rob PM, Lebeau A, Nobiling R, et al. Magnesium metabolism: basic aspects and implications of ciclosporine toxicity in rats. Nephron. 1996;72(1):59–66.

77. Lote CJ, Thewles A, Wood JA, et al. The hypomagnesaemic action of FK506: urinary excretion of magnesium and calcium and the role of parathyroid hormone. Clin Sci (Lond). 2000;99(4):285–92.

78. Chang CT, Hung CC, Tian YC, et al. Ciclosporin reduces paracellin-1 expression and magnesium transport in thick ascending limb cells. Nephrol Dial Transplant. 2007;22(4):1033–40.

79. Nijenhuis T, Hoenderop JG, Bindels RJ. Downregulation of Ca(2+) and Mg(2+) transport proteins in the kidney explains tacrolimus (FK506)-induced hypercalciuria and hypomagnesemia. J Am Soc Nephrol. 2004;15(3):549–57.

80. Goel M, Garcia R, Estacion M, et al. Regulation of drosophila TRPL channels by immunophilin FKBP59. J Biol Chem. 2001;276(42):38762–73.

81. Mervaala EM, Müller DN, Park JK, et al. Monocyte infiltration and adhesion molecules in a rat model of high human renin hypertension. Hypertension. 1999;33(1 Pt 2):389–95.

82. Miura K, Nakatani T, Asai T, et al. Role of hypomagnesemia in chronic cyclosporine nephropathy. Transplantation. 2002;73(3):340–7.

83. Groenestege WM, Thébault S, van der Wijst J, et al. Impaired basolateral sorting of pro-EGF causes isolated recessive renal hypomagnesemia. J Clin Invest. 2007;117(8):2260–7.

84. Tejpar S, Piessevaux H, Claes K, et al. Magnesium wasting associated with epidermal-growth-factor receptor-targeting antibodies in colorectal cancer: a prospective study. Lancet Oncol. 2007;8(5):387–94.

85. Cao Y, Liao C, Tan A, et al. Meta-analysis of incidence and risk of hypomagnesemia with cetuximab for advanced cancer. Chemotherapy. 2010;56(6):459–65.

86. Cundy T, Mackay J. Proton pump inhibitors and severe hypomagnesaemia. Curr Opin Gastroenterol. 2011;27(2):180–5.

87. Epstein M, McGrath S, Law F. Proton-pump inhibitors and hypomagnesemic hypoparathyroidism. N Engl J Med. 2006;355(17):1834–6.

88. Shabajee N, Lamb EJ, Sturgess I, et al. Omeprazole and refractory hypomagnesaemia. BMJ. 2008;337:a425.

89. Ahmad ASR. Disorders of magnesium metabolism. The kidney: physiology and pathophysiology. New York: Raven Press; 2000. p. 1732–48.

90. Agus ZS. Hypomagnesemia. J Am Soc Nephrol. 1999;10(7):1616–22.

91. Koo W, Tsang RC. Calcium and magnesium homeostasis. In: Avery G, Fletcher M, MacDonald M, editors. Neonatology – pathophysiology and management of the newborn. 5th ed. Philadelphia/Baltimore/New York: Lippincott Williams & Wilkins; 1999. p. 730.

92. Cronan K, Norman ME. Renal and electrolyte emergencies. In: Fleisher G, Ludwig S, editors. Pediatric emergency medicine. 4th ed. Philadelphia/Baltimore/New York: Lippincott Williams & Wilkins; 2000.

93. Gal P, Reed M. Medications. In: Behrman R, Kliegman R, Jenson H, editors. Textbook of pediatrics. 16th ed. Philadelphia/Toronto/London: WB Saunders; 2000.

94. Ranade VV, Somberg JC. Bioavailability and pharmacokinetics of magnesium after administration of magnesium salts to humans. Am J Ther. 2001;8(5):345–57.

95. Ryan MP. Magnesium and potassium-sparing diuretics. Magnesium. 1986;5(5–6):282–92.

96. Netzer T, Knauf H, Mutschler E. Modulation of electrolyte excretion by potassium retaining diuretics. Eur Heart J. 1992;13(Suppl G):22–7.

97. Colussi G, Rombola G, De Ferrari ME, et al. Correction of hypokalemia with antialdosterone therapy in Gitelman's syndrome. Am J Nephrol. 1994;14(2):127–35.

98. Bundy JT, Connito D, Mahoney MD, et al. Treatment of idiopathic renal magnesium wasting with amiloride. Am J Nephrol. 1995;15(1):75–7.

99. Simon DB, Lu Y, Choate KA, et al. Paracellin-1, a renal tight junction protein required for paracellular Mg2+ resorption. Science. 1999;285(5424):103–6.

100. Konrad M, Schaller A, Seelow D, et al. Mutations in the tight-junction gene claudin 19 (CLDN19) are associated with renal magnesium wasting, renal failure, and severe ocular involvement. Am J Hum Genet. 2006;79(5):949–57.

101. Michelis MF, Drash AL, Linarelli LG, et al. Decreased bicarbonate threshold and renal magnesium wasting in a sibship with distal renal tubular acidosis. (Evaluation of the pathophysiological role of parathyroid hormone). Metabolism. 1972; 21(10):905–20.

102. Praga M, Vara J, González-Parra E, et al. Familial hypomagnesemia with hypercalciuria and nephrocalcinosis. Kidney Int. 1995;47(5):1419–25.

103. Weber S, Schneider L, Peters M, et al. Novel paracellin-1 mutations in 25 families with familial hypomagnesemia with hypercalciuria and nephrocalcinosis. J Am Soc Nephrol. 2001;12(9):1872–81.

104. Godron A, Harambat J, Boccio V, et al. Familial hypomagnesemia with hypercalciuria and nephrocalcinosis: phenotype-genotype correlation and outcome in 32 patients with CLDN16 or CLDN19 mutations. Clin J Am Soc Nephrol. 2012;7(5):801–9.

105. Claverie-Martin F, Garcia-Nieto V, Loris C, et al. Claudin-19 mutations and clinical phenotype in Spanish patients with familial hypomagnesemia with hypercalciuria and nephrocalcinosis. PLoS ONE. 2013;8(1):e53151.

106. Zimmermann B, Plank C, Konrad M, et al. Hydrochlorothiazide in CLDN16 mutation. Nephrol Dial Transplant. 2006;21(8):2127–32.

107. Rodriguez-Soriano J, Vallo A, Garcia-Fuentes M. Hypomagnesaemia of hereditary renal origin. Pediatr Nephrol. 1987;1(3):465–72.

108. Colegio OR, Van Itallie C, Rahner C, et al. Claudin extracellular domains determine paracellular charge selectivity and resistance but not tight junction fibril architecture. Am J Physiol Cell Physiol. 2003;284(6):C1346–54.

109. Ohba Y, Kitagawa H, Kitoh K, et al. A deletion of the paracellin-1 gene is responsible for renal tubular dysplasia in cattle. Genomics. 2000;68(3):229–36.

110. Will C, Breiderhoff T, Thumfart J, et al. Targeted deletion of murine Cldn16 identifies extra- and intrarenal compensatory mechanisms of Ca2+ and Mg2+ wasting. Am J Physiol Renal Physiol. 2010;298(5):F1152–61.

111. Konrad M, Hou J, Weber S, et al. CLDN16 genotype predicts renal decline in familial hypomagnesemia with hypercalciuria and nephrocalcinosis. J Am Soc Nephrol. 2008;19(1):171–81.

112. Blanchard A, Jeunemaitre X, Coudol P, et al. Paracellin-1 is critical for magnesium and calcium reabsorption in the human thick ascending limb of Henle. Kidney Int. 2001;59(6):2206–15.

113. Müller D, Kausalya PJ, Claverie-Martin F, et al. A novel claudin 16 mutation associated with childhood hypercalciuria abolishes binding to ZO-1 and results in lysosomal mistargeting. Am J Hum Genet. 2003;73(6):1293–301.

114. Knoers NV, Levtchenko EN. Gitelman syndrome. Orphanet J Rare Dis. 2008;3:22.

115. Simon DB, Nelson-Williams C, Bia MJ, et al. Gitelman's variant of Bartter's syndrome, inherited hypokalaemic alkalosis, is caused by mutations in the thiazide-sensitive Na-Cl cotransporter. Nat Genet. 1996;12(1):24–30.

116. Gitelman HJ, Graham JB, Welt LG. A new familial disorder characterized by hypokalemia and hypomagnesemia. Trans Assoc Am Physicians. 1966; 79:221–35.

117. Peters N, Bettinelli A, Spicher I, et al. Renal tubular function in children and adolescents with Gitelman's syndrome, the hypocalciuric variant of Bartter's syndrome. Nephrol Dial Transplant. 1995;10(8):1313–9.

118. Bettinelli A, Bianchetti MG, Girardin E, et al. Use of calcium excretion values to distinguish two forms of primary renal tubular hypokalemic alkalosis: Bartter and Gitelman syndromes. J Pediatr. 1992; 120(1):38–43.

119. Peters M, Jeck N, Reinalter S, et al. Clinical presentation of genetically defined patients with hypokalemic salt-losing tubulopathies. Am J Med. 2002;112(3):183–90.

120. Tammaro F, Bettinelli A, Cattarelli D, et al. Early appearance of hypokalemia in Gitelman syndrome. Pediatr Nephrol. 2010;25(10):2179–82.

121. Bettinelli A, Tosetto C, Colussi G, et al. Electrocardiogram with prolonged QT interval in Gitelman disease. Kidney Int. 2002;62(2):580–4.

122. Calo L, Punzi L, Semplicini A. Hypomagnesemia and chondrocalcinosis in Bartter's and Gitelman's syndrome: review of the pathogenetic mechanisms. Am J Nephrol Switzerland. 2000;20:347–50.

123. Luthy C, Bettinelli A, Iselin S, et al. Normal prostaglandinuria E2 in Gitelman's syndrome, the hypocalciuric variant of Bartter's syndrome. Am J Kidney Dis. 1995;25(6):824–8.

124. Bockenhauer D, Feather S, Stanescu HC, et al. Epilepsy, ataxia, sensorineural deafness, tubulopathy, and KCNJ10 mutations. N Engl J Med. 2009;360(19):1960–70.

125. Scholl UI, Choi M, Liu T, et al. Seizures, sensorineural deafness, ataxia, mental retardation, and electrolyte imbalance (SeSAME syndrome) caused by mutations in KCNJ10. Proc Natl Acad Sci U S A. 2009;106(14):5842–7.

126. Neusch C, Rozengurt N, Jacobs RE, et al. Kir4.1 potassium channel subunit is crucial for oligodendrocyte development and in vivo myelination. J Neurosci. 2001;21(15):5429–38.

127. Paunier L, Radde IC, Kooh SW, et al. Primary hypomagnesemia with secondary hypocalcemia in an infant. Pediatrics. 1968;41(2):385–402.

128. Shalev H, Phillip M, Galil A, et al. Clinical presentation and outcome in primary familial hypomagnesaemia. Arch Dis Child. 1998;78(2):127–30.

129. Lombeck I, Ritzl F, Schnippering HG, et al. Primary hypomagnesemia. I. Absorption studies. Z Kinderheilkd. 1975;118(4):249–58.

130. Milla PJ, Aggett PJ, Wolff OH, et al. Studies in primary hypomagnesaemia: evidence for defective carrier-mediated small intestinal transport of magnesium. Gut. 1979;20(11):1028–33.

131. Matzkin H, Lotan D, Boichis H. Primary hypomagnesemia with a probable double magnesium transport defect. Nephron. 1989;52(1):83–6.

132. Walder RY, Shalev H, Brennan TM, et al. Familial hypomagnesemia maps to chromosome 9q, not to the X chromosome: genetic linkage mapping and analysis of a balanced translocation breakpoint. Hum Mol Genet. 1997;6(9):1491–7.

133. Schlingmann KP, Weber S, Peters M, et al. Hypomagnesemia with secondary hypocalcemia is caused by mutations in TRPM6, a new member of the TRPM gene family. Nat Genet. 2002;31(2):166–70.

134. Walder RY, Landau D, Meyer P, et al. Mutation of TRPM6 causes familial hypomagnesemia with secondary hypocalcemia. Nat Genet. 2002;31(2):171–4.

135. Jalkanen R, Pronicka E, Tyynismaa H, et al. Genetic background of HSH in three polish families and a patient with an X;9 translocation. Eur J Hum Genet. 2006;14(1):55–62.

136. Guran T, Akcay T, Bereket A, et al. Clinical and molecular characterization of Turkish patients with familial hypomagnesaemia: novel mutations in TRPM6 and CLDN16 genes. Nephrol Dial Transplant. 2012;27(2):667–73.

137. Lainez S, Schlingmann KP, van der Wijst J, et al. New TRPM6 missense mutations linked to hypomagnesemia with secondary hypocalcemia. Eur J Hum Genet. 2014;22(4):497–504.

138. Chubanov V, Schlingmann KP, Wäring J, et al. Hypomagnesemia with secondary hypocalcemia due to a missense mutation in the putative pore-forming region of TRPM6. J Biol Chem. 2007;282(10):7656–67.

139. Ryazanova LV, Dorovkov MV, Ansari A, et al. Characterization of the protein kinase activity of TRPM7/ChaK1, a protein kinase fused to the transient receptor potential ion channel. J Biol Chem. 2004;279(5):3708–16.

140. Nadler MJ, Hermosura MC, Inabe K, et al. LTRPC7 is a Mg.ATP-regulated divalent cation channel required for cell viability. Nature. 2001;411(6837):590–5.

141. Cole DE, Kooh SW, Vieth R. Primary infantile hypomagnesaemia: outcome after 21 years and treatment with continuous nocturnal nasogastric magnesium infusion. Eur J Pediatr. 2000;159(1–2):38–43.

142. Chubanov V, Waldegger S, Mederos y Schnitzler M, et al. Disruption of TRPM6/TRPM7 complex formation by a mutation in the TRPM6 gene causes hypomagnesemia with secondary hypocalcemia. Proc Natl Acad Sci U S A. 2004;101(9):2894–9.

143. Schmitz C, Dorovkov MV, Zhao X, et al. The channel kinases TRPM6 and TRPM7 are functionally nonredundant. J Biol Chem. 2005;280(45):37763–71.

144. Voets T, Nilius B, Hoefs S, et al. TRPM6 forms the Mg2+ influx channel involved in intestinal and renal Mg2+ absorption. J Biol Chem. 2004;279(1):19–25.

145. Li M, Jiang J, Yue L. Functional characterization of homo- and heteromeric channel kinases TRPM6 and TRPM7. J Gen Physiol. 2006;127(5):525–37.

146. Zhang Z, Yu H, Huang J, et al. The TRPM6 kinase domain determines the Mg.ATP sensitivity of TRPM7/M6 heteromeric ion channels. J Biol Chem. 2014;289(8):5217–27.

147. Meij IC, Koenderink JB, van Bokhoven H, et al. Dominant isolated renal magnesium loss is caused by misrouting of the Na(+), K(+)-ATPase gamma-subunit. Nat Genet. 2000;26(3):265–6.

148. Geven WB, Monnens LA, Willems HL, et al. Renal magnesium wasting in two families with autosomal dominant inheritance. Kidney Int. 1987;31(5):1140–4.

149. Sweadner KJ, Arystarkhova E, Donnet C, et al. FXYD proteins as regulators of the Na, K-ATPase in the kidney. Ann N Y Acad Sci. 2003;986:382–7.

150. Arystarkhova E, Wetzel RK, Sweadner KJ. Distribution and oligomeric association of splice forms of Na(+)-K(+)-ATPase regulatory gamma-subunit in rat kidney. Am J Physiol Renal Physiol. 2002;282(3):F393–407.

151. Arystarkhova E, Donnet C, Asinovski NK, et al. Differential regulation of renal Na, K-ATPase by splice variants of the gamma subunit. J Biol Chem. 2002;277(12):10162–72.

152. Meij IC, van den Heuvel LP, Hemmes S, et al. Exclusion of mutations in FXYD2, CLDN16 and SLC12A3 in two families with primary renal Mg2+ loss. Nephrol Dial Transplant. 2003;18(3):512–6.

153. Glaudemans B, van der Wijst J, Scola RH, et al. A missense mutation in the Kv1.1 voltage-gated potassium channel-encoding gene KCNA1 is linked to human autosomal dominant hypomagnesemia. J Clin Invest. 2009;119(4):936–42.

154. Browne DL, Gancher ST, Nutt JG, et al. Episodic ataxia/myokymia syndrome is associated with point mutations in the human potassium channel gene, KCNA1. Nat Genet. 1994;8(2):136–40.

155. van der Wijst J, Glaudemans B, Venselaar H, et al. Functional analysis of the Kv1.1 N255D mutation associated with autosomal dominant hypomagnesemia. J Biol Chem. 2010;285(1):171–8.

156. Geven WB, Monnens LA, Willems JL, et al. Isolated autosomal recessive renal magnesium loss in two sisters. Clin Genet. 1987;32(6):398–402.

157. Thebault S, Alexander RT, Tiel Groenestege WM, et al. EGF increases TRPM6 activity and surface expression. J Am Soc Nephrol. 2009;20(1):78–85.

158. Stuiver M, Lainez S, Will C, et al. CNNM2, encoding a basolateral protein required for renal Mg2+ handling, is mutated in dominant hypomagnesemia. Am J Hum Genet. 2011;88(3):333–43.

159. Goytain A, Quamme GA. Functional characterization of ACDP2 (ancient conserved domain protein), a divalent metal transporter. Physiol Genomics. 2005;22(3):382–9.

160. Meyer TE, Verwoert GC, Hwang SJ, et al. Genome-wide association studies of serum magnesium, potassium, and sodium concentrations identify six Loci influencing serum magnesium levels. PLoS Genet. 2010;6(8):e1001045.

161. Arjona FJ, de Baaij JH, Schlingmann KP, et al. CNNM2 mutations cause impaired brain development and seizures in patients with hypomagnesemia. PLoS Genet. 2014;10(4):e1004267.

162. Wang CY, Shi JD, Yang P, et al. Molecular cloning and characterization of a novel gene family of four ancient conserved domain proteins (ACDP). Gene. 2003;306:37–44.

163. de Baaij JH, Stuiver M, Meij IC, et al. Membrane topology and intracellular processing of cyclin M2 (CNNM2). J Biol Chem. 2012;287(17):13644–55.

164. Horikawa Y, Iwasaki N, Hara M, et al. Mutation in hepatocyte nuclear factor-1 beta gene (TCF2) associated with MODY. Nat Genet. 1997;17(4):384–5.

165. Lindner TH, Njolstad PR, Horikawa Y, et al. A novel syndrome of diabetes mellitus, renal dysfunction and genital malformation associated with a partial deletion of the pseudo-POU domain of hepatocyte nuclear factor-1beta. Hum Mol Genet. 1999;8(11):2001–8.

166. Faguer S, Decramer S, Chassaing N, et al. Diagnosis, management, and prognosis of HNF1B nephropathy in adulthood. Kidney Int. 2011;80(7):768–76.

167. Heidet L, Decramer S, Pawtowski A, et al. Spectrum of HNF1B mutations in a large cohort of patients who harbor renal diseases. Clin J Am Soc Nephrol. 2010;5(6):1079–90.

168. Adalat S, Woolf AS, Johnstone KA, et al. HNF1B mutations associate with hypomagnesemia and renal magnesium wasting. J Am Soc Nephrol. 2009;20(5): 1123–31.

169. Ferre S, de Baaij JH, Ferreira P, et al. Mutations in PCBD1 cause hypomagnesemia and renal magnesium wasting. J Am Soc Nephrol. 2014;25(3): 574–86.

170. Wilson FH, Hariri A, Farhi A, et al. A cluster of metabolic defects caused by mutation in a mitochondrial tRNA. Science. 2004;306(5699):1190–4.

Disorders of Phosphorus Metabolism

35

Dieter Haffner and Siegfried Waldegger

Introduction

The underlying pathophysiological mechanisms of hypophosphatemic disorders have been unraveled during the last decade, although some puzzles remain to be solved. In 1937, Albright first reported on a patient with rickets and severe hypophosphatemia not responding to high doses of vitamin D. The term vitamin D resistant rickets was coined, and later the disease was named X-linked hypophosphatemic rickets (XLHR) [1].

In recent years several underlying genes have been identified in distinct forms of hypophosphatemic rickets [2]. Rickets is a disease of the growth plate and therefore only growing children are affected. Whereas in the past rickets was thought to be a disease of calcium and vitamin D metabolism, there is growing evidence that rickets is due to insufficient availability of phosphate which is required for normal bone metabolism [3].

In principle, phosphate deficiency may result from inappropriate absorption in the gut or reabsorption in the kidney. The latter situation can be further divided between defects in the tubular reabsorption apparatus and abnormalities of circulating factors which regulate phosphate reabsorption [4]. The major breakthrough in our understanding of hypophosphatemic disorders was the discovery of fibroblast growth factor 23 (FGF23), a member of the FGF family, which mediates the combined renal tubular defects in phosphate reabsorption and altered vitamin D metabolism observed in patients with hypophosphatemic rickets.

Currently, specific disease-causing mutations in genes involved in the regulation of phosphate homeostasis can be identified in approx. 85 % of familial or sporadic cases of hypophosphatemic rickets [5–7]. This chapter focuses on the etiology, pathogenesis, clinical presentation, differential diagnosis and treatment of hypophosphatemic disorders due to a reduction of renal tubular reabsorption.

Phosphate Homeostasis

Inorganic phosphate (Pi) is a key player in cellular metabolism and skeletal mineralization. It accounts for about 0.61 and 1 % of body weight of a neonate and an adult, respectively. Approximately 85 % of total body Pi content is deposited as hydroxyl-apatite $[Ca_5(PO_4)_3OH]$ in the skeleton and the teeth. About 14 % distributes within the intracellular compartment. There,

D. Haffner
Department of Pediatric Kidney, Liver, and Metabolic Diseases, Hannover Medical School,
Hannover, Germany
e-mail: haffner.dieter@mh-hannover.de

S. Waldegger
Department of Pediatrics, University Hospital Innsbruck, Innsbruck, Austria
e-mail: siegfried.waldegger@tirol-kliniken.at

© Springer-Verlag Berlin Heidelberg 2016
D.F. Geary, F. Schaefer (eds.), *Pediatric Kidney Disease*, DOI 10.1007/978-3-662-52972-0_35

Pi participates in as diverse cellular processes as cell membrane function (phospholipids), energy metabolism (ATP), cell signaling (phosphorylation by kinases), and DNA- or RNA-biosynthesis (phosphorylated nucleotides). Only 1 % of the total body Pi content is found as a soluble fraction in the extracellular compartment. There, Pi contributes to the acid-base buffering capacity of the plasma and even more important of the urine. Solely this tip of the iceberg is amenable to conventional laboratory investigations from blood and urine samples. Moreover, circulatory Pi is the central mediator between bone, the parathyroid glands, the gut and the kidneys, which are fine-tuned by numerous hormonal signals to keep the serum phosphate concentration within close limits.

In a steady state condition, as it is the case after completion of skeletal growth, the serum Pi concentration is determined by the balance between intestinal absorption of phosphate from the diet (16 mg/kg per day), bone-turnover of phosphate in the skeleton (3 mg/kg per day), and excretion of phosphate through the urine (16 mg/kg per day), (Fig. 35.1). In growing individuals, the balance of Pi must be positive to meet the needs of skeletal growth and consolidation. A typical Western diet commonly provides plenty of alimentary Pi, most of which provided by protein-rich foods like meat, milk and eggs. In contrast to plant-derived phosphate in the form of phytate (hexa-phospho-inosite), the animal derived phosphate is easily absorbed by the intestine, where roughly two thirds of the ingested phosphate are absorbed. Intestinal Pi absorption in growing infants is higher than in adults and can exceed 90 % of dietary intake. Absorbed Pi first distributes in the extracellular

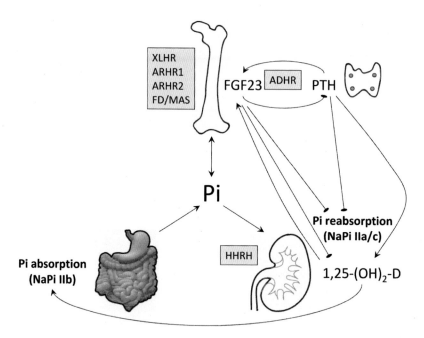

Fig. 35.1 Regulation of phosphate homeostasis. FGF23 and PTH reduce renal tubular phosphate reabsorption via a decrease in apical expression of the sodium-phosphate cotransporters NaPi IIa and NaPi IIc. In contrast to FGF23, which inhibits 1,25-(OH)₂D synthesis, PTH stimulates 1,25-(OH)₂D production. 1,25-(OH)₂D increases intestinal absorption of dietary Pi via increased expression of NaPi IIb and activates FGF23 production. PTH and FGF23 affect each other's production through a negative feed back loop that is not yet fully elucidated. The sites of defect of the different genetic forms of hypophosphatemic disorders are given. *XLHR* X-linked dominant hypophosphatemic rickets, *ARHR1/2* autosomal recessive hypophosphatemic rickets 1/2, *FD/MAS* Fibrous dysplasia/McCune-Albright syndrome, *HHRH* hereditary hypophosphatemic rickets with hypercalciuria, *ADHR* X-linked dominant hypophosphatemic rickets. * = FGF23 protein resistant to degradation

compartment and then equilibrates with the bone and intracellular compartment. Within the kidney, Pi is freely filtered at the glomerular capillaries and is reabsorbed mainly along the proximal nephrons according to the actual requirements of the organism. The majority of the transepithelial Pi transport in the intestine and the kidney is mediated by the type II family of sodium-coupled phosphate transporters, i.e., NaPi-IIa (NPT2a; *SLC34A1*), NaPi-IIb (NPT2b; *SLC34A2*), and NaPi-IIc (NPT2c; *SLC34A3*) [8]. NaPi-IIa is primarily localized at the brush border of proximal tubular epithelial cells and accounts for roughly 90 % of renal phosphate reabsorption. Reabsorption of the remaining 10 % is accomplished by NaPi-IIc exclusively expressed along proximal tubules of deep nephrons. Its critical contribution to Pi homeostasis is demonstrated by loss-of-function mutations, which leads to renal phosphate wasting resulting in the rare syndrome of hypophosphatemic rickets with hypercalcemia (HHRH) [9].

In contrast to NaPi-IIa and NaPi-IIc, NaPi-IIb shows a broader expression pattern including pulmonary alveolar type II cells, where it participates in Pi uptake from the alveolar fluid for surfactant production. *SLC34A2* mutations cause pulmonary alveolar microlithiasis, a disease characterized by the deposition of calcium-phosphate crystals throughout the lungs [10]. In the intestine, NaPi-IIb is expressed in the brush border membrane of enterocytes and mediates absorption of ingested phosphate.

Regulators of Phosphate Homeostasis

The amount of intestinal phosphate absorption directly correlates with dietary supply. Only 30 % of intestinal Pi absorption occurs in a regulated, 1,25-dihydroxyvitamin D [1,25-(OH)$_2$D] dependent manner. This poor regulation at the uptake level contrasts with the meticulous regulation of phosphate excretion within the kidney. Proximal tubular reabsorption of phosphate, mainly via regulation of expression of NaPi-IIa and NaPi-IIc within proximal tubular brush border membranes, thus plays a key role in maintaining serum phosphate homeostasis. The amount of renal phosphate reabsorption is tightly regulated primarily by dietary Pi intake, parathyroid hormone (PTH) and fibroblast growth factor 23 (FGF23). Other factors like insulin, human growth hormone, and possibly FGF7 also affect renal phosphate handling, but their actions are less well understood [11].

Dietary Pi intake directly affects the amount of renal phosphate reabsorption. An increase or decrease in dietary Pi induces an increase or decrease, respectively, in renal Pi excretion independent of vitamin D, PTH or FGF23. Part of this effect might be explained by a phosphate-responsive element in the promoter of the *SLC34A1* gene [12].

Parathyroid hormone is a major hormonal regulator of proximal tubular Pi reabsorption. PTH synthesis and secretion are up-regulated by low serum calcium and increased serum phosphate levels, and down-regulated by increased serum calcium and 1,25(OH)$_2$D levels. Its binding to proximal tubular PTH receptors results in an inhibition of NaPi-cotransport through mechanisms that involve rapid clearance of NaPi-IIa from the tubular epithelial brush border membrane [13]. On the other hand, PTH stimulates the synthesis of 1,25-(OH)$_2$D. The net effect of these actions is an increase of serum calcium levels and a decrease in serum phosphate levels.

Fibroblast Growth Factor 23 is a glycoprotein primarily synthesized in osteocytes and osteoblasts. FGF23 expression is induced by increased serum phosphate and 1,25(OH)$_2$D levels. In the presence of Klotho, a membrane bound protein with ß-glucuronidase activity, FGF23 binds with high affinity to the FGF receptor FGFR1 [11]. Klotho/FGFR1 mediated renal effects of FGF23 result in inhibition of proximal tubular Pi reabsorption and 1,25(OH)$_2$D synthesis. Its net effect thus is a reduction in serum phosphate and 1,25-(OH)$_2$D levels, which may result in hypocalcemia (Fig. 35.1).

See Table 35.1 for genetic disorders of phosphate regulation.

Table 35.1 Genetic disorders of phosphate regulation

Definition	Abbreviation	MIM ID	Location	Gene/locus involved	Pathogenesis
X-linked dominant hypophosphatemic rickets	XLHR	307800	Xp22.1	*PHEX*	FGF23 expression in bone ↑
Autosomal dominant hypophosphatemic rickets	ADHR	193100	12p13.32	*FGF23*	FGF23 protein resistant to degradation
Autosomal recessive hypophosphatemic rickets 1	ARHR1	241520	4q.22.1	*DMP1*	FGF23 expression in bone ↑
Autosomal recessive hypophosphatemic rickets 2	ARHR2	613312	6q23.2	*ENPP1*	FGF23 expression in bone ↑
Hereditary hypophosphatemic rickets with hypercalciuria	HHRH	241530	9q34.3	*SLC34A3*	Loss of function of NaPi2c in the proximal tubule
X-linked recessive hypophosphatemic rickets	–	300554	Xp11.23-p11.22	*CLCN5*	Loss of function of CLCN5 in the proximal tubule
Hypophosphatemic rickets and Hyperparathyroidism	–	612089	13q13.1	Translocation with Klotho	unknown
Fibrous dysplasia/ McCune-Albright syndrome	FD/MAS	174800	20q13.32	*GNAS1*	FGF23 expression in bone lesions ↑
Autosomal recessive Fanconi syndrome, hypophosphatemic rickets	–	182309	5q35.3	*NaPi2a*	Loss of function of NaPi2a in the proximal tubule

Hypophosphatemic Disorders

Clinical, Biochemical, and Radiological Manifestations

Clinical Findings

Clinical and radiological features of the various types of hypophosphatemic rickets are similar, although not identical. In children the primary clinical symptoms are skeletal pain and deformity, bone fractures, disproportionate short stature, and dental abscesses (Figs. 35.2a, b and 35.3). In adults, osteomalacia, bone pain and stiffness and enthesopathy are typical findings [15]. With medical therapy these abnormalities can be improved, but usually do not entirely resolve [14]. Most children with hypophosphatemic rickets are identified in the first year of life if there is a known family history of the disorder. By 6 months of age, classic skeletal deformities may already appear including frontal bossing with flattening at the back of the head. In the absence of a family history, children often present between ages 2 and 3 years with progressive lower extremity deformities (bow-legged). Common misdiagnoses are metaphyseal dysplasia and nutritional rickets. Long-term outcomes are substantially better when treatment is applied at an early age, i.e., in the first year of life [16–18]. In contrast to hypophosphatemic rickets the clinical signs of phosphopenic osteomalacia are non-descript and often overlooked. Patients may report on diffuse skeletal pain and muscle weakness resulting in a waddling gait. Skeletal pain frequently worsens with activity and sometimes results in an antalgic gait. The occurrence of

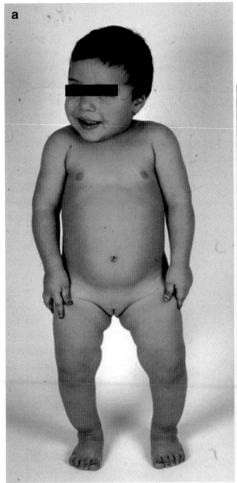

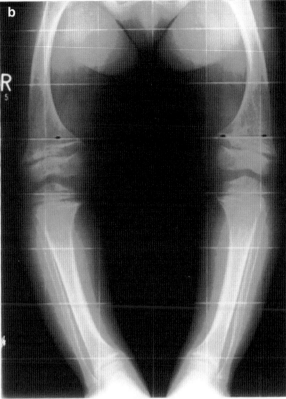

Fig. 35.2 Photograph (**a**) and radiograph of the lower extremities (**b**) of a 3 year old girl with X-linked hypophosphatemic rickets. The patient shows disproportionate stunting with bowed legs. The radiograph reveals severe leg bowing, partial fraying and irregularity of the distal femoral and proximal tibial growth plates

fractures of the long bones, the ribs and vertebral bodies may result in progressive deformities in addition to pain.

Bone histology is influenced by the pathophysiology of the disease. In general, pure hypophosphatemia results in accumulation of unmineralized osteoid (Fig. 35.4), while the concomitant presence of hyperparathyroidism adds the component of enhanced bone resorption by osteoclasts [20]. However, establishing a diagnosis of phosphopenic osteomalacia requires histopathological proof that the abundant osteoid results from abnormal mineralization and not increased osteoid production. Thus, histopathological detection of an increase in the bone-forming cell surface by incompletely cov-

ered mineralized osteoid, an increase in osteoid volume and thickness and a decrease in the mineralization front (the percentage of osteoid-covered bone-forming surface undergoing calcification) or the mineral apposition rate is a prerequisite [21].

In addition to these skeletal defects, dental abnormalities contribute to considerable clinical morbidity. Tooth eruption may be delayed and teeth may exhibit inadequate dentine calcification [22]. As a result, the pulp chambers expand, and the overall barrier to external pathogens is compromised, thereby predisposing to dental abscesses. The prevalence of dental abscesses is about 25 % in children and more than 85 % in adults [23]. Individuals who present with one abscess usually

Fig. 35.3 Mean standard deviation scores (SDS) and 95 % confidence intervals (CI) of stature, sitting height, and arm and leg length in 76 children with X-linked hypophosphatemic rickets. Patients showed disproportionate stunting. Leg length was the most impaired and trunk length the most preserved linear body dimension (Used with permission of Springer Science + Business Media from Zivicnjak et al. [14])

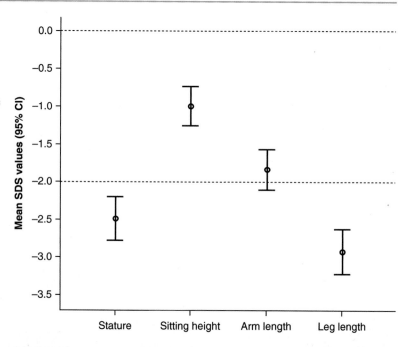

Fig. 35.4 Bone biopsy in a patient with X-linked hypophosphatemic rickets showing abundance of unmineralized osteoid (*orange*), and decreased mineralization of trabecular and cortical bone (Used with permission of Springer Science + Business Media from Schnabel and Haffner [19])

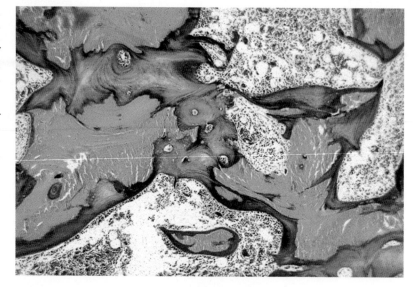

develop multiple abscesses during follow-up, indicating that the development of one abscess predicts future abscesses. It is important to note that dental abscesses usually occur in the absence of caries. Finally, hypertension, left ventricular hypertrophy, nephrocalcinosis, craniosynostosis, and hearing loss have been identified in patients suffering from hypophosphatemic rickets, although it is not clear if these abnormalities are due to the disease itself or to the treatment [24–26].

Radiological Findings

The rachitic abnormalities in children with phosphopenic disease result in a variety of characteristic radiological findings in the skeleton. The growth plates of the long bones are cupped and show increased thickness and irregular, hazy appearance at the diaphyseal line (Fig. 35.2). The latter is due to an irregular invasion of recently calcified cartilage in bone tissue. These abnormalities preferentially occur at sites of rapid growth. Therefore, widening of the forearm at the wrist and thickening of the costochondral junctions frequently occur. For clinical confirmation, an x-ray of the knees and/or the wrist is usually sufficient to diagnose rickets. In addition, other typical signs of rickets such as rachitic rosary and Harrison's groove may also develop. Rapid growth of the long bones also results in bowing of the lower extremities and of the skull, i.e., parietal flattening, frontal bossing and widened sutures.

Biochemical Findings

In general the primary diagnosis of rickets is based on typical clinical and radiological findings (see above) in combination with an elevated serum alkaline phosphatase activity. Physicians often overlook the latter abnormality in children, since normal levels in young children are high. On the other hand in some affected patients, normal alkaline phosphatase activity might be observed. Moreover, in adults, the alkaline phosphatase levels are often inexplicably normal. For differential diagnosis of the various forms of rickets, additional biochemical parameters are needed. Based on the supposition of phosphorus as the common denominator of all types of rickets, a new differential diagnosis of rickets was recently proposed [3, 4, 20]. This diagnostic approach focuses on the mechanisms leading to hypophosphatemia, i.e., (i) high PTH activity, (ii) inadequate phosphate absorption from the gut, or (iii) renal phosphaturia. The latter may be due to either tubular defects or high circulating FGF23 levels (Fig. 35.5).

Renal phosphate loss can be evaluated through the tubular reabsorption of phosphate per glomerular filtration rate (TmP/GFR) as: TmP/GFR $= P_p - (U_p \times P_{cr}/U_{cr})$, where P_p, U_p, P_{cr} and U_{cr} refer to plasma and urine concentration of phosphate and creatinine, respectively. All values must be expressed in the same units, e.g., in milligrams per deciliter [27]. The normal range of TmP/GFR in infants and children (6 months–6 years) ranges from 1.2 to 2.6 mmol/l and in adults from 0.6 to 1.7 mmol/l. An important pitfall to recognize is that in patients with insufficient intake or absorption of phosphate from the gut TmP/GFR might be falsely low when serum phosphate levels have not been restored to normal. This can usually be assumed in the presence of low urinary phosphate levels. In such cases, TmP/GFR should only be calculated after phosphate supplementation when serum and urine phosphate concentrations are raised.

Typically in cases of hypophosphaetmic rickets due to renal tubular abnormalities or elevated serum levels of FGF23, serum concentrations of calcium and PTH are normal before

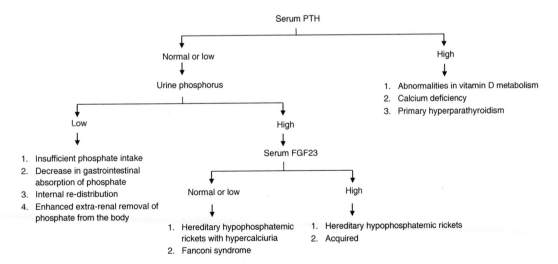

Fig. 35.5 Algorithm for the evaluation of the child with rickets. Further details of individual entities can be found in Tables 35.1 and 35.2: FGF-23, fibroblast growth factor 23 (Used with permission of Springer Science + Business Media from Penido and Alon [4])

Table 35.2 Biochemical characteristics of the various forms of hypophosphatemic rickets due to pertubations in proximal tubule phosphate reabsorption compared to vitamin D deficiency rickets

Disorder	Ca	P	AP	U_{ca}	TmP/GFR	FGF23	PTH	25-OH-D$^\$$	1,25(OH)$_2$D
Vitamin D deficiency rickets	N, ↓	N, ↓	↑	↓	↓	N, ↓	↑	↓	Varies
X-linked hypophosphatemic rickets	N	↓	↑	N	↓	↑	N	N	N°
Autosomal dominant hypophosphatemic rickets	N	↓	↑	N	↓	↑	N	N	N°
Autosomal recessive hypophosphatemic rickets 1	N	↓	↑	N	↓	↑	N	N	N°
Autosomal recessive hypophosphatemic rickets 2	N	↓	↑	N	↓	↑	N	N	N°
Fibrous dysplasia/tumor-induced osteomalacia	N	↓	↑	N	↓	↑	N, ↓	N	N°
Hereditary hypophosphatemic rickets with hypercalciuria	N	↓	↑	↑	↓	N, ↓	↓	N	↑
X-linked recessive hypophosphatemic rickets	N	↓	↑	↑	↓	Varies	Varies	N	↑
Hypophosphatemic rickets and hyperparathyroidism	N	↓	↑	N	↓	↑	↑	N	N°
Fanconi syndrome	N	↓	↑	Varies	↓	N, ↓	↓	N	Varies

Ca serum calcium, *P* serum phosphate, *AP* alkaline phosphatase, U_{ca} urinary calcium excretion, *TmP/GFR* maximum rate of renal tubular reabsorption of phosphate normalized to the glomerular filtration rate, *FGF23* fibroblast growth factor 23, *PTH* parathyroid hormone, *1,25(OH)$_2$D* 1,25-dihydroxyvitamin, ° decreased relative to the serum phosphate concentration, $^\$$ cave: prevalence of vitamin D deficiency was reported to be up-to 50 % in healthy children

initiation of treatment. Circulating levels of 1,25-dihydroxyvitamin D (1,25(OH)$_2$D) levels are low or inappropriately normal in the setting of hypophosphatemia. Plasma FGF23 levels are usually elevated with the exception of HHRH patients. Measurement of serum 1,25(OH)$_2$D levels may be a useful tool for diagnosis in HHHR patients. In Table 35.2, the main biochemical features of the various forms of hypophosphatemic rickets due to perturbations in proximal tubule phosphate reabsorption compared to vitamin D deficiency rickets are summarized.

Hypophosphatemic Disorders with Increased FGF23 Activity

XLHR (PHEX Mutation)

X-linked hypophosphatemic rickets (XLHR) is the most frequent inherited phosphate wasting disorder, accounting for about 80 % of familial cases with an incidence of 1:20,000 individu-

als. It typically presents within the first 2 years of life. Males usually show the full manifestation of the disease and females show a wide spectrum ranging from one identical to males to one with no clinical symptoms but only isolated hypophosphatemia. The characteristic laboratory results are hypophosphatemia, hyperphosphaturia, hyperphosphatasia and normocalcemia. Serum levels of 25(OH)D and of 1,25(OH)$_2$D levels are in the normal range. However, the level of the latter appears to be decreased relative to the diminished serum phosphate concentrations. Elevated serum levels of FGF23 and mutations in the *PHEX* gene (phosphate regulating gene with homologies to endopeptidases on the X-chromosome) can be found in most patients [7, 28]. In the case of a positive family history, affected patients can be detected between the ages of 4–6 months by increased alkaline phosphatase activity. In 2011, Morey et al. showed a phenotype-genotype correlation between PHEX gene mutations and disease pattern in 46 individuals with XLHR. Patients with clearly deleterious *PHEX* mutations had lower TmP/GFR and 1,25(OH)$_2$D levels, suggesting that the type of *PHEX* mutation might predict the severity of phenotype expression [29]. However, this could not be confirmed in a later study. In a study on 23 XLHR patients treated with phosphate and calcitriol from childhood onwards a weak positive correlation between final adult height and TmP/GFR at the time of diagnosis was reported [23].

Although the genetic cause of XLHR is well established, the exact pathogenic mechanisms of how mutations in the PHEX gene result in elevated plasma FGF23 levels remains to be elucidated. PHEX encodes for a membrane-bound endopeptidase and is primarily expressed in osteoblasts, osteocytes, odontoblasts, muscle, lung and ovary [30]. The finding that hypophosphatemia recurs in XLHR patients undergoing kidney transplantation with prior parathyreoidectomy strongly suggests a circulating factor causing phosphate wasting in the kidney transplant which was labelled "phosphatonin" [31]. Likewise, studies in *Hyp* mice, an orthologic animal model of XLHR employing parabiosis and cross-transplantation of the kidneys between *Hyp* and normal mice, also showed recurrence of hypophosphatemia [32]. After it became clear that FGF23 is the cause of ADHR, FGF23 levels were measured in patients with XLHR and *Hyp* mice. The majority of XLHR patients as well as *Hyp* mice show elevated FGF23 levels [33, 34]. The finding that some XLHR patients present "normal" FGF23 serum levels might be viewed as inappropriately high in relation to the degree of hypohosphatemia. Administration of neutralizing antibodies to FGF23 corrects the hypophosphatemia and decreases 1,25(OH)$_2$D levels in *Hyp* mice and thus confirms the pathogenic role of FGF23 in XLHR [35]. FGF23 was once thought to be substrate of PHEX but this finding could not be confirmed in other studies [36]. It is not yet clear how *PHEX* mutations result in elevated FGF23 levels.

ADHR (FGF23 Mutation)

Autosomal-dominant hypophosphatemic rickets (ADHR) is a rare disorder that was first described by Bianchine et al. in 1971 [37]. ADHR and XLHR have marked clinical similarities but differ in their modes of inheritance. ADHR is due to activating mutations of the *FGF23* gene. The mutated protein is resistant to cleavage by proteolytic activity, which in turn leads to elevated, circulating FGF23 levels [38]. Elevated FGF23 levels result in phosphaturia, hypophosphatemia, and inappropriately low levels of 1,25(OH)$_2$D. The penetrance of ADHR is incomplete, with a highly variable phenotype and, thus, variable symptomatology and biological findings. In contrast to XLHR, patients suffering from ADHR may become symptomatic in adolescence or even during adulthood. During childhood the clinical symptoms are similar to that observed in XLHR, i.e., rickets with bone deformities, disproportionately short stature, and dental abnormalities (abscesses) [39]. If patients become symptomatic after puberty, complications due to osteomalacia, e.g., weakness, fatigue, bone pain and fractures are the major symptoms. Adults present with symptoms similar to those with tumor induced osteomalacia (TIO), as discussed below. Interestingly, some children show improvement of phosphate wasting during puberty [40]. Recent studies in ADHR mice and humans suggest that iron status may regulate FGF23 metabolic pathways [41, 42]. Therefore, the onset of ADHR is the product of gene-environment interactions. In ADHR patients' serum iron was negatively associated with both c-terminal FGF23 and intact FGF23. Similarly, a negative correlation between serum iron and c-terminal FGF23 was observed in healthy subjects, indicating increased expression and cleavage of FGF23 in the setting of a low iron status.

ARHR (1, DMP1 Mutation; 2, ENPP1 Mutation)

The finding of hypophosphatemic rickets in consanguineous kindreds suggested an autosomal recessive form of hypophosphatemia (ARHR) [43]. Clinical symptoms are similar to those observed in XLHR patients and affected individuals present with elevated FGF23 serum levels, renal phosphate wasting and inappropriately normal levels of 1,25(OH)$_2$D. One characteristic radiological feature of this disorder is the relatively high bone density of the vertebral bodies. ARHR is either due to mutations in the *DMP1* gene encoding for dentin matrix acidic phosphoprotein 1 (ARHR1) or to mutations in the *ENPP1* gene encoding for ectonucleotide pyrophosphatase/phosphodiesterase 1 (ARHR2) [44–47]. DMP1 is a member of the short integrin-binding ligand interacting N-linked glycoprotein (SIBLING) family of skeletal matrix proteins and is highly expressed in mineralized tissues, e.g., in osteoblasts and osteocytes. It is an important regulator of the development of bone, cartilage, and teeth. How mutations in DMP1 result in elevated FGF23 serum levels in ADHR1 patients is unclear. Levi-Litan et al. identified an inactivating mutation in the *ENPP1* gene (later named ARHR2) that caused ARHR in a Bedouin family [47]. ENPP1 is a cell surface protein that catalyzes phosphoester cleavage of adenosine triphosphate, generating the mineralization inhibitor pyrophosphate. Mutations in *ENPP1* were initially reported in patients with infantile arterial calcifications [48]. It remains to be elucidated how inactivating *ENPP1* gene mutations result in increased FGF23 synthesis from bone.

Tumor-Induced Osteomalacia and Tumor-Induced Rickets (TIO)

Tumor-induced osteomalacia (TIO), also called tumor-induced rickets, is a rare disorder characterized by hypophosphatemia, hyperphosphaturia, low $1,25(OH)_2D$ serum levels, and osteomalacia which develops in previously healthy individuals [49, 50]. Therefore, in any patients presenting with hypophosphatemic rickets beyond the second year of life TIO should be excluded. Clinical symptoms are similar to that in XLHR or ADHR patients. TIO is caused by usually small, often difficult to locate, tumors. Most histologic diagnoses have been classified as phosphaturic mesenchymal tumors of the mixed connective tissue type. A characteristic histologic feature of these tumors is a background of spindle cells that tend to have low mitotic activity [51]. Once the tumor is removed, the clinical symptoms quickly resolve, which has led to the notion that circulating factors produced by the

tumor (phosphatonins) are causing renal phosphate loss in these patients. Later, TIO tumors were shown to contain high levels of FGF23 mRNA and protein, and TIO patients revealed elevated circulating FGF23 levels, which rapidly declined after removal of the tumor in parallel with resolution of clinical symptoms [52]. The tumors are benign, but may recur. The paranasal sinuses, neck and mandible are common sites of these tumors. Newer imaging techniques such as nuclear magnetic resonance and positron emission tomography are helpful in establishing diagnosis of TIO [49].

Hypophosphatemic Rickets and Hyperparathyroidism

This is an extremely rare disorder caused by increased synthesis of α-Klotho. Patients reveal both hypophosphatemic rickets and hyperparathyroidism due to parathyroid hyperplasia. It is caused by *de novo* translocation resulting in elevated plasma α-Klotho levels [53]. Recently it was demonstrated that α-Klotho enhances FGF23-stimulated FGF receptor activation, and consequently inhibition of sodium phosphate transporter and hyperphosphaturia [54]. It is thought that the concomitant suppression of calcitriol production by α-Klotho/FGF23 action may cause increased production of FGF23 and PTH in these patients.

Fibrous Dysplasia (FD) and McCune-Albright Syndrome (MAS)

Fibrous dysplasia (FD) is characterized by fibrous skeletal lesions and localized mineralization defects. Patients may present with solitary or multiple bone lesions. When the skeletal findings occur in combination with abnormal skin pigmentation (e.g., café-au-lait spots), premature sexual development and/or thyrotoxicosis, the disease is called McCune-Albright syndrome (MAS) [55]. FD/MAS is a rare disorder due to post-zygotic gain-of-function mutations in the *GNAS1* gene, encoding for the α subunit of a stimulatory G protein [56]. G proteins function to couple specific receptors to intracellular signaling molecules. Phosphate wasting is due to increased secretion of FGF23 from bone lesions and the severity of hypophosphatemia correlates with the number of fibrous dysplasia lesions. However, how *GNAS1* mutations result in elevated FGF23 secretion is currently unknown.

Hypophosphatemic Disorders with Normal or Suppressed FGF23 Activity

HHRH (SLC34A3 Mutation)

In 1985 Tieder et al. described an unusual case of hypophosphatemic rickets in a consanguineous Bedouin tribe [57]. In contrast to XLHR, hypophosphatemia and phosphate wasting was associated with elevated 1,25(OH)₂D serum levels resulting in hypercalciuria and suppressed PTH plasma concentrations. The disorder was later shown to be caused by mutations in the *SLC34A3* gene encoding for the NaPi-IIc renal phosphate cotransporter in the proximal tubule, and many more patients were identified [58]. The reported mutations were all loss-of-function mutations and, most likely, reduced renal phosphate absorption through decreasing the apical membrane expression of NaPi-IIc or the uncoupling of sodium-phosphate co-transport in the proximal tubule [59]. Thus, in contrast to XLHR and ADHR hypophosphatemia is not due to enhanced FGF23 serum levels in HHRH. The normal physiological reaction to hypophosphatemia resulting in increased serum elevated 1,25(OH)₂D levels results in increased intestinal calcium absorption, hypercalciuria and suppression of PTH. Consequent to hypercalciuria, patients developed nephrocalcinosis and nephrolithiasis. Milder forms may be under-diagnosed and therefore careful evaluation of urinary calcium excretion before and during medical treatment is strongly recommended in all patients with hypophosphatemic rickets, especially in those without a proven underlying genetic cause.

Nephrolithiasis and Osteoporosis Associated with Hypophosphatemia

Two different heterozygous mutations (A48P and V147M) in *NPT2a*, a gene encoding a sodium dependent phosphate transporter, have been reported in patients suffering from urolithiasis or osteoporosis and persistent hypophosphatemia due to decreased tubular phosphate reabsorption [60].

Fanconi Syndrome

Fanconi syndrome is characterized by generalized proximal tubular dysfunction with impaired ability to absorb water, phosphate, glucose, urate, amino acids and low molecular weight proteins. Other common features include increased excretion of sodium, potassium, calcium and bicarbonate. Clinical consequences result mainly from hypophosphatemia and metabolic acidosis, i.e., rickets and osteomalacia. The syndrome may be due to both genetic defects and acquired disorders (see Chap. 32).

Treatment of XLHR

Current treatment of patients with FGF23-dependent hypophosphatemic rickets is based on the combined treatment with active vitamin D metabolites (calcitriol or alfacalcidol) and oral inorganic phosphate salts [61]. The disease spectrum, and thus the magnitude of medication, is variable – some individuals are only minimally affected even without treatment. Adults need less treatment than children or even no treatment depending on the clinical symptoms.

Patients requiring high doses of calcitriol and phosphate are at risk of developing complications such as nephrocalcinosis and secondary hyperparathyroidism. Therefore medical treatment must be carefully balanced between undertreatment and occurrence of side effects. Medical treatment in patients with hypophosphatemic rickets is mainly based on the results in XLHR patients. Other forms of FGF23-dependent hypophosphatemic rickets like ADHR are usually treated similarly. However, some disorders require disease-specific approaches (see below).

Children with XLHR

Most children with XLHR require treatment with active vitamin D metabolites and oral phosphate supplementation from the time of diagnosis until attainment of final height. Children in affected families should therefore be screened for abnormal serum and urine phosphorus levels and serum alkaline phosphatase activity within the first month of life and at 3 and 6 months. In case of abnormal biochemical findings a radiological examination should be performed. If rickets is present, therapy with calcitriol and phosphate should be started immediately. In patients with negative family history for XLHR, hypercalciuria should be excluded before initiation of calcitriol treatment. The latter would suggest the diagnosis of HHRH where calcitriol treatment is contraindicated.

Administration of phosphate increases the plasma phosphate concentration, which lowers the plasma ionized calcium concentration, and further reduces the plasma calcitriol concentration (by removing the hypophosphatemic stimulus of its synthesis). This causes secondary hyperparathyroidism [62]. The latter can aggravate the bone disease and increase urinary phosphate excretion, thereby defeating the aim of phosphate therapy. Secondary hyperparathyroidism can be prevented by additional treatment with calcitriol. Calcitriol increases intestinal calcium absorption, and to a lesser degree phosphate, and consequently suppresses secondary hyperparathyroidism. In addition it also directly suppresses PTH release.

Initial Treatment

The recommended starting dose of elemental phosphorus is 30 mg/kg/day, with a maximum of 100 mg/kg/day not to exceed 3 g/day, increasing gradually according to the biochemical profile of the patient. Phosphorus is administered in four to five doses that are evenly spaced throughout a 24-h period. Especially in infants and young children, a nighttime dose is important to achieve satisfactory results. Liquid formulations may improve adherence and allow for more precise dosing in young children. Powders and crushed tablets may also be employed. Powders/tablets can be dissolved in water and the child may drink the solution at intervals during the day. It is important not to administer the phosphate

preparation with dairy products, since their calcium content interferes with intestinal phosphate absorption. In general, phosphorus absorption is slower in capsule or tablet formulations than in liquid ones. Therefore, when possible, it is better to use the former. Transient side effects related to phosphate medication are abdominal pain and osmotic diarrhea. Calcitriol is usually given at a starting dose of 25 ng/kg/day, e.g., 0.25 μg for an infant, administered in two doses per day. In case uneven doses of calcitriol are required, the higher dose should be given at night in order to reduce calcitriol-induced intestinal calcium absorption, which is higher during daytime due to nutritional intake. Alternatively alfacalcidol can be given in similar doses.

Monitoring and Dose Adjustments

The primary goals of treatment are to correct or minimize rickets/osteomalacia, as assessed by clinical, biochemical and radiological findings. Serum alkaline phosphatase activity is a useful surrogate marker for bone healing. With adequate treatment, serum levels of alkaline phosphatase decrease, reaching normal or slightly elevated levels. A common misconception is that successful treatment requires normalization of serum phosphate concentration, which is not a practical goal in these patients, since this could only be reached by excessive phosphate doses and paying the price of severe side effects like nephrocalcinosis and secondary hyperparathyroidism. Therefore, important measurement of therapeutic efficacy include enhanced growth velocity, improvement in lower extremity bowing and associated abnormalities, and radiological evidence of epiphyseal healing. Children should be seen every 2–4 months to monitor growth, serum concentrations of calcium, phosphate, alkaline phosphatase activity, creatinine, PTH and urinary calcium excretion. A random "spot" urine collection in infants and small children, and 24-h urine collections if possible, can be used to monitor urinary calcium excretion. The goal is to maintain a spot calcium/creatinine ratio <0.3 mg/mg or <4 mg of calcium per kg body weight per day. Renal ultrasound should be performed at yearly intervals to detect nephrocalcinosis. The etiology of nephrocalcinosis, shown by kidney biopsies to be composed of calcium phosphate precipitates, was thought to be due either to hypercalciuria, hyperphosphaturia, hyperoxaluria, hyperparathyroidism or any combination of these [63–65]. However, the reported prevalence of nephrocalcinosis in XLHR patients ranges between 17 and 80 % and is clearly related to the dose of phosphate medication [66, 67]. In addition, other soft-tissue calcifications, e.g., ocular, myocardial, and aortic valve calcifications, have been reported in XLHR patients with persistent hyperparathyroidism and/or high dose treatment [24].

Therefore, the calcitriol doses should be adjusted according to the serum levels of PTH and urinary calcium excretion. A high PTH level requires an increase in the calcitriol dose and/or a decrease of the phosphate dose (Table 35.3). The main side effect of an excessive dose of calcitriol is the development of hypercalciuria. In the presence of hypercalciuria the calcitriol dose should be reduced or thiazide diuretics added. The latter not only reduces urinary calcium excretion but also raises the TmP/GFR, most likely secondary to some degree of volume contraction. Calcitriol and phosphate treatment was shown to increase FGF23 synthesis and consequently serum FGF23 levels in humans with XLHR and in Hyp mice, thereby further stimulating urinary phosphate excretion [68]. Therefore, high dose treatment should not only be avoided to prevent hypercalciuria and nephrocalcinosis but also to prevent a vicious circle of therapy driven phosphate wasting. When secondary hyperparathyroidism cannot be adequately controlled by calcitriol treatment, i.e., persistent hypercalcemia and/or hypercalciuria, autonomous (tertiary) hyperparathyroidism can occur, necessitating surgical intervention. Finally, it is often necessary to increase dosages of phosphate and calcitriol during the pubertal growth spurt as this may result in greater mineral demands and worsening of bowing defects so that a transient increase in dosage can be advantageous. Therapy with phosphate and calcitriol is maintained as long as the growth plates are open.

Table 35.3 General guidelines for the treatment of XLHR and other forms of hypophosphatemic conditions associated with elevated FGF23 and low/inappropriately low $1,25(OH)_2D$ levels, e.g., ADHR

Clinical finding	Intervention
Lack of radiographic response or inappropriate growth retardation	↑ Calcitriol, and/or ↑ phosphate; consider growth hormone treatment
Continued osteomalacic pain	↑ Calcitriol and/or ↑ phosphate as tolerated
Hypophosphatemia	This is generally not an indication to increase phosphate dose as PTH ↑
Hypercalciuria, normal serum calcium	↓ Calcitriol, and/or add thiazide
Hypercalcemia with suppressed PTH	Discontinue all medication until serum Ca normalized
↑ PTH, normal serum calcium	↑ Calcitriol, and/or ↓ phosphate; consider cinacalcet
↑ PTH, hypercalcemia	Discontinue all medication; consider cinacalcet

Adults with XLHR

In contrast to children, the goal of therapy is mainly to manage bone pain if it occurs, and to cure any non-union fractures [15, 69]. In the light of the complexity of therapy, possible side effects, and lack of increased risk of fracture in patients without pseudo-fractures, asymptomatic patients should not be treated. Adults who are treated are prescribed medications based on symptomatology. Adults who require treatment are usually commenced on calcitriol doses of 0.75–1.0 µg per day, given in two doses per day. In addition, phosphate is given in a dose of 1–4 g per day in three to four doses. Patients should be treated with the minimal dose to allow for a pain free status. It is known that plasma phosphate of the fetus is determined by diffusion across the placenta. Therefore, is seems reasonable to maintain a higher level of phosphate in affected women who become pregnant. However, this point is still controversial and studies are underway to determine if hypophosphatemia during pregnancy affects bone mineralization or development of the fetus. Many adults with XLHR suffer from enthesopathy, which may lead to spinal cord compression and debilitating pain. Unfortunately, calcitriol and phosphate treatment does not prevent or improve this complication. It is important to note that in mice transgenic for human FGF23, treatment with calcitriol and phosphate even exacerbated the mineralization of fibrochondrocytes that define the bone spur of the Achilles insertion [70]. Therefore, innovative interventions targeted at limiting the actions of FGF23 and minimizing both the toxicities and potential morbidities associated with standard therapy, are much required.

Adjunctive Therapies

Human Growth Hormone

Although an impairment of the growth hormone (GH) insulin-like growth factor-1 axis is not the primary cause of short stature in XLHR patients, the physiological antiphosphaturic effect of GH

by stimulation of phosphate retention may be a useful adjunct to conventional treatment in improving growth in poorly growing XLHR patients. Several mostly uncontrolled studies and a placebo-controlled randomized trial have documented stimulation of growth velocity, and most likely adult height, in short XLHR patients [71–76]. In the latter trial, mean growth velocity was −1.9 SDS and 4.0 SDS during placebo and GH treatment, respectively (p<0.001). However, concern was raised that GH might aggravate the preexisting body disproportion in XLHR [73, 74]. Recently, Zivicnjak et al. reported on a European multicenter randomized trial on 3-year GH treatment in severely short (< −2.5 SDS) prepubertal XLHR patients [76]. Standardized height was increased in the GH group by 1.1 SDS with no change in body disproportion, whereas no significant change in standardized height was noted in controls (Fig. 35.6a, b). In line with previous uncontrolled studies, a transient rise in TmP/GFR, and consequently of serum phosphate

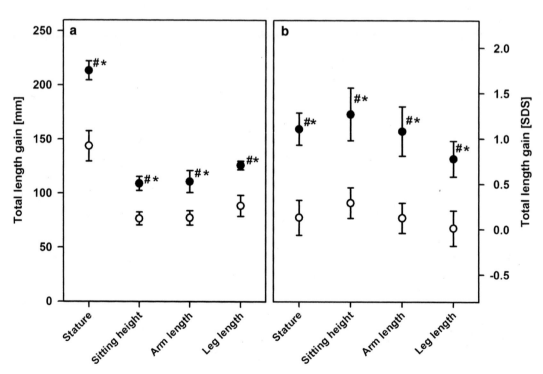

Fig. 35.6 Change in absolute values – mm (**a**) and standardized values – SDS (**b**) of stature, sitting height, and arm and leg length within 3 years in children with XLHR treated with growth hormone (GH) (●) vs. untreated controls (○). Data are given as mean ± SEM. *, P<0.01, GH vs. controls; #, P<0.01, GH vs. age-matched healthy children (Used with permission from Zivicnjak et al. [14])

concentrations, was noted during the first 6 months of GH treatment but not in controls. Importantly, the degree of leg bowing tended to be higher in GH treated patients. Therefore administration of GH might be considered in XLHR patients with persistent short stature despite adequate metabolic control. However, the possibility of worsening of leg deformities needs to be discussed as a legitimate risk of GH therapy in these patients.

Calcimimetics

The calcimimetic agent cinacalcet was shown to reduce PTH levels in XLHR patients, leading to increases in TmP/GFR and serum phosphate [77, 78]. The cinacalcet-induced decrease in serum PTH was accompanied by a slight decrease in serum-ionized calcium concentrations and was not associated with clinical symptoms. Similarly, Geller et al. proved the efficacy of cinacalcet in increasing serum phosphate levels in patients with TIO [79]. It has been suggested that long-term adjunctive treatment of XLHR patients with cinacalcet may allow for lower doses of phosphate and calcitriol and thus may minimize the risk of secondary hyperparathyroidism, hypercalcemia, hypercalciuria and nephrocalcinosis caused by high-dose phosphate and calcitriol treatment. However, randomized controlled trials on the long-term efficacy and safety of this drug in XLHR patients are lacking.

Blockade of FGF23 Action

Studies in *Hyp* mice showed that the inhibition of FGF23 overproduction by anti-FGF23 neutralizing antibodies, targeting either the FGF receptor or the α-Klotho-binding domain, resulted in normalization of serum phosphate levels, renal tubular phosphate reabsorption and marked improvement in bone mineralization, muscle weakness and longitudinal growth [35, 80]. Therefore, inhibition of FGF23 activity seems to be a promising novel therapeutic approach for FGF23-dependent forms of hypophosphatemic rickets. Early clinical studies in adult XLHR patients are currently underway in order to prove the efficacy and safety of anti-FGF23 antibody therapy. Long-term trials are going to be needed to ensure that dosage regimens

do not result in FGF23 activity being reduced to such an extent as to cause hyperphosphatemia and ectopic calcification. Another possible therapeutic approach may be to use the C-terminal tail of FGF23 to block FGF23 activity in XLHR [81]. However, this concept remains to be proven.

Surgical and Dental Care

Some patients require surgical corrections of severe bowing, regardless of adequate medical treatment. In general, candidates for osteotomy in childhood should have severe bowing, with the projection that irreversible progression of the defect cannot be avoided as growth continues. Corrective osteotomies are not usually performed in children aged less than 6 years, as medical therapy often improves bone deformities in this age group [82]. Newer, less-invasive approaches include epiphysiodesis, which induces corrective differential growth of the growth plate. Obviously, an orthopedic surgeon with experience in procedures in children with XLHR should be consulted before any intervention, and medical expertise throughout the course of surgical intervention and healing is necessary. Calcitriol medication should be adjusted during times of immobilization to avoid hypercalcemic episodes.

Unfortunately, the globular nature of dentin and under-mineralization does not appear to be improved by medical treatment. Therefore, dental abscesses might occur in XLHR patients despite adequate metabolic control [15]. Rigorous dental hygiene is recommended, including brushing two to three times daily and regular dental hygiene visits [83]. Some dentists have suggested sealant application.

Expected Outcomes

Children with XLHR have normal length at birth and show growth retardation, hypophosphatemia and rickets during the first year of life. With treatment, growth and skeletal deformities generally improve. Height velocity commonly increases during the first year of treatment. Leg deformities may correct spontaneously obviating the need for surgery, although this is not always the case. Despite general growth improvement during treatment, correction is limited and adult height is often compromised. Median adult height in XLHR patients on calcitriol and phosphate supplements (median age at start 2.3 years) published during the last two decades amounted to −2.3 SDS (range −2.7 to −1.2 SDS) [14, 15, 17, 23, 84]. However, growth outcome is significantly better if treatment is initiated early (<1 year). In two recently published studies the mean standardized height after treatment periods of approx. 10 years was substantially higher in XLHR patients with early compared to late treatment (−0.7 SDS versus −2.0 SDS, p<0.01; −1.3 SDS versus −2.0 SDS, p=0.06; Fig. 35.7) [17, 18]. However, even early treatment does not completely normalize skeletal development, and the main effect of early treatment was the prevention of a severe height deficit during early childhood.

Recently, Zivicnjak et al. reported on age-related stature and linear body dimensions in 76 children with XLHR [14]. Despite calcitriol and phosphate treatment XLHR patients showed progressive stunting and body disproportion during childhood, which was mainly due to diminished growth in the legs; growth of the trunk was less affected (Fig. 35.8a, b). This resulted in an ever-increasing sitting height index (i.e., ratio between sitting height to stature). Thus, despite medical treatment XLHR patients show uncoupled growth of legs and trunk during childhood, which in turn aggravates the pre-existent disproportion between trunk and leg length. Important to note, the degree of leg bowing was only weakly associated with leg length, explaining approximately 15 % of the overall variability. The finding that the lower limbs are more severely affected than the upper limbs and spine in XLHR most likely reflects the fact that legs, as weight-bearing extremities, are usually exposed to higher mechanical stress loads than the upper limbs and the spine. Furthermore, growth plate activity, which in turn determines the rate of endochondral bone formation and thus bone length, is usually highest around the knees. Thus, this region is also highly prone to the development of rickets and growth impairment.

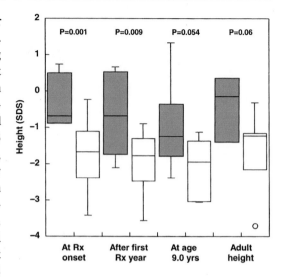

Fig. 35.7 Height z-scores in XLHR patients started on calcitriol and phosphate treatment within the first 12 months of life (■) and after the age of 12 months (□) at treatment onset, at the end of first treatment year, at age 9 years, and at final height (adult height or predicted adult height). The *bottom* of each box indicates the 25th, the cross line the 50th, and the top the 75th percentile; the *bottom* and *top lines* indicate the minimum and maximum values. P values refer to the difference between groups. *Rx* Treatment (Used with permission of Makitie et al. [17])

Notably, average serum phosphate levels and stature SDS exhibit a weak, though significant, positive correlation in children with XLHR. Recently, Jehan et al. showed that the growth outcome in XLHR patients treated from early childhood with phosphate and alphacalcidiol was associated with the presence of one or two alleles of the Hap1 haplotype in the vitamin D promoter region [85]. Therefore, the vitamin D promoter genotype appears to provide valuable information for adjusting treatment and for deciding upon utility of adjuvant therapies such as GH.

Treatment of Other Forms of Hypophosphatemic Rickets

Limited experience is available in the treatment of other forms of hypophosphatemic rickets. In general hypophosphatemic conditions associated with elevated FGF23 and low/inappropriately low $1,25(OH)_2D$ levels, i.e., ADHR and ARHR

a

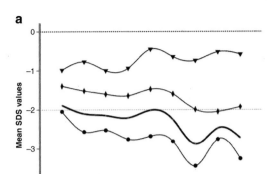

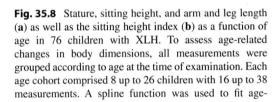

b

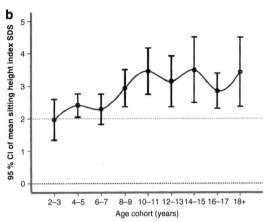

Fig. 35.8 Stature, sitting height, and arm and leg length (**a**) as well as the sitting height index (**b**) as a function of age in 76 children with XLH. To assess age-related changes in body dimensions, all measurements were grouped according to age at the time of examination. Each age cohort comprised 8 up to 26 children with 16 up to 38 measurements. A spline function was used to fit age-related changes. Unmarked solid line: stature; solid line with filled *circles*: leg length; solid line with filled rhombuses: arm length; solid line with filled inverted *triangles*: sitting height. The 95 % CI is indicated for sitting height index (Used with permission of Springer Science + Business Media from Zivicnjak et al. [14])

are treated similarly as XLHR. In patients with FD/MAS treatment with bisphosphonates results in decreased serum FGF23 levels and improves TmP/GFR [86]. Recently, treatment with bisphosphonates in combination with cabergoline, a ₃ynthetic ergot alkaloid, which acts as a long-acting D2-selective dopamine agonist, was shown to successfully arrest both dysplastic bone growth and endocrine malfunction in a female patient with FD/MAS and severe facial involvement [87]. This approach might be a suitable option in order to circumvent surgical interventions that might be of particular risk in patients suffering from polyostotic FD involving the skull base.

In patients with TIO, tumor removal usually results in a rapid clinical improvement but tumors might recur. Before surgery, patients are treated similarly to XLHR patients. Cinacalcet was successfully used in TIO patients resulting in increased TmP/GFR and serum phosphate concentrations, thereby allowing the use of significantly lower doses of phosphate and calcitriol before surgery [79].

Treatment of HHRH usually requires the administration of phosphate salts alone. In fact, treatment with calcitriol may lead to development of nephrocalcinosis and chronic renal fail-

ure. The treatment goal is to provide sufficient phosphorus to improve mineralization of osteoid, and to decrease the circulating 1,25(OH)₂D level, thereby reducing intestinal calcium resorption.

References

1. Winters RW, Graham JB, Williams TF, McFalls VW, Burnett CH. A genetic study of familial hypophosphatemia and vitamin D resistant rickets with a review of the literature. Medicine (Baltimore). 1958;37(2): 97–142.
2. Carpenter TO. The expanding family of hypophosphatemic syndromes. J Bone Miner Metab. 2012; 30(1):1–9.
3. Tiosano D, Hochberg Z. Hypophosphatemia: the common denominator of all rickets. J Bone Miner Metab. 2009;27(4):392–401.
4. Penido MG, Alon US. Hypophosphatemic rickets due to perturbations in renal tubular function. Pediatr Nephrol. 2014;29(3):361–73.
5. Gaucher C, Walrant-Debray O, Nguyen TM, Esterle L, Garabedian M, Jehan F. PHEX analysis in 118 pedigrees reveals new genetic clues in hypophosphatemic rickets. Hum Genet. 2009;125(4):401–11.
6. A gene (PEX) with homologies to endopeptidases is mutated in patients with X-linked hypophosphatemic rickets. The HYP consortium. Nat Genet. 1995;11(2): 130–6.
7. Beck-Nielsen SS, Brixen K, Gram J, Brusgaard K. Mutational analysis of PHEX, FGF23, DMP1,

SLC34A3 and CLCN5 in patients with hypophosphatemic rickets. J Hum Genet. 2012;57(7):453–8.

8. Biber J, Hernando N, Forster I. Phosphate transporters and their function. Annu Rev Physiol. 2013;75:535–50.

9. Bergwitz C, Roslin NM, Tieder M, et al. SLC34A3 mutations in patients with hereditary hypophosphatemic rickets with hypercalciuria predict a key role for the sodium-phosphate cotransporter NaPi-IIc in maintaining phosphate homeostasis. Am J Hum Genet. 2006;78(2):179–92.

10. Huqun, Izumi S, Miyazawa H, et al. Mutations in the SLC34A2 gene are associated with pulmonary alveolar microlithiasis. Am J Respir Crit Care Med. 2007;175(3):263–8.

11. Bergwitz C, Juppner H. Regulation of phosphate homeostasis by PTH, vitamin D, and FGF23. Annu Rev Med. 2010;61:91–104.

12. Kido S, Miyamoto K, Mizobuchi H, et al. Identification of regulatory sequences and binding proteins in the type II sodium/phosphate cotransporter NPT2 gene responsive to dietary phosphate. J Biol Chem. 1999;274(40):28256–63.

13. Murer H, Biber J. Molecular mechanisms of renal apical na/phosphate cotransport. Annu Rev Physiol. 1996;58:607–18.

14. Zivicnjak M, Schnabel D, Billing H, et al. Age-related stature and linear body segments in children with X-linked hypophosphatemic rickets. Pediatr Nephrol. 2011;26(2):223–31.

15. Beck-Nielsen SS, Brusgaard K, Rasmussen LM, et al. Phenotype presentation of hypophosphatemic rickets in adults. Calcif Tissue Int. 2010;87(2):108–19.

16. Kruse K, Hinkel GK, Griefahn B. Calcium metabolism and growth during early treatment of children with X-linked hypophosphataemic rickets. Eur J Pediatr. 1998;157(11):894–900.

17. Makitie O, Doria A, Kooh SW, Cole WG, Daneman A, Sochett E. Early treatment improves growth and biochemical and radiographic outcome in X-linked hypophosphatemic rickets. J Clin Endocrinol Metab. 2003;88(8):3591–7.

18. Quinlan C, Guegan K, Offiah A, et al. Growth in PHEX-associated X-linked hypophosphatemic rickets: the importance of early treatment. Pediatr Nephrol. 2012;27(4):581–8.

19. Schnabel D, Haffner D. Rickets. Diagnosis and therapy. Orthopade. 2005;34(7):703–14; quiz 715–6.

20. Penido MG, Alon US. Phosphate homeostasis and its role in bone health. Pediatr Nephrol. 2012;27(11):2039–48.

21. Frame B, Parfitt AM. Osteomalacia: current concepts. Ann Intern Med. 1978;89(6):966–82.

22. Andersen MG, Beck-Nielsen SS, Haubek D, Hintze H, Gjorup H, Poulsen S. Periapical and endodontic status of permanent teeth in patients with hypophosphatemic rickets. J Oral Rehabil. 2012;39(2):144–50.

23. Berndt M, Ehrich JH, Lazovic D, et al. Clinical course of hypophosphatemic rickets in 23 adults. Clin Nephrol. 1996;45(1):33–41.

24. Sun GE, Suer O, Carpenter TO, Tan CD, Li-Ng M. Heart failure in hypophosphatemic rickets: complications from high-dose phosphate therapy. Endocr Pract. 2013;19(1):e8–11.

25. Fishman G, Miller-Hansen D, Jacobsen C, Singhal VK, Alon US. Hearing impairment in familial X-linked hypophosphatemic rickets. Eur J Pediatr. 2004;163(10):622–3.

26. Alon US, Monzavi R, Lilien M, Rasoulpour M, Geffner ME, Yadin O. Hypertension in hypophosphatemic rickets – role of secondary hyperparathyroidism. Pediatr Nephrol. 2003;18(2):155–8.

27. Brodehl J, Krause A, Hoyer PF. Assessment of maximal tubular phosphate reabsorption: comparison with direct measurement with the nomogram of bijvoet. Pediatr Nephrol. 1988;2(2):183–9.

28. Carpenter TO, Insogna KL, Zhang JH, et al. Circulating levels of soluble klotho and FGF23 in X-linked hypophosphatemia: circadian variance, effects of treatment, and relationship to parathyroid status. J Clin Endocrinol Metab. 2010;95(11):E352–7.

29. Morey M, Castro-Feijoo L, Barreiro J, et al. Genetic diagnosis of X-linked dominant hypophosphatemic rickets in a cohort study: tubular reabsorption of phosphate and 1,25(OH)2D serum levels are associated with PHEX mutation type. BMC Med Genet. 2011;12:116. 2350-12-116.

30. Du L, Desbarats M, Viel J, Glorieux FH, Cawthorn C, Ecarot B. cDNA cloning of the murine pex gene implicated in X-linked hypophosphatemia and evidence for expression in bone. Genomics. 1996;36(1):22–8.

31. Morgan JM, Hawley WL, Chenoweth AI, Retan WJ, Diethelm AG. Renal transplantation in hypophosphatemia with vitamin D-resistant rickets. Arch Intern Med. 1974;134(3):549–52.

32. Meyer Jr RA, Tenenhouse HS, Meyer MH, Klugerman AH. The renal phosphate transport defect in normal mice parabiosed to X-linked hypophosphatemic mice persists after parathyroidectomy. J Bone Miner Res. 1989;4(4):523–32.

33. Liu S, Zhou J, Tang W, Jiang X, Rowe DW, Quarles LD. Pathogenic role of Fgf23 in hyp mice. Am J Physiol Endocrinol Metab. 2006;291(1):E38–49.

34. Yamazaki Y, Okazaki R, Shibata M, et al. Increased circulatory level of biologically active full-length FGF-23 in patients with hypophosphatemic rickets/osteomalacia. J Clin Endocrinol Metab. 2002;87(11):4957–60.

35. Aono Y, Yamazaki Y, Yasutake J, et al. Therapeutic effects of anti-FGF23 antibodies in hypophosphatemic rickets/osteomalacia. J Bone Miner Res. 2009;24(11):1879–88.

36. Gattineni J, Baum M. Regulation of phosphate transport by fibroblast growth factor 23 (FGF23): implications for disorders of phosphate metabolism. Pediatr Nephrol. 2010;25(4):591–601.

37. Bianchine JW, Stambler AA, Harrison HE. Familial hypophosphatemic rickets showing autosomal dominant

inheritance. Birth Defects Orig Artic Ser. 1971;7(6): 287–95.

38. Gribaa M, Younes M, Bouyacoub Y, et al. An autosomal dominant hypophosphatemic rickets phenotype in a tunisian family caused by a new FGF23 missense mutation. J Bone Miner Metab. 2010;28(1): 111–5.

39. Econs MJ, McEnery PT. Autosomal dominant hypophosphatemic rickets/osteomalacia: clinical characterization of a novel renal phosphate-wasting disorder. J Clin Endocrinol Metab. 1997;82(2):674–81.

40. Kruse K, Woelfel D, Strom TM. Loss of renal phosphate wasting in a child with autosomal dominant hypophosphatemic rickets caused by a FGF23 mutation. Horm Res. 2001;55(6):305–8.

41. Farrow EG, Yu X, Summers LJ, et al. Iron deficiency drives an autosomal dominant hypophosphatemic rickets (ADHR) phenotype in fibroblast growth factor-23 (Fgf23) knock-in mice. Proc Natl Acad Sci U S A. 2011;108(46):E1146–55.

42. Imel EA, Peacock M, Gray AK, Padgett LR, Hui SL, Econs MJ. Iron modifies plasma FGF23 differently in autosomal dominant hypophosphatemic rickets and healthy humans. J Clin Endocrinol Metab. 2011; 96(11):3541–9.

43. Perry W, Stamp TC. Hereditary hypophosphataemic rickets with autosomal recessive inheritance and severe osteosclerosis. A report of two cases. J Bone Joint Surg (Br). 1978;60-B(3):430–4.

44. Feng JQ, Ward LM, Liu S, et al. Loss of DMP1 causes rickets and osteomalacia and identifies a role for osteocytes in mineral metabolism. Nat Genet. 2006; 38(11):1310–5.

45. Lorenz-Depiereux B, Bastepe M, Benet-Pages A, et al. DMP1 mutations in autosomal recessive hypophosphatemia implicate a bone matrix protein in the regulation of phosphate homeostasis. Nat Genet. 2006;38(11):1248–50.

46. Lorenz-Depiereux B, Schnabel D, Tiosano D, Hausler G, Strom TM. Loss-of-function ENPP1 mutations cause both generalized arterial calcification of infancy and autosomal-recessive hypophosphatemic rickets. Am J Hum Genet. 2010;86(2):267–72.

47. Levy-Litan V, Hershkovitz E, Avizov L, et al. Autosomal-recessive hypophosphatemic rickets is associated with an inactivation mutation in the ENPP1 gene. Am J Hum Genet. 2010;86(2):273–8.

48. Rutsch F, Ruf N, Vaingankar S, et al. Mutations in ENPP1 are associated with 'idiopathic' infantile arterial calcification. Nat Genet. 2003;34(4):379–81.

49. Chong WH, Andreopoulou P, Chen CC, et al. Tumor localization and biochemical response to cure in tumor-induced osteomalacia. J Bone Miner Res. 2013;28(6):1386–98.

50. Weidner N, Santa Cruz D. Phosphaturic mesenchymal tumors. A polymorphous group causing osteomalacia or rickets. Cancer. 1987;59(8):1442–54.

51. Chong WH, Molinolo AA, Chen CC, Collins MT. Tumor-induced osteomalacia. Endocr Relat Cancer. 2011;18(3):R53–77.

52. White KE, Jonsson KB, Carn G, et al. The autosomal dominant hypophosphatemic rickets (ADHR) gene is a secreted polypeptide overexpressed by tumors that cause phosphate wasting. J Clin Endocrinol Metab. 2001;86(2):497–500.

53. Brownstein CA, Adler F, Nelson-Williams C, et al. A translocation causing increased alpha-klotho level results in hypophosphatemic rickets and hyperparathyroidism. Proc Natl Acad Sci U S A. 2008;105(9): 3455–60.

54. Kovesdy CP, Quarles LD. Fibroblast growth factor-23: what we know, what we don't know, and what we need to know. Nephrol Dial Transplant. 2013;28(9): 2228–36.

55. Boyce AM, Glover M, Kelly MH, et al. Optic neuropathy in McCune-albright syndrome: effects of early diagnosis and treatment of growth hormone excess. J Clin Endocrinol Metab. 2013;98(1): E126–34.

56. Narumi S, Matsuo K, Ishii T, Tanahashi Y, Hasegawa T. Quantitative and sensitive detection of GNAS mutations causing mccune-albright syndrome with next generation sequencing. PLoS ONE. 2013;8(3): e60525.

57. Tieder M, Modai D, Samuel R, et al. Hereditary hypophosphatemic rickets with hypercalciuria. N Engl J Med. 1985;312(10):611–7.

58. Lorenz-Depiereux B, Benet-Pages A, Eckstein G, et al. Hereditary hypophosphatemic rickets with hypercalciuria is caused by mutations in the sodium-phosphate cotransporter gene SLC34A3. Am J Hum Genet. 2006;78(2):193–201.

59. Jaureguiberry G, Carpenter TO, Forman S, Juppner H, Bergwitz C. A novel missense mutation in SLC34A3 that causes hereditary hypophosphatemic rickets with hypercalciuria in humans identifies threonine 137 as an important determinant of sodium-phosphate cotransport in NaPi-IIc. Am J Physiol Renal Physiol. 2008;295(2):F371–9.

60. Prie D, Huart V, Bakouh N, et al. Nephrolithiasis and osteoporosis associated with hypophosphatemia caused by mutations in the type 2a sodium-phosphate cotransporter. N Engl J Med. 2002;347(13):983–91.

61. Carpenter TO, Imel EA, Holm IA, Jan de Beur SM, Insogna KL. A clinician's guide to X-linked hypophosphatemia. J Bone Miner Res. 2011;26(7):1381–8.

62. Schmitt CP, Mehls O. The enigma of hyperparathyroidism in hypophosphatemic rickets. Pediatr Nephrol. 2004;19(5):473–7.

63. Reusz GS, Latta K, Hoyer PF, Byrd DJ, Ehrich JH, Brodehl J. Evidence suggesting hyperoxaluria as a cause of nephrocalcinosis in phosphate-treated hypophosphataemic rickets. Lancet. 1990;335(8700): 1240–3.

64. Patzer L, van't Hoff W, Shah V, et al. Urinary supersaturation of calcium oxalate and phosphate in patients with X-linked hypophosphatemic rickets and in healthy schoolchildren. J Pediatr. 1999;135(5):611–7.

65. Alon U, Donaldson DL, Hellerstein S, Warady BA, Harris DJ. Metabolic and histologic investigation of

the nature of nephrocalcinosis in children with hypophosphatemic rickets and in the hyp mouse. J Pediatr. 1992;120(6):899–905.

66. Friedman NE, Lobaugh B, Drezner MK. Effects of calcitriol and phosphorus therapy on the growth of patients with X-linked hypophosphatemia. J Clin Endocrinol Metab. 1993;76(4):839–44.

67. Verge CF, Lam A, Simpson JM, Cowell CT, Howard NJ, Silink M. Effects of therapy in X-linked hypophosphatemic rickets. N Engl J Med. 1991;325(26): 1843–8.

68. Imel EA, DiMeglio LA, Hui SL, Carpenter TO, Econs MJ. Treatment of X-linked hypophosphatemia with calcitriol and phosphate increases circulating fibroblast growth factor 23 concentrations. J Clin Endocrinol Metab. 2010;95(4):1846–50.

69. Sullivan W, Carpenter T, Glorieux F, Travers R, Insogna K. A prospective trial of phosphate and 1,25-dihydroxyvitamin D3 therapy in symptomatic adults with X-linked hypophosphatemic rickets. J Clin Endocrinol Metab. 1992;75(3):879–85.

70. Karaplis AC, Bai X, Falet JP, Macica CM. Mineralizing enthesopathy is a common feature of renal phosphate-wasting disorders attributed to FGF23 and is exacerbated by standard therapy in hyp mice. Endocrinology. 2012;153(12):5906–17.

71. Wilson DM. Growth hormone and hypophosphatemic rickets. J Pediatr Endocrinol Metab. 2000;13 Suppl 2:993–8.

72. Baroncelli GI, Bertelloni S, Ceccarelli C, Saggese G. Effect of growth hormone treatment on final height, phosphate metabolism, and bone mineral density in children with X-linked hypophosphatemic rickets. J Pediatr. 2001;138(2):236–43.

73. Haffner D, Nissel R, Wuhl E, Mehls O. Effects of growth hormone treatment on body proportions and final height among small children with X-linked hypophosphatemic rickets. Pediatrics. 2004;113(6): e593–6.

74. Reusz GS, Miltenyi G, Stubnya G, et al. X-linked hypophosphatemia: effects of treatment with recombinant human growth hormone. Pediatr Nephrol. 1997;11(5):573–7.

75. Seikaly MG, Brown R, Baum M. The effect of recombinant human growth hormone in children with X-linked hypophosphatemia. Pediatrics. 1997;100(5): 879–84.

76. Zivicnjak M, Schnabel D, Staude H, et al. Three-year growth hormone treatment in short children with X-linked hypophosphatemic rickets: effects on linear growth and body disproportion. J Clin Endocrinol Metab. 2011;96(12):E2097–105.

77. Yavropoulou MP, Kotsa K, Gotzamani Psarrakou A, et al. Cinacalcet in hyperparathyroidism secondary to X-linked hypophosphatemic rickets: case report and brief literature review. Hormones (Athens). 2010;9(3): 274–8.

78. Alon US, Levy-Olomucki R, Moore WV, Stubbs J, Liu S, Quarles LD. Calcimimetics as an adjuvant treatment for familial hypophosphatemic rickets. Clin J Am Soc Nephrol. 2008;3(3):658–64.

79. Geller JL, Khosravi A, Kelly MH, Riminucci M, Adams JS, Collins MT. Cinacalcet in the management of tumor-induced osteomalacia. J Bone Miner Res. 2007;22(6):931–7.

80. Wohrle S, Henninger C, Bonny O, et al. Pharmacological inhibition of fibroblast growth factor (FGF) receptor signaling ameliorates FGF23-mediated hypophosphatemic rickets. J Bone Miner Res. 2013;28(4):899–911.

81. Goetz R, Nakada Y, Hu MC, et al. Isolated C-terminal tail of FGF23 alleviates hypophosphatemia by inhibiting FGF23-FGFR-klotho complex formation. Proc Natl Acad Sci U S A. 2010;107(1):407–12.

82. Petje G, Meizer R, Radler C, Aigner N, Grill F. Deformity correction in children with hereditary hypophosphatemic rickets. Clin Orthop Relat Res. 2008;466(12):3078–85.

83. Chaussain-Miller C, Sinding C, Wolikow M, Lasfargues JJ, Godeau G, Garabedian M. Dental abnormalities in patients with familial hypophosphatemic vitamin D-resistant rickets: prevention by early treatment with 1-hydroxyvitamin D. J Pediatr. 2003;142(3):324–31.

84. Haffner D, Weinfurth A, Manz F, et al. Long-term outcome of paediatric patients with hereditary tubular disorders. Nephron. 1999;83(3):250–60.

85. Jehan F, Gaucher C, Nguyen TM, et al. Vitamin D receptor genotype in hypophosphatemic rickets as a predictor of growth and response to treatment. J Clin Endocrinol Metab. 2008;93(12):4672–82.

86. Silverman SL. Bisphosphonate use in conditions other than osteoporosis. Ann N Y Acad Sci. 2011; 1218:33–7.

87. Classen CF, Mix M, Kyank U, Hauenstein C, Haffner D. Pamidronic acid and cabergoline as effective long-term therapy in a 12-year-old girl with extended facial polyostotic fibrous dysplasia, prolactinoma and acromegaly in McCune-albright syndrome: a case report. J Med Case Rep. 2012;6:32. 1947-6-32.

Renal Tubular Acidosis

36

R. Todd Alexander and Detlef Bockenhauer

Introduction

Plasma pH is maintained in a very tight range, from 7.35 to 7.45, via multiple regulatory mechanisms including buffering, altered respiration and ultimately fine regulation by the kidney. This tight control of plasma pH is essential for many physiological functions including but not limited to: proper folding and functioning of proteins, neural transmission and cardiac contractility. Typically perturbations in plasma pH are caused by alterations in respiration or the presence of exogenous acids, which overwhelm the remarkable underlying capacity of the body to regulate plasma pH. However, less commonly, excess loss of bicarbonate from the gut or kidney or the failure of the renal tubule to excrete acid is at fault. It is these less common causes of metabolic acidosis that are the subject of this chapter.

In order to understand the molecular pathogenesis of renal tubular acidosis, it is a prerequisite to know both the role of the kidney in the maintenance and regulation of plasma pH and its interrelation to other processes that participate in acid-base homeostasis. Proteins and phosphate mediate buffering in the cell. In the extracellular compartment bicarbonate is the predominant buffer preventing decreases in pH in response to an acid load. This is followed by an increase in respiratory rate and depth (respiratory compensation). Finally the kidneys respond by increasing bicarbonate reabsorption, a process that leads to increased ammonia genesis and ultimately facilitates increased acid secretion from the distal nephron. A detailed discussion of buffering and respiratory control of acid-base status is beyond the scope of this chapter. However, in order to inform the discussion of the pathophysiology of altered tubular handling of acid, we will begin by detailing the current understanding of how the kidney participates in acid-base homeostasis.

Physiology of Renal Acid-Base Handling

Bicarbonate Reabsorption

A significant amount of bicarbonate is filtered and consequently reabsorbed daily in order to preserve extracellular buffering capacity [1, 2]. Assuming a GFR of 120 mL/min in the average adult male and a plasma bicarbonate concentration of 24 mM, this amounts to approximately 4,150 mMoles of bicarbonate that is filtered

R.T. Alexander (✉)
Department of Pediatrics and Physiology, Stollery Children's Hospital, 11405-87 Avenue, Edmonton, Alberta T6G 1C9, Canada
e-mail: todd2@ualberta.ca

D. Bockenhauer
Department of Nephrology, Great Ormond Street Hospital for Children NHS Foundation Trust, Great Ormond Street, London WC1N 3JH, UK
e-mail: d.bockenhauer@ucl.ac.uk

© Springer-Verlag Berlin Heidelberg 2016
D.F. Geary, F. Schaefer (eds.), *Pediatric Kidney Disease*, DOI 10.1007/978-3-662-52972-0_36

daily. Under normal circumstances the urine is free of bicarbonate, which means that all filtered bicarbonate is reabsorbed by the nephron [3] (Fig. 36.1). The vast majority is reabsorbed from the proximal tubule [4, 5]. Animal experiments provide evidence for bicarbonate reabsorption also in the thick ascending limb and the collecting duct, albeit to a much lesser degree [6–11]. The relative amount of bicarbonate absorbed from these sites varies depending on physiological status but in normal physiologic conditions is never more than a fraction of the proximal tubule's contribution to this process [3].

Proximal Tubule

There is no known bicarbonate transporter in the apical membrane of the proximal tubule. Consequently filtered bicarbonate is converted to water and carbon dioxide by a brush border membrane carbonic anhydrase [12]. Carbonic anhydrase IV and likely also the transmembrane isoform carbonic anhydrase XIV mediate this function [13–15]. The water channel, aquaporin-1, permits the rapid influx of water into the proximal tubular epithelial cell [16–19] and may also facilitate the permeation of carbon dioxide [20–22], which is membrane permeable and can also diffuse along its concentration gradient [23]. Cytoplasmic carbonic anhydrase II then converts intracellular water and carbon dioxide back into bicarbonate and a proton (through the intermediate carbonic acid) [24–28]. The proton is exchanged for a sodium ion, predominantly by the apical sodium proton exchanger isoform 3 (NHE3) [29–32], while the bicarbonate is extruded back into the circulation across the basolateral membrane via the electrogenic sodium dependent bicarbonate transporter (NBCe1) [33, 34]. The importance of these transporters is demonstrated by the fact that mutations in any of the encoding genes cause proximal renal tubular acidosis [35, 36].

There is also a proton pump, H^+ ATPase which effluxes protons into the lumen of the proximal tubule [37, 38], although its contribution to proximal tubular bicarbonate reabsorption is minimal relative to that of NHE3 [31]. The majority of bicarbonate transport occurs in the first part of the proximal tubule [39]. This results in a slightly lumen negative transepithelial potential difference, which is believed to be responsible for driving paracellular chloride reabsorption from the latter part of the proximal tubule [40, 41].

Thick Ascending Limb of Henle's Loop

NHE3, the epithelial sodium proton exchanger, is also expressed in the apical membrane of the thick ascending limb of Henle's loop (TAL) [42]. Consequently bicarbonate reabsorption from this segment is felt to occur via a similar process as in the proximal tubule [43, 44]. The absence of aquaporin-1 from this segment may explain the decreased efficiency of bicarbonate reabsorption from the thick ascending limb relative to the proximal tubule [16]. Efflux across the basolateral membrane is mediated by the anion exchanger isoform 2 [45–47].

Collecting Duct

Any remaining bicarbonate reaching the collecting duct is reabsorbed by an analogous process [7, 8]. Efflux of a proton into the lumen permits the titration of bicarbonate back into carbonic acid and then carbon dioxide and water. Proton efflux is achieved via a luminally situated V-type H^+ ATPase, also called a proton pump [48]. Apically expressed proton pumps are only found in α-intercalated cells [37, 49, 50], whose apical membranes are largely impermeable to water, although carbon dioxide could diffuse into the epithelial cells of the collecting duct including α-intercalated cells. Intracellular carbon dioxide is hydrated, generating a proton and bicarbonate. This is achieved by cytosolic carbonic anhydrase II [50, 51]. The de novo generated bicarbonate is then extruded into the circulation via the basolateral anion-exchanger (AE1) [52]. This is the same mechanism permitting the trapping of ammonium in the distal nephron described below.

Acid Secretion

Acid secretion is achieved in the collecting duct via the mechanism described above for the titration of bicarbonate. The luminal H^+ ATPase in

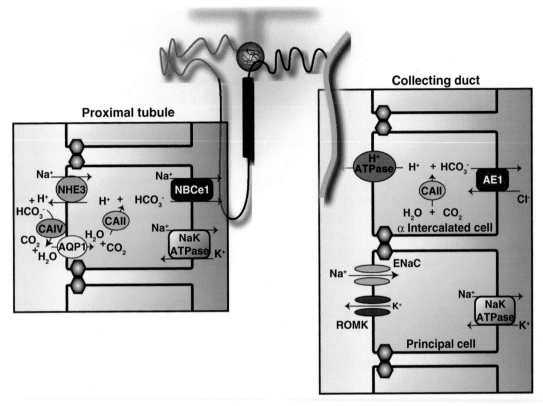

Fig. 36.1 Renal handling of bicarbonate and acid. The majority of filtered bicarbonate (HCO_3^-) is reabsorbed from the proximal tubule, after enzymatic (carbonic anhydrase IV, CAIV) conversion to water and carbon dioxide (CO_2). This is facilitated by proton excretion through the sodium proton exchanger isoform 3 (NHE3). In the cytosol carbonic anhydrase II (CAII), converts the water and CO_2 back into a proton, which is recycled through NHE3, and HCO_3^-, which is effluxed back into the blood through the sodium bicarbonate cotransporter NBCe1. In the collecting duct, H^+ is secreted from the α-intercalated cell via the apically expressed H^+ATPase. The proton is generated via the catalysis, by CAII, of water and CO_2. This also generates HCO_3^-, which is exchanged for Cl^- by the basolateral anion exchanger (AE1). In principle, cell sodium is reabsorbed through the epithelial sodium channel (ENaC). As this is an electrogenic process, either potassium (K^+) secretion trough ROMK or proton secretion via the H^+ATPase is required to maintain a permissive potential difference across the luminal membrane

α-intercalated cells secretes a proton that is trapped by converting ammonia into ammonium, or by titrating another acid [53, 54]. These so called titratable acids include: bicarbonate, phosphate and sulphate. The proton is generated from cytosolic carbon dioxide and water via the action of carbonic anhydrase II [24, 51]. The bicarbonate generated by this process is extruded back into the circulation in exchange for a chloride via AE1 [55, 56]. Moreover there is a potassium-proton pump in the apical membrane of collecting duct α-intercalated cells, which also participates in acid secretion although to a lesser extent [57–59].

Beta-intercalated cells exhibit essentially reverse polarity to α-intercalated cells and thus have an opposite function, as they can generate and secrete bicarbonate into the urine and a proton back into the circulation [8, 37, 49]. They contain a chloride bicarbonate exchanger in their apical membrane, Pendrin, and a proton pump in the basolateral membrane [50, 60–62]. They also contain a cytosolic carbonic anhydrase, CAII [56, 60]. Importantly, recent evidence has implicated this cell type in sodium and chloride reabsorption [63, 64]. ß-intercalated cells nearly completely lack the expression of the Na^+/K^+ ATPase, instead the basolateral H^+ ATPase appears to drive transport across this cell type [65]. This facilitative role of the H⁺ ATPase may contribute to the polyuria and volume contraction often observed in patients with distal renal tubular acidosis due to mutations in this pump [66, 67].

Ammonia Genesis and Recycling

Ammonia (NH3) is the major urinary buffer and consequently its protonation to ammonium (NH_4^+) is essential for the efficient urinary excretion of acid [53, 68].

Ammonia Genesis

Ammonium is produced in the proximal tubule from glutamine and then secreted into the lumen [69]. Free circulating glutamine in the plasma enters the proximal tubular epithelial cell across the basolateral membrane via the LAT2 amino acid transporter [70]. Glutamine in the cytosol then enters the mitochondria via an electroneutral uniporter [71] where it is first converted to glutamate by glutaminase, then to ammonium by a glutamate dehydrogenase [72]. These enzyme-catalyzed reactions produce bicarbonate, which is returned to the circulation via the sodium-dependent bicarbonate transporter NBCe1.

Ammonia Recycling

Ammonium is thought to be secreted into the proximal tubule by substituting for sodium on the apical sodium proton exchanger NHE3 [73–76]. However, a recent study employing a proximal tubular NHE3 knockout mouse argues against this role for the exchanger [77]. Alternatively, another EIPA (Ethylisopropyl-amiloride) sensitive sodium proton exchanger that is expressed in the apical membrane of the proximal tubule such as NHE8 may play this role [31, 78, 79], or free ammonia may diffuse into the lumen where proton excretion may trap it by conversion to ammonium.

Luminal ammonium then travels down the thin descending limb. In TAL, a nephron segment largely impermeant to ammonia, luminal ammonium is absorbed into the tubular epithelial cell across the apical membrane via the sodium potassium chloride co-transporter NKCC2 [80].

Ammonium is approximately the size of potassium and consequently substitutes for it. It is for this reason that hyperkalemia is felt to inhibit ammonium excretion, as increased luminal concentrations of potassium will compete with ammonium for the transport site on NKCC2, preventing its influx into the tubular epithelial cell [81, 82]. Once transported across the luminal membrane of TAL cells, it diffuses across the basolateral membrane into the interstitium in the form of ammonia. Accumulation in the interstitium occurs as the apical membrane is impermeable to ammonia, preventing a back leak of ammonia into the tubular lumen [83].

This medullary interstitial accumulation of ammonia is essential to the efficient excretion of acid as it provides a concentration difference, from interstitium to lumen of the collecting duct for ammonia diffusion into the lumen. Consequently ammonia diffuses into the lumen of the collecting duct where it is trapped via the excretion of protons as ammonium [84, 85]. The collecting duct is relatively impermeable to ammonium [86]. Recent evidence has implicated RhCG, a rhesus glycoprotein homologue, in this process as it forms a pore in the apical and basolateral membranes of the collecting duct epithelial cells permitting the passage of ammonia, but not ammonium [87–90]. Proton excretion is achieved as described above via apically expressed ATPases, predominantly the V-type H⁺ ATPase and to a lesser extent the H⁺K⁺-ATPase. Ultimately, ammonium generation in the proximal tubule, recycling in the loop of Henle and finally trapping in the collecting duct permit significant and efficient proton excretion in the urine (Fig. 36.2).

Pathophysiology of Renal-Acid Base Handling

Definitions

The principles of renal tubular acid-base handling discussed above provide the foundation of the classification of renal tubular acidosis. Defects in bicarbonate reabsorption, which occurs predominantly in the proximal nephron, are referred to as proximal

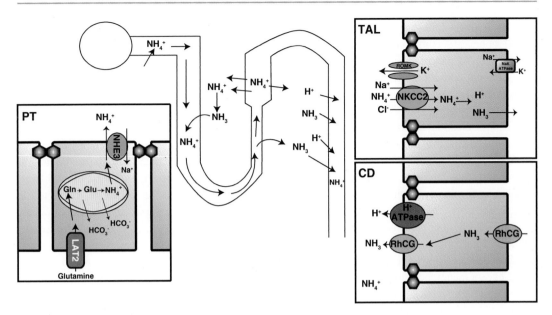

Fig. 36.2 Ammonia generation and recycling. Ammonium is generated in the proximal tubule (PT) and secreted into the lumen in exchange for sodium (Na$^+$) by the sodium proton exchanger isoform 3 (NHE3). It then travels down the nephron to the thick ascending limb (TAL) where it is reabsorbed by the sodium potassium chloride cotransporter, (NKCC2). Ammonia then diffuses into the interstitium where it either undergoes recycling in the loop or permeates the collecting duct through RhCG and is trapped by a proton secreted through the H$^+$-ATPase

renal tubular acidosis, or pRTA [91]. Historically, pRTA has also been classified as type II RTA. Defects in distal tubular proton secretion are referred to as distal renal tubular acidosis, dRTA [91]. This type of RTA has also been referred to as Type I. Clinical syndromes with features of both proximal and distal renal tubular acidosis, i.e., a failure to reclaim both filtered bicarbonate and excrete acid in the urine, are known as mixed renal tubular acidosis or type III RTA. All these types of RTA are typically accompanied by normal or low plasma potassium levels, and are distinguished by the presence of bicarbonaturia and/or the failure to acidify the urine in the presence of an acid load. Due to the molecular link between sodium and acid-base homeostasis, RTA can also occur as a secondary consequence of impaired sodium reabsorption in the collecting duct, as sodium uptake by ENaC provides a favorable electrical gradient for proton secretion. The salt-wasting tubulopathy related to impaired ENaC activity is also referred to as aldosterone insufficient or resistant RTA, or type IV RTA. Since ENaC activity also facilitates potassium secre-

tion, this type of RTA is distinguished from the other types by being associated with hyperkalemia. All forms of RTA are associated with a non-anion gap acidosis, consistent with loss of bicarbonate. For pRTA, this is obvious, as bicarbonate reabsorption is impaired. In dRTA the mechanism is indirect: bicarbonate is used up to buffer the protons the distal tubule fails to excrete.

Proximal Renal Tubular Acidosis (Type II RTA)

Clinical Presentations

Isolated proximal renal tubular acidosis is a rare condition, which is almost exclusively due to a single gene defect in the sodium dependent bicarbonate transporter, NBCe1 [92–94]. This genetic form of pRTA is inherited in an autosomal recessive pattern [95]. Given that the renal isoform of NBCe1 is also expressed in the eye it is not surprising that affected individuals commonly display band cataracts, glaucoma or band keratopathy [95–97]. As with all untreated renal tubular acidosis, failure to thrive and hypomineralized bones are common at presentation [95]. There are also pancreatic and brain isoforms of NBCe1 and consequently, some patients with mutations affecting these isoforms also have increased circulating amylase levels (without evidence of pancreatitis) and there are reports of associated intellectual impairment [95].

Autosomal dominant pRTA has been described in two separate families. The responsible gene accounting for this syndrome has yet to be determined. The first family identified is Costa Rican. One affected brother presented with short stature, bilateral coloboma and subaortic stenosis, while another brother showed limited clinical symptoms, except metabolic acidosis with a urinary pH <5.0 as did the affected sibling [98]. They both had evidence of hypomineralized bones. The other family described includes a father and all four of his children who have metabolic acidosis with increased bicarbonate excretion following bicarbonate loading. Despite sequencing a number of candidate genes the cause of their disease is yet to be defined [93]. Surprisingly, mutations in NHE3 have yet to be reported to cause pRTA, likely because this phenotype would be masked by bicarbonate losing diarrhea, as NHE3 is important for water and bicarbonate reabsorption from the gut [30, 99]. These patients would also be predicted to have hypercalciuria and/or nephrolithiasis [100].

Other genetic and acquired forms of pRTA usually occur as part of the renal Fanconi syndrome [101], which is characterized by complex proximal tubular dysfunction due to genetic defects or proximal tubular toxicity from a drug, toxin or metabolite. pRTA causes are listed and described in Chap. 32.

Diagnosis

Patients with pRTA typically demonstrate a hyperchloremic non-anion gap metabolic acidosis, accompanied by hypokalemia. Urinary pH is typically alkaline due to bicarbonate wasting. However, since the ability to acidify urine is preserved, patients with pRTA can lower their urine pH to less than 5.5 when plasma bicarbonate levels are lower than their renal threshold for tubular bicarbonate absorption. This distinguishes pRTA

from dRTA. A definitive means of diagnosing pRTA is by assessing renal tubular bicarbonate absorption (or the fractional excretion of bicarbonate) across a range of plasma bicarbonate levels. A fractional excretion of bicarbonate greater than 15 % in the context of a metabolic acidosis definitively diagnoses pRTA [101, 102]. Some authors have suggested an even lower cut off level, i.e., 5 % [37]. In case of doubt, the diagnosis can be ascertained by assessing tubular bicarbonate handling as an alkali is given to the patient, resulting in a gradual increase in plasma pH [103]. Practically this can be done by measuring the fractional excretion of bicarbonate repeatedly while normalizing plasma bicarbonate levels with increasing doses of alkali (e.g., administration of intravenous bicarbonate at a rate predicted to increase blood bicarbonate by 2 mmol/L/h, until urine pH is >6.8 [104]). A marked increase in urinary bicarbonate excretion normally occurs at a specific serum bicarbonate level. This is called the bicarbonate threshold. The bicarbonate threshold is around 22 mmol/l in infants and 25 mmol/l in older children/adults [104]. A bicarbonate threshold less than 20 indicates pRTA. In practical terms, a pRTA patient with a bicarbonate threshold of 16 will stop wasting bicarbonate and be able to acidify their urine to <5.0 at a plasma bicarbonate at or below 16 [105].

When working up a patient for pRTA, renal Fanconi syndrome should be considered by assessment of glycosuria, phosphaturia, low molecular weight proteinuria and amino aciduria. In patients with isolated recessive pRTA with typical eye findings, a genetic diagnosis can be established by screening of *SLC4A4* [92]. An algorithm for the diagnosis of RTA is presented in Fig. 36.3.

Although decreased bone mineralization and nephrocalcinosis is less common in pRTA than in dRTA, one should consider these possibilities and assess with imaging. Exclusion of nephrocalcinosis and hypercalciuria, while not precluding pRTA, will direct the differential diagnosis towards dRTA.

Treatment

For treatment of renal Fanconi syndrome, please see Chap. 32. For isolated pRTA, alkali replace-

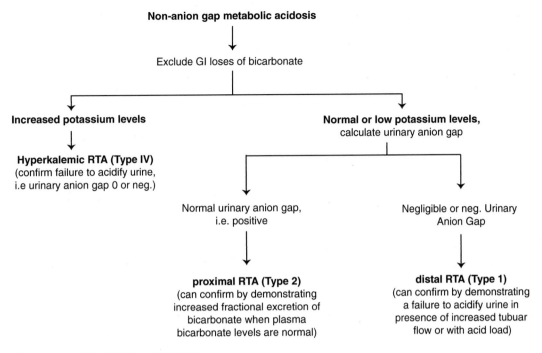

Non-anion gap metabolic acidosis

Exclude GI loses of bicarbonate

Increased potassium levels

Normal or low potassium levels,
calculate urinary anion gap

Hyperkalemic RTA (Type IV)
(confirm failure to acidify urine,
i.e urinary anion gap 0 or neg.)

Normal urinary anion gap,
i.e. positive

Negligible or neg. Urinary
Anion Gap

proximal RTA (Type 2)
(can confirm by demonstrating
increased fractional excretion of
bicarbonate when plasma
bicarbonate levels are normal)

distal RTA (Type 1)
(can confirm by demonstrating
a failure to acidify urine in
presence of increased tubuar
flow or with acid load)

Fig. 36.3 Algorithm for diagnosis of RTA

ment is the main line of therapy [106, 107]. This is especially important in prepubertal children as persistent metabolic acidosis will impair growth [106]. Given the pathophysiology causing bicarbonate wasting when plasma bicarbonate levels are above the threshold, it is not surprising that prodigious quantities (5–15 mEq/kg) of bicarbonate are required to normalize plasma pH [101]. Co-administration of a thiazide diuretic has been shown to decrease the amount of bicarbonate required [108]. The proposed mechanism is thought to be due to mild volume contraction caused by the diuretic with consequent increased bicarbonate absorption from the loop and proximal tubule. An unfortunate side effect of this therapy is the aggravation of hypokalemia, as increased sodium delivery to the collecting duct will increase sodium absorption in this nephron segment driving potassium excretion. Consequently potassium should be carefully monitored when these therapies are used together and potassium should be supplemented. This is easily accomplished by administering either a mixture of sodium and potassium alkali salts such as polycitra or simply potassium citrate.

Prognosis

Due to the rarity of the disease, little information on the long-term outcomes of children with isolated pRTA is available. So far, renal failure has not been reported in contrast to dRTA, and growth can be improved by normalizing plasma pH [106, 109]. Nevertheless, due the severely decreased threshold for bicarbonate reabsorption in pRTA, maintaining normal plasma bicarbonate levels is challenging, as the increased filtered load mostly leads to increased urinary losses [110]. With respect to acquired causes, removal of the inciting agent often leads to recovery; however, it does not always, especially with alkylating agents such as ifosfamide [111].

Distal Renal Tubular Acidosis (Type I RTA)

Clinical Presentation

Distal renal tubular acidosis is more common than the proximal form. Biochemically, it also presents as a hyperchloremic non-anion-gap metabolic acidosis, typically in association with hypokalemia, hypercalciuria and nephrocalcinois, although these features are not always present [112].

Mutations in at least three different genes have been identified and found to cause dRTA [113]. Moreover, a number of conditions, drugs and toxins can cause dRTA (see Table 36.1). In particular drugs targeting the distal nephron, autoimmune diseases and conditions characterized by hypercalciuria can be associated with dRTA [114].

Genotype-Phenotype Associations

Mutations in the anion exchanger isoform 1, AE1, have been found to cause dRTA [115–117]. The encoding gene, *SLC4A1*, is expressed in both red blood cells as well as in α-intercalated cells of the collecting duct [118]. Some mutations in AE1 cause congenital forms of anemia including hereditary spherocytosis and ovalocytosis [119–123]. Interestingly mutations in AE1 that cause blood dyscrasias generally do not result in dRTA and conversely mutations causing dRTA often do not cause anemia. Red blood cells express glycophorin and other chaperones responsible for trafficking AE1 to the plasma membrane that are absent in renal epithelial cells. This explains how some mutations cause dRTA and not anemia [124]. The converse explanation, i.e., specific renal chaperones, might explain exclusively hematological manifestations. In addition, the isoforms of AE1 expressed in red cells and kidney are different, the latter lacking the first 65 amino acids, so that mutations in this region would not be expected to cause kidney disease [125]. In a minority of patients both dRTA and anemia is present [126–130].

Mutations in AE1 were originally reported to only be transmitted in an autosomal dominant fashion [115]. Families with disease of this type have been reported globally [115–117, 127, 131, 132]. Autosomal dominant mutations can cause complete or incomplete dRTA (note incomplete dRTA is evidence of a failure to acidify urine when challenged with an acid load in an individual *without* metabolic acidosis) [133]. Typically patients with autosomal dominant dRTA present in adolescence or even at adult age. In general, hypokalemia is less severe than in patients with mutations

Table 36.1 Causes of distal renal tubular acidosis

Genetic
H$^+$ATPase, α4 (*ATPV0A4*)
H$^+$ATPase, ß1 (*ATPV1B1*)
AE1 (*SLC4A1*)
CAII (*CA2*)[a]
Autoimmune
Cryoglobulinemia
Sjorgren syndrome
Thyroiditis
HIV-nephropathy
Chronic active hepatitis
Primary bilary cirrhosis
Polyarthritis nodosa
Hypercalciuria/nephrocalcinosis
Primary hyperparathyroidism
Hypothyroidism
Medullary sponge kidney
Drug induced
Amphotericin B
Cyclamate
Vanadate
Ifosfamide
Toluene
Mercury
Lithium
Foscarnet
Analgesic nephropathy
Miscellaneous causes
Sickle cell disease
Marfan syndrome
Ehlers-Danlos syndrome
Carnitine palmitoyltransferase deficiency

[a]CAII deficiency causes a combined pRTA and dRTA, i.e., type III RTA

in the H$^+$-ATPase. Hypercalciuria, nephrocalcinosis and nephrolithiasis have been associated with this disease [117, 124, 132]. The frequency of these associations appears to increase with patient age.

Later, patients with mutations in AE1 inherited in an autosomal recessive fashion were reported [122, 124, 134–138]. Typically, although not always, these patients display hemolytic anemia, most commonly ovalocytosis of the southeast Asian variety. Complete dRTA has been exclusively reported. Besides the typical hypokalemic metabolic acidosis, the patients usually suffer from nephrocalcinosis and rachitic bony abnormalities.

Mutations in at least two of the subunits of the vacuolar H^+-ATPase also cause dRTA [66, 139–143]. This 14-subunit proton pump is expressed in the luminal membrane of the α-intercalated cell and is responsible for the secretion of protons into the pro-urine. Mutations in the α4 and ß1 subunit have been reported to cause complete dRTA [143]. Given the known expression of these subunits in both the kidney and inner ear it is not surprising that dRTA due to mutations in the H^+-ATPase have been associated with sensorineural hearing loss [143]. Interestingly, all children with mutations in the ß1 subunit displayed hearing loss at diagnosis, while children with mutations in the α4 subunit did not demonstrate impaired hearing [66, 144]. However, audiological testing of older patients with dRTA due to mutations in the α4 subunit also demonstrates hearing impairment [140, 143]. The majority of patients with mutations in the H^+ATPase demonstrate or develop nephrocalcinosis and or nephrolithiasis.

Diagnosis

The presence of a hypokalemic, hyperchloremic, non-anion gap metabolic acidosis in the absence of diarrhea and in the presence of a normal GFR should make one suspect RTA [113, 145]. Notably, reduced GFR can cause a metabolic acidosis due to insufficient nephron mass to excrete sufficient protons to maintain normal plasma pH. While technically this is identical to dRTA, this form of metabolic acidosis associated with renal failure has not traditionally been labeled as dRTA, and can be easily distinguished by assessment of global renal function and the presence of the other clinical consequences of kidney disease.

Urinary pH will be inappropriately elevated with dRTA. Unfortunately this finding can also be observed with pRTA when plasma pH is above the bicarbonate threshold. Definitive diagnosis of dRTA is made by demonstrating an inability to acidify the urine. Since ammonium is the major component of acid secretion is should be measured either directly or indirectly. The simplest means of measuring urinary ammonia excretion indirectly is to calculate the urinary anion gap

[146]. This is the difference in the sum of urinary cations and anions:

$$U_{AG} = \left[\left[Cl^-\right]_U + \left[HCO_3^-\right]_U\right] - \left[\left[Na^+\right]_U + \left[K^+\right]\right]$$

The unmeasured urinary anions sulphate and phosphate are generally constant and at low levels. Similarly the urinary excretion of calcium and magnesium is relatively low and constant relative to sodium and potassium. Consequently the urinary excretion of ammonia, (NH_4^+) represents the greatest unmeasured urinary cation, making this equation a useful estimate of ammonia excretion. In the presence of metabolic acidosis there should be significant urinary ammonia excretion and consequently a positive anion gap. An alkaline urine pH in the presence of a large urinary anion gap is consistent with the diagnosis of pRTA. A negligible or negative anion gap reflects the inappropriate absence of ammonium excretion and supports a diagnosis of dRTA.

It is important to remember that protons and bicarbonate are in equilibrium with water and carbon dioxide and that the latter can easily diffuse off when urine is exposed to air. Thus, urine pH and bicarbonate should be measured in a fresh sample, ideally collected under oil, which of course may be difficult to obtain in younger children. Exposure of the sample to air will result in decreased bicarbonate levels and increased pH.

Most patients with dRTA will present with the classical biochemical findings, easily establishing the diagnosis. Yet in milder (incomplete) forms the diagnosis may be more challenging and requires further diagnostic procedures to assess distal acidification. Two such procedures are commonly employed to this end. The first is the administration of an acid load typically as ammonia [147]. Patients with dRTA will not be able to acidify their urine and in patients with incomplete dRTA this may induce an actual metabolic acidosis. Alternatively, one can increase distal sodium uptake by administration of a loop diuretic, such as furosemide. Sodium reabsorption via the epithelial sodium channel ENaC (Fig. 36.1) provides a favorable electrical gradient for acid secretion in the collecting duct. To mitigate differences in response of individuals due to altered sodium ingestion the test is best performed by coadministration of a mineralocorticoid, such as fludrocortisone [148, 149]. In patients with normal distal tubular function this results in an acidification of the urine (as sodium absorption will be stimulated necessitating the secretion of a counter ion, i.e., H^+ and K^+). Patients with dRTA will not acidify their urine under these conditions either. The latter study is better tolerated and is therefore preferable for the diagnosis of dRTA, as ammonia is foul tasting and often induces vomiting. The tests are described in Fig. 36.4.

Once a diagnosis of dRTA has been made, identification of clinical conditions and/or toxins causing dRTA is important and their treatment or removal often effective therapy. If primary dRTA is suspected, a thorough hearing examination is useful. Patients with mutations in AE1 will have normal hearing; patients with mutations in carbonic anhydrase II will have conductive hearing loss, while patients with mutations in the H^+ ATPase often have sensorineural hearing loss, especially those with mutations in the ß1 subunit [66, 150]. This can aid in decision making regarding targeted genetic testing.

Treatment

The goal of therapy is to ensure adequate growth while preventing bony abnormalities, nephrolithiasis and nephrocalcinosis [113]. Importantly this

latter complication is thought to cause renal insufficiency in some patients [151]. Since children with dRTA also demonstrate hypocitruria [151], alkali therapy should be provided as a citrate salt. A mixture of sodium and potassium citrate, i.e., polycitra is preferred as this also takes care of the associated mild salt wasting and hypokalemia [152, 153]. The dose of alkali equivalents to compensate alkalosis is typically much lower than in pRTA (i.e., <5 meq/kg/day) [113]. Some authors have recommended the addition of amiloride as a potassium sparing diuretic in cases where persistent hypokalemia is an issue [113]. Finally the management of kidney stones, coexisting hearing loss or anemia may require other subspecialty support.

Prognosis

If the diagnosis is made early and alkali therapy provided consistently the prognosis is good, with improved growth and preserved global kidney function [154]. Unfortunately, due to the non-specific nature of presenting symptoms, diagnosis is often delayed [155] and in these or non-compliant patients progression to renal failure and or significant growth impairment can occur [154, 156]. Importantly, alkali therapy does not prevent hearing loss [157]. Despite treatment of autoimmune conditions and or removal of an offending agent, acquired dRTA may persist in some individuals.

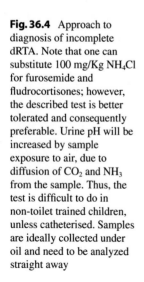

Fig. 36.4 Approach to diagnosis of incomplete dRTA. Note that one can substitute 100 mg/Kg NH_4Cl for furosemide and fludrocortisones; however, the described test is better tolerated and consequently preferable. Urine pH will be increased by sample exposure to air, due to diffusion of CO_2 and NH_3 from the sample. Thus, the test is difficult to do in non-toilet trained children, unless catheterised. Samples are ideally collected under oil and need to be analyzed straight away

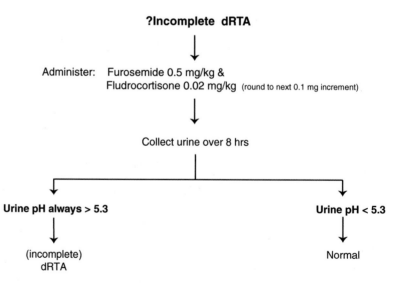

Mixed Proximal and Distal Renal Tubular Acidosis (Type III RTA)

Carbonic anhydrase II is a metalloenzyme that catalyzes the reversible hydration of carbon dioxide into a proton and bicarbonate. This cytosolic enzyme is expressed in renal tubular epithelial cells along the nephron. The highest level of expression is in the intercalated cells with reduced levels of expression in the proximal tubule and thick ascending limb. In both the proximal tubule and the α-intercalated cells it provides protons for secretion into the lumen (via NHE3 and the H^+-ATPase, respectively). Its other product bicarbonate is effluxed into the peritubular interstitium via NBCe1 and AE1 respectively. Mutations in this enzyme lead to mixed proximal and distal RTA, or Type III RTA [36, 158]. Carbonic anhydrase II is also essential for osteoclast function, and loss-of-function is therefore associated with excessive mineralization (osteopetrosis) accompanied by cerebral calcification, developmental delay, facial dysmorphism (low set ears, hypertelorism and a depressed nasal bridge), nephrocalcinosis, kidney stones, conductive hearing loss and cognitive impairment [139, 159–161]. The condition is inherited in an autosomal recessive fashion and is most common in the Middle East [162]. Bone marrow transplantation has been used to prevent the progression of osteopetrosis although it may not be completely curative [163]. Alkali supplementation remains the mainstay of treatment for metabolic acidosis.

Hyperkalemic Renal Tubular Acidosis (Type IV RTA)

Clinical Presentation

Hyperkalemic renal tubular acidosis is typically the result of actual or functional hypoaldosteronism [164]. This condition is primarily a salt-wasting tubulopathy of the collecting duct. Since sodium reabsorption and potassium and proton secretion are coupled in this nephron segment, hyperkalemic acidosis occurs as a secondary consequence. Aldosterone is required for sodium reabsorption through the epithelial sodium channel, ENaC, which generates the negative transmembrane potential required to drive both potassium and proton secretion across this nephron segment. While several rare genetic disorders are associated with hyperkalemic RTA, this type of RTA more commonly results from acquired causes such as renal damage from obstructive uropathy, post renal transplantation, due to an autoimmune disorder, drug therapy or interstitial renal disease (Table 36.2).

Notably, hyperkalemia in type IV RTA is not only a consequence of impaired distal sodium

Table 36.2 Causes of hyperkalemic renal tubular acidosis

Genetic
Pseudohypoaldosteronism type 1: MR
ENaC, α, ß and γ subunits
Pseudohypoaldosteronism type 2: WNK1 (PHA2)
WNK4 (PHA2)
Bartter syndrome type 2[a]: ROMK (Bartter type 2)
Congenital adrenal insufficiency: 21 hydroxylase deficiency
Drug induced
Spironolactone
Heparin
Amiloride
Prostaglandin inhibitors
Triamtere
ACE inhibitors and ARBs
Calcineurin inhibitors
Methicillin
Intrinsic renal disease
Obstructive uropathy
Pylonephritis
Interstitial nephritis
Nephrosclerosis
Post renal transplant
Lupus nephritis
Renal amyloidosis
Miscellaneous causes
Adison's disease
Conn's disease
Diabetes
Gout
Renal venous thrombosis

[a]Note ROM K mutations can cause type IV RTA in infancy that evolves into a hypokalemic metabolic alkalosis as a young child

reabsorption, due to aldosterone insufficiency or resistance. Hyperkalemia also appears to inhibit ammonia production in the proximal tubule, thereby reducing ammonium excretion and exacerbating the renal tubular acidosis [165, 166].

An important cause of hyperkalemic RTA is pseudohypoaldosteronism, both type 1 and type 2 [167]. Type 1 is associated with lower blood pressure, hyponatremia and renal salt wasting, despite elevated circulating levels of aldosterone and renin. The condition results from mineralcorticoid resistance. Patients typically present as infants with dehydration, hypotension, weight loss and vomiting. There are two clinically and genetically distinct subtypes of this disorder. A milder renal-limited form, which is inherited in an autosomal dominant fashion, is due to loss-of-function mutations in the mineralocorticoid receptor [168, 169]. Interestingly patients with this disease may undergo spontaneous remission as they age. The more severe form is inherited in an autosomal recessive fashion and often displays evidence of multiple organ dysfunction, including increased sodium concentration in sweat, saliva and airway liquid which often leads to the erroneous diagnosis of cystic fibrosis [170]. This form of pseudohypoaldosteronism type 1 is caused by mutations in one of the three epithelial sodium channel subunits, α, ß or γ [171–174].

Pseudohypoaldosteronism type II, also known as hyperkalemic hypertension or Gordon's syndrome, describes a disorder characterized by hyperkalemic renal tubular acidosis and hypertension with variable aldosterone and low renin levels. This disorder demonstrates chloride dependent sodium retention and is highly sensitive to therapy with thiazide diuretics, whose target is the apically expressed sodium chloride co-transporter, NCC. Mutations in several genes have been identified to cause this disorder including, *WNK1*, *WNK4*, *CUL3* and *KLHL3* [175–177], and Table 36.3. The complicated signaling network of the WNK kinases is still being elucidated: it is thought that WNK4 directly regulates NCC and is itself regulated by WNK1, whereas CUL3 and KLHL3 are thought to be important in the degradation of the WNK4 [178]. The final consequence of the mutations identified in affected individuals is increased cell surface expression of NCC and increased sodium reabsorption. The volume expansion caused by increased NCC activity suppresses renin and impairs the distal secretion of potassium and protons leading to a hyperkalemic metabolic acidosis. Aldosterone levels are typically low, but can be variable, as aldosterone is also stimulated by hyperkalaemia.

Diagnosis

The initial diagnosis of type IV RTA is rather straightforward. A hyperchloremic non-anion gap metabolic acidosis in the absence of grastrointestinal losses with hyperkalemia is consistent with the diagnosis. The urinary anion gap is negative in type IV RTA due to the failure of the distal nephron to excrete protons. Further investigations to determine the underlying cause will be guided by patient history and physical examination and include serum and urinary biochemistry to screen for nephritis as well as renal ultrasound to assess urinary tract obstruction. Potential inciting drugs should be identified. Evaluation of blood pressure and plasma renin and aldosterone concentrations will help establishing the diagnosis of pseudohypoaldosteronism, although the latter are variable in PHAII. Ambiguous genitalia point to congenital adrenal hyperplasia. Targeted genetic testing should be sought whenever available to confirm hereditary disorders.

Treatment

The treatment of type IV RTA is largely etiology dependent. Offending drugs should be discontinued and any underlying renal disease treated. In the case of obstructive uropathy adequate urinary flow should be achieved by catheterization or an appropriate urologic procedure.

Alkali should be administered as sodium salts to permit a normal plasma pH and when salt wasting is present to correct plasma sodium levels and intravascular volume. This will often necessitate the concurrent administration of sodium chloride. In the case of pseudohyperaldosteronism type II, thiazide diuretics are very effective [179–181].

Table 36.3 Genetic causes of RTA

Gene name	Protein name	MIM #	Inheritance	Typical clinical features	Type of RTA
SLC4A4	NBCe1	603345, 604278	AR	Glaucoma, cataracts, band keratopathy	pRTA, type II
?	?	?179830	AD	Short stature?	pRTA, type II
ATP6V1B1	ß1 subunit of the H$^+$ATPase	267300	AR	Sensorineural hearing loss, nephrocalcinosis or nephrolithiasis	dRTA, type I
ATP6V0A4	α4 subunit of H$^+$ATPase	602722, 605239	AR	Late onset sensorineural hearing loss, nephrocalcinosis or nephrolithiasis	dRTA, type I
SLC4A1	AE1	109270, 179800, 611590	AD (less commonly AR)	Nephrocalcinosis, osteomalacia, hemolytic anemia with AR inheritance	dRTA, type I
CA2	CAII	611492, 259730	AR	Osteopetrosis	Mixed or type III
NR3C2[a]	Mineralo-corticoid receptor	600983, 177735	AD	Pseudo-hypoaldosteronism type 1	Hyperkalemic RTA, type IV
SCNN1A[a], *SCNN1B*[a], *SCNN1G*[a]	α, ß, or γ subunit of ENaC	264350, 600228, 600761, 600760	AR	Pseuodo-hypoaldosterism Type 1	Hyperkalemic RTA, type IV
WNK1[a]	WNK1	6052323, 614492	AD	Pseuodo-hypoaldosterism Type 2, hypertension	Hyperkalemic RTA, type IV
WNK4[a]	WNK4	145260	AD	Pseuodo-hypoaldosterism Type 2, hypertension	Hyperkalemic RTA, type IV
CUL3[a]	Cullin 3	603136, 614496	AD	Pseuodo-hypoaldosterism Type 2, hypertension	Hyperkalemic RTA, Type IV
KLHL3[a]	Kelch-Like 3	614495	AD	Pseuodo-hypoaldosterism Type 2, hypertension	Hyperkalemic RTA, type IV

[a]Mutations of the genes in grey are primarily disorders of renal sodium handling and may not always cause RTA

References

1. Maren TH. Chemistry of the renal reabsorption of bicarbonate. Can J Physiol Pharmacol. 1974;52(6): 1041–50.
2. Rector Jr FC. Renal regulation of acid-base balance. Aust NZ J Med. 1981;11 Suppl 1:1–5.
3. DuBose Jr TD. Reclamation of filtered bicarbonate. Kidney Int. 1990;38(4):584–9.
4. Cogan MG, Maddox DA, Lucci MS, Rector Jr FC. Control of proximal bicarbonate reabsorption in normal and acidotic rats. J Clin Invest. 1979;64(5): 1168–80.
5. Cogan MG. Disorders of proximal nephron function. Am J Med. 1982;72(2):275–88.
6. Lombard WE, Kokko JP, Jacobson HR. Bicarbonate transport in cortical and outer medullary collecting tubules. Am J Phys. 1983;244(3):F289–96.
7. McKinney TD, Burg MB. Bicarbonate transport by rabbit cortical collecting tubules. Effect of acid and alkali loads in vivo on transport in vitro. J Clin Invest. 1977;60(3):766–8.
8. Atkins JL, Burg MB. Bicarbonate transport by isolated perfused rat collecting ducts. Am J Phys. 1985;249(4 Pt 2):F485–9.
9. Capasso G, Unwin R, Agulian S, Giebisch G. Bicarbonate transport along the loop of Henle. I. Microperfusion studies of load and inhibitor sensitivity. J Clin Invest. 1991;88(2):430–7.
10. Good DW. Sodium-dependent bicarbonate absorption by cortical thick ascending limb of rat kidney. Am J Phys. 1985;248(6 Pt 2):F821–9.
11. Good DW, Knepper MA, Burg MB. Ammonia and bicarbonate transport by thick ascending limb of rat kidney. Am J Phys. 1984;247(1 Pt 2):F35–44.
12. Rector Jr FC, Carter NW, Seldin DW. The mechanism of bicarbonate reabsorption in the proximal and distal tubules of the kidney. J Clin Invest. 1965; 44:278–90.
13. Brown D, Zhu XL, Sly WS. Localization of membrane-associated carbonic anhydrase type IV in kidney epithelial cells. Proc Natl Acad Sci U S A. 1990;87(19):7457–61.
14. Zhu XL, Sly WS. Carbonic anhydrase IV from human lung. Purification, characterization, and comparison

with membrane carbonic anhydrase from human kidney. J Biol Chem. 1990;265(15):8795–801.

15. Kaunisto K, Parkkila S, Rajaniemi H, Waheed A, Grubb J, Sly WS. Carbonic anhydrase XIV: luminal expression suggests key role in renal acidification. Kidney Int. 2002;61(6):2111–8.

16. Nielsen S, Smith BL, Christensen EI, Agre P. Distribution of the aquaporin CHIP in secretory and resorptive epithelia and capillary endothelia. Proc Natl Acad Sci U S A. 1993;90(15):7275–9.

17. Preston GM, Carroll TP, Guggino WB, Agre P. Appearance of water channels in Xenopus oocytes expressing red cell CHIP28 protein. Science. 1992; 256(5055):385–7.

18. Schnermann J, Chou CL, Ma T, Traynor T, Knepper MA, Verkman AS. Defective proximal tubular fluid reabsorption in transgenic aquaporin-1 null mice. Proc Natl Acad Sci U S A. 1998;95(16):9660–4.

19. Vallon V, Verkman AS, Schnermann J. Luminal hypotonicity in proximal tubules of aquaporin-1-knockout mice. Am J Physiol Ren Physiol. 2000; 278(6):F1030–3.

20. Cooper GJ, Boron WF. Effect of PCMBS on CO2 permeability of Xenopus oocytes expressing aquaporin 1 or its C189S mutant. Am J Phys. 1998;275(6 Pt 1):C1481–6.

21. Endeward V, Musa-Aziz R, Cooper GJ, Chen LM, Pelletier MF, Virkki LV, et al. Evidence that aquaporin 1 is a major pathway for CO2 transport across the human erythrocyte membrane. FASEB J Off Publ Fed Am Soc Exp Biol. 2006;20(12):1974–81.

22. Nakhoul NL, Davis BA, Romero MF, Boron WF. Effect of expressing the water channel aquaporin-1 on the CO2 permeability of Xenopus oocytes. Am J Phys. 1998;274(2 Pt 1):C543–8.

23. de Groot BL, Hub JS. A decade of debate: significance of CO2 permeation through membrane channels still controversial. Chemphyschem Eur J Chem Phys Phys Chem. 2011;12(5):1021–2.

24. Spicer SS, Sens MA, Tashian RE. Immunocytochemical demonstration of carbonic anhydrase in human epithelial cells. J Histochem Cytochem Off J Histochem Soc. 1982;30(9):864–73.

25. Sly WS, Hewett-Emmett D, Whyte MP, Yu YS, Tashian RE. Carbonic anhydrase II deficiency identified as the primary defect in the autosomal recessive syndrome of osteopetrosis with renal tubular acidosis and cerebral calcification. Proc Natl Acad Sci U S A. 1983;80(9):2752–6.

26. Sly WS, Whyte MP, Sundaram V, Tashian RE, Hewett-Emmett D, Guibaud P, et al. Carbonic anhydrase II deficiency in 12 families with the autosomal recessive syndrome of osteopetrosis with renal tubular acidosis and cerebral calcification. N Engl J Med. 1985;313(3):139–45.

27. Pitts RF, Lotspeich WD. Bicarbonate and the renal regulation of acid base balance. Am J Phys. 1946; 147:138–54.

28. Pitts RF, Lotspeich WD. The renal excretion and reabsorption of bicarbonate. Fed Proc. 1946;5(1 Pt 2):82.

29. Lorenz JN, Schultheis PJ, Traynor T, Shull GE, Schnermann J. Micropuncture analysis of single-nephron function in NHE3-deficient mice. Am J Phys. 1999;277(3 Pt 2):F447–53.

30. Schultheis PJ, Clarke LL, Meneton P, Miller ML, Soleimani M, Gawenis LR, et al. Renal and intestinal absorptive defects in mice lacking the NHE3 Na+/H+ exchanger. Nat Genet. 1998;19(3):282–5.

31. Wang T, Yang CL, Abbiati T, Schultheis PJ, Shull GE, Giebisch G, et al. Mechanism of proximal tubule bicarbonate absorption in NHE3 null mice. Am J Phys. 1999;277(2 Pt 2):F298–302.

32. Berry CA, Warnock DG, Rector Jr FC. Ion selectivity and proximal salt reabsorption. Am J Phys. 1978;235(3):F234–45.

33. Krapf R, Alpern RJ, Rector Jr FC, Berry CA. Basolateral membrane Na/base cotransport is dependent on CO2/HCO3 in the proximal convoluted tubule. J Gen Physiol. 1987;90(6):833–53.

34. Damkier HH, Nielsen S, Praetorius J. Molecular expression of SLC4-derived Na+ -dependent anion transporters in selected human tissues. Am J Physiol Regul Integr Comp Physiol. 2007;293(5):R2136–46.

35. Igarashi T, Sekine T, Inatomi J, Seki G. Unraveling the molecular pathogenesis of isolated proximal renal tubular acidosis. J Am Soc Nephrol JASN. 2002;13(8):2171–7.

36. Alper SL. Familial renal tubular acidosis. J Nephrol. 2010;23 Suppl 16:S57–76.

37. Brown D, Hirsch S, Gluck S. Localization of a proton-pumping ATPase in rat kidney. J Clin Invest. 1988;82(6):2114–26.

38. Zimolo Z, Montrose MH, Murer H. H+ extrusion by an apical vacuolar-type H+-ATPase in rat renal proximal tubules. J Membr Biol. 1992;126(1):19–26.

39. Liu FY, Cogan MG. Axial heterogeneity of bicarbonate, chloride, and water transport in the rat proximal convoluted tubule. Effects of change in luminal flow rate and of alkalemia. J Clin Invest. 1986;78(6):1547–57.

40. Fromter E, Rumrich G, Ullrich KJ. Phenomenologic description of Na+, Cl- and HCO-3 absorption from proximal tubules of rat kidney. Pflugers Arch – Eur J Physiol. 1973;343(3):189–220.

41. Rector Jr FC. Sodium, bicarbonate, and chloride absorption by the proximal tubule. Am J Phys. 1983;244(5):F461–71.

42. Biemesderfer D, Rutherford PA, Nagy T, Pizzonia JH, Abu-Alfa AK, Aronson PS. Monoclonal antibodies for high-resolution localization of NHE3 in adult and neonatal rat kidney. Am J Phys. 1997;273(2 Pt 2):F289–99.

43. Capasso G, Rizzo M, Pica A, Ferrara D, Di Maio FS, Morelli F, et al. Physiology and molecular biology of tubular bicarbonate transport. Nephrol Dial Transplant Off Publ Eur Dial Transplant Assoc Eur Ren Assoc. 2000;15 Suppl 6:36–8.

44. Capasso G, Unwin R, Rizzo M, Pica A, Giebisch G. Bicarbonate transport along the loop of Henle: molecular mechanisms and regulation. J Nephrol. 2002;15 Suppl 5:S88–96.

45. Quentin F, Eladari D, Frische S, Cambillau M, Nielsen S, Alper SL, et al. Regulation of the Cl⁻/HCO⁻₃ exchanger AE2 in rat thick ascending limb of Henle's loop in response to changes in acid-base and sodium balance. J Am Soc Nephrol JASN. 2004; 15(12):2988–97.

46. Alper SL, Stuart-Tilley AK, Biemesderfer D, Shmukler BE, Brown D. Immunolocalization of AE2 anion exchanger in rat kidney. Am J Phys. 1997;273(4 Pt 2):F601–14.

47. Leviel F, Eladari D, Blanchard A, Poumarat JS, Paillard M, Podevin RA. Pathways for HCO⁻₃ exit across the basolateral membrane in rat thick limbs. Am J Phys. 1999;276(6 Pt 2):F847–56.

48. Bastani B, Haragsim L. Immunocytochemistry of renal H-ATPase. Miner Electrolyte Metab. 1996;22(5–6):382–95.

49. Brown D, Hirsch S, Gluck S. An H⁺-ATPase in opposite plasma membrane domains in kidney epithelial cell subpopulations. Nature. 1988;331(6157):622–4.

50. Teng-umnuay P, Verlander JW, Yuan W, Tisher CC, Madsen KM. Identification of distinct subpopulations of intercalated cells in the mouse collecting duct. J Am Soc Nephrol JASN. 1996;7(2):260–74.

51. Brown D, Roth J, Kumpulainen T, Orci L. Ultrastructural immunocytochemical localization of carbonic anhydrase. Presence in intercalated cells of the rat collecting tubule. Histochemistry. 1982; 75(2):209–13.

52. Stehberger PA, Shmukler BE, Stuart-Tilley AK, Peters LL, Alper SL, Wagner CA. Distal renal tubular acidosis in mice lacking the AE1 (band3) Cl⁻/HCO⁻₃ exchanger (slc4a1). J Am Soc Nephrol JASN. 2007;18(5):1408–18.

53. Hamm LL, Simon EE. Roles and mechanisms of urinary buffer excretion. Am J Phys. 1987;253(4 Pt 2):F595–605.

54. Wagner CA, Devuyst O, Bourgeois S, Mohebbi N. Regulated acid-base transport in the collecting duct. Pflugers Arch Eur J Physiol. 2009;458(1):137–56.

55. Han JS, Kim GH, Kim J, Jeon US, Joo KW, Na KY, et al. Secretory-defect distal renal tubular acidosis is associated with transporter defect in H⁺-ATPase and anion exchanger-1. J Am Soc Nephrol JASN. 2002; 13(6):1425–32.

56. Kim J, Kim YH, Cha JH, Tisher CC, Madsen KM. Intercalated cell subtypes in connecting tubule and cortical collecting duct of rat and mouse. J Am Soc Nephrol JASN. 1999;10(1):1–12.

57. Campbell-Thompson ML, Verlander JW, Curran KA, Campbell WG, Cain BD, Wingo CS, et al. In situ hybridization of H-K-ATPase beta-subunit mRNA in rat and rabbit kidney. Am J Phys. 1995;269(3 Pt 2):F345–54.

58. Nakamura S. H⁺-ATPase activity in selective disruption of H⁺-K⁺-ATPase alpha 1 gene of mice under normal and K-depleted conditions. J Lab Clin Med. 2006;147(1):45–51.

59. Lynch IJ, Rudin A, Xia SL, Stow LR, Shull GE, Weiner ID, et al. Impaired acid secretion in cortical collecting duct intercalated cells from H-K-ATPase-deficient mice: role of HKalpha isoforms. Am J Physiol Ren Physiol. 2008;294(3):F621–7.

60. Kim YH, Kwon TH, Frische S, Kim J, Tisher CC, Madsen KM, et al. Immunocytochemical localization of pendrin in intercalated cell subtypes in rat and mouse kidney. Am J Physiol Ren Physiol. 2002;283(4):F744–54.

61. Wall SM, Hassell KA, Royaux IE, Green ED, Chang JY, Shipley GL, et al. Localization of pendrin in mouse kidney. Am J Physiol Ren Physiol. 2003; 284(1):F229–41.

62. Wagner CA, Mohebbi N, Capasso G, Geibel JP. The anion exchanger pendrin (SLC26A4) and renal acid-base homeostasis. Cell Physiol Biochem Int J Exp Cell Physiol Biochem Pharmacol. 2011;28(3):497–504.

63. Leviel F, Hubner CA, Houillier P, Morla L, El Moghrabi S, Brideau G, et al. The Na⁺-dependent chloride-bicarbonate exchanger SLC4A8 mediates an electroneutral Na⁺ reabsorption process in the renal cortical collecting ducts of mice. J Clin Invest. 2010;120(5):1627–35.

64. Gueutin V, Vallet M, Jayat M, Peti-Peterdi J, Corniere N, Leviel F, et al. Renal beta-intercalated cells maintain body fluid and electrolyte balance. J Clin Invest. 2013;123(10):4219–31.

65. Chambrey R, Kurth I, Peti-Peterdi J, Houillier P, Purkerson JM, Leviel F, et al. Renal intercalated cells are rather energized by a proton than a sodium pump. Proc Natl Acad Sci U S A. 2013;110(19):7928–33.

66. Karet FE, Finberg KE, Nelson RD, Nayir A, Mocan H, Sanjad SA, et al. Mutations in the gene encoding B1 subunit of H⁺-ATPase cause renal tubular acidosis with sensorineural deafness. Nat Genet. 1999;21(1):84–90.

67. Smith AN, Skaug J, Choate KA, Nayir A, Bakkaloglu A, Ozen S, et al. Mutations in ATP6N1B, encoding a new kidney vacuolar proton pump 116-kD subunit, cause recessive distal renal tubular acidosis with preserved hearing. Nat Genet. 2000;26(1):71–5.

68. Eladari D, Chambrey R. Ammonium transport in the kidney. J Nephrol. 2010;23 Suppl 16:S28–34.

69. Good DW, Burg MB. Ammonia production by individual segments of the rat nephron. J Clin Invest. 1984;73(3):602–10.

70. Rossier G, Meier C, Bauch C, Summa V, Sordat B, Verrey F, et al. LAT2, a new basolateral 4F2hc/CD98-associated amino acid transporter of kidney and intestine. J Biol Chem. 1999;274(49):34948–54.

71. Sastrasinh S, Sastrasinh M. Glutamine transport in submitochondrial particles. Am J Phys. 1989;257(6 Pt 2):F1050–8.

72. Taylor L, Curthoys NP. Glutamine metabolism: role in acid-base balance*. Biochem Mol Biol Educ Bimonthly Publ Int Union Biochem Mol Biol. 2004;32(5):291–304.

73. Aronson PS, Suhm MA, Nee J. Interaction of external H⁺ with the Na⁺-H⁺ exchanger in renal microvillus membrane vesicles. J Biol Chem. 1983;258(11):6767–71.

74. Kinsella JL, Aronson PS. Interaction of NH₄⁺ and Li⁺ with the renal microvillus membrane Na⁺-H⁺ exchanger. Am J Phys. 1981;241(5):C220–6.

75. Nagami GT. Luminal secretion of ammonia in the mouse proximal tubule perfused in vitro. J Clin Invest. 1988;81(1):159–64.

76. Nagami GT. Net luminal secretion of ammonia by the proximal tubule. Contrib Nephrol. 1988;63:1–5.

77. Li HC, Du Z, Barone S, Rubera I, McDonough AA, Tauc M, et al. Proximal tubule specific knockout of the Na$^+$/H$^+$ exchanger NHE3: effects on bicarbonate absorption and ammonium excretion. J Mol Med. 2013;91(8):951–63.

78. Choi JY, Shah M, Lee MG, Schultheis PJ, Shull GE, Muallem S, et al. Novel amiloride-sensitive sodium-dependent proton secretion in the mouse proximal convoluted tubule. J Clin Invest. 2000;105(8):1141–6.

79. Baum M, Twombley K, Gattineni J, Joseph C, Wang L, Zhang Q, et al. Proximal tubule Na$^+$/H$^+$ exchanger activity in adult NHE8$^{-/-}$, NHE3$^{-/-}$, and NHE3$^{-/-}$/NHE8$^{-/-}$ mice. Am J Physiol Ren Physiol. 2012;303(11):F1495–502.

80. Good DW. Ammonium transport by the thick ascending limb of Henle's loop. Annu Rev Physiol. 1994;56:623–47.

81. Good DW. Effects of potassium on ammonia transport by medullary thick ascending limb of the rat. J Clin Invest. 1987;80(5):1358–65.

82. Good DW. Active absorption of NH$_4$+ by rat medullary thick ascending limb: inhibition by potassium. Am J Phys. 1988;255(1 Pt 2):F78–87.

83. Kikeri D, Sun A, Zeidel ML, Hebert SC. Cell membranes impermeable to NH3. Nature. 1989;339(6224):478–80.

84. Flessner MF, Wall SM, Knepper MA. Permeabilities of rat collecting duct segments to NH3 and NH$_4$+. Am J Phys. 1991;260(2 Pt 2):F264–72.

85. Flessner MF, Wall SM, Knepper MA. Ammonium and bicarbonate transport in rat outer medullary collecting ducts. Am J Phys. 1992;262(1 Pt 2):F1–7.

86. Flessner MF, Knepper MA. Ammonium transport in collecting ducts. Miner Electrolyte Metab. 1990;16(5):299–307.

87. Liu Z, Chen Y, Mo R, Hui C, Cheng JF, Mohandas N, et al. Characterization of human RhCG and mouse Rhcg as novel nonerythroid Rh glycoprotein homologues predominantly expressed in kidney and testis. J Biol Chem. 2000;275(33):25641–51.

88. Yip KP, Kurtz I. NH3 permeability of principal cells and intercalated cells measured by confocal fluorescence imaging. Am J Phys. 1995;269(4 Pt 2):F545–50.

89. Biver S, Belge H, Bourgeois S, Van Vooren P, Nowik M, Scohy S, et al. A role for Rhesus factor Rhcg in renal ammonium excretion and male fertility. Nature. 2008;456(7220):339–43.

90. Bourgeois S, Bounoure L, Christensen EI, Ramakrishnan SK, Houillier P, Devuyst O, et al. Haploinsufficiency of the ammonia transporter Rhcg predisposes to chronic acidosis: Rhcg is critical for apical and basolateral ammonia transport in the mouse collecting duct. J Biol Chem. 2013;288(8):5518–29.

91. Rodriguez-Soriano J, Edelmann Jr CM. Renal tubular acidosis. Annu Rev Med. 1969;20:363–82.

92. Seki G, Horita S, Suzuki M, Yamazaki O, Usui T, Nakamura M, et al. Molecular mechanisms of renal and extrarenal manifestations caused by inactivation of the electrogenic Na-HCO cotransporter NBCe1. Front Physiol. 2013;4:270.

93. Katzir Z, Dinour D, Reznik-Wolf H, Nissenkorn A, Holtzman E. Familial pure proximal renal tubular acidosis – a clinical and genetic study. Nephrol Dial Transplant Off Publ Eur Dial Transplant Assoc Eur Ren Assoc. 2008;23(4):1211–5.

94. Inatomi J, Horita S, Braverman N, Sekine T, Yamada H, Suzuki Y, et al. Mutational and functional analysis of SLC4A4 in a patient with proximal renal tubular acidosis. Pflugers Arc Eur J Physiol. 2004;448(4):438–44.

95. Igarashi T, Inatomi J, Sekine T, Cha SH, Kanai Y, Kunimi M, et al. Mutations in SLC4A4 cause permanent isolated proximal renal tubular acidosis with ocular abnormalities. Nat Genet. 1999;23(3):264–6.

96. Demirci FY, Chang MH, Mah TS, Romero MF, Gorin MB. Proximal renal tubular acidosis and ocular pathology: a novel missense mutation in the gene (SLC4A4) for sodium bicarbonate cotransporter protein (NBCe1). Mol Vis. 2006;12:324–30.

97. Dinour D, Chang MH, Satoh J, Smith BL, Angle N, Knecht A, et al. A novel missense mutation in the sodium bicarbonate cotransporter (NBCe1/SLC4A4) causes proximal tubular acidosis and glaucoma through ion transport defects. J Biol Chem. 2004;279(50):52238–46.

98. Lemann Jr J, Adams ND, Wilz DR, Brenes LG. Acid and mineral balances and bone in familial proximal renal tubular acidosis. Kidney Int. 2000;58(3):1267–77.

99. Gawenis LR, Stien X, Shull GE, Schultheis PJ, Woo AL, Walker NM, et al. Intestinal NaCl transport in NHE2 and NHE3 knockout mice. Am J Physiol Gastrointest Liver Physiol. 2002;282(5):G776–84.

100. Pan W, Borovac J, Spicer Z, Hoenderop JG, Bindels RJ, Shull GE, et al. The epithelial sodium/proton exchanger, NHE3, is necessary for renal and intestinal calcium (re)absorption. Am J Physiol Ren Physiol. 2012;302(8):F943–56.

101. Haque SK, Ariceta G, Batlle D. Proximal renal tubular acidosis: a not so rare disorder of multiple etiologies. Nephrol Dial Transplant Off Publ Eur Dial Transplant Assoc Eur Ren Assoc. 2012;27(12):4273–87.

102. McSherry E, Sebastian A, Morris Jr RC. Renal tubular acidosis in infants: the several kinds, including bicarbonate-wasting, classic renal tubular acidosis. J Clin Invest. 1972;51(3):499–514.

103. Soriano JR, Boichis H, Edelmann Jr CM. Bicarbonate reabsorption and hydrogen ion excretion in children with renal tubular acidosis. J Pediatr. 1967;71(6):802–13.

104. Edelmann CM, Soriano JR, Boichis H, Gruskin AB, Acosta MI. Renal bicarbonate reabsorption and

hydrogen ion excretion in normal infants. J Clin Invest. 1967;46(8):1309–17.

105. Rodriguez Soriano J. Renal tubular acidosis: the clinical entity. J Am Soc Nephrol JASN. 2002; 13(8):2160–70.

106. McSherry E, Morris Jr RC. Attainment and maintenance of normal stature with alkali therapy in infants and children with classic renal tubular acidosis. J Clin Invest. 1978;61(2):509–27.

107. Nash MA, Torrado AD, Greifer I, Spitzer A, Edelmann Jr CM. Renal tubular acidosis in infants and children. Clinical course, response to treatment, and prognosis. J Pediatr. 1972;80(5):738–48.

108. Rampini S, Fanconi A, Illig R, Prader A. Effect of hydrochlorothiazide on proximal renal tubular acidosis in a patient with idiopathic "de toni-debre-fanconi syndrome". Helv Paediatr Acta. 1968;23(1): 13–21.

109. Shiohara M, Igarashi T, Mori T, Komiyama A. Genetic and long-term data on a patient with permanent isolated proximal renal tubular acidosis. Eur J Pediatr. 2000;159(12):892–4.

110. Kari J, El Desoky S, Singh AK, Gari M, Kleta R, Bockenhauer D. Renal tubular acidosis and eye findings. Kidney Int. 2014;86(1):217–8.

111. Skinner R. Chronic ifosfamide nephrotoxicity in children. Med Pediatr Oncol. 2003;41(3):190–7.

112. Rodriguez-Soriano J, Vallo A. Renal tubular acidosis. Pediatr Nephrol. 1990;4(3):268–75.

113. Batlle D, Haque SK. Genetic causes and mechanisms of distal renal tubular acidosis. Nephrol Dial Transplant Off Publ Eur Dial Transplant Assoc Eur Ren Assoc. 2012;27(10):3691–704.

114. Reddy P. Clinical approach to renal tubular acidosis in adult patients. Int J Clin Pract. 2011;65(3):350–60.

115. Karet FE, Gainza FJ, Gyory AZ, Unwin RJ, Wrong O, Tanner MJ, et al. Mutations in the chloride-bicarbonate exchanger gene AE1 cause autosomal dominant but not autosomal recessive distal renal tubular acidosis. Proc Natl Acad Sci U S A. 1998;95(11):6337–42.

116. Bruce LJ, Cope DL, Jones GK, Schofield AE, Burley M, Povey S, et al. Familial distal renal tubular acidosis is associated with mutations in the red cell anion exchanger (Band 3, AE1) gene. J Clin Invest. 1997;100(7):1693–707.

117. Jarolim P, Shayakul C, Prabakaran D, Jiang L, Stuart-Tilley A, Rubin HL, et al. Autosomal dominant distal renal tubular acidosis is associated in three families with heterozygosity for the R589H mutation in the AE1 (band 3) Cl⁻/ HCO⁻₃ exchanger. J Biol Chem. 1998;273(11):6380–8.

118. Fejes-Toth G, Chen WR, Rusvai E, Moser T, Naray-Fejes-Toth A. Differential expression of AE1 in renal HCO3-secreting and -reabsorbing intercalated cells. J Biol Chem. 1994;269(43):26717–21.

119. Jarolim P, Rubin HL, Liu SC, Cho MR, Brabec V, Derick LH, et al. Duplication of 10 nucleotides in the erythroid band 3 (AE1) gene in a kindred with hereditary spherocytosis and band 3 protein defi-

ciency (band 3PRAGUE). J Clin Invest. 1994;93(1): 121–30.

120. Maillet P, Vallier A, Reinhart WH, Wyss EJ, Ott P, Texier P, et al. Band 3 Chur: a variant associated with band 3-deficient hereditary spherocytosis and substitution in a highly conserved position of transmembrane segment 11. Br J Haematol. 1995;91(4): 804–10.

121. Mohandas N, Winardi R, Knowles D, Leung A, Parra M, George E, et al. Molecular basis for membrane rigidity of hereditary ovalocytosis. A novel mechanism involving the cytoplasmic domain of band 3. J Clin Invest. 1992;89(2):686–92.

122. Jarolim P, Palek J, Amato D, Hassan K, Sapak P, Nurse GT, et al. Deletion in erythrocyte band 3 gene in malaria-resistant Southeast Asian ovalocytosis. Proc Natl Acad Sci U S A. 1991;88(24):11022–6.

123. Tanner MJ, Bruce L, Martin PG, Rearden DM, Jones GL. Melanesian hereditary ovalocytes have a deletion in red cell band 3. Blood. 1991;78(10):2785–6.

124. Tanphaichitr VS, Sumboonnanonda A, Ideguchi H, Shayakul C, Brugnara C, Takao M, et al. Novel AE1 mutations in recessive distal renal tubular acidosis. Loss-of-function is rescued by glycophorin A. J Clin Invest. 1998;102(12):2173–9.

125. Parker MD, Boron WF. The divergence, actions, roles, and relatives of sodium-coupled bicarbonate transporters. Physiol Rev. 2013;93(2):803–959.

126. Vasuvattakul S, Yenchitsomanus PT, Vachuanichsanong P, Thuwajit P, Kaitwatcharachai C, Laosombat V, et al. Autosomal recessive distal renal tubular acidosis associated with Southeast Asian ovalocytosis. Kidney Int. 1999;56(5):1674–82.

127. Bruce LJ, Wrong O, Toye AM, Young MT, Ogle G, Ismail Z, et al. Band 3 mutations, renal tubular acidosis and South-East Asian ovalocytosis in Malaysia and Papua New Guinea: loss of up to 95 % band 3 transport in red cells. Biochem J. 2000;350(Pt 1):41–51.

128. Chu C, Woods N, Sawasdee N, Guizouarn H, Pellissier B, Borgese F, et al. Band 3 Edmonton I, a novel mutant of the anion exchanger 1 causing spherocytosis and distal renal tubular acidosis. Biochem J. 2010;426(3):379–88.

129. Shmukler BE, Kedar PS, Warang P, Desai M, Madkaikar M, Ghosh K, et al. Hemolytic anemia and distal renal tubular acidosis in two Indian patients homozygous for SLC4A1/AE1 mutation A858D. Am J Hematol. 2010;85(10):824–8.

130. Fawaz NA, Beshlawi IO, Al Zadjali S, Al Ghaithi HK, Elnaggari MA, Elnour I, et al. dRTA and hemolytic anemia: first detailed description of SLC4A1 A858D mutation in homozygous state. Eur J Haematol. 2012;88(4):350–5.

131. Rungroj N, Devonald MA, Cuthbert AW, Reimann F, Akkarapatumwong V, Yenchitsomanus PT, et al. A novel missense mutation in AE1 causing autosomal dominant distal renal tubular acidosis retains normal transport function but is mistargeted in polarized epithelial cells. J Biol Chem. 2004;279(14):13833–8.

132. Cheidde L, Vieira TC, Lima PR, Saad ST, Heilberg IP. A novel mutation in the anion exchanger 1 gene is associated with familial distal renal tubular acidosis and nephrocalcinosis. Pediatrics. 2003;112(6 Pt 1): 1361–7.

133. Rysava R, Tesar V, Jirsa Jr M, Brabec V, Jarolim P. Incomplete distal renal tubular acidosis coinherited with a mutation in the band 3 (AE1) gene. Nephrol Dial Transplant Off Publ Eur Dial Transplant Assoc Eur Ren Assoc. 1997;12(9):1869–73.

134. Ribeiro ML, Alloisio N, Almeida H, Gomes C, Texier P, Lemos C, et al. Severe hereditary spherocytosis and distal renal tubular acidosis associated with the total absence of band 3. Blood. 2000;96(4): 1602–4.

135. Sritippayawan S, Sumboonnanonda A, Vasuvattakul S, Keskanokwong T, Sawasdee N, Paemanee A, et al. Novel compound heterozygous SLC4A1 mutations in Thai patients with autosomal recessive distal renal tubular acidosis. Am J Kidney Dis Off J Natl Kidney Found. 2004;44(1):64–70.

136. Yenchitsomanus PT, Sawasdee N, Paemanee A, Keskanokwong T, Vasuvattakul S, Bejrachandra S, et al. Anion exchanger 1 mutations associated with distal renal tubular acidosis in the Thai population. J Hum Genet. 2003;48(9):451–6.

137. Choo KE, Nicoli TK, Bruce LJ, Tanner MJ, Ruiz-Linares A, Wrong OM. Recessive distal renal tubular acidosis in Sarawak caused by AE1 mutations. Pediatr Nephrol. 2006;21(2):212–7.

138. Kittanakom S, Cordat E, Akkarapatumwong V, Yenchitsomanus PT, Reithmeier RA. Trafficking defects of a novel autosomal recessive distal renal tubular acidosis mutant (S773P) of the human kidney anion exchanger (kAE1). J Biol Chem. 2004; 279(39):40960–71.

139. Borthwick KJ, Kandemir N, Topaloglu R, Kornak U, Bakkaloglu A, Yordam N, et al. A phenocopy of CAII deficiency: a novel genetic explanation for inherited infantile osteopetrosis with distal renal tubular acidosis. J Med Genet. 2003;40(2):115–21.

140. Feldman M, Prikis M, Athanasiou Y, Elia A, Pierides A, Deltas CC. Molecular investigation and long-term clinical progress in Greek Cypriot families with recessive distal renal tubular acidosis and sensorineural deafness due to mutations in the ATP6V1B1 gene. Clin Genet. 2006;69(2):135–44.

141. Hahn H, Kang HG, Ha IS, Cheong HI, Choi Y. ATP6B1 gene mutations associated with distal renal tubular acidosis and deafness in a child. Am J Kidney Dis Off J Natl Kidney Found. 2003; 41(1):238–43.

142. Ruf R, Rensing C, Topaloglu R, Guay-Woodford L, Klein C, Vollmer M, et al. Confirmation of the ATP6B1 gene as responsible for distal renal tubular acidosis. Pediatr Nephrol. 2003;18(2):105–9.

143. Stover EH, Borthwick KJ, Bavalia C, Eady N, Fritz DM, Rungroj N, et al. Novel ATP6V1B1 and ATP6V0A4 mutations in autosomal recessive distal renal tubular acidosis with new evidence for hearing loss. J Med Genet. 2002;39(11):796–803.

144. Karet FE, Finberg KE, Nayir A, Bakkaloglu A, Ozen S, Hulton SA, et al. Localization of a gene for autosomal recessive distal renal tubular acidosis with normal hearing (rdRTA2) to 7q33-34. Am J Hum Genet. 1999;65(6):1656–65.

145. Unwin RJ, Capasso G. The renal tubular acidoses. J R Soc Med. 2001;94(5):221–5.

146. Batlle DC, Hizon M, Cohen E, Gutterman C, Gupta R. The use of the urinary anion gap in the diagnosis of hyperchloremic metabolic acidosis. N Engl J Med. 1988;318(10):594–9.

147. Wrong O, Davies HE. The excretion of acid in renal disease. Q J Med. 1959;28(110):259–313.

148. Walsh SB, Shirley DG, Wrong OM, Unwin RJ. Urinary acidification assessed by simultaneous furosemide and fludrocortisone treatment: an alternative to ammonium chloride. Kidney Int. 2007; 71(12):1310–6.

149. Smulders YM, Frissen PH, Slaats EH, Silberbusch J. Renal tubular acidosis. Pathophysiology and diagnosis. Arch Intern Med. 1996;156(15):1629–36.

150. Batlle D, Ghanekar H, Jain S, Mitra A. Hereditary distal renal tubular acidosis: new understandings. Annu Rev Med. 2001;52:471–84.

151. Caruana RJ, Buckalew Jr VM. The syndrome of distal (type 1) renal tubular acidosis. Clinical and laboratory findings in 58 cases. Medicine. 1988;67(2): 84–99.

152. Domrongkitchaiporn S, Khositseth S, Stitchantrakul W, Tapaneya-olarn W, Radinahamed P. Dosage of potassium citrate in the correction of urinary abnormalities in pediatric distal renal tubular acidosis patients. Am J Kidney Dis Off J Natl Kidney Found. 2002;39(2):383–91.

153. Tapaneya-Olarn W, Khositseth S, Tapaneya-Olarn C, Teerakarnjana N, Chaichanajarernkul U, Stitchantrakul W, et al. The optimal dose of potassium citrate in the treatment of children with distal renal tubular acidosis. J Med Assoc Thai Chotmaihet thangphaet. 2002;85 Suppl 4:S1143–9.

154. Santos F, Chan JC. Renal tubular acidosis in children. Diagnosis, treatment and prognosis. Am J Nephrol. 1986;6(4):289–95.

155. Vivante A, Lotan D, Pode-Shakked N, Landau D, Svec P, Nampoothiri S, et al. Familial autosomal recessive renal tubular acidosis: importance of early diagnosis. Nephron Physiol. 2011;119(3):P31–9.

156. Bajpai A, Bagga A, Hari P, Bardia A, Mantan M. Long-term outcome in children with primary distal renal tubular acidosis. Indian Pediatr. 2005;42(4): 321–8.

157. Bajaj G, Quan A. Renal tubular acidosis and deafness: report of a large family. Am J Kidney Dis Off J Natl Kidney Found. 1996;27(6):880–2.

158. Bolt RJ, Wennink JM, Verbeke JI, Shah GN, Sly WS, Bokenkamp A. Carbonic anhydrase type II deficiency. Am J Kidney Dis Off J Natl Kidney Found. 2005;46(5):A50, e71-3.

159. Shah GN, Bonapace G, Hu PY, Strisciuglio P, Sly WS. Carbonic anhydrase II deficiency syndrome (osteopetrosis with renal tubular acidosis and brain

calcification): novel mutations in CA2 identified by direct sequencing expand the opportunity for genotype-phenotype correlation. Hum Mutat. 2004;24(3):272.

160. Ismail EA, Abul Saad S, Sabry MA. Nephrocalcinosis and urolithiasis in carbonic anhydrase II deficiency syndrome. Eur J Pediatr. 1997;156(12):957–62.

161. Muzalef A, Alshehri M, Al-Abidi A, Al-Trabolsi HA. Marble brain disease in two Saudi Arabian siblings. Ann Trop Paediatr. 2005;25(3):213–8.

162. Fathallah DM, Bejaoui M, Lepaslier D, Chater K, Sly WS, Dellagi K. Carbonic anhydrase II (CA II) deficiency in Maghrebian patients: evidence for founder effect and genomic recombination at the CA II locus. Hum Genet. 1997;99(5):634–7.

163. McMahon C, Will A, Hu P, Shah GN, Sly WS, Smith OP. Bone marrow transplantation corrects osteopetrosis in the carbonic anhydrase II deficiency syndrome. Blood. 2001;97(7):1947–50.

164. Karet FE. Mechanisms in hyperkalemic renal tubular acidosis. J Am Soc Nephrol JASN. 2009; 20(2):251–4.

165. DuBose Jr TD, Good DW. Effects of chronic hyperkalemia on renal production and proximal tubule transport of ammonium in rats. Am J Phys. 1991;260(5 Pt 2):F680–7.

166. Jaeger P, Bonjour JP, Karlmark B, Stanton B, Kirk RG, Duplinsky T, et al. Influence of acute potassium loading on renal phosphate transport in the rat kidney. Am J Phys. 1983;245(5 Pt 1):F601–5.

167. Riepe FG. Pseudohypoaldosteronism. Endocr Dev. 2013;24:86–95.

168. Geller DS, Rodriguez-Soriano J, Vallo Boado A, Schifter S, Bayer M, Chang SS, et al. Mutations in the mineralocorticoid receptor gene cause autosomal dominant pseudohypoaldosteronism type I. Nat Genet. 1998;19(3):279–81.

169. Sartorato P, Lapeyraque AL, Armanini D, Kuhnle U, Khaldi Y, Salomon R, et al. Different inactivating mutations of the mineralocorticoid receptor in fourteen families affected by type I pseudohypoaldosteronism. J Clin Endocrinol Metab. 2003;88(6):2508–17.

170. Hanukoglu A, Bistritzer T, Rakover Y, Mandelberg A. Pseudohypoaldosteronism with increased sweat and saliva electrolyte values and frequent lower respiratory tract infections mimicking cystic fibrosis. J Pediatr. 1994;125(5 Pt 1):752–5.

171. Chang SS, Grunder S, Hanukoglu A, Rosler A, Mathew PM, Hanukoglu I, et al. Mutations in subunits of the epithelial sodium channel cause salt wasting with hyperkalaemic acidosis, pseudohypoaldosteronism type 1. Nat Genet. 1996;12(3): 248–53.

172. Kerem E, Bistritzer T, Hanukoglu A, Hofmann T, Zhou Z, Bennett W, et al. Pulmonary epithelial sodium-channel dysfunction and excess airway liquid in pseudohypoaldosteronism. N Engl J Med. 1999;341(3):156–62.

173. Saxena A, Hanukoglu I, Saxena D, Thompson RJ, Gardiner RM, Hanukoglu A. Novel mutations responsible for autosomal recessive multisystem pseudohypoaldosteronism and sequence variants in epithelial sodium channel alpha-, beta-, and gamma-subunit genes. J Clin Endocrinol Metab. 2002; 87(7):3344–50.

174. Strautnieks SS, Thompson RJ, Gardiner RM, Chung E. A novel splice-site mutation in the gamma subunit of the epithelial sodium channel gene in three pseudohypoaldosteronism type 1 families. Nat Genet. 1996;13(2):248–50.

175. Wilson FH, Disse-Nicodeme S, Choate KA, Ishikawa K, Nelson-Williams C, Desitter I, et al. Human hypertension caused by mutations in WNK kinases. Science. 2001;293(5532):1107–12.

176. Boyden LM, Choi M, Choate KA, Nelson-Williams CJ, Farhi A, Toka HR, et al. Mutations in kelch-like 3 and cullin 3 cause hypertension and electrolyte abnormalities. Nature. 2012;482(7383): 98–102.

177. Louis-Dit-Picard H, Barc J, Trujillano D, Miserey-Lenkei S, Bouatia-Naji N, Pylypenko O, et al. KLHL3 mutations cause familial hyperkalemic hypertension by impairing ion transport in the distal nephron. Nat Genet. 2012;44(4):456–60, S1-3.

178. Shibata S, Zhang J, Puthumana J, Stone KL, Lifton RP. Kelch-like 3 and Cullin 3 regulate electrolyte homeostasis via ubiquitination and degradation of WNK4. Proc Natl Acad Sci U S A. 2013;110(19): 7838–43.

179. Achard JM, Disse-Nicodeme S, Fiquet-Kempf B, Jeunemaitre X. Phenotypic and genetic heterogeneity of familial hyperkalaemic hypertension (Gordon syndrome). Clin Exp Pharmacol Physiol. 2001; 28(12):1048–52.

180. Gordon RD, Geddes RA, Pawsey CG, O'Halloran MW. Hypertension and severe hyperkalaemia associated with suppression of renin and aldosterone and completely reversed by dietary sodium restriction. Australas Ann Med. 1970;19(4):287–94.

181. Schambelan M, Sebastian A, Rector Jr FC. Mineralocorticoid-resistant renal hyperkalemia without salt wasting (type II pseudohypoaldosteronism): role of increased renal chloride reabsorption. Kidney Int. 1981;19(5):716–27.

Diabetes Insipidus

37

Detlef Bockenhauer and Daniel G. Bichet

History

Diabetes insipidus derives from the Greek word *diabinein* for "flow-through" and the Latin word *insapere* for "non-sweet tasting," separating it from another polyuric disorder, diabetes mellitus ("like honey"). A familial form affecting "chiefly males on the female side of the house" was first described by McIlraith in 1892 [1]. De Lange in 1935 reported a family with diabetes insipidus and no male-to-male transmission unresponsive to injections of posterior lobe extracts [2]. Forssman [3] and Waring [4] in 1945 recognized the disorder in these families as a renal problem. In 1947 Williams and Henry established the unresponsiveness to arginine-vasopressin (AVP) in these patients and coined the term nephrogenic diabetes insipidus (NDI) [5]. In 1969 the "Hopewell-Hypothesis" was proposed by Bode and Crawford, proposing that most cases of NDI in the USA and Canada could be traced to descendants of Ulster Scots, who arrived on the ship Hopewell in Novia Scotia in 1761 [6]. Bichet later refuted this by molecular analysis [7]. In 1992 the *AVPR2* gene encoding the AVP2 receptor was cloned and mutations identified in patients with x-linked NDI [8–11]. Shortly after, the *AQP2* gene encoding the vasopressin-regulated water channel aquaporin-2 (*AQP2*) was cloned [12, 13] and in 1994 mutations in *AQP2* were found to underlie autosomal recessive DI [14].

Clinic

Presentation in Infancy

Patients with congenital NDI typically present in the first weeks to months of life with dehydration. Sometimes, patients receive repeated investigations for sepsis, as the dehydration can be associated with low-grade temperatures, until a set of serum electrolytes is obtained, revealing hypernatraemia. Failure-to-thrive with irritability are further symptoms. Often, patients suck vigorously, but develop vomiting shortly after starting to feed. Vomiting may be due to reflux exacerbated by the large volumes of fluid necessary to compensate for the renal losses. Interestingly, breast-fed infants with NDI typically thrive better than formula-fed ones, as breast milk presents a lower osmolar load than most standard formulas (see below). Of note, pregnancies with babies afflicted with NDI are not complicated by polyhydramnios, since the AVP-dependent mechanisms for urinary concentration

D. Bockenhauer (✉)
UCL Centre for Nephrology, Great Ormond Street Hospital for Children, Rowland Hill Street, London NW3 2PF, UK
e-mail: d.bockenhauer@ucl.ac.uk

D.G. Bichet
Research Center, Hopital du Sacre-Coeur de Montreal, 5400, Boulevard Gouin Ouest, Montreal, Quebec H4J 1C5, Canada
e-mail: daniel.bichet@umontreal.ca

© Springer-Verlag Berlin Heidelberg 2016
D.F. Geary, F. Schaefer (eds.), *Pediatric Kidney Disease*, DOI 10.1007/978-3-662-52972-0_37

are not fully developed until after birth and the osmolar load is cleared by the placenta [15].

Symptoms During Childhood and Infancy

Symptoms typically improve with advancing age, especially once food intake has changed to mainly solids, so that caloric intake and fluid intake are separated. Free access to water allows for self-regulation of serum osmolality. Patients remain polyuric, however, and typical problems include constipation and nocturnal enuresis. The frequency of voiding and drinking, especially during the night is useful information to assess the severity of the problem. Parents also often report problems with concentration and attention span in their children and in one study almost half the patients were diagnosed with attention deficit hyperactivity disorder [16]. The reason for this is unclear, but maybe partly due to the constant need to drink and void.

With treatment, patients with NDI can function well [16]. Untreated, patients typically have persistent failure to thrive, probably because the constant intake of fluids limits their appetite. In addition, impaired mental development used to be a common feature, likely due to the repeated episodes of hypernatraemic dehydration [17–19]. Some patients develop dilatation of the urinary tract from the high urinary flow, especially if they have poor voiding habits [17, 20, 21]. However, in those with hydronephrosis, anatomic causes of obstruction need also be considered, as these are potentially remediable and even minor impediments to flow can cause severe dilatation in this polyuric disorder [22].

Physiologic Principles

Tubular Concentration/Dilution Mechanism (Counter Current Mechanism with Figure)

The kidney creates a concentration gradient via a so-called countercurrent multiplication system [23, 24]. The tonicity (osmolality) of urine as it proceeds along the nephron is depicted in Fig. 37.1. In the proximal tubule the urine remains isotonic to plasma because of the high water permeability of this segment, mediated by aquaporin 1 (AQP1) [25–27]. Urine then enters the tubular segment most important for countercurrent multiplication: the loop of Henle. First, urine is concentrated as it descends the thin descending limb (TDL). The precise mechanisms of concentration are still debated: initially, it was thought that the TDL also expresses AQP1, allowing water exit into the medullary interstitium [28]. More recent data, however, show that only about 10–15 % of TDL (the "long-looped" nephrons) express AQP1, whereas the other ones do not [29]. Consequently, concentration of the tubular fluid in TDL of these nephrons is assumed to occur via passive sodium influx [30]. Urine subsequently enters the thick ascending limb (TAL), which is impermeable for water, but actively removes sodium chloride, via the co-transporter NKCC2 [31]. Therefore, urine is diluted on its way up the TAL by active removal of solutes. The accumulation of solutes in the interstitium in turn generates the driving force for the removal of water from the thin descending limb (in the long-looped nephrons) and the entry of sodium chloride (into the short-looped majority of nephrons), completing the countercurrent multiplier.

There is further removal of sodium chloride in the distal convoluted tubule via the thiazide-sensitive co-transporter NCC and at entry in the collecting duct, urinary osmolality is typically around 50–100 mosm/kg. The final osmolality of the urine is now solely dependent on the water permeability of the collecting duct and thus the availability of water channels. If water channels are present, water will exit the tubule following the interstitial concentration gradient and the urine is concentrated. If no water channels are present, dilute urine will be excreted.

AVP Effects in the Kidney

The availability of water channels in the collecting duct is under the control of AVP. The final

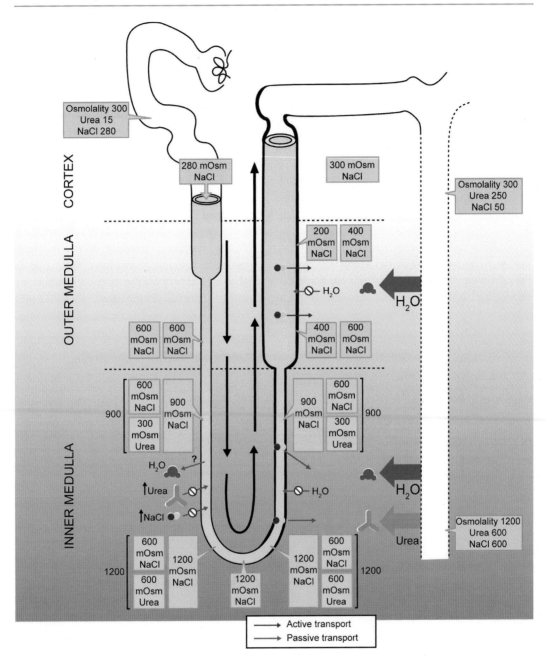

Fig. 37.1 Tubular and interstitial osmolalities in the loop of Henle of a deep nephron during antidiuresis. The numbers in the pink boxes refer to osmolality due to NaCl in the tubular lumen. The numbers in the green boxes refer to osmolality due to NaCl or urea in the interstitium. The "forbidden" icon (*red circle with slash*) indicates a lack of permeability. The thin descending limb of the loop of Henle of deep nephrons is highly permeable to water but poorly permeable to urea or NaCl. The question mark indicates that aquaporin-1 is not expressed in the last part of the descending limbs of short loop nephrons in rats and mice. By contrast, the thin and thick ascending limbs of the loop of Henle are impermeable to water since they do not express any water channel and reabsorb NaCl (Used with permission of Elsevier from Boron WF, Boulpaep EL eds. Medical Physiology. Elsevier; 2005.)

regulated step is the insertion of AQP2 into the apical (urine-facing) side of the membrane of principal cells in the collecting duct [32]. Figure 37.2 shows a model of a principal cell. AVP binds to the vasopressin receptor (AVPR2) on the basolateral (blood-facing) side. AVPR2 is a G-protein coupled receptor that upon activation stimulates adenylate cyclase, thus raising cAMP production [33–36]. Protein kinase A (PKA) is stimulated by cAMP and phosphorylates AQP2 at a consensus site in the cytoplasmic carboxy-terminal tail of the protein, serine 256 (S256) [12, 37, 38]. Unphosphorylated AQP2 is present in intracellular vesicles, which upon phosphorylation at S256 are fused in the apical membrane [39]. Of note, AQP2 water channels are homotetramers, i.e., consisting of four subunits. In vitro

evidence suggests that minimally three subunits need to be phosphorylated for the channel to be fused in the plasma membrane [40].

After insertion of AQP2 in the apical membrane water can enter from the tubular lumen into the cell and exit via the basolateral water channels AQP3 and AQP4. While AQP4 appears to be constitutively expressed in collecting duct, there is some evidence that AVP may also regulate the expression of AQP3 [41–43].

Extrarenal Effects of AVP

The vasopressive and glycogenolytic effects of AVP are mediated through AVP1 receptors expressed in vasculature and liver [44], while the renal effects, especially the increase in water permeability of the CD are mediated by AVPR2 [45].

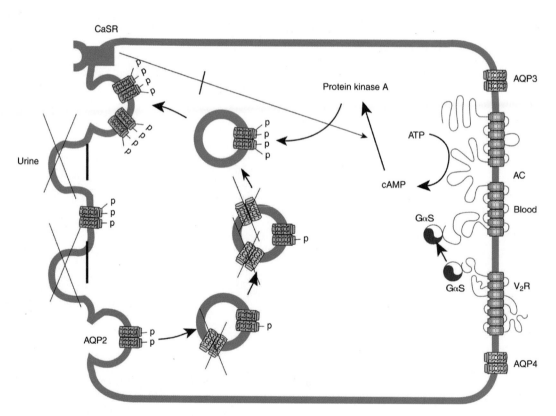

Fig. 37.2 Diagram of a principal cell. Depicted is a schematic of a principal cell with relevant proteins for water transport. AVP binds to the AVR2 receptor (depicted in *green*), expressed on the basolateral side of the cell. AVPR2 is a G-protein-coupled receptor and AVP binding releases the stimulatory G-protein GαS, which, in turn, stimulates adenylcyclase. The increased production of cycline adenosine monophosphate (cAMP) stimulates

protein kinase A (PKA), which phosphorylates the water channel AQP2, leading to insertion of these channels into the apical membrane. Water can then enter the cell from the tubular lumen and exit into the interstitium via the constitutively expressed water channels AQP3 and AQP4 (Used with permission of The American Physiological Society from Nielsen et al. [32].)

Interestingly, administration of the AVPR2-specific agonist 1-Desamino-8-D-Arginine Vasopressin (DDAVP) results not only in an increase in urine osmolality, but also has extrarenal effects, including:

1. a small depression of blood pressure with a concomitant increase in heart rate and increase in plasma renin activity [46, 47];
2. an increase in factor VIIIc and von Willebrand factor with a decrease in bleeding time [46, 48, 49].

These extrarenal effects are abolished in patients with X-linked NDI, suggesting that AVPR2 is expressed beyond the kidney. Clinically, this can be used to differentiate between X-linked and autosomal recessive NDI (see below).

Diagnosis

The presence of inappropriately dilute urine in the face of an elevated serum osmolality defines DI. Dehydration in a child with good urine output should always prompt consideration of a urinary concentrating defect. The diagnosis is easily made by obtaining serum and urine biochemistries. Maximal urinary concentrating ability increases with age, but a urine osmolality below plasma osmolality in a dehydrated child establishes a diagnosis of DI [50]. In classic NDI the urine osmolality is always below 200 mosm/kg.

Diagnostic Procedures

DDAVP Test

The kidney concentrates the urine in response to the pituitary hormone AVP. Failure to concentrate can therefore be due to a deficiency in AVP (central DI or CDI) or an inability of the kidney to respond to it (NDI). AVP effects are mediated via two different receptors: (1) the vasoconstriction ("vasopressin") is mediated by AVP receptor 1 (AVPR1), while the antidiuretic response is mediated by receptor type 2 (AVPR2). DDAVP has a high specificity for AVPR2 and can therefore be used to assess the renal response while avoiding the systemic effects mediated by AVPR1. Different protocols exist in the literature with respect to dosage and route of administration of DDAVP. Some authors use intranasal DDAVP, others oral, subcutaneous (sc), intramuscular (im) or intravenous (iv) administration [46, 51, 52]. While oral or intranasal DDAVP is less invasive, absorption is less reliable. Thus, if the result of the test is inconclusive, it may need to be repeated using injected DDAVP. DDAVP given iv requires a shorter observation period (2 h) than other modes of administration (4–6 h), where absorption is more protracted. Moreover, DDAVP at the dose commonly used in von Willebrand disease (0.3 mcg/kg iv) induces some systemic side effects in the form of a mild decrease in blood pressure and concomitant increase in heart rate via AVPR2 (see above). Consequently, patients with mutated AVPR2 (X-linked NDI) do not experience these haemodynamic changes, while patients with intact AVPR2, but mutated AQP2 (autosomal DI) do. The DDAVP test can therefore help differentiate between these two forms. A typical protocol, modified from [46] is given in Table 37.1. A commonly feared, but actually rare complication of the DDAVP test is hyponatraemia. Patients with intact thirst mechanism who respond to DDAVP will stop drinking water, due to their stable serum osmolality. Yet patients with habitual polydipsia, who will keep on drinking despite lowered serum osmolality, and infants, who continue to be fed by their caregivers throughout the test are at risk for hyponatraemia. Thus, close observation and strict limitation of fluid intake to a volume equal to urine output during the test period is critical to prevent this complication.

A urine osmolality after DDAVP below 200 mosm/kg is consistent with a diagnosis of NDI, while patients with intact urinary concentrating ability typically achieve urine osmolalities greater than 800 mosm/kg (>300 in infants) [50]. Patients with intermediate values should be assessed for inaccurate test results (especially when DDAVP was administered intranasally) or intrinsic renal disease limiting the urinary concentrating capacity (including chronic renal failure and obstructive uropathy, see below).

Table 37.1 Protocol of a DDAVP test

Time	−30	−15	0	10	15	20	30	40	50	60	75	90	110	130	150
Actual time (example: 09 : 00)	_:_	_:_	_:_	_:_	_:_	_:_	_:_	_:_	_:_	_:_	_:_	_:_	_:_	_:_	_:_
dDAVP infusion															
Blood pressure (mmHg)															
Pulse (b/min)															
Fluid intake (ml)															
Urine: volume (ml)															
Osmolality															
Na															
Plasma: U&E															
Osmolality															

Patients should be observed for a minimum of 2 h (iv) to 6 h (oral and nasal) after DDAVP administration. Volume of fluid intake during the test must be limited to the volume of urine produced in order to avoid hyponatremia. See text for more information and interpretation of results

Water Deprivation Test

The aim of the water-deprivation test is to induce mild dehydration and thus challenge the kidney to preserve water. Water is withheld until serum osmolality is just above the upper limit of normal (>295 mosm/kg). Obviously, no child presenting with hypernatraemia and inappropriately dilute urine needs to undergo this test, as the challenge had already presented naturally. A water deprivation test carries the risk of severe hypernatraemic dehydration, especially in infants, as there may be delays in obtaining and reacting to laboratory results. It is useful to distinguish habitual polydipsia from central DI in patients with a good response to DDAVP, and is usually reserved for those particular patients: those with habitual polydipsia will be able to increase urine osmolality with water deprivation, whilst those with central DI will not. For a first assessment, a simple and informal water deprivation test is to ask the parents to obtain the first morning urine on their child and note the last time the child has drunk (water should not be withheld from the child). This can be used as an initial screening test in polyuric patients, as a concentrated urine excludes a diagnosis of DI.

Differential Diagnosis

Central DI

A urinary concentrating defect can be due to a lack of AVP (central DI) or the inability of the kidney to respond to it (NDI). A DDAVP test helps to differentiate between the two (see above). Central DI is most commonly the consequence of head trauma, or other diseases affecting the hypothalamus or pituitary, but there are some rare cases of hereditary DI due to mutations in the gene encoding *AVP* [53–55].

X-Linked and Autosomal NDI

A careful family history and assessment of systemic effects in the DDAVP test can discriminate the more common X-linked (90% of patients with identified mutations) from the rare autosomal NDI (10%). In approximately 10% of patients with presumed primary NDI, no mutation in either AVPR2 or AQP2 is identified [56]. Thus, these patients either have mutations in genes not yet identified to cause primary NDI, or have mutations in regions of the two known genes not assayed (e.g., introns or promoter), or have been misdiagnosed and actually have a secondary form of NDI (see below).

Partial NDI

An intermediate urine osmolality, that is between 200 and 800 mosm/kg after administration of DDAVP is referred to as partial NDI. As discussed above, children less than 3 years of age, and especially in the first months of life, may not be able to maximally concentrate their urine yet and a value below 800 can be physiologic [50]. Further, technical problems with the DDAVP test should be excluded, especially if administration was intranasally, before a diagnosis of partial NDI is considered.

Inherited forms of partial DI are typically due to mutations in the *AVPR2* gene, that allow proper expression of the receptor at the cell membrane, but decrease the affinity to AVP, thus shifting the dose-response curve and requiring higher amounts of AVP to increase urinary concentration [57, 58]. However, mutations in *AQP2* with some retained urinary concentrating ability have also been identified [59]. Obviously, since these patients have a partially retained ability to concentrate their urine, their clinical symptoms are milder.

Secondary NDI

The defining feature of NDI is a pathologic deficiency of AQP2 in the apical membrane of the collecting duct. This can be primary inherited, i.e., due to mutations in either *AQP2* itself or in *AVPR2*, or occur as a secondary phenomenon: as a side effect of medications, anatomical problems or in the context of other tubulopathies [60]. The distinction is important, as misclassification as primary NDI may miss the opportunity to identify a remediable cause, such as urinary obstruction, or to make the correct diagnosis, which may result in potentially harmful treatment. Thus, in any patient with clinical NDI who displays unusual features, such as a history of polyhydramnios or hypercalciuria/nephrocalcinosis or hypokalaemia (before thiazide treatment), a secondary form of NDI should be considered and consequently a primary diagnosis sought.

Secondary Inherited NDI

A secondary form of NDI has been observed in other inherited tubulopathies, which can lead to misdiagnosis [61]. This seems to occur most commonly in Bartter syndrome types 1 and 2 [62–64]. Whilst isosthenuria (i.e., an impaired ability to either concentrate or dilute the urine with a urine osmolality similar to that of plasma) is an expected feature of Bartter syndrome (see Bartter syndrome below), some of the affected patients clearly have hyposthenuria (i.e., a urine osmolality persistently below that of plasma). Indeed, in the laboratory in Montreal, the genes underlying type 1 and type 2 Bartter syndrome, *NKCC2* and *KCNJ1*, are tested next if no mutations were identified in *AVPR2* or *AQP2* in the DNA of patients referred with a clinical diagnosis of NDI [60].

Secondary NDI has also been described in many other inherited diseases affecting the kidney, including renal Fanconi syndromes, especially cystinosis, distal renal tubular acidosis (dRTA), apparent mineralocorticoid excess (AME) and ciliopathies [60, 61].

The precise etiology of this secondary NDI is unclear, but may be related to the electrolyte abnormalities inherent in these disorders, especially hypercalciuria and hypokalaemia (see below). Regardless of the etiology, establishing the correct diagnosis is obviously important: some of the primary disorders can be treated specifically (e.g., cytinosis, dRTA or AME). Moreover, the thiazide treatment commonly used in NDI could compound the defect in tubular salt reabsorption inherent to some of these disorders (e.g., renal Fanconi syndromes, Bartter syndrome) resulting potentially in serious hypovolaemia.

Obstructive Uropathy

Polyuria after release of urinary tract obstruction is a well-recognized phenomenon (post-obstructive diuresis). However, if obstruction is incomplete, it is often associated with polyuria, as well. Animal studies show a decreased level of AQP2 expression with bilateral ureteric obstruction [65]. Experiments with unilateral obstruction show a marked decrease in AQP2 in the obstructed kidney, consistent with the view that local factors, such as increased pressure, affect AQP2 expression [66]. Supporting this view is also the fact that other signs of distal tubular dysfunction are usually present in obstructive uropathies, like hyperkalaemia and acidosis. The downregulation of AQP2 persists up to 30 days after release of obstruction, explaining the post-obstructive diuresis [32].

Interstitial Renal Disease

Polyuria is frequently seen in renal failure, especially if the underlying aetiology primarily affects the interstitium, such as in renal dysplasia (see Chap. 10), nephronophthisis (see Chap. 13) or tubulointerstitial nephritis (see Chap. 38). It is also commonly seen after ischemic renal failure [67, 68]. However, these patients will typically have isosthenuria. This is in contrast to the hyposthenuria, i.e., a urine osmolality persistently below that of plasma that characterizes NDI.

Lithium

While rarely used in children, lithium therapy is a common treatment for manic-depressive disease in adults and roughly a fifth of patients develop polyuria [69]. Animal studies have shown decreased expression of AQP2 in principal cells, probably due to inhibition of cAMP formation in the collecting duct [35, 70–72]

Hypercalcaemia and Hypercalciuria

Hypercalcaemia can be associated with polyuria and two mechanisms have been proposed to explain the AVP-resistant concentrating defect; both likely involving the calcium-sensing receptor (CaSR). This receptor is expressed on the basolateral (blood) side of thick ascending limb cells and indirectly inhibits the NKCC2 cotransporter, thus impairing the generation of a medullary concentration gradient [73–75]. Second, this receptor is also expressed on the luminal (urine) side of collecting duct cells and thought to affect AQP2 trafficking [76, 77]. The latter mechanism would thus be mediated by hypercalciuria and has been proposed to constitute a protective measure against the formation of calcium-containing stones [78]. It would also provide an explanation for the hypercalciuric forms of secondary NDI, such as Bartter syndrome (see above). However, doubts have been raised about the clinical relevance of this mechanism, as the protection against stones would come at the risk of dehydration. Indeed, in normal control subjects the highest urine calcium concentrations were found in the most concentrated urine samples, arguing against a clinically relevant effect of urine calcium on urine concentration [79].

Hypokalaemia

Hypokalaemia causes an AVP-resistant concentration defect. As in the other forms of acquired NDI, reduced expression of AQP2 has been demonstrated [80]. Thus, downregulation of AQP2 seems to be a common feature in acquired NDI [32]. However, the mechanism by which hypokalaemia affects this remains to be elucidated.

Disorders Impairing the Generation of a Medullary Concentration Gradient

Bartter Syndrome

As discussed above, the loop of Henle and active salt reabsorption in thick ascending limb are necessary for the generation of a medullary concentration gradient. Therefore, factors impairing salt reabsorption in the thick ascending limb will lead to a urinary concentration defect (hypo- or isosthenuria). Patients with Bartter syndrome have inherited defects in thick ascending limb salt transport and symptoms include polyuria and episodes of hypernatraemic dehydration (see Chaps. 30 and 31), similar to patients with NDI. However, the presence of a hypokalaemic alkalosis and elevated urinary electrolytes, particularly chloride, help differentiate it from NDI, although the former may be absent in young infants [63]. A history of polyhydramnios further helps to exclude a diagnosis of NDI.

Urea Transporter

Urea is an important constituent of the medullary interstitial concentration gradient. Urea is a bipolar molecule and thus can only diffuse slowly through membranes [81]. Diffusion is facilitated by urea transporters and two genes encoding these transporters have been identified in humans [82]. A mild urinary concentrating defect has been described in patients not expressing the minor blood group antigen Kidd (Jk) [83]. Later, this antigen was identified to be identical with the urea transporter UT-1, encoded by *SLC14A1* and several mutations in this gene have been identified in Kidd-negative individuals [84–86]. Recent evidence suggests that UT-1 is also expressed in the endothelium of the vasa recta and that the combined defect in red cell and vascular urea diffusion impairs countercurrent concentration [87, 88]. Interestingly, no mutations have been found so far in the gene encoding the urea transporter expressed in renal tubule UT-2 (*SLC14A2*).

Genetics

AVPR2

The majority of cases of NDI (90%) are due to mutations in the *AVPR2* gene [89, 90]. The gene is located on chromosome region Xq28 and the mode of inheritance is X-linked recessive. Therefore, the majority of patients with NDI are male, but due to skewed X-inactivation (lionization), females can be affected with variable degrees of polyuria and polydipsia [17, 91–93]. Indeed, in some families, X-inactivation is strongly biased leading to a pseudo-dominant inheritance pattern [94]. X-inactivation may be strongly biased because of a) chance, b) a co-existent mutation on the affected X-chromosome affecting cell survival or c) a co-existing mutation in a gene regulating X-inactivation [95].

So far, more than 211 distinct putative disease-causing mutations have been described in more than 326 families [89, 96]. When investigated in vitro, these mutations can be classified according to their effect [97–114]:

Class 1 mutations result in frame-shifts, premature stop-codons and aberrant splicing and prevent translation of the receptor protein.

Class 2 mutations are missense mutations that allow for translation of the protein, but lead to aberrant trafficking. Typically, these mutations induce improper folding with subsequent trapping in the endoplasmatic reticulum (ER).

Class 3 mutations allow the mutated protein to reach the cell-surface, but impair the receptor's signaling, typically by affecting binding of AVP.

The majority of mutations identified in X-linked NDI belong to class 2 [115]. Conversely, mutations identified in inherited partial NDI fall into class 3: these mutated receptors reach the cell membrane, but have a decreased affinity for AVP [51, 57].

Interestingly, three distinct class 3 mutations have been identified in the *AVPR2* gene, leading to gain-of-function with constitutive activation of the receptor and thus to a "nephrogenic syndrome of inappropriate antidiuresis" [116, 117].

AQP2

The analysis of a pedigree with affected females and the presence of intact extrarenal responses to DDAVP in some patients with NDI lead to the postulation of an autosomal inherited "post-receptor" defect in these individuals [118–120]. The molecular basis for this distinct form of NDI was identified in 1994 to be the water channel aquaporin-2, which is expressed in collecting

duct [14]. Approximately 10 % of all patients with NDI carry mutations in the AQP2. As expected for a loss-of-function defect, inheritance is usually recessive and –similar to AVPR2- the majority of mutations fall into class 2 with retention in the endoplasmic reticulum [115, 121]. Interestingly, there are some families with autosomal dominant inheritance of NDI. Molecular analysis has shown that affected members carry mutations in the c-terminus of AQP2 [40, 122–124]. So why does this lead to a dominant inheritance? The final water-channel is a homotetramer, meaning it consists of four AQP2 subunits (Fig. 37.2). Dominant mutations in the C-terminus lead to aberrant trafficking (class 2), but are able to oligomerize with wild-type protein to form the tetramer. As tetramerization takes place before export to the plasma membrane, these mutations exert a dominant-negative effect on AQP2 function, by misguiding trafficking of the assembled tetramer. Interestingly, specific mutations direct AQP2 trafficking to distinct cellular compartments, such as the Golgi complex [40], late endosomes/lysosomes [122] or the basolateral membrane [124, 125].

Treatment

General Aspects of Treatment

The importance of prompt treatment of NDI is highlighted by the fact that mental retardation used to be an invariable feature, but can be completely prevented by proper treatment. Caring for a patient with NDI is most difficult during infancy, when the babies are dependent on their caregivers for access to fluids. Therefore fluids should be offered in 2-h intervals, placing a considerable burden on the caregivers, particularly at night. Feeding per nasogastric tube is often helpful in this period. A continuous overnight feed delivered by a pump will provide fluid and calories to the baby and much needed rest to the parents. Families also need to be instructed to bring the child to immediate medical attention, when there are increased extra-renal fluid losses, such as when diarrhoea, vomiting, or fever is present. It is often helpful for the parents to have a letter detailing the condition of their child and the need for prompt physical and biochemical assessment so that they can present this in these instances in order to avoid being sent home by medical personnel with no experience in this condition. There should be a low threshold for admission and intravenous hydration in these instances to prevent dehydration. When in hospital, hypotonic fluids, such as 5% Dextrose or 0.22% saline are usually appropriate for intravenous hydration, because of the obligate water losses in the urine. Replacement fluids with a higher osmolality than urine osmolality will exacerbate hypernatraemia. For instance, 0.45% saline results in an osmotic load of 154 mosm/l (77 mosm Na and 77 mosm Cl). A patient with a maximal urine osmolality of 100 mosm/kg will need to excrete 1.54 l of urine for each litre of 0.45% saline received in order to excrete the osmotic load presented by the replacement fluid (see below). Thus, in patients with NDI, the administration of fluids that are hypertonic compared to urine can lead to hypernatraemic dehydration, even though the fluid may be hypotonic to plasma. However, if there are increased salt losses, as can occur with diarrhea, or if hypotonic fluids are administered at a rate higher than the urine losses, hyponatraemia could ensue. Close monitoring of the patient with respect to weight, fluid balance, clinical symptoms and biochemistries is therefore imperative to prevent complications.

Osmotic Load Reduction

The most important part in the treatment of patients with NDI is a reduction in their osmotic load, also called renal solute load, which determines urine volume. Therefore close involvement of a dietician with experience in the management of children with kidney problems is necessary. The osmotic load consists of osmotically active substances that need to be excreted in the urine, i.e., proteins, as they are metabolized to urea, and salts. A typical western diet contains about 800 mosm per day. Thus, an individual with a urine osmolality of 800 mosm/kg only needs 1 l of water to excrete that load. Yet a patient with NDI and a maximal urine osmolality

of 100 mosm/kg needs at least 8 l of water for excretion and if the urine osmolality is 50 mosm/kg then 16 l of water are required. One gram of table salt is equivalent to about 18 mmol NaCl, providing an osmolar load of 36 mosm (18 mosm Na and 18 mosm Cl). Consequently, for a patient with a urine osmolality of 100 mosm/kg, each gram of salt ingested increases obligatory urine output by 360 ml. The osmolar load of a diet can be roughly estimated by the following formula: twice the millimolar amount of sodium and potassium (to account for the accompanying anions) plus protein [g] times 4 (as metabolisation of each g of protein yields approximately 4 mmol of urea [126]. Since lipids and sugars are metabolized without byproducts requiring renal excretion, only protein intake needs to be limited, but should still meet the recommended daily allowance to enable normal growth and development. A reasonable goal is a diet containing about 15 mosm/kg/d. A child with a urine osmolality of 100 mOsm will need a fluid intake of 150 ml/kg/d to be able to excrete that load, which is achievable. Enriching the fluid intake with carbohydrates will provide additional calories without increasing the osmolar load.

Diuretics

The use of a diuretic in a polyuric disorder appears at first glance counterintuitive, but does make physiologic sense. The successful use of thiazides in NDI with a subsequent increase in urine osmolality and concomitant decrease in urine output was first reported in 1959 [127, 128]. Thiazides inhibit reabsorption of sodium and chloride in the distal convoluted tubule (part of the urinary dilution mechanism-see above) and thus increase the salt concentration and osmolality of the urine. The increased salt losses decrease intravascular volume with a subsequent up-regulation of proximal tubular reabsorption of salt and water. Consequently, less volume is delivered to the collecting duct and lost in the urine. Typically used is hydrochlorothiazide at 2 mg/kg/day in two divided doses. The more longer acting Bendroflumethiazide

(50–100 mcg/kg/d) can be given as a single daily dose. Hypokalaemia is a common complication of thiazide administration, but supplementation with potassium salts increases the osmolar load. Therefore, combination of the thiazide with a potassium-sparing diuretic, such as amiloride (0.1–0.3 mg/kg/day) is advantageous, but the latter can cause gastrointestinal side effects, especially nausea.

Prostaglandin Synthesis Inhibitors

Like in many other tubular disorders prostaglandin synthesis inhibitors are used in NDI with the aim to reduce GFR and thus provide a "partial chemical nephrectomy" to minimize losses. However, experiments in animals and humans suggest that prostaglandin synthesis inhibitors can increase urine osmolality without decreasing GFR. The exact mechansim remains to be elucidated, but appears to be ADH-independent [129–131]. Some evidence suggests that activation of basolateral prostaglandin receptors by prostaglandin E2 inhibits Adenylcyclase and/or the shuttling of AQP2 to the apical membrane [132–134].

Typically used is Indomethacin (1–3 mg/kg/day in three to four divided doses). The long-term use of this drug is associated with deterioration of renal function and haematological, as well as gastro-intestinal side effects including life-threatening haemorrhage [135, 136]. The latter may be avoided by using a selective COX-2 inhibitor and the successful use of these in NDI has been reported [137, 138]. However, there are concerns about cardiotoxic side effects of these drugs, as evident by the removal of Rofecoxib from the marketplace [139]. In our experience, the combination of Hydrochlorothiazide with Indomethacin is useful during the first years of life, with a subsequent switch to Bendroflumethiazide with or without Amiloride. Key is the close observation of the individual patient for side effects and for changes in urine output or growth percentiles.

The use of anti-gastrointestinal reflux medications, such as a histamine H2-antagonists, (e.g., Ranitidine 2–4 mg/kg/dose twice daily) and a pro-kinetic (e.g., Domperidone 250–500 mcg/kg three to four times daily) can help with the vomiting often seen in infants with NDI and help prevent gastro-intestinal side effects of Indomethacin.

Future Perspectives

An increasing understanding of the molecular mechanisms of the (patho)physiology of urinary concentration opens up perspectives for novel treatments [140].

Molecular Chaperones

The vast majority of mutations identified in the AVPR2 gene lead to improper folding of the resultant protein with entrapment in the endoplasmic reticulum (see AVPR2 above). Retention is dependent on specialized endoplasmic reticulum proteins, many of which require calcium for optimal function. Therefore, depletion of endoplasmic reticulum calcium stores by inhibiting the sarcoplasmatic calcium pump may be useful to overcome entrapment [141]. Indeed, this approach has been successfully used in vitro to induce surface expression of an AVPR2 mutant [142]. Even more promising, and more specific, is the idea to use small pharmacological chaperones that can enter the cell, bind to the mutant receptor and thus induce proper folding with subsequent release from the endoplasmic reticulum [143, 144]. With the development of small membrane-permeable AVPR2-receptor antagonists, designed to fit neatly into the binding fold of the receptor, this approach has become feasible and indeed successful in vitro [145–147]. More importantly, a recent trial of a AVP antagonist in five patients with NDI, bearing either the mutation del62-64, R137H or W164S (all of which lead to ER retention), has shown a significant decrease in urine output with a concomitant increase in urine osmolality [148]. Total 24-h urine volume decreased from a mean of 11.9–8.2 l and mean urine osmolality rose from 98–170 mosm/kg and thus the observed effect was modest. Nevertheless, these results hold the promise of a targeted, mutation-specific therapy in patients with NDI.

Prostaglandin Receptor Agonists

The identification of cAMP as a key messenger in urinary concentration has led to the search for compounds that could increase cAMP in the principal cell independent of AVPR2. Recently, it was shown that agonists for the prostaglandin receptor EP2 and EP4, such as prostaglandin E2 could provide such an alternative pathway [149]. Indeed, in a rat model of NDI these compounds were able to reduce urine output significantly. Yet, giving prostaglandins to treat NDI is in apparent contradiction to the clinically proven efficacy of prostaglandin synthesis inhibition (see above) and more data are needed to resolve this conundrum.

References

1. McIlraith CH. Notes on some cases of diabetes insipidus with marked family and hereditary tendencies. Lancet. 1892;2:767.
2. de Lange C. Ueber erblichen diabetes insipidus. Jahrbuch Fuer Kinderheilkunde. 1935;145(1):135.
3. Forssman HH. On hereditary diabets insipidus. Acta Med Scand. 1945;121 Suppl 159:9.
4. Waring AJ, Kajdi L, Tappan V. A congenital defect of water metabolism. Am J Dis Child. 1945;69:323–4.
5. Williams RH, Henry C. Nephrogenic diabetes insipidus: transmitted by females and appearing during infancy in males. Ann Intern Med. 1947;27:84–95.
6. Bode HH, Crawford JD. Nephrogenic diabetes insipidus in North America – the hopewell hypothesis. NEJM. 1967;280:750–4.
7. Seibold A, Rosenthal W, Bichet DG, Birnbaumer M. The vasopressin type 2 receptor gene. Chromosomal localization and its role in nephrogenic diabetes insipidus. Regul Pept. 1993;45(1–2):67–71.
8. Lolait SJ, O'Carroll AM, McBride OW, Konig M, Morel A, Brownstein MJ. Cloning and characterization of a vasopressin V2 receptor and possible link to nephrogenic diabetes insipidus. Nature. 1992;357 (6376):336–9.
9. Rosenthal W, Seibold A, Antaramian A, Lonergan M, Arthus MF, Hendy GN, et al. Molecular identification of the gene responsible for congenital nephrogenic diabetes insipidus. Nature. 1992;359(6392):233–5.
10. van den Ouweland AM, Dreesen JC, Verdijk M, Knoers NV, Monnens LA, Rocchi M, et al. Mutations in the vasopressin type 2 receptor gene (AVPR2) associated with nephrogenic diabetes insipidus. Nat Genet. 1992;2(2):99–102.
11. Pan Y, Metzenberg A, Das S, Jing B, Gitschier J. Mutations in the V2 vasopressin receptor gene are associated with X-linked nephrogenic diabetes insipidus. Nat Genet. 1992;2(2):103–6.
12. Fushimi K, Uchida S, Hara Y, Hirata Y, Marumo F, Sasaki S. Cloning and expression of apical membrane water channel of rat kidney collecting tubule. Nature. 1993;361(6412):549–52.
13. Sasaki S, Fushimi K, Saito H, Saito F, Uchida S, Ishibashi K, et al. Cloning, characterization, and chromosomal mapping of human aquaporin of collecting duct. J Clin Invest. 1994;93(3):1250–6.
14. Deen PM, Verdijk MA, Knoers NV, Wieringa B, Monnens LA, van Os CH, et al. Requirement of human renal water channel aquaporin-2 for vasopressin-dependent concentration of urine. Science. 1994;264(5155):92–5.
15. Bonilla-Felix M. Development of water transport in the collecting duct. Am J Physiol Renal Physiol. 2004;287(6):F1093–101.
16. Hoekstra JA, van Lieburg AF, Monnens LA, Hulstijn-Dirkmaat GM, Knoers VV. Cognitive and psychosocial functioning of patients with congenital nephrogenic diabetes insipidus. Am J Med Genet. 1996;61(1):81–8.
17. van Lieburg AF, Knoers NV, Monnens LA. Clinical presentation and follow-up of 30 patients with congenital nephrogenic diabetes insipidus. J Am Soc Nephrol. 1999;10(9):1958–64.
18. Hillman DA, Neyzi O, Porter P, Cushman A, Talbot NB. Renal (vasopressin-resistant) diabetes insipidus; definition of the effects of a homeostatic limitation in capacity to conserve water on the physical, intellectual and emotional development of a child. Pediatrics. 1958;21(3):430–5.
19. Vest M, Talbot NB, Crawford JD. Hypocaloric dwarfism and hydronephrosis in diabetes insipidus. Am J Dis Child. 1963;105:175–81.
20. Yoo TH, Ryu DR, Song YS, Lee SC, Kim HJ, Kim JS, et al. Congenital nephrogenic diabetes insipidus presented with bilateral hydronephrosis: genetic analysis of V2R gene mutations. Yonsei Med J. 2006;47(1):126–30.
21. Stevens S, Brown BD, McGahan JP. Nephrogenic diabetes insipidus: a cause of severe nonobstructive urinary tract dilatation. J Ultrasound Med. 1995;14(7):543–5.
22. Jaureguiberry G, Van't Hoff W, Mushtaq I, Desai D, Mann NP, Kleta R, et al. A patient with polyuria and hydronephrosis: question. Pediatr Nephrol. 2011;26(11):1977–8, 9–80.
23. Stephenson JL. Concentration of urine in a central core model of the renal counterflow system. Kidney Int. 1972;2(2):85–94.
24. Kokko JP, Rector Jr FC. Countercurrent multiplication system without active transport in inner medulla. Kidney Int. 1972;2(4):214–23.
25. Zhang R, Skach W, Hasegawa H, van Hoek AN, Verkman AS. Cloning, functional analysis and cell localization of a kidney proximal tubule water transporter homologous to CHIP28. J Cell Biol. 1993; 120(2):359–69.

26. Sabolic I, Valenti G, Verbavatz JM, Van Hoek AN, Verkman AS, Ausiello DA, et al. Localization of the CHIP28 water channel in rat kidney. Am J Physiol. 1992;263(6 Pt 1):C1225–33.

27. Nielsen S, Smith BL, Christensen EI, Knepper MA, Agre P. CHIP28 water channels are localized in constitutively water-permeable segments of the nephron. J Cell Biol. 1993;120(2):371–83.

28. Nielsen S, Pallone T, Smith BL, Christensen EI, Agre P, Maunsbach AB. Aquaporin-1 water channels in short and long loop descending thin limbs and in descending vasa recta in rat kidney. Am J Physiol. 1995;268(6 Pt 2):F1023–37.

29. Zhai XY, Fenton RA, Andreasen A, Thomsen JS, Christensen EI. Aquaporin-1 is not expressed in descending thin limbs of short-loop nephrons. J Am Soc Nephrol. 2007;18(11):2937–44.

30. Halperin ML, Kamel KS, Oh MS. Mechanisms to concentrate the urine: an opinion. Curr Opin Nephrol Hypertens. 2008;17(4):416–22.

31. Obermuller N, Kunchaparty S, Ellison DH, Bachmann S. Expression of the Na-K-2Cl cotransporter by macula densa and thick ascending limb cells of rat and rabbit nephron. J Clin Invest. 1996;98(3):635–40.

32. Nielsen S, Frokiaer J, Marples D, Kwon TH, Agre P, Knepper MA. Aquaporins in the kidney: from molecules to medicine. Physiol Rev. 2002;82(1):205–44.

33. Eggena P, Christakis J, Deppisch L. Effect of hypotonicity on cyclic adenosine monophosphate formation and action in vasopressin target cells. Kidney Int. 1975;7(3):161–9.

34. Edwards RM, Jackson BA, Dousa TP. ADH-sensitive cAMP system in papillary collecting duct: effect of osmolality and PGE2. Am J Physiol. 1981;240(4):F311–8.

35. Nielsen S, Chou CL, Marples D, Christensen EI, Kishore BK, Knepper MA. Vasopressin increases water permeability of kidney collecting duct by inducing translocation of aquaporin-CD water channels to plasma membrane. Proc Natl Acad Sci U S A. 1995;92(4):1013–7.

36. Knepper MA, Nielsen S, Chou CL, DiGiovanni SR. Mechanism of vasopressin action in the renal collecting duct. Semin Nephrol. 1994;14(4):302–21.

37. Katsura T, Gustafson CE, Ausiello DA, Brown D. Protein kinase A phosphorylation is involved in regulated exocytosis of aquaporin-2 in transfected LLC-PK1 cells. Am J Physiol. 1997;272(6 Pt 2): F817–22.

38. Fushimi K, Sasaki S, Marumo F. Phosphorylation of serine 256 is required for cAMP-dependent regulatory exocytosis of the aquaporin-2 water channel. J Biol Chem. 1997;272(23):14800–4.

39. Christensen BM, Zelenina M, Aperia A, Nielsen S. Localization and regulation of PKA-phosphorylated AQP2 in response to V(2)-receptor agonist/antagonist treatment. Am J Physiol Renal Physiol. 2000;278(1):F29–42.

40. Mulders SM, Bichet DG, Rijss JP, Kamsteeg EJ, Arthus MF, Lonergan M, et al. An aquaporin-2 water channel mutant which causes autosomal dominant nephrogenic diabetes insipidus is retained in the Golgi complex. J Clin Invest. 1998;102(1):57–66.

41. Ecelbarger CA, Terris J, Frindt G, Echevarria M, Marples D, Nielsen S, et al. Aquaporin-3 water channel localization and regulation in rat kidney. Am J Physiol. 1995;269(5 Pt 2):F663–72.

42. Terris J, Ecelbarger CA, Nielsen S, Knepper MA. Long-term regulation of four renal aquaporins in rats. Am J Physiol. 1996;271(2 Pt 2):F414–22.

43. Terris J, Ecelbarger CA, Marples D, Knepper MA, Nielsen S. Distribution of aquaporin-4 water channel expression within rat kidney. Am J Physiol. 1995;269(6 Pt 2):F775–85.

44. Hua Li J, Jain S, McMillin SM, Cui Y, Gautam D, Sakamoto W, et al. A novel experimental strategy to assess the metabolic effects of selective activation of a Gq-coupled receptor in hepatocytes in vivo. Endocrinology. 2013;154(10):3539–51.

45. Holmes CL, Landry DW, Granton JT. Science review: vasopressin and the cardiovascular system part 1 – receptor physiology. Crit Care. 2003;7(6): 427–34.

46. Bichet DG, Razi M, Lonergan M, Arthus MF, Papukna V, Kortas C, et al. Hemodynamic and coagulation responses to 1-desamino[8-D-arginine] vasopressin in patients with congenital nephrogenic diabetes insipidus. N Engl J Med. 1988;318(14): 881–7.

47. Williams TD, Lightman SL, Leadbeater MJ. Hormonal and cardiovascular responses to DDAVP in man. Clin Endocrinol (Oxf). 1986;24(1):89–96.

48. Mannucci PM, Canciani MT, Rota L, Donovan BS. Response of factor VIII/von Willebrand factor to DDAVP in healthy subjects and patients with haemophilia A and von Willebrand's disease. Br J Haematol. 1981;47(2):283–93.

49. Mannucci PM, Aberg M, Nilsson IM, Robertson B. Mechanism of plasminogen activator and factor VIII increase after vasoactive drugs. Br J Haematol. 1975;30(1):81–93.

50. Winberg J. Determination of renal concentration capacity in infants and children without renal disease. Acta Paediatr. 1958;48:318–28.

51. Vargas-Poussou R, Forestier L, Dautzenberg MD, Niaudet P, Dechaux M, Antignac C. Mutations in the vasopressin V2 receptor and aquaporin-2 genes in 12 families with congenital nephrogenic diabetes insipidus. J Am Soc Nephrol. 1997;8(12):1855–62.

52. Monnens L, Smulders Y, van Lier H, de Boo T. DDAVP test for assessment of renal concentrating capacity in infants and children. Nephron. 1981; 29(3-4):151–4.

53. Ito M, Mori Y, Oiso Y, Saito H. A single base substitution in the coding region for neurophysin II associated with familial central diabetes insipidus. J Clin Invest. 1991;87(2):725–8.

54. Ghirardello S, Malattia C, Scagnelli P, Maghnie M. Current perspective on the pathogenesis of central diabetes insipidus. J Pediatr Endocrinol Metab. 2005;18(7):631–45.

55. Christensen JH, Rittig S. Familial neurohypophyseal diabetes insipidus – an update. Semin Nephrol. 2006;26(3):209–23.

56. Sasaki S, Chiga M, Kikuchi E, Rai T, Uchida S. Hereditary nephrogenic diabetes insipidus in Japanese patients: analysis of 78 families and report of 22 new mutations in AVPR2 and AQP2. Clin Exp Nephrol. 2013;17(3):338–44.

57. Sadeghi H, Robertson GL, Bichet DG, Innamorati G, Birnbaumer M. Biochemical basis of partial nephrogenic diabetes insipidus phenotypes. Mol Endocrinol. 1997;11(12):1806–13.

58. Bockenhauer D, Carpentier E, Rochdi D, Van't Hoff W, Breton B, Bernier V, et al. Vasopressin type 2 receptor V88M mutation: molecular basis of partial and complete nephrogenic diabetes insipidus. Nephron Physiol. 2009;114(1):p1–10.

59. Canfield MC, Tamarappoo BK, Moses AM, Verkman AS, Holtzman EJ. Identification and characterization of aquaporin-2 water channel mutations causing nephrogenic diabetes insipidus with partial vasopressin response. Hum Mol Genet. 1997;6(11):1865–71.

60. Bockenhauer D, Bichet DG. Inherited secondary nephrogenic diabetes insipidus: concentrating on humans. Am J Physiol Renal Physiol. 2013; 304(8):F1037–42.

61. Bockenhauer D, van't Hoff W, Dattani M, Lehnhardt A, Subtirelu M, Hildebrandt F, et al. Secondary nephrogenic diabetes insipidus as a complication of inherited renal diseases. Nephron Physiol. 2010; 116(4):23–9.

62. Bockenhauer D, Cruwys M, Kleta R, Halperin LF, Wildgoose P, Souma T, et al. Antenatal Bartter's syndrome: why is this not a lethal condition? QJM. 2008;101(12):927–42.

63. Bettinelli A, Ciarmatori S, Cesareo L, Tedeschi S, Ruffa G, Appiani AC, et al. Phenotypic variability in Bartter syndrome type I. Pediatr Nephrol. 2000;14(10-11):940–5.

64. Lee EH, Heo JS, Lee HK, Han KH, Kang HG, Ha IS, et al. A case of Bartter syndrome type I with atypical presentations. Kor J Pediatr. 2010;53(8):809–13.

65. Frokiaer J, Marples D, Knepper MA, Nielsen S. Bilateral ureteral obstruction downregulates expression of vasopressin-sensitive AQP-2 water channel in rat kidney. Am J Physiol. 1996;270(4 Pt 2):F657–68.

66. Frokiaer J, Christensen BM, Marples D, Djurhuus JC, Jensen UB, Knepper MA, et al. Downregulation of aquaporin-2 parallels changes in renal water excretion in unilateral ureteral obstruction. Am J Physiol. 1997;273(2 Pt 2):F213–23.

67. Kwon TH, Frokiaer J, Fernandez-Llama P, Knepper MA, Nielsen S. Reduced abundance of aquaporins in rats with bilateral ischemia-induced acute renal failure: prevention by alpha-MSH. Am J Physiol. 1999;277(3 Pt 2):F413–27.

68. Johnston PA, Rennke H, Levinsky NG. Recovery of proximal tubular function from ischemic injury. Am J Physiol. 1984;246(2 Pt 2):F159–66.

69. Boton R, Gaviria M, Batlle DC. Prevalence, pathogenesis, and treatment of renal dysfunction associated with chronic lithium therapy. Am J Kidney Dis. 1987;10(5):329–45.

70. Carney SL, Ray C, Gillies AH. Mechanism of lithium-induced polyuria in the rat. Kidney Int. 1996;50(2):377–83.

71. Christensen S, Kusano E, Yusufi AN, Murayama N, Dousa TP. Pathogenesis of nephrogenic diabetes insipidus due to chronic administration of lithium in rats. J Clin Invest. 1985;75(6):1869–79.

72. Trepiccione F, Christensen BM. Lithium-induced nephrogenic diabetes insipidus: new clinical and experimental findings. J Nephrol. 2010;23 Suppl 16:S43–8.

73. Watanabe S, Fukumoto S, Chang H, Takeuchi Y, Hasegawa Y, Okazaki R, et al. Association between activating mutations of calcium-sensing receptor and Bartter's syndrome. Lancet. 2002;360(9334):692–4.

74. Hebert SC. Bartter syndrome. Curr Opin Nephrol Hypertens. 2003;12(5):527–32.

75. Wang W, Kwon TH, Li C, Frokiaer J, Knepper MA, Nielsen S. Reduced expression of Na-K-2Cl cotransporter in medullary TAL in vitamin D-induced hypercalcemia in rats. Am J Physiol Renal Physiol. 2002;282(1):F34–44.

76. Sands JM, Naruse M, Baum M, Jo I, Hebert SC, Brown EM, et al. Apical extracellular calcium/polyvalent cation-sensing receptor regulates vasopressin-elicited water permeability in rat kidney inner medullary collecting duct. J Clin Invest. 1997;99(6):1399–405.

77. Earm JH, Christensen BM, Frokiaer J, Marples D, Han JS, Knepper MA, et al. Decreased aquaporin-2 expression and apical plasma membrane delivery in kidney collecting ducts of polyuric hypercalcemic rats. J Am Soc Nephrol. 1998;9(12):2181–93.

78. Hebert SC, Brown EM, Harris HW. Role of the Ca(2+)-sensing receptor in divalent mineral ion homeostasis. J Exp Biol. 1997;200(Pt 2):295–302.

79. Lam GS, Asplin JR, Halperin ML. Does a high concentration of calcium in the urine cause an important renal concentrating defect in human subjects? Clin Sci (Lond). 2000;98(3):313–9.

80. Marples D, Frokiaer J, Dorup J, Knepper MA, Nielsen S. Hypokalemia-induced downregulation of aquaporin-2 water channel expression in rat kidney medulla and cortex. J Clin Invest. 1996;97(8): 1960–8.

81. Gallucci E, Micelli S, Lippe C. Non-electrolyte permeability across thin lipid membranes. Arch Int Physiol Biochim. 1971;79(5):881–7.

82. Sands JM. Renal urea transporters. Curr Opin Nephrol Hypertens. 2004;13(5):525–32.

83. Gillin AG, Sands JM. Urea transport in the kidney. Semin Nephrol. 1993;13(2):146–54.

84. Sidoux-Walter F, Lucien N, Nissinen R, Sistonen P, Henry S, Moulds J, et al. Molecular heterogeneity of the Jk(null) phenotype: expression analysis of the Jk(S291P) mutation found in Finns. Blood. 2000;96(4):1566–73.

85. Lucien N, Sidoux-Walter F, Olives B, Moulds J, Le Pennec PY, Cartron JP, et al. Characterization of the gene encoding the human Kidd blood group/urea transporter protein. Evidence for splice site mutations in Jknull individuals. J Biol Chem. 1998;273(21):12973–80.

86. Olives B, Mattei MG, Huet M, Neau P, Martial S, Cartron JP, et al. Kidd blood group and urea transport function of human erythrocytes are carried by the same protein. J Biol Chem. 1995;270(26):15607–10.

87. Pallone TL, Turner MR, Edwards A, Jamison RL. Countercurrent exchange in the renal medulla. Am J Physiol Regul Integr Comp Physiol. 2003;284(5):R1153–75.

88. Promeneur D, Rousselet G, Bankir L, Bailly P, Cartron JP, Ripoche P, et al. Evidence for distinct vascular and tubular urea transporters in the rat kidney. J Am Soc Nephrol. 1996;7(6):852–60.

89. Sands JM, Bichet DG. Nephrogenic diabetes insipidus. Ann Intern Med. 2006;144(3):186–94.

90. Bichet DG, Oksche A, Rosenthal W. Congenital nephrogenic diabetes insipidus. J Am Soc Nephrol. 1997;8(12):1951–8.

91. Sato K, Fukuno H, Taniguchi T, Sawada S, Fukui T, Kinoshita M. A novel mutation in the vasopressin V2 receptor gene in a woman with congenital nephrogenic diabetes insipidus. Intern Med. 1999;38(10):808–12.

92. Arthus MF, Lonergan M, Crumley MJ, Naumova AK, Morin D, De Marco LA, et al. Report of 33 novel AVPR2 mutations and analysis of 117 families with X-linked nephrogenic diabetes insipidus. J Am Soc Nephrol. 2000;11(6):1044–54.

93. Kinoshita K, Miura Y, Nagasaki H, Murase T, Bando Y, Oiso Y. A novel deletion mutation in the arginine vasopressin receptor 2 gene and skewed X chromosome inactivation in a female patient with congenital nephrogenic diabetes insipidus. J Endocrinol Invest. 2004;27(2):167–70.

94. Friedman E, Bale AE, Carson E, Boson WL, Nordenskjold M, Ritzen M, et al. Nephrogenic diabetes insipidus: an X chromosome-linked dominant inheritance pattern with a vasopressin type 2 receptor gene that is structurally normal. Proc Natl Acad Sci U S A. 1994;91(18):8457–61.

95. Puck JM, Willard HF. X inactivation in females with X-linked disease. N Engl J Med. 1998;338(5):325–8.

96. Spanakis E, Milord E, Gragnoli C. AVPR2 variants and mutations in nephrogenic diabetes insipidus: review and missense mutation significance. J Cell Physiol. 2008;217(3):605–17.

97. Holtzman EJ, Kolakowski Jr LF, Geifman-Holtzman O, O'Brien DG, Rasoulpour M, Guillot AP, et al. Mutations in the vasopressin V2 receptor gene in two families with nephrogenic diabetes insipidus. J Am Soc Nephrol. 1994;5(2):169–76.

98. Pan Y, Wilson P, Gitschier J. The effect of eight V2 vasopressin receptor mutations on stimulation of adenylyl cyclase and binding to vasopressin. J Biol Chem. 1994;269(50):31933–7.

99. Tsukaguchi H, Matsubara H, Mori Y, Yoshimasa Y, Yoshimasa T, Nakao K, et al. Two vasopressin type 2 receptor gene mutations R143P and delta V278 in patients with nephrogenic diabetes insipidus impair ligand binding of the receptor. Biochem Biophys Res Commun. 1995;211(3):967–77.

100. Tsukaguchi H, Matsubara H, Inada M. Expression studies of two vasopressin V2 receptor gene mutations, R202C and 804insG, in nephrogenic diabetes insipidus. Kidney Int. 1995;48(2):554–62.

101. Tsukaguchi H, Matsubara H, Taketani S, Mori Y, Seido T, Inada M. Binding-, intracellular transport-, and biosynthesis-defective mutants of vasopressin type 2 receptor in patients with X-linked nephrogenic diabetes insipidus. J Clin Invest. 1995;96(4):2043–50.

102. Yokoyama K, Yamauchi A, Izumi M, Itoh T, Ando A, Imai E, et al. A low-affinity vasopressin V2-receptor gene in a kindred with X-linked nephrogenic diabetes insipidus. J Am Soc Nephrol. 1996;7(3):410–4.

103. Oksche A, Schulein R, Rutz C, Liebenhoff U, Dickson J, Muller H, et al. Vasopressin V2 receptor mutants that cause X-linked nephrogenic diabetes insipidus: analysis of expression, processing, and function. Mol Pharmacol. 1996;50(4):820–8.

104. Wenkert D, Schoneberg T, Merendino Jr JJ, Rodriguez Pena MS, Vinitsky R, Goldsmith PK, et al. Functional characterization of five V2 vasopressin receptor gene mutations. Mol Cell Endocrinol. 1996;124(1-2):43–50.

105. Sadeghi HM, Innamorati G, Birnbaumer M. An X-linked NDI mutation reveals a requirement for cell surface V2R expression. Mol Endocrinol. 1997;11(6):706–13.

106. Schoneberg T, Schulz A, Biebermann H, Gruters A, Grimm T, Hubschmann K, et al. V2 vasopressin receptor dysfunction in nephrogenic diabetes insipidus caused by different molecular mechanisms. Hum Mutat. 1998;12(3):196–205.

107. Ala Y, Morin D, Mouillac B, Sabatier N, Vargas R, Cotte N, et al. Functional studies of twelve mutant V2 vasopressin receptors related to nephrogenic diabetes insipidus: molecular basis of a mild clinical phenotype. J Am Soc Nephrol. 1998;9(10):1861–72.

108. Wildin RS, Cogdell DE, Valadez V. AVPR2 variants and V2 vasopressin receptor function in nephrogenic diabetes insipidus. Kidney Int. 1998;54(6):1909–22.

109. Pasel K, Schulz A, Timmermann K, Linnemann K, Hoeltzenbein M, Jaaskelainen J, et al. Functional characterization of the molecular defects causing nephrogenic diabetes insipidus in eight families. J Clin Endocrinol Metab. 2000;85(4):1703–10.

110. Albertazzi E, Zanchetta D, Barbier P, Faranda S, Frattini A, Vezzoni P, et al. Nephrogenic diabetes insipidus: functional analysis of new AVPR2 mutations identified in Italian families. J Am Soc Nephrol. 2000;11(6):1033–43.

111. Postina R, Ufer E, Pfeiffer R, Knoers NV, Fahrenholz F. Misfolded vasopressin V2 receptors caused by extracellular point mutations entail congential nephrogenic diabetes insipidus. Mol Cell Endocrinol. 2000;164(1-2):31–9.

112. Knoers NV, Deen PM. Molecular and cellular defects in nephrogenic diabetes insipidus. Pediatr Nephrol. 2001;16(12):1146–52.

113. Hermosilla R, Oueslati M, Donalies U, Schonenberger E, Krause E, Oksche A, et al. Disease-causing V(2) vasopressin receptors are retained in different compartments of the early secretory pathway. Traffic. 2004;5(12):993–1005.

114. Robben JH, Knoers NV, Deen PM. Characterization of vasopressin V2 receptor mutants in nephrogenic diabetes insipidus in a polarized cell model. Am J Physiol Renal Physiol. 2005;289(2):F265–72.

115. Fujiwara TM, Bichet DG. Molecular biology of hereditary diabetes insipidus. J Am Soc Nephrol. 2005;16(10):2836–46.

116. Feldman BJ, Rosenthal SM, Vargas GA, Fenwick RG, Huang EA, Matsuda-Abedini M, et al. Nephrogenic syndrome of inappropriate antidiuresis. N Engl J Med. 2005;352(18):1884–90.

117. Carpentier E, Greenbaum LA, Rochdi D, Abrol R, Goddard 3rd WA, Bichet DG, et al. Identification and characterization of an activating F229V substitution in the V2 vasopressin receptor in an infant with NSIAD. J Am Soc Nephrol. 2012;23(10):1635–40.

118. Brenner B, Seligsohn U, Hochberg Z. Normal response of factor VIII and von Willebrand factor to 1-deamino-8D-arginine vasopressin in nephrogenic diabetes insipidus. J Clin Endocrinol Metab. 1988; 67(1):191–3.

119. Knoers N, Monnens LA. A variant of nephrogenic diabetes insipidus: V2 receptor abnormality restricted to the kidney. Eur J Pediatr. 1991;150(5):370–3.

120. Langley JM, Balfe JW, Selander T, Ray PN, Clarke JT. Autosomal recessive inheritance of vasopressin-resistant diabetes insipidus. Am J Med Genet. 1991;38(1):90–4.

121. Marr N, Bichet DG, Hoefs S, Savelkoul PJ, Konings IB, De Mattia F, et al. Cell-biologic and functional analyses of five new Aquaporin-2 missense mutations that cause recessive nephrogenic diabetes insipidus. J Am Soc Nephrol. 2002;13(9):2267–77.

122. Marr N, Bichet DG, Lonergan M, Arthus MF, Jeck N, Seyberth HW, et al. Heteroligomerization of an Aquaporin-2 mutant with wild-type Aquaporin-2 and their misrouting to late endosomes/lysosomes explains dominant nephrogenic diabetes insipidus. Hum Mol Genet. 2002;11(7):779–89.

123. Kuwahara M, Iwai K, Ooeda T, Igarashi T, Ogawa E, Katsushima Y, et al. Three families with autosomal dominant nephrogenic diabetes insipidus caused by aquaporin-2 mutations in the C-terminus. Am J Hum Genet. 2001;69(4):738–48.

124. Kamsteeg EJ, Bichet DG, Konings IB, Nivet H, Lonergan M, Arthus MF, et al. Reversed polarized delivery of an aquaporin-2 mutant causes dominant nephrogenic diabetes insipidus. J Cell Biol. 2003; 163(5):1099–109.

125. Bichet DG, el Tarazi A, Matar J, Lussier Y, Arthus MF, Lonergan M, et al. Aquaporin-2: new mutations responsible for autosomal-recessive nephrogenic diabetes insipidus—update and epidemiology. Clin Kidney J. 2012;5:195–202.

126. Coleman J. Diseases of organ system: the kidney. In: Shaw V, Lawson M, editors. Clinical paediatric dietetics. 2nd ed. Oxford: Blackwell Science Ltd; 2001.

127. Kennedy GC, Crawford JD. Treatment of diabetes insipidus with hydrochlorothiazide. Lancet. 1959; 1(7078):866–7.

128. Crawford JD, Kennedy GC. Chlorothiazid in diabetes insipidus. Nature. 1959;183(4665):891–2.

129. Stoff JS, Rosa RM, Silva P, Epstein FH. Indomethacin impairs water diuresis in the DI rat: role of prostaglandins independent of ADH. Am J Physiol. 1981;241(3):F231–7.

130. Walker RM, Brown RS, Stoff JS. Role of renal prostaglandins during antidiuresis and water diuresis in man. Kidney Int. 1982;21(2):365–70.

131. Usberti M, Pecoraro C, Federico S, Cianciaruso B, Guida B, Romano A, et al. Mechanism of action of indomethacin in tubular defects. Pediatrics. 1985; 75(3):501–7.

132. Tamma G, Wiesner B, Furkert J, Hahm D, Oksche A, Schaefer M, et al. The prostaglandin E2 analogue sulprostone antagonizes vasopressin-induced antidiuresis through activation of Rho. J Cell Sci. 2003;116(Pt 16):3285–94.

133. Huber TB, Simons M, Hartleben B, Sernetz L, Schmidts M, Gundlach E, et al. Molecular basis of the functional podocin-nephrin complex: mutations in the NPHS2 gene disrupt nephrin targeting to lipid raft microdomains. Hum Mol Genet. 2003;12(24): 3397–405.

134. Hebert RL, Breyer RM, Jacobson HR, Breyer MD. Functional and molecular aspects of prostaglandin E receptors in the cortical collecting duct. Can J Physiol Pharmacol. 1995;73(2):172–9.

135. Langman MJ, Weil J, Wainwright P, Lawson DH, Rawlins MD, Logan RF, et al. Risks of bleeding peptic ulcer associated with individual non-steroidal anti-inflammatory drugs. Lancet. 1994;343(8905): 1075–8.

136. Garcia Rodriguez LA, Jick H. Risk of upper gastrointestinal bleeding and perforation associated with individual non-steroidal anti-inflammatory drugs. Lancet. 1994;343(8900):769–72.

137. Soylu A, Kasap B, Ogun N, Ozturk Y, Turkmen M, Hoefsloot L, et al. Efficacy of COX-2 inhibitors in a case of congenital nephrogenic diabetes insipidus. Pediatr Nephrol. 2005;20(12):1814–7.

138. Pattaragarn A, Alon US. Treatment of congenital nephrogenic diabetes insipidus by hydrochlorothiazide and cyclooxygenase-2 inhibitor. Pediatr Nephrol. 2003;18(10):1073–6.

139. Dogne JM, Hanson J, Supuran C, Pratico D. Coxibs and cardiovascular side-effects: from light to shadow. Curr Pharm Des. 2006;12(8):971–5.

140. Bockenhauer D, Bichet DG. Urinary concentration: different ways to open and close the tap. Pediatr Nephrol. 2014;29(8):1297–303.

141. Egan ME, Glockner-Pagel J, Ambrose C, Cahill PA, Pappoe L, Balamuth N, et al. Calcium-pump inhibitors induce functional surface expression of Delta F508-CFTR protein in cystic fibrosis epithelial cells. Nat Med. 2002;8(5):485–92.

142. Robben JH, Sze M, Knoers NV, Deen PM. Rescue of vasopressin V2 receptor mutants by chemical chaperones: specificity and mechanism. Mol Biol Cell. 2006;17(1):379–86.

143. Romisch K. A cure for traffic jams: small molecule chaperones in the endoplasmic reticulum. Traffic. 2004;5(11):815–20.

144. Ulloa-Aguirre A, Janovick JA, Brothers SP, Conn PM. Pharmacologic rescue of conformationally-defective proteins: implications for the treatment of human disease. Traffic. 2004;5(11):821–37.

145. Morello JP, Salahpour A, Laperriere A, Bernier V, Arthus MF, Lonergan M, et al. Pharmacological chaperones rescue cell-surface expression and function of misfolded V2 vasopressin receptor mutants. J Clin Invest. 2000;105(7):887–95.

146. Tan CM, Nickols HH, Limbird LE. Appropriate polarization following pharmacological rescue of V2 vasopressin receptors encoded by X-linked nephrogenic diabetes insipidus alleles involves a conformation of the receptor that also attains mature glycosylation. J Biol Chem. 2003;278(37):35678–86.

147. Wuller S, Wiesner B, Loffler A, Furkert J, Krause G, Hermosilla R, et al. Pharmacochaperones post-translationally enhance cell surface expression by increasing conformational stability of wild-type and mutant vasopressin V2 receptors. J Biol Chem. 2004;279(45):47254–63.

148. Bernier V, Morello JP, Zarruk A, Debrand N, Salahpour A, Lonergan M, et al. Pharmacologic chaperones as a potential treatment for X-linked nephrogenic diabetes insipidus. J Am Soc Nephrol. 2006;17(1):232–43.

149. Olesen ET, Rutzler MR, Moeller HB, Praetorius HA, Fenton RA. Vasopressin-independent targeting of aquaporin-2 by selective E-prostanoid receptor agonists alleviates nephrogenic diabetes insipidus. Proc Natl Acad Sci U S A. 2011;108(31):12949–54.